Surgical Procedures and Anesthetic Implications

A HANDBOOK FOR NURSE ANESTHESIA PRACTICE

Lynn Fitzgerald Macksey, MSN, RN, CRNA
Raleigh, North Carolina
with
William Sowka | Eric Cipcic
Patricia E. Kaufman | Freda D. Callaway

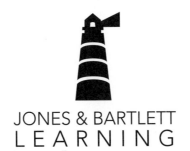

JONES & BARTLETT
LEARNING

World Headquarters
Jones & Bartlett Learning
5 Wall Street
Burlington, MA 01803
978-443-5000
info@jblearning.com
www.jblearning.com

Jones & Bartlett Learning books and products are available through most bookstores and online booksellers. To contact Jones & Bartlett Learning directly, call 800-832-0034, fax 978-443-8000, or visit our website, www.jblearning.com.

Production Credits

Publisher: Kevin Sullivan
Acquisitions Editor: Amanda Harvey
Editorial Assistant: Rachel Shuster
Production Manager: Carolyn F. Rogers
Marketing Manager: Meagan Norlund
V.P., Manufacturing and Inventory Control:
  Therese Connell

Composition: diacriTech
Cover Design: Scott Moden
Cover Image: © Bocos Benedict/ShutterStock, Inc.
Printing and Binding: Edwards Brothers Malloy
Cover Printing: Edwards Brothers Malloy

Library of Congress Cataloging-in-Publication Data

Macksey, Lynn Fitzgerald.
  Surgical procedures and anesthetic implications: a handbook for nurse anesthesia practice / Lynn Fitzgerald Macksey.
      p. ; cm.
  Includes bibliographical references and index.
  ISBN 978-0-7637-8057-9 (pbk.)
  1. Nurse anesthetists—Handbooks, manuals, etc. I. Title.
  [DNLM: 1. Anesthesia—methods—Handbooks. 2. Anesthesia—nursing—Handbooks. 3. Operating Room Nursing—methods—Handbooks. 4. Safety Management—methods—Handbooks. WY 49 M156s 2011]
  RD82.M33 2011
  617.9'6—dc22
                          2010021816

6048

Printed in the United States of America
16 15 14   10 9 8 7 6 5 4 3

This book is dedicated to Sandy Sell, CRNA
Teacher, mentor, friend
and to
Keith, Kevin, and Kimberly
My heart's prayer realized

Contents

Acknowledgments xv

Contributors. xvii

Preface xxi

Preoperative Testing Guidelines. xxiii

Operating Room Pearls: Hints from the Trenches xxix

Chapter 1   Safety Concerns 1
             Airway Safety with Laser and Cautery Use 1
             Electrocautery: Electric Surgical Unit (ESU) 3
             Fires and Burns in the Operating Room 4
             Magnetic Resonance Imaging 6
             Radiation 7

Chapter 2   Positioning and Patient Effect .9
             Introduction 9
             Supine Position 11
             Prone Position 11
             Trendelenburg Position 12
             Reverse Trendelenburg Position 13
             Lithotomy Position 13
             Sitting or Beach-Chair (Semi-Fowler) Position 13
             Jack-Knife Position 14
             Lateral Decubitus Position 14
             Flexed Lateral Decubitus Position .15
             Patient Positioning on a Fracture Table 16

Chapter 3   Special Techniques and Concepts in Anesthesia 17

Anesthesia and the Pregnant Patient 17

Aortic Cross-Clamping, Spinal Cord Issues, and Aortic Shunting 18

Spinal Cord Injury and Aortic Cross-Clamping 19

Blood Products 20

Carcinoid Syndrome 21

Cardiopulmonary Bypass 22

Cerebral Protection 22

Common Allergies, Asthma, and Histamine in the
    Operating Room 25

Deep Hypothermic Cardiac Arrest 26

Double-Lumen Endobronchial Tube 28

Embolism 30

Hemodialysis Catheter Access and Flush Guidelines .33

High-Frequency Jet Ventilation 33

Laparoscopic Issues 34

Mask (Ventilator) Strap Facial Injuries 35

Methylmethacrylate Bone Cement 36

Mixed Venous Oxygen Content 36

Intraoperative Neurologic Monitoring by the Electrophysiologist 37

Neurophysiologic Monitoring 37

Electroencephalography 37

Evoked Potentials 39

Electromyography 44

Wake-Up Test 44

Anesthetics and Body States Influencing Intraoperative
    Neurologic Monitoring 45

Postoperative Visual Loss 46

Pulmonary Hypertension 47

Tourniquet Issues 47

Chapter 4   Special Drugs and Concepts in Anesthesia 51

Anesthesia and Lung Function 51

Nausea and Vomiting 56

Blood Glucose and Insulin 57

Coagulation and Anticoagulation 58

Corticosteroids, Glucocorticoids, and Mineralocorticoids 66

NSAID Preoperative Protocol 66

Precedex (Dexmedetomidine) Worksheet 67

Remifentanil (Ultiva) Infusion 67

Total Intravenous Anesthesia 68

Neuromuscular Diseases and Anesthesia 70

Drugs for Cardiovascular Surgeries 82

Heart Setup 87

How to Use the Cardiovascular Drug Table 88

Chapter 5   Neurovascular Surgery **331**

Neurosurgery Pearls 331

Postoperative Nausea and Vomiting 331

Two Diseases Commonly Associated with Neurosurgery 332

Brain and Spinal Cord Anatomy Basics 332

Ventricular System and Cerebrospinal Fluid 333

Cranial Nerves 337

Vasomotor Center 340

Glasgow Coma Scale 343

Goals in Neuroanesthesia 343

Types of Neurosurgical Cases 346

Neurosurgery 349

Brain and Cranium: Intracranial Neurosurgery 351

Posterior Fossa Surgery 383

Neuroperipheral Nerve Surgery Pearls 389

Peripheral Nerve Surgery 389

Sympathectomy 390

Spine Surgery Pearls 392

Vertebrae of the Spinal Column, Sensory Levels, and Associated Injuries 393

Spinal Surgery 396

Chapter 6   Craniofacial Surgery **409**

Craniofacial Surgery Pearls 409

Craniofacial Surgery 409

Chapter 7   **Ophthalmic Surgery** **417**

Important Eye Anatomy and Terms Related to Ophthalmic Surgery 417

Ophthalmic Surgery Pearls 418

Anesthesia for Ophthalmic Surgery 419

Oculocardiac Reflex 420

Postoperative Nausea and Vomiting 421

Ophthalmic Surgery: Eyelids 421

Ophthalmic Surgery: Lacrimal Gland 426

Ophthalmic Surgery: Globe and Orbit 428

Ophthalmic Surgery: Conjunctiva 436

Ophthalmic Surgery: Cornea 437

Ophthalmic Surgery: Transplantation 437

Ophthalmic Surgery: Glaucoma 439

Ophthalmic Surgery: Lens 441

Ophthalmic Surgery: Retina 442

Ophthalmic Surgery: Vitreous 443

Laser Therapy and Photocoagulation 444

Refractive Eye Surgery 447

Chapter 8   **Ear Surgery** **449**

Ear Surgery Pearls 449

Postoperative Nausea and Vomiting 449

Ear Surgery 449

Chapter 9   **Sinus and Rhinologic Surgery** **459**

Sinus and Rhinologic Surgery Pearls 459

Postoperative Nausea and Vomiting 461

Sinus Surgery 461

Rhinologic Surgery 467

Chapter 10   **Mouth Surgery** **471**

Mouth Surgery Pearls 471

Mouth Surgery 471

Chapter 11   **Endocrine Surgery** **479**

Endocrine Surgery Pearls 479

Endocrine Disorders 479

Endocrine Surgery 482

Chapter 12   **Neck and Laryngologic Surgery** **489**

    Neck and Laryngologic Surgery Pearls 489

    Postoperative Nausea and Vomiting 490

    Tracheostomy Considerations 490

    Neck and Laryngologic Surgery 490

Chapter 13   **Breast Surgery** **503**

    Breast Surgery Pearls 503

    Postoperative Nausea and Vomiting 503

    Breast Surgery 504

    Reconstruction of the Breast 510

Chapter 14   **Thoracic Surgery** **515**

    Thoracic Surgery Pearls 515

    Anesthesia for Thoracic Surgeries: Key Points 516

    Thoracic Endoscopy 517

    Lung Surgery 523

    Thoracic Surgery 537

    Transplantation 540

Chapter 15   **Cardiac Surgery** **543**

    Cardiac Surgery Pearls 543

    Key Cardiac Surgery Definitions 543

    Heart Pressures 543

    Formulas 544

    Anesthetics and the Heart 545

    Conduction Disturbances 545

    Heart Blocks 550

    Bundle Branch Blocks 550

    Hemiblocks 551

    Cardiac Surgery: Permanent Pacing and AICD 551

    Cardiac Surgery: Temporary Pacing 554

    Cardiac Surgery: Coronary Artery Disease 556

    Heart Valves 570

    Cardiac Surgery: Aortic Valve 571

    Cardiac Surgery: Mitral Valve 573

    Pericardial Surgery 576

Cardiac Surgery: Thoracic Aorta 577

Transplantation 582

Chapter 16   Abdominal and Gastrointestinal Surgery **589**

Abdominal and Gastrointestinal Surgery Pearls 589

Esophagus Surgery 590

Stomach Surgery 595

Bariatric Surgery 601

Small Intestine Surgery 605

Large Bowel Surgery 608

Rectum Surgery 613

Chapter 17   Endoscopy Surgery **617**

Endoscopy Surgery Pearls 617

Colonoscopy 618

Endoscopic Retrograde Cholangiopancreatography 619

Esophagogastroduodenoscopy 620

Esophagoscopy: Upper Gastrointestinal Endoscopy 621

Gastroscopy 622

Sigmoidoscopy 623

Small Bowel Enteroscopy 623

Chapter 18   Liver, Biliary Tract, Gallbladder, Pancreas, and Spleen Surgery **625**

Liver Surgery Pearls 625

Functions of the Liver 625

Sphincter of Oddi 626

Liver Blood Flow 626

Liver Disease 627

Anesthetics in Patients with Liver Disease or During
    Hepatic Surgery 627

Anesthetic Considerations in Patients with Liver Disease or
    During Hepatic Surgery 627

Viral Hepatitis 628

Hepatic Surgery 628

Liver Transplantation 630

Biliary Tract and Gallbladder Surgery 636

Pancreas Surgery 638

Spleen Surgery 642

Chapter 19　**Genitourinary and Renal Surgery** 643

　　Genitourinary and Renal Surgery Pearls 643

　　Functions of the Kidney 643

　　Basic Anatomy of the Kidneys 644

　　Diuretic Agents 644

　　Renal Disease 644

　　GU/Renal Surgery for Patients without Renal Disease .646

　　Anesthesia in Patients with Renal Disease 646

　　GU/Renal Scope Procedures 649

　　Penis and Urethra Surgery 650

　　Scrotum and Testicles Surgery 652

　　Prostate Gland Surgery 656

　　Bladder and Urethra Surgery 665

　　Urinary Diversions 668

　　Surgery for Urinary Incontinence 669

　　Kidney and Ureter Surgery 672

　　Dialysis Access 679

　　Transplantation 680

Chapter 20　**Gynecological Surgery** 683

　　Gynecological Surgery Pearls 683

　　Postoperative Nausea and Vomiting 683

　　Preemptive analgesia 684

　　Drugs to Have Available for Gynecological Surgery 684

　　Vulva Surgery 684

　　Vaginal Approach 686

　　Abdominal Approach 696

　　Obstetric Surgery 703

Chapter 21　**Orthopedic Surgery** 709

　　Orthopedic Surgery Pearls 709

　　Fat Embolism Syndrome 710

　　Rhabdomyolysis 710

　　Definitions 711

　　Levels of Orthopedic Surgery 712

　　Anesthetics for Orthopedic Procedures 712

　　Orthopedic Surgery: Shoulder Girdle 713

Orthopedic Surgery: Humerus, Radius, and Ulna 722

Orthopedic Surgery: Hand and Wrist 727

Orthopedic Transplantation 731

Orthopedic Surgery: Pelvis 731

Orthopedic Surgery: Hip 733

Orthopedic Surgery: Femur 735

Orthopedic Surgery: Knee 738

Orthopedic Surgery: Lower Leg 743

Orthopedic Surgery: Ankle and Foot 744

Amputation of the Lower Extremity 748

Orthopedic Surgery: Total Joint Replacement 750

Orthopedic Arthroscopy 756

Orthopedic Surgery: Spinal Column 759

Chapter 22   **Vascular Surgery** **765**

Vascular Surgery Pearls 765

Vascular Surgery 767

Distal Revascularization 780

Inflow Reconstruction 781

Outflow Reconstruction 783

Chapter 23   **Plastic Surgery** **787**

Plastic Surgery Pearls 787

Face and Ears 790

Neck 799

Breast 800

Abdomen 807

Liposuction 808

Extremity 810

Skin and Flap Grafting 810

Chapter 24   **Pediatric Surgery** **813**

Neonate Surgery Pearls 813

Neonate Anesthesia and Issues 814

Pediatric Surgery Pearls 816

Pediatric Anesthesia and Issues 817

Temperature Issues with Neonate and Pediatric Patents 819

Down Syndrome: Anesthetic Implications 819

Cerebral Palsy: Anesthetic Implications 820

Mandibular Hypoplasia (Micrognathia): Anesthetic Implications 820

Neurosurgery 821

Ear, Nose, and Throat Surgery 824

Pediatric Thoracic Surgery 831

Cardiovascular Surgery 836

Gastrointestinal Disorder Repair 849

Orthopedic Surgery 864

Genitourinary Surgery 865

Plastic and Reconstructive Surgery 870

Chapter 25   **Hernia Surgery** . . . . **.873**

Hernia Surgery Pearls 873

Hernia Surgery 874

Chapter 26   **Miscellaneous Surgery** . . . . **.877**

Electroconvulsant Therapy 877

Organ Donor Management 879

Shock States 880

Trauma Resuscitation 882

Fluid Resuscitation in Trauma Patients 886

Resuscitation Markers 888

Trauma Resuscitation Recommendations 889

Anesthesia on Trauma Patients 889

Abbreviations . . . . **.891**

Spanish–English Anesthesia Translator . . . . **.895**

Sources . . . . **.907**

Index . . . . **.909**

Acknowledgments

- Kevin Warrick Fitzgerald
- Martha Anne Whiteley Marsden
- Mary Lou Tucker Taylor, CRNA
- Bill Sowka, CRNA
- Allison Roach, CRNA, Sara Zucco, CRNA, and David Kilduff, CRNA—call-partners extraordinaire
- For all the people in the Preservation in Glenshaw Society who have been the greatest friends and support, especially Cheryl and Pete Larimer, Mark and Donna Mastandrea, and Andy and Linda Hartman.
- My thanks to those who helped me get *into* anesthesia school: Lou Guzzi, MD; Jim Molinaro, CRNA; David Hartson MD; Joe Gallo, MD; and especially Martha LeVeque, CRNA, whose friendship and encouragement gave me the courage.
- My undying thanks to those who helped me get *through* school: Pam Gill, CRNA; Patti Kaufman, CRNA; April Hassler, CRNA; Kelly Wiltse, CRNA; Shelly Boyce, CRNA; Pete Machi, CRNA; Meghan Connelly, CRNA; David Caragein, CRNA; Scott Pearson, CRNA; Karen Pelch; Sandy Sell, CRNA; Laura Palmer, CRNA; John O'Donnell, CRNA; Rick Henker, CRNA; Bettina Dixon, CRNA; Karen Ferguson, CRNA; and Sharon Doolin, CRNA.
- Also, Phyllis (Eve) Overton, Mary Boutieller, Cindy Percival, Tammy Fleming Smith, Kathy Miller, Carla Gregg, Penny Obrecht, Sara LoVerde, Tammy and Eric Cipcic, Stu Napshin and Evelyn Orenbuch, Freda Callaway, Susan Andrews, Donielle Stone, Harry Anderson, Bert Fisher, Sandi Higgins, Darcey Harnage, Pam Jacobson, and Maaike Clark.

Contributors

William Atkinson, MD
Cardiothoracic Surgery
Raleigh, North Carolina

Kenneth J. Benson, DDS
Oral and Maxillofacial Surgery
Apex, North Carolina

Hillary Brainard, RN, BSN
Raleigh, North Carolina

Tony Bray, RN, BSN, CNOR
WakeMed Health and Hospitals
Raleigh, North Carolina

Julie Brewer, CRNA
American Anesthesiology

Timothy Bukowski, MD
Pediatric Urology of North Carolina

Tiffany Burke, CRNA
American Anesthesiology

Grant Buttram, MD
Raleigh Neurosurgical Clinic, Inc.
Raleigh, North Carolina

Mike Caskey, CRNA
American Anesthesiology

Jonathan D. Chappell, MD
Wake Orthopaedics, LLC
Raleigh, North Carolina

Lord Kirk Charles, MD
Vascular Surgery
Raleigh, North Carolina

Sam Chawla, MD
Fellow of American Board Urology
WakeMed Specialty Physicians

Eric Cipcic, CRNA, MSN
Pennsylvania

Christine Cutter, CRNA
American Anesthesiology

Michael G. DeLissio, MD
Gastroenterology, Private Practice
Raleigh, North Carolina

Catherine Dingman, MD
Obstetrics and Gynecology
Raleigh, North Carolina

Dean Dornic, MD
Ophthalmology
Raleigh, North Carolina

Melissa Farmer, SRNA
Raleigh School of Nurse Anesthesia
Raleigh, North Carolina

Kelly Fitzgerald, CRNA
American Anesthesiology

Pamela Fitzpatrick, RN
University of Massachusetts Memorial
Endoscopy Center
Worcester, Massachusetts

Jonathon Francis, RN, BSN, SRNA
Raleigh School of Nurse Anesthesia

David L. Froelich, RN, CNOR, CRNFA
Raleigh, North Carolina

Renee Gamble, CRNA
American Anesthesiology

Laura Garilli, CRNA
American Anesthesiology

Kelly Gignac, CRNA
Dunn, North Carolina

Noel E. Hamm RN, BSN, CNOR
Staff Nurse IV, Operating Room,
    Neuro-Vascular Service
WakeMed Health and Hospitals,
    Raleigh Campus
Raleigh, North Carolina

Timothy Harris, MD
Wake Orthopaedics, LLC
Raleigh, North Carolina

Douglas K. Holmes, MD
Otolaryngology
Raleigh, North Carolina

Daniel Ingram, MHS, PA-C
Raleigh, North Carolina

Shavone Johnson, CRNA
American Anesthesiology

Patti Kaufman, CRNA
Pennsylvania

David Kilduff, CRNA
American Anesthesiology

William Killinger, MD
Cardiothoracic surgery
Raleigh, North Carolina

Andrew Lutz, MD
Anesthesiologist
American Anesthesiology

Keith P. Mankin, MD, FAAP
Pediatric Orthopaedic Service
Raleigh Orthopaedic Clinic
Raleigh, North Carolina

Scott McGowan, CRNA
American Anesthesiology

Timothy Naomi, DDS
Raleigh, North Carolina

Michael Neville, MD
Anesthesiologist
American Anesthesiology

Kelly Wiltse Nicely, CRNA, MSN
Philadelphia, Pennsylvania

Ivelca Nintzel, CRNA
Georgia

W. Fred Obrecht, MD
Anesthesiologist
Coastal Carolina Anesthesiologists
Whiteville, North Carolina

John O'Dell, CRNA
American Anesthesiology

Sandra M. Ouellette, CRNA, MED, FAAN
Durham, North Carolina

J. Duncan Phillips, MD
Surgeon-in-Chief
WakeMed Children's Hospital
Raleigh, North Carolina

Richard M. Pino, MD
Associate Professor of Anesthesia
Harvard Medical School
Associate Anesthesiologist
Massachusetts General Hospital
Boston, Massachusetts

Jeremy Reading, MD
Anesthesiologist
American Anesthesiology

Brandon Roy, MD
General and Trauma Surgeon
Raleigh, North Carolina

Karl Schwarz, MD
Plastic Surgeon
Raleigh, North Carolina

Sandy Sell, CRNA, MSN
Pittsburgh, Pennsylvania

Tim Settlemeyer, Perfusionist
WakeMed Health and Hospitals
Raleigh, North Carolina

William Sowka, CRNA, MS
Staff CRNA
Central Massachusetts Anesthesia Affiliates

Tim Suttles, CRNA, MSN
American Anesthesiology

Sonja Sutton, CRNA, MSN
North Carolina

Preface

Certainly, there is an enormous amount of information to be found in the literature on every surgery. In this book, I have tried to identify the "core" information for each procedure. Some cases the most common ones—go into more specifics. This book does not include all of the specific surgical details—that is, the name of each ligated nerve, every severed muscle, or all instruments used. Instead, it excludes edetails that do not affect the anesthetic plan. The surgical details included here will, I hope, help the CRNA understand the general progression of each case.

While not all encompassing for each major body system, the "pearls" listed in each surgical chapter are the information I find most useful in the operating room and the material that is highlighted in anesthesia review books.

Any anesthesia drugs listed in this book are simply suggestions. Follow your institutional guidelines.

Some drugs (such as halothane) have been discontinued in the United States. However, information on these agents is included in these chapters for international practitioners.

Please email me at LFMacksey@gmail.com with any questions or edits. If you find any incorrect or outdated information, please let me know and cite your sources. I welcome your comments and suggestions.

Preoperative Testing Guidelines

Screening tests are not commonly performed preoperatively without, at least to some extent, being based on the patient, the surgery, and the anesthesia. To be useful, the preoperative test result should provide information to the caregiver that affects how the anesthesia is given or that offers an idea of perioperative risk if the result is abnormal. The following points should be considered:

- *The age, gender, likelihood of pregnancy, and reliability of the patient.* For example, older or less reliable patients may be more likely to have an unsuspected abnormality picked up by a "screening" test and may need more extensive testing than would otherwise be indicated.
- *The surgical procedure.* Major procedures are associated with significant physiologic stress. Existing medical conditions that may be of little concern during a brief and minor procedure may cause major problems during (and after) a long and complex surgery. Testing should reflect this need for an increased level of preparedness and monitoring.
- *The type of anesthesia.* For some procedures done *without* general anesthesia, fewer tests *may* be needed. Even so, the anesthetic plan should take into account the possibility that a conversion to a general anesthetic may occur due to unforeseen circumstances.

Some lab tests—usually a hematocrit level—are needed before *any* surgery. Others may be needed in specific cases. Follow your institutional guidelines and use good judgment. The laboratory or preoperative tests recommended with the surgeries profiled in this book are suggestions only; more or fewer tests may be needed for a particular patient.

An HCG pregnancy test should be done preoperatively, either on blood or urine, on a woman of child-bearing age.

PREOPERATIVE TESTING GUIDELINES: GENERAL INFORMATION AND SUGGESTED TESTS

Pre-op	WBC	CBC	H&H	PT/INR/PTT	Platelets	Serum Chem	BUN/Cr	Glucose	Ca++	CXR	EKG	T&S/T&C	PFT	UA
Procedure with blood loss		X	X			X						X		
Neonate			X					X						
< 40 years			Female											
41–50 yrs			Female								Male			
51–60 years			Female								X			
> 60 years		X	X					X			X			
CNS disease	X	X				X					X			
Cardiovascular disease	X	X		X	X	X		X		X	X			
Diabetes						X	X	X			X			
Hypertension							X				X			
Liver disease (including hepatitis)	X			X	X	X								
Parathyroid disease						X	X		X		X			X
Pulmonary disease					X					X	X		X	
Renal disease	X			X	X	X; especially Na+, K+	X	X		X	X			
Rheumatoid arthritis			X							X	X			
Thyroid disease			X		X	X		X	X		X			
Bleeding history	X			X	X									
UTI														X

Condition						
Smoker						X
Older than 40 years	X					X
Possible pregnancy						X
Diuretic use			X; especially Na$^+$, K$^+$			
Anticoagulant use	X	X				
Antihypertensive			X; especially Na$^+$, K$^+$			
Digoxin			X; especially Na$^+$, K$^+$			X
Coumadin	X					
Steroid use			X			X
Malignancy	X	X	X	X	X	
Obese	X		X		X	
Asthmatic						X
Congestive heart failure		X	X	X	X	
TURP or hysteroscopy			X; especially Na$^+$, K$^+$			
For upper abdominal/thoracic procedures	X		X	X	X	X
Invasive surgery	X	X	X	X	X	X

Chem = chemistry; BUN/Cr = blood urea nitrogen/creatinine; Ca^{++} = calcium; CXR = chest X-ray; T&S/T&C = type and screen/type and cross-match; PFT = pulmonary function tests; UA = urinalysis; Na$^+$ = sodium; K$^+$ = potassium.

PRIOR TEST RESULTS

- *Chest X-ray* within 1 year; if it was normal or showed a stable condition and if there has been no intervening clinical event
- *EKG* within 6 months; if it was normal or showed a stable condition and if there has been no intervening clinical event
- *Blood tests* within 30 days; if they were normal or showed a stable condition and if there has been no intervening clinical event

Preoperative Risk Factors

- Myocardial infarction within 1 month and evidence of CHF.
- Severe aortic or mitral stenosis: considered an acceptable contraindication to elective surgery

MEDICATIONS FOR PATIENT ON THE MORNING OF SURGERY: SHOULD TAKE (UNLESS OTHERWISE INSTRUCTED)

- Antihypertensive medications
- Medications for asthma or emphysema
- Antiseizure medications
- Cardiac medications
- Anti-reflux (GERD) medications

MEDICATIONS FOR PATIENT ON THE MORNING OF SURGERY: SHOULD NOT TAKE (UNLESS OTHERWISE INSTRUCTED)

- Oral hypoglycemic agents

MEDICATIONS FOR PATIENT ON THE MORNING OF SURGERY: SHOULD TAKE HALF OF THE NORMAL DOSE (UNLESS OTHERWISE INSTRUCTED)

- Subcutaneous injected insulin

GENERAL QUESTIONS TO ASK OR TO ASSESS PREOPERATIVELY PER BODY SYSTEM

- General: exercise tolerance, weakness, fatigue, weight change, fever, blood-borne diseases.
- Skin: rashes, sores, lesions.
- Head: frequent headaches, head injury, patient alert and good historian; stroke or seizure history.
- Eyes: double vision, loss of vision, cataracts, glaucoma. Implanted lens(es) present?
- Ears: limited hearing, tinnitus, vertigo, pain, discharge.
- Nose and throat: sinusitis, sore throat, epistaxis, dysphagia.

- Mouth: lesions, bleeding gums, Mallampati score.
- Cardiac: history of hypertension, myocardial infarction, congestive heart failure, rheumatic heart fever, heart murmurs, angina, palpitations, dyspnea, orthopnea. Ever had heart work-up: stress test, cardiac catheterization? Increased risk is present if the patient is unable to climb two flights of stairs.
- Respiratory: cough, sputum, hemoptysis, asthma, wheezing, bronchitis, emphysema, smoking history, pneumonia, history of or current tuberculosis.
- GI: hiatal hernia, gastroesophageal reflux disease, peptic ulcer disease, heartburn, nausea or vomiting, diarrhea, constipation, hematemesis, melena, jaundice, hepatitis.

HISTORY OF PRESENT ILLNESS

- Onset/chronology: date and mode
- Symptoms: nature and course
- Precipitating factors
- Frequency and severity
- Current manifestations
- Character (quality)
- System(s) involved; pertinent family history

Organ systems involved also include those that are significant or pertinent to the presenting problem.

CLINICAL PREDICTORS OF INCREASED PERIOPERATIVE CARDIOVASCULAR RISK OR REINFARCTION RISK

Major Risk (requires intensive management including delay of surgery)

- Unstable angina
- Decompensated heart failure
- Severe valvular disease
- Acute (less than 7 days) or recent myocardial infarction (within 7–30 days) with evidence of important ischemic risk by clinical symptoms or noninvasive study
- High-grade atrioventricular block
- Symptomatic ventricular arrhythmias in the presence of underlying heart disease
- Supraventricular arrhythmias with uncontrolled ventricular rate

Intermediate Risk

- Current, mild angina pectoris
- Previous myocardial infarction by history or pathological Q waves
- Compensated or prior heart failure
- Very limited exercise tolerance; 1–3 MET levels
- Diabetes mellitus (particularly insulin-dependent)
- Renal insufficiency, chronic (serum creatinine > 2 mg/100 mL)

Minor Risk

- Advanced age
- Abnormal EKG (left ventricular hypertrophy, left bundle branch block, ST-T abnormalities)
- Rhythm other than sinus (e.g., atrial fibrillation)
- Low functional capacity (e.g., inability to climb one flight of stairs with a bag of groceries); 3–5 MET levels
- History of stroke
- Uncontrolled systemic hypertension

MET SCORE

MET: metabolic equivalent and exercise tolerance. This scale is adapted from the Duke Activity Status Index and AHA Exercise Standards. Left ventricular function determines exercise tolerance.

Can you take care of yourself? Eat, dress, or use the toilet? Walk indoors around the house? Walk a block or two on level ground at 2–3 mph or 3.2–4.8 km/hr?	1 MET	
Do light work around the house like dusting or washing dishes? Climb a flight of stairs or walk up a hill? Walk on level ground at 4 mph or 6.4 km/hr?	4 METs	
Run a short distance? Do heavy work around the house like scrubbing floors or lifting or moving heavy furniture? Participate in moderate recreational activities like golf, bowling, dancing, doubles tennis, or throwing a baseball or football? Participate in strenuous sports like swimming, singles tennis, football, basketball, or skiing?	10 METs	

Operating Room Pearls: Hints from the Trenches

- Always monitor lead II and V_5 for P-wave and ST-segment changes.
  - Three-lead placement:
    - White lead: on the right shoulder
    - Black lead: on the left shoulder
    - Red lead: on the left mid-axillary line around T8
    - These may be either anterior or posterior on the shoulders.
  - Five-lead placement:
    - White lead: on the right shoulder
    - Green lead: on the right mid-axillary line around T8
    - Black lead: on the left shoulder
    - Brown lead: on the right of the patient's sternum around T7
    - Red lead: on the left mid-axillary line around T8
- No antecubital IVs should be established in patients who will be placed in the prone position.
- When inserting an orogastric tube into the throat, lift the patient's lower jaw forward. The head should be flexed to help ease insertion of the tube into the esophagus behind the trachea. Once the distal tip is past the tongue and hypopharynx, let go of the lower jaw and pinch around the neck while inserting the tube; this helps to narrow the throat to keep the tube from coiling. If all else fails, do all the same maneuvers with the patient's head turned to the right or use a laryngoscope blade to help with insertion.
- Normal saline 0.9% should be give at a rate of 30 mL/hr in patients undergoing renal surgery. It is such a small amount of fluid going in that a fluid warmer is not necessary.
- Hearing the surgeon ask for a specific size of suture can give you an idea where the team is in the case: Suturing deep tissues uses a bigger thread; superficial and skin sutures are very small. Think of suture sizes as a line of numbers with "zero" in the middle:

$$3.0-2.0-1.0-\mathbf{0}-1-2-3-4$$

The whole numbers to the right of zero are big sutures; a "4" is like a wire. The numbers to the left of zero become smaller the farther left they go. These sizes are called "three-Os" (OOO) or "two-Os" (OO)—meaning small. A three-O is commonly used to close bowel; a two-O is commonly used to close fascia; a ten-O is an ophthalmic stitch.

- Hearing the circulators counting equipment is another way to know that the team is winding up the procedure.
- Preoperatively, when interviewing the patient before surgery, write the procedure side (right or left) on the anesthetic record on the "Procedure" line. You will probably remember that the surgery is to be a hernia repair, but you may not remember the side when doing "time-out." By documenting this information, you can look on your anesthetic record to confirm the side. (You usually do not have the surgical consent form available in the OR, so the anesthetic record notation can help clarify the side to be operated on for anesthesia time-out.)
- Once the patient is brought into the operating room and moved over to the table, put the pulse oximeter probe on first (a sedative or anxiolytics will likely have been given in the preoperative area), then put the blood pressure cuff on and start taking the pressure, and then put the EKG leads on. With this sequence, while you are placing the monitors, you will at least know whether the patient has a pulse and where the oxygen level is.
- If someone else is pushing the induction medications while you control the airway for intubation, once you have checked for "lash" and have started bagging the patient, let the other person know whether you are adequately ventilating the patient. Say "Ventilating," which cues your partner to give succinylcholine or a nondepolarizing muscle relaxant (these medications should not be given until you know you can ventilate the patient with a mask).
- *Intubation hint:* Once the patient is deep enough into anesthesia with induction drugs, pick up the blade and handle, open it, and hold it in your left hand. With your left thumb, pull down the patient's lower jaw. With your right hand, put your "scissored fingers" as far back on the right as you can and "scissor" the jaw open. Using your left hand, insert the blade into the mouth to the back of the throat on the right side of the tongue. Once the blade is in, you can remove your right fingers. The blade is in and being held with your left hand at this point. Using your right hand, pull the patient's upper and lower lips away from the teeth and the blade. You can start to insert and reposition the laryngoscope blade deeper into the throat, sweeping the tongue up and to the left as you insert it. Your right hand is essentially free and can help to push cricoid pressure or lift the back of the head slightly to improve the angle to view "the cords."
- At the end of the case, as the surgeon is finishing the suture line, start to take down the temperature connector, warming blanket hose, and anything else that is still attached to the patient and is no longer necessary. This will help you be ready for wake-up.
- Once the dressing or surgical glue is placed over the incision line, you can start to take the surgical drapes down.

- The big plastic bag that is placed over the C-arm on the X-ray machine is sterile—so watch out when you are walking by it. The radiology staff never laughs when you touch the plastic covering.
- When the surgeon asks for local anesthetic and cites a percentage solution ("¼%" or "½%") the medication is usually marcaine. If the surgeon asks for a whole-number local anesthetic, the medication is usually lidocaine. If the surgeon says "0.25% with," it means "marcaine 0.25% with epinephrine"; "1% plain" means "lidocaine 1% without epinephrine."
- When applying an oxygen face mask to a patient who is having upper chest or shoulder surgery, turn the mask upside down and paper-tape the tubing onto the patient's forehead. This practice allows mask oxygen to flow to the patient while the tubing stays out of the surgical field.
- When a throat pack is placed, write "throat pack" on a piece of tape and stick it over the face mask. At the end of the case, when you pick up the mask for extubation, you will be reminded to make sure the throat pack has been removed and documented on the anesthesia record.
- Leave the pulse oximeter on the patient's finger until you actually leave the operating room and are heading to the recovery room. It gives you so much information: You know the patient has a pulse and you can hear the patient's saturation level. Put simply, you know the patient is safe while you gather your papers for transport.
- When you pick up the mask attached to circuit tubing to place it on the patient's face, first check to make sure "pop-off" valve is open (set at 0).

AIRWAY SAFETY WITH LASER AND CAUTERY USE

Common Sites of Operating Room Fires

- 34% airway
- 28% head or face
- 38% elsewhere on or inside patient

An oxygen-enriched atmosphere was a contributing factor in a majority of cases.

Methods to Protect the Patient

If using a nasal cannula during a procedure involving a laser or cautery:

- Drapes should be arranged to avoid trapping high concentrations of O_2 within them.
- Place a suction catheter under drapes to help pull trapped exhaled gases away.

When using a laser or cautery in the airway:

- All lubricants used in the airway should be water-soluble types.
- Use an oxygen/air combination that includes the minimum O_2 concentration needed to support clinically acceptable arterial saturation (30% or less).
- Do not use nitrous oxide—it is combustible.

Endotracheal Tubes, Circuit Tubing, and Fire Prevention

A polyvinyl chloride (PVC) endotracheal tube (ETT) is highly flammable. Specific laser-retardant ETTs (flexible metal laser ETTs) should be used during oral, tracheal, or esophageal laser procedures that require supplemental oxygen.

Filling the endotracheal balloon with saline can help to put out any fire or spark that arises. Alternatively, the balloon can be filled with a mixture of saline and methylene blue to indicate if the balloon's patency has been compromised at any time during the surgery. Also employ the following precautions:

- Metallic wrap around a PVC endotracheal tube
- Tape around the patient's mouth or face—3M Blenderm (paper and adhesive tape can ignite)
- Breathing circuit—covered with foil and wet towels
- Saline-soaked pledgets—can be placed around the ETT for an airway laser procedure
- Bottle of sterile water—kept at the work area to extinguish any fire if it occurs

Minimizing Oxygen Concentration in the Field

Oxygen and nitrous oxide vastly increase the flammability potential of a surgical area. Even air supports combustion, albeit to a lesser degree. Use an air/O_2 combination in ignition-prone cases; avoid the use of nitrous oxide.

Keep the FiO_2 as low as possible. If the patient's oxygen saturation falls, notify the surgeon, who can stop the laser. Increase the FiO_2 and manually ventilate the patient to increase the saturation level. The surgeon can begin to use the laser again when the FiO_2 is back down to 30%.

Low flow of oxygen is better than higher flow; use the lowest required concentration of inspired oxygen. Concentrations of oxygen greater than 21% are considered "enriched."

When using oxygen prongs during facial surgery performed under local anesthesia, the surgeon may instruct the anesthetist to turn off the oxygen, and wait at least 60 seconds for the oxygen to dissipate before using the cautery unit. The oxygen flow can be resumed when the electrical surgical unit (ESU) is no longer needed. Regulate the oxygen at the lowest setting that keeps the patient's oxygen saturation at a safe level; usually 2 to 3 liters per minute is usually all that is needed. Stop oxygen flow at least 1 minute before the use of an ESU, if possible.

You can "blend" the gases with this nasal cannula setup—that is, an adaptor is placed at the end of the circuit, allowing a nasal cannula to be connected (see Figure 1-1). You can dial in a percentage FiO_2 with this system. Whatever method you choose, make sure you have a safe delivery of the oxygen/air mixture to the patient in an "oxygen-enriched environment." You do not need to use the nasal cannula outlet for these cases.

Many institutions do not use oxygen supplementation except for rescue. Other considerations include the patient's ASA status and the level of sedation needed for the procedure. Let the surgeon know if you cannot maintain an oxygen saturation level that is greater than 92%.

If oxygen is needed by the patient, it is generally safe to place the prongs in the patient's mouth when operating on the upper face. The tubing should be taped to keep it in place.

Extreme vigilance must be maintained to be sure the prongs stay in place so that oxygen never blows openly over the field. If it does, there is a risk of igniting a fire on the patient's face.

In summary, be aware of possible oxygen enrichment (the accumulation of oxygen or nitrous oxide) under the drapes near the surgical site, especially during head and neck surgery (from the nipples up). Arrange drapes (tenting to allow room air circulation and avoid oxygen trapping) to minimize oxygen buildup underneath; put suction tubing under the drapes to suction excess flow. Also, maintain lower

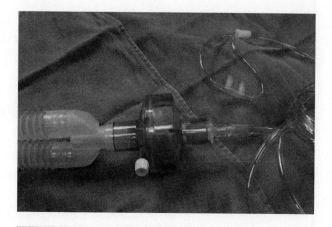

Figure 1-1 *Nasal Cannula*

flows of oxygen, if it is needed at all. With an outlet around the drapes, gravity will assist in pulling oxygen to the floor and away from the patient.

Management of Airway Fires

The mnemonic DIVER can help you remember the steps for managing an airway fire. At the first sign of a tracheal tube fire, rapidly take the following actions:

Disconnect the breathing circuit from the tracheal tube and extubate the patient. Disconnect the O_2 source at the Y-piece and remove burning objects from airway (i.e., remove the ETT, ensuring that the entire tube is removed).

Irrigate the site with water if fire is still smoldering.

Ventilate the patient by mask or reintubate; deliver the lowest possible O_2 concentration.

Examine the patient's mouth and oral cavity. Evaluate the injury by bronchoscope and laryngoscopy, looking for burns in the trachea and bronchial tree; remove foreign bodies and debris.

Reintubate or manage the patient accordingly.

ELECTROCAUTERY: ELECTRIC SURGICAL UNIT (ESU)

Electrocautery is the process of burning or cutting through tissue by using a small probe (the ESU) with a radio-frequency electrical current running through it. It has become a popular surgical tool for cutting or coagulating away unwanted tissue and slowing or stopping hemorrhage.

Types of Electrocautery

In **monopolar ESU** (also known as unipolar ESU), the active electrode is the surgical site; the current passes through the patient to a collecting electrode or a dispersive plate (placed somewhere else on the patient's body), thereby completing the electrical circuit back to its source. The energy is then returned to the generator.

An argon beam coagulator (unipolar ESU) uses a stream of argon gas to support the electric current, which avoids charring of the instrument tip. This technique was developed to effectively control large amounts of bleeding in surgery. The flow of gas blows away debris from the surgical field and produces a more uniform coagulated surface with less smoke. Thus surgeons are able to stop bleeding faster.

Bipolar ESU uses two electrodes that look like forceps; a dispersive pad and collecting electrode are unnecessary because the energy flows from one tine of the forceps to the other (completing the electrical circuit), passing through the patient's tissue as it flows. The energy is then returned to the generator. This technique, which uses less energy than unipolar ESU, is used mostly for ophthalmic surgery and neurosurgery.

Fire Hazards Associated with ESU

The ESU is a common OR ignition source. The same cautions and procedures to prevent surgical/airway fires for laser surgery are applicable to the ESU.

With an ESU, the cautery tip is heated to a temperature of several hundred degrees Fahrenheit; the unit produces heat by concentrating electric current at the tip of the electrode.

Characteristics of the ESU

- The ESU operates by generating megahertz frequency currents (radio-frequency range) of anywhere from 500,000 Hz to more than 1 million Hz.
- Voltage is as high as 3000 volts.
- An ESU can produce nearly 400 watts of power.
- Heat is produced at the tip to cauterize a blood vessel or cut tissue.
- Energy is focused on a small area. Current enters the patient, is dispersed through a grounding pad, and must complete a circle

back to the unit. Current will seek to return through other conductors (patient or surgeon) if a dispersive plate or grounding pad is not properly placed.

Correct Placement of a Grounding Pad

- Close to the operative site
- As far away as possible from the EKG pads
- In conjunction with adequate gel and sufficient skin contact
- Not placed over scar tissue, hair, or implants

Injuries with ESU

Skin burns are a potential hazard when ESU is used. They can result from problems with the following elements:

- Return-plate connection—must cover a large area so that the current density is below a level that will cause burns
- Inadequate or improper application of the pad
- Disruption of the return wire—newer units have a double return wire with impedance monitoring
- Insufficient conductive gel (dry dispersive plate)
- Wet patients—from electrolyte solution or blood; may form electrical contacts with equipment

Nitrous oxide and oxygen are both highly flammable. Use a mixture of oxygen and air if the ESU is in use.

ESU and Pacemakers

ESUs can reprogram pacemakers or automatic implantable cardioverter-defibrillator (AICD) units or cause microshock. To avoid these problems:

- Place the pad below the thorax.
- Have equipment (magnet, external pacemaker, and defibrillator) and drugs ready for an emergency.

The AICD may interpret the ESU signal as an arrhythmia and trigger a defibrillation, possibly causing ventricular tachycardia and ventricular fibrillation.

Given these potential problems, an AICD should be deprogrammed (by a technician) prior to the patient undergoing an elective procedure.

FIRES AND BURNS IN THE OPERATING ROOM

Communication with the surgeon and surgical team is *essential* to prevent fires! If a laser or cautery is used, have a bottle of normal saline or water nearby to use in case of a fire. Three elements are required to have a fire:

- An ignition source (heat): electrocautery, lasers, static electricity, fiberoptic sources, defibrillators (primarily under the control of the surgeon)
- A fuel source: hair, skin, body tissue, intestinal gases, chemicals, endotracheal tubes, drapes, sheets, gown, towels, sponges (primarily under the control of the OR personnel)
- A source of oxygen (oxidizer): oxygen and nitrous oxide vastly increase flammability; medical air and ambient air are also oxidizers (primarily under the control of the anesthesia provider)

Common Operating Room Ignition Sources

- Electric surgical unit (68%)
- ESU grounding pad
- Lasers (13%)
- Static electricity
- High-intensity fiberoptic light source (Tip temperature is well above the ignition temperature of most surgical drapes.)
- Argon beam coagulator
- Defibrillator paddles—if used incorrectly
- Heated IV fluids, lights or compresses, warming blankets—can cause thermal injuries

Methods to Protect Patients from Ignition Sources

- Keep the cautery tip in its holder.
- Turn off the fiberoptic light source when it is not in use; do not set it down when it is turned on.

- Do not fire defibrillator paddles into open air.
- Do not use a warming blanket hose without the warming blanket.

Common Operating Room Fuel Sources

- Drapes
- Hair
- Intestinal gas
- Skin prep solutions (especially alcohol based)

Water-based preps such as Betadine, Soloprep, and Pharmaseal contain no alcohol and are considered nonflammable. A water-soluble lubricant (K-Y Jelly) should be used instead of petrolatum on the surgical field because it is not flammable.

Preps such as iodophor (Duraprep) and chlorhexidine digluconate (Hibitane) contain alcohol but in an aqueous solution, which is less flammable.

Any solution labeled "tincture" by definition is suspended in alcohol and is, therefore, extremely combustible. Benzoin, Mastisol, and merthiolate (Thimerosal) all contain alcohol. These dangerously flammable solutions should be used with the utmost caution in the OR. Petroleum jelly (Vaseline) and petroleum-based ointments can ignite in the presence of oxygen. Caution is also advised when using other materials that are flammable, such as degreasers (acetone and ether), aerosols, paraffin, and wax.

Methods to Protect Patients from Fuel Sources

- Do not drape the patient until all flammable prep fluids have fully dried.
- Use fire-retardant surgical drapes.
- The prepping solution should be applied with minimal dripping to avoid forming pools of liquid on, under, or around the body. Any pools that do form, especially in the umbilicus and cricoid notch, should be blotted. Allow thorough drying of applied solutions (this may take 2 to 3 minutes or as long as 10 minutes) before draping, and ensure dissipation of alcohol vapors before using any heat source

near the patient. A completely dry prep ensures that potentially flammable ethanol vapors from alcohol-based preparations will not be trapped beneath the drapes. Only then can an ESU or laser be used without fear of igniting the alcohol.

- Avoid petroleum-based compounds near an ignition source.
- Keep drapes and the patient's skin moist (but not with prepping solutions) around the surgical site.
- Protect hair near the surgical site by coating it with Surgilube or K-Y Jelly (water-based gels).
- Have the patient wash his or her hair before the procedure to remove any hairspray.

Common Operating Room Oxygen Sources

Oxygen and nitrous oxide vastly increase the flammability of the surgical area. Even air supports combustion, albeit to a lesser degree. Use an air/O_2 mixture in ignition-prone cases; avoid the use of nitrous oxide.

Methods to Protect Patients from Oxygen Sources

Minimize the oxygen concentration in the surgical field. Keep the FiO_2 as low as possible. If the patient's oxygen saturation falls, notify the surgeon, who can stop the laser. Increase the FiO_2 and manually ventilate the patient to increase the saturation level. The surgeon can begin to use the laser again when the delivered FiO_2 returns to 30%.

A low flow of oxygen is better than a higher flow; use the lowest required concentration of inspired oxygen. Concentrations of oxygen greater than 21% are considered "enriched."

Types of Fire Extinguishers

Class A (*ash*): for wood, paper, cloth fires

Class B (*boils*): grease, flammable liquid fires

Class C (*current*): electrical fires

ABC: dry chemical, fights all types of fires

Carbon dioxide (CO_2): used for Class B and C fires; doesn't leave a harmful residue

Surgeries in Which Fires Commonly Occur

- Bowel surgery with bowel gas ignition: To protect against this type of fire, vent the bowel before entering it surgically, and do not enter the bowel with an ESU.
- Oropharyngeal surgery: To protect against the risk of fire, use moist sponges to pack the patient's throat and fill ETT balloon with saline or methylene blue-dyed water.
- Tracheostomy: The tracheal tube can catch on fire when an ESU is used to enter the trachea. To protect against this risk, use a fire-resistant ETT tube, monitor the surgical method used to enter the trachea, and be extremely vigilant about recognizing an airway fire if an ESU is used.

Fire on a Patient in the Operating Room (Oxygen-Enriched Environment): What You Do

1. Remove what is burning to protect against direct burns.
2. Smother any remaining flames or extinguish the fire with water or saline if an electrical source is not involved. If electrical equipment is involved, do *not* attempt to extinguish it with water or saline; instead, disconnect the power source and use a Class C fire extinguisher.
3. Turn off all oxygen sources.
4. Alert others to start the fire plan.
5. Rescue the patient from danger, and move him or her to a safe area.
6. Provide medical treatment as required.
   - Control bleeding.
   - Deal with further injuries.

MAGNETIC RESONANCE IMAGING

Magnetic resonance imaging (MRI) is based on absorption and emission of energy in the radio-frequency range of the electromagnetic spectrum.

MRI Safety Considerations

There are three main problem areas in MRI:

- Magnetic field
- Radio frequency (potential for heating and burns; use reinforced anode ETTs and PA catheter thermistor wires to reduce this risk)
- Time-varied magnetic fields

Other difficulties may be related to the MRI unit's noise level, which should not exceed 140 db. Also, although MRI is not considered hazardous to a fetus, caution is recommended when using this imaging modality during the first trimester of pregnancy.

Metal Objects

A "missile effect" occurs when MRI is used in the presence of metal objects because the static magnetic field has the capacity to attract ferromagnetic objects. Everyone entering the area should be questioned and asked to remove the following items:

- Purse, wallet, money clip, credit cards, cards with magnetic strips
- Electronic devices (e.g., beepers or cell phones)
- Hearing aids
- Metal jewelry, mechanical watches
- Pens, paper clips, keys, coins
- Hair barrettes, hairpins
- Any article of clothing that has a metal zipper, buttons, snaps, hooks, underwire, or metal threads
- Shoes, belt buckles, safety pins

Foreign bodies are contraindicated in an MRI because they could create a health hazard. This includes *any* ferromagnetic electronic, magnetic, or mechanically activated implants that have the possibility of moving in the body once the patient is inside the MRI machine. Examples include a neurostimulator, AICD, pacemaker, catheter with metal components (poses a risk of burn injury), aneurysm clip, implanted infusion pump, or cochlear implant. The risk depends on the possibility of movement and dislodgment in the body. X-rays should be done first if the patient's body is suspected to contain any metal.

Transfer the patient into the MRI suite with an *aluminum* oxygen tank. Brass pipes hold tubing and circuits that are used to pass through MRI wall into the control room.

RADIATION

Radiation is used extensively in the operating room, such as in fluoroscopy, portable X-ray, and radiation implants. Because lead absorbs X-rays, healthcare providers are advised to protect themselves from radiation by wearing a lead apron and thyroid shield.

The occupational limit of radiation exposure is mandated to be less than 5000 mrem (roentgen-equivalent for man) or 50 millisieverts (mSv) annually. The occupational limit of exposure for pregnant women is 500 mrem (5 mSv). The unit dose of equivalence is based on the absorbed dose (radiation absorbed dose [RAD]), where 1 milliroentgen (mrem) = 1/1000 rem.

Sources of Radiation Exposure

- Flat films: One chest X-ray = 25 mrem to patient
- Routine angiography: approximately 8000 mrem
- Fluoroscopy with video display: may be greater than 75,000 mrem; amount depends on how long the beam is on
  - X-rays can be scattered and reflected from surfaces.
  - Backward scatter occurs in the direction opposite that of the gun.

The dose of radiation received may be reduced by moving approximately 6 feet away; being 6 feet away from the X-ray source is equivalent to the protection from wearing a 0.5-mm-thick lead sheet.

The intensity of any radiation is inversely proportional to the square distance from the source: Double the distance and cut the exposure by 75%. The farther away you are from the X-ray, the better protected you are.

Positioning and Patient Effect

2

INTRODUCTION

Surgical procedures that require the use of anesthesia (both general and conscious sedation) render patients vulnerable to potential injury and unable to protect themselves fully or at all. Each position carries some degree of risk, which is magnified in the anesthetized patient. Accordingly, the operating room personnel must provide for total protection of the patient. Specific attention to bony prominences, joint position, and dependent portions of the patient's body are of utmost importance. Dependent portions at risk for compression injury include the following body parts:

- Eyes/ears
- Penis/scrotum
- Breasts
- Fingers
- Pendulous tissue (table-related injury)

The aim of optimal positioning for surgery is to provide the best surgical access while minimizing potential risk to the patient. However, there is an increased risk of nerve damage in *any* position if the surgery lasts more than 4 hours, if the patient's body mass index (BMI) is less than 20, or if the patient has diabetes or is a smoker.

Patient positioning can affect all systems, but especially the following areas.

Circulatory System

- Impaired autonomic/sympathetic nervous systems
- Loss of vasomotor tone
- Depressed cardiac output
- Gravity effects and redistribution of circulating volume
- Compression of extremities or great vessels
- Ischemia/decreased venous return

Pulmonary System

- Barriers to thoracic excursion
- Loss of hypoxic pulmonary vasoconstriction (HPV)
- Alteration in ventilation/perfusion (V/Q) ratio

Peripheral Nerves

Nerve injury risk is high; nerve injury is one of the most common causes of surgery-related lawsuits. Ischemia of the nerve sheath can be due to either direct injury (e.g., compression of the nerve) or indirect injury (e.g., compartment syndrome). The brachial plexus (C4–T2) may be stretched, resulting in potential injury, when any of the following manipulations occurs:

- Neck extension
- Opposite arm rotation
  - 90° abduction of an extremity
  - External rotation of the arm

Surgical Position and Effects on Functional Residual Capacity

When the patient is *supine*, the abdominal contents force the diaphragm toward the head and will decrease functional residual capacity (FRC). Lithotomy and use of Trendelenburg position further reduce FRC. In the *steep* Trendelenburg position, most of the lung may be below the left atrium (zone 3 or 4 condition) and the lung is susceptible to development of pulmonary interstitial edema.

The effects of the lateral decubitus surgical position on FRC vary:

- FRC is decreased in the dependent lung.
- FRC is increased in the nondependent lung.
- The dependent lung is prone to atelectasis and fluid accumulation because it is below the left atrium.

Not all surgical positions decrease FRC. The prone position may actually *increase* FRC.

Migration of Endotracheal Tubes: Potential Causes Related to Patient Position and Surgery

Always assess breath sounds for endotracheal tube (ETT) placement after changes in the patient position.

- Migration of the ETT can occur after head movement or repositioning of the patient.
- A tube that had been previously positioned in the trachea can enter a bronchus or exit the vocal cords.
- Flexion of the head causes caudad (deeper insertion) movement of the ETT.
- Extension of the head causes cephalad (pulls up and out) movement of the ETT.
- Trendelenburg position can cause a cephalad shift of the diaphragm and carina.
- Cephalad movement of the diaphragm and carina may follow insufflation.
- Endotracheal tube movement must be suspected after any sudden desaturation.

Cerebral Perfusion Pressure and Transducer Levels Associated with Patient Positioning

Cerebral perfusion pressure (CPP) and mean arterial blood pressure (MAP) are related as follows:

$$CPP = MAP - ICP \text{ (or CVP)}$$

where ICP is the intracranial pressure and CVP is the central venous pressure.

New research indicates that the lower limit of cerebral autoregulation should be maintained within the range of 70–93 mm Hg (with a mean of ± 80) and with 150 mm Hg as the upper limit. The old value cited for the lower limit (mm Hg 50) is simply too low and leaves no margin for error; severe cerebral perfusion compromise can result.

Cerebral perfusion pressure decreases by 15% in the sitting non-anesthetized patient and can further decrease during anesthesia due to vasodilation and myocardial depression. *MAP is uniform among the brain, heart, and arm in the supine or lateral patient but can change drastically in the patient in a heads-up position.*

The arterial blood pressure transducer can be zeroed and calibrated at the *phlebostatic axis*: The stopcock is placed level with the phlebostatic axis, a common physical reference point; the phlebostatic axis is located at the fourth intercostal space and at half the anterior–posterior (AP) diameter of the chest. This approximates the location of the right atrium. After zeroing the transducer, it is raised and maintained at the level of the external auditory meatus to obtain a meaningful index of CPP.

Alternatively, the arterial blood pressure transducer can be zeroed at the level of the *external auditory meatus* and kept there to transduce at the brain level to obtain a meaningful index of CPP.

The MAP should be maintained at a minimum level of 60 mm Hg in healthy patients. This level is increased for elderly patients, patients with hypertension, and patients with known cerebral vascular disease.

If the sitting patient's pressure is measured by a blood pressure cuff, it is crucial to know the vertical distance between the brain and the blood pressure cuff (this difference is the hydrostatic pressure gradient between the heart and the brain). The blood pressure for *the base of the brain* should be calculated by decreasing the cuff MAP by *0.75 mm Hg for every 1 cm of vertical height* above the site of cuff measurement; this will be the mean arterial blood pressure the base of the brain "sees." Moreover, the pressure difference between the base of the brain (circle of Willis) and the very top of the brain can be as much as 9 mm Hg. If leg blood pressures must be used, a MAP less than 75–80% of preoperative values should be treated aggressively.

Maintaining adequate cerebral perfusion during surgery is critical. Keep in mind that there may be a huge difference between the arterial blood pressure at the level of the brain and the blood pressure reading by cuff placed on a leg.

SUPINE POSITION

In the supine position (also called the dorsal position), the patient lies on his or her back; the knees are flexed on a pillow. *With the patient flat (either supine or lateral), the blood pressure is uniform throughout.*

- **Cardiac issues:** aortocaval compression may occur in obese patients.
- **Pulmonary issues:** the abdominal contents force the diaphragm toward the head and will decrease functional residual capacity.
- **Nerve issues:** ulnar nerve injury (ulnar groove at the posterior edge of the medial epicondyle) may occur. Laying the arm supine is the best prevention for ulnar nerve injury.

The *supine position with shoulder roll* may be used in anterior cervical, neck, and jaw surgeries. This position supports the head, and doesn't let it dangle.

PRONE POSITION

In the prone position, the patient lies face down with arms either flexed at the elbow or tucked at the patient's sides and shoulders at less than a 90-degree angle.

Following insertion of a peripheral IV (not in the antecubital fossa, unless the arms are to be positioned tucked at the patient's sides) and endotracheal intubation, the patient is turned onto the operating room table in the prone position. With the elbows flexed, the arms are extended on armboards angled toward the head of the bed with the shoulders less than 90 degrees and supported so they are not hanging, and the hands pronated ("swimmer's position"). Pillows are placed under the ankles. Padding is placed under the elbows and knees. A safety strap is secured across the patient's thighs. The neck should be in a neutral position. The eyes and the tip of the nose should be checked and charted on the anesthesia record at least every 15 minutes to make sure no pressure is applied to these areas.

- **Cardiac issues:** Potential problems may include lower extremity/gut pooling of blood, inferior vena cava compression, and epidural engorgement.
- **Pulmonary issues:** Use chest rolls, as the lungs must have free excursion. The prone position may actually *increase* FRC. If the chest is not free, there is decreased compliance with high peak pressures and ventilation/perfusion problems.
- **Nerve issues:** Damage to the brachial plexus is possible. The arms should be in the swimmer's position or tucked at the sides, with the shoulders still at an angle less than 90 degrees.

Prone Position Checklist

- Eyes/ears
- Taped closed/padded eyes
- All extremities
- Penis/breasts in the clear—move breasts inward medially
- Clear catheter tubing
- Chest rolls in good position, below the clavicle and below the inguinal space
- Brachial plexus checks
- Clavicle/mandible checks
- Check eyes and nose for no pressure every 15 minutes; document

Postoperative Visual Loss

Complete or partial blindness is a potentially devastating complication for a patient in the prone position; postoperative visual loss (POVL) is most often associated with long-duration spinal surgery with instrumentation. Commonly, these patients have surgery in the prone position lasting several hours and develop hypotension with considerable blood loss replaced only with crystalloid fluids with low urinary output.

POVL is thought to be due to multiple factors, including elevated central venous pressure from retarded drainage from the ophthalmic veins, and the head spending a prolonged period in the down-tilt position, causing decreased venous outflow from the cranium. Interventions to help prevent POVL include slight reverse Trendelenburg (head-up) position, transfusion of blood products to maintain preoperative hematocrit (HCT) levels, normothermia, euglycemia, and urinary output minimum of 0.5 mL/kg/h.

Prone Position on Andrews Frame

In this position, the patient is prone with the hips bent down and the patient kneeling. This position raises concerns for the following areas:

- Eyes
- Knee/ankles/toes (padding is needed)
- Penis/breasts (should be kept free)
- Chest excursion
- Venous pooling

TRENDELENBURG POSITION

In the Trendelenburg position, the head of the bed is lowered by 15 degrees or more.

- **Brain issues:** Trendelenburg position increases cerebral blood flow and intracranial pressure.
- **Cardiac issues:** Baroreceptors are activated and compensate with vasodilation. Increased pulmonary artery wedge pressures, mean arterial pressures, and mixed venous oxygen levels may occur. Stroke volume is decreased. Left atrial pressure is increased. Other potential cardiac problems include congestive heart failure, pulmonary edema, and facial engorgement.
- **Pulmonary issues:** Functional residual capacity decreases by 20%; abdominal contents shift cephalad. Vital capacity is decreased, as is pulmonary compliance. Pulmonary engorgement may occur. In the *steep* Trendelenburg position, most of the lung may be below the left atrium and the lung is

susceptible to the development of pulmonary interstitial edema.

- **Nerve issues:** There is no specific nerve risk with the Trendelenburg position.

REVERSE TRENDELENBURG POSITION

In the reverse Trendelenburg position, the head of the bed is raised by 15 degrees or more.

- **Cardiac issues:** Cardiac problems associated with this position include hypotension and venous pooling.
- **Pulmonary issues:** There is increased functional residual capacity and increased compliance. Oxygenation is improved with adequate cardiac output.
- **Nerve issues:** There is no specific nerve risk associated with the reverse Trendelenburg position.

LITHOTOMY POSITION

In the lithotomy position, the patient is on his or her back, with hips flexed and legs apart. Strap-stirrups or boot-style stirrups (used to support the foot and the calf, thereby relieving pressure on the popliteal space) are used to support the legs and feet. After lithotomy, the feet are brought together and then lowered to decrease the lumbar torsion; check the patient's blood pressure after lowering the legs.

In the *exaggerated lithotomy* position, the hips are aggressively flexed so that bent knees are closer to shoulders than chest.

- **Cardiac issues:** These issues are minimal if the patient is not pregnant, does not have an abdominal mass, and is not obese. Approximately 600 ml auto-infusion of blood occurs when the legs are lifted into the lithotomy position. Cardiac output is decreased.
- **Pulmonary issues:** An abdominal shift occurs; FRC is decreased by 20%; vital capacity is decreased; and hypoventilation occurs in the spontaneously breathing patient.

- **Nerve issues:** Damage to the *peroneal* nerve is the most common injury in the lithotomy position, caused by nerve compression at the head of the fibula (i.e., the leg in a stirrup with the outer leg pressing against the stirrup); this injury causes foot drop and leaves the patient unable to dorsiflex the foot and with sensory deficits. Damage to the *sciatic* nerve may occur during the lithotomy position with thigh and leg external rotation causing traction; its symptom is foot drop. Damage to the *saphenous* nerve may occur when the nerve is compressed by the leg holder and the tibia, causing medial sensory deficits. Damage to the *femoral obturator* may occur because of calf pressure from the leg holder. Damage to the *femoral* nerve may occur when excessive thigh flexion causes the nerve to be pressured by the pubic ramus. Damage to the *popliteal fossa* may occur when pressure leads to development of compartment syndrome. Risk of nerve damage is increased for the patient in the lithotomy position if surgery lasts longer than 4 hours, the patient's body mass index (BMI) is less than 20, and/or patient is a diabetic or a smoker.

Patients in the lithotomy position are also at a higher risk of deep venous thrombosis (DVT). For this reason, it is important they have DVT prophylaxis (e.g., compression stockings, inflating stockings, and mini-dose heparin).

Special vigilance is needed regarding hand and finger positions when lowering or raising the foot of the bed.

SITTING OR BEACH-CHAIR (SEMI-FOWLER) POSITION

In the semi-Fowler position, patients are placed in a seated position with the head of the bed 30–90 degrees above the horizontal plane. The chin must be 1–2 finger breadths from the chest; otherwise, this position can strain the C5 vertebra.

- **Brain issues:** Advantages of the sitting position include facilitation of venous blood drainage from the brain and decreasing ICP and CSF pressure.

- **Cardiac issues:** The patient may develop decreased mean arterial pressure (MAP) and central venous pressure (CVP), impaired venous return from a reduced stroke volume, and decreased cardiac output (by 20%). There is massive venous pooling in the lower extremities (especially in a head-up position greater than 60 degrees).
- **Pulmonary issues:** Functional residual capacity increases with increased compliance. Decreased pulmonary artery pressures with increased pulmonary vascular resistance.
- **Nerve issues:** Affected nerves may include the sciatic (lack of knee flexion in the sitting position), ulnar, and cervical nerves.

Pressure points in the sitting position include the occipit, scapula, elbow, sacrum, ischial tuberosities, and heels.

Advantages of Sitting Position

- Better surgical exposure
- Blood and cerebral spinal fluid drainage
- Potential advantage of improved hemostasis

Disadvantages of Sitting Position

- Hypotension, postural; decreased blood return to the heart (Avoid this by changing the patient's position gradually.)
- Decreased cerebral perfusion
- Venous air emboli (43%); especially with surgery involving bone (e.g., skull)
- Pneumocephalus (presence of air or gas within the cranium) because of the open sinuses and large veins
- Ocular compression
- Mid-cervical tetraplegia
- Edema or macroglossia
- Increased potential to lose airway

The risk of quadriplegia, paraplegia, peripheral nerve injuries, and facial/glossal edema have been reported to be increased when patients are placed in the sitting position.

Avoid use of nitrous oxide with a patient in the sitting position, as it increases the bubble size if venous air embolism (VAE) occurs.

JACK-KNIFE POSITION

In the jack-knife position, the patient lies in the prone position with the buttocks raised.

- **Cardiac issues:** These problems may include venous pooling, mesenteric/epidural engorgement, and decreased cardiac output.
- **Pulmonary issues:** Visceral shift occurs; FRC is decreased by 20% or more; decreased compliance occurs. Care should be taken to provide for free chest excursion. Hypoventilation may occur in a spontaneously breathing patient.
- **Nerve issues:** Guard against damage to the brachial plexus; arms should be placed in the swimmer's position or tucked at sides, with the shoulders still at an angle less than 90 degrees.

LATERAL DECUBITUS POSITION

The lateral decubitus position is a side-lying position.

With the patient on either the right or left side; clarify that the neck is in straight alignment with the spine and the head by placing folded towels or blankets under the foam head ring. There should be a two finger-breadths gap between the sternum and the chin. Check the "down" ear to make sure the pinna is flat and not folded. An axillary roll is placed under the dependent axilla; it is positioned slightly caudad to the axilla to provide an outlet and prevent compression of the brachial plexus. *Caution: An axillary roll can cut off circulation.*

The arm on the unaffected side (down side) is extended on an armboard with the shoulder at an angle less than 90 degrees, through use of a Velcro strap or taped to secure it. The arm on the affected side (up side) is supported on 1–2 pillows with the shoulder at an angle less than 90 degrees.

Two-inch tape can be used to secure the upper arm with pillows to the bed frame; protect the upper arm skin with a pad of gauze or a towel before taping it. The torso may be stabilized by kidney rests, pillows, or sandbags. The leg on the unaffected side is extended and the uppermost leg is flexed with a pillow placed between the legs. Adequate padding is needed for the ankles, feet, and knees. Protect and pad all bony prominences. This position is secured by use of wide adhesive tape at the shoulder, thighs, and legs, fastened to the underside of the table.

Equipment needed for this patient position includes beanbags, special hip pads, pillows, and overhead armboard for upper arm, and axillary rolls (blankets, foam).

- **Cardiac issues:** Minimal alterations are usually necessary unless the patient is hypovolemic. Check the pulse/capillary refill on the patient's lower arm/hand.
- **Pulmonary issues:** Ventilation/perfusion (V/Q) ratio mismatching may occur. The FRC is decreased in the dependent lung and increased in the nondependent (upper) lung; the dependent lung is prone to atelectasis and fluid accumulation because it is below the left atrium. Lower lung excursion may be aided with axillary rolls, which lifts the chest and decreases pressure on brachial plexus.

Lateral Decubitus Position: Awake, Spontaneous Breather

- V/Q ratio is *not* greatly altered!
- Ventilation and perfusion are increased proportionately to the dependent lung.
- The distribution of the V/Q ratios of the two lungs is not greatly altered when the awake patient is in the lateral decubitus position.
- The V/Q ratio decreases from the non-dependent to the dependent lung, just as it does in upright and supine lungs.

Lateral Decubitus Position: Anesthetized Patient, Not Spontaneously Breathing

- The distribution of the V/Q ratios of the two lungs *is* altered when the anesthetized patient is in the lateral decubitus position.
- The dependent lung continues to receive more blood flow.
- The dependent lung receives significantly less ventilation because it is less compliant, has a lower FRC, and is weighed down by the abdomen and mediastinum.
- **Nerve issues:** There is a risk of brachial plexus injury or suprascapular nerve injury with the lateral decubitus position. Brachial plexus injury is a frequent complaint after lateral positioning. Traction and stretching of the brachial plexus comes from rotating the head away from the surgical field, elevating the ipsilateral shoulder and placing traction on the arm. Make sure the suprascapular neurovascular bundle is not stretching in the lateral position.

A patient in the lateral position is at increased risk for nerve damage and is at significant risk for injuries to neurovascular structures along with injuries to soft tissues. Pressure on the dependent eye, exacerbated by intraoperative hypotension, can cause retinal artery thrombosis, resulting in postoperative vision loss.

FLEXED LATERAL DECUBITUS POSITION

In the flexed lateral decubitus position, the patient is in a side-lying position with the bed flexed so that the head and feet are lower than the patient's mid-section. The break in the bed should be at the flat area of the iliac crest. This position spreads the thorax and costal margin to iliac crest distance.

- **Cardiac issues:** increased venous pooling.
- **Pulmonary issues:** similar to issues for the lateral decubitus position unless the patient is positioned incorrectly.
- **Nerve issues:** brachial plexus injury, suprascapular nerve injury.

PATIENT POSITIONING ON A FRACTURE TABLE

The fracture table is a special table used for reconstructive and reparative orthopedic surgeries; it contains radiolucent abductor bars and a perineal post (Figure 2-1). The patient is placed in the supine position; his or her feet are secured in foot boots with Velcro taping. Traction is applied to the affected leg, raised at an upward tilt of 10 degrees. The nonsurgical leg is relaxed and kept as low as possible. The perineal post is well padded to prevent pudendal nerve injury and skin necrosis, but fits snugly against genitalia to secure the patient's body. A C-arm machine is used to take X-rays intraoperatively.

For a male patient, the scrotum may need to be padded, pulled gently upward, and adhered to the abdomen to prevent lateral X-ray imaging.

- **Cardiac issues:** aortocaval compression with obesity.
- **Pulmonary issues:** decreased functional residual capacity.

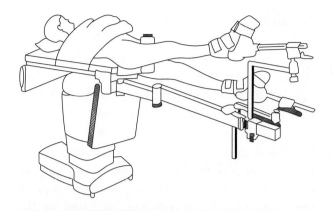

Figure 2-1   *Fracture Table*

- **Nerve issues:** vulvar or penile/testicular injury can occur from the fracture table post placed between legs.

Special Techniques and Concepts in Anesthesia

ANESTHESIA AND THE PREGNANT PATIENT

Postpone all elective surgery until 6 weeks following delivery. The risks of teratogenesis and/or preterm labor are too high to consider elective surgery prior to delivery.

Depending on the severity or emergent nature of an operative procedure, fetal and uterine monitoring may be warranted (e.g., in women who are more than 16 weeks pregnant) throughout the surgery, with plans and preparation for an emergency cesarean section (C-section) if necessary.

Later in pregnancy, the goal is to prevent fetal asphyxia by maintaining a maximum delivery of oxygen to the mother and, therefore, the fetus via the placenta. Maintain maternal blood pressure to ensure adequate placental perfusion. In evaluating laboratory values, the total blood volume will be increased; therefore, one would expect a reduction in hemoglobin and hematocrit values. Blood gases normally show a respiratory acidosis.

Use left uterine displacement (LUD) to prevent compression on the aorta when the mother is in the supine position (in women who are more than 16–20 weeks pregnant).

Tocolytics are drugs that suppress onset of premature labor and should be available when giving anesthesia to any pregnant patient. They include the following medications:

- Magnesium sulfate: first-line agent; calcium antagonist
- Ritodrine: beta-2 agonist; decreases levels of free calcium
- Terbutaline: beta-2 agonist
- Calcium-channel blockers: nifedipine, verapamil

Anesthetics in Pregnancy

General anesthesia helps to block uterine contractions. Use lower doses of all medications. Short-acting agents are preferred and minimize overall exposure to all anesthetic agents.

Narcotics cross the placental barrier and affect the fetus.

Muscle relaxants do *not* cross the placental barrier as readily as narcotics.

Avoid benzodiazepines (owing to the increased incidence of deformities in the fetus) and nitrous oxide in any pregnant patient.

Regional anesthesia is preferred because it minimizes fetal exposure to the anesthetic agents and reduces the risk of maternal aspiration.

AORTIC CROSS-CLAMPING, SPINAL CORD ISSUES, AND AORTIC SHUNTING

Application and Withdrawal of an Aortic Cross-Clamp

The higher the cross-clamp on the aorta (at the suprarenal or supraceliac levels), the more severe the effects. Fewer hemodynamic changes occur when cross-clamping the infra-renal aorta.

Prior to Clamp Placement

The systolic blood pressure (SBP) should be 90 mm Hg prior to clamp placement. Minimize the effects of clamping with nitroprusside, nitroglycerin, betablockers, fenoldopam, nicardipine, and/or inhalational agents.

After Clamp Is Applied

Marked hypertension occurs in the proximal aortic segment (above the clamp).

- MAP increases by 40%.
- Acute elevations in left ventricular pressure occur.
- Cardiac output is decreased.
- CVP increases by approximately 4 mm Hg.
- Left atrial pressure (LAP) and pulmonary capillary wedge pressure (PCWP) increase 12 mm Hg or more.
- Coronary blood flow increases by 40%.
- Systemic vascular resistance (SVR) increases by 100%.
- Levels of catecholamines, renin, and angiotensin increase, leading to vasoconstriction.

Hypotension occurs in the distal aortic segment (below the clamp), with MAP decreasing by 15%. Spinal blood flow decreases:

Proximal and distal clamp placement to isolate the diseased aortic segment may include critical intercostal vessels that provide flow to the cord; this loss is not compensated for by distal perfusion. The following measures are directed at protecting the spinal cord when the cross-clamp is on:

- Maintain MAP at 40–60 mm Hg.
- Use somatosensory evoked potentials (SSEPs) to monitor dorsal column function (sensory tracts). *Anterior cord function (i.e., motor tracts) is not monitored with SSEP.*
- Motor evoked potentials (MEPs) can accurately monitor anterior horn function. However, *muscle relaxants cannot be given* when monitoring MEPs.
- Hypothermia (decreasing core temperature to 33–34°C) will lower the patient's metabolic rate. This can be accomplished with application of ice and administration of cold blood. Care must be taken as the myocardium becomes irritable at 32°C.
- Spinal drains can be used to relieve pressure. The pressure exerted by the cerebrospinal fluid (CSF) increases during cross-clamping.
- Give steroids to further protect the spinal cord.

Renal and intestinal blood flow decreases:

To prevent renal failure and gut ischemia, keep the patient's BP up with good perfusion. Give Mannitol (0.5 mg/kg), furosemide, and IV infusion of low-dose dopamine or fenoldopam for renal protection. Even if aortic shunting is used, the distribution changes in renal blood flow make these interventions prudent.

Before Clamp Is Removed

Check the volume load. The patient may need vasopressors prior to removal of the cross-clamp.

Aortic Cross-Clamp Removal Effects

Declamping shock is a possibility. Severe hypotension—a decline in BP of as much as 70%—may occur due to hypovolemia (combined with bleeding), with this abrupt decrease in after load. The release of vasodilating acid metabolites from the ischemic lower body into the general circulation (noted as an increase in $ETCO_2$), the release of vasodilator substances, and an increase in the vascular space all cause a severe decrease in ventricular preload. Declamping shock is also associated with hyperkalemia and hypocalcemia.

Removal of the cross-clamp may also lead to decreased contractility and cardiac output. The severity of this effect is influenced by the duration of clamping, existence of adequate preload, and influence of circulating drugs.

Treat cross-clamp removal effects by decreasing the anesthetic levels, decreasing or discontinuing vasodilators, and administering volume (crystalloids, colloids, cell saver, blood products), and calcium chloride. May also need to give phenylephrine, epinephrine, or norepinephrine to maintain the BP. Increasing the ventilation rate will help decrease acidosis, though it may be necessary to give sodium bicarbonate as well. The surgeon may need to remove the cross-clamp slowly to minimize these effects.

Renal blood flow decreases by 50% when the cross-clamp is removed. To compensate for this effect, keep the patient hydrated and keep the BP within normal limits.

- The spinal cord must also be protected from severe hypotension *after* removing the aortic cross-clamp by maintaining the BP within normal limits.

SPINAL CORD INJURY AND AORTIC CROSS-CLAMPING

Spinal cord perfusion in the thoracolumbar area is derived from the artery of Adamkiewicz (the principal arterial supply of the anterior spinal cord).

The artery of Adamkiewicz joins the anterior spinal artery in sending flow to the lower thoracic and lumbar segments T8–L4: the celiac artery at T12 (gastric, splenic, hepatic branches), the superior mesenteric artery at L1, and the inferior mesenteric artery at L3. The lateral aortic branches are the suprarenal and renal branches at L1 and the gonadal branch at L2. The posterolateral artery contains the inferior phrenic and lumbar branches. Maintaining perfusion in these areas can be important, particularly in thoracoabdominal aneurysm repair, where the cross-clamp is applied above these structures.

The most feared major complication of aortic cross-clamping is paraplegia from prolonged spinal cord ischemia as a consequence of hypotension and surgical interruption of the blood supply to the artery of Adamkiewicz. Along with paraplegia, there is a risk of mesenteric/bowel ischemia/infarction, renal ischemia/failure, and hepatic ischemia. Coagulopathy can occur if thoracolumbar blood flow is decreased when systemic pressures are low. Maintaining a distal perfusion pressure mean of 70 mm Hg or higher will minimize the incidence of paraplegia and organ ischemia/failure.

As far as aortic cross-clamp time goes, a simple rule applies: Shorter is better. The duration of aortic cross-clamping is directly related to the risk of complications; cross-clamping the aorta for more than 30 minutes increases their incidence.

Spinal Cord Protection During Aortic Cross-Clamping

Protective measures during aortic cross-clamping aim to stabilize cell membranes, prevent release of chemical mediators, and scavenge oxygen-free radicals. These measures are summarized here:

- Thiopental IV
- Intrathecal Papaverine (3 mL of 1% strength)
- Corticosteroids (methylprednisone)
- Magnesium sulfate
- Mannitol
- Betablockers

- Drain 20–25 mL CSF prior to clamping to decrease intrathecal pressure.
- Maintain MAP at greater than 70 mm Hg intraoperatively and postoperatively.

The MAP distal to the aortic clamp is decreased and the distal spinal cord will be at risk of ischemia. Several techniques can increase the distal arterial perfusion pressure, such as the placement of a simple shunt (a shunt is placed above and below the cross-clamp) or a partial (femoral vein to femoral artery) or full cardiopulmonary bypass (left atrium to femoral artery). Heparin is given with these techniques.

Administration of nitroprusside can be detrimental to spinal cord perfusion by decreasing systemic vascular resistance and shunting blood away from the spinal cord vessels and collateral branches.

Cross-clamping the aorta below the left common carotid increases the proximal systemic pressure, which in turn increases the CSF pressure. This increased CSF pressure can increase the incidence of paraplegia and careful drainage of CSF can be beneficial.

Spinal cord perfusion = anterior spinal artery
pressure (SCPP)   pressure (distal aortic
                       MAP) − CSF pressure

To increase SCPP, either increase the distal aortic MAP or lower the CSF pressure. SCPP should be maintained at a level higher than 15 mm Hg.

Hypothermia at 24–32°C decreases spinal cord oxygen requirement, decreases tissue metabolism, and increases tolerance to anoxia.

It is important to prevent hyperglycemia when aortic cross-clamping is used. Maintain blood glucose levels between 80 and 120 mg/dL.

Prolonged latency or reduced amplitude of SSEPs and MEPs indicates spinal cord ischemia, although this relationship is not always reliable. SSEPs monitor sensory neurons in dorsal root ganglia to the posterior column; MEPs monitor motor neurons in the anterior horn cells and is more sensitive to ischemia.

Aortic Shunt

Placement of a shunt may be used to bypass the cross-clamped aorta. In this case, the proximal end of the shunt is placed in the ascending aorta and the distal end in the descending thoracic aorta past the aneurysm. Shunt flow should be approximately 2.5 L/min, with distal MAP being maintained at more than 70 mm Hg.

Nevertheless, the spinal cord and kidneys cannot be assumed to be "protected" when a shunt or bypass is used. Even with these measures, atherosclerosis may prevent significant flow to the kidneys and spinal cord.

Distal shunt placement advantages include the ability to attenuate proximal hypertension by sending blood down past the clamps via the shunt. This approach may lead to perfusion of the vascular beds distal to clamp. The placement of such a shunt minimizes the risk of paraplegia, attenuates metabolic acidosis, and relieves hypotension.

BLOOD PRODUCTS

Whole blood: 500 mL. Contains red blood cells (RBCs), plasma, white blood cells (WBCs), and platelets, along with 63 mL anticoagulant/preservative. Given to increase red cell mass and plasma volume.

Packed red blood cells (PRBCs): 300 mL. Contains RBCs, WBCs, platelets, and some plasma. Each unit will raise the hematocrit (HCT) by one-third or hemoglobin (HGB) by 1 g/dL. PRBCs are deficient in Factors V and VIII.

RBC washed: 175 mL. Has no plasma; has increased RBC mass; confers a reduced risk of allergy to plasma proteins.

RBC leukocyte poor: 250 mL. Has no plasma; has increased RBC mass; confers a reduced risk of febrile reaction due to leukocyte antibodies.

Platelets: 50 mL/unit. Don't put on ice or heat, as such a temperature change affects platelet function. Consists of platelets and plasma; each unit will increase the platelet count by 7500 to 10,000. Controls bleeding associated with decreased platelet number or function.

- A male older than age 18 can receive any Rh and type.
- A female of child-bearing age must receive Rh-appropriate platelets but any type is acceptable.
- A child younger than age 18 must receive an exact match in terms of Rh and type.

Fresh frozen plasma (FFP): 200 mL. Must be ABO compatible with the recipient's RBCs; Rh matching need not be considered. FFP reverses the effects of Coumadin (warfarin). FFP contains all coagulation factors in normal amounts; it has no platelets, leukocytes, or RBCs. FFP is made from plasma removed from a unit of whole blood and frozen; it is not a concentrate of clotting factors. One unit of FFP increases clotting factors by 2%.

Cryoprecipitate: 15 mL/unit. Contains fibrinogen F1, von Willebrand's Factor VII, and fibrin F13. Cryoprecipitate is given for hemophilia and hypofibrinogenemia; it is also given to correct factor deficiencies. One bag contains 100 units of Factor VIII and 250 mg of fibrinogen.

Autologous blood does not need a filter.
Scavenged cell saver blood (BRAT) needs a filter.
Platelets can use regular tubing or blood tubing.
PRBC, cryoprecipitate, and FFP can use blood tubing.
All products can be put through a fluid warmer except platelets,
which should not be cooled or warmed.

CARCINOID SYNDROME

Carcinoid syndrome refers to an array of symptoms that occur when a proliferation of cells secrete several vasoactive substances (e.g., serotonin, bradykinin, histamine, prostaglandins, and polypeptide hormones) from malignant carcinoid tumors. These tumors arise from endocrine cells situated in the ileum, although they can also arise from anywhere in the gastrointestinal (GI) tract, pancreas, gonads, or the bronchi. Serotonin release causes a syndrome of episodic cutaneous flushing, diarrhea, bronchospasm, supraventricular dysrhythmias, hyperglycemia, and valvular heart disease and, less commonly, asthma.

The current treatment of choice for significant cardiovascular complications or bronchospasm with suspected carcinoid syndrome is:

- Octreotide (Sandostatin) IV neutralizes serotonin, gastrin, insulin, glucagon, and vasoactive intestinal peptide (VIP). It is a universal inhibitor of GI motility that acts by binding to somatostatin receptors in the GI tract.
- Histamine (H_1 and H_2) blockers help the histamine-related symptoms.
- Phenoxybenzamine and phenothiazines control flushing from bradykinin release.
- Glucocorticoids, indomethacin, and nonsteroidal anti-inflammatory drugs (NSAIDs) inhibit the bradykinin system and control flushing.
- Aminophylline and steroids ease bronchospasm (secondary to bradykinin).
- Ondansetron can relieve nausea and diarrhea.
- Digitalis and diuretics may help with congestive heart failure secondary to valve malfunction.

Carcinoid Crisis

Carcinoid crisis occurs in patients with 5-HIAA levels greater than 200 mg/day and is precipitated by stressful events (e.g., anesthesia, manipulation, chemotherapy, hepatic artery embolization). Patients can experience flushing, severe abdominal pain, explosive diarrhea, CNS depression, CV instability, profound hypotension, CV collapse, severe hypertension, tachycardia, and bronchospasm.

Treat carcinoid crisis with Octreotide 50–100 mcg IV over 30 minutes, fluid resuscitation, and direct-acting vasopressors.

Surgical Resection of Carcinoid Tumor

Intraoperative management includes the following measures:

- Hydrate the patient well and consistently maintain blood volume.
- Monitor the CVP and urine output.
- Monitor the blood pressure by arterial line.
- Place a pulmonary artery catheter if the patient has advanced cardiac disease.
- Avoid drugs that release histamine, such as morphine and atracurium.
- Use succinylcholine with caution: It increases intra-abdominal pressure, but has been used safely in these surgeries.
- Check glucose levels intermittently, maintain glucose levels between 80–120 mg/dL.

Postoperative treatment consists of chemotherapy with 5-fluoruracil (5-FU) and doxorubicin.

CARDIOPULMONARY BYPASS
Why Off-Pump Is Done

As the serious complications associated with traditional coronary artery bypass graft (CABG) and cardiopulmonary bypass (CPB) were increasingly identified, and cardiac stabilization devices were developed, performing coronary bypass without the use of cardiopulmonary bypass found new popularity.

Some of the many complications of traditional CABG and CPB include microembolization with resultant strokes and cerebral dysfunction; platelet consumption or sequestration and endothelial dysfunction, causing coagulopathy and anemia requiring blood product transfusion; aortic cannulation;

systemic inflammatory response and activation of fibrinolysis; sternal wound infections; and respiratory insufficiency. There is a higher incidence of renal failure after CPB as the kidneys operate best with pulsatile flow.

On-Pump Issues

Cardiopulmonary bypass allows the heart muscle to be still while the patient's blood is diverted, oxygenated, and then reperfused. CPB can be either total or partial. Three components of CPB are hemodilution, hypothermia, and anticoagulation; these three components contribute to the complications associated with CPB.

CPB must be established so that blood can be taken from the body and returned. Blood is usually diverted from the body at the right atrium, the femoral vein, or the inferior vena cava. Blood is usually returned to the body by an artery—ascending aorta, femoral, or subclavian.

Weaning off bypass may need to be gradual if the patient's blood pressure is too low. The perfusionist will partially occlude the venous line, allowing the heart to fill; the arterial flow from the pump is then decreased and ejection begins. It is also possible to use "parallel circulation" (the patient's own circulation along with bypass support) during CPB. Time spent in parallel circulation is directly related to the risk of myocardial dysfunction.

If the patient has increased BP, the bypass flow should be shut off completely.

If the patient has decreased BP, it is recommended to maintain partial CPB (parallel circulation) and begin appropriate infusions. Continue to assess blood pressure and contractility, titrate volume, and give appropriate drugs during further attempts to reduce CPB flow.

CEREBRAL PROTECTION
Cerebral protection: $\downarrow$ CPP = $\downarrow$ CBV = $\downarrow$ ICP = $\downarrow$ CBF

Cerebral blood flow (CBF) is normally auto regulated with the body maintaining a mean arterial pressure (MAP) between 50 and 150 mm Hg (newer data suggest that this range is 70–150 mm Hg); vascular resistance changes in response to pressure changes. Patients who have shifted to the right (chronically hypertensive patients in whom auto regulation occurs in a higher MAP range) have adapted to higher pressures and will not tolerate hypotension.

To protect the patient's brain, it is essential to maintain good cerebral blood flow, normocapnia, blood sugar levels, oxygenation levels, and carrying capacity.

Pharmacologic Methods of Cerebral Protection

Cerebral Vasoconstrictor

Cerebral metabolism may be reduced by administration of a *barbiturate* (e.g., sodium thiopental [Pentothal]), which is a potent cerebral vasoconstrictor that decreases CBF, cerebral blood volume, $CMRO_2$ (cerebral metabolic rate of oxygen), and ICP. The cerebral metabolism reduction dose of thiopental is 4 mg/kg (2–5 g range dose). Pentothal is the only drug proven to save an ischemic brain. Barbiturates are thought to enhance gamma-aminobutyric acid (GABA) activity and antagonize the N-methyl-D-aspartate receptor, thereby reducing ischemic excitotoxicity.

Propofol and etomidate are also potent cerebral vasoconstrictors. The use of this technique must be weighed against the potential complications if the symptoms of cerebral ischemia are present, because the possible hypotension can compound the ischemia.

Burst Suppression

Barbiturates are also used for burst suppression because they follow a pattern of initial EEG activation followed by dose-related depression. Eventually high doses lead to lengthening periods of suppression alternating with periods of activity. Pentothal burst suppression doses consist of 10–30 mg/kg total dose and can reduce EEG electrical activity (in a dose-dependent manner) by as much as 50%.

Propofol will induce burst suppression in a dose-dependent fashion and has the potential to be as beneficial as thiopental. Furthermore, this agent is metabolized quickly, providing a more predictable wake-up time for the patient.

See this chapter, "Neuro-physiologic Monitoring," for more information.

Fluid restriction is rarely used to lower ICP for purposes of cerebral protection, as it can cause hypovolemia, resulting in hypotension with anesthesia induction.

Loop diuretics used for cerebral protection include furosemide 0.3 mg/kg (or 10–20 mg IV), Edecrin, or Bumex. These medications decrease blood volume; the onset of action occurs in 10–30 minutes. Lasix (furosemide) lowers BP by reducing intravascular volume and cardiac output; it may require as long as 30 minutes to lower ICP.

An *osmotic diuretic*, Mannitol 0.5–2 g/kg (or 25–50 g) increases urinary output, acts as a free-radical scavenger, and decreases ICP. The surgeon will often order a specific amount in total to be given, such as 50 g mannitol. (25% is 12.5 g in 50 mL) to be given over 15–30 minutes. Mannitol crystallizes and should be drawn up through a filter needle; an administration set with a filter should be used for infusions containing 20% or more of this agent. Mannitol acts within 10–15 minutes and its effect last as long as 2 hours.

Mannitol can cause a triphasic hemodynamic response:

Phase 1: transient (1–2 minutes) hypotension after rapid administration. Mannitol causes vasodilation, the extent of which is dependent on the dose and the rate of administration.

Phase 2: transient increase in blood volume, cardiac index, and PCWP. The maximum increase occurs shortly after termination of infusion.

Phase 3: 30 minutes after infusion, blood volume returns to normal; PCWP and cardiac index drop to below normal levels because of peripheral vascular pooling. Due to mannitol's potent diuretic effect, excessive administration of this agent may result in systemic hypotension and cerebral hypoperfusion.

Mannitol can also have a biphasic effect on ICP:

Phase 1: transient increase in ICP due to increased CBF and CBV. This increase in blood volume and ICP may be attenuated by giving Lasix beforehand.

Phase 2: maximal reduction of ICP within 10 minutes of administration, an effect that persists for 3–4 hours. Mannitol increases serum osmolarity, which creates an osmotic gradient across an intact blood–brain barrier (BBB), drawing water out of the brain parenchyma. (e.g., from interstitial and intracellular spaces into the intravascular system).

Corticosteroids stabilize cell membranes, prevent release of chemical mediators, decrease edema, and act as free radical scavengers. These agents also reduce swelling around tumors, improve pulmonary compliance, and decrease pulmonary vascular resistance. Although it may take many hours or days before the ICP is reduced, the advantage associated with use of corticosteroids is that these agents may restore the BBB. Examples include Decadron 10 mg IV or methylprednisolone (also known as methylprednisone or SoluMedrol) 1 g IV or 30 mg/kg.

While administration of steroids is useful in reducing cerebral edema, the associated hyperglycemia can be detrimental to the ischemic brain. Insulin infusions should be used to help reduce blood glucose to normoglycemic levels when corticosteroids are given.

Other pharmacologic methods of cerebral protection include *judicious use of anesthetic agents* and good skeletal *muscle relaxation. Antiseizure medication* may also confer this kind of protection, such as Dilantin (phenytoin) 1 gram IV piggyback drip. Give Dilantin very slowly as an IV medication, as its administration can cause profound hypotension and arrhythmias. Seizure activity produces increases in both CBF and $CMRO_2$ by "supranormal" energy demand.

Magnesium may act as a free-radical scavenger; it may exert beneficial effects during brain ischemia by dilating cerebral vascular smooth muscle.

Calcium-channel blockers such as nimodipine may exert beneficial effects during brain ischemia by acting on cerebral vascular smooth muscle.

Interventions in Cerebral Protection

A simple mnemonic to remember in terms of cerebral protection is the "30-31-32 rule": keep the head of bed (HOB) up 30 degrees—hematocrit $\geq$ 31%—body temperature at 32°C.

Carbon dioxide (hypercarbia) is a potent cerebral vasodilator. Low normal $ETCO_2$ (30–34 mm Hg) is ideal. At that level, CBF is decreased by approximately 10%. CBF decreases 4% if the $PaCO_2$ decreases from 34 to 33 mm Hg.

Hyperventilation is still the fastest way to decrease brain bulk by blowing off carbon dioxide; decreases in carbon dioxide cause cerebral arterial vasoconstriction and reductions in CBF and CBV. Vasoconstriction occurs so quickly with hyperventilation because CO_2 crosses the BBB without limitation. The effect may last only 6–8 hours before the body's balancing mechanisms kick in (metabolic; bicarbonate levels change). One disadvantage of hyperventilation is that the decrease in CBF can cause ischemia in brain tissue.

Hyperventilation Benefits
- Cerebral vasoconstriction and reductions in CBF, $CMRO_2$, CBV, and ICP.
- Increased pH decreases acidosis.
- Inverse steal to feed injured tissue.
- Decreased brain bulk.
- Reduction in brain tissue bulk increases exposure for surgeon.

Hyperventilation should not be used in patients with possible focal ischemia because of the "steal" phenomenon: During periods of cerebral ischemia, blood flow is increased in *normal* areas of the brain but not in ischemic areas.

A mild decrease in *body temperature* to 32–33°C is most effective in providing cerebral protection; it decreases both basal and metabolic requirements.

$CMRO_2$ decreases 7% for every 1°C decrease in temperature. This is due to a reduction in the transmembrane ion flux and basal energy expenditure, which produces a neuron-sparing effect. To use this approach to provide cerebral protection, passively expose patient to decrease body temperature, or lay the patient on a cooling blanket but turn it on only if necessary. At the end of the procedure, use a warming blanket to prevent shivering. Hypothermia can cause platelet dysfunction.

Blood viscosity can also be used to provide cerebral protection. The optimal hematocrit range is 30–33. Anemia increases CBF; polycythemia decreases CBF. A hematocrit of 33 decreases viscosity, which in turn decreases CBF but still provides good oxygen-carrying capacity.

Postural changes (e.g., raising the head of the bed up to approximately 30 degrees) are associated with increased venous drainage and a lower ICP. Keep the patient's neck straight to facilitate venous outflow.

Planned CSF drainage from a ventricular catheter or lumbar drain can also be used to protect the brain. The collection device is placed at a scale that allows for drainage. The drainage device is placed at a certain level (say, 15 cm H_2O), and the CSF drains only when pressure is above that level. A scale too high would impede drainage, whereas a scale too low would allow too much CSF to flow out. Strict parameters of CSF removal, including how much and how often, have been established. If a lumbar drain is inserted in a patient with increased ICP, there is a chance the brain tissue will herniate through the foramen magnum.

With this technique, a ventriculostomy drain to monitor ICP or drain CSF is placed in lateral horn of the lateral ventricle near the foramen of Monroe in the brain. The transducer is leveled at the tragus of the ear (or external auditory meatus). A ventriculostomy catheter can be used to drain CSF, although one should never remove more than 10 mL at a time or as much as 50 mL in total.

Normotension alterations—namely, induced hypotension—is implemented only at surgeon's request; it is rarely used for cerebral protection purposes (hypertension causes an increase in CBV). Deliberate hypotension may be utilized as a means to decrease blood loss and hyperemic complications (cerebral edema or hemorrhage).

Good oxygenation (hyperoxia) is based on the following premises: A PaO_2 less than 60 mm Hg profoundly increases CBF and causes anaerobic metabolism. The condition worsens ischemia by releasing free radicals and worsening neurologic injury. Studies show that a marked improvement in the survival of cortical neurons occurs if PaO_2 kept above 200 mm Hg.

Blood glucose concentration is also important during episodes of ischemia. It is thought that hyperglycemia, in the presence of hypoxia, will increase intracellular acidosis. Insulin has a direct protective effect on ischemic neural tissue. Insulin and glucose infusions should be used to bring the patient to a normoglycemic level.

Deep hypothermic circulatory arrest (DHCA) for cerebral protection is discussed later in this chapter.

COMMON ALLERGIES, ASTHMA, AND HISTAMINE IN THE OPERATING ROOM

Agents Associated with Anaphylaxis

1. Muscle relaxants: rocuronium, succinylcholine, atracurium
2. Latex
3. Antibiotics: penicillin, cephalosporin, vancomycin
4. Colloids
5. Hypnotic/induction agents: propofol, thiopental, midazolam

Asthmatic Patients

Drugs to avoid with asthmatic patients include beta-2 blockers (e.g., propranolol, labetalol) and histamine-releasing drugs. Histamine-releasing anesthetic drugs include trimethaphan (Arfonad), succinylcholine, mivacurium, atracurium, opioids (MSO_4), Demerol, thiopental, and curare.

Histamine release from mast cells results in bronchospasm, hypotension from peripheral vasodilation, and skin flushing. The effects of histamine can be minimized by slow opioid infusion, adequate IV volume, or pretreatment with H_1 or H_2 antagonists. True antibody-mediated allergic reactions are extremely rare. Histamine release is associated with signs and symptoms including flushing, itching, and even wheezing. Hypotension can occur; it is especially likely to occur in a hypovolemic patient, in whom it may lead to orthostatic hypotension. Nausea, vomiting, and retching due to stimulation of chemoreceptor trigger zone (parasellar region lateral medulla) by the opioid are possible as well and may be exacerbated by movement (e.g., vestibular stimulation).

Histamine blockers come in two varieties: H_1 blockers, such as Benadryl (diphenhydramine), and H_2 blockers, such as Tagamet, Zantac, Axid, and Pepcid.

DEEP HYPOTHERMIC CARDIAC ARREST

Deep hypothermic cardiac arrest (DHCA) is used in pediatric intracardiac defect surgery (e.g., transposition of great arteries, hypoplastic left heart syndrome), major adult vascular procedures such as aortic arch reconstruction, removal of hepatic and renal tumors, intracranial surgery, and cardiac surgery. The goal in using DHCA is to lower body temperature, thereby lowering the patient's metabolic rate and oxygen demand to the point where blood flow and oxygen delivery can be completely stopped for an extended period of 45–60 minutes.

Initiation of cooling is done once cardiopulmonary bypass is established. Pharmacologic cerebral protection is implemented prior to initiating hypothermic arrest.

The perfusionist decreases the core body temperature to 14–18°C; that temperature is maintained until approximately 20 minutes prior to circulatory arrest. The period of hypothermic circulatory arrest with minimal cerebral complications is approximately 45 minutes at 18°C and 1 hour at 15°C.

In addition to the cooling implemented by the perfusionist, the anesthetist packs the patient's head in ice, over towels (to protect the skin, nose, eyes, and earlobes from frostbite). The head temperature is monitored with a nasal or tympanic probe. The best estimate of the brain temperature is measured in the nasopharyngeal area. The rectal temperature measures the body temperature.

The following monitors are commonly used in DHCA:

- Right radial arterial line
- Right femoral arterial line
- Pulmonary artery catheter
- Separate CVP line to monitor retrograde cerebral flow
- Transesophageal echocardiography (TEE) monitor

Cerebral Protection with Hypothermic Blood Flow

Both antegrade cerebral perfusion (ACP) and retrograde cerebral perfusion (RCP) allow for continued hypothermic blood flow to the brain while maintaining a bloodless field.

Antegrade Cerebral Perfusion

ACP is a technique utilized to maintain selective cerebral perfusion during total-body DHCA. Once DHCA has been established, depending on the surgeon's aortic cannula placement (generally through the carotid or brachiocephalic artery), the cannula is either removed or clamped. The dissected/aneurysmal aorta is opened. Ballooned retrograde perfusion catheters are then placed into the innominate artery (to access the right carotid) and directly into the left carotid; these catheters are attached to individual pump heads on the CPB machine. A flow rate of 500–700 mL/min of cold blood at 20°C is delivered; thus the brain is perfused with cold blood while the patient is maintained in DHCA. Distal and arch vessels are anastomosed to the replacement aortic tube graft;

ACP is terminated and the balloon catheters are deflated and removed. The new graft is flushed and de-aired with trickle blood flow from the arterial cannula. Once the new graft is de-aired, total body perfusion is reinitiated and rewarming begins.

ACP has several notable advantages. For example, cerebral flow provides uniform cooling in a normal flow direction, and metabolic substrate delivery tends to have more favorable outcomes. ACP has also been shown to be a more effective cerebral protector than retrograde flow. Disadvantages include the complexity of the procedure, the presence of an extra cannula on the surgical field, an increased risk of emboli, problems with fragile vessels, and the difficulty level of performing this procedure.

Retrograde Cerebral Perfusion

RCP, with deep hypothermic circulatory arrest, will increase the safe arrest time. Due to the greater fragility of the venous system (compared to the arterial system), RCP is maintained at a pressure of 20–25 mm Hg at 8–14°C (flow rates depend on pressures but are usually approximately 500–800 mL/min). The patient is placed in the steep Trendelenburg position to ensure brain perfusion.

After DHCA is initiated, the arterial perfusion line is connected to the SVC cannula and low perfusion flow is initiated backward or retrograde through the brain. The brain is perfused in retrograde fashion with cold, oxygen-rich blood with 100% oxygen saturation via SVC to jugular vein; the blood will come back through the carotid and innominate arteries and is recovered by suction.

Advantages of RCP include effective global cerebral cooling; decreased cerebral embolization; ability to wash out air bubbles, embolic debris, and metabolic waste products; use of simpler system; avoidance of fragile vessels; and delivery of oxygen and nutritional substrates to brain tissue. Moreover, use of RCP decreases strokes and neurologic injury.

Disadvantages of RCP include increased cerebral edema from over-perfusion; the fact that substrate delivery is *not* reliable, as only 20–60% of the brain is perfused with retrograde flow; ability of venous valves to alter flow; ability of collateral veins to divert the flow; and ability of drainage from the RCP catheter to affect the surgical view.

Anesthesia Considerations with DHCA

- Prolonged effect of anesthesia agents due to slowed drug metabolism and elimination
- Decreased minimal alveolar concentration (MAC) of inhalational agents
- Need for a narcotic, amnestic, and nondepolarizing muscle relaxant (NDMR) when the patient is rewarmed to 34°C.
- Positioning and padding must be meticulous as DHCA leaves the patient more susceptible to nerve and tissue injury
- Monitor urine output every 30 minutes and report it to the perfusionist

Surgical Considerations with DHCA

DHCA provides for a bloodless field. There is also no need for aortic cross-clamping, thereby reducing the risks associated with embolization sequelae.

Systemic Effects from DHCA

Cerebral Effects

- Rapid core cooling to 15–18°C. EEG becomes flat at 18°C.
- Protection with metabolic suppression occurs by severe reduction of body temperature, reducing intracellular enzymatic reactions and thereby reducing oxygen demand and cerebral blood flow.
- Fewer cerebral intracellular enzymatic reactions.
- Proportionate reduction in cerebral oxygen requirements and blood flow.
- Brain tissue protectant—preserves pH and ATP stores.
- Decreased cerebral oxygen consumption. The patient is able to tolerate anoxia longer.

- Edema, which can occur after hypothermia due to cellular membrane permeability.
- An isoelectric EEG and bispectral analysis monitor (BIS) reading of 0—used to gauge the degree of hypothermia necessary to prevent neurologic damage. Different areas of the brain have varying abilities to tolerate a lack of oxygen: Some regions tolerate very short ischemic times, whereas others can sustain function for longer periods under these conditions. The amount of time the brain can tolerate ischemia depends on its tissue energy stores and the rate of energy consumption. The rate of energy consumption depends on temperature, metabolic rate, brain activity, and the use of anesthetics.
- Hypothermia: $CMRO_2$ is decreased by approximately 7% per 1°C decrease in temperature. A mild body temperature decrease to 32–34°C is most effective; it decreases both basal and metabolic requirements.
- Blood viscosity: Optimal hematocrit is 30–35%.
- Injection of Papaverine into subdural space— can be done to dilate the anterior spinal artery to preserve blood flow.

Cardiovascular Effects

- Oxyhemoglobin dissociation curve: shifts to the left with oxygen less readily available to the tissues. The reduced oxygen demand from core cooling usually mitigates this effect.
- Decreased heart rate.
- Increased SVR with decreased cardiac output and decreased LV compliance.
- Prolonged refractory period.
- Heart: most susceptible to ventricular fibrillation when the body is warmed to 30°C.

Hematological Effects

- Coagulopathy from the profound cooling—due to clotting factor and platelet dysfunction and activation (of platelets) with release of granules. Hemodilution is needed to prevent increased viscosity of the patient's blood at these extremely cold temperatures, which also helps increase the tissue perfusion.
- Cerebral macro-circulatory obstruction occurrence from coagulopathy.
- Impaired enzymatic activity of clotting factors, promoting abnormal clot formation; a slowed coagulation cascade; decreased platelet number and function. DHCA contributes to greater blood product requirements.
- Decreased heparin metabolism.
- Hyperglycemia: Requires monitoring of glucose levels, maintain between 80–120 mg/dL.

Metabolic Effects

- Change of 1°C = 7% metabolic decrease.
- Carbon dioxide production—decreased due to the decreased metabolic rate. CO_2 levels should be adjusted to maintain a $PaCO_2$ of 40 mm Hg to help prevent cerebral injury.
- Metabolic acidosis due to peripheral hypoperfusion; increased production of lactic acid with cold body temperature. $ETCO_2$ levels will rise with the reperfusion after blood flow is restored.

DOUBLE-LUMEN ENDOBRONCHIAL TUBE

One-lung ventilation allows for the collapse of the operative lung; it facilitates surgical exposure. With a double-lumen endobronchial tube (DLEBT), the following settings are used:

- Proximal tracheal cuff: 10–20 mL air (high volume, low pressure)
- Bronchial cuff: 3 mL only

The tube and stylet should be coated liberally with a water-soluble lubricant (or spray).

DLEBT Sizing in Adult Patients

- Height of 170 cm (approximately 5 feet, 5 inches): 29 cm at central incisors; advance or withdraw the tube by 1 cm for each 10-cm height difference.

< 165 cm (less than 5 feet, 3 inches): 35–37 Fr

165–179 cm (5 feet, 3 inches to 5 feet, 8 inches): 37–39 Fr

> 179 cm (greater than 5 feet, 8 inches): 39–41 Fr

- Females: typically use DLEBT 35–39; *place the largest device you can to decrease resistance*
- Males: typically use DLEBT 39–43

DLEBT Sizing in Pediatric Patients

	Preemie	Birth	6 mo	1 y	2 y	3 y	4 y	5 y	6 y	7 y	8 y	10 y	12 y	> 15 y
kg	1.5	3.5	7	10	12	14	17		20		25	33	40	50+
lb	3.5	7.5	15	22	26	31	37	40	44	49	55	73	88	
DLEBT size											26	26–28	32	35

For all patients, it is important to *remove the stylet before rotating and advancing the DLEBT to avoid tracheal or bronchial lacerations.* Once the tube is thought to be placed properly, the tracheal cuff should be inflated and equal ventilation of both lungs established. (Is it through the vocal cords and in trachea?)

To check for proper position, go into the tracheal lumen first. In pediatric patients, use a *pediatric flexible fiber optic bronchoscope.*

Obtain a baseline ABG on two-lung ventilation; remeasure ABG after 15 minutes on one-lung ventilation.

When going from two-lung to one-lung ventilation:

- Go to 100% FiO_2.
- Decrease the tidal volume.
- Increase the respiratory rate.
- Clamp the tube to the nondependent lung.
- Open the pop-cap to the air.
- Avoid peak airway pressures greater than 40 mm Hg.

In case of decreasing SaO_2 with DLEBT with one-lung ventilation:

- Notify the surgeon. Discuss which modality is most advantageous for the patient and least likely to interfere with the surgery.
- Administer 100% FiO_2.
- Check tube position and make sure the cuff has not moved.

- Deliver continuous positive airway pressure (CPAP) on the *deflated* lung (surgical lung).
- Deliver positive end-expiratory pressure (PEEP) on the inflated lung.
- Jet ventilation may be helpful with low driving pressure and an increased respiratory rate.
- Allow the patient to desaturate to a certain level, have the surgeon stop the procedure, inflate both lungs and oxygenate the patient to the desirable level, and then clamp lung again (until the patient desaturates again).
- Band the pulmonary artery (PA) to stop blood flow to the surgical lung. This step can be taken only if the surgical team is performing a total pneumonectomy.

Indications and Contraindications for DLEBT

Absolute indications (to isolate one lung from the other): Infection, massive hemorrhage, bronchopleural fistula, bronchopleural cutaneous fistula, washout for alveolar proteinosis, bronchial disruption or trauma, unilateral cyst, or bullous. Video-assisted thoracoscopic surgery (VATS) requires lung separation and is becoming the most common indication for one-lung ventilation.

Relative Indications: Surgical exposure for thoracic aortic aneurysm; pneumonectomy; upper, middle, or lower lobectomy; or esophageal surgery.

Contraindications: Airway lesion, poor laryngeal visualization, or patients so unstable that short periods of apnea would be life-threatening.

EMBOLISM

Venous Air Embolism

Air embolism is the abnormal presence of air or carbon dioxide in the vena cava and right atrium, resulting in obstruction of the flow of blood through the heart. *Venous air embolism* (VAE) is related to a mass of foamy bubbles that interfere with the right heart venous outflow tract; blood cannot get into the heart (venous return) and, therefore, cannot get into the lungs because of all the air. Cardiac output will fall and circulatory collapse may result. One-third of 1 mL air can cause problems; *50 mL air is lethal.* The latter condition causes air lock in heart (air cannot flow into lungs) accompanied by a foamy, incompressible mass.

The physiologic consequences of VAE depend on the volume of air, the rate of air entry, and the presence or absence of a patent foramen ovale (PFO). A PFO can facilitate passage of air into arterial circulation (paradoxical air embolism), especially when the normal transatrial (left→right) pressure gradient is reversed. Reversal of this gradient is favored by hypovolemia and perhaps by PEEP. Potential end-organ damage can also occur from paradoxical air emboli to the microvascular circulation.

VAE can occur when the pressure within an open vein is subatmospheric. This pressure gradient develops when the surgical site is higher than the right atrium (approximately 2-torr pressure difference for 1-inch difference in height). These conditions may exist in any position (and during any procedure) whenever the wound is above the level of the heart:

- Sitting craniotomies (highest incidence of VAE, at 25–50%), especially with open bone
- Severe barotrauma associated with mechanical ventilation

- Open sinuses
- Open, large veins
- Cement impaction in orthopedic surgeries, when air is forced into vessels
- Sitting position
- Side-lying posterior fossa procedures (Brain surgery is dealing with highly vascular membranes; e.g., the dura can entrain air when cut.)
- Low central venous pressures (especially from positioning the legs too low)
- Inadvertent opening of a large-bore venous catheter
- Accidental IV bolus of air
- Traumatically, as by a puncture wound

Nitrous oxide can markedly accentuate the effects of even small amounts of air.

Monitors for VAE

The monitors for VAE are presented here in order of decreasing sensitivity.

Transesophageal echocardiography (TEE): Transesophageal two-dimensional echocardiography is the most sensitive intraoperative monitor but some consider it "too sensitive" due to the potential for false positives. TEE "sees" every bubble. Some argue though that detecting even small amounts of venous air embolism is important because it allows surgical control of the entry site before additional air is entrained. TEE has the added benefits of detecting the amount of bubbles and their transatrial passage, as well as evaluating cardiac function. TEE is expensive and requires trained personnel to be continually available for interpretation. There is also potential for injury to the esophagus or larynx; there have been reports of esophageal rupture and recurrent laryngeal nerve injury with TEE use.

Precordial Doppler: The monitor is placed over the right atrium/ventricle at the second through sixth intercostal spaces at the right sternal border. Interruption of regular swishing of the Doppler signal by sporadic roaring sounds or a high-pitched whoosh (called mill-wheel murmur) indicates venous embolism. Even 0.25–0.5 mL of air can be detected. Precordial Doppler is considered the best air embolism monitor, because it is sensitive but does not generate a lot of false positives.

ETCO$_2$ monitoring: A sudden decrease in expired carbon dioxide may indicate VAE.

Signs of VAE
The following signs also have air emboli as a differential diagnosis. *These signs can occur with anaphylaxis, acute myocardial infarction, and pulmonary embolism.*

- Sudden hypotension
- Decreased SaO$_2$/PaO$_2$
- Change in heart sounds, cardiac murmur
- EKG changes and dysrhythmias; tachycardia
- Sudden decrease in expired carbon dioxide (ETCO$_2$): decreases due to a fall in cardiac output and increased dead space
- Appearance of nitrogen in the expired gas
- Increased pulmonary artery pressure (PAP) and central venous pressure (CVP)
- Sudden appearance of vigorous spontaneous ventilation despite continuing mechanical ventilation

Signs of VAE are often not apparent until large amounts of air have been entrained. Rapid entrainment of large amounts of air can produce sudden circulatory arrest by obstructing right ventricular outflow.

Treatment of VAE
- Inform everyone.
- Immediately cease insufflation and release the pneumoperitoneum.
- Hyperventilate with 100% oxygen; discontinue nitrous oxide if it is being used.

- The surgeon will flood the surgical field with normal saline and apply bone wax.
- Aspirate the central venous line/PA line in an attempt to retrieve the entrained air. Note that the aspirate may appear foamy.
- Occlude the neck veins; discontinue pressurized gas.
- Place the patient in steep Trendelenburg or left lateral position.
- Vasopressors should be given to correct hypotension.
- Give intravascular volume infusion to increase central venous pressure.
- Use PEEP/CPAP to increase CVP (although there are some arguments against doing this).
- Undertake cardiopulmonary resuscitation, if necessary.

Prevention of VAE
Prevent hydrostatic gradient development by limiting positions where the operative site is above the right atrium. Maintain vigilance for VAE in high-risk situations.

Carbon Dioxide Gas Embolism

There is a risk of carbon dioxide embolus during a laparoscopic procedure; gas may enter the circulation through any opening in an injured vessel. This type of embolism is the most dangerous complication associated with laparoscopy. It develops principally during induction of a pneumoperitoneum. With carbon dioxide embolus, "gas lock" occurs in the vena cava and right atrium; venous return is obstructed. Blood cannot go into pulmonary artery. Cardiac output will fall and circulatory collapse may result.

Signs of Gas Embolism
Signs of carbon dioxide embolus include a sudden decrease in expired carbon dioxide (ETCO$_2$; ETCO$_2$ *decreases* due to the fall in cardiac output and increased dead space), unexplained tachycardia, EKG changes and dysrhythmias, sudden hypotension,

increased PAP and CVP, a change in heart sounds, a cardiac murmur, the appearance of nitrogen in the expired gas, and decreased SaO_2/PaO_2.

Treatment of Gas Embolism
- Immediately cease insufflation and release the pneumoperitoneum.
- Position the patient in a steep head-down and left lateral decubitus position.
- Hyperventilate with 100% O_2.
- Aspirate gas if a CVP catheter is in place.

Fat Embolism Syndrome

Fat embolism syndrome (FES) is a rare clinical condition in which embolized and circulating fat particles are deposited in the pulmonary capillary beds and brain tissue and lead to multisystem dysfunction in the skin, lungs, blood, and brain. Microvascular plugging of these fat droplets produces local ischemia, causing the release of inflammatory mediators and platelet aggregation.

Implicated procedures and causes include long bone fractures, multiple fractures with pelvic injury, total joint replacement, intra-abdominal surgery, liposuction, bone marrow transplant, and burns. A factor increasing the risk of FES is aggressive reaming or nailing of the bone's medullary cavity. Mobilized fat particles occur to some degree in most long bone fractures.

Symptoms may be subclinical or masked by general anesthesia; manifestations of FES may occur 12–72 hours after injury.

Signs and Symptoms of FES
FES has three main symptoms: dyspnea, confusion, and petechiae. All together, the following signs can be seen with FES:

Skin

- Petechiae (transient cutaneous pin-point sized red dots in the axilla, conjunctiva, neck, shoulders, chest, arms)

Lungs

- Dyspnea
- Increased $PaCO_2$
- Decreased PaO_2 and oxygen saturation
- Decreased $ETCO_2$ and arterial hypoxemia
- ARDS (interstitial edema, alveolar collapse, decreased compliance)
- Sudden increase in peak inspiratory pressures

Neurological

- Level of consciousness (LOC) changes
- Confusion
- Seizures
- Coma

Heart

- EKG changes (dysrhythmias, tachycardia, ischemic changes)

Blood

- Thrombocytopenia
- Anemia
- Coagulopathy
- Disseminated intravascular coagulation (DIC)
- Increased lipase
- Triglyceride levels
- Fat globules in urine and sputum
- Decreased serum calcium levels (calcium binds with free fatty acids)

Diagnostic Tests for FES
- Fat globules in urine and sputum
- Complete blood count: anemia and thrombocytopenia
- Increased lipase and triglyceride levels
- Low calcium levels (calcium binds with free fatty acids)

Supportive Measures for FES
- Adequate hydration
- Oxygenation

- Early splinting of fracture especially long bones
- Give albumin to provide free fatty acid binding sites

High-dose steroids have not been proved effective for treatment of FES.

HEMODIALYSIS CATHETER ACCESS AND FLUSH GUIDELINES

This section outlines the authors' practice policy and is just one example of dialysis catheter access guidelines. Check your institution's policy for your specific guidelines.

- A physician's order *must* be written on the chart before the provider can access a dialysis catheter.
- Use a dialysis catheter *only* if you are unable to get any other vascular access.
- Use sterile technique when accessing these ports!
- Wear sterile gloves and clean the ports using sterile technique. Cleanse with Betadine solution for 30 seconds on the caps. Aspirate out the heparin flush and discard it; flush the port with normal saline (NS); and connect the port to the NS fluids.
- Have the circulator order heparin 5000 units/mL from the pharmacy so you will have it ready. If the dialysis catheter is *not* your only access, then you should discontinue IV fluids in the OR and flush with the previously described heparin solution. If this catheter is your *only* access, then take the heparin with you; the hemodialysis catheter can be flushed in the PACU.

HIGH-FREQUENCY JET VENTILATION

There is no bulk flow of gases with high-frequency jet ventilation (HFJV); it is referred to as coaxial flow in the larger airways. Following are the usual setting ranges for HFJV:

Rate = 60–600 cycles per minute (cpm)

- Lower cpm: < 60 cpm will increase inspiratory time (improves CO_2 elimination)

- Extremely high cpm: > 400 cpm may decrease inspiratory time (worsens CO_2 elimination)

Tidal volume (VT) = less than dead space (2–5 mL/kg)

CO_2 = eliminated by passive expirations through an open system/exhalation takes place continuously

ETT with special connector; attaches to any tube with a 15-mm connector

Factors Affecting Ventilation during HFJV

Driving Pressure
Driving pressure (DP) is measured in pounds/square inch (psi). It is the pressure of the force of inhaled gases: air/O_2 or N_2O/O_2 (*not* inhalation agents). In the Venturi effect, velocity of airflow increases through a small orifice, resulting in a decreased pressure; this effect causes a decrease in the pressure at the outflow of the jet injector, and gas will be entrained, increasing the tidal volume at 10–20%. This volume must be humidified for cases where surgery lasts more than 45 minutes or in ICUs.

Percent Inspiratory Time with HFJV
Increasing the inspiratory to expiratory ratio (I:E) ratio will increase tidal volume and minute ventilation. The range is usually set between 30% and 50%. Minute ventilation is most dependent on DP and the I:E ratio.

Jet Catheter Size and Configuration
The bigger the catheter, the greater the jet volume and minute ventilation. It is best to have two side holes for entrained volume: jet velocity or tip velocity from the nozzle.

Cycle Rates
Generally, changing the cycle rate does not change minute ventilation. The exception occurs when delivering HFJV at rates < 60 cpm and > 400 cpm.

FiO₂

The FiO_2 percent used is a matter of choice and depends on the case and technique employed. Blenders are used for O_2, air, or N_2O.

Humidity

Humidity can be delivered using a small saline bag and infusion line with some ventilators. The recommended rate is 15 cc/h 0.9% NS or 0.45% NS. This technique may not be used in the OR; it is associated with fog buildup if the surgeon is working with airway scopes.

LAPAROSCOPIC ISSUES

Laparoscopic surgery involves the introduction of a laparoscope through a single or multiple ports placed through a body wall into a cavity. Usually several 2- to 3-cm slits are made across the skin surface where ports are placed, specimens retrieved, and surgery performed. Laparoscopic surgery is done for exploration, diagnosis, and treatment purposes. To visualize an internal surface, the external body surface is distended away from the internal organs by establishing insufflation with carbon dioxide.

With abdominal laparoscopy, the parietal wall is distended away from the internal organs by establishing a pneumoperitoneum with CO_2. Before insufflating the area, the anesthetist inserts an orogastric or nasogastric tube and suctions out the stomach contents. A urethral catheter should also be placed by the OR staff.

When the trocar pierces a body cavity, the anesthetist should monitor viewing screens to look for any internal trauma (e.g., the trocar piercing an internal organ).

Insufflation pressures used are usually between 5 mm Hg and 14–16 mm Hg and can decrease cardiac output, venous return, and the lung's functional residual capacity (FRC). Increased abdominal pressure from insufflation can also stimulate vagal nerve activity, and the patient's heart rate can become bradycardic to asystolic. Notify the surgeon if the patient becomes severely bradycardic; team members can decrease insufflation pressures a little or completely until the heart rate increases. IV glycopyrrolate may need to be given to increase the heart rate. If glycopyrrolate is ineffective, IV atropine should be given. Have epinephrine 1:10,000 immediately available for severe bradycardia unresponsive to vagolytics medications.

Carbon dioxide gases can increase end-tidal carbon dioxide ($ETCO_2$) but should level out after 30–45 minutes. This increase can be offset by increasing the minute ventilations to keep the $ETCO_2$ in appropriate ranges (32–39 mm Hg). If $ETCO_2$ continues to rise, check for subcutaneous emphysema; the insufflation pressure may need to be reduced and ventilation increased dramatically.

Once pneumoperitoneum is achieved, setting the ventilator on *pressure-controlled ventilations* can help decrease airway pressures while maintaining oxygenation, lung expansion, and $ETCO_2$ while the pneumoperitoneum lasts. Tidal volumes may need to be decreased to allow adequate pneumoperitoneum. The anesthetist must be constantly aware of the presence of the pneumoperitoneum. The surgeon may decrease or desufflate at any time; if the ventilator is set on pressure ventilation and the pneumoperitoneum is lost, the patient's lung volumes may increase dramatically.

The patient may be moved from Trendelenburg position to reverse Trendelenburg position several times during surgery to change internal organ positioning so as to facilitate organ exposure for surgeon. If the patient's arms are secured on padded armboards, be sure to secure both the forearm and the upper arm to eliminate the chance of the arms rolling off the boards.

Urine output tends to diminish with insufflation of the abdomen. Nausea and vomiting are more common following laparoscopic procedures.

Patients may complain of right shoulder/shoulder blade pain after a laparoscopic surgery. This effect is thought to be due to carbon dioxide insufflation causing chemical irritation to the diaphragm.

Carbon dioxide gas embolism, pneumothorax, pneumomediastinum, subcutaneous emphysema, and hypercarbia with ensuing acidosis are potential risks of CO_2 insufflation. Air can enter the thorax through weakened areas in the diaphragm. Immediate chest tube decompression is required for any clinical evidence of a tension pneumothorax.

Effects of Abdominal Laparoscopic Surgery on the Respiratory System

Intraperitoneal insufflation of CO_2 creates a pneumoperitoneum that results in ventilatory and respiratory changes:

- Decreases thoraco-pulmonary compliance.
- Decreases lung compliance by 30–50%.
- During uneventful laparoscopy, $PaCO_2$ progressively increases and reaches a plateau 15–30 minutes after insufflation. The increase in $PaCO_2$ depends on the intra-abdominal pressure.
- Once the pneumoperitoneum is created and kept constant, compliance is not affected by patient tilting or changes in minute ventilation.

Respiratory Complications from Abdominal Insufflation

Endobronchial Intubation

Cephalad displacement of the diaphragm during pneumoperitoneum also results in cephalad movement of the carina; this effect may occur even in laparoscopic cases in which the patient is in a head-up position. If the patient's oxygen saturation decreases after insufflation of the abdomen, check for bilateral breath sounds. The tracheal tube can go into the right mainstem bronchus, with the pressure of insufflation pushing the diaphragm upward. If breath sounds are decreased on the left side, pull the endotracheal tube back until breath sounds are audible bilaterally and retape the endotracheal tube.

Pneumothorax

Pneumothorax may occur due to a defect in the diaphragm or as a result of a pleural tear. If rupture of preexisting bullae occurs in the lung, causing air to escape into the thorax, the pneumothorax will not resolve spontaneously. A thoracentesis (pleural tap) must be done to remove the air in the pleural space. Capnothorax (carbon dioxide in the pleural space) without pulmonary trauma will spontaneously resolve 30–60 minutes after ex-sufflation. Treatment of CO_2 or venous air pneumothorax consists of adding PEEP and reducing all intra-abdominal pressure.

Carbon Dioxide Gas Embolism

See the discussion of this condition presented earlier in this chapter.

CO_2-Subcutaneous Emphysema

This condition develops secondary to extraperitoneal insufflation. It results in increased carbon dioxide levels after $ETCO_2$ has plateaued. Hypercapnia becomes unresponsive to adjustment of ventilation. To resolve this condition, laparoscopy should be temporarily interrupted to allow for CO_2 elimination.

MASK (VENTILATOR) STRAP FACIAL INJURIES

Direct pressure on the patient's brow from the ventilator face mask can cause hair loss or nerve damage. The facial nerve can also be affected, specifically at the following branches (all branches are listed):

- Temporal branch. Supraorbital pressure, especially by the ETT connector, can cause eye pain, photophobia, and/or forehead numbness.
- Zygomatic branch.
- Buccal branch. This branch innervates the orbicularis oris around the mouth; damage to this branch can cause loss of motor ability (e.g., no puckering of lips).

- Mandibular branch. Damage to this branch can cause motor loss and minimal sensory loss to the mandible.
- Cervical branch.

METHYLMETHACRYLATE BONE CEMENT

Methylmethacrylate (MMA) is a self-polymerizing bone cement that is used to secure a prosthesis inside the bone/joint. It is part of an exothermic reaction that leads to cement hardening and expansion against prosthetic components. This expansion can exert pressure in excess of 500 mm Hg in the intramedullary space. MMA can embolize fat, clot, air, cement, marrow, and bone chips. Its reaction may also trigger tissue thromboplastin, causing small clots to travel to the lung. Unpolymerized monomer can be absorbed into the circulation. Pressurization of the bone canal with cement is also associated with hemodynamic changes.

Complications of MMA Use

The following problems are associated with MMA use:

- **Hypotension**
  - MMA may be a direct vasodilator/myocardial depressant.
  - Severity: usually related to volume (could result from a pulmonary embolism [PE] or anaphylactoid reaction).
  - Onset: 30 seconds to 10 minutes.
  - Termination: usually spontaneous within 5 minutes.
  - Treatment: adequate hydration to full support.
- **Desaturation**
  - Result: In one study, 34% of patients had desaturation with a baseline FiO_2 of 33%.
  - Treatment: increase FiO_2 to at least 50% during cementing.
- **Fat embolism**
  - Result: arterial hypoxemia, ARDS, coagulopathy, fever confusion, coma, seizures;

petechiae on the neck, shoulders, and chest.
  - Treatment: supportive, oxygenation, corticosteroids, immobilize long bones.
- **Ambient contamination: fumes**
  - MMA should be mixed in a vented hood.
  - Liquid monomer is highly flammable.
  - Contact lenses and other plastics can be affected by MMA vapors.
  - Vapors can cause irritation of the eyes and respiratory tract.
- **Mortality**
  - Deaths can occur intraoperatively or post-operatively due to pulmonary embolism.
  - PE may result from the impact from surgical instrumentation and the expansion/pressure of the cement against the femoral shaft.

MMA use can also cause significant increases in PVR and pulmonary wedge pressure and decreases in SVR, CO, and MAP pressures. Hypotension, hypoxia, cardiovascular collapse and arrest, and pulmonary embolus following prosthesis insertion have been reported.

Prevention of MMA-Related Complications

- Better surgical lavage helps to avoid complications.
- Maintain vigilance for potential problems.
- Use 100% oxygen (FiO_2) when using MMA.

MIXED VENOUS OXYGEN CONTENT

Mixed venous oxygen content (MVO_2), also known as *saturated venous oxygen content* (SVO_2), is an index of cardiac output and overall tissue perfusion. Its ongoing measurement allows minute-to-minute assessment of total tissue oxygen balance (delivery versus consumption) at the tissue level.

MVO_2 varies directly with cardiac output, hemoglobin levels, and oxygen saturation. It varies inversely with tissue oxygen requirements and oxygen consumption (VO_2). Normal MVO_2 is considered to be in the range of 65–75%; 25% extracted and utilized in body tissues. In other words, under normal conditions, if 1000 mL of oxygen is available, 350 mL of oxygen is used by the body's tissues and 650 mL is returned to the lungs; thus the normal SVO_2 is 65%.

Increased MVO_2 may be caused by a wedged Swan-Ganz catheter (common cause), increased FiO_2, methemoglobinemia, sepsis, hypothermia, an elevated cardiac output with left to right shunts, neuromuscular paralysis (muscles less active), or excessive inotropic drugs.

Decreased MVO_2 may be caused by a decreased hemoglobin level, a low oxygen saturation (arterial hypoxia), low cardiac output with myocardial damage, congestive heart failure, hypovolemia, hypoxia, or inadequate pulmonary gas exchange. It may also reflect increased tissue demand owing to malignant hyperthermia, thyroid storm, shivering, fever, exercise, or agitation.

If the MVO_2 falls below 30%, the oxygen balance is compromised and anaerobic metabolism ensues.

INTRAOPERATIVE NEUROLOGIC MONITORING BY THE ELECTROPHYSIOLOGIST

1. EEG (electroencephalography):
   - BIS
   - PSA 4000
2. Evoke potentials:
   - Somatosensory (SSEP)
   - Auditory (BAER)
   - Visual (VEP)
   - Dermatome (trigeminal)
   - Motor (MEP)
3. Electromyography
4. Wake-up test

NEUROPHYSIOLOGIC MONITORING

Electrophysiological measurements are done to detect adequate cerebral perfusion and proper neuronal functioning; protect and monitor the functional integrity of "at risk" neural structures; monitor the effects of anesthetic agents and other CNS drugs; and identify pathophysiologic conditions that can alter neurologic function. Such monitoring allows for intraoperative detection of cerebral ischemia, which may require a change in surgical technique to improve or restore perfusion. It can also be indicated when temporary occlusion of a vessel is planned, to determine the duration of tolerance, or for titration of anesthetic agents when pharmacologic metabolic suppression is desired.

The impact of anesthetic agents on neurophysiologic monitoring increases with the number of synapses in the pathway being monitored. This relationship arises because all anesthetic agents produce their effects by altering neuronal excitability via changes in synaptic function or axonal conduction.

ELECTROENCEPHALOGRAPHY

EEG has long been regarded as the "gold standard" for assessing cerebral ischemia during cerebrovascular procedures and is used as a guide for tolerable hypotensive techniques. The EEG is a recording of unstimulated brain waves (cortical activity) that results from spontaneous, continuous electrical activity of the brain; it measures electrical activity of the neurons of the cerebral cortex. Thus, EEG may be used as a marker for detection of ischemia due to inadequate cerebral blood flow (CBF). The character of the EEG waves depends on the level of metabolic activity of the cerebral cortex and level of wakefulness.

EEG involves continuous intraoperative monitoring. The EEG technician reads the EEG monitor and analyzes the summative numerical value. Changes in the EEG are characterized by *alterations in both frequency and amplitude* as the cerebral cortex becomes increasingly ischemic. Changes range from subtle changes, such as mild loss of beta/theta activity with a mild increase in delta frequencies, to isoelectric recordings. Summation of all electrical activity and conversion into characteristic waveforms (see Figure 3-1) is of key interest to the EEG technician:

- Beta waves: presence of increased mental stimulation and with eye opening; 12–42 Hz
- Alpha waves: typical of an awake, resting patient with the eyes closed; 8–12 Hz
- Theta waves: occur during general anesthesia and in healthy children while sleeping; 4–8 Hz
- Delta waves: occur in deep sleep, general anesthesia, and organic brain disease; less than 4 Hz

EEG is now used for the detection of depth of anesthesia (via BIS) technology.

Cerebral Blood Flow

Normal CBF is 50 mL/100 g/min.

CBF $\geq$ 20 mL/100 g/min: normal amplitude and latency components of cortical evoked potentials are maintained.

CBF < 18 mL/100 g/min: has been associated with significant alterations in EEG signaling. Amplitude measures decline to 50% with CBF of approximately 16 mL/100 g/min; waveforms are completely abolished at levels below 12 mL/100 g/min.

CBF < 6 mL/100 g/min: irreversible changes in EEG signaling.

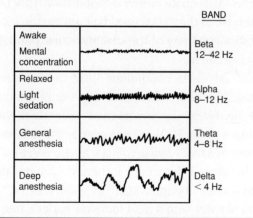

Figure 3-1   *EEG Waves, Bands*

Mean Arterial Pressure

50 mm Hg: EEG slows

25–40 mm Hg: flat EEG

< 20 mm Hg: irreversible damage in normothermic patient

Other Uses of EEG

EEG can be used intraoperatively as a means by which to detect abnormal activity such as spike and wave interictal events and epileptiform discharge. These types of recording are commonly performed before and after resection of epileptic foci or temporal lobectomy. *Don't use propofol in these cases, as this agent raises the seizure threshold.*

EEG monitoring is especially useful to evaluate cerebral perfusion with clamping of major vessels. Is also used as a guide with use of hypotensive surgical techniques.

EEG Burst Suppression

Monitored by an EEG, drug-induced burst suppression is a reversible decrease in cortical neuronal metabolic function ($CMRO_2$). It is used as a cerebral protection technique. Burst suppression pattern also occurs with ischemic encephalopathy.

The characteristic signal of EEG burst suppression is often recognized with deepening of anesthesia. This pattern consists of high voltage periods of bursts and low voltage periods of suppression, each lasting from 1.5 to 6 seconds. During suppression, low-voltage mixed frequency activity can be seen. EEG findings during the suppression phase are not isoelectric.

EEG burst suppression may be seen with any anesthetic when combined with hypothermic technique.

- **General anesthetics:** Potent inhaled gases (isoflurane, sevoflurane, enflurane, desflurane) follow the basic anesthesia-related EEG pattern. Burst suppression occurs at approximately

1.5 MAC for isoflurane, desflurane, and sevoflurane. Enflurane shows burst suppression at 2–3 MAC. Sevoflurane and enflurane bursts can turn into epileptic seizure activity.

- **Barbiturates and propofol:** These drugs follow a pattern of initial EEG activation followed by dose-related depression. Eventually high doses lead to lengthening periods of suppression alternating with periods of activity (burst suppression). Pentothal burst suppression doses are in the range of 10–30 mg/kg total dose. Barbiturates reduce EEG electrical activity (in a dose-dependent manner) by as much as 50%.
- **Ischemic brain damage:** Hypoxia leads to slowing of EEG activity, with electrical activity potentially ceasing altogether depending on the severity of the event. Cerebral blood flow below 18 mL/100 g/min has been associated with significant alterations in EEG signaling.
- **Hypothermia:** Complete EEG suppression occurs at 15–18°C. Additive effects are noted with other suppressive factors (e.g., inhaled gases, barbiturates, ischemia).
- **Hyperventilation:** Hyperventilation can activate excitable seizure foci (burst).
- **Ventilation/oxygenation:** Hypoxemia can result in evoked potential deterioration.

Burst suppression on EEG can be multifactorial in origin, given that we utilize many classes of drugs and other intraoperative factors influence the EEG.

Note that the background EEG activity of neonates is much less regular than that for older children and adults.

The following medications are *not* associated with burst suppression: ketamine, benzodiazepines, opiates, halothane.

BISMonitor: Bispectral Analysis

Bispectral analysis requires fewer electrodes and gives a global assessment of EEG rather than evaluation of specific areas of the brain. It is used by anesthesia specialists to assess the level of hypnosis and possible awareness. This technique does not measure anesthetic depth.

Measurements are calculated over 15–30 seconds. A time delay may occur in rapidly changing states.

Electrode placement is provided via a prepackaged electrode setup, which is applied to the patient's forehead and temple. The machine sets itself up automatically and tests conduction.

Advantages of BIS
- Reduced risk of awareness
- Better management of responses to surgical stimulation
- Faster wake-up
- More cost-effective use of drugs

BIS readings are affected by electrocautery, pacer spikes, and patient movement.

BIS Data Interpretation
100: awake

70: light hypnotic effects

60: moderate hypnotic effects

40: deep hypnotic effects

0: EEG suppression

Under general anesthesia, 40–60 is the desired range

There is no guarantee the patient will have no awareness or recall. Research indicates that levels above 70 have an increased risk of recall.

BIS is not affected by neuromuscular paralysis.

PSA 4000: Patient State Analysis

PSA 4000 analyzes a four-channel processed EEG continuously over regions of the brain. This technology uses quantitative EEG; it removes artifacts—both physiologic and environmental—as well.

EVOKED POTENTIALS

Evoked potentials (EP), measured from either the cortex or periphery, are generated in response to some stimulus or behavior. This information is valuable for monitoring the functional integrity of the ascending (sensory) or descending (motor) pathways.

How sensitive are evoked potentials to anesthesia?

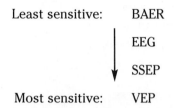

Least sensitive: BAER

EEG

SSEP

Most sensitive: VEP

In general, evoked potentials differ in their sensitivity to anesthetic agents depending on the neurologic pathways involved and the agent being used. The impact of anesthetic agents on neurophysiologic monitoring increases with the number of synapses in the pathway being monitored. This relationship arises because all anesthetic agents produce their effects by altering neuronal excitability via changes in synaptic function or axonal conduction.

Sensory Pathways: Ascending

Somatosensory Evoked Potentials

While best known for monitoring during spinal surgery, somatosensory evoked potentials (SSEP) have been used to monitor for ischemia in cortical tissue. They are used to determine the adequacy of collateral blood flow, tolerance of vessel occlusion, and tolerance of hypotensive technique during intracranial surgery. A change in SSEP cortical amplitude is the most sensitive indication of ischemia.

For SSEP monitoring, the stimulating electrodes are placed at a peripheral nerve while the response is recorded at the contralateral sensory cortex via scalp electrodes. *Because the pathway is afferent, it goes **into** the brain from the periphery.* Use of multiple recording sites allows for coverage along the entire neural axis, from peripheral stimulus to the primary somatosensory cortex.

The choice of electrode placement for recording evoked potentials from the scalp will be dictated by the site of stimulation (see Figure 3-2). The critical electrode for detecting the evoked potential after stimulation of the tibial nerve must be placed over the primary sensory cortex at the midline of the scalp. If the ulnar nerve is stimulated, the electrode must be placed over the primary sensory cortex, somewhat laterally from midline.

The integrity of the gracilis and cuneatus tracts of the posterior spinal cord is assessed by SSEP. If posterior cord or brain ischemia is present, transmission of action potentials through the posterior cord or brain will be diminished, thereby reducing the intensity and delaying the arrival of action potentials in reaching the cerebral cortex. Stimulation of a peripheral nerve results in an ascending volley of action potentials, which travels ipsilaterally via the fasiculus gracilis or cuneatus in the dorsal columns and first synapses at the dorsal column nuclei at the cervico-medullary junction. At this point the volley crosses the midline via the medial lemniscal pathway, traverses the brain stem, and synapses at the thalamus. From here, the volley ultimately synapses in the primary somatosensory cortex or post-central gyrus.

Noninvasive measurement of the brain stem's response to repetitive stimulation of a distal sensory peripheral nerve is possible with SSEP. This technology assesses the integrity of the sensory pathway in the posterior column of the spinal cord. SSEP monitoring measures sensory perception and does not ensure intact motor response. For SSEP monitoring to be useful, the surgery must place neural tissue at risk and options for intervention must exist.

The most common peripheral nerves monitored are the median (wrist), common peroneal (knee), or the posterior tibial (ankle). SSEP monitoring measures both latency (how long) and amplitude (how big) of the waveform. A change in SSEP cortical amplitude is the most sensitive indicator of ischemia or some interruption in the posterior

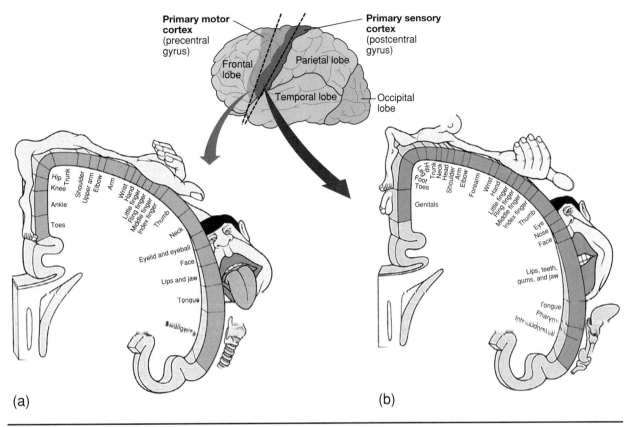

Figure 3-2 *Primary Motor (a) and Sensory (b) Areas of the Cerebrum*

column pathway. A greater than 50% decrease in amplitude or a greater than 10% increase in latency indicates an interruption of the posterior spinal cord pathway. Elevated ICP is associated with reductions in amplitude and increases in latency of cortically generated SSEPs; by virtue of its effect on cortical structures, this increase in ICP produces a pressure-related decrease in cortical SSEP responses.

SSEP monitoring is used to determine the adequacy of collateral blood flow, tolerance of vessel occlusion, and tolerance of hypotensive technique during intracranial surgery. While it is best known for its utility during spinal surgery (especially spinal fusion), this type of monitoring has also been used to check for ischemia in cortical tissue during surgery in the posterior fossae (especially that requiring retraction of the brain stem), during surgery near the primary somatosensory cortex and during supratentorial surgeries. Moreover, it is valuable in assessing lumbar and sacral nerve roots in posterior interbody fusion, lumbar fusion with instrumentation, and cauda equine surgeries; during carotid endarterectomy, scoliosis repair, aortic aneurysm repair, and spinal cord tumor surgeries; in cervical surgery with instrumentation; and in cardiac procedures where cardiopulmonary bypass is used.

Anesthetic Agents and SSEP Monitoring

It is essential to communicate changes in anesthesia level to neurophysiology staff. It is best to keep anesthesia at constant levels, especially during critical points of surgery. Neurophysiology personnel will determine which agents may or may not be used and what their dose limits are.

SSEP monitoring offers intermediate sensitivity to anesthetics. In general, an anesthetic technique involving the use of a low-dose inhalational agent (at "half-MAC": minimum alveolar concentration.) along with a narcotic infusion and nitrous oxide at 66% with oxygen at 33% provides the most stable and optimal conditions for monitoring nerve function.

Volatile Anesthetics N_2O and inhaled anesthetics have the greatest effects to SSEP. Nevertheless, all anesthetic agents depress SSEP amplitude in dose-dependent manner, including nitrous oxide. This effect varies from isoflurane (most potent) to enflurane (intermediate potency) to halothane (least potent). Sevoflurane and desflurane have similar effects to isoflurane when the patient is at a steady state; however, because of their more rapid onset and offset of effect (both are more insoluble than isoflurane), they may appear to be more potent during periods when concentrations are increasing.

Good SSEP monitoring is compatible with 0.5–1 MAC isoflurane and 60% N_2O and oxygen, after which the waveforms are lost.

Systemic Factors

Blood pressure: Mean arterial pressures below the threshold for cerebral auto regulation via blood loss or drug effects result in progressive decreases in amplitude until loss of the waveform occurs (but no changes in latency). Hypotension considered "safe" combined with surgical manipulation can result in spinal cord ischemia.

Temperature: Hyperthermia leads to decreased amplitude of SSEPs, with loss of waves occurring at 42°C.

Blood gases/hematocrit: Hypoxia and severe drops in HCT have been reported to lead to decreased amplitude of SSEPs.

IV Agents

- Barbiturates cause dose-dependent reduction of SSEP amplitude and increased latency, but waveforms are still present at doses high enough to suppress the EEG.
- Propofol decreases SSEP amplitude and increases SSEP latency.
- Opioids cause dose-dependent decreased amplitude and increased latency. High-dose fentanyl (60 mcg/kg) is still compatible with SSEP monitoring. Morphine has effects similar to those of fentanyl. Avoid large boluses at moments of potential neural compromise. Meperidine can decrease or increase SSEP amplitude.
- Benzodiazepines also decrease SSEP amplitude. Midazolam has no effect on latency.
- Droperidol has varying effects on SSEPs but can decrease their amplitude.
- Drugs that can increase amplitude include etomidate (can be used to enhance SSEPs), ketamine, meperidine, and methohexital.
- Muscle relaxants have no effect on SSEPs. However, these agent cannot be used if the team is evaluating motor evoked potentials.

Brain Stem Auditory Evoked Responses

Brain stem auditory evoked responses (BAER), also known as brain stem auditory evoked potentials (BAEP), record data from the scalp that are generated in response to an auditory stimulus applied to the ear via an external or insert earphone. This placement monitors posterior fossa and brain stem activity for cranial nerve VIII (auditory). BAERs are generated in response to depolarization of the cochlear nerve and are processed almost entirely in the three divisions of the brain stem. Such a potential can arise secondary to compression or ischemia to the nerve or brain stem. BAERs are reflected as changes in both amplitude and latency in high-frequency deflections termed

Jewett waves. Each wave has a specific site of generation along the auditory axis and can provide the interpreter with information about specific sites of pathology.

BAERs are very resistant to (essentially unaffected by) anesthetics. BAER monitoring is a good choice for surgeries on posterior fossae or in which the brain stem at risk; it is also effective in cases involving acoustic neuroma, vestibular nerve resection, posterior fossae masses, vertebral-basilar aneurysms, brain stem lesions (meningioma), or posterior circulation aneurysms.

Visual Evoked Potentials

Visual evoked potentials (VEP) are recorded from the scalp in response to a visual stimulus provided in the form of either a flash or a changing checkerboard pattern. In the operating room, a flash stimulus is delivered via either a strobe lamp or fiber optic leads or goggles fitted very close to the patient's eyes. A potential is recorded from electrodes placed over the occipital cortex. Changes in latency, phase, and amplitude of the VEP can be used to assess the visual pathway integrity. The primary visual pathway consists of the retina (receptor), the optic nerves/tracts (pathway), and the pathway from the thalamus to the primary visual cortex.

VEPs are extremely (most) sensitive to anesthetic agents; they are obliterated with inhaled agents. VEP monitoring is useful for surgery near the optic pathway, especially during pituitary surgery; surgery targeting supra- and infra-sellar tumors; surgery focused on optic nerve tumors and decompression; surgery on occipital cortical masses; and pallidotomy, which involves destruction of part of the globus pallidus, a region of the brain involved with the control of movement.

Dermatome Evoked Potentials

Sensory evoked potentials can also be useful in evaluating a single segmental (dermatome) nerve root function; this technique focuses on dermatome evoked potentials (DEP), also known as trigeminal evoked potentials. Stimulation of a single dermatome results in the depolarization of a single nerve root and subsequent ascending conduction of a signal via the dorsal column pathways to the primary somatosensory cortex. SSEPs and other evoked potentials assess a mixed nerve root and do not provide information on individual nerve roots. Input to the spinal cord via, for example, the median nerve is distributed over several nerve root levels.

In DEP monitoring, electrodes are placed several centimeters apart within a single dermatome. The key problem with this technique is that overlap exists between dermatomes. Anatomical pathways and alarm criteria with regard to changes in DEPs are the same as with SSEPs.

Dermatome monitoring is used during surgery on lesions of specific nerve roots, brachial plexus explorations, and spina bifida/tethered cord releases.

Motor Pathways: Descending

Motor Evoked Potentials

Motor evoked potential (MEP) monitoring tests for the adequacy of perfusion of ventral spinal cord and the motor pathways. MEPs monitor activation of motor pathways (proximal to the surgical site) while recording motor responses (distal to the surgical site) from the arms and legs. They are recorded as nerve action potentials from peripheral nerves or from the distal musculature (compound muscle action potential). Once these potentials are activated, information flows to the ipsilateral thalamus and subsequently to lower motor neurons after crossing over at the level of the brain stem. These same pathways can be activated via stimulation of the brain stem or stimulation of the spinal cord directly.

MEP monitoring is used in procedures involving anterior approaches to the spinal cord, abdominal aortic aneurysms, scoliosis repair, intradural and intramedullary spinal cord tumors, spinal decompression and fusion.

Anesthesia during MEP monitoring:

- MEPs recorded from the musculature are abolished easily by halogenated inhalational agents.
- Transcranially elicited MEPs are interfered with markedly by anesthetics.
- *Muscle relaxants cannot be used with MEP monitoring.* Muscle relaxation will reduce the ability to detect nerve irritation and quantify functional integrity.
- When recordable, MEPs may occur only at low concentrations (e.g., 0.2–0.5%).
- The effect of the inhalational agent is likely the result of depression of synaptic transmission either in the anterior horn cell synapses on motor neurons or in the cortex at the level of the interneuronal connections.
- As with the barbiturates, midazolam produces a prolonged, marked depression of MEPs.

ELECTROMYOGRAPHY

Electromyography (EMG) provides real-time information about the integrity of the cranial nerves and their underlying brain stem nuclei, the muscles innervated by cranial nerves, and the muscles innervated by spinal nerve roots. EMG monitoring is especially useful if there is any potential for inadvertent resection of cranial nerves V, VII, IX, and X during brain surgery. It is typically recorded by placing bipolar pairs of needle electrodes in the muscle groups of interest.

An alarm criterion for EMG recording is simply the presence of a signal. A baseline or "normal" situation is the absence of spontaneous muscle activity. Different grades of spontaneous activity results in different levels of alert (i.e., neurotonic discharges or injury potentials). Significant change is often unilateral and typically abrupt; it is not necessarily correlative to a particular surgical maneuver.

Neuromuscular junction stimulation is essential for EMG. Thus one cannot use this type of monitoring when muscle relaxants have been administered; one can use total intravenous anesthesia (TIVA) and inhalation at low doses, however. EMG monitoring is especially used for facial nerve and some spinal surgeries; it can be used in such cases to detect muscle and nerve disorders. Profound neuromuscular blockade will prevent recording of EMG activity during MEP recordings.

MEP cranial nerve monitoring can be used during procedures related to acoustic neuromas, microvascular decompression, posterior fossae tumors, facial nerve surgery, spinal surgery, skull base procedures, and ENT procedures (tympanomastoidectomy, cochlear implants). It is also useful for peripheral nerve explorations, including brachial plexus explorations, sciatic nerve explorations, and lumbosacral explorations and fusions (e.g., pedicle screw fusions, tethered cord releases, dorsal rhizotomy, and interbody cage fusions).

WAKE-UP TEST

The wake-up test is intended to measure the patient's motor function. The surgeon will indicate when a patient should be awakened during surgery. The patient will be asked to wiggle his or her toes on command upon wakening from anesthesia and will then be put back to sleep.

Desflurane, which offers a quick wake-up profile, is a volatile anesthesia option that is commonly used in today's OR. If nerve paralysis is used, it is allowed to resolve before wake-up occurs. Use of small amounts of propofol and a narcotic can help keep the patient sleepy (and not coughing and bucking), yet still able to follow commands. Dexmedetomidine is also helpful in that patients remain sedated but easily awaken to voice commands.

It is important for patients to have thorough preoperative teaching and explanation to prepare them for having a "wake-up test." The patient should not be in severe pain and will be immediately put back under general anesthesia after checking motor function.

ANESTHETICS AND BODY STATES INFLUENCING INTRAOPERATIVE NEUROLOGIC MONITORING

The effects of anesthetic agents result from one of two mechanisms of action:

- Inhibition of synaptic pathways
- Indirect action on pathways by changing the balance of inhibitory and excitatory influences

While most anesthetics depress evoked response amplitude and increase latency, some anesthetic agents (etomidate, methohexital, ketamine) enhance both SSEP and MEP amplitudes. This phenomenon is thought to occur via a mechanism whereby inhibition is attenuated.

Intravenous induction and sedation agents interact at a number of different receptors. For example, barbiturates, etomidate, propofol, and benzodiazepines primarily act by enhancing the inhibitory effects of gamma-aminobutyric acid (GABA). Binding and activation of the GABA-a receptor results in an increase in chloride conductance and a subsequent hyperpolarization resulting in synaptic inhibition.

Some intravenous agents work by blocking the excitatory effects of glutamate via antagonism of a variety of receptor subtypes: NMDA, kainate, and quisqualate. For example, ketamine appears to have its major action by inhibiting the NMDA receptor and subsequently reducing sodium flux and intracellular calcium levels. Other intravenous anesthetic agents activate opioid receptors (mu, kappa, and delta).

Ketamine can enhance cortical SSEP amplitude and MEP amplitude. Its effects on subcortical and peripheral SSEP responses are minimal. Although this agent is ideal for cases involving intraoperative monitoring, increases in intracranial pressure are associated with ketamine, and

this medication can produce hallucinations in some patients.

Thiopental, a popular barbiturate induction agent, results in a transient decrease in amplitude and an increase in latency of cortical responses occurring immediately after induction. Minimal effects are seen on the subcortical and peripheral responses.

MEPs are unusually sensitive to barbiturates, with a prolonged effect being observed when these agents are used. *Methohexital* is the exception: It has been found to increase the amplitudes of cortical SSEPs.

Midazolam, a benzodiazepine, has desirable properties of amnesia. When administered at moderate doses, it produces a mild depression of cortical SSEPs. Like the barbiturates, midazolam produces a prolonged, marked depression of MEPs.

Like ketamine, *etomidate* increases the amplitude of cortical SSEP components and increases the amplitude of MEPs.

Like thiopental, *propofol* produces amplitude depression in cortical SSEPs with rapid recovery after termination of infusion due to rapid metabolism. MEPs have demonstrated a similar depressive effect on response amplitude.

The *neuromuscular blocking agents* act at the acetylcholine receptors found at the neuromuscular junction. Because muscle relaxants exert the majority of their action at the neuromuscular junction, they have little effect on electrophysiologic recordings such as SSEPs, which are not derived from muscle activity. However, profound neuromuscular blockade will prevent recording of EMG activity during MEP recordings. Partial neuromuscular blockade has the benefit of reducing a substantial portion of patient movement and facilitates surgical procedures when muscle relaxation is needed for retraction of tissues.

Nitrous oxide reduces SSEP cortical amplitude and increases latency when used alone or when combined with halogenated inhalational agents or opioid agents. When anesthetic agents are compared at equipotent concentrations, nitrous oxide produces more profound changes in cortical SSEPs and MEPs than any other inhalational agent.

Opioids depress electroexcitability by increasing inward potassium ion (K^+) current and depressing outward sodium ion current via a G-protein mechanism linking the receptors to ion channels. The effects of opioid analgesics (e.g., alfentanil, fentanyl, remifentanil, sufentanil) on SSEPs and MEPs are weaker than those associated with inhalational agents. The opioids produce minimal changes in spinal or subcortical SSEP recordings, although there is some depression of amplitude and an increase of latency in the cortical responses. Spinal application of morphine or fentanyl for postoperative pain management produces minimal changes in SSEPs and MEPs.

Blood Flow

Local factors may produce regional ischemia not predicted by systemic blood pressure. For example, during spinal surgery, the effects of hypotension may be aggravated by spinal distraction, such that an acceptable limit of systemic hypotension cannot be determined without monitoring. Regional effects include peripheral nerve ischemia from positioning, tourniquets, or vascular interruption secondary to vasospasm. MEPs and SSEPs are both sensitive to spinal cord events produced by vascular ischemia (carotid cross-clamping) or mechanical compression. These types of potentials may show differential sensitivity to ischemic events.

Intracranial Pressure

Elevated ICP is associated with reductions in amplitude and increases in latency of SSEPs, leading to a loss of brain stem responses with uncal herniation. For MEPs, a gradual increase in the onset latency occurs with a gradual complete abolishment of responses.

Blood Rheology

Changes in hematocrit can alter both oxygen-carrying capacity and blood viscosity. Maximum oxygen delivery is thought to occur with a midrange hematocrit (30–32%). Evoked response changes with hematocrit are consistent within this optimal range.

Ventilation/Oxygenation

Hypoxemia can result in evoked potential deterioration before other clinical parameters show any changes. Alterations in carbon dioxide levels are known to affect spinal cord and cortical blood flow. Remarkable SSEP changes occur when the CO_2 tension is extremely low, suggesting that excessive vasoconstriction may produce ischemia (< 20 mm Hg).

Temperature

SSEP and MEP changes can be observed with hypothermia. These changes are consistent with those seen with ischemia and anesthesia, in that they are more significant in the cortically recorded responses as opposed to the subcortical potentials. MEPs exhibit a gradual increase in onset latency due to slowed conduction time along the neural axis. An increase in activation threshold latencies is also seen.

POSTOPERATIVE VISUAL LOSS

No single factor has been identified as a cause of postoperative visual loss (POVL), although several risk factors are commonly observed:

- Eye pressure (small risk)
- Elevated central venous pressure from retarded drainage from ophthalmic veins
- Hypotension, hypovolemia: may be partially causative
- Increased intraocular pressure (IOP):
  - In the prone position the risk of POVL increases dramatically if: surgery lasts

more than 5 hours and if in a prolonged head down (Trendelenburg) position causing decreased venous outflow from cranium.
  - With administration of increased amounts of IV fluids
  - With increased intra-abdominal pressure (increases epidural vein pressure)
- Increased serum blood glucose levels: affects neurons
- Hypothermia: a decreased temperature increases the viscosity of blood, decreasing blood flow to the eye.
- Repeat spine surgery in the prone position.
- Preoperative donation of blood; hematocrit low, anemic patient.
- Smoking, obesity

Preoperative/Anesthetic Management
- Blood replacement should be timely to maintain hematocrit.
- IV fluid balance should be maintained carefully. Infusion of colloid is an alternative to infusion of multiple liters of crystalloid. Avoid hemodilution.
- Keep the patient's head at or above the level of the heart.
- Avoid abdominal compression.
- Keep blood glucose within "tight control"; serum blood glucose 80–120 mg/dL.
- Pad the eyes
- Urinary output should be maintained at a rate of 1 mL/kg/h or more.
- Conduct surgery in the minimal amount of time when the patient is in the prone position.
- Maintain an adequate mean arterial blood pressure; maintain adequate perfusion pressure to the optic nerve.

PULMONARY HYPERTENSION

Normal pulmonary circulation is a high-flow, low-pressure circuit. Progressive increases in pulmonary vascular resistance (PVR) initially result in right ventricular hypertrophy (RVH) but will eventually lead to right heart failure, defined as pulmonary artery pressures that exceed 30/10 mm Hg. Pulmonary hypertension may be caused by obstruction of the vascular bed, pulmonary vasoconstriction, chronic hypoxia, collagen vascular disease, sickle cell disease, congenital heart disease, portal hypertension, high altitude, allergic alveolitis, or acidosis.

Treatment
- Identify and treat the underlying cause.
- Reduce vascular tone.
- Optimize right ventricular function.

Anesthesia Management if the Patient Has Pulmonary Hypertension
- Pre-oxygenation is crucial, as the patient will have a decreased FRC. A decreased FRC subjects the patient to rapid oxygen desaturation and hypoxemia.
- Inspired oxygen concentration may be lowered to maintain a SpO_2 greater than 91% to reduce the risk of O_2 toxicity.
- Avoid barotrauma with mechanical ventilation; ventilation should be maintained with decreased tidal volumes and increased respiratory rate.

TOURNIQUET ISSUES

The primary objective of tourniquet use in surgical settings is the creation of a bloodless operative field; this is achieved by applying circumferential pressure on the arterial and venous circulation. In certain situations, tourniquets may be useful for preventing the undesirable escape of vascular fluids into body areas or to confine local anesthetics to an extremity. Orthopedics and plastic surgery are two specialties that frequently utilize pneumatic tourniquets.

Prior to Tourniquet Inflation

Check to make sure the antibiotic has been given before the Esmarch bandage and the tourniquet are applied. An adhesive occlusive dressing should be applied over any open skin before padding and the tourniquet are applied. Wrapping the skin (e.g., with cuff padding, cast padding, or soft cotton wrap) to protect it from the tourniquet itself helps to prevent damage to the skin and subcutaneous tissue.

Multiple sizes of tourniquets should be available to ensure an adequate size to encircle the limb with enough overlap in the cuff—minimum 3 inches and maximum 6 inches. The overlap itself should lie on the outside of the extremity to avoid nerve sheath compression. Palpate the patient's distal extremity pulses before inflation to assess baseline pulses.

The cuff should be positioned over the largest amount of soft tissue. The cuff should not apply pressure to the bend of the elbow or of the knee when inflated.

Elevate the operative extremity to drain blood passively, and then wrap extremity tightly with an Esmarch bandage (or equivalent).

Tourniquet Inflation

It is the surgeon's responsibility to dictate the tourniquet pressure setting. The setting is based on the patient's systolic blood pressure, age, and limb size. Usually, the inflation setting is 50–100 mm Hg greater than the patient's systolic pressure. The inflation pressure maximum is usually 300 mm Hg in the upper extremity and 400 mm Hg in the lower extremity.

Over-pressurization may cause pain at the tourniquet cuff site; muscle weakness; compression injuries to blood vessels, nerve, muscle, or skin; or extremity paralysis. *Under-pressurization* may result in blood in the surgical field, passive congestion of the limb, shock, and hemorrhagic infiltration of a nerve.

- Pale coloring is indicative of adequate exsanguination.
- Extensive mottling is indicative of inadequate exsanguination.

Tourniquet Pain

After inflation of the pneumatic tourniquet for 30–60 minutes, patients may experience "tourniquet pain," accompanied by an increase in heart rate and blood pressure. Pain should be assessed and managed. A sympathetic response can occur even when the patient is under general anesthesia. Tourniquet pain frequency occurs, with intensity depending on the type of anesthesia administered: IV regional > epidural > spinal > general anesthesia.

Treatment of tourniquet pain includes regional analgesics, opioids, hypnotics for a patient under local anesthesia, and change in sedation technique. Local hypothermia appears to be a safe and effective method of decreasing the adverse effects of tourniquet ischemia and allowing continuous tourniquet inflation time to extend safely beyond the customary 2-hour limit.

While the tourniquet is inflated, be mindful of how much narcotic is administered for tourniquet pain. As soon as the tourniquet is deflated, this noxious stimulus will be removed and presence of excessive narcotic may affect the return of spontaneous ventilation for patients under general anesthesia.

Tourniquet Time: Safe Duration

Tourniquets may be applied for a maximum of 2 hours. Tourniquets have been used up to 4 hours with intermittent deflation of the cuff. The *minimum time of application should be 20 minutes* to prevent release of the local anesthetic into the general circulation.

Damage from tourniquet use can affect the extremity vessels, nerves, or muscle. Direct cuff pressure can cause ischemia with muscle dysfunction. Any damage to vessels, nerves, and skeletal muscle is usually reversible for tourniquet inflations of 1–2 hours.

Deflation of the Tourniquet

When the tourniquet is deflated, a decrease in blood pressure occurs as blood is shunted to the extremity. Products of anaerobic metabolism and newly released acid metabolites enter the circulation upon deflation of the tourniquet cuff, causing transient increases in end-tidal carbon dioxide, metabolic acidosis, and a decrease in oxygen saturation. The time for clearance of the metabolites depends on the patient's physiologic status, the extremity involved, and the duration of tourniquet inflation.

Special Drugs and Concepts in Anesthesia

4

ANESTHESIA AND LUNG FUNCTION

Decrease in Functional Residual Capacity

A decrease in functional residual capacity (FRC) of 15–20% occurs on induction of anesthesia. The effect occurs regardless of whether ventilation is spontaneous or controlled. General anesthesia alone causes most of the decrease in FRC secondary to the following mechanisms:

- Loss of end-expiratory tone in the diaphragm
- Loss of normal distending force
- Shifting of the abdominal contents in a cephalad direction when the patient is put in a head-down position

See Chapter 2, "Positioning and Patient Effect," for more information.

Note that administration of a muscle relaxant does not significantly change the FRC if the patient is already anesthetized.

Effect of Anesthesia on Postoperative FRC

FRC decreases approximately 15% after lower abdominal surgery, 30% after upper abdominal surgery, and 25% after a thoracotomy. Approximately 80% of pulmonary function is recovered by postoperative day 3.

Effect of Positive End-Expiratory Pressure on FRC

Positive end-expiratory pressure (PEEP) increases FRC, arterial oxygenation, and pulmonary compliance. It expands previously collapsed but perfused alveoli. In addition, PEEP decreases intrapulmonary shunt.

Not all PEEP is helpful, however. PEEP increases alveolar pressure and may increase zone 1 dead space. It may also decrease cardiac output: Normal lungs will transmit the pressure to the vasculature causing decreased cardiac output and hypotension.

Continuous positive airway pressure (CPAP) provides constant airway pressure to lung, without ventilation. CPAP is another frequently used adjuvant therapy during thoracic surgery for poor oxygenation. Peak airway pressures are lowered while mean pressures are increased; these effects are accomplished through prolonged inspiratory times and shortened expiratory time. CPAP decreases the potential for airway closure. Peak airway pressure does not exceed the preset level.

Anesthesia Type and Respiratory Patterns or Function

All *volatile agents* decrease all lung volumes and increase respiratory rate in a dose-dependent manner (i.e., produce rapid, shallow breathing). Overall, hypoventilation occurs that is proportional to anesthetic depth. Reduction of lung volumes also results in a decreased caliber of airways with a tendency toward airway collapse.

Inhalational agents do not measurably affect normal airway tone; however, they do affect *increased*

airway resistance. Volatile agents decrease airway resistance by exerting direct relaxant effects on airway smooth muscle mainly by decreasing vagal tone (vagal stimulation affects smaller airways more than large airways).

Use of an endotracheal tube (ETT), anesthesia circuit, or pharyngeal or laryngeal obstruction all increase the work of breathing to some degree. Airway resistance from commonly used breathing circuits and endotracheal tubes can be significant: Work of breathing may increase threefold.

Inhalational agents (including nitrous oxide) depress the ventilatory response to hypoxemia. Normally mediated by the carotid bodies, this reflex is blunted 50–70% by as little as 0.1 MAC of a volatile anesthetic; 1.1 MAC will cause a 100% depression ventilatory response to hypoxemia.

Narcotics decrease the respiratory rate and increase tidal volume (produce slower, deeper breathing). *The narcotic level will affect the patient's ability to ventilate spontaneously.*

Administration of a muscle relaxant *increases* chest wall compliance. This effect can be appreciated

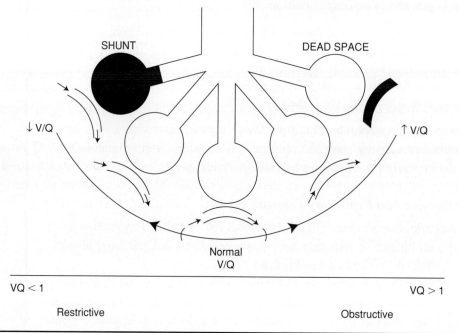

Figure 4-1 *Shunt and Dead Space Conditions*

by observing the decrease in peak inspiratory pressures (PIP).

Manipulation of End-Tidal Carbon Dioxide Level

- *To lower the end-tidal carbon dioxide ($ETCO_2$) on a spontaneously ventilating patient:* Assisting a spontaneously ventilating patient to lower the $ETCO_2$ will only cause apnea because of the apneic threshold; providers must decrease the anesthetic depth to lower the $ETCO_2$.
- *To raise the $ETCO_2$ and initiate spontaneous ventilation after mechanical ventilation:* $PaCO_2$ will rise 5–6 mm Hg in the first minute of apnea; it will rise 3–4 mm Hg every minute thereafter.
- *To slowly increase the $ETCO_2$:* Decrease the respiratory rate and/or tidal volume so that $ETCO_2$ increases to at least 3–5 mm Hg lower than the $PaCO_2$.

The deeper the anesthetic, the longer the period of apnea necessary before the patient will begin to breathe. Continue to mechanically ventilate the patient and progressively decrease the volatile agents. This management will decrease the apneic threshold.

Absorption Atelectasis

Absorption atelectasis occurs when high alveolar oxygen concentrations cause alveolar collapse. Normally, nitrogen splints alveoli open. When a high FiO_2 is given, nitrogen is washed out, causing the alveoli to become filled with only oxygen. In some conditions, oxygen is absorbed (into the blood) faster than ventilation can replace it; this causes the alveoli to shrink until they collapse. Conditions favoring absorption atelectasis include the following:

- Long exposure time to $FiO_2 > 50\%$
- Low V/Q ratio

- Low mixed venous PvO_2
- Nitrogen in alveoli replaced by oxygen

Ventilation/Perfusion Matching and General Anesthesia

The distribution of *ventilation* is influenced by posture and the type of ventilation. Induction of general anesthesia does affect the distribution of ventilation.

Distribution of *blood flow* depends on gravity. Induction of general anesthesia does not significantly change the distribution of blood flow, but keep the following points in mind:

- Use of positive-pressure ventilation can increase lung zone I areas.
- Positive-pressure ventilation causes an increase in alveolar pressure.
- When alveolar pressure exceeds pulmonary capillary pressures, capillaries collapse.
- Positive-pressure ventilation will preferentially ventilate the non-dependent lung.

Lateral Decubitus Position and Ventilation/Perfusion Matching

In the lateral decubitus position, when the patient is awake and breathing spontaneously, the V/Q ratio is *not* greatly altered. Ventilation and perfusion are both increased proportionately to the dependent lung.

The distribution of the V/Q ratios of the two lungs *is* altered in the anesthetized patient. The dependent lung continues to receive more blood flow but receives significantly less ventilation for the following reasons:

- It is less compliant. Any position that decreases FRC decreases compliance.
- It has a lower FRC due to cephalad displacement of the diaphragm.
- It is weighed down by the abdomen and mediastinum.

With opening of the chest wall and pleural cavity, a loss of negative intrapleural pressure causes the full weight of the mediastinum to be transmitted to the dependent lung.

Hypoxic Pulmonary Vasoconstriction

Hypoxic pulmonary vasocontriction (HPV) is an adaptive mechanism that increases pulmonary vascular resistance when there is a decrease in alveolar oxygen tension (PAO_2). In this scenario, blood flow is diverted away from hypoxic regions of the lung due to an increase in pulmonary artery pressure. By shifting blood flow from poorly to better ventilated regions of the lung, oxygenation is improved and hypoxemia is decreased. HPV has a rapid onset with alveolar hypoxia and can last for several hours.

Inhibition of regional HPV can impair arterial oxygenation by allowing for an increased venous admixture from hypoxic or atelectatic areas of the lung (decreasing oxygen levels). Antagonists to HPV include any condition that increases the pressure against which the vessels must constrict. This kind of antagonism results in increased flow to the hypoxic region. Examples of antagonists include the following:

- Direct vasodilating drugs (e.g., nitrates, nitric oxide, betablockers, calcium-channel blockers)
- Nitroprusside (decreases pulmonary vascular resistance, thereby reducing arterial oxygen levels)
- Inhaled anesthetics
- Hypocapnia
- Lung infections
- Mitral stenosis
- Volume overload

Potentiators of HPV include prostaglandin inhibitors (NSAIDs), and propofol.

Drugs with no effects on HPV include barbiturates, Propofol, benzodiazepines, narcotics, and muscle relaxants.

Hypercapnia: Causes During Anesthesia

- Hypoventilation
- Increased dead space ventilation

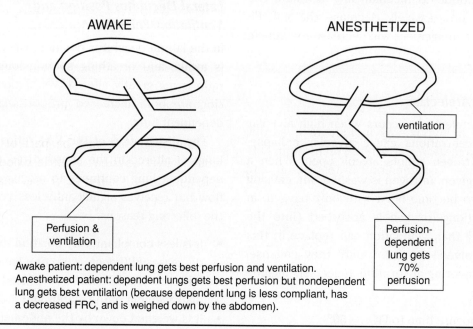

AWAKE

ANESTHETIZED

ventilation

Perfusion & ventilation

Perfusion-dependent lung gets 70% perfusion

Awake patient: dependent lung gets best perfusion and ventilation.
Anesthetized patient: dependent lungs gets best perfusion but nondependent lung gets best ventilation (because dependent lung is less compliant, has a decreased FRC, and is weighed down by the abdomen).

Figure 4-2 *Awake vs. Anesthetized Patient Abdomen*

- Increased CO_2 production (without increased ventilation)
- Impaired CO_2 absorbent

Hypoventilation may occur in the spontaneously ventilating patient for any of the following reasons:

- The patient is less willing to breathe and hypoventilates because the chemical control of breathing is significantly altered during moderate to deep levels of anesthesia.
- The patient finds it difficult to breath and hypoventilates because of increased airway resistance, decreased lung compliance, or residual muscle relaxant.

Increased dead space may result from the following causes:

- Decreased pulmonary artery pressure
- Increased mean airway pressure (PEEP)
- Pulmonary embolus

Hypocapnia: Causes During Anesthesia

- Hyperventilation
- Mechanical hyperventilation (most common cause of hypocapnia during general anesthesia)
- Decreased CO_2 production due to deep anesthesia, hypothermia, or hypotension

Hypoxemia

Early signs of hypoxemia include tachycardia, tachypnea, agitation, and altered mentation. Late signs include hypotension, bradycardia, and obtundation.

Nitric Oxide

Nitric oxide (NO) is a naturally produced endogenous compound synthesized by an enzyme called nitric oxide synthase (NOS); this enzyme is produced in numerous cells throughout the body, including neurons, macrophages, and the endothelial cells in the lining of the lumen of blood vessels.

With each heart contraction, the endothelial cells within the blood vessels release nitric oxide, causing the vessels to relax and dilate.

Nitric oxide (NO) or inhaled nitric oxide (INO) is a commercially available, nonflammable gas used for therapeutic inhalation. It aids in pulmonary vasodilation, inhibition of platelet aggregation, renal perfusion, neurotransmission, and many other physiologic functions. Inhalation of NO can cause selective pulmonary vasodilation in aerated lung regions (in conditions associated with reversible vasoconstriction and pulmonary hypertension) and may be beneficial in the treatment of various forms of pulmonary hypertension and respiratory distress due to V/Q mismatch. NO has been shown to improve gas exchange and right ventricular performance. INO is approved for the treatment of preterm infants (more than 34 weeks gestation) and term neonates who are experiencing hypoxic respiratory failure associated with persistent pulmonary hypertension (PPHN) and who have not responded to conventional therapies.

NO is absorbed systemically after inhalation by combining with hemoglobin and subsequent conversion to nitrites and nitrates. It is then excreted in the urine.

NO is given in conjunction with ventilatory support. This compound, which is unstable in air, undergoes spontaneous oxidation to nitrogen dioxide (NO_2).

Three monitors must be part of every nitric oxide delivery system: a nitric oxide administration apparatus, a nitric oxide gas analyzer, and a nitrogen dioxide gas analyzer.

Helium (Heliox): Use in Pediatric Patients

Helium has a lower density (in relation to oxygen) and allows more laminar gas flow through areas of turbulence; this effect may decrease the resistance in the conducting airways and facilitate breathing. Helium is used as a temporary measure to decrease the work of breathing, delay respiratory failure in upper airway obstruction (e.g., croup), or lower airway obstruction (e.g., asthma).

The combination of helium and oxygen may be used to improve air flow through a small ETT. The use of helium requires the oxygen concentration to be at or less than 30%. The patient's oxygen saturation is the key to identifying the optimal oxygen/helium mixture concentration. Heliox can be attached to the ventilator air inlet.

NAUSEA AND VOMITING

Nausea and vomiting occur when stimuli from peripheral organs/tissues are carried by afferent neurons of the vagus nerve to the emetic center in the midbrain, medulla, and near the nucleus of the solitary tract in close proximity to the chemoreceptor trigger zone (CTZ) in area postrema. Neuronal pathways connect the cerebral cortex (associated with balance, salivation, respiration, and vasomotor responses) to the emetic center. The area postrema contains serotonin receptors (5-HT_3). Histaminic and muscarinic-cholinergic (Ach) are predominant in the nucleus of the solitary tract.

Antiemetics

Antiemetic agents may be given on the following schedule:

- Preoperatively: Pepcid 10 mg IV.
- Intraoperatively: Phenergan 12.5 mg IM; dexamethasone 4–10 mg IV (steroid). These options have a synergistic effect when given with ondansetron.
- Within 30 to 60 minutes of emergence: ondansetron 4–8 mg IV (5-HT_3 blocker).

Droperidol (25 mcg/kg intravenously) has also been shown to be very effective as an antiemetic for procedures involving the osseous labyrinth of the ear. However, its sedative effects coupled with a recent finding that droperidol causes QT-wave prolongation and possibly torsades de pointes have made this a less appealing therapy for postoperative nausea and vomiting.

Propofol has also been shown to have significant antiemetic properties.

Antiemetic drug effects are potentiated by Decadron.

Some key antiemetics are profiled here:

Ondansetron (Zofran)
Selective 5-HT_3 (serotonin) receptor antagonist
IV 4–8 mg in a single or divided dose administered over 1–2 minutes
Give at least 30 minutes prior to emergence from anesthesia

Dolasetron (Anzemet)
Selective 5-HT_3 (serotonin) receptor antagonist
Advocated as a single IV 12.5 mg dose
Give at least 30 minutes prior to emergence from anesthesia

Cimetidine, ranitidine, nizatidine
H_2 blockers

Famotidine (Pepcid)
IV 20 mg
Best given in advance of induction
Selective and reversible inhibition of H_2-receptor-mediated secretion of acidic gastric fluid

Metoclopramide (Reglan)
Dopamine antagonist
IV 10 mg: Check with surgeon before giving for *any* GI case
Promotes gastric emptying (prokinetic); increases lower esophageal sphincter tone
Contraindications: bowel obstruction (can perforate), Parkinson's disease, QT prolongation

Droperidol (Inapsine)

Dopamine antagonist that carries a *black box warning*

Very low dose is needed: 0.625–1.25 mg IV 30 minutes prior to emergence from anesthesia

Need higher doses to *treat* vomiting; higher doses are also used for sedation

Antacids (sodium citrate; Bicitra):

Must be *non*-particulate

15–30 mL PO 30 minutes before induction

Persons with Increased Risk of Postoperative Nausea and Vomiting

- Females
- Motion sickness history
- Pediatrics: 6–10 years of age (34% PONV occurrence)
- 11–14 years of age (35–50% PONV occurrence)
- Nonsmokers
- Anxiety

Types of Surgery with Increased Risk of Postoperative Nausea and Vomiting

- Surgery length > 45–60 minutes
- Breast surgery
- Abdominal surgery: endoscopy and laparotomy
- Ear, nose, and throat surgery
- Ophthalmic surgery
- Neurologic surgery
- Gynecological surgery

BLOOD GLUCOSE AND INSULIN

The normal blood glucose (BG) serum is in the range of 80 to 110 mg/dL. The HbA_{1c} (glycosylated hemoglobin) level reflects the adequacy of glucose control over the preceding 1–3 months. For non-diabetic patients, HbA_{1c} levels are in the range of 5–7% of total hemoglobin; for diabetics with poor long-term glucose control, the HbA_{1c} may exceed 8%.

Preoperative Guidelines Regarding Hypoglycemic Agents

This is a suggested protocol. You should follow your own institution's guidelines.

Oral hypoglycemic agents: Other oral agents should not be taken the morning of surgery. If the patient is taking Diabenese (which has a really long half-life), he or she should stop taking this medication 48–72 hours preoperatively.

Subcutaneous insulin preparations: The patient should be instructed to take half of the normal dose on the morning of surgery.

Insulin: Patients with type 1 diabetes should receive some insulin perioperatively to maintain adequate metabolic control, to limit protein catabolism, and to prevent the development of ketoacidosis.

Hypoglycemia Normals and Treatment (BG < 80 mg/dL)

Hypoglycemia treatment: 1 mL $D_{50}W$ increases BG by approximately 2 mg/dL

1 amp $D_{50}W$ = 50 mL

½ amp $D_{50}W$ IV push should raise BG level by approximately 50 mg/dL

1 amp $D_{50}W$ IV push should raise BG level by approximately 100 mg/dL

Hypoglycemia treatment in non-acute situation

D_5W IV drip at 100–200 mL/h

$D_{10}W$ IV drip at 50–100 mL/h

Hyperglycemia Normals and Treatment (BG > 110 mg/dL)

Hyperglycemia treatment: 1 unit of regular insulin lowers BG by approximately 25–30 mg/dL

Insulin infusion: 250 units regular insulin in 250 mL 0.9% normal saline. Divide the BG level by 150 to find the rate to run the insulin drip (example: 300 ÷ 150 = 2; run the insulin drip at 2 units/hour).

Subcutaneous regular insulin injection:

BLOOD GLUCOSE	UNITS OF REGULAR INSULIN BY SUBCUTANEOUS INJECTION
150–200	2 units
201–250	4 units
251–300	6 units
301–350	8 units
> 350	10 units

Tight BG control in the critically ill patient certainly reduces morbidity and most likely reduces overall mortality through the following effects: improved wound healing, decreased infection rate, and improved neurologic outcome with central nervous system ischemic injury.

Normal Levels of Glucose Needed (Basal Cerebral Requirement)

The *cerebral metabolic rate of glucose consumption* (CMRGlc) is 5 mg/100 g brain tissue per minute; this is the basal requirement. This brain demand must be met by adequate delivery of glucose. If the patient is diabetic, or if his or her serum glucose level is outside the normal range, insulin or glucose IV infusions should be titrated to maintain the patient at a normoglycemic level.

Healthy adult: 0.25–0.4 units/g glucose (1.25 to 4 units per hour)

Sick adult (increased basal needs): 0.4–0.8 units/g glucose (2 to 8 units per hour)

When giving insulin, be aware of its effects on electrolytes:

- *Acidosis* causes a shift of potassium from the intracellular space of cells into the plasma; thus there is a "base deficit" (indicates an acidotic state). If the patient is in a hypoperfused state, give fluids and treat the cause.
- *Alkalosis* causes a shift of potassium from the plasma into cells.
- Insulin is the first-line defense against *hyperkalemia.* A rise in plasma potassium stimulates insulin release by the pancreas. Insulin, in turn, enhances potassium uptake into the cells, returning plasma potassium to normal levels.

COAGULATION AND ANTICOAGULATION

Coagulation Tests

PT: tests primarily Factor VII. Secondarily tests Factors II, IX, and X. Normal < 12 seconds

PTT: tests primarily Factors VIII through XI. Secondarily tests Factors II, V, and X. Normal < 30 seconds

ACT: tests extrinsic and final common coagulation pathway. Normal 90–120 seconds

TEG (thrombelastography): measures platelet function, not just platelet number. It gives a rapid picture of the fibrinolytic process.

- *r:* length from start of test until line begins to widen; primarily correlates with PTT.
- *alpha:* angle between the line and the widened part; primarily correlates with fibrinogen.
- *M:* maximum width reached; primarily correlates with functional platelet count.

Platelet function test (PFA-100): a laboratory test designed to measure platelet function. Adequate platelet function depends on the platelets' ability to adhere to the site of endothelial injury, activate surface receptors to attract other platelets, and aggregate (clump together) to form a platelet plug.

Chronic Anticoagulation Therapy

Patients on warfarin (Coumadin) usually have atrial fibrillation, a prosthetic heart valve, and/or a history of venous thromboembolism. Treatment with warfarin presents a problem if patients with these indications need surgery or a neuraxial block, because the interruption of anticoagulant therapy increases the risk of thromboembolism.

After warfarin therapy is stopped, it takes approximately 4–5 days for the international normalized ratio (INR) to reach 1.5 in almost all patients, which is the point when surgery can be safely performed. Depending on the risk of thromboembolism, bridge therapy with prophylactic low-molecular-weight heparin (LMWH; enoxaparin [Lovenox]) or unfractionated heparin may be necessary in the interim period prior to surgery. After warfarin is restarted, it takes about three days for the INR to reach 2.0.

If the thromboembolic risk is deemed high, anticoagulation can be stopped the day before surgery and reversed with vitamin K and/or fresh frozen plasma (FFP). If the procedure is an emergency and anticoagulation therapy has not been stopped, FFP at 15–20 mL/kg can be administered prior to the procedure in both instances. Intravenous heparin therapy can then be initiated 12–24 hours postoperatively once surgical hemostasis is adequate.

Anticoagulants delay or prevent clotting but do not affect a thrombus.

Oral Anticoagulants

Warfarin (Coumadin)

Warfarin affects both the intrinsic and extrinsic pathways of the coagulation cascade. It inhibits vitamin K, which is a cofactor in the production of Factors II, VII, IX, and X and proteins C and S.

Adequate suppression of all factors is not achieved until 4–6 days after starting regular dosing of warfarin. If a patient is receiving high-dose warfarin (15–30 mg PO for 2–3 days), the PT/INR will increase to anticoagulation levels within 48–72 hours. Low doses of warfarin affect Factor VII (i.e., the extrinsic pathway); higher doses affect Factors II, IX, and X (i.e., the intrinsic pathway). After warfarin is restarted, it takes approximately 3 days for the INR to (increase) reach 2.0.

Lab values for warfarin measure the extrinsic clotting pathway:

Prothrombin time (PT): Range 12–15 seconds

INR range: 0.8–1.2 seconds

PTT: altered at high warfarin dosage

The effects of warfarin can be immediately reversed by giving fresh frozen plasma and giving vitamin K (Aqua-Mephyton) sub-Q, IV, IM, or PO.

Parenteral Anticoagulants

Heparin IV

1 mg = 100 units

Heparin attaches to antithrombin III; it irreversibly blocks the effect of thrombin and blood clotting factors, thereby prolonging coagulation times. The half-life of heparin is 90–120 minutes.

Lab values measured include PTT (normal range 25–35 seconds), activated partial thromboplastin (APTT), activated clotting time (ACT), or thromboelastography (TEG).

The effects of heparin are reversed by giving protamine.

Antithrombin III (Thrombate III)

Antithrombin III can be given if the patient is less sensitive to heparin and his or her coagulation time is slow or does not respond to heparin. This agent is a major inhibitor of thrombin, which works by inhibiting prothrombin's conversion to thrombin; it inactivates Factor X.

Dose: units required (IU) = [(desired – baseline AT-III level in %)] [weight in kg]/1.4

Supplied: 500 IU and 1000 IU; reconstituted with sterile water for injection, brought to room temperature prior to administration. Should be drawn up through a sterile filter needle (supplied in the package) and should be administered within 3 hours following reconstitution. Infused over 10–20 minutes IV.

The effects of antithrombin III are reversed by giving protamine.

Low-Molecular-Weight Heparin (Enoxaparin [Lovenox])

LMWH is made of fragments of the unfractionated heparin molecule. Enoxaparin binds to and accelerates antithrombin III activity, prolonging coagulation time by preventing the start of the coagulation cascade. Its half-life is 3–6 hours when it is administered by subcutaneous injection.

Enoxaparin does not increase PT, INR, or PTT times; its effects are difficult to monitor. Enoxaparin is resistant to protamine reversal.

Low dose LMWH: 20 mg once a day

High dose LMWH: Enoxaparin 1 mg/kg every 12 hours

> Enoxaparin 1.5 mg/kg daily
> Dalteparin 120 U/kg every 12 hours
> Dalteparin 200 U/kg daily
> Tinzaparin 175 U/kg daily

Direct Thrombin Inhibitors

Direct thrombin inhibitor agents are frequently used in patients when heparin is contraindicated. Many of these agents have prolonged half-lives and are difficult to reverse without administration of blood components. Three such drugs are available for clinical use:

- Bivalirudin (Angiomax)
- Lepirudin (Refludan or Hirudin; from leeches): used in the treatment of

thrombosis in patients with heparin-induced thrombocytopenia (HIT).
- Argatroban: used in the treatment of thrombosis in patients with HIT. Half-life is 50 minutes; monitored by PTT.

Antiplatelet Drugs

There is no one lab test available to guide all antiplatelet therapy. Platelet count may be normal, yet these drugs may still have an antiplatelet effect.

Dextran 40/70: decreases platelet aggregation and fibrin polymerization.

Cyclooxygenase inhibitors: irreversibly inhibit thromboxane A_2 (platelet aggregate stimulator and vasoconstrictor); lifetime of platelets is 7–10 days.

- **Aspirin** (acetylsalicylic acid)

Nonsteroidal anti-inflammatory agents: influence aggregation of platelets for 1 to 3 days after stopping therapy. The use of NSAIDs does not increase the risk of hematoma, although the combination of NSAIDs and other anticoagulants may increase this risk.

- **Anaprox, Aleve** (naproxen)
- **Feldene** (piroxicam)
- **Motrin** (ibuprofen)

Adenosine diphosphate (ADP) receptor inhibitors:
- **Plavix** (clopidogrel bisulfate): prototype antiplatelet
- **Ticlid** (ticlopidine)
- **Effient** (prasugrel): more potent than Plavix

Phosphodiesterase inhibitors
- **Pletal** (cilostazol)

Glycoprotein IIB/IIIA inhibitors: exert a profound effect on platelet aggregation.

- **ReoPro** (abciximab): takes 24–48 hours for normal platelet function to return after this agent is administered.

- **Integrilin** (eptifibatide): takes 4–8 hours for normal platelet function to return after this agent is administered.
- **Aggrastat** (tirofiban): takes 4–8 hours for normal platelet function to return after this agent is administered.

Adenosine reuptake inhibitors:
- *Persantine (dipyridamole)*

Thrombolytics and Fibrinolytics
- Streptokinase (Streptase)
- Activase (tissue plasminogen activator [t-PA])
- Urokinase (Abbokinase)
- Reteplase (Retavase)
- Tenecteplase (TNKase)
- Anistreplase (Eminase)

These drugs work by activating free plasmin and have a profound effect on hemostasis. Serious hemorrhagic events can occur if a patient undergoes an invasive procedure after receiving a thrombolytic/fibrinolytic.

Heparin Reversal: Protamine
Dose: 1–1.3 mg for every 100 units of circulating heparin (ACT guided)

Protamine side effects include hypotension (give slowly to avoid this problem) and pulmonary hypertension. *Protamine use may result in anaphylaxis* owing to histamine release and mast cell degranulation after basic drug administration. Allergic reactions more common in patients who are sensitized to protamine, including members of the following groups:

- Patients with a fish allergy: 24.5-fold risk increase for allergic reaction
- Diabetics maintained on neutral protamine Hagedorn (NPH) insulin
- Allergy to any drug: 3-fold risk increase for allergic reaction

- Patients with previous exposure to protamine (e.g., previous cardiac catheterization or hemodialysis)
- Vasectomized males

Anaphylaxis is mediated by immunoglobulin E antibodies, which bind to the surface of mast cells and basophils. Prior sensitization to protamine is needed to create these antibodies. With re-exposure to protamine, these cells release histamine, prostaglandins, and chemotactic factors, resulting in vascular collapse.

Anaphylactoid reaction is non-immunologic; its occurrence does not require prior exposure to protamine. In this reaction, the complement system is activated, including generation of anaphylatoxins and thromboxane. Patient reactions may range from mild hypotension to acute cardiovascular collapse, decreased SVR, marked pulmonary hypertension, and increased CVP.

Prothrombotics

Desmopressin (DDAVP)
DDAVP is a synthetic analogue of L-arginine vasopressin (ADH) that increases platelet aggregation. It is used to promote the release of von Willebrand factor and for patients with thrombocytopenia.

The dose for bleeding is 0.3 mcg/kg in 50–100 ml 0.9% NS. This agent causes hypotension, so it should be given slowly. Doses sufficient to provide hemostasis will have an antidiuretic effect for 8–20 hours.

DDAVP shortens the prolonged APTT and the bleeding time by increasing the plasma levels of Factor VIII and von Willebrand factor 3 to 5 times above basal levels within 30–60 minutes. This agent provides for nonspecific platelet function augmentation.

Topical Hemostatics

Topical hemostatics include Gelfoam, Oxycel, Surgicel, Avitene, and Thrombin. These agents work by providing a lattice or structure for clot to form to or to stimulate the coagulation cascade (thrombin). When left in the wound, they provide microvascular hemostasis, but they can become infected.

Antifibrinolytics

Antifibrinolytics are used to prevent excessive blood loss. They inhibit the activation of plasminogen to plasmin; plasmin is responsible for the degradation of fibrin (fibrin is the main component in blood clots). When an antifibrinolytic is given, the clot does not break down, spilling out fibrin split products.

Fibrinolysis is the process wherein a fibrin clot is broken down. Its main enzyme plasmin cuts the fibrin mesh at various places, leading to the production of circulating fragments.

- **Amicar (aminocaproic acid):** 5 g = 20 mL syringe; usually 5 g load, then 1–2 g/h (250 mg/mL; 1 g = 4 mL; 2 g = 8 mL)
- **Tranexamic acid (Cyklokapron)**

Serum BUN and creatinine should be normal when these dosages are used.

Neuraxial Anesthesia and Anticoagulants

There is a risk of hematoma formation around the spinal cord in any patient who is anticoagulated with a spinal or epidural. See the American Society of Regional Anesthesia (ASRA) guidelines at http://www.asra.com/consensus-statements/2.html for further guidance regarding anticoagulants and neuraxial anesthesia.

As per the ASRA website, "The decision to perform spinal or epidural anesthesia/analgesia and the timing of catheter removal in a patient receiving antithrombotic therapy should be made on an individual basis, weighing the small, though definite risk of spinal hematoma with the benefits of regional anesthesia for a specific patient."

Concurrent anticoagulation therapies (e.g., taking antiplatelets with LMWH) may increase the risk of spinal hematoma and other bleeding complications.

See the ASRA guidelines regarding traumatic needle or catheter placement.

ANTICOAGULANTS

ROUTE	DRUG	LAB TEST	AFTER ANTICOAGULANT GIVEN: TO PLACE NEURAXIAL CATHETER	AFTER ANTICOAGULANT GIVEN: TO REMOVE NEURAXIAL CATHETER	TO GIVE ANTICOAGULANT: ONCE A SPINAL OR EPIDURAL HAS BEEN PLACED	TO GIVE ANTICOAGULANT: AFTER REMOVING A SPINAL OR EPIDURAL	REVERSAL
PO	Warfarin (Coumadin)	PT/INR	Document normal INR (≤ 1.5) prior to insertion of spinal or epidural; caution must be used (*see ASRA guidelines*)	INR (≤ 1.25–1.5)			Vitamin K, fresh frozen plasma (FFP)
IV	Heparin	APTT		Wait 2–4 hours and evaluate coagulation status	Wait ≥ 1 hour to give heparin	Wait ≥ 1 hour to give heparin	Protamine
SQ	Heparin	APTT	No contraindication to neuraxial techniques with subcutaneous dosed heparin				
IV	LMWH (enoxaparin) (lower-dose)	—	Wait 10–12 hours to place	Wait ≥ 10–12 hours to remove catheter after last dose of LMWH	Wait ≥ 6–8 hours to give first dose of LMWH; wait 24 hours for the second dose	Wait at least 2 hours to give first dose of LMWH after catheter removal	Resistant to protamine
IV	LMWH (enoxaparin) (higher-dose) *See LMWH information for dosing examples*	—	Wait 24 hours to place; higher dose is associated with an increased risk of spinal hematoma		Wait 24 hours postoperatively to give first dose of LMWH, no matter what anesthetic technique and only if adequate hemostasis has been achieved	Wait at least 2 hours to give first dose of LMWH after catheter removal	

(continues)

ROUTE	DRUG	LAB TEST	AFTER ANTICOAGULANT GIVEN: TO PLACE NEURAXIAL CATHETER	AFTER ANTICOAGULANT GIVEN: TO REMOVE NEURAXIAL CATHETER	TO GIVE ANTICOAGULANT ONCE A SPINAL OR EPIDURAL HAS BEEN PLACED	TO GIVE ANTICOAGULANT: AFTER REMOVING A SPINAL OR EPIDURAL	REVERSAL
ANTIPLATELETS (Platelet count may be normal but will still have antiplatelet effects from these drugs)							
IV	Dextran 40/70	Platelet function	*See ASRA guidelines*				Influences aggregation of platelets for 1–3 days after stopping therapy
PO	NSAIDs (naproxen, piroxicam, ibuprofen)	Platelet function	"NSAIDs represent no added significant risk for the development of spinal hematoma in patients having epidural or spinal anesthesia. The use of NSAIDs alone does not create a level of risk that will interfere with the performance of neuraxial blocks. There do not seem to be specific concerns as to the timing of single-shot or catheter techniques in relationship to the dosing of NSAIDs, postoperative monitoring, or the timing of neuraxial catheter removal" (Horlocker et al., 2003, p. 187).				
CYCLOOXYGENASE INHIBITORS							
PO	Aspirin (acetylsalicylic acid)	Platelet function					Irreversible, effect for platelet life span of approximately 7 days
ADENOSINE DIPHOSPHATE (ADP) RECEPTOR INHIBITORS							
PO	Plavix (clopidogrel bisulfate)	Platelet function	7-day wait between giving Plavix and neuraxial block is suggested				Irreversible, effect for platelet life span of approximately 7 days
PO	Ticlid (ticlopidine HCl)		14-day wait between giving Ticlid and neuraxial block is suggested				
	Effient	Information not available at this time; listed as "more potent" than Plavix					

PHOSPHODIESTERASE INHIBITORS

| PO | Pletal (cilostazol) | Information not available at this time; refer to current ASRA guidelines. | |

GLYCOPROTEIN IIB/IIIA INHIBITORS

IV	ReoPro (abciximab)	Neuraxial techniques should be avoided until platelet function has recovered. Glycoprotein IIB/IIIA inhibitors are contraindicated within 4 weeks of surgery	Decreases platelet aggregation; takes 24–48 hours for normal platelet function to return
IV	Integrilin (eptifibatide)		Takes 4–8 hours for normal platelet function to return
IV	Aggrastat (tirofiban)		Takes 4–8 hours for normal platelet function to return

ADENOSINE REUPTAKE INHIBITORS

| PO | Persantine (dipyridamole) | Platelet function | Platelet inhibitor |
| PO | Herbal therapy | Platelet function | *See ASRA guidelines* |

Note: Always refer to the current ASRA guidelines before working with neuraxial anesthesia and anticoagulants.

Source: Adapted from American Society of Regional Anesthesia and Pain Medication (ASRA). (n.d.). *Publications Consensus statements.* Retrieved September 10, 2010, from http://www.asra.com/publications.php

CORTICOSTEROIDS, GLUCOCORTICOIDS, AND MINERALOCORTICOIDS

Chronic Steroid Use

Most experts recommend perioperative steroid coverage for patients who are receiving more than 5 mg/day of prednisone or an equivalent and for patients who have recently stopped long-term steroid therapy. The stress dose should be proportionate to the severity of surgical stress and should be given for no longer than 1 to 3 days perioperatively.

The physiologic rationale for steroid coverage is that long-term corticosteroid therapy, or as little as 5 mg/day for more than 5 days, suppresses the hypothalamic–pituitary–adrenal (HPA) axis. In normal patients, severe illness, trauma, stress, and surgery are accompanied by activation of the HPA axis. Patients with HPA axis suppression from long-term corticosteroid therapy may be unable to produce this physiologic response to stress, resulting in an acute adrenal crisis.

Stress doses are not required for patients who have recently received short bursts of corticosteroids (therapy lasting 5 days or less), because in these patients, HPA function recovers within 1 week.

Examples of Stress Doses

- Hydrocortisone 100 mg IV
- Solu-Medrol 125 mg IV

Glucocorticoids

- Betamethasone (Diprosone, Diprolene)
- Dexamethasone (Decadron)
- Fluprednisolone (Fluprednidene)
- Hydrocortisone
- Methylprednisolone (Solu-Medrol)
- Paramethasone (Haldrone)
- Prednisolone (cortisol)
- Prednisone (cortisone)

Cortisol is the main steroid secreted by the adrenal cortex middle zone (zona fasiculata). Cortisol is a glucocorticoid that increases blood glucose levels and is essential for the body to secrete when faced with stress. In supraphysiologic doses, glucocorticoids have an anti-inflammatory effect. The body naturally produces cortisol at a rate of 20 mg/kg/day.

Mineralocorticoids

Mineralocorticoids include aldosterone and progesterone.

NSAID PREOPERATIVE PROTOCOL

Gabapentin (Neurontin) 1200 mg PO × 1

Celecoxib (Celebrex) 400 mg PO × 1

Acetaminophen (Tylenol) 1000 mg PO × 1

Do not exceed 4000 mg acetaminophen in 24 hours; consider *all* sources. In patients who have liver impairment or chronic liver disease, do not exceed 2000 mg in 24 hours.

Recommendation for Perioperative Hydrocortisone Dosage for Patients on Long-Term Steroid Therapy	
SURGERY TYPE	**STRESS DOSE**
Minor	25 mg
Moderate	50–75 mg
Major	100–150 mg

Source: Adapted from Olyaei, A. (2004). *Perioperative steroid coverage (stress dose).* Retrieved September 10, 2010, from http://www.ohsu.edu/medicine/residency/handouts/pharmpearls/Endocrine/SteroidsStressDose.pdf

PRECEDEX (DEXMEDETOMIDINE) WORKSHEET

Mix 400 mcg in 96 mL NSS = 4 mcg/mL = 100 mL total

Loading dose: 1 mcg/kg over 20 min

Patient weight in kg ____ (#1) × 1 mcg/kg = ____ (#2) ____ mcg (#2) ÷ 4 mcg/mL = ____ mL (#3) ____ mL (#3) × 3 ____ mL/h (#4)

Set IV pump rate at #4 with volume limit #3

Maintenance range: 0.2–0.7 mcg/kg/h

0.4 mcg/kg (#5) × ____ kg (#1) = ____ mcg (#6) ÷ by 4 mcg/mL = ____ mL/h

---

or
Patient weight in kg × 0.1 = ____ mL/h
to run at 0.4 mcg/kg/h

Precedex is a centrally acting alpha-2 agonist with sedative, hypnotic, analgesic, anxiolytic, and sympatholytic properties. It has a synergistic effect with anesthetics, opioids, and benzodiazepines that may significantly reduce their dosage requirement. Precedex usage is not associated with respiratory depression, but this medication can cause hypotension, bradycardia, or cardiovascular depression. *Caution:* Do not use Precedex in a patient with second- or third-degree heart block.

REMIFENTANIL (ULTIVA) INFUSION

Mix 2 mg in 40 mL mixture (50 mcg/mL); titrate to patient response. Alternatively, mix 1 mg in 20 mL.

Remifentanil is an ultra-short-acting opioid. Its onset of action is 1–3 minutes; its half-life is 3–10 minutes. This medication is metabolized by ester hydrolysis.

Remifentanil: Adult Dosage

Induction: 0.1–1 mcg/kg over 30–60 seconds

Remifentanil infusion only: 0.1 mcg/kg 90 seconds before stimulation, then 0.05 mcg/kg/min infusion (range 0.025–0.2 mcg/kg/min)

Maintenance with other anesthetic:
- Nitrous oxide 70%: range 0.1–0.2 mcg/kg/min
- Propofol 100–200 mcg/kg/min: 0.25 mcg/kg/min (range 0.05–2 mcg/kg/min)

Induction and maintenance of anesthesia with coronary artery bypass surgery: 1 mcg/kg/min (range 0.125–4 mcg/kg/min)

Postoperatively for analgesia: Range 0.05–1 mcg/kg/min

Remifentanil Dosage: Pediatric Age 1–12 Years

Initial dose: 1 mcg/kg may be administered over 30–60 seconds

Maintenance with 1 MAC of halothane, sevoflurane, or isoflurane: 0.25 mcg/kg/min (range 0.05–1.3 mcg/kg/min)

Maintenance with nitrous oxide 70%: 0.4 mcg/kg/min

Remifentanil Dosage: Pediatric Age Birth to 12 Months

Maintenance with nitrous oxide 70%: 0.4 mcg/kg/min (range 0.4–1 mcg/kg/min)

TOTAL INTRAVENOUS ANESTHESIA

Total Intravenous Anesthesia (TIVA) entails the use of IV agent(s) given exclusively to provide a complete anesthetic. No volatile inhaled anesthetics are used. TIVA can be given as a single dose, as multiple doses, or as a continuous IV infusion. This involves achieving the desired elements of the three components of general anesthesia (the *three A's*):

- **A**mnesia (anxiolysis, ataraxia)
- **A**utonomic areflexia (cardiovascular, respiratory, gastrointestinal)
- **A**nalgesia

A combination of drugs is required, as no single available agent provides complete general anesthesia. Most IV anesthetics provide only amnesia and autonomic areflexia. The major exception is ketamine; the most complete of the IV agents, it provides all three A's. *However, combining drugs with different mechanisms creates a synergy associated with less toxicity, faster recovery, and reduced costs.*

Hypnotics that may be used in TIVA include propofol, ketamine, benzodiazepines, etomidate, and barbiturates. Analgesics that may be used in TIVA include fentanyl, remifentanil, sufentanil, alfentanil, morphine, and methadone. A propofol–analgesic (opioid) synergy markedly reduces the propofol requirement when opioids are used in conjunction with this hypnotic. No apparent pharmacokinetic interaction occurs between propofol and opioids.

Precedex (dexmedetomidine) usually not used in TIVA owing to the side effects of bradycardia, sinus arrest, and hypotension.

General TIVA Information

- Run the maintenance fluid in line with TIVA.
- Avoid dead space in IV tubing. The TIVA should not enter the tubing more than a few inches from the IV insertion site at the patient's vein. When you turn off the drug, a large amount of drug should not be present in the IV line, waiting to be infused.
- The patient can receive muscle relaxation with TIVA if needed.
- Use BIS monitoring.

Examples of TIVA

Example 1
Presedation with midazolam 1–5 mg IV.

Example 2: Propofol
Supplied: 10 mg/mL

Bolus: 0.25–1.5 mg/kg IV

Infusion: 100–150 mcg/kg/min; titrate to hemodynamic response. Have bolus dose available (0.25–1 mcg/kg). Titrate bolus as needed. Discontinue 5–8 minutes before extubation.

Example 3: Propofol AND Remifentanil OR Fentanyl OR Alfentanil
Remifentanil
Supplied: 2 mg remifentanil vial; mix in 40 mL 0.09% normal saline in a 60 mL syringe (50 mcg/mL).

Induction boluses: 0.1–1 mcg/kg 30–60 seconds before direct laryngoscopy or stimulation.

Maintenance infusions: titrate to hemodynamic response.

Remifentanil infusion only for MAC case: 1 mcg/kg/min IV bolus, then 0.05 mcg/kg/min infusion (range 0.025–0.2 mcg/kg/min)

Remifentanil infusion with propofol infusion at 100–200 mcg/kg/min: 0.25 mcg/kg/min (range 0.05–2 mcg/kg/min)

Bolus: 1 mcg/kg as needed

Fentanyl
Supplied: provided in ampules; do not mix.

Induction bolus: 50–100 mcg IV.

Maintenance infusions: 1–3 mcg/kg/hr infusion if plan is to extubate the patient; 1–15 mcg/kg/hr if the patient will remain intubated.

Alfentanil

Supplied: 500 mcg/mL in ampules.

Induction boluses: 0.5–1 mcg/kg on induction; insert oral endotracheal tube (OETT) or laryngeal mask airway (LMA) 90 seconds after bolus.

Maintenance infusions:

> For anesthetic time 30 minutes:
> Alfentanil infusion alone: 0.5–1 mcg/kg/min (total dose < 40 mcg/kg)
> Alfentanil in combination with propofol 100–200 mcg/kg/min; 0.25 mcg/kg/min

> For anesthetic time > 45 minutes: after first hour of alfentanil at maintenance rate, decrease infusion rate by 30–50%.
> Alfentanil infusion alone: 0.5–3 mcg/kg/min; maximum 4 mcg/kg/min
> Alfentanil in combination with propofol 100–200 mcg/kg/min: 0.25 mcg/kg/min

If patient is spontaneously breathing, titrate alfentanil to respiratory rate of 8–12.

Stop alfentanil 10 minutes prior to removing the ETT or LMA in a spontaneously breathing patient.

Alfentanil infusion does not require additional opioid.

Onset: immediate; peak effect in 1.5 minutes; half-life is 60–120 minutes.

15 minutes Prior to Planned Extubation

- Get patient back breathing spontaneously, if not already doing so.
- Give narcotics based on respiratory rate and minute ventilation; *minute ventilation: tidal volume* × *respiratory rate.*
- Consider ketorolac (Toradol) for postoperative pain control.

- Encourage infiltration of local anesthesia by surgeon.

TIVA and the Elderly

- Smaller volume of distribution
- Decreased clearance
- Decrease bolus dosage of all drugs, usually by 50%
- Decrease maintenance dosages of all drugs usually by one third
- Give slowly; there is an increased time to peak effect of 2–3 minutes due to slower circulation times.

Advantages of TIVA

- Eliminates anesthesia machine and waste gases
- Eliminates malignant hyperthermia risk
- Can do motor evoked potential monitoring and other neurologic monitoring

Disadvantages of TIVA

- Need infusion pumps
- Increased drug costs
- Limited clinical training/experience
- Wider variety of response
- Possibly increased awareness

Toradol (Ketorolac)

Toradol inhibits platelet aggregation and may prolong bleeding time. It is dosed as follows:

- 30 mg IM or IV if patient weight > 50 kg
- 15 mg IM if patient weight < 50 kg

Decrease the dosage if the patient has renal insufficiency or is elderly. Toradol is contraindicated in patients with ulcers or GI bleeding, with coronary artery bypass surgery, strokes, bleeding risk, during labor and delivery, and in nursing mothers.

NEUROMUSCULAR DISEASES AND ANESTHESIA

NEUROMUSCULAR DISEASES AND OTHER CONDITIONS	DESCRIPTION	ANESTHETIC	SUCCINYLCHOLINE	NONPOLARIZING MUSCLE RELAXANT (NDMAR)	DAILY MEDICATIONS	NOTES
MUSCLE DISEASES						
Lambert-Eaton syndrome (myasthenic syndrome)	Decreased release of acetylcholine by nerve stimulation (presynaptic junction); fluctuating strength and weakness of extremity muscles.	Maintain normothermia. May need ventilator support post-op.	Avoid succinylcholine; very sensitive. Will increase potassium levels.	Very sensitive; decrease dose or don't give at all. Antagonism with an anticholinesterase may be inadequate.	Continue medications to time of surgery.	Autoimmune disease. Fluctuating weakness, which improves with exercise. May need ventilator post-op. Frequently seen with small-cell lung carcinoma. Consider this disease in patients with known lung cancers.
Muscular dystrophy (MD) (Duchenne MD)	*Muscular dystrophy* is a term used to describe a number of inherited muscle-destroying disorders characterized by progressive weakness and wasting of the muscles. These diseases vary in inheritance pattern, age of onset,	Patients with MD are extremely susceptible to malignant hyperthermia, especially when given the inhaled agent halothane. These patients can be sensitive to *all* anesthetic agents. Regional anesthesia can be safely used.	Succinylcholine has been used successfully in patients with Duchenne MD, but it is best avoided to prevent a severe hyperkalemic response or triggering malignant hyperthermia. Can cause rhabdomyolysis or cardiac arrest.	Very sensitive; 3–6 times longer duration of action with vecuronium and atricurium. If NDMR is required, use the shortest-acting agent available and only give one-fourth to one-fifth the usual dose. Cholinesterase inhibitors may carry additional risks.		Cardiac issues are a large consideration: Many forms of MD affect the myocardium, leading to cardiomyopathy; arrhythmias are common. A pacemaker may be needed. Weakness of the diaphragm and ventilatory muscles may be present with a decreased ability to cough, with a predisposition to aspiration and

	location of involved muscles, and the rate of progression.				atelectasis; there is a decreased FRC. May need to remain ventilated post-op.
Myasthenia gravis (MG)	Downregulation of acetylcholine receptors at the motor end plate (post-synaptic neuromuscular junction). MG is known for exacerbations and remissions of skeletal muscle weakness, characterized by rapid exhaustion, especially after repetitive muscle use. Exacerbations occur from stress, emotions, and/or heat.	Sedation is acceptable, although patients may become apneic after receiving opioids, benzodiazepines, and inhalation agents. Aminoglycosides can potentiate muscle weakness. Procainamide, quinidine, phenothiazines, and tranquilizers can aggravate MG.	Unpredictable or resistant to succinylcholine, may need increased dose. If on anticholinesterase medications, plasma cholinesterase activity may be impaired and the succinylcholine effect may be prolonged.	Extremely sensitive; reduce dose by one-half to one-third. Best to avoid if possible. When use of NDMR is necessary, always keep one-fourth twitches. Use only a short-acting NDMR. Consider these patients to be already three-fourths muscle relaxed.	Continue medications to time of surgery. May hold anticholinergic medication on the morning of surgery. Determine steroid use within the past year prior to surgery. Abrupt deterioration in patient condition is usually caused by under-dosing of usual anticholinesterase medications, called myasthenia crisis (causes paralysis of respiratory muscles). Usual medications include Mestinon, Pyridostigmine, Neostigmine, and Edrophonium. Pharyngeal/laryngeal muscles are weak; respiratory and swallowing difficulties are present, with risk of aspiration. Skeletal muscle weakness worsens with exercise and improves with rest. Arrhythmias due to myocarditis; may have cardiomyopathy. Be certain the patient can meet the extubation criteria before extubating (e.g., head lift for 5 seconds, tidal volume > 5 mL/kg, regular respirations, strong hand grip). May need ventilator post-op. May present for thymectomy. To differentiate between myasthenic crisis and cholinergic crisis, give Edrophonium 2 mg every 2 minutes to a maximum dose of

(continues)

NEUROMUSCULAR DISEASES AND OTHER CONDITIONS	DESCRIPTION	ANESTHETIC	SUCCINYLCHOLINE	NONPOLARIZING MUSCLE RELAXANT (NDMAR)	DAILY MEDICATIONS	NOTES
MUSCLE DISEASES					*Goal of anticholinesterase medications is to provide more acetylcholine to the reduced number of receptors so as to increase neuromuscular transmission interaction. Overdose of usual medications can lead to cholinergic crisis (diarrhea, vomiting, difficulty breathing, swallowing; increased bronchial secretions), which is treated with anticholinergic (atropine, robinul).*	10 mg (Tensilon test). If it helps and muscle weakness is reduced, the problem was a myasthenic crisis. If muscle weakness persists, the patient is in cholinergic crisis and needs treatment with an anticholinergic agent (atropine, robinul).

| Myotonia (myotonic dystrophy) | A symptom of a small number of disorders characterized by the slow relaxation of a skeletal muscle after contraction (voluntary or electrical stimulation). Caused by an abnormality in the sodium channels of a muscle membrane. | Succinylcholine and all inhaled volatile agents have potentially lethal (malignant hyperthermia) or serious (myocardial depression) adverse affects. Safe anesthetic agents that can be used with myotonia include propofol, pentothal, etomidate, ketamine, narcotics, nitrous oxide, local anesthetics, anticholinergics, and anticholinesterase. | Avoid; can lead to malignant hyperthermia or myotonic reaction. | Normal response or hypersensitive. Use smaller dose of NDMR. | Myotonia can affect any and all muscle groups. Monitor the patient's temperature. Patients are predisposed to aspiration. Kyphoscoliosis (with restrictive lung disease) and skeletal muscle necrosis occur; death usually occurs by 25 years of age due to congestive heart failure or pneumonia. Myocardial dysfunction; decreased pulmonary reserve with retention of secretions; delayed gastric emptying. |
| Periodic paralysis, hyperkalemic (familial periodic paralysis) | Disorder that affects sodium channels in muscle cells and the ability to regulate potassium levels in the blood; causes intermittent episodes of extreme muscle weakness. | Careful EKG monitoring is essential to watch for arrhythmias and detect attacks. | Avoid; do not use succinylcholine if the hyperkalemic type of periodic paralysis is present. | Possible sensitivity | Acute episodes of skeletal muscle weakness or paralysis. Infuse glucose solution during fasting; maintain normothermia; monitor EKG. |

(continues)

NEUROMUSCULAR DISEASES AND OTHER CONDITIONS

CONDITIONS	DESCRIPTION	ANESTHETIC	SUCCINYLCHOLINE	NONPOLARIZING MUSCLE RELAXANT (NDMAR)	DAILY MEDICATIONS	NOTES
MUSCLE DISEASES						
Periodic paralysis hypokalemic (familial periodic paralysis)	Disorder that affects calcium channels in muscle cells and the ability to regulate potassium levels in the blood, causing hypokalemia. Causes intermittent episodes of extreme muscle weakness.	Careful EKG monitoring is essential to watch for arrhythmias and detect attacks.	*No information on using succinyl-cholin with hypokalemic periodic paralysis is available.*	Sensitive. Response is unpredictable.		Acute episodes of skeletal muscle weakness or paralysis. Avoid strenuous exercise or hypothermia. Must correct potassium levels before surgery. Avoid metabolic alkalosis or glucose infusions; these treatments lower potassium levels even further.
DEMYLINATING DISEASES						
Guillain-Barré syndrome	Acute idiopathic polyneuritis, diffuse inflammation in peripheral nervous system with demyelination of dorsal and ventral roots. Characterized by acute flaccid paralysis	Mechanical ventilation, plasmapheresis. Regional anesthesia can be used.	Avoid; associated with hyperkalemia.	Sensitive; a sensitivity to muscle relaxants can last for 4 years.	Determine steroid use within the past year prior to surgery. Alpha and betablockers.	ANS dysfunction with wide swings in BP, tachycardia, dysrhythmias, and cardiac arrest. Bronchial and salivary secretions; paralytic ileus; pneumonia. Bilateral facial paralysis with difficulty in swallowing and coughing; may need

Disorder	Pathophysiology	Anesthetic Considerations	Succinylcholine	NDMR	Medications	Other
(continued)	that usually progresses from the legs upward (distal to proximal progression). Regional anesthesia is controversial.					ventilation post-op. Autonomic dysfunction leads to cardiovascular instability; sudden death can occur.
Multiple sclerosis (MS)	Multiple sites of demyelination of corticospinal tract neurons in the brain and spinal cord. May exhibit limb paresthesia and weakness (legs more than arms).	Good sedation to prevent stress. *Do not* use warming blanket. General anesthetic usually preferred. Peripheral nerve blocks can be done. Spinal anesthesia is not recommended, although epidurals are used in obstetrics. Demyelination renders the spinal cord susceptible to the neurotoxic effects of local anesthetics; use decreased dosages.	May exacerbate symptoms. Avoid; associated with hyperkalemia.	Associated with both resistant and prolonged response to NDMR; need increased doses.	Continue medications to time of surgery. Use of antispasmodics and phenytoin for seizure prophylaxis is common. Determine steroid use within the past year prior to surgery.	Treat even a slight increase in temperature; heat can block conduction in demyelinated nerves. Symptoms of MS can be exacerbated in the postoperative period. Avoid stress.

(continues)

NEUROMUSCULAR DISEASES AND OTHER CONDITIONS	DESCRIPTION	ANESTHETIC	SUCCINYLCHOLINE	NONPOLARIZING MUSCLE RELAXANT (NDMAR)	DAILY MEDICATIONS	NOTES
NEURODEGENERATIVE DISEASES						
Alzheimer's disease	Cortical atrophy. Complex degenerative disorder characterized by generalized atrophy of the cerebral cortex.	Avoid sedation to decrease mental confusion; use robinul (does not cross blood–brain barrier). Use agents with rapid elimination.	Use appears acceptable.	Use appears acceptable.		Fewer nicotinic cholinergic receptors and decreased acetylcholine synthesis. Centrally acting anticholinergics may make the patient more confused. Glycopyrrolate does not cross the blood–brain barrier and is the drug of choice as a neuromuscular reversal agent.
Amyotrophic lateral sclerosis (ALS) (Lou Gehrig's disease)	Degenerative disease of motor cells; upper and lower motor neurons involved. Characterized by increased heart rate and increased norepinephrine and epineph-rine levels.	Use caution with the airway on induction and extubation, owing to weak bulbar muscles. Epidural anesthetic has been used successfully.	Succinylcholine causes hyperkalemia; contraindicated.	Sensitivity and prolonged effect; use reduced doses.		With progression, most skeletal muscles (including tongue, pharynx, larynx, and chest skeletal muscles) fasciculate. Have dysphagia with pulmonary aspiration. Restrictive lung disease. Expect hypovolemia.

Creutzfeldt-Jakob disease (spongiform encephalopathy; mad cow disease)	Subacute human spongiform encephalopathy. Non-inflammatory disease of CNS. Caused by infectious pathogen "prion"; differs from viruses in that prions lack RNA/DNA. Incubation period is months to years.	Abnormal CV response to anesthesia and vasoactive drugs.	Avoid; may be contraindicated.	Avoid; may be contraindicated.	No specific drug treatment.	*Disease is transmissable!* Myoclonic and EEG changes; impaired swallowing and decreased laryngeal reflexes. Reusable equipment must be sterilized in sodium hypochlorite. Full protective equipment must be worn; staff should be kept to a minimum to minimize exposure to the disease.
Huntington's chorea (Huntington's disease, Huntington's major)	Marked atrophy of basal ganglia; decreased GABA and acetylcholine levels in the brain. Progressive dementia combined with movement disorders (choreiform movements: involuntary, disordered facial and limb movements).	Give less Versed. All intravenous or inhaled anesthetics are acceptable, except note that delayed awakening and tonic spasms have occurred after Thiopental was given. A normal response with rapid recovery occurs with propofol. NO_2 and volatile anesthetics are all acceptable.	Avoid; incidence of decreased pseudocholinesterase activity is substantially higher in Huntington's disease and may prolong the succinylcholine effect.	Sensitive.	Treated with phenothiazines (Haldol and droperidol).	Risk of aspiration increases as disease progresses.

(continues)

NEUROMUSCULAR DISEASES AND OTHER CONDITIONS

NEURODEGENERATIVE DISEASES

NEUROMUSCULAR DISEASES AND OTHER CONDITIONS	DESCRIPTION	ANESTHETIC	SUCCINYLCHOLINE	NONPOLARIZING MUSCLE RELAXANT (NDMAR)	DAILY MEDICATIONS	NOTES
Parkinsonism (Parkinson's disease)	Degenerative changes of CNS caused by loss of dopaminergic fibers in basal ganglia. Dopamine is depleted; there is a decreased inhibition of the extrapyramidal motor system and unopposed action of acetylcholine. Resting tremor; skeletal muscle rigidity; diaphragmatic spasms.	Do rapid-sequence induction. Avoid Droperidol, Reglan (dopamine-receptor antagonist in basal ganglia), halothane, alfentanil, ketamine, phenothiazines (Compazine), buyrophenones. Acceptable to give Zofran.	Avoid; may increase potassium release.	Use appears acceptable.	Continue medications to time of surgery. Dopamine agonists: Levodopa (L-dopa). Symmetrel; anticholinergics, and/or monoamine oxidase (MAO) inhibitors. Acceptable to use Benadryl for sedation.	Treatment for Parkinson's disease is aimed at blocking the acetylcholine effect by use of anticholinergic drugs or by enhancing dopaminergic transmission. Patients on Levodopa are prone to dysrhythmias, labile blood pressures, and ANS dysfunction. These patients have delayed gastric emptying, altered gag, and excessive salivation. Anticipate hypotension; treat with Neosynephrine. Patient should be wide awake for extubation. May present for pallidotomy.

Condition	Description	Management	Succinylcholine	Nondepolarizing relaxants	Comments
Shy-Drager syndrome (multiple system atrophy)	Multiple system atrophy (brainstem, basal ganglia, and cerebellum) with autonomic effects.	Goal is to maintain blood pressure. Pre-op assessment of sympathetic function and degree of neurologic involvement. Maintain normovolemia, using colloid and crystalloid solutions to maintain BP. Phenylephrine is acceptable, may need low-dose infusion. Arterial line or PA catheter should be considered.	Avoid; should be avoided in muscle wasting.	Avoid; abnormal reactions have been reported.	Patients have dysphagia, sleep apnea, orthostatic hypotension, rigid muscles, and autonomic neuropathy—that is, reduced ANS activity. Direct-acting sympathomimetics can cause severe hypertension (denervation hypersensitivity). Bradycardia best treated with Atropine.

OTHER DISEASES OR CONDITIONS WITH AN ALTERED RESPONSE TO MUSCLE RELAXANTS

Condition	Description	Management	Succinylcholine	Nondepolarizing relaxants	Comments
Burns			Avoid; can result in hyperkalemia.	Resistant to muscle relaxants.	
Cerebral palsy (CP)	Due to nonprogressive motor disorder.		Avoid; can be hypersensitive.	Resistant.	CP patients can have impairment of laryngeal and pharyngeal reflexes with reflux and risk of aspiration. They are often on antispasmodics (e.g., Dantrolene

(continues)

OTHER DISEASES OR CONDITIONS WITH AN ALTERED RESPONSE TO MUSCLE RELAXANTS

NEUROMUSCULAR DISEASES AND OTHER CONDITIONS	DESCRIPTION	ANESTHETIC	SUCCINYLCHOLINE	NONPOLARIZING MUSCLE RELAXANT (NDMAR)	DAILY MEDICATIONS	NOTES
						and Baclofen—both skeletal muscle relaxants). May experience increased sedation and muscle weakness when given anesthetics.
Epilepsy	Seizures are a temporary, abnormal synchronization of electrical activity of a group of neurons.	*Methohexital* has been reported to produce seizures in epileptics, especially children, by lowering the seizure threshold. *Etomidate* has the potential to elicit seizures. Avoid *ketamine.* Some inhaled agents, including *nitrous oxide* and *enflurane,* can produce seizures and cause EEG changes; *sevoflurane,* in high induction doses, has	Appears to be acceptable to give succinylcholine to a patient with epilepsy.	Resistant to muscle relaxants if on anti-seizure medication. Avoid atricurium and cisatricurium; both have a pro-convulsant metabolite, laudanosine.	Maintain normal medications preoperatively.	High doses of fentanyl/sufentanil induce skeletal muscle rigidity; can be confused with a seizure. Epileptics who have been taking anti-seizure medications may have increased activity of the CYP-450 system (drug-induced enzyme induction) and be resistant to many anesthetics, requiring higher dosages or more frequent dosing (e.g., with narcotics and muscle relaxants). Coexisting sedation produced by

antiseizure medication can be exacerbated by anesthetic drugs. Prevent seizure: Dilantin 20mg/kg IV over 20 minutes.

also caused seizures.

Emergent treatment for seizure: pentobarbita , thiopental, diazepam, midazolam. Thiobarbiturates, opioids, benzodiazepines, and isoflurane seem to be acceptable anesthetics.

Hemiplegia	Avoid; can result in hyperkalemia.	Resistance on affected side.	
Muscle denervation	Avoid; should be avoided in patient with muscle contractures; can result in hyperkalemia.	Resistant to a normal response.	Denervation may be due to a disease (e.g., polio) where the death of motor neurons causes the denervation of muscle fibers; alternatively, it may derive from a surgical procedure designed to remove the nerve pathways that are transmitting a pain signal.

DRUGS FOR CARDIOVASCULAR SURGERIES

Amicar (Aminocaproic Acid)

Supplied: 5 g in 20 mL

Mix: 5 g in 20 mL 0.9% NS by syringe: give though syringe as secondary on IV pump;

Amount per mL: 250 mg/mL; 1 g = 4 mL/h; 2 g = 8 mL/h

OR

5 g in 100 mL in D_5W or NS and infuse by IV bag and tubing

Amount per mL: 50 mg/mL; 1 g = 20 mL/h; 2 g = 40 mL/h

Dose:

    Load: 5–10 g over 20–60 minutes

    Infusion range: 1–2 g/h, usually for 5 hours

Action: antifibrinolytic—enhances hemostasis when fibrinolysis contributes to bleeding. Inhibits activation of plasminogen.

Side effects: hypotension, bradycardia, and serious/fatal thrombus formation in disseminated intravascular coagulation (DIC).

Notes: may not give if serum creatinine levels are increased or patient in acute/chronic renal failure.

**This drug not included in IV drip chart.*

Aminophylline

Supplied: 25 mg/mL

Mix: 500 mg/250 mL D_5W or 0.9% NS

Amount per mL: 2 mg/mL

Dose:

    Load: 5–6 mg/kg over 20–30 minutes

    Infusion range: 0.5–1 mg/kg/h

Action: smooth-muscle relaxation (bronchodilation) to treat asthma. Respiratory and myocardial stimulant.

Side effects: use with extreme caution in patients with seizure disorders or history of cardiac arrhythmias.

Notes: do not give by IV push.

Amiodarone (Cordarone)

Supplied: 50 mg/mL in 3, 9, and 18 mL vials

Mix: in D_5W or NS; administer through filter *[in order: IV bag–IV pump tubing–filter–patient]*

Dose:

    Load: mix 150 mg in 100 mL and infuse over 10 minutes

    Amount per mL: 1.5 mg/mL

    OR

    Mix 900 mg in 500 mL and infuse at *500 mL/h × 83 mL*

    Infusion range: mix 900 mg in 500 mL

Amount per mL: 1.8 mg/mL. Run at 1 mg/min = 33 mL/h × 6 hours; next 0.5 mg/min = 17 mL/h × 18 hours.

Action: antiarrhythmic; prolongs action potential; for break-through ventricular tachycardia or fibrillation. Can cause bradycardia and atrioventricular block.

Side effects: arrhythmias, bradycardia, hypotension.

Notes: do not give by IV push.

Amrinone (Inocor)

Supplied: 5 mg/mL

Mix: 300 mg/60 mL (total volume 120 mL) 0.45% or 0.9% NS only

Amount per mL: 2490 mcg/mL or 2.5 mg/mL

Dose:

    Load: 0.75 mg/kg (or 750 mcg/kg) IV over 10 minutes. May be given by IV push over 2–3 minutes. May be repeated in 30 minutes if necessary.

    Infusion range: 5–10 mcg/kg/min; maximum 10 mg/kg/24 h.

Action: to treat congestive heart failure and left ventricular dysfunction. Increases cardiac output and contractility with positive inotrope; decreases preload, afterload, and pulmonary vascular resistance (PVR) by vascular smooth-muscle dilation.

Side effects: arrhythmias, hypotension, hypokalemia.

Notes: do not use if patient has hypertrophic obstructive cardiomyopathy (HOCM).

Antithrombin III (AT III; Thrombate III)

Supplied: in international units (IU). Should be reconstituted with sterile water for injection; should be filtered through a supplied sterile filter needle and given intravenously within 3 hours of reconstitution.

Mix: 500 IU/10 mL 0.9% NS

Amount per mL: variable

Dose:

Bolus: give over 10–20 minutes

Infusion: 45 IU/kg/min

Action: inactivates thrombin, plasmin, and other products of coagulation. May give if patient is suspected to be heparin resistant due to hereditary or acquired antithrombin III deficiency. Risk of hemorrhage may be increased.

Notes: product is prepared from pooled human plasma and carries a risk of viral transmission.

**This drug not included in IV drip chart.*

Brevibloc (Esmolol)

Supplied: 10 mg/mL in 10 mL vial

Mix: 2.5 g/250 mL D$_5$W

Amount per mL: 10 mg/mL or 10,000 mcg/mL

Dose:

Load: 250 mcg/kg over 1 minute, slow IV push

Infusion range: 50–100 mcg/kg/min; maximum 200 mcg/kg/min × 48 hours.

Action: beta blocker; to treat tachyarrhythmia.

Side effects: decreases blood pressure and heart rate.

Notes: do not give to patient with asthma, bradycardia, or heart block.

Cardene (Nicardipine)

Supplied: 25 mg/mL in 10 mL vial

Mix: 25 mg/240 mL (total 250 mL) D$_5$W or 0.9% NS

Amount per mL: 0.1 mg/mL

Dose:

Infusion range: 0.5–10 mg/h, start at 5 mg/h (50 mL/h) and titrate to effect. Maximum 15 mg/h (150 mL/h).

Action: calcium-channel blocker; relaxes coronary arteries, vasodilates vasculature, decreases blood pressure.

Side effects: arrhythmias, congestive heart failure.

Cardizem (Diltiazem)

Supplied: 5 mg/mL in 5, 10, and 25 mL vials

Mix: 50 mg/100 mL D$_5$W or 0.9% NS

Amount per mL: 0.5 mg/mL

Dose:

Load: 0.25 mg/kg over 20 min; may repeat in 15 minutes with a 0.35 mg/kg dose

Infusion range: 5–15 mg/h

Action: calcium-channel blocker; relaxes coronary arteries, vasodilates vasculature, decreases blood pressure.

Side effects: arrhythmias, congestive heart failure.

Notes: during radial artery harvest: 1–2 mg/h (2–4 mL/h)

Desmopressin (DDAVP)

Supplied: 4 mcg/mL

Mix: 0.3 mcg/kg in 50–100 mL 0.9% NS

Dose: 0.3 mcg/kg over 30 minutes.

Action: control of bleeding; increases Factors VIII and XII, and von Willebrand factor.

Notes: causes hypotension. Use regular tubing.

Dobutamine (Dobutrex)

Supplied: premix: 250 mg/125 mL, 250 mg/250 mL, 500 mg/500 mL, 500 mg/250 mL, 1000 mg/250 mL; in D$_5$W or 0.9% NS

Mix: premix

Amount per mL: 250 mg/125 mL = 2 mg/mL or 2000 mcg/mL

Dose:

Infusion range: 2–20 mcg/kg/min; maximum 40 mcg/kg/min.

Action: positive inotrope; mainly beta-1 but also has weak beta-2 and alpha properties. Coronary artery vasodilator. Used in cardiac failure, and low cardiac output states. Increases cardiac output without significantly increasing heart rate.

Side effects: hypertension, increased heart rate, premature ventricular contractions.

Notes: no major change in heart rate, SVR, or myocardial oxygen consumption.

Dopamine (Intropin)

Supplied: premix: 200 mg/250 mL, 400 mg/250 mL, 800 mg/250 mL, 800 mg/500 mL D_5W

Mix: premix

Amount per mL: 400 mg/250 mL = 1600 mcg/mL

Dose:

   Infusion range: 2–20 mcg/kg/min

Action: positive inotrope. 1–5 mcg/kg: affects renal vasculature, improving renal blood flow. 5–10 mcg/kg: beta-1 and -2 effect; increases SVR and cardiac output. > 10 mcg/kg: alpha-2 effect; increases cardiac output and blood pressure.

Side effects: arrhythmias, hypotension, myocardial ischemia.

Ephedrine

Supplied: 50 mg/mL vial

Mix: 50 mg in 4 mL 0.9% NS = total 5 mL

Amount per mL: 10 mg/mL

Dose:

   Infusion range: 5–25 mg bolus; maximum 150 mg/ 24 hours

Action: alpha-1 sympathomimetic; used for hypotension. Increases blood pressure, heart rate, cardiac output, contractility.

Notes: increases heart rate. Minimal effect on uterine blood flow.

**This drug not included in IV drip chart.*

Epinephrine (Adrenalin)

Supplied: 1:1000 = 1 mg/mL vial; 1:10,000 = 0.1 mg/mL

Mix: 4 mg/250 mL D_5W or 0.9% NS

Amount per mL: 16 mcg/mL

Dose:

   Load: 0.1–0.25 mg IV over 5–15 minutes

   Infusion range: 1–4 mcg/min; maximum 20 mcg/min.

Action: positive inotrope; direct alpha-1, beta-1 and -2 adrenergic agonists; vasoconstrictor.

Side effects: arrhythmias, tachycardia, hypertension, myocardial ischemia.

Notes: causes tremendous increase in myocardial oxygen consumption. Used to increase myocardial contractility and in cardiac failure/low cardiac output states; used in cardiac arrest. Bronchodilator and treatment for allergic reaction.

Factor VII

Notes: 90 mcg/kg

Dose: bolus over 5 minutes.

Mix: mix in sterile water.

Fenoldapam (Corlopam)

Supplied: 10 mg/mL in 1 mL or 2 mL ampules

Mix: 10 mg/250 mL D_5W or 0.9% NS

Amount per mL: 40 mcg/mL

Dose:

   Infusion: 0.01–1.6 mcg/kg/min

Action: rapid decrease of blood pressure; used to treat hypertension, including hypertension in malignant hyperthermia. Dopa-1 agonist; also binds to alpha receptors.

Notes: half-life of 9 minutes. Do not bolus; give by infusion only. Can see reflex tachycardia.

Heparin

Supplied (units per mL): 10, 100, 1000, 5000, 7500, 10,000, 20,000, or 40,000 units/mL

Mix: given IV without dilution

Range: 200–400 units/kg in cases where vascular procedures and coronary bypass is used. Give through central line if possible. May cause hypotension.

Insulin (Regular)

Supplied: 1 unit/mL

Mix: 250 units in 250 mL NS (1:1 ratio)

Amount per mL: 1 unit/mL

Dose: titrate to maintain blood glucose in the range of 80–110 mg/dL.

Notes: hang with special tubing that does not absorb insulin.

Isoproterenol (Isuprel)

Supplied: 0.02 mg/mL (20 mcg/mL), or 0.2 mg/mL (200 mcg/mL) vials

Mix: 1 mg/250 mL in 0.9% NS

Amount per mL: 4 mcg/mL

Dose:

    Bolus: 0.02 mg

    Infusion range: 5 mcg/min

Action: direct-acting pure beta stimulant, positive inotrope: increases cardiac output and systolic BP. Decreases mean arterial pressure due to decreased SVR and diastolic BP. Positive chronotrope: increases heart rate; "chemical pacemaker." Bronchodilator; decreases pulmonary vascular resistance. Used with congestive heart failure, bradycardia, pulmonary hypertension.

Notes: if arrhythmia occurs, must decrease or discontinue infusion.

Lidocaine

Supplied: premix 2 g/250 mL D_5W

Mix: premix

Amount per mL: 8 mg/mL

Dose:

    Load: 1–1.5 mg/kg; maximum 300 mg in first hour

    Infusion range: 1–4 mg/min; maximum 3 mg/kg/h; 1 mg/min = 7.5 mL/h

Action: treatment of ventricular arrhythmias; suppresses automaticity; shortens effective refractory period and duration of the action potential. Can cause central nervous system depression, bradycardia, hypotension, respiratory depression, vomiting.

Notes: avoid in patients with Wolf-Parkinson-White syndrome. Can decrease blood pressure.

Nitroglycerin (Tridil; NTG)

Supplied: premix 50 mg/250 mL, 50 mg/500 mL, 100 mg/250 mL, 200 mg/500 mL

Mix: premix

Amount per mL: 50 mg/250 mL = 200 mcg/mL

Dose: titrate to effect

    Infusion rage: 3–200 mcg/min; 1 mL/h = 3 mcg/min; 60 mL/h = 200 mcg/min

Action: smooth-muscle relaxant; greater venous dilation than arterial dilation. Coronary artery dilator; decreases SVR and PVR. Reduces myocardial oxygen consumption.

Side effects: tachycardia, hypotension.

Notes: effect in 2–3 minutes.

Nitroprusside (Sodium Nitroprusside; SNP)

Supplied: 25 mg/mL in 2 mL vials

Mix: 100 mg/250 mL D_5W

Amount per mL: 400 mcg/mL

Dose: titrate to effect

    Infusion rage: 5–300 mcg/min or 0.5–10 mcg/kg/min; 1 mL/h = 6.66 mcg/min

Action: to control hypertension; for heart failure or cardiogenic shock. Vasodilates by acting on venous and arterial smooth muscle. Greater arterial dilation than venous dilation.

Notes: effect in 1–2 minutes. Must keep IV fluid bag (not tubing) covered with opaque material to protect from light. Cyanide poisoning is possible with infusions lasting more than 24 hours.

Norepinephrine (Levophed)

Supplied: 1 mg/mL in 4 mL ampules

Mix: 4 mg/250 mL D_5W, *avoid mixing with 0.9% NS*

Amount per mL: 16 mcg/mL

Dose:

    Infusion range: 2–20 mcg/min; titrate to blood pressure and cardiac output.

Action: positive inotrope, arterial vasoconstrictor. Alpha-1 and -2, weak beta-1, minimal beta-2.

Side effects: arrhythmias, myocardial ischemia, hypertension, bradycardia.

Notes: avoid subcutaneously. Used for hypotensive states, shock with sepsis, given to increase blood pressure, cardiac output, and systemic vascular resistance. Baroreceptor-mediated bradycardia reflex.

Phenylephrine (Neosynephrine)

Supplied: 1% in 1 mL vials = 10 mg/mL

Mix: 20 mg/250 mL D_5W or 0.9% NS

Amount per mL: 80 mcg/mL

Range: 10–200 mcg/min or 0.15–4 mcg/kg/min; 1 mL/h = 1.3 mcg/min

Dose: titrate to effect; 1 mL/h = 1.3 mcg/min or 10 mcg/min = 7.5 mL/h

Action: direct-acting alpha-1 agonist; used for hypotension—increases blood pressure and SVR by direct vasoconstriction of blood vessels.

Side effects: arrhythmias, bradycardia, hypertension.

Notes: slows heart rate (baroreceptor-mediated reflex bradycardia).

Primacor (Milrinone)

Supplied: 1 mg/mL in 10, 20, and 50 mL vials; premix 20 mg/100 mL, 40 mg/200 mL, or 50 mg/250 mL in D_5W or NS

Mix: 40 mg/200 mL D_5W or 0.9% NS

Amount per mL: 200 mcg/mL

Dose:

   Load: 0.05 mg/kg (50 mcg/kg) over 10 minutes; can be given undiluted.

   Infusion: 0.5 mcg/kg/min

Action: positive inotrope and positive chronotrope; vasodilator; to treat congestive heart failure and left ventricular dysfunction. Decreases preload and afterload by directly dilating vascular smooth muscle. Increases cardiac output.

Side effects: ventricular arrhythmias, decreased potassium.

Notes: will precipitate with furosemide.

Protamine Sulfate

Supplied: 10 mg/mL in 5 and 25 mL vials

Mix: surgeon may give directly into vessel at surgical opening; or mix dose into 100 mL NS.

Amount per mL: varies

Dose: 1 mg Protamine/100 units of heparin given. If given more than 30 minutes after heparin dose, give 0.5 mg/100 units of heparin.

Notes: give slowly, as can cause significant hypotension (has negative inotropic effect). Give through central line if possible.

**This drug not included in IV drip chart.*

Trimethaphan (Arfonad)

Supplied: 50 mg/mL

Mix: 500 mg/500 mL of D_5W (only)

Amount per mL: 1 mg/mL

Dose:

   Load: 3–4 mg/min

   Infusion range: 0.3–6 mg/min; titrate to effect

Action: to rapidly decrease blood pressure; decreases cardiac output and PVR. Trimethaphan is a nicotinic ganglionic blocking agent that prevents stimulation of postsynaptic receptors by competing with acetylcholine.

Side effects: tachycardia, urticaria, hypotension.

Notes: takes effect in 1–2 minutes, duration of action 10–15 minutes. Can cause release of histamine and vasodilation. By infusion only, do not bolus by syringe.

Vasopressin (Pitressin)

Supplied: 20 units/mL in 0.5 and 1 mL ampules

Mix: 40 units/100 mL or 100 units/100 mL in 0.9% NS or D_5W

Amount per mL: 40 units/100 mL = 0.4 unit/mL; 100 units/100 mL = 1 unit/mL

Range: 0.1–0.4 unit/min

Dose: 0.02 unit/min = 3 mL/h; 0.04 unit/min = 6 mL/h

   Load: 20 units over 20–30 minutes; do not give bolus

Infusion range for vasopressor: 0.2–1 unit/min
Action: potent vasopressor; can decrease coronary blood flow.
Notes: used to decrease blood loss, vasopressor for vasodilatory shock, antidiuretic effect with diabetes insipidus.

Abbreviations

D_5W: dextrose 5% in water IV fluid
h: hour
min: = minutes
mL: milliliter
NS: 0.9% normal saline
PVR: pulmonary vascular resistance
SVR: systemic vascular resistance
u: units
*Side effects listed are short-term side effect issues in the OR.

HEART SETUP

Succinylcholine 200 mg
Pentothal 4 mg/kg used for induction primarily or Etomidate 0.3 mg/kg given if CO < 30% or patient has aortic stenosis

Vecuronium 2 mg/mL (10 mL syringe) or Pavulon (*give if patient needs a vagolytic*): maintenance 0.007–0.015 mg/kg; 2 mg/mL
Fentanyl 20 mL × 2; *75–150 mcg/kg for cardiac anesthesia*
Versed 10–15 mg
Atropine 1 mg
Ephedrine 50 mg/4 mL sterile H_2O
Neosynephrine 80 mcg/mL
Lidocaine 100 mg syringe
Calcium chloride 1% 20 mL (2 g)
Heparin 1000 u/mL in 60 mL syringe; give through central line
Epinephrine 10 mcg/mL
Ancef 2 g (if not allergic) – 1 g q 4 h
Protamine 50 mL in 50 mL syringe; give through central line. Give slowly as it can cause hypotension and PA hypertension.
Amicar 5 g in 20 mL
Volatile inhaled agent at ½ MAC and give Fentanyl for anesthesia. Never use N_2O; increases bubble size.
Redo heart? Have blood ready in room.
Preop: read BP from both arms; 20% difference = ? subclavian stenosis. Put arterial line in the arm with higher BP.

PRELOAD		CONTRACTILITY		AFTERLOAD	
CVP	PCWP	SVI	LVSWI	PVR	SVR
low	high	low	high	low	high
volume	dilators	+ Inotrope	beta block	vasopressor	dilator
- colloids	- NTG	- Dobutamine	- Esmolol	- Epi	- Nipride
- blood	diuretic	- Dopamine	- Metoprolol	- Norepi	- Amrinone
- crystalloids		- Epinephine	- Labetalol	- Dopa	- Milrinone
		- Inocor		IABP 1:1	IABP 1:1
		- Levophed			
		- Neosynephine			
		- Primacor			

HOW TO USE THE CARDIOVASCULAR DRUG TABLE

In the following charts, the **drug index number** (in shaded box) has already been calculated for infusions ordered in micrograms per kilogram per minute (mcg/kg/min).

The calculation to find the drug index number:
  mcg/cc ÷ 60 ÷ kg weight = drug index number

For Loading Doses

The ordered milligram amount has already been calculated and listed under "total dose to give." Then, based on the drug mixture and resulting amount of drug per milliliter, the calculation has already been made for how many total milliliters to give, at what rate, and for how many milliliters (total volume to give).

For example, for the 45-kg patient, the first loading dose in the chart is aminophylline 5 mg/kg over 20 minutes. In this case, 5 mg has been multiplied by the patient's weight (in kilograms) and the total amount to give is shown: 225 mg. The drug mixture is 500 mg in 250 mL of fluid, giving 2 mg/mL. The calculation shows that 113 mL of the mixture should be given over 20 minutes. 113 mL × (60 min ÷ 20 min) means the IV pump should be set at 337.5 × 20 minutes **or** 337.5 for a total volume given of 113 mL.

IV infusion formulas are written for each drug if the dose is listed in a range and could not be calculated.

IV Infusion Calculations

To find the rate (mL/h) to set on IV pump:

Ordered at **mg/kg/h**
  Ordered mg dose × kg weight ÷ mg/mL of mixture = mL/h to set on IV pump

Ordered at **mg/h**
  Ordered mg dose ÷ mg/mL = mL/h to set on IV pump

Ordered at **mg/min**
  Ordered mg dose ÷ mg/mL × 60 min/h = mL/h to set on IV pump

Ordered at **mcg/kg/min**
  Ordered mcg dose × 60 min/h × kg weight ÷ mcg/mL = mL/h to set on IV pump

Ordered at **mcg/min**
  Ordered mcg dose ÷ mcg/mL × 60 min/h = mL/h to set on IV pump

What is your drug dose if you know the mL/h?
  mg/min = mg/mL × mL/h ÷ 60 min/h
  mcg/kg/min = mcg/mL × mL/h ÷ kg weight × 60 min/h

Another way to find mcg/mL in solution and other IV drip calculations:

- Multiply mg in solution by 1000 = mcg/solution
- Divide mcg/solution by amount of original solution = mcg/mL
- Multiply mcg/mL by mL/h = mcg/h
- Divide mcg/h by 60 min = mcg/min
- Divide mcg/min by patient's kg weight = mcg/kg/min

Calculations if you already know the drug index number:

To find how many mL/h to set on pump when mcg/kg/min ordered,
take dose you want in mcg ÷ **drug index #** = mL/h on pump

To find dose in mcg if you already know mL/h on pump,
mL × **drug index #** = dose in mcg/kg/min

45 kg

DRUG	ORDERED AMOUNT	TOTAL DOSE TO GIVE	DRUG INDEX NUMBER	DIRECTIONS	INFUSION RANGE	DRUG MIXTURE	AMOUNT	DRUG/mL	RUN AT	mL/h
Aminophylline	5 mg/kg =	225 mg		Give mg/kg load over 20 min		500 mg/ 250 mL	2 mg/mL		
	mg to give ÷ mg/mL =	113 mL			113	mL × (60 min/h ÷ 20 min) =		**337.5**	mL/h × 20 min
	Infusion				0.5–1 mg/kg/h	500 mg/ 250 mL	2 mg/mL		
						mg dose ordered × kg ÷ mg/mL =		___	mL/h
Amiodarone	Loading dose			Load **150 mg** over 10 min		900 mg/ 500 mL	1.8 mg/mL		
				Ordered mg load dose (150 mg) ÷ mg/mL (1.8 mg/mL) = 83 mL to give × (60 min/h ÷ 10 min) = mL/h to set on pump				**500**	mL/h × 83 mL
	Infusion			Run at **1 mg/ min** × 6 h		900 mg/ 500 mL	1.8 mg/mL		
				Ordered mg dose (1 mg/min) ÷ mg/mL (1.8 mg/mL) = × 60 min/h = mL/h to set on pump				**33**	mL/h × 6 h
	Infusion			Run at **0.5 mg/ min** × 18 h		900 mg/ 500 mL	1.8 mg/mL		
				Ordered mg dose (0.5 mg/min) ÷ mg/mL (1.8 mg/mL) = ___ × 60 min/h = mL/h to set on pump				**17**	mL/h × 18 h
Amrinone	0.75 mg/kg =	33.75 mg		Give mg/kg load over 10 min		300 mg/ 120 mL	2.5 mg/mL		
	mg to give ÷ mg/mL =	14 mL			13.5	mL × (60 min/h ÷ 10 min) =		**81**	mL/h × 10 min
	Infusion		0.92		5–10 mcg/ kg/min	300 mg/ 120 mL	2500 mcg/mL	___	mL/h
				Take dose you want in mcg ÷ by drug index number = mL/h on pump					
Brevibloc	Infusion		3.70		50–100 mcg/ kg/min	2.5 g/ 250 mL	10,000 mcg/mL	___	mL/h
				Take dose you want in mcg ÷ by drug index number = mL/h on pump					
Cardene	Infusion				0.5–10 mg/h	25 mg 250 mL	0.1 mg/mL		
				Ordered mg dose ÷ mg/mL = mL/h to set on pump				___	mL/h
Cardizem	0.25 mg/kg =	11.25 mg		Give mg/kg load over 20 min		50 mg/ 100 mL	0.5 mg/mL		
	mg to give ÷ mg/mL =	23 mL			22.5	mL × (60 min/h ÷ 20 min) =		**68**	mL/h
	0.35 mg/kg =	15.75 mg		May repeat loading dose in 15 min			0.5 mg/mL		
	mg to give ÷ mg/mL =	32 mL			31.5	mL × (60 min/h ÷ 20 min) =		**95**	mL/h
	Infusion				5–15 mg/h				
				Ordered mg dose ÷ mg/mL = mL/h to set on pump				___	mL/h
Desmopressin	0.3 mcg/kg =	14 mcg		Give dose over 20–30 min			4 mcg/vial		
Dobutamine	Infusion		0.74		2.5–40 mcg/kg/ min	250 mg/ 125 mL	2000 mcg/mL	___	mL/h
				Take dose you want in mcg ÷ by drug index number = mL/h on pump					

(continues)

45 kg (continued)

DRUG	ORDERED AMOUNT	TOTAL DOSE TO GIVE	DRUG INDEX NUMBER	DIRECTIONS	INFUSION RANGE	DRUG MIXTURE	AMOUNT	DRUG/ mL	RUN AT	mL/h
Dopamine	Infusion		0.59		1–20 mcg/ kg/min	400 mg/ 250 mL	1600	mcg/mL	___	mL/h
	Take dose you want in mcg ÷ by drug index number = mL/h on pump									
Epinephrine	Infusion	1 mcg/min = 4 mL/h 2 mcg/min = 8 mL/h 3 mcg/min = 11 mL/h 4 mcg/min = 15 mL/h			1–4 mcg/min	4 mg/ 250 mL	16	mcg/mL		
		Ordered mcg dose/min ÷ mcg/mL × 60 min/h =							___	mL/h
Fenoldapam	Infusion		0.0149		0.01–1.6 mcg/ kg/min	10 mg/ 250 mL	40	mcg/mL	___	mL/h
	Take dose you want in mcg ÷ by drug index number = mL/h on pump									
Heparin	100 u/kg = 4500 u 200 u/kg = 9000 u 300 u/kg = 13,500 u 400 u/kg = 18,000 u									
Isoproterenol	Infusion				5 mcg/min	1 mg/ 250 mL	4	mcg/mL		
		Ordered mcg dose/min ÷ mcg/mL × 60 min/h =							75	mL/h
Lidocaine	Infusion	1 mg/min = 7.5 mL/h			1–4 mg/min	2 g/ 250 mL	8	mg/mL		
		Ordered mg/min ÷ mg/mL × 60 min/h =							___	mL/h
Nitroglycerin	Infusion	3 mcg/min = 1 mL/h			3–200 mcg/min	50 mg/ 250 mL	200	mcg/mL		
		Ordered mcg/min ÷ mcg/mL × 60 min/h =							___	mL/h
Nitroprusside	Infusion	6.7 mcg/min = 1 mL/h			5–300 mcg/min	100 mg/ 250 mL	400	mcg/mL		
		Ordered mcg/min ÷ mcg/mL × 60 min/h =							___	mL/h
Norepinephrine	Infusion	1 mcg/min = 4 mL/h 2 mcg/min = 8 mL/h 3 mcg/min = 11 mL/h 4 mcg/min = 15 mL/h 5 mcg/min = 19 mL/h			2–20 mcg/min	4 mg/ 250 mL	16	mcg/mL		
		Ordered mcg dose/min ÷ mcg/mL × 60 min/h =							___	mL/h
Phenylephrine	Infusion	1.3 mcg/min = 1 mL/h			10–200 mcg/min	20 mg/ 250 mL	80	mcg/mL		
		Ordered mcg/min ÷ mcg/mL × 60 min/h =							___	mL/h
Primacor	0.05 mg/kg = 2.25 mg			Give load over 10 min		40 mg/ 200 mL	0.2	mg/mL		
	mg to give ÷ mg/mL =	11 mL			11	mL × (60 min/h ÷ 10 min) =			67.5	mL/h × 10 min
	Infusion		0.074		0.5 mcg/ kg/min	40 mg/ 200 mL	200	mcg/mL	___	mL/h
	Take dose you want in mcg ÷ by drug index number = mL/h on pump									
Trimethaphan	Infusion				0.3–6 mg/min	500 mg/ 500 mL	1	mg/mL		
		Ordered mg/min ÷ mg/mL × 60 min/h =							___	mL/h
Vasopressin		0.02 u/min = 3 mL/h 0.04 u/min = 6 mL/h				40 u/ 100 mL	400	u/mL		

46 kg

DRUG	ORDERED AMOUNT	TOTAL DOSE TO GIVE	DRUG INDEX NUMBER	DIRECTIONS	INFUSION RANGE	DRUG MIXTURE	AMOUNT	DRUG/mL	RUN AT	mL/h
Aminophylline	5 mg/kg =	230 mg		Give mg/kg load over 20 min		500 mg/ 250 mL	2 mg/mL			
	mg to give ÷ mg/mL =	115 mL			115	mL × (60 min/h ÷ 20 min) =			345	mL/h × 20 min
	Infusion				0.5–1 mg/kg/h	500 mg/ 250 mL	2 mg/mL			
					mg dose ordered × kg ÷ mg/mL =				___	mL/h
Amiodarone	Loading dose			Load **150 mg** over 10 min		900 mg/ 500 mL	1.8 mg/mL	___		
				Ordered mg load dose (150 mg) ÷ mg/mL (1.8 mg/mL) = 83 mL to give × (60 min/h ÷ 10 min) = mL/h to set on pump					500	mL/h × 83 mL
	Infusion			Run at **1 mg/ min** × 6 h		900 mg/ 500 mL	1.8 mg/mL			
				Ordered mg dose (1 mg/min) ÷ mg/mL (1.8 mg/mL) ____ × 60 min/h mL/h to set on pump					33	mL/h × 6 h
	Infusion			Run at **0.5 mg/ min** × 18 h		900 mg/ 500 mL	1.8 mg/mL			
				Ordered mg dose (0.5 mg/min) ÷ mg/mL (1.8 mg/mL) = ____ × 60 min/h = mL/h to set on pump					17	mL/h × 18 h
Amrinone	0.75 mg/kg =	34.5 mg		Give mg/kg load over 10 min		300 mg/ 120 mL	2.5 mg/mL	___		
	mg to give ÷ mg/mL =	14 mL			13.8	mL × (60 min/h ÷ 10 min) =			82.8	mL/h × 10 min
	Infusion		0.90		5–10 mcg/ kg/min	300 mg/ 120 mL	2500 mcg/mL			
				Take dose you want in mcg ÷ by drug index number = mL/h on pump						
Brevibloc	Infusion		3.62		50–100 mcg/ kg/min	2.5 g/ 250 mL	10,000 mcg/mL	___	mL/h	
				Take dose you want in mcg ÷ by drug index number = mL/h on pump						
Cardene	Infusion		—		0.5–10 mg/h	25 mg 250 mL	0.1 mg/mL	___		
				Ordered mg dose ÷ mg/mL = mL/h to set on pump					___	mL/h
Cardizem	0.25 mg/kg =	11.5 mg		Give mg/kg load over 20 min		50 mg/ 100 mL	0.5 mg/mL	___		
	mg to give ÷ mg/mL =	23 mL			23	mL × (60 min/h ÷ 20 min) =			69	mL/h
	0.35 mg/kg =	16.1 mg		May repeat loading dose in 15 min			0.5 mg/mL	___		
	mg to give ÷ mg/mL =	32 mL			32.2	mL × (60 min/h ÷ 20 min) =			97	mL/h
	Infusion				5–15 mg/h				___	
				Ordered mg dose ÷ mg/mL = mL/h to set on pump					___	mL/h
Desmopressin	0.3 mcg/kg =	14 mcg		Give dose over 20–30 min			4 mcg/vial			
Dobutamine	Infusion		0.72		2.5–40 mcg/kg/ min	250 mg/ 125 mL	2000 mcg/mL			
				Take dose you want in mcg ÷ by drug index number = mL/h on pump						

(continues)

46 kg (continued)

DRUG	ORDERED AMOUNT	TOTAL DOSE TO GIVE	DRUG INDEX NUMBER	DIRECTIONS	INFUSION RANGE	DRUG MIXTURE	AMOUNT	DRUG/mL	RUN AT	mL/h
Dopamine	Infusion		0.58		1–20 mcg/kg/min	400 mg/250 mL	1600	mcg/mL		
			Take dose you want in mcg ÷ by drug index number = mL/h on pump							
Epinephrine	Infusion	1 mcg/min = 4 mL/h 2 mcg/min = 8 mL/h 3 mcg/min = 11 mL/h 4 mcg/min = 15 mL/h			1–4 mcg/min	4 mg/250 mL	16	mcg/mL		
				Ordered mcg dose/min ÷ mcg/mL × 60 min/h =					___	mL/h
Fenoldapam	Infusion		0.0146		0.01–1.6 mcg/kg/min	10 mg/250 mL	40	mcg/mL		
			Take dose you want in mcg ÷ by drug index number = mL/h on pump							
Heparin	100 u/kg = 4600 u 200 u/kg = 9200 u 300 u/kg = 13,800 u 400 u/kg = 18,400 u									
Isoproterenol	Infusion				5 mcg/min	1 mg/250 mL	4	mcg/mL		
				Ordered mcg dose/min ÷ mcg/mL × 60 min/h =					75	mL/h
Lidocaine	Infusion	1 mg/min = 7.5 mL/h			1–4 mg/min	2 g/250 mL	8	mg/mL	___	
				Ordered mg/min ÷ mg/mL × 60 min/h =					___	mL/h
Nitroglycerin	Infusion	3 mcg/min = 1 mL/h			3–200 mcg/min	50 mg/250 mL	200	mcg/mL	___	
				Ordered mcg/min ÷ mcg/mL × 60 min/h =					___	mL/h
Nitroprusside	Infusion	6.7 mcg/min = 1 mL/h			5–300 mcg/min	100 mg/250 mL	400	mcg/mL	___	
				Ordered mcg/min ÷ mcg/mL × 60 min/h =					___	mL/h
Norepinephrine	Infusion	1 mcg/min = 4 mL/h 2 mcg/min = 8 mL/h 3 mcg/min = 11 mL/h 4 mcg/min = 15 mL/h 5 mcg/min = 19 mL/h			2–20 mcg/min	4 mg/250 mL	16	mcg/mL		
				Ordered mcg dose/min ÷ mcg/mL × 60 min/h =					___	mL/h
Phenylephrine	Infusion	1.3 mcg/min = 1 mL/h			10–200 mcg/min	20 mg/250 mL	80	mcg/mL		
				Ordered mcg/min ÷ mcg/mL × 60 min/h =					___	mL/h
Primacor	0.05 mg/kg = 2.3 mg			Give load over 10 min		40 mg/200 mL	0.2	mg/mL		
	mg to give ÷ mg/mL = 12 mL				12	mL × (60 min/h ÷ 10 min) =			69	mL/h × 10 min
	Infusion		0.072391304		0.5 mcg/kg/min	40 mg/200 mL	200	mcg/mL	___	
			Take dose you want in mcg ÷ by drug index number = mL/h on pump							
Trimethaphan	Infusion		___		0.3–6 mg/min	500 mg/500 mL	1	mg/mL	___	
				Ordered mg/min ÷ mg/mL × 60 min/h =					___	mL/h
Vasopressin		0.02 u/min = 3 mL/h 0.04 u/min = 6 mL/h				40 u/100 mL	400	u/mL		

47 kg									
DRUG	**ORDERED AMOUNT**	**TOTAL DOSE TO GIVE**	**DRUG INDEX NUMBER**	**DIRECTIONS**	**INFUSION RANGE**	**DRUG MIXTURE**	**AMOUNT**	**DRUG/ mL**	**RUN AT** **mL/h**
Aminophylline	5 mg/kg = 235 mg			Give mg/kg load over 20 min		500 mg/ 250 mL	2 mg/mL	
	mg to give ÷ mg/mL = 118 mL				118	mL × (60 min/h ÷ 20 min) =		**352.5** mL/h × 20 min
	Infusion				0.5–1 mg/kg/h	500 mg/ 250 mL	2 mg/mL	
					mg dose ordered × kg ÷ mg/mL =			___ mL/h
Amiodarone	Loading dose			Load **150 mg** over 10 min		900 mg/ 500 mL	1.8 mg/mL	___
				Ordered mg load dose (150 mg) ÷ mg/mL (1.8 mg/mL) = 83 mL to give × (60 min/h ÷ 10 min) = mL/h to set on pump				**500** mL/h × 83 mL
	Infusion			Run at **1 mg/ min** × 6 h		900 mg/ 500 mL	1.8 mg/mL	
				Ordered mg dose (1 mg/min) ÷ mg/mL (1.8 mg/mL) = ___ × 60 min/h = mL/h to set on pump				**33** mL/h × 6 h
	Infusion			Run at **0.5 mg/ min** × 18 h		900 mg/ 500 mL	1.8 mg/mL	
				Ordered mg dose (0.5 mg/min) ÷ mg/mL (1.8 mg/mL) = ___ × 60 min/h = mL/h to set on pump				**17** mL/h × 18 h
Amrinone	0.75 mg/kg = 35.25 mg			Give mg/kg load over 10 min		300 mg/ 120 mL	2.5 mg/mL	___
	mg to give ÷ mg/mL = 14 mL				14.1	mL × (60 min/h ÷ 10 min) =		**84.6** mL/h × 10 min
	Infusion		0.89		5–10 mcg/ kg/min	300 mg/ 120 mL	2500 mcg/mL	___
				Take dose you want in mcg ÷ by drug index number = mL/h on pump				
Brevibloc	Infusion		3.54		50–100 mcg/ kg/min	2.5 g/ 250 mL	10,000 mcg/mL	___ mL/h
				Take dose you want in mcg ÷ by drug index number = mL/h on pump				
Cardene	Infusion		___		0.5–10 mg/h	25 mg 250 mL	0.1 mg/mL	___
				Ordered mg dose ÷ mg/mL = mL/h to set on pump				___ mL/h
Cardizem	0.25 mg/kg = 11.75 mg			Give mg/kg load over 20 min		50 mg/ 100 mL	0.5 mg/mL	___
	mg to give ÷ mg/mL = 24 mL				23.5	mL × (60 min/h ÷ 20 min) =		**71** mL/h
	0.35 mg/kg = 16.45 mg			May repeat loading dose in 15 min			0.5 mg/mL	___
	mg to give ÷ mg/mL = 33 mL				32.9	mL × (60 min/h ÷ 20 min) =		**99** mL/h
	Infusion				5–15 mg/h			___
				Ordered mg dose ÷ mg/mL = mL/h to set on pump				___ mL/h
Desmopressin	0.3 mcg/kg = 14 mcg			Give dose over 20–30 min			4 mcg/vial	
Dobutamine	Infusion		0.71		2.5–40 mcg/kg/ min	250 mg/ 125 mL	2000 mcg/mL	
				Take dose you want in mcg ÷ by drug index number = mL/h on pump				

(continues)

47 kg (continued)

DRUG	ORDERED AMOUNT	TOTAL DOSE TO GIVE	DRUG INDEX NUMBER	DIRECTIONS	INFUSION RANGE	DRUG MIXTURE	AMOUNT	DRUG/ mL	RUN AT	mL/h
Dopamine	Infusion		0.57		1–20 mcg/ kg/min	400 mg/ 250 mL	1600	mcg/mL		
					Take dose you want in mcg ÷ by drug index number = mL/h on pump					
Epinephrine	Infusion	1 mcg/min = 4 mL/h 2 mcg/min = 8 mL/h 3 mcg/min = 11 mL/h 4 mcg/min = 15 mL/h			1–4 mcg/min	4 mg/ 250 mL	16	mcg/mL		
					Ordered mcg dose/min ÷ mcg/mL × 60 min/h =				___	mL/h
Fenoldapam	Infusion		0.0143		0.01–1.6 mcg/ kg/min	10 mg/ 250 mL	40	mcg/mL		
					Take dose you want in mcg ÷ by drug index number = mL/h on pump					
Heparin	100 u/kg = 4700 u 200 u/kg = 9400 u 300 u/kg = 14,100 u 400 u/kg = 18,800 u									
Isoproterenol	Infusion				5 mcg/min	1 mg/ 250 mL	4	mcg/mL		
					Ordered mcg dose/min ÷ mcg/mL × 60 min/h =				75	mL/h
Lidocaine	Infusion	1 mg/min = 7.5 mL/h			1–4 mg/min	2 g/ 250 mL	8	mg/mL	___	
					Ordered mg/min ÷ mg/mL × 60 min/h =				___	mL/h
Nitroglycerin	Infusion	3 mcg/min = 1 mL/h			3–200 mcg/min	50 mg/ 250 mL	200	mcg/mL	___	
					Ordered mcg/min ÷ mcg/mL × 60 min/h =				___	mL/h
Nitroprusside	Infusion	6.7 mcg/min = 1 mL/h			5–300 mcg/min	100 mg/ 250 mL	400	mcg/mL	___	
					Ordered mcg/min ÷ mcg/mL × 60 min/h =				___	mL/h
Norepinephrine	Infusion	1 mcg/min = 4 mL/h 2 mcg/min = 8 mL/h 3 mcg/min = 11 mL/h 4 mcg/min = 15 mL/h 5 mcg/min = 19 mL/h			2–20 mcg/min	4 mg/ 250 mL	16	mcg/mL		
					Ordered mcg dose/min ÷ mcg/mL × 60 min/h =				___	mL/h
Phenylephrine	Infusion	1.3 mcg/min = 1 mL/h			10–200 mcg/min	20 mg/ 250 mL	80	mcg/mL		
					Ordered mcg/min ÷ mcg/mL × 60 min/h =				___	mL/h
Primacor	0.05 mg/kg = 2.35 mg			Give load over 10 min		40 mg/ 200 mL	0.2	mg/mL		
	mg to give ÷ mg/mL = 12 mL				12 mL × (60 min/h ÷ 10 min) =				70.5	mL/h × 10 min
	Infusion		0.070851064		0.5 mcg/ kg/min	40 mg/ 200 mL	200	mcg/mL	___	
					Take dose you want in mcg ÷ by drug index number = mL/h on pump					
Trimethaphan	Infusion	___			0.3–6 mg/min	500 mg/ 500 mL	1	mg/mL	___	
					Ordered mg/min ÷ mg/mL × 60 min/h =				___	mL/h
Vasopressin		0.02 u/min = 3 mL/h 0.04 u/min = 6 mL/h				40 u/ 100 mL	400	u/mL		

48　kg

DRUG	ORDERED AMOUNT	TOTAL DOSE TO GIVE	DRUG INDEX NUMBER	DIRECTIONS	INFUSION RANGE	DRUG MIXTURE	AMOUNT	DRUG/ mL	RUN AT	mL/h
Aminophylline	5　mg/kg =	240　mg		Give mg/kg load over 20 min		500 mg/ 250 mL	2　mg/mL		
	mg to give ÷ mg/mL =	120　mL			120	mL × (60 min/h ÷ 20 min) =			**360**	mL/h × 20 min
	Infusion				0.5–1 mg/kg/h	500 mg/ 250 mL	2　mg/mL		
					mg dose ordered × kg ÷ mg/mL =				____	mL/h
Amiodarone	Loading dose			Load **150 mg** over 10 min		900 mg/ 500 mL	1.8　mg/mL		____
				Ordered mg load dose (150 mg) ÷ mg/mL (1.8 mg/mL) = 83 mL to give × (60 min/h ÷ 10 min) = mL/h to set on pump					**500**	mL/h × 83 mL
	Infusion			Run at **1 mg/ min** × 6 h		900 mg/ 500 mL	1.8　mg/mL		
				Ordered mg dose (1 mg/min) ÷ mg/mL (1.8 mg/mL) = ____ × 60 min/h = mL/h to set on pump					**33**	mL/h × 6 h
	Infusion			Run at **0.5 mg/ min** × 18 h		900 mg/ 500 ml	1.8　mg/mL		
				Ordered mg dose (0.5 mg/min) ÷ mg/mL (1.8 mg/mL) = ____ × 60 min/h = mL/h to set on pump					**17**	mL/h × 18 h
Amrinone	0.75　mg/kg =	36　mg		Give mg/kg load over 10 min		300 mg/ 120 mL	2.5　mg/mL		____
	mg to give ÷ mg/mL =	14　mL			14.4	mL × (60 min/h ÷ 10 min) =			**86.4**	mL/h × 10 min
	Infusion		**0.87**		5–10 mcg/ kg/min	300 mg/ 120 mL	2500　mcg/mL		
				Take dose you want in mcg ÷ by drug index number = mL/h on pump					
Brevibloc	Infusion		**3.47**		50–100 mcg/ kg/min	2.5 g/ 250 mL	10,000　mcg/mL		____ mL/h
				Take dose you want in mcg ÷ by drug index number = mL/h on pump					
Cardene	Infusion		____		0.5–10 mg/h	25 mg 250 mL	0.1　mg/mL		____
				Ordered mg dose ÷ mg/mL = mL/h to set on pump					____	mL/h
Cardizem	0.25　mg/kg =	12　mg		Give mg/kg load over 20 min		50 mg/ 100 mL	0.5　mg/mL		____
	mg to give ÷ mg/mL =	24　mL			24	mL × (60 min/h ÷ 20 min) =			**72**	mL/h
	0.35　mg/kg =	16.8　mg		May repeat loading dose in 15 min			0.5　mg/mL		
	mg to give ÷ mg/mL =	34　mL			33.6	mL × (60 min/h ÷ 20 min) =			**101**	mL/h
	Infusion				5–15 mg/h				____
				Ordered mg dose ÷ mg/mL = mL/h to set on pump					____	mL/h
Desmopressin	0.3　mcg/kg =	14　mcg		Give dose over 20–30 min			4　mcg/vial		
Dobutamine	Infusion		**0.69**		2.5–40 mcg/kg/ min	250 mg/ 125 mL	2000　mcg/mL		
				Take dose you want in mcg ÷ by drug index number = mL/h on pump					

(continues)

48 kg (continued)

DRUG	ORDERED AMOUNT	TOTAL DOSE TO GIVE	DRUG INDEX NUMBER	DIRECTIONS	INFUSION RANGE	DRUG MIXTURE	AMOUNT	DRUG/mL	RUN AT	mL/h
Dopamine	Infusion		0.56		1–20 mcg/ kg/min	400 mg/ 250 mL	1600	mcg/mL		
		Take dose you want in mcg ÷ by drug index number = mL/h on pump								
Epinephrine	Infusion	1 mcg/min = 4 mL/h 2 mcg/min = 8 mL/h 3 mcg/min = 11 mL/h 4 mcg/min = 15 mL/h			1–4 mcg/min	4 mg/ 250 mL	16	mcg/mL		
		Ordered mcg dose/min ÷ mcg/mL × 60 min/h =							___	mL/h
Fenoldapam	Infusion		0.0140		0.01–1.6 mcg/ kg/min	10 mg/ 250 mL	40	mcg/mL		
		Take dose you want in mcg ÷ by drug index number = mL/h on pump								
Heparin	100 u/kg = 4800 u 200 u/kg = 9600 u 300 u/kg = 14,400 u 400 u/kg = 19,200 u									
Isoproterenol	Infusion				5 mcg/min	1 mg/ 250 mL	4	mcg/mL		
		Ordered mcg dose/min ÷ mcg/mL × 60 min/h =							75	mL/h
Lidocaine	Infusion	1 mg/min = 7.5 mL/h			1–4 mg/min	2 g/ 250 mL	8	mg/mL	___	
		Ordered mg/min ÷ mg/mL × 60 min/h =							___	mL/h
Nitroglycerin	Infusion	3 mcg/min = 1 mL/h			3–200 mcg/min	50 mg/ 250 mL	200	mcg/mL	___	
		Ordered mcg/min ÷ mcg/mL × 60 min/h =							___	mL/h
Nitroprusside	Infusion	6.7 mcg/min = 1 mL/h			5–300 mcg/min	100 mg/ 250 mL	400	mcg/mL	___	
		Ordered mcg/min ÷ mcg/mL × 60 min/h =							___	mL/h
Norepinephrine	Infusion	1 mcg/min = 4 mL/h 2 mcg/min = 8 mL/h 3 mcg/min = 11 mL/h 4 mcg/min = 15 mL/h 5 mcg/min = 19 mL/h			2–20 mcg/min	4 mg/ 250 mL	16	mcg/mL		
		Ordered mcg dose/min ÷ mcg/mL × 60 min/h =							___	mL/h
Phenylephrine	Infusion	1.3 mcg/min = 1 mL/h			10–200 mcg/min	20 mg/ 250 mL	80	mcg/mL		
		Ordered mcg/min ÷ mcg/mL × 60 min/h =							___	mL/h
Primacor	0.05 mg/kg = 2.4 mg			Give load over 10 min		40 mg/ 200 mL	0.2	mg/mL		
	mg to give ÷ mg/mL = 12 mL				12	mL × (60 min/h ÷ 10 min) =			72	mL/h × 10 min
	Infusion		0.069375		0.5 mcg/ kg/min	40 mg/ 200 mL	200	mcg/mL	___	
		Take dose you want in mcg ÷ by drug index number = mL/h on pump								
Trimethaphan	Infusion		___		0.3–6 mg/min	500 mg/ 500 mL	1	mg/mL	___	
		Ordered mg/min ÷ mg/mL × 60 min/h =							___	mL/h
Vasopressin		0.02 u/min = 3 mL/h 0.04 u/min = 6 mL/h				40 u/ 100 mL	400	u/mL		

49 kg										
DRUG	**ORDERED AMOUNT**	**TOTAL DOSE TO GIVE**	**DRUG INDEX NUMBER**	**DIRECTIONS**	**INFUSION RANGE**	**DRUG MIXTURE**	**AMOUNT**	**DRUG/ mL**	**RUN AT**	**mL/h**
Aminophylline	5 mg/kg = 245 mg			Give mg/kg load over 20 min		500 mg/ 250 mL	2 mg/mL			
	mg to give ÷ mg/mL = 123 mL				123	mL × (60 min/h ÷ 20 min) =			367.5	mL/h × 20 min
	Infusion				0.5–1 mg/kg/h	500 mg/ 250 mL	2 mg/mL			
						mg dose ordered × kg ÷ mg/mL =			___	mL/h
Amiodarone	Loading dose			Load **150 mg** over 10 min		900 mg/ 500 mL	1.8 mg/mL		___	
				Ordered mg load dose (150 mg) ÷ mg/mL (1.8 mg/mL) = 83 mL to give × (60 min/h ÷ 10 min) = mL/h to set on pump					500	mL/h × 83 mL
	Infusion			Run at **1 mg/ min** × 6 h		900 mg/ 500 mL	1.8 mg/mL			
				Ordered mg dose (1 mg/min) ÷ mg/mL (1.8 mg/ml) = ___ × 60 min/h = mL/h to set on pump					33	mL/h × 6 h
	Infusion			Run at **0.5 mg/ min** × 18 h		900 mg/ 500 mL	1.8 mg/mL			
				Ordered mg dose (0.5 mg/min) ÷ mg/mL (1.8 mg/mL) = ___ × 60 min/h = mL/h to set on pump					17	mL/h × 18 h
Amrinone	0.75 mg/kg = 36.75 mg			Give mg/kg load over 10 min		300 mg/ 120 mL	2.5 mg/mL		___	
	mg to give ÷ mg/mL = 15 mL				14.7	mL × (60 min/h ÷ 10 min) =			88.2	mL/h × 10 min
	Infusion		0.85		5–10 mcg/ kg/min	300 mg/ 120 mL	2500 mcg/mL		___	
				Take dose you want in mcg ÷ by drug index number = mL/h on pump						
Brevibloc	Infusion		3.40		50–100 mcg/ kg/min	2.5 g/ 250 mL	10,000 mcg/mL		___	mL/h
				Take dose you want in mcg ÷ by drug index number = mL/h on pump						
Cardene	Infusion		___		0.5–10 mg/h	25 mg 250 mL	0.1 mg/mL		___	
				Ordered mg dose ÷ mg/mL = mL/h to set on pump					___	mL/h
Cardizem	0.25 mg/kg = 12.25 mg			Give mg/kg load over 20 min		50 mg/ 100 mL	0.5 mg/mL			
	mg to give ÷ mg/mL = 25 mL				24.5	mL × (60 min/h ÷ 20 min) =			74	mL/h
	0.35 mg/kg = 17.15 mg			May repeat loading dose in 15 min			0.5 mg/mL			
	mg to give ÷ mg/mL = 34 mL				34.3	mL × (60 min/h ÷ 20 min) =			103	mL/h
	Infusion				5–15 mg/h				___	
				Ordered mg dose ÷ mg/mL = mL/h to set on pump					___	mL/h
Desmopressin	0.3 mcg/kg = 15 mcg			Give dose over 20–30 min			4 mcg/vial			
Dobutamine	Infusion		0.68		2.5–40 mcg/kg/ min	250 mg/ 125 mL	2000 mcg/mL			
				Take dose you want in mcg ÷ by drug index number = mL/h on pump						

(continues)

49 kg (continued)

DRUG	ORDERED AMOUNT		TOTAL DOSE TO GIVE		DRUG INDEX NUMBER	DIRECTIONS	INFUSION RANGE	DRUG MIXTURE	AMOUNT	DRUG/ mL	RUN AT	mL/h
Dopamine	Infusion				0.54		1–20 mcg/ kg/min	400 mg/ 250 mL	1600	mcg/mL		
	Take dose you want in mcg ÷ by drug index number = mL/h on pump											
Epinephrine	Infusion		1 mcg/min = 4 mL/h 2 mcg/min = 8 mL/h 3 mcg/min = 11 mL/h 4 mcg/min = 15 mL/h				1–4 mcg/min	4 mg/ 250 mL	16	mcg/mL		
			Ordered mcg dose/min ÷ mcg/mL × 60 min/h =								___	mL/h
Fenoldapam	Infusion				0.0137		0.01–1.6 mcg/ kg/min	10 mg/ 250 mL	40	mcg/mL		
	Take dose you want in mcg ÷ by drug index number = mL/h on pump											
Heparin	100 u/kg = 200 u/kg = 300 u/kg = 400 u/kg =	4900 u 9800 u 14,700 u 19,600 u										
Isoproterenol	Infusion						5 mcg/min	1 mg/ 250 mL	4	mcg/mL		
			Ordered mcg dose/min ÷ mcg/mL × 60 min/h =								75	mL/h
Lidocaine	Infusion		1 mg/min = 7.5 mL/h				1–4 mg/min	2 g/ 250 mL	8	mg/mL	___	
			Ordered mg/min ÷ mg/mL × 60 min/h =								___	mL/h
Nitroglycerin	Infusion		3 mcg/min = 1 mL/h				3–200 mcg/min	50 mg/ 250 mL	200	mcg/mL	___	
			Ordered mcg/min ÷ mcg/mL × 60 min/h =								___	mL/h
Nitroprusside	Infusion		6.7 mcg/min = 1 mL/h				5–300 mcg/min	100 mg/ 250 mL	400	mcg/mL	___	
			Ordered mcg/min ÷ mcg/mL × 60 min/h =								___	mL/h
Norepinephrine	Infusion		1 mcg/min = 4 mL/h 2 mcg/min = 8 mL/h 3 mcg/min = 11 mL/h 4 mcg/min = 15 mL/h 5 mcg/min = 19 mL/h				2–20 mcg/min	4 mg/ 250 mL	16	mcg/mL		
			Ordered mcg dose/min ÷ mcg/mL × 60 min/h =								___	mL/h
Phenylephrine	Infusion		1.3 mcg/min = 1 mL/h				10–200 mcg/min	20 mg/ 250 mL	80	mcg/mL		
			Ordered mcg/min ÷ mcg/mL × 60 min/h =								___	mL/h
Primacor	0.05 mg/kg =	2.45 mg				Give load over 10 min		40 mg/ 200 mL	0.2	mg/mL		
	mg to give ÷ mg/mL =	12 mL							12 mL × (60 min/h ÷ 10 min) =		73.5	mL/h × 10 min
	Infusion				0.067959184		0.5 mcg/ kg/min	40 mg/ 200 mL	200	mcg/mL	___	
	Take dose you want in mcg ÷ by drug index number = mL/h on pump											
Trimethaphan	Infusion				—		0.3–6 mg/min	500 mg/ 500 mL	1	mg/mL	___	
			Ordered mg/min ÷ mg/mL × 60 min/h =								___	mL/h
Vasopressin			0.02 u/min = 3 mL/h 0.04 u/min = 6 mL/h					40 u/ 100 mL	400	u/mL		

50 kg

DRUG	ORDERED AMOUNT	TOTAL DOSE TO GIVE	DRUG INDEX NUMBER	DIRECTIONS	INFUSION RANGE	DRUG MIXTURE	AMOUNT	DRUG/mL	RUN AT	mL/h
Aminophylline	5 mg/kg =	**250** mg		Give mg/kg load over 20 min		500 mg/ 250 mL	2 mg/mL			
	mg to give ÷ mg/mL =	**125** mL			125	mL × (60 min/h ÷ 20 min) =			**375**	mL/h × 20 min
	Infusion				0.5–1 mg/kg/h	500 mg/ 250 mL	2 mg/mL			
					mg dose ordered × kg ÷ mg/mL =				___	mL/h
Amiodarone	Loading dose			Load **150 mg** over 10 min		900 mg/ 500 mL	1.8 mg/mL		—	
				Ordered mg load dose (150 mg) ÷ mg/mL (1.8 mg/mL) = 83 mL to give × (60 min/h ÷ 10 min) = mL/h to set on pump					**500**	mL/h × 83 mL
	Infusion			Run at **1 mg/ min** × 6 h		900 mg/ 500 mL	1.8 mg/mL			
				Ordered mg dose (1 mg/min) ÷ mg/mL (1.8 mg/mL) = ___ × 60 min/h = mL/h to set on pump					**33**	mL/h × 6 h
	Infusion			Run at **0.5 mg/ min** × 18 h		900 mg/ 500 mL	1.0 mg/mL			
				Ordered mg dose (0.5 mg/min) ÷ mg/mL (1.8 mg/mL) = ___ × 60 min/h = mL/h to set on pump					**17**	mL/h × 18 h
Amrinone	0.75 mg/kg =	**37.5** mg		Give mg/kg load over 10 min		300 mg/ 120 mL	2.5 mg/mL		—	
	mg to give ÷ mg/mL =	**15** mL			15	mL × (60 min/h ÷ 10 min) =			**90**	mL/h × 10 min
	Infusion		**0.83**		5–10 mcg/ kg/min	300 mg/ 120 mL	2500 mcg/mL		—	
				Take dose you want in mcg ÷ by drug index number = mL/h on pump						
Brevibloc	Infusion		**3.33**		50–100 mcg/ kg/min	2.5 g/ 250 mL	10,000 mcg/mL		___	mL/h
				Take dose you want in mcg ÷ by drug index number = mL/h on pump						
Cardene	Infusion			—	0.5–10 mg/h	25 mg 250 mL	0.1 mg/mL		—	
				Ordered mg dose ÷ mg/mL = mL/h to set on pump					___	mL/h
Cardizem	0.25 mg/kg =	**12.5** mg		Give mg/kg load over 20 min		50 mg/ 100 mL	0.5 mg/mL		—	
	mg to give ÷ mg/mL =	**25** mL			25	mL × (60 min/h ÷ 20 min) =			**75**	mL/h
	0.35 mg/kg =	**17.5** mg		May repeat loading dose in 15 min			0.5 mg/mL		—	
	mg to give ÷ mg/mL =	**35** mL			35	mL × (60 min/h ÷ 20 min) =			**105**	mL/h
	Infusion				5–15 mg/h				—	
				Ordered mg dose ÷ mg/mL = mL/h to set on pump					___	mL/h
Desmopressin	0.3 mcg/kg =	**15** mcg		Give dose over 20–30 min			4 mcg/vial			
Dobutamine	Infusion		**0.67**		2.5–40 mcg/kg/ min	250 mg/ 125 mL	2000 mcg/mL			
				Take dose you want in mcg ÷ by drug index number = mL/h on pump						

(continues)

50 kg (continued)

DRUG	ORDERED AMOUNT	TOTAL DOSE TO GIVE	DRUG INDEX NUMBER	DIRECTIONS	INFUSION RANGE	DRUG MIXTURE	AMOUNT	DRUG/ mL	RUN AT	mL/h
Dopamine	Infusion		0.53		1–20 mcg/ kg/min	400 mg/ 250 mL	1600	mcg/mL		
			Take dose you want in mcg ÷ by drug index number = mL/h on pump							
Epinephrine	Infusion	1 mcg/min = 4 mL/h 2 mcg/min = 8 mL/h 3 mcg/min = 11 mL/h 4 mcg/min = 15 mL/h			1–4 mcg/min	4 mg/ 250 mL	16	mcg/mL		
				Ordered mcg dose/min ÷ mcg/mL × 60 min/h =					___	mL/h
Fenoldapam	Infusion		0.0134		0.01–1.6 mcg/ kg/min	10 mg/ 250 mL	40	mcg/mL		
			Take dose you want in mcg ÷ by drug index number = mL/h on pump							
Heparin	100 u/kg = 5000 u 200 u/kg = 10,000 u 300 u/kg = 15,000 u 400 u/kg = 20,000 u									
Isoproterenol	Infusion				5 mcg/min	1 mg/ 250 mL	4	mcg/mL		
				Ordered mcg dose/min ÷ mcg/mL × 60 min/h =					75	mL/h
Lidocaine	Infusion	1 mg/min = 7.5 mL/h			1–4 mg/min	2 g/ 250 mL	8	mg/mL	___	
				Ordered mg/min ÷ mg/mL × 60 min/h =					___	mL/h
Nitroglycerin	Infusion	3 mcg/min = 1 mL/h			3–200 mcg/min	50 mg/ 250 mL	200	mcg/mL	___	
				Ordered mcg/min ÷ mcg/mL × 60 min/h =					___	mL/h
Nitroprusside	Infusion	6.7 mcg/min = 1 mL/h			5–300 mcg/min	100 mg/ 250 mL	400	mcg/mL	___	
				Ordered mcg/min ÷ mcg/mL × 60 min/h =					___	mL/h
Norepinephrine	Infusion	1 mcg/min = 4 mL/h 2 mcg/min = 8 mL/h 3 mcg/min = 11 mL/h 4 mcg/min = 15 mL/h 5 mcg/min = 19 mL/h			2–20 mcg/min	4 mg/ 250 mL	16	mcg/mL		
				Ordered mcg dose/min ÷ mcg/mL × 60 min/h =					___	mL/h
Phenylephrine	Infusion	1.3 mcg/min = 1 mL/h			10–200 mcg/min	20 mg/ 250 mL	80	mcg/mL		
				Ordered mcg/min ÷ mcg/mL × 60 min/h =					___	mL/h
Primacor	0.05 mg/kg = 2.5 mg			Give load over 10 min		40 mg/ 200 mL	0.2	mg/mL		
	mg to give ÷ mg/mL = 13 mL				13	mL × (60 min/h ÷ 10 min) =			75	mL/h × 10 min
	Infusion		0.0666		0.5 mcg/ kg/min	40 mg/ 200 mL	200	mcg/mL	___	
			Take dose you want in mcg ÷ by drug index number = mL/h on pump							
Trimethaphan	Infusion		—		0.3–6 mg/min	500 mg/ 500 mL	1	mg/mL	___	
				Ordered mg/min ÷ mg/mL × 60 min/h =					___	mL/h
Vasopressin		0.02 u/min = 3 mL/h 0.04 u/min = 6 mL/h				40 u/ 100 mL	400	u/mL		

51 kg

DRUG	ORDERED AMOUNT	TOTAL DOSE TO GIVE	DRUG INDEX NUMBER	DIRECTIONS	INFUSION RANGE	DRUG MIXTURE	AMOUNT	DRUG/mL	RUN AT	mL/h
Aminophylline	5 mg/kg =	255 mg		Give mg/kg load over 20 min		500 mg/ 250 mL	2 mg/mL			
	mg to give ÷ mg/mL =	128 mL			128	mL × (60 min/h ÷ 20 min) =			382.5	mL/h × 20 min
	Infusion				0.5–1 mg/kg/h	500 mg/ 250 mL	2 mg/mL			
					mg dose ordered × kg ÷ mg/mL =				___	mL/h
Amiodarone	Loading dose			Load **150 mg** over 10 min		900 mg/ 500 mL	1.8 mg/mL		___	
				Ordered mg load dose (150 mg) ÷ mg/mL (1.8 mg/mL) = 83 mL to give × (60 min/h ÷ 10 min) = mL/h to set on pump					500	mL/h × 83 mL
	Infusion			Run at **1 mg/ min** × 6 h		900 mg/ 500 mL	1.8 mg/mL			
				Ordered mg dose (1 mg/min) ÷ mg/ml (1.8 mg/ml) = ___ × 60 min/h = mL/h to set on pump					33	mL/h × 6 h
	Infusion			Run at **0.5 mg/ min** × 18 h		900 mg/ 500 mL	1.8 mg/mL			
				Ordered mg dose (0.5 mg/min) ÷ mg/mL (1.8 mg/mL) = ___ × 60 min/h = mL/h to set on pump					17	mL/h × 18 h
Amrinone	0.75 mg/kg =	38.25 mg		Give mg/kg load over 10 min		300 mg/ 120 mL	2.5 mg/mL		___	
	mg to give ÷ mg/mL =	15 mL			15.3	mL × (60 min/h ÷ 10 min) =			91.8	mL/h × 10 min
	Infusion		0.82		5–10 mcg/ kg/min	300 mg/ 120 mL	2500 mcg/mL		___	
				Take dose you want in mcg ÷ by drug index number = mL/h on pump						
Brevibloc	Infusion		3.27		50–100 mcg/ kg/min	2.5 g/ 250 mL	10,000 mcg/mL		___	mL/h
				Take dose you want in mcg ÷ by drug index number = mL/h on pump						
Cardene	Infusion		—		0.5–10 mg/h	25 mg 250 mL	0.1 mg/mL		___	
				Ordered mg dose ÷ mg/mL = mL/h to set on pump					___	mL/h
Cardizem	0.25 mg/kg =	12.75 mg		Give mg/kg load over 20 min		50 mg/ 100 mL	0.5 mg/mL		___	
	mg to give ÷ mg/mL =	26 mL			25.5	mL × (60 min/h ÷ 20 min) =			77	mL/h
	0.35 mg/kg =	17.85 mg		May repeat loading dose in 15 min			0.5 mg/mL		___	
	mg to give ÷ mg/mL =	36 mL			35.7	mL × (60 min/h ÷ 20 min) =			107	mL/h
	Infusion				5–15 mg/h				___	
				Ordered mg dose ÷ mg/mL = mL/h to set on pump					___	mL/h
Desmopressin	0.3 mcg/kg =	15 mcg		Give dose over 20–30 min			4 mcg/vial			
Dobutamine	Infusion		0.65		2.5–40 mcg/kg/ min	250 mg/ 125 mL	2000 mcg/mL			
				Take dose you want in mcg ÷ by drug index number = mL/h on pump						

(continues)

51 kg (continued)

DRUG	ORDERED AMOUNT	TOTAL DOSE TO GIVE	DRUG INDEX NUMBER	DIRECTIONS	INFUSION RANGE	DRUG MIXTURE	AMOUNT	DRUG/ mL	RUN AT	mL/h
Dopamine	Infusion		0.52		1–20 mcg/ kg/min	400 mg/ 250 mL	1600	mcg/mL		
			Take dose you want in mcg ÷ by drug index number = mL/h on pump							
Epinephrine	Infusion	1 mcg/min = 4 mL/h 2 mcg/min = 8 mL/h 3 mcg/min = 11 mL/h 4 mcg/min = 15 mL/h			1–4 mcg/min	4 mg/ 250 mL	16	mcg/mL		
				Ordered mcg dose/min ÷ mcg/mL × 60 min/h =						___ mL/h
Fenoldapam	Infusion		0.0131		0.01–1.6 mcg/ kg/min	10 mg/ 250 mL	40	mcg/mL		
			Take dose you want in mcg ÷ by drug index number = mL/h on pump							
Heparin	100 u/kg = 5100 u 200 u/kg = 10,200 u 300 u/kg = 15,300 u 400 u/kg = 20,400 u									
Isoproterenol	Infusion				5 mcg/min	1 mg/ 250 mL	4	mcg/mL		
				Ordered mcg dose/min ÷ mcg/mL × 60 min/h =					75	mL/h
Lidocaine	Infusion	1 mg/min = 7.5 mL/h			1–4 mg/min	2 g/ 250 mL	8	mg/mL		___
				Ordered mg/min ÷ mg/mL × 60 min/h =						___ mL/h
Nitroglycerin	Infusion	3 mcg/min = 1 mL/h			3–200 mcg/min	50 mg/ 250 mL	200	mcg/mL		___
				Ordered mcg/min ÷ mcg/mL × 60 min/h =						___ mL/h
Nitroprusside	Infusion	6.7 mcg/min = 1 mL/h			5–300 mcg/min	100 mg/ 250 mL	400	mcg/mL		___
				Ordered mcg/min ÷ mcg/mL × 60 min/h =						___ mL/h
Norepinephrine	Infusion	1 mcg/min = 4 mL/h 2 mcg/min = 8 mL/h 3 mcg/min = 11 mL/h 4 mcg/min = 15 mL/h 5 mcg/min = 19 mL/h			2–20 mcg/min	4 mg/ 250 mL	16	mcg/mL		
				Ordered mcg dose/min ÷ mcg/mL × 60 min/h =						___ mL/h
Phenylephrine	Infusion	1.3 mcg/min = 1 mL/h			10–200 mcg/min	20 mg/ 250 mL	80	mcg/mL		
				Ordered mcg/min ÷ mcg/mL × 60 min/h =						___ mL/h
Primacor	0.05 mg/kg = 2.55 mg			Give load over 10 min		40 mg/ 200 mL	0.2	mg/mL		
	mg to give ÷ mg/mL = 13 mL				13 mL × (60 min/h ÷ 10 min) =				76.5	mL/h × 10 min
	Infusion		0.065294118		0.5 mcg/ kg/min	40 mg/ 200 mL	200	mcg/mL		___
			Take dose you want in mcg ÷ by drug index number = mL/h on pump							
Trimethaphan	Infusion		___		0.3–6 mg/min	500 mg/ 500 mL	1	mg/mL		___
				Ordered mg/min ÷ mg/mL × 60 min/h =						___ mL/h
Vasopressin		0.02 u/min = 3 mL/h 0.04 u/min = 6 mL/h				40 u/ 100 mL	400	u/mL		

52　kg

DRUG	ORDERED AMOUNT	TOTAL DOSE TO GIVE	DRUG INDEX NUMBER	DIRECTIONS	INFUSION RANGE	DRUG MIXTURE	AMOUNT DRUG/mL	RUN AT mL/h
Aminophylline	5　mg/kg =	260　mg		Give mg/kg load over 20 min		500 mg/250 mL	2　mg/mL	
	mg to give ÷ mg/mL =	130　mL			130	mL × (60 min/h ÷ 20 min) =		**390** mL/h × 20 min
	Infusion				0.5–1 mg/kg/h	500 mg/250 mL	2　mg/mL	
				mg dose ordered × kg ÷ mg/mL =				___ mL/h
Amiodarone	Loading dose			Load **150 mg** over 10 min		900 mg/500 mL	1.8　mg/mL	___
				Ordered mg load dose (150 mg) ÷ mg/mL (1.8 mg/mL) = 83 mL to give × (60 min/h ÷ 10 min) = mL/h to set on pump				**500** mL/h × 83 mL
	Infusion			Run at **1 mg/ min** × 6 h		900 mg/500 mL	1.8　mg/mL	
				Ordered mg dose (1 mg/min) ÷ mg/mL (1.8 mg/mL) = ___ × 60 min/h = mL/h to set on pump				**33** mL/h × 6 h
	Infusion			Run at **0.5 mg/ min** × 18 h		900 mg/500 mL	1.8　mg/mL	
				Ordered mg dose (0.5 mg/min) ÷ mg/mL (1.8 mg/mL) = ___ × 60 min/h = mL/h to set on pump				**17** mL/h × 18 h
Amrinone	0.75　mg/kg =	39　mg		Give mg/kg load over 10 min		300 mg/120 mL	2.5　mg/mL	___
	mg to give ÷ mg/mL =	16　mL			15.6	mL × (60 min/h ÷ 10 min) =		**93.6** mL/h × 10 min
	Infusion		0.80		5–10 mcg/kg/min	300 mg/120 mL	2500　mcg/mL	___
				Take dose you want in mcg ÷ by drug index number = mL/h on pump				
Brevibloc	Infusion		3.20		50–100 mcg/kg/min	2.5 g/250 mL	10,000　mcg/mL	___ mL/h
				Take dose you want in mcg ÷ by drug index number = mL/h on pump				
Cardene	Infusion		—		0.5–10 mg/h	25 mg/250 mL	0.1　mg/mL	___
				Ordered mg dose ÷ mg/mL = mL/h to set on pump				___ mL/h
Cardizem	0.25　mg/kg =	13　mg		Give mg/kg load over 20 min		50 mg/100 mL	0.5　mg/mL	___
	mg to give ÷ mg/mL =	26　mL			26	mL × (60 min/h ÷ 20 min) =		**78** mL/h
	0.35　mg/kg =	18.2　mg		May repeat loading dose in 15 min			0.5　mg/mL	___
	mg to give ÷ mg/mL =	36　mL			36.4	mL × (60 min/h ÷ 20 min) =		**109** mL/h
	Infusion				5–15 mg/h			___
				Ordered mg dose ÷ mg/mL = mL/h to set on pump				___ mL/h
Desmopressin	0.3　mcg/kg =	16　mcg		Give dose over 20–30 min			4　mcg/vial	
Dobutamine	Infusion		0.64		2.5–40 mcg/kg/min	250 mg/125 mL	2000　mcg/mL	
				Take dose you want in mcg ÷ by drug index number = mL/h on pump				

(continues)

52 kg (continued)

DRUG	ORDERED AMOUNT		TOTAL DOSE TO GIVE		DRUG INDEX NUMBER	DIRECTIONS	INFUSION RANGE	DRUG MIXTURE	AMOUNT	DRUG/ mL	RUN AT	mL/h
Dopamine	Infusion				0.51		1–20 mcg/ kg/min	400 mg/ 250 mL	1600	mcg/mL		
						Take dose you want in mcg ÷ by drug index number = mL/h on pump						
Epinephrine	Infusion		1 mcg/min = 4 mL/h 2 mcg/min = 8 mL/h 3 mcg/min = 11 mL/h 4 mcg/min = 15 mL/h				1–4 mcg/min	4 mg/ 250 mL	16	mcg/mL		
							Ordered mcg dose/min ÷ mcg/mL × 60 min/h =				___	mL/h
Fenoldapam	Infusion				0.0129		0.01–1.6 mcg/ kg/min	10 mg/ 250 mL	40	mcg/mL		
						Take dose you want in mcg ÷ by drug index number = mL/h on pump						
Heparin	100 u/kg = 200 u/kg = 300 u/kg = 400 u/kg =	5200 u 10,400 u 15,600 u 20,000 u										
Isoproterenol	Infusion						5 mcg/min	1 mg/ 250 mL	4	mcg/mL		
							Ordered mcg dose/min ÷ mcg/mL × 60 min/h =				75	mL/h
Lidocaine	Infusion		1 mg/min = 7.5 mL/h				1–4 mg/min	2 g/ 250 mL	8	mg/mL	___	
							Ordered mg/min ÷ mg/mL × 60 min/h =				___	mL/h
Nitroglycerin	Infusion		3 mcg/min = 1 mL/h				3–200 mcg/min	50 mg/ 250 mL	200	mcg/mL	___	
							Ordered mcg/min ÷ mcg/mL × 60 min/h =				___	mL/h
Nitroprusside	Infusion		6.7 mcg/min = 1 mL/h				5–300 mcg/min	100 mg/ 250 mL	400	mcg/mL	___	
							Ordered mcg/min ÷ mcg/mL × 60 min/h =				___	mL/h
Norepinephrine	Infusion		1 mcg/min = 4 mL/h 2 mcg/min = 8 mL/h 3 mcg/min = 11 mL/h 4 mcg/min = 15 mL/h 5 mcg/min = 19 mL/h				2–20 mcg/min	4 mg/ 250 mL	16	mcg/mL		
							Ordered mcg dose/min ÷ mcg/mL × 60 min/h =				___	mL/h
Phenylephrine	Infusion		1.3 mcg/min = 1 mL/h				10–200 mcg/min	20 mg/ 250 mL	80	mcg/mL		
							Ordered mcg/min ÷ mcg/mL × 60 min/h =				___	mL/h
Primacor	0.05 mg/kg =	2.6 mg				Give load over 10 min		40 mg/ 200 mL	0.2	mg/mL		
	mg to give ÷ mg/mL =	13 mL					13	mL × (60 min/h ÷ 10 min) =			78	mL/h × 10 min
	Infusion				0.064038462		0.5 mcg/ kg/min	40 mg/ 200 mL	200	mcg/mL	___	
						Take dose you want in mcg ÷ by drug index number = mL/h on pump						
Trimethaphan	Infusion		___				0.3–6 mg/min	500 mg/ 500 mL	1	mg/mL	___	
							Ordered mg/min ÷ mg/mL × 60 min/h =				___	mL/h
Vasopressin			0.02 u/min = 3 mL/h 0.04 u/min = 6 mL/h					40 u/ 100 mL	400	u/mL		

53 kg

DRUG	ORDERED AMOUNT	TOTAL DOSE TO GIVE	DRUG INDEX NUMBER	DIRECTIONS	INFUSION RANGE	DRUG MIXTURE	AMOUNT	DRUG/ mL	RUN AT	mL/h
Aminophylline	5 mg/kg =	**265 mg**		Give mg/kg load over 20 min		500 mg/ 250 mL		2 mg/mL		
	mg to give ÷ mg/mL =	**133 mL**					**133** mL × (60 min/h ÷ 20 min) =		<u>397.5</u>	mL/h × 20 min
	Infusion				0.5–1 mg/kg/h	500 mg/ 250 mL		2 mg/mL		
						mg dose ordered × kg ÷ mg/mL =			___	mL/h
Amiodarone	Loading dose			Load **150 mg** over 10 min		900 mg/ 500 mL		1.8 mg/mL	—	
				Ordered mg load dose (150 mg) ÷ mg/mL (1.8 mg/mL) = 83 mL to give × (60 min/h ÷ 10 min) = mL/h to set on pump					<u>500</u>	mL/h × 83 mL
	Infusion			Run at **1 mg/ min** × 6 h		900 mg/ 500 mL		1.8 mg/mL		
				Ordered mg dose (1 mg/min) ÷ mg/mL (1.0 mg/mL) = ___ × (60 min/h) = mL/h to set on pump					<u>33</u>	mL/h × 6 h
	Infusion			Run at **0.5 mg/ min** × 18 h		900 mg/ 500 mL		1.0 mg/mL		
				Ordered mg dose (0.5 mg/min) ÷ mg/mL (1.8 mg/mL) = ___ × 60 min/h = mL/h to set on pump					<u>17</u>	mL/h × 18 h
Amrinone	0.75 mg/kg =	**39.75 mg**		Give mg/kg load over 10 min		300 mg/ 120 mL		2.5 mg/mL	—	
	mg to give ÷ mg/mL =	**16 mL**					**15.9** mL × (60 min/h ÷ 10 min) =		<u>95.4</u>	mL/h × 10 min
	Infusion		**0.78**		5–10 mcg/ kg/min	300 mg/ 120 mL		2500 mcg/mL		
				Take dose you want in mcg ÷ by drug index number = mL/h on pump						
Brevibloc	Infusion		**3.14**		50–100 mcg/ kg/min	2.5 g/ 250 mL		10,000 mcg/mL		mL/h
				Take dose you want in mcg ÷ by drug index number = mL/h on pump						
Cardene	Infusion		—		0.5–10 mg/h	25 mg 250 mL		0.1 mg/mL		
				Ordered mg dose ÷ mg/mL = mL/h to set on pump					___	mL/h
Cardizem	0.25 mg/kg =	**13.25 mg**		Give mg/kg load over 20 min		50 mg/ 100 mL		0.5 mg/mL		
	mg to give ÷ mg/mL =	**27 mL**					**26.5** mL × (60 min/h ÷ 20 min) =		<u>80</u>	mL/h
	0.35 mg/kg =	**18.55 mg**		May repeat loading dose in 15 min				0.5 mg/mL		
	mg to give ÷ mg/mL =	**37 mL**					**37.1** mL × (60 min/h ÷ 20 min) =		<u>111</u>	mL/h
	Infusion				5–15 mg/h				—	
				Ordered mg dose ÷ mg/mL = mL/h to set on pump					___	mL/h
Desmopressin	0.3 mcg/kg =	**16 mcg**		Give dose over 20–30 min				4 mcg/vial		
Dobutamine	Infusion		**0.63**		2.5–40 mcg/kg/ min	250 mg/ 125 mL		2000 mcg/mL		
				Take dose you want in mcg ÷ by drug index number = mL/h on pump						

(continues)

53 kg (continued)

DRUG	ORDERED AMOUNT		TOTAL DOSE TO GIVE		DRUG INDEX NUMBER	DIRECTIONS	INFUSION RANGE	DRUG MIXTURE	AMOUNT	DRUG/ mL	RUN AT	mL/h
Dopamine	Infusion				0.50		1–20 mcg/ kg/min	400 mg/ 250 mL	1600	mcg/mL		
					Take dose you want in mcg ÷ by drug index number = mL/h on pump							
Epinephrine	Infusion		1 mcg/min = 4 mL/h 2 mcg/min = 8 mL/h 3 mcg/min = 11 mL/h 4 mcg/min = 15 mL/h				1–4 mcg/min	4 mg/ 250 mL	16	mcg/mL		
						Ordered mcg dose/min ÷ mcg/mL × 60 min/h =						___ mL/h
Fenoldapam	Infusion				0.0126		0.01–1.6 mcg/ kg/min	10 mg/ 250 mL	40	mcg/mL		
					Take dose you want in mcg ÷ by drug index number = mL/h on pump							
Heparin	100 u/kg = 200 u/kg = 300 u/kg = 400 u/kg =	5300 u 10,600 u 15,900 u 21,200 u										
Isoproterenol	Infusion						5 mcg/min	1 mg/ 250 mL	4	mcg/mL		
						Ordered mcg dose/min ÷ mcg/mL × 60 min/h =						75 mL/h
Lidocaine	Infusion		1 mg/min = 7.5 mL/h				1–4 mg/min	2 g/ 250 mL	8	mg/mL		—
						Ordered mg/min ÷ mg/mL × 60 min/h =						___ mL/h
Nitroglycerin	Infusion		3 mcg/min = 1 mL/h				3–200 mcg/min	50 mg/ 250 mL	200	mcg/mL		—
						Ordered mcg/mL ÷ mcg/mL × 60 min/h =						___ mL/h
Nitroprusside	Infusion		6.7 mcg/min = 1 mL/h				5–300 mcg/min	100 mg/ 250 mL	400	mcg/mL		—
						Ordered mcg/mL ÷ mcg/mL × 60 min/h =						___ mL/h
Norepinephrine	Infusion		1 mcg/min = 4 mL/h 2 mcg/min = 8 mL/h 3 mcg/min = 11 mL/h 4 mcg/min = 15 mL/h 5 mcg/min = 19 mL/h				2–20 mcg/min	4 mg/ 250 mL	16	mcg/mL		
						Ordered mcg dose/min ÷ mcg/mL × 60 min/h =						___ mL/h
Phenylephrine	Infusion		1.3 mcg/min = 1 mL/h				10–200 mcg/min	20 mg/ 250 mL	80	mcg/mL		
						Ordered mcg/min ÷ mcg/mL × 60 min/h =						___ mL/h
Primacor	0.05 mg/kg =	2.65 mg				Give load over 10 min		40 mg/ 200 mL	0.2	mg/mL		
	mg to give ÷ mg/mL =	13 mL					13	mL × (60 min/h ÷ 10 min) =			79.5	mL/h × 10 min
	Infusion				0.062830189		0.5 mcg/ kg/min	40 mg/ 200 mL	200	mcg/mL		—
					Take dose you want in mcg ÷ by drug index number = mL/h on pump							
Trimethaphan	Infusion				—		0.3–6 mg/min	500 mg/ 500 mL	1	mg/mL		—
						Ordered mg/min ÷ mg/mL × 60 min/h =						___ mL/h
Vasopressin			0.02 u/min = 3 mL/h 0.04 u/min = 6 mL/h					40 u/ 100 mL	400	u/mL		

54 kg

DRUG	ORDERED AMOUNT	TOTAL DOSE TO GIVE	DRUG INDEX NUMBER	DIRECTIONS	INFUSION RANGE	DRUG MIXTURE	AMOUNT	DRUG/mL	RUN AT	mL/h
Aminophylline	5 mg/kg = 270 mg			Give mg/kg load over 20 min		500 mg/ 250 mL	2 mg/mL			
	mg to give ÷ mg/mL = 135 mL				135	mL × (60 min/h ÷ 20 min) =			**405**	mL/h × 20 min
	Infusion				0.5–1 mg/kg/h	500 mg/ 250 mL	2 mg/mL			
				mg dose ordered × kg ÷ mg/mL =					___	mL/h
Amiodarone	Loading dose			Load **150 mg** over 10 min		900 mg/ 500 mL	1.8 mg/mL		—	
				Ordered mg load dose (150 mg) ÷ mg/mL (1.8 mg/mL) = 83 mL to give × (60 min/h ÷ 10 min) = mL/h to set on pump					**500**	mL/h × 83 mL
	Infusion			Run at **1 mg/ min** × 6 h		900 mg/ 500 mL	1.8 mg/mL			
				Ordered mg dose (1 mg/min) ÷ mg/mL (1.8 mg/mL) = ___ × 60 min/h = mL/h to set on pump					**33**	mL/h × 6 h
	Infusion			Run at **0.5 mg/ min** × 18 h		900 mg/ 500 mL	1.8 mg/mL			
				Ordered mg dose (0.5 mg/min) ÷ mg/mL (1.8 mg/mL) = ___ × 60 min/h = mL/h to set on pump					**17**	mL/h × 18 h
Amrinone	0.75 mg/kg = 40.5 mg			Give mg/kg load over 10 min		300 mg/ 120 mL	2.5 mg/mL		—	
	mg to give ÷ mg/mL = 16 mL				16.2	mL × (60 min/h ÷ 10 min) =			**97.2**	mL/h × 10 min
	Infusion		0.77		5–10 mcg/ kg/min	300 mg/ 120 mL	2500 mcg/mL			
				Take dose you want in mcg ÷ by drug index number = mL/h on pump						
Brevibloc	Infusion		3.09		50–100 mcg/ kg/min	2.5 g/ 250 mL	10,000 mcg/mL		___	mL/h
				Take dose you want in mcg ÷ by drug index number = mL/h on pump						
Cardene	Infusion		—		0.5–10 mg/h	25 mg 250 mL	0.1 mg/mL			
				Ordered mg dose ÷ mg/mL = mL/h to set on pump					___	mL/h
Cardizem	0.25 mg/kg = 13.5 mg			Give mg/kg load over 20 min		50 mg/ 100 mL	0.5 mg/mL			
	mg to give ÷ mg/mL = 27 mL				27	mL × (60 min/h ÷ 20 min) =			**81**	mL/h
	0.35 mg/kg = 18.9 mg			May repeat loading dose in 15 min			0.5 mg/mL			
	mg to give ÷ mg/mL = 38 mL				37.8	mL × (60 min/h ÷ 20 min) =			**113**	mL/h
	Infusion				5–15 mg/h				—	
				Ordered mg dose ÷ mg/mL = mL/h to set on pump					___	mL/h
Desmopressin	0.3 mcg/kg = 16 mcg			Give dose over 20–30 min			4 mcg/vial			
Dobutamine	Infusion		0.62		2.5–40 mcg/kg/ min	250 mg/ 125 mL	2000 mcg/mL			
				Take dose you want in mcg ÷ by drug index number = mL/h on pump						

(continues)

54 kg (continued)

DRUG	ORDERED AMOUNT	TOTAL DOSE TO GIVE	DRUG INDEX NUMBER	DIRECTIONS	INFUSION RANGE	DRUG MIXTURE	AMOUNT	DRUG/ mL	RUN AT	mL/h
Dopamine	Infusion		0.49		1–20 mcg/kg/min	400 mg/250 mL	1600	mcg/mL		
			Take dose you want in mcg ÷ by drug index number = mL/h on pump							
Epinephrine	Infusion	1 mcg/min = 4 mL/h 2 mcg/min = 8 mL/h 3 mcg/min = 11 mL/h 4 mcg/min = 15 mL/h			1–4 mcg/min	4 mg/250 mL	16	mcg/mL		
				Ordered mcg dose/min ÷ mcg/mL × 60 min/h =					___	mL/h
Fenoldapam	Infusion		0.0124		0.01–1.6 mcg/kg/min	10 mg/250 mL	40	mcg/mL		
			Take dose you want in mcg ÷ by drug index number = mL/h on pump							
Heparin	100 u/kg = 5400 u 200 u/kg = 10,800 u 300 u/kg = 16,200 u 400 u/kg = 21,600 u									
Isoproterenol	Infusion				5 mcg/min	1 mg/250 mL	4	mcg/mL		
				Ordered mcg dose/min ÷ mcg/mL × 60 min/h =					<u>75</u>	mL/h
Lidocaine	Infusion	1 mg/min = 7.5 mL/h			1–4 mg/min	2 g/250 mL	8	mg/mL		
				Ordered mg/min ÷ mg/mL × 60 min/h =					___	mL/h
Nitroglycerin	Infusion	3 mcg/min = 1 mL/h			3–200 mcg/min	50 mg/250 mL	200	mcg/mL		
				Ordered mcg/min ÷ mcg/mL × 60 min/h =					___	mL/h
Nitroprusside	Infusion	6.7 mcg/min = 1 mL/h			5–300 mcg/min	100 mg/250 mL	400	mcg/mL		
				Ordered mcg/min ÷ mcg/mL × 60 min/h =					___	mL/h
Norepinephrine	Infusion	1 mcg/min = 4 mL/h 2 mcg/min = 8 mL/h 3 mcg/min = 11 mL/h 4 mcg/min = 15 mL/h 5 mcg/min = 19 mL/h			2–20 mcg/min	4 mg/250 mL	16	mcg/mL		
				Ordered mcg dose/min ÷ mcg/mL × 60 min/h =					___	mL/h
Phenylephrine	Infusion	1.3 mcg/min = 1 mL/h			10–200 mcg/min	20 mg/250 mL	80	mcg/mL		
				Ordered mcg/min ÷ mcg/mL × 60 min/h =					___	mL/h
Primacor	0.05 mg/kg = 2.7 mg			Give load over 10 min		40 mg/200 mL	0.2	mg/mL		
	mg to give ÷ mg/mL = 14 mL				14 mL × (60 min/h ÷ 10 min) =				<u>81</u>	mL/h × 10 min
	Infusion		0.061666667		0.5 mcg/kg/min	40 mg/200 mL	200	mcg/mL		—
			Take dose you want in mcg ÷ by drug index number = mL/h on pump							
Trimethaphan	Infusion		—		0.3–6 mg/min	500 mg/500 mL	1	mg/mL		—
				Ordered mg/min ÷ mg/mL × 60 min/h =					___	mL/h
Vasopressin		0.02 u/min = 3 mL/h 0.04 u/min = 6 mL/h				40 u/100 mL	400	u/mL		

55 kg

DRUG	ORDERED AMOUNT	TOTAL DOSE TO GIVE	DRUG INDEX NUMBER	DIRECTIONS	INFUSION RANGE	DRUG MIXTURE	AMOUNT	DRUG/ mL	RUN AT	mL/h
Aminophylline	5 mg/kg = **275 mg**			Give mg/kg load over 20 min		500 mg/ 250 mL	2 mg/mL		
	mg to give ÷ mg/mL = **138 mL**				**138**	mL × (60 min/h ÷ 20 min) =			**412.5**	mL/h × 20 min
	Infusion				0.5–1 mg/kg/h	500 mg/ 250 mL	2 mg/mL		
						mg dose ordered × kg ÷ mg/mL =			___	mL/h
Amiodarone	Loading dose			Load **150 mg** over 10 min		900 mg/ 500 mL	1.8 mg/mL	___	
				Ordered mg load dose (150 mg) ÷ mg/mL (1.8 mg/mL) = 83 mL to give × (60 min/h ÷ 10 min) = mL/h to set on pump					**500**	mL/h × 83 mL
	Infusion			Run at **1 mg/ min** × 6 h		900 mg/ 500 mL	1.8 mg/mL		
				Ordered mg dose (1 mg/min) ÷ mg/mL (1.8 mg/mL) = × 60 min/h = mL/h to set on pump					**33**	mL/h × 6 h
	Infusion			Run at **0.5 mg/ min** × 18 h		900 mg/ 500 mL	1.8 mg/mL		
				Ordered mg dose (0.5 mg/min) ÷ mg/mL (1.8 mg/mL) = ____ × 60 min/h = mL/h to set on pump					**17**	mL/h × 18 h
Amrinone	0.75 mg/kg = **41.25 mg**			Give mg/kg load over 10 min		300 mg/ 120 mL	2.5 mg/mL	___	
	mg to give ÷ mg/mL = **17 mL**				**16.5**	mL × (60 min/h ÷ 10 min) =			**99**	mL/h × 10 min
	Infusion		0.76		5–10 mcg/ kg/min	300 mg/ 120 mL	2500 mcg/mL	___	
				Take dose you want in mcg ÷ by drug index number = mL/h on pump						
Brevibloc	Infusion		3.03		50–100 mcg/ kg/min	2.5 g/ 250 mL	10,000 mcg/mL	___ mL/h	
				Take dose you want in mcg ÷ by drug index number = mL/h on pump						
Cardene	Infusion		___		0.5–10 mg/h	25 mg 250 mL	0.1 mg/mL	___	
				Ordered mg dose ÷ mg/mL = mL/h to set on pump					___ mL/h	
Cardizem	0.25 mg/kg = **13.75 mg**			Give mg/kg load over 20 min		50 mg/ 100 mL	0.5 mg/mL		
	mg to give ÷ mg/mL = **28 mL**				**27.5**	mL × (60 min/h ÷ 20 min) =			**83** mL/h	
	0.35 mg/kg = **19.25 mg**			May repeat loading dose in 15 min			0.5 mg/mL		
	mg to give ÷ mg/mL = **39 mL**				**38.5**	mL × (60 min/h ÷ 20 min) =			**116** mL/h	
	Infusion				5–15 mg/h				___	
				Ordered mg dose ÷ mg/mL = mL/h to set on pump					___ mL/h	
Desmopressin	0.3 mcg/kg = **17 mcg**			Give dose over 20–30 min			4 mcg/vial		
Dobutamine	Infusion		0.61		2.5–40 mcg/kg/ min	250 mg/ 125 mL	2000 mcg/mL		
				Take dose you want in mcg ÷ by drug index number = mL/h on pump						

(continues)

55 kg (continued)

DRUG	ORDERED AMOUNT	TOTAL DOSE TO GIVE	DRUG INDEX NUMBER	DIRECTIONS	INFUSION RANGE	DRUG MIXTURE	AMOUNT	DRUG/ mL	RUN AT	mL/h
Dopamine	Infusion		0.49		1–20 mcg/ kg/min	400 mg/ 250 mL	1600	mcg/mL		
			Take dose you want in mcg ÷ by drug index number = mL/h on pump							
Epinephrine	Infusion	1 mcg/min = 4 mL/h 2 mcg/min = 8 mL/h 3 mcg/min = 11 mL/h 4 mcg/min = 15 mL/h			1–4 mcg/min	4 mg/ 250 mL	16	mcg/mL		
				Ordered mcg dose/min ÷ mcg/mL × 60 min/h =					___	mL/h
Fenoldapam	Infusion		0.0122		0.01–1.6 mcg/ kg/min	10 mg/ 250 mL	40	mcg/mL		
			Take dose you want in mcg ÷ by drug index number = mL/h on pump							
Heparin	100 u/kg = 5500 u 200 u/kg = 11,000 u 300 u/kg = 16,500 u 400 u/kg = 22,000 u									
Isoproterenol	Infusion				5 mcg/min	1 mg/ 250 mL	4	mcg/mL		
				Ordered mcg dose/min ÷ mcg/mL × 60 min/h =					75	mL/h
Lidocaine	Infusion	1 mg/min = 7.5 mL/h			1–4 mg/min	2 g/ 250 mL	8	mg/mL	___	
				Ordered mg/min ÷ mg/mL × 60 min/h =					___	mL/h
Nitroglycerin	Infusion	3 mcg/min = 1 mL/h			3–200 mcg/min	50 mg/ 250 mL	200	mcg/mL	___	
				Ordered mcg/min ÷ mcg/mL × 60 min/h =					___	mL/h
Nitroprusside	Infusion	6.7 mcg/min = 1 mL/h			5–300 mcg/min	100 mg/ 250 mL	400	mcg/mL	___	
				Ordered mcg/min ÷ mcg/mL × 60 min/h =					___	mL/h
Norepinephrine	Infusion	1 mcg/min = 4 mL/h 2 mcg/min = 8 mL/h 3 mcg/min = 11 mL/h 4 mcg/min = 15 mL/h 5 mcg/min = 19 mL/h			2–20 mcg/min	4 mg/ 250 mL	16	mcg/mL		
				Ordered mcg dose/min ÷ mcg/mL × 60 min/h =					___	mL/h
Phenylephrine	Infusion	1.3 mcg/min = 1 mL/h			10–200 mcg/min	20 mg/ 250 mL	80	mcg/mL		
				Ordered mcg/min ÷ mcg/mL × 60 min/h =					___	mL/h
Primacor	0.05 mg/kg = 2.75 mg			Give load over 10 min		40 mg/ 200 mL	0.2	mg/mL		
	mg to give ÷ mg/mL = 14 mL				14 mL × (60 min/h ÷ 10 min) =				82.5	mL/h × 10 min
	Infusion		0.06		0.5 mcg/ kg/min	40 mg/ 200 mL	200	mcg/mL	___	
			Take dose you want in mcg ÷ by drug index number = mL/h on pump							
Trimethaphan	Infusion		___		0.3–6 mg/min	500 mg/ 500 mL	1	mg/mL	___	
				Ordered mg/min ÷ mg/mL × 60 min/h =					___	mL/h
Vasopressin	0.02 u/min = 3 mL/h 0.04 u/min = 6 mL/h					40 u/ 100 mL	400	u/mL		

56 kg

DRUG	ORDERED AMOUNT	TOTAL DOSE TO GIVE	DRUG INDEX NUMBER	DIRECTIONS	INFUSION RANGE	DRUG MIXTURE	AMOUNT DRUG/mL	RUN AT mL/h
Aminophylline	5 mg/kg =	280 mg		Give mg/kg load over 20 min		500 mg/ 250 mL	2 mg/mL	
	mg to give ÷ mg/mL =	140 mL				140	mL × (60 min/h ÷ 20 min) =	420 mL/h × 20 min
	Infusion				0.5–1 mg/kg/h	500 mg/ 250 mL	2 mg/mL	
					mg dose ordered × kg ÷ mg/mL =			___ mL/h
Amiodarone	Loading dose			Load **150 mg** over 10 min		900 mg/ 500 mL	1.8 mg/mL	___
				Ordered mg load dose (150 mg) ÷ mg/mL (1.8 mg/mL) = 83 mL to give × (60 min/h ÷ 10 min) = mL/h to set on pump				500 mL/h × 83 mL
	Infusion			Run at **1 mg/ min** × 6 h		900 mg/ 500 mL	1.8 mg/mL	
				Ordered mg dose (1 mg/min) ÷ mg/mL (1.8 mg/mL) = _____ × 60 min/h = mL/h to set on pump				33 mL/h × 6 h
	Infusion			Run at **0.5 mg/ min** × 18 h		900 mg/ 500 mL	1.8 mg/mL	
				Ordered mg dose (0.5 mg/min) ÷ mg/mL (1.8 mg/mL) = _____ × 60 min/h = mL/h to set on pump				17 mL/h × 18 h
Amrinone	0.75 mg/kg =	42 mg		Give mg/kg load over 10 min		300 mg/ 120 mL	2.5 mg/mL	___
	mg to give ÷ mg/mL =	17 mL				16.8	mL × (60 min/h ÷ 10 min) =	100.8 mL/h × 10 min
	Infusion		0.74		5–10 mcg/ kg/min	300 mg/ 120 mL	2500 mcg/mL	___
				Take dose you want in mcg ÷ by drug index number = mL/h on pump				
Brevibloc	Infusion		2.98		50–100 mcg/ kg/min	2.5 g/ 250 mL	10,000 mcg/mL	___ mL/h
				Take dose you want in mcg ÷ by drug index number = mL/h on pump				
Cardene	Infusion		___		0.5–10 mg/h	25 mg 250 mL	0.1 mg/mL	___
				Ordered mg dose ÷ mg/mL = mL/h to set on pump				___ mL/h
Cardizem	0.25 mg/kg =	14 mg		Give mg/kg load over 20 min		50 mg/ 100 mL	0.5 mg/mL	___
	mg to give ÷ mg/mL =	28 mL				28	mL × (60 min/h ÷ 20 min) =	84 mL/h
	0.35 mg/kg =	19.6 mg		May repeat loading dose in 15 min			0.5 mg/mL	___
	mg to give ÷ mg/mL =	39 mL				39.2	mL × (60 min/h ÷ 20 min) =	118 mL/h
	Infusion				5–15 mg/h			___
				Ordered mg dose ÷ mg/mL = mL/h to set on pump				___ mL/h
Desmopressin	0.3 mcg/kg =	17 mcg		Give dose over 20–30 min			4 mcg/vial	
Dobutamine	Infusion		0.59		2.5–40 mcg/kg/ min	250 mg/ 125 mL	2000 mcg/mL	
				Take dose you want in mcg ÷ by drug index number = mL/h on pump				

(continues)

56   kg (continued)

DRUG	ORDERED AMOUNT	TOTAL DOSE TO GIVE	DRUG INDEX NUMBER	DIRECTIONS	INFUSION RANGE	DRUG MIXTURE	AMOUNT	DRUG/ mL	RUN AT	mL/h
Dopamine	Infusion		0.48		1–20 mcg/ kg/min	400 mg/ 250 mL	1600	mcg/mL		
				Take dose you want in mcg ÷ by drug index number = mL/h on pump						
Epinephrine	Infusion	1 mcg/min = 4 mL/h 2 mcg/min = 8 mL/h 3 mcg/min = 11 mL/h 4 mcg/min = 15 mL/h			1–4 mcg/min	4 mg/ 250 mL	16	mcg/mL		
				Ordered mcg dose/min ÷ mcg/mL × 60 min/h =					___	mL/h
Fenoldapam	Infusion		0.0120		0.01–1.6 mcg/ kg/min	10 mg/ 250 mL	40	mcg/mL		
				Take dose you want in mcg ÷ by drug index number = mL/h on pump						
Heparin	100 u/kg = 5600 u 200 u/kg = 11,200 u 300 u/kg = 16,800 u 400 u/kg = 22,400 u									
Isoproterenol	Infusion				5 mcg/min	1 mg/ 250 mL	4	mcg/mL		
				Ordered mcg dose/min ÷ mcg/mL × 60 min/h =					**75**	mL/h
Lidocaine	Infusion	1 mg/min = 7.5 mL/h			1–4 mg/min	2 g/ 250 mL	8	mg/mL	___	
				Ordered mg/min ÷ mg/mL × 60 min/h =					___	mL/h
Nitroglycerin	Infusion	3 mcg/min = 1 mL/h			3–200 mcg/min	50 mg/ 250 mL	200	mcg/mL	___	
				Ordered mcg/min ÷ mcg/mL × 60 min/h =					___	mL/h
Nitroprusside	Infusion	6.7 mcg/min = 1 mL/h			5–300 mcg/min	100 mg/ 250 mL	400	mcg/mL	___	
				Ordered mcg/min ÷ mcg/mL × 60 min/h =					___	mL/h
Norepinephrine	Infusion	1 mcg/min = 4 mL/h 2 mcg/min = 8 mL/h 3 mcg/min = 11 mL/h 4 mcg/min = 15 mL/h 5 mcg/min = 19 mL/h			2–20 mcg/min	4 mg/ 250 mL	16	mcg/mL		
				Ordered mcg dose/min ÷ mcg/mL × 60 min/h =					___	mL/h
Phenylephrine	Infusion	1.3 mcg/min = 1 mL/h			10–200 mcg/min	20 mg/ 250 mL	80	mcg/mL		
				Ordered mcg/min ÷ mcg/mL × 60 min/h =					___	mL/h
Primacor	0.05 mg/kg = 2.8 mg			Give load over 10 min		40 mg/ 200 mL	0.2	mg/mL		
	mg to give ÷ mg/mL = 14 mL				14	mL × (60 min/h ÷ 10 min) =			**84**	mL/h × 10 min
	Infusion		0.06		0.5 mcg/ kg/min	40 mg/ 200 mL	200	mcg/mL	___	
				Take dose you want in mcg ÷ by drug index number = mL/h on pump						
Trimethaphan	Infusion		—		0.3–6 mg/min	500 mg/ 500 mL	1	mg/mL	___	
				Ordered mg/min ÷ mg/mL × 60 min/h =					___	mL/h
Vasopressin		0.02 u/min = 3 mL/h 0.04 u/min = 6 mL/h				40 u/ 100 mL	400	u/mL		

57 kg

DRUG	ORDERED AMOUNT	TOTAL DOSE TO GIVE	DRUG INDEX NUMBER	DIRECTIONS	INFUSION RANGE	DRUG MIXTURE	AMOUNT DRUG/mL	RUN AT mL/h
Aminophylline	5 mg/kg = **285** mg			Give mg/kg load over 20 min		500 mg/ 250 mL	2 mg/mL	
	mg to give ÷ mg/mL = **143** mL				**143**	mL × (60 min/h ÷ 20 min) =		**427.5** mL/h × 20 min
	Infusion				0.5–1 mg/kg/h	500 mg/ 250 mL	2 mg/mL	
					mg dose ordered × kg ÷ mg/mL =			___ mL/h
Amiodarone	Loading dose			Load **150 mg** over 10 min		900 mg/ 500 mL	1.8 mg/mL	___
				Ordered mg load dose (150 mg) ÷ mg/mL (1.8 mg/mL) = 83 mL to give × (60 min/h ÷ 10 min) = mL/h to set on pump				**500** mL/h × 83 mL
	Infusion			Run at **1 mg/ min** × 6 h		900 mg/ 500 mL	1.8 mg/mL	
				Ordered mg dose (1 mg/min) ÷ mg/mL (1.8 mg/mL) = _____ × 60 min/h = mL/h to set on pump				**33** mL/h × 6 h
	Infusion			Run at **0.5 mg/ min** × 18 h		900 mg/ 500 mL	1.8 mg/mL	
				Ordered mg dose (0.5 mg/min) ÷ mg/mL (1.8 mg/mL) = _____ × 60 min/h = mL/h to set on pump				**17** mL/h × 18 h
Amrinone	0.75 mg/kg = **42.75** mg			Give mg/kg load over 10 min		300 mg/ 120 mL	2.5 mg/mL	___
	mg to give ÷ mg/mL = **17** mL				**17.1**	mL × (60 min/h ÷ 10 min) =		**102.6** mL/h × 10 min
	Infusion		0.73		5–10 mcg/ kg/min	300 mg/ 120 mL	2500 mcg/mL	___
				Take dose you want in mcg ÷ by drug index number = mL/h on pump				
Brevibloc	Infusion		2.92		50–100 mcg/ kg/min	2.5 g/ 250 mL	10,000 mcg/mL	___ mL/h
				Take dose you want in mcg ÷ by drug index number = mL/h on pump				
Cardene	Infusion		—		0.5–10 mg/h	25 mg 250 mL	0.1 mg/mL	
				Ordered mg dose ÷ mg/mL = mL/h to set on pump				___ mL/h
Cardizem	0.25 mg/kg = **14.25** mg			Give mg/kg load over 20 min		50 mg/ 100 mL	0.5 mg/mL	___
	mg to give ÷ mg/mL = **29** mL				**28.5**	mL × (60 min/h ÷ 20 min) =		**86** mL/h
	0.35 mg/kg = **19.95** mg			May repeat loading dose in 15 min			0.5 mg/mL	___
	mg to give ÷ mg/mL = **40** mL				**39.9**	mL × (60 min/h ÷ 20 min) =		**120** mL/h
	Infusion				5–15 mg/h			
				Ordered mg dose ÷ mg/mL = mL/h to set on pump				___ mL/h
Desmopressin	0.3 mcg/kg = **17** mcg			Give dose over 20–30 min			4 mcg/vial	
Dobutamine	Infusion		0.58		2.5–40 mcg/kg/ min	250 mg/ 125 mL	2000 mcg/mL	
				Take dose you want in mcg ÷ by drug index number = mL/h on pump				

(continues)

57 kg (continued)

DRUG	ORDERED AMOUNT	TOTAL DOSE TO GIVE	DRUG INDEX NUMBER	DIRECTIONS	INFUSION RANGE	DRUG MIXTURE	AMOUNT	DRUG/mL	RUN AT	mL/h
Dopamine	Infusion		0.47		1–20 mcg/kg/min	400 mg/250 mL	1600	mcg/mL		
	Take dose you want in mcg ÷ by drug index number = mL/h on pump									
Epinephrine	Infusion	1 mcg/min = 4 mL/h 2 mcg/min = 8 mL/h 3 mcg/min = 11 mL/h 4 mcg/min = 15 mL/h			1–4 mcg/min	4 mg/250 mL	16	mcg/mL		
		Ordered mcg dose/min ÷ mcg/mL × 60 min/h =							___	mL/h
Fenoldapam	Infusion		0.0118		0.01–1.6 mcg/kg/min	10 mg/250 mL	40	mcg/mL		
	Take dose you want in mcg ÷ by drug index number = mL/h on pump									
Heparin	100 u/kg = 5700 u 200 u/kg = 11,400 u 300 u/kg = 17,100 u 400 u/kg = 22,800 u									
Isoproterenol	Infusion				5 mcg/min	1 mg/250 mL	4	mcg/mL		
		Ordered mcg dose/min ÷ mcg/mL × 60 min/h =							**75**	mL/h
Lidocaine	Infusion	1 mg/min = 7.5 mL/h			1–4 mg/min	2 g/250 mL	8	mg/mL		
		Ordered mg/min ÷ mg/mL × 60 min/h =							___	mL/h
Nitroglycerin	Infusion	3 mcg/min = 1 mL/h			3–200 mcg/min	50 mg/250 mL	200	mcg/mL		
		Ordered mcg/min ÷ mcg/mL × 60 min/h =							___	mL/h
Nitroprusside	Infusion	6.7 mcg/min = 1 mL/h			5–300 mcg/min	100 mg/250 mL	400	mcg/mL		
		Ordered mcg/min ÷ mcg/mL × 60 min/h =							___	mL/h
Norepinephrine	Infusion	1 mcg/min = 4 mL/h 2 mcg/min = 8 mL/h 3 mcg/min = 11 mL/h 4 mcg/min = 15 mL/h 5 mcg/min = 19 mL/h			2–20 mcg/min	4 mg/250 mL	16	mcg/mL		
		Ordered mcg dose/min ÷ mcg/mL × 60 min/h =							___	mL/h
Phenylephrine	Infusion	1.3 mcg/min = 1 mL/h			10–200 mcg/min	20 mg/250 mL	80	mcg/mL		
		Ordered mcg/min ÷ mcg/mL × 60 min/h =							___	mL/h
Primacor	0.05 mg/kg = 2.85 mg			Give load over 10 min		40 mg/200 mL	0.2	mg/mL		
	mg to give ÷ mg/mL = 14 mL				14	mL × (60 min/h ÷ 10 min) =			85.5	mL/h × 10 min
	Infusion		0.06		0.5 mcg/kg/min	40 mg/200 mL	200	mcg/mL		
	Take dose you want in mcg ÷ by drug index number = mL/h on pump									
Trimethaphan	Infusion			—	0.3–6 mg/min	500 mg/500 mL	1	mg/mL		
		Ordered mg/min ÷ mg/mL × 60 min/h =							___	mL/h
Vasopressin		0.02 u/min = 3 mL/h 0.04 u/min = 6 mL/h				40 u/100 mL	400	u/mL		

58 kg

DRUG	ORDERED AMOUNT	TOTAL DOSE TO GIVE	DRUG INDEX NUMBER	DIRECTIONS	INFUSION RANGE	DRUG MIXTURE	AMOUNT	DRUG/ mL	RUN AT	mL/h
Aminophylline	5 mg/kg =	**290** mg		Give mg/kg load over 20 min		500 mg/ 250 mL		2 mg/mL		
	mg to give ÷ mg/mL =	**145** mL				145	mL × (60 min/h ÷ 20 min) =		**435**	mL/h × 20 min
	Infusion				0.5–1 mg/kg/h	500 mg/ 250 mL		2 mg/mL		
						mg dose ordered × kg ÷ mg/ml =			___ mL/h	
Amiodarone	Loading dose			Load **150 mg** over 10 min		900 mg/ 500 mL		1.8 mg/mL	—	
				Ordered mg load dose (150 mg) ÷ mg/mL (1.8 mg/mL) = 83 mL to give × (60 min/h ÷ 10 min) = mL/h to set on pump					**500**	mL/h × 83 mL
	Infusion			Run at **1 mg/ min** × 6 h		900 mg/ 500 mL		1.8 mg/mL		
				Ordered mg dose (1 mg/min) ÷ mg/mL (1.8 mg/mL) = ___ × 60 min/h = mL/h to set on pump					**33**	ml/h × 6 h
	Infusion			Run at **0.5 mg/ min** × 18 h		900 mg/ 500 mL		1.8 mg/mL		
				Ordered mg dose (0.5 mg/min) ÷ mg/mL (1.8 mg/mL) = ___ × 60 min/h = mL/h to set on pump					**17**	mL/h × 18 h
Amrinone	0.75 mg/kg =	**43.5** mg		Give mg/kg load over 10 min		300 mg/ 120 mL		2.5 mg/mL	—	
	mg to give ÷ mg/mL =	**17** mL				17.4	mL × (60 min/h ÷ 10 min) =		**104.4**	mL/h × 10 min
	Infusion		0.72		5–10 mcg/ kg/min	300 mg/ 120 mL		2500 mcg/mL	—	
				Take dose you want in mcg ÷ by drug index number = mL/h on pump						
Brevibloc	Infusion		2.87		50–100 mcg/ kg/min	2.5 g/ 250 mL		10,000 mcg/mL	___ mL/h	
				Take dose you want in mcg ÷ by drug index number = mL/h on pump						
Cardene	Infusion		—		0.5–10 mg/h	25 mg 250 mL		0.1 mg/mL		
				Ordered mg dose ÷ mg/mL = mL/h to set on pump					___ mL/h	
Cardizem	0.25 mg/kg =	**14.5** mg		Give mg/kg load over 20 min		50 mg/ 100 mL		0.5 mg/mL		
	mg to give ÷ mg/mL =	**29** mL				29	mL × (60 min/h ÷ 20 min) =		**87** mL/h	
	0.35 mg/kg =	**20.3** mg		May repeat loading dose in 15 min				0.5 mg/mL	—	
	mg to give ÷ mg/mL =	**41** mL				40.6	mL × (60 min/h ÷ 20 min) =		**122** mL/h	
	Infusion				5–15 mg/h				—	
				Ordered mg dose ÷ mg/mL = mL/h to set on pump					___ mL/h	
Desmopressin	0.3 mcg/kg =	**17** mcg		Give dose over 20–30 min				4 mcg/vial		
Dobutamine	Infusion		0.57		2.5–40 mcg/kg/ min	250 mg/ 125 mL		2000 mcg/mL		
				Take dose you want in mcg ÷ by drug index number = mL/h on pump						

(continues)

58 kg (continued)

DRUG	ORDERED AMOUNT	TOTAL DOSE TO GIVE	DRUG INDEX NUMBER	DIRECTIONS	INFUSION RANGE	DRUG MIXTURE	AMOUNT	DRUG/mL	RUN AT	mL/h
Dopamine	Infusion		0.46		1–20 mcg/kg/min	400 mg/250 mL	1600	mcg/mL		
			Take dose you want in mcg ÷ by drug index number = mL/h on pump							
Epinephrine	Infusion	1 mcg/min = 4 mL/h 2 mcg/min = 8 mL/h 3 mcg/min = 11 mL/h 4 mcg/min = 15 mL/h			1–4 mcg/min	4 mg/250 mL	16	mcg/mL		
			Ordered mcg dose/min ÷ mcg/mL × 60 min/h =						___	mL/h
Fenoldapam	Infusion		0.0116		0.01–1.6 mcg/kg/min	10 mg/250 mL	40	mcg/mL		
			Take dose you want in mcg ÷ by drug index number = mL/h on pump							
Heparin	100 u/kg =	5800 u								
	200 u/kg =	11,600 u								
	300 u/kg =	17,400 u								
	400 u/kg =	23,200 u								
Isoproterenol	Infusion				5 mcg/min	1 mg/250 mL	4	mcg/mL		
			Ordered mcg dose/min ÷ mcg/mL × 60 min/h =						**75**	mL/h
Lidocaine	Infusion	1 mg/min = 7.5 mL/h			1–4 mg/min	2 g/250 mL	8	mg/mL	___	
			Ordered mg/min ÷ mg/mL × 60 min/h =						___	mL/h
Nitroglycerin	Infusion	3 mcg/min = 1 mL/h			3–200 mcg/min	50 mg/250 mL	200	mcg/mL	___	
			Ordered mcg/min ÷ mcg/mL × 60 min/h =						___	mL/h
Nitroprusside	Infusion	6.7 mcg/min = 1 mL/h			5–300 mcg/min	100 mg/250 mL	400	mcg/mL	___	
			Ordered mcg/min ÷ mcg/mL × 60 min/h =						___	mL/h
Norepinephrine	Infusion	1 mcg/min = 4 mL/h 2 mcg/min = 8 mL/h 3 mcg/min = 11 mL/h 4 mcg/min = 15 mL/h 5 mcg/min = 19 mL/h			2–20 mcg/min	4 mg/250 mL	16	mcg/mL		
			Ordered mcg dose/min ÷ mcg/mL × 60 min/h =						___	mL/h
Phenylephrine	Infusion	1.3 mcg/min = 1 mL/h			10–200 mcg/min	20 mg/250 mL	80	mcg/mL		
			Ordered mcg/min ÷ mcg/mL × 60 min/h =						___	mL/h
Primacor	0.05 mg/kg =	2.9 mg		Give load over 10 min		40 mg/200 mL	0.2	mg/mL		
	mg to give ÷ mg/mL =	15 mL			15	mL × (60 min/h ÷ 10 min) =			**87**	mL/h × 10 min
	Infusion		0.06		0.5 mcg/kg/min	40 mg/200 mL	200	mcg/mL	___	
			Take dose you want in mcg ÷ by drug index number = mL/h on pump							
Trimethaphan	Infusion		—		0.3–6 mg/min	500 mg/500 mL	1	mg/mL	___	
			Ordered mg/min ÷ mg/mL × 60 min/h =						___	mL/h
Vasopressin		0.02 u/min = 3 mL/h 0.04 u/min = 6 mL/h				40 u/100 mL	400	u/mL		

59 kg

DRUG	ORDERED AMOUNT	TOTAL DOSE TO GIVE	DRUG INDEX NUMBER	DIRECTIONS	INFUSION RANGE	DRUG MIXTURE	AMOUNT	DRUG/mL	RUN AT	mL/h
Aminophylline	5 mg/kg =	295 mg		Give mg/kg load over 20 min		500 mg/ 250 mL	2 mg/mL		
	mg to give ÷ mg/mL =	148 mL			148	mL × (60 min/h ÷ 20 min) =		<u>442.5</u>	mL/h × 20 min
	Infusion				0.5–1 mg/kg/h	500 mg/ 250 mL	2 mg/mL		
					mg dose ordered × kg ÷ mg/mL =			___ mL/h
Amiodarone	Loading dose			Load **150 mg** over 10 min		900 mg/ 500 mL	1.8 mg/mL	—	
				Ordered mg load dose (150 mg) ÷ mg/mL (1.8 mg/mL) = 83 mL to give × (60 min/h ÷ 10 min) = mL/h to set on pump				<u>500</u>	mL/h × 83 mL
	Infusion			Run at **1 mg/ min** × 6 h		900 mg/ 500 mL	1.8 mg/mL		
				Ordered mg dose (1 mg/min) ÷ mg/mL (1.8 mg/mL) = ___ × 60 min/h = mL/h to set on pump				<u>33</u>	mL/h × 6 h
	Infusion			Run at **0.5 mg/ min** × 18 h		900 mg/ 500 mL	1.8 mg/mL		
				Ordered mg dose (0.5 mg/min) ÷ mg/mL (1.8 mg/mL) = ___ × 60 min/h = mL/h to set on pump				<u>17</u>	mL/h × 18 h
Amrinone	0.75 mg/kg =	44.25 mg		Give mg/kg load over 10 min		300 mg/ 120 mL	2.5 mg/mL	—	
	mg to give ÷ mg/mL =	18 mL			17.7	mL × (60 min/h ÷ 10 min) =		<u>106.2</u>	mL/h × 10 min
	Infusion		0.71		5–10 mcg/ kg/min	300 mg/ 120 mL	2500 mcg/mL	—	
				Take dose you want in mcg ÷ by drug index number = mL/h on pump					
Brevibloc	Infusion		2.82		50–100 mcg/ kg/min	2.5 g/ 250 mL	10,000 mcg/mL	___ mL/h	
				Take dose you want in mcg ÷ by drug index number = mL/h on pump					
Cardene	Infusion		—		0.5–10 mg/h	25 mg 250 mL	0.1 mg/mL	—	
				Ordered mg dose ÷ mg/mL = mL/h to set on pump				___ mL/h	
Cardizem	0.25 mg/kg =	14.75 mg		Give mg/kg load over 20 min		50 mg/ 100 mL	0.5 mg/mL		
	mg to give ÷ mg/mL =	30 mL			29.5	mL × (60 min/h ÷ 20 min) =		<u>89</u> mL/h	
	0.35 mg/kg =	20.65 mg		May repeat loading dose in 15 min			0.5 mg/mL	—	
	mg to give ÷ mg/mL =	41 mL			41.3	mL × (60 min/h ÷ 20 min) =		<u>124</u> mL/h	
	Infusion				5–15 mg/h			—	
				Ordered mg dose ÷ mg/mL = mL/h to set on pump				___ mL/h	
Desmopressin	0.3 mcg/kg =	18 mcg		Give dose over 20–30 min			4 mcg/vial		
Dobutamine	Infusion		0.56		2.5–40 mcg/kg/ min	250 mg/ 125 mL	2000 mcg/mL		
				Take dose you want in mcg ÷ by drug index number = mL/h on pump					

(continues)

59 kg (continued)

DRUG	ORDERED AMOUNT	TOTAL DOSE TO GIVE	DRUG INDEX NUMBER	DIRECTIONS	INFUSION RANGE	DRUG MIXTURE	AMOUNT	DRUG/mL	RUN AT	mL/h
Dopamine	Infusion		0.45		1–20 mcg/kg/min	400 mg/250 mL	1600	mcg/mL		
	Take dose you want in mcg ÷ by drug index number = mL/h on pump									
Epinephrine	Infusion	1 mcg/min = 4 mL/h 2 mcg/min = 8 mL/h 3 mcg/min = 11 mL/h 4 mcg/min = 15 mL/h			1–4 mcg/min	4 mg/250 mL	16	mcg/mL		
		Ordered mcg dose/min ÷ mcg/mL × 60 min/h =							___	mL/h
Fenoldapam	Infusion		0.0114		0.01–1.6 mcg/kg/min	10 mg/250 mL	40	mcg/mL		
	Take dose you want in mcg ÷ by drug index number = mL/h on pump									
Heparin	100 u/kg = 5900 u 200 u/kg = 11,800 u 300 u/kg = 17,700 u 400 u/kg = 23,600 u									
Isoproterenol	Infusion				5 mcg/min	1 mg/250 mL	4	mcg/mL		
	Ordered mcg dose/min ÷ mcg/mL × 60 min/h =								75	mL/h
Lidocaine	Infusion	1 mg/min = 7.5 mL/h			1–4 mg/min	2 g/250 mL	8	mg/mL	___	
		Ordered mg/min ÷ mg/mL × 60 min/h =							___	mL/h
Nitroglycerin	Infusion	3 mcg/min = 1 mL/h			3–200 mcg/min	50 mg/250 mL	200	mcg/mL	___	
		Ordered mcg/min ÷ mcg/mL × 60 min/h =							___	mL/h
Nitroprusside	Infusion	6.7 mcg/min = 1 mL/h			5–300 mcg/min	100 mg/250 mL	400	mcg/mL	___	
		Ordered mcg/min ÷ mcg/mL × 60 min/h =							___	mL/h
Norepinephrine	Infusion	1 mcg/min = 4 mL/h 2 mcg/min = 8 mL/h 3 mcg/min = 11 mL/h 4 mcg/min = 15 mL/h 5 mcg/min = 19 mL/h			2–20 mcg/min	4 mg/250 mL	16	mcg/mL		
		Ordered mcg dose/min ÷ mcg/mL × 60 min/h =							___	mL/h
Phenylephrine	Infusion	1.3 mcg/min = 1 mL/h			10–200 mcg/min	20 mg/250 mL	80	mcg/mL		
		Ordered mcg/min ÷ mcg/mL × 60 min/h =							___	mL/h
Primacor	0.05 mg/kg = 2.95 mg			Give load over 10 min		40 mg/200 mL	0.2	mg/mL		
	mg to give ÷ mg/mL = 15 mL					15 mL × (60 min/h ÷ 10 min) =			88.5	mL/h × 10 min
	Infusion		0.06		0.5 mcg/kg/min	40 mg/200 mL	200	mcg/mL	___	
	Take dose you want in mcg ÷ by drug index number = mL/h on pump									
Trimethaphan	Infusion		___		0.3–6 mg/min	500 mg/500 mL	1	mg/mL	___	
		Ordered mg/min ÷ mg/mL × 60 min/h =							___	mL/h
Vasopressin		0.02 u/min = 3 mL/h 0.04 u/min = 6 mL/h				40 u/100 mL	400	u/mL		

60 kg

DRUG	ORDERED AMOUNT	TOTAL DOSE TO GIVE	DRUG INDEX NUMBER	DIRECTIONS	INFUSION RANGE	DRUG MIXTURE	AMOUNT	DRUG/mL	RUN AT	mL/h
Aminophylline	5 mg/kg =	300 mg		Give mg/kg load over 20 min		500 mg/250 mL		2 mg/mL		
	mg to give ÷ mg/mL =	150 mL			150	mL × (60 min/h ÷ 20 min) =			450	mL/h × 20 min
	Infusion				0.5–1 mg/kg/h	500 mg/250 mL		2 mg/mL		
				mg dose ordered × kg ÷ mg/mL =						___ mL/h
Amiodarone	Loading dose			Load **150 mg** over 10 min		900 mg/500 mL		1.8 mg/mL	—	
				Ordered mg load dose (150 mg) ÷ mg/mL (1.8 mg/mL) = 83 mL to give × (60 min/h ÷ 10 min) = mL/h to set on pump					500	mL/h × 83 mL
	Infusion			Run at **1 mg/min** × 6 h		900 mg/500 mL		1.8 mg/mL		
				Ordered mg dose (1 mg/min) ÷ mg/mL (1.8 mg/mL) = × 60 min/h = mL/h to set on pump					33	mL/h × 6 h
	Infusion			Run at **0.5 mg/min** × 18 h		900 mg/500 mL		1.8 mg/mL		
				Ordered mg dose (0.5 mg/min) ÷ mg/mL (1.8 mg/mL) = ___ × 60 min/h = mL/h to set on pump					17	mL/h × 18 h
Amrinone	0.75 mg/kg =	45 mg		Give mg/kg load over 10 min		300 mg/120 mL		2.5 mg/mL	—	
	mg to give ÷ mg/mL =	18 mL			18	mL × (60 min/h ÷ 10 min) =			108	mL/h × 10 min
	Infusion		0.69		5–10 mcg/kg/min	300 mg/120 mL	2500 mcg/mL		—	
				Take dose you want in mcg ÷ by drug index number = mL/h on pump						
Brevibloc	Infusion		2.78		50–100 mcg/kg/min	2.5 g/250 mL	10,000 mcg/mL			___ mL/h
				Take dose you want in mcg ÷ by drug index number = mL/h on pump						
Cardene	Infusion			—	0.5–10 mg/h	25 mg/250 mL	0.1 mg/mL		—	
				Ordered mg dose ÷ mg/mL = mL/h to set on pump						___ mL/h
Cardizem	0.25 mg/kg =	15 mg		Give mg/kg load over 20 min		50 mg/100 mL	0.5 mg/mL			
	mg to give ÷ mg/mL =	30 mL			30	mL × (60 min/h ÷ 20 min) =			90	mL/h
	0.35 mg/kg =	21 mg		May repeat loading dose in 15 min			0.5 mg/mL			
	mg to give ÷ mg/mL =	42 mL			42	mL × (60 min/h ÷ 20 min) =			126	mL/h
	Infusion				5–15 mg/h				—	
				Ordered mg dose ÷ mg/mL = mL/h to set on pump						___ mL/h
Desmopressin	0.3 mcg/kg =	18 mcg		Give dose over 20–30 min			4 mcg/vial			
Dobutamine	Infusion		0.56		2.5–40 mcg/kg/min	250 mg/125 mL	2000 mcg/mL			
				Take dose you want in mcg ÷ by drug index number = mL/h on pump						

(continues)

60 kg (continued)

DRUG	ORDERED AMOUNT	TOTAL DOSE TO GIVE	DRUG INDEX NUMBER	DIRECTIONS	INFUSION RANGE	DRUG MIXTURE	AMOUNT	DRUG/mL	RUN AT	mL/h
Dopamine	Infusion		0.45		1–20 mcg/kg/min	400 mg/250 mL	1600	mcg/mL		
		Take dose you want in mcg ÷ by drug index number = mL/h on pump								
Epinephrine	Infusion	1 mcg/min = 4 mL/h 2 mcg/min = 8 mL/h 3 mcg/min = 11 mL/h 4 mcg/min = 15 mL/h			1–4 mcg/min	4 mg/250 mL	16	mcg/mL		
				Ordered mcg dose/min ÷ mcg/mL × 60 min/h =					___	mL/h
Fenoldapam	Infusion		0.0112		0.01–1.6 mcg/kg/min	10 mg/250 mL	40	mcg/mL		
		Take dose you want in mcg ÷ by drug index number = mL/h on pump								
Heparin	100 u/kg = 6000 u 200 u/kg = 12,000 u 300 u/kg = 18,000 u 400 u/kg = 24,000 u									
Isoproterenol	Infusion				5 mcg/min	1 mg/250 mL	4	mcg/mL		
				Ordered mcg dose/min ÷ mcg/mL × 60 min/h =					75	mL/h
Lidocaine	Infusion	1 mg/min = 7.5 mL/h			1–4 mg/min	2 g/250 mL	8	mg/mL	___	
				Ordered mg/min ÷ mg/mL × 60 min/h =					___	mL/h
Nitroglycerin	Infusion	3 mcg/min = 1 mL/h			3–200 mcg/min	50 mg/250 mL	200	mcg/mL	___	
				Ordered mcg/min ÷ mcg/mL × 60 min/h =					___	mL/h
Nitroprusside	Infusion	6.7 mcg/min = 1 mL/h			5–300 mcg/min	100 mg/250 mL	400	mcg/mL	___	
				Ordered mcg/min ÷ mcg/mL × 60 min/h =					___	mL/h
Norepinephrine	Infusion	1 mcg/min = 4 mL/h 2 mcg/min = 8 mL/h 3 mcg/min = 11 mL/h 4 mcg/min = 15 mL/h 5 mcg/min = 19 mL/h			2–20 mcg/min	4 mg/250 mL	16	mcg/mL		
				Ordered mcg dose/min ÷ mcg/mL × 60 min/h =					___	mL/h
Phenylephrine	Infusion	1.3 mcg/min = 1 mL/h			10–200 mcg/min	20 mg/250 mL	80	mcg/mL		
				Ordered mcg/min ÷ mcg/mL × 60 min/h =					___	mL/h
Primacor	0.05 mg/kg = 3 mg			Give load over 10 min		40 mg/200 mL	0.2	mg/mL		
	mg to give ÷ mg/mL = 15 mL				15 mL × (60 min/h ÷ 10 min) =				90	mL/h × 10 min
	Infusion		0.06		0.5 mcg/kg/min	40 mg/200 mL	200	mcg/mL	___	
		Take dose you want in mcg ÷ by drug index number = mL/h on pump								
Trimethaphan	Infusion		___		0.3–6 mg/min	500 mg/500 mL	1	mg/mL	___	
				Ordered mg/min ÷ mg/mL × 60 min/h =					___	mL/h
Vasopressin		0.02 u/min = 3 mL/h 0.04 u/min = 6 mL/h				40 u/100 mL	400	u/mL		

61 kg

DRUG	ORDERED AMOUNT	TOTAL DOSE TO GIVE	DRUG INDEX NUMBER	DIRECTIONS	INFUSION RANGE	DRUG MIXTURE	AMOUNT	DRUG/mL	RUN AT	mL/h
Aminophylline	5 mg/kg = 305 mg			Give mg/kg load over 20 min		500 mg/ 250 mL	2 mg/mL			
	mg to give ÷ mg/mL = 153 mL				153	mL × (60 min/h ÷ 20 min) =			457.5	mL/h × 20 min
	Infusion				0.5–1 mg/kg/h	500 mg/ 250 mL	2 mg/mL			
						mg dose ordered × kg ÷ mg/mL =			___	mL/h
Amiodarone	Loading dose			Load **150 mg** over 10 min		900 mg/ 500 mL	1.8 mg/mL		___	
				Ordered mg load dose (150 mg) ÷ mg/mL (1.8 mg/mL) = 83 mL to give × (60 min/h ÷ 10 min) = mL/h to set on pump					500	mL/h × 83 mL
	Infusion			Run at **1 mg/ min** × 6 h		900 mg/ 500 mL	1.8 mg/mL			
				Ordered mg dose (1 mg/min) ÷ mg/mL (1.8 mg/mL) = _____ × 60 min/h = mL/h to set on pump					33	mL/h × 6 h
	Infusion			Run at **0.5 mg/ min** × 18 h		900 mg/ 500 mL	1.8 mg/mL			
				Ordered mg dose (0.5 mg/min) ÷ mg/mL (1.8 mg/mL) = _____ × 60 min/h = mL/h to set on pump					17	mL/h × 18 h
Amrinone	0.75 mg/kg = 45.75 mg			Give mg/kg load over 10 min		300 mg/ 120 mL	2.5 mg/mL		___	
	mg to give ÷ mg/mL = 18 mL				18.3	mL × (60 min/h ÷ 10 min) =			109.8	mL/h × 10 min
	Infusion		0.68		5–10 mcg/ kg/min	300 mg/ 120 mL	2500 mcg/mL		___	
				Take dose you want in mcg ÷ by drug index number = mL/h on pump						
Brevibloc	Infusion		2.73		50–100 mcg/ kg/min	2.5 g/ 250 mL	10,000 mcg/mL		___	mL/h
				Take dose you want in mcg ÷ by drug index number = mL/h on pump						
Cardene	Infusion			___	0.5–10 mg/h	25 mg 250 mL	0.1 mg/mL		___	
				Ordered mg dose ÷ mg/mL = mL/h to set on pump					___	mL/h
Cardizem	0.25 mg/kg = 15.25 mg			Give mg/kg load over 20 min		50 mg/ 100 mL	0.5 mg/mL			
	mg to give ÷ mg/mL = 31 mL				30.5	mL × (60 min/h ÷ 20 min) =			92	mL/h
	0.35 mg/kg = 21.35 mg			May repeat loading dose in 15 min			0.5 mg/mL			
	mg to give ÷ mg/mL = 43 mL				42.7	mL × (60 min/h ÷ 20 min) =			128	mL/h
	Infusion				5–15 mg/h				___	
				Ordered mg dose ÷ mg/mL = mL/h to set on pump					___	mL/h
Desmopressin	0.3 mcg/kg = 18 mcg			Give dose over 20–30 min			4 mcg/vial			
Dobutamine	Infusion		0.55		2.5–40 mcg/kg/ min	250 mg/ 125 mL	2000 mcg/mL			
				Take dose you want in mcg ÷ by drug index number = mL/h on pump						

(continues)

61 kg (continued)

DRUG	ORDERED AMOUNT	TOTAL DOSE TO GIVE	DRUG INDEX NUMBER	DIRECTIONS	INFUSION RANGE	DRUG MIXTURE	AMOUNT	DRUG/ mL	RUN AT	mL/h
Dopamine	Infusion		0.44		1–20 mcg/ kg/min	400 mg/ 250 mL	1600	mcg/mL		
	Take dose you want in mcg ÷ by drug index number = mL/h on pump									
Epinephrine	Infusion	1 mcg/min = 4 mL/h 2 mcg/min = 8 mL/h 3 mcg/min = 11 mL/h 4 mcg/min = 15 mL/h			1–4 mcg/min	4 mg/ 250 mL	16	mcg/mL		
	Ordered mcg dose/min ÷ mcg/mL × 60 min/h =								___	mL/h
Fenoldapam	Infusion		0.0110		0.01–1.6 mcg/ kg/min	10 mg/ 250 mL	40	mcg/mL		
	Take dose you want in mcg ÷ by drug index number = mL/h on pump									
Heparin	100 u/kg = 6100 u 200 u/kg = 12,200 u 300 u/kg = 18,300 u 400 u/kg = 24,400 u									
Isoproterenol	Infusion				5 mcg/min	1 mg/ 250 mL	4	mcg/mL		
	Ordered mcg dose/min ÷ mcg/mL × 60 min/h =								75	mL/h
Lidocaine	Infusion	1 mg/min = 7.5 mL/h			1–4 mg/min	2 g/ 250 mL	8	mg/mL	___	
	Ordered mg/min ÷ mg/mL × 60 min/h =								___	mL/h
Nitroglycerin	Infusion	3 mcg/min = 1 mL/h			3–200 mcg/min	50 mg/ 250 mL	200	mcg/mL	___	
	Ordered mcg/min ÷ mcg/mL × 60 min/h =								___	mL/h
Nitroprusside	Infusion	6.7 mcg/min = 1 mL/h			5–300 mcg/min	100 mg/ 250 mL	400	mcg/mL	___	
	Ordered mcg/min ÷ mcg/mL × 60 min/h =								___	mL/h
Norepinephrine	Infusion	1 mcg/min = 4 mL/h 2 mcg/min = 8 mL/h 3 mcg/min = 11 mL/h 4 mcg/min = 15 mL/h 5 mcg/min = 19 mL/h			2–20 mcg/min	4 mg/ 250 mL	16	mcg/mL		
	Ordered mcg dose/min ÷ mcg/mL × 60 min/h =								___	mL/h
Phenylephrine	Infusion	1.3 mcg/min = 1 mL/h			10–200 mcg/min	20 mg/ 250 mL	80	mcg/mL		
	Ordered mcg/min ÷ mcg/mL × 60 min/h =								___	mL/h
Primacor	0.05 mg/kg = 3.05 mg			Give load over 10 min		40 mg/ 200 mL	0.2	mg/mL		
	mg to give ÷ mg/mL = 15 mL				15 mL × (60 min/h ÷ 10 min) =				91.5	mL/h × 10 min
	Infusion		0.05		0.5 mcg/ kg/min	40 mg/ 200 mL	200	mcg/mL	___	
	Take dose you want in mcg ÷ by drug index number = mL/h on pump									
Trimethaphan	Infusion		—		0.3–6 mg/min	500 mg/ 500 mL	1	mg/mL	___	
	Ordered mg/min ÷ mg/mL × 60 min/h =								___	mL/h
Vasopressin	0.02 u/min = 3 mL/h 0.04 u/min = 6 mL/h					40 u/ 100 mL	400	u/mL		

62 kg									
DRUG	**ORDERED AMOUNT**	**TOTAL DOSE TO GIVE**	**DRUG INDEX NUMBER**	**DIRECTIONS**	**INFUSION RANGE**	**DRUG MIXTURE**	**AMOUNT**	**DRUG/ mL**	**RUN AT mL/h**
Aminophylline	5 mg/kg =	310 mg		Give mg/kg load over 20 min		500 mg/ 250 mL	2 mg/mL		—
	mg to give ÷ mg/mL =	155 mL			155	mL × (60 min/h ÷ 20 min) =			**465** mL/h × 20 min
	Infusion				0.5–1 mg/kg/h	500 mg/ 250 mL	2 mg/mL		
						mg dose ordered × kg ÷ mg/mL =			___ mL/h
Amiodarone	Loading dose			Load **150 mg** over 10 min		900 mg/ 500 mL	1.8 mg/mL		—
				Ordered mg load dose (150 mg) ÷ mg/mL (1.8 mg/mL) = 83 mL to give × (60 min/h ÷ 10 min) = mL/h to set on pump					**500** mL/h × 83 mL
	Infusion			Run at **1 mg/ min** × 6 h		900 mg/ 500 mL	1.8 mg/mL		
				Ordered mg dose (1 mg/min) ÷ mg/mL (1.8 mg/mL) = ___ × 60 min/h = mL/h to set on pump					**33** mL/h × 6 h
	Infusion			Run at **0.5 mg/ min** × 18 h		900 mg/ 500 mL	1.8 mg/mL		
				Ordered mg dose (0.5 mg/min) ÷ mg/mL (1.8 mg/mL) = ___ × 60 min/h = mL/h to set on pump					**17** mL/h × 18 h
Amrinone	0.75 mg/kg =	46.5 mg		Give mg/kg load over 10 min		300 mg/ 120 mL	2.5 mg/mL		—
	mg to give ÷ mg/mL =	19 mL			18.6	mL × (60 min/h ÷ 10 min) =			**111.6** mL/h × 10 min
	Infusion		0.67		5–10 mcg/ kg/min	300 mg/ 120 mL	2500 mcg/mL		—
				Take dose you want in mcg ÷ by drug index number = mL/h on pump					
Brevibloc	Infusion		2.69		50–100 mcg/ kg/min	2.5 g/ 250 mL	10,000 mcg/mL		___ mL/h
				Take dose you want in mcg ÷ by drug index number = mL/h on pump					
Cardene	Infusion		—		0.5–10 mg/h	25 mg 250 mL	0.1 mg/mL		—
				Ordered mg dose ÷ mg/mL = mL/h to set on pump					___ mL/h
Cardizem	0.25 mg/kg =	15.5 mg		Give mg/kg load over 20 min		50 mg/ 100 mL	0.5 mg/mL		
	mg to give ÷ mg/mL =	31 mL			31	mL × (60 min/h ÷ 20 min) =			**93** mL/h
	0.35 mg/kg =	21.7 mg		May repeat loading dose in 15 min			0.5 mg/mL		—
	mg to give ÷ mg/mL =	43 mL			43.4	mL × (60 min/h ÷ 20 min) =			**130** mL/h
	Infusion				5–15 mg/h				—
				Ordered mg dose ÷ mg/mL = mL/h to set on pump					___ mL/h
Desmopressin	0.3 mcg/kg =	19 mcg		Give dose over 20–30 min			4 mcg/vial		
Dobutamine	Infusion		0.54		2.5–40 mcg/kg/ min	250 mg/ 125 mL	2000 mcg/mL		
				Take dose you want in mcg ÷ by drug index number = mL/h on pump					

(continues)

62 kg (continued)

DRUG	ORDERED AMOUNT	TOTAL DOSE TO GIVE	DRUG INDEX NUMBER	DIRECTIONS	INFUSION RANGE	DRUG MIXTURE	AMOUNT	DRUG/ mL	RUN AT	mL/h
Dopamine	Infusion		0.43		1–20 mcg/ kg/min	400 mg/ 250 mL	1600	mcg/mL		
	Take dose you want in mcg ÷ by drug index number = mL/h on pump									
Epinephrine	Infusion	1 mcg/min = 4 mL/h 2 mcg/min = 8 mL/h 3 mcg/min = 11 mL/h 4 mcg/min = 15 mL/h			1–4 mcg/min	4 mg/ 250 mL	16	mcg/mL		
	Ordered mcg dose/min ÷ mcg/mL × 60 min/h =								___	mL/h
Fenoldapam	Infusion		0.0108		0.01–1.6 mcg/ kg/min	10 mg/ 250 mL	40	mcg/mL		
	Take dose you want in mcg ÷ by drug index number = mL/h on pump									
Heparin	100 u/kg = 6200 u 200 u/kg = 12,400 u 300 u/kg = 18,600 u 400 u/kg = 24,800 u									
Isoproterenol	Infusion				5 mcg/min	1 mg/ 250 mL	4	mcg/mL		
	Ordered mcg dose/min ÷ mcg/mL × 60 min/h =								75	mL/h
Lidocaine	Infusion	1 mg/min = 7.5 mL/h			1–4 mg/min	2 g/ 250 mL	8	mg/mL	___	
	Ordered mg/min ÷ mg/mL × 60 min/h =								___	mL/h
Nitroglycerin	Infusion	3 mcg/min = 1 mL/h			3–200 mcg/min	50 mg/ 250 mL	200	mcg/mL	___	
	Ordered mcg/min ÷ mcg/mL × 60 min/h =								___	mL/h
Nitroprusside	Infusion	6.7 mcg/min = 1 mL/h			5–300 mcg/min	100 mg/ 250 mL	400	mcg/mL	___	
	Ordered mcg/min ÷ mcg/mL × 60 min/h =								___	mL/h
Norepinephrine	Infusion	1 mcg/min = 4 mL/h 2 mcg/min = 8 mL/h 3 mcg/min = 11 mL/h 4 mcg/min = 15 mL/h 5 mcg/min = 19 mL/h			2–20 mcg/min	4 mg/ 250 mL	16	mcg/mL		
	Ordered mcg dose/min ÷ mcg/mL × 60 min/h =								___	mL/h
Phenylephrine	Infusion	1.3 mcg/min = 1 mL/h			10–200 mcg/min	20 mg/ 250 mL	80	mcg/mL		
	Ordered mcg/min ÷ mcg/mL × 60 min/h =								___	mL/h
Primacor	0.05 mg/kg = 3.1 mg			Give load over 10 min		40 mg/ 200 mL	0.2	mg/mL		
	mg to give ÷ mg/mL = 16 mL				16	mL × (60 min/h ÷ 10 min) =			93	mL/h × 10 min
	Infusion		0.05		0.5 mcg/ kg/min	40 mg/ 200 mL	200	mcg/mL	___	
	Take dose you want in mcg ÷ by drug index number = mL/h on pump									
Trimethaphan	Infusion		___		0.3–6 mg/min	500 mg/ 500 mL	1	mg/mL	___	
	Ordered mg/min ÷ mg/mL × 60 min/h =								___	mL/h
Vasopressin		0.02 u/min = 3 mL/h 0.04 u/min = 6 mL/h				40 u/ 100 mL	400	u/mL		

63 kg

DRUG	ORDERED AMOUNT	TOTAL DOSE TO GIVE	DRUG INDEX NUMBER	DIRECTIONS	INFUSION RANGE	DRUG MIXTURE	AMOUNT	DRUG/mL	RUN AT	mL/h
Aminophylline	5 mg/kg =	315 mg		Give mg/kg load over 20 min		500 mg/ 250 mL	2 mg/mL		
	mg to give ÷ mg/mL =	158 mL			158	mL × (60 min/h ÷ 20 min) =			472.5	mL/h × 20 min
	Infusion				0.5–1 mg/kg/h	500 mg/ 250 mL	2 mg/mL		
				mg dose ordered × kg ÷ mg/mL =					___	mL/h
Amiodarone	Loading dose			Load **150 mg** over 10 min		900 mg/ 500 mL	1.8 mg/mL		___
				Ordered mg load dose (150 mg) ÷ mg/mL (1.8 mg/mL) = 83 mL to give × (60 min/h ÷ 10 min) = mL/h to set on pump					**500**	mL/h × 83 mL
	Infusion			Run at **1 mg/ min** × 6 h		900 mg/ 500 mL	1.8 mg/mL		
				Ordered mg dose (1 mg/min) ÷ mg/mL (1.8 mg/mL) = ___ × 60 min/h = mL/h to set on pump					33	mL/h × 6 h
	Infusion			Run at **0.5 mg/ min** × 18 h		900 mg/ 500 mL	1.8 mg/mL		
				Ordered mg dose (0.5 mg/min) ÷ mg/mL (1.8 mg/mL) = ___ × 60 min/h = mL/h to set on pump					17	mL/h × 18 h
Amrinone	0.75 mg/kg =	47.25 mg		Give mg/kg load over 10 min		300 mg/ 120 mL	2.5 mg/mL		___
	mg to give ÷ mg/mL =	19 mL			18.9	mL × (60 min/h ÷ 10 min) =			**113.4**	mL/h × 10 min
	Infusion		**0.66**		5–10 mcg/ kg/min	300 mg/ 120 mL	2500 mcg/mL		
				Take dose you want in mcg ÷ by drug index number = mL/h on pump					
Brevibloc	Infusion		**2.64**		50–100 mcg/ kg/min	2.5 g/ 250 mL	10,000 mcg/mL		___ mL/h
				Take dose you want in mcg ÷ by drug index number = mL/h on pump					
Cardene	Infusion		—		0.5–10 mg/h	25 mg 250 mL	0.1 mg/mL		___
				Ordered mg dose ÷ mg/mL = mL/h to set on pump						___ mL/h
Cardizem	0.25 mg/kg =	15.75 mg		Give mg/kg load over 20 min		50 mg/ 100 mL	0.5 mg/mL		___
	mg to give ÷ mg/mL =	32 mL			31.5	mL × (60 min/h ÷ 20 min) =			95	mL/h
	0.35 mg/kg =	22.05 mg		May repeat loading dose in 15 min			0.5 mg/mL		___
	mg to give ÷ mg/mL =	44 mL			44.1	mL × (60 min/h ÷ 20 min) =			132	mL/h
	Infusion				5–15 mg/h				___
				Ordered mg dose ÷ mg/mL = mL/h to set on pump						___ mL/h
Desmopressin	0.3 mcg/kg =	19 mcg		Give dose over 20–30 min			4 mcg/vial		
Dobutamine	Infusion		**0.53**		2.5–40 mcg/kg/ min	250 mg/ 125 mL	2000 mcg/mL		
				Take dose you want in mcg ÷ by drug index number = mL/h on pump					

(continues)

63 kg (continued)

DRUG	ORDERED AMOUNT	TOTAL DOSE TO GIVE	DRUG INDEX NUMBER	DIRECTIONS	INFUSION RANGE	DRUG MIXTURE	AMOUNT	DRUG/mL	RUN AT	mL/h
Dopamine	Infusion		0.42		1–20 mcg/kg/min	400 mg/250 mL	1600	mcg/mL		
	Take dose you want in mcg ÷ by drug index number = mL/h on pump									
Epinephrine	Infusion	1 mcg/min = 4 mL/h 2 mcg/min = 8 mL/h 3 mcg/min = 11 mL/h 4 mcg/min = 15 mL/h			1–4 mcg/min	4 mg/250 mL	16	mcg/mL		
		Ordered mcg dose/min ÷ mcg/mL × 60 min/h =							___	mL/h
Fenoldapam	Infusion		0.0106		0.01–1.6 mcg/kg/min	10 mg/250 mL	40	mcg/mL		
	Take dose you want in mcg ÷ by drug index number = mL/h on pump									
Heparin	100 u/kg = 6300 u 200 u/kg = 12,600 u 300 u/kg = 18,900 u 400 u/kg = 25,200 u									
Isoproterenol	Infusion				5 mcg/min	1 mg/250 mL	4	mcg/mL		
		Ordered mcg dose/min ÷ mcg/mL × 60 min/h =							75	mL/h
Lidocaine	Infusion	1 mg/min = 7.5 mL/h			1–4 mg/min	2 g/250 mL	8	mg/mL	___	
		Ordered mg/min ÷ mg/mL × 60 min/h =							___	mL/h
Nitroglycerin	Infusion	3 mcg/min = 1 mL/h			3–200 mcg/min	50 mg/250 mL	200	mcg/mL	___	
		Ordered mcg/min ÷ mcg/mL × 60 min/h =							___	mL/h
Nitroprusside	Infusion	6.7 mcg/min = 1 mL/h			5–300 mcg/min	100 mg/250 mL	400	mcg/mL	___	
		Ordered mcg/min ÷ mcg/mL × 60 min/h =							___	mL/h
Norepinephrine	Infusion	1 mcg/min = 4 mL/h 2 mcg/min = 8 mL/h 3 mcg/min = 11 mL/h 4 mcg/min = 15 mL/h 5 mcg/min = 19 mL/h			2–20 mcg/min	4 mg/250 mL	16	mcg/mL		
		Ordered mcg dose/min ÷ mcg/mL × 60 min/h =							___	mL/h
Phenylephrine	Infusion	1.3 mcg/min = 1 mL/h			10–200 mcg/min	20 mg/250 mL	80	mcg/mL		
		Ordered mcg/min ÷ mcg/mL × 60 min/h =							___	mL/h
Primacor	0.05 mg/kg = 3.15 mg			Give load over 10 min		40 mg/200 mL	0.2	mg/mL		
	mg to give ÷ mg/mL = 16 mL				16 mL × (60 min/h ÷ 10 min) =				94.5	mL/h × 10 min
	Infusion		0.05		0.5 mcg/kg/min	40 mg/200 mL	200	mcg/mL	___	
	Take dose you want in mcg ÷ by drug index number = mL/h on pump									
Trimethaphan	Infusion		___		0.3–6 mg/min	500 mg/500 mL	1	mg/mL	___	
		Ordered mg/min ÷ mg/mL × 60 min/h =							___	mL/h
Vasopressin		0.02 u/min = 3 mL/h 0.04 u/min = 6 mL/h				40 u/100 mL	400	u/mL		

64 kg

DRUG	ORDERED AMOUNT	TOTAL DOSE TO GIVE	DRUG INDEX NUMBER	DIRECTIONS	INFUSION RANGE	DRUG MIXTURE	AMOUNT	DRUG/mL	RUN AT	mL/h
Aminophylline	5 mg/kg =	320 mg		Give mg/kg load over 20 min		500 mg/ 250 mL	2 mg/mL		
	mg to give ÷ mg/mL =	160 mL			160	mL × (60 min/h ÷ 20 min) =			**480**	mL/h × 20 min
	Infusion				0.5–1 mg/kg/h	500 mg/ 250 mL	2 mg/mL			
					mg dose ordered × kg ÷ mg/mL =				___	mL/h
Amiodarone	Loading dose			Load **150 mg** over 10 min		900 mg/ 500 mL	1.8 mg/mL		—	
				Ordered mg load dose (150 mg) ÷ mg/mL (1.8 mg/mL) = 83 mL to give × (60 min/h ÷ 10 min) = mL/h to set on pump					**500**	mL/h × 83 mL
	Infusion			Run at **1 mg/ min** × 6 h		900 mg/ 500 mL	1.8 mg/mL			
				Ordered mg dose (1 mg/min) ÷ mg/mL (1.0 mg/mL) ___ × 60 min/h = mL/h to set on pump					**33**	mL/h × 6 h
	Infusion			Run at **0.5 mg/ min** × 18 h		900 mg/ 500 mL	1.8 mg/ml			
				Ordered mg dose (0.5 mg/min) ÷ mg/mL (1.8 mg/mL) = ___ × 60 min/h = mL/h to set on pump					**17**	mL/h × 18 h
Amrinone	0.75 mg/kg =	48 mg		Give mg/kg load over 10 min		300 mg/ 120 mL	2.5 mg/mL		—	
	mg to give ÷ mg/mL =	19 mL			19.2	mL × (60 min/h ÷ 10 min) =			**115.2**	mL/h × 10 min
	Infusion		**0.65**		5–10 mcg/ kg/min	300 mg/ 120 mL	2500 mcg/mL		—	
				Take dose you want in mcg ÷ by drug index number = mL/h on pump						
Brevibloc	Infusion		**2.60**		50–100 mcg/ kg/min	2.5 g/ 250 mL	10,000 mcg/mL		___	mL/h
				Take dose you want in mcg ÷ by drug index number = mL/h on pump						
Cardene	Infusion			—	0.5–10 mg/h	25 mg 250 mL	0.1 mg/mL		—	
				Ordered mg dose ÷ mg/mL = mL/h to set on pump					___	mL/h
Cardizem	0.25 mg/kg =	16 mg		Give mg/kg load over 20 min		50 mg/ 100 mL	0.5 mg/mL		—	
	mg to give ÷ mg/mL =	32 mL			32	mL × (60 min/h ÷ 20 min) =			**96**	mL/h
	0.35 mg/kg =	22.4 mg		May repeat loading dose in 15 min			0.5 mg/mL		—	
	mg to give ÷ mg/mL =	45 mL			44.8	mL × (60 min/h ÷ 20 min) =			**134**	mL/h
	Infusion				5–15 mg/h				—	
				Ordered mg dose ÷ mg/mL = mL/h to set on pump					___	mL/h
Desmopressin	0.3 mcg/kg =	19 mcg		Give dose over 20–30 min			4 mcg/vial			
Dobutamine	Infusion		**0.52**		2.5–40 mcg/kg/ min	250 mg/ 125 mL	2000 mcg/mL			
				Take dose you want in mcg ÷ by drug index number = mL/h on pump						

(continues)

64 kg (continued)

DRUG	ORDERED AMOUNT	TOTAL DOSE TO GIVE	DRUG INDEX NUMBER	DIRECTIONS	INFUSION RANGE	DRUG MIXTURE	AMOUNT	DRUG/mL	RUN AT	mL/h
Dopamine	Infusion		0.42		1–20 mcg/kg/min	400 mg/250 mL	1600	mcg/mL		
				Take dose you want in mcg ÷ by drug index number = mL/h on pump						
Epinephrine	Infusion	1 mcg/min = 4 mL/h 2 mcg/min = 8 mL/h 3 mcg/min = 11 mL/h 4 mcg/min = 15 mL/h			1–4 mcg/min	4 mg/250 mL	16	mcg/mL		
				Ordered mcg dose/min ÷ mcg/mL × 60 min/h =					___	mL/h
Fenoldapam	Infusion		0.0105		0.01–1.6 mcg/kg/min	10 mg/250 mL	40	mcg/mL		
				Take dose you want in mcg ÷ by drug index number = mL/h on pump						
Heparin	100 u/kg = 6400 u 200 u/kg = 12,800 u 300 u/kg = 19,200 u 400 u/kg = 25,600 u									
Isoproterenol	Infusion				5 mcg/min	1 mg/250 mL	4	mcg/mL		
				Ordered mcg dose/min ÷ mcg/mL × 60 min/h =					75	mL/h
Lidocaine	Infusion	1 mg/min = 7.5 mL/h			1–4 mg/min	2 g/250 mL	8	mg/mL	___	
				Ordered mg/min ÷ mg/mL × 60 min/h =					___	mL/h
Nitroglycerin	Infusion	3 mcg/min = 1 mL/h			3–200 mcg/min	50 mg/250 mL	200	mcg/mL	___	
				Ordered mcg/min ÷ mcg/mL × 60 min/h =					___	mL/h
Nitroprusside	Infusion	6.7 mcg/min = 1 mL/h			5–300 mcg/min	100 mg/250 mL	400	mcg/mL		
				Ordered mcg/min ÷ mcg/mL × 60 min/h =					___	mL/h
Norepinephrine	Infusion	1 mcg/min = 4 mL/h 2 mcg/min = 8 mL/h 3 mcg/min = 11 mL/h 4 mcg/min = 15 mL/h 5 mcg/min = 19 mL/h			2–20 mcg/min	4 mg/250 mL	16	mcg/mL		
				Ordered mcg dose/min ÷ mcg/mL × 60 min/h =					___	mL/h
Phenylephrine	Infusion	1.3 mcg/min = 1 mL/h			10–200 mcg/min	20 mg/250 mL	80	mcg/mL		
				Ordered mcg/min ÷ mcg/mL × 60 min/h =					___	mL/h
Primacor	0.05 mg/kg = 3.2 mg			Give load over 10 min		40 mg/200 mL	0.2	mg/mL		
	mg to give ÷ mg/mL = 16 mL				16 mL × (60 min/h ÷ 10 min) =				96	mL/h × 10 min
	Infusion		0.05		0.5 mcg/kg/min	40 mg/200 mL	200	mcg/mL	___	
				Take dose you want in mcg ÷ by drug index number = mL/h on pump						
Trimethaphan	Infusion		___		0.3–6 mg/min	500 mg/500 mL	1	mg/mL	___	
				Ordered mg/min ÷ mg/mL × 60 min/h =					___	mL/h
Vasopressin		0.02 u/min = 3 mL/h 0.04 u/min = 6 mL/h				40 u/100 mL	400	u/mL		

65　kg

DRUG	ORDERED AMOUNT	TOTAL DOSE TO GIVE	DRUG INDEX NUMBER	DIRECTIONS	INFUSION RANGE	DRUG MIXTURE	AMOUNT	DRUG/mL	RUN AT	mL/h
Aminophylline	5　mg/kg = 325　mg			Give mg/kg load over 20 min		500 mg/ 250 mL	2　mg/mL			
	mg to give ÷ mg/mL = 163　mL				163	mL × (60 min/h ÷ 20 min) =			**487.5**	mL/h × 20 min
	Infusion				0.5–1 mg/kg/h	500 mg/ 250 mL	2　mg/mL			
					mg dose ordered × kg ÷ mg/mL =				___	mL/h
Amiodarone	Loading dose			Load **150 mg** over 10 min		900 mg/ 500 mL	1.8　mg/mL		—	
				Ordered mg load dose (150 mg) ÷ mg/mL (1.8 mg/mL) = 83 mL to give × (60 min/h ÷ 10 min) = mL/h to set on pump					**500**	mL/h × 83 mL
	Infusion			Run at **1 mg/ min** × 6 h		900 mg/ 500 mL	1.8　mg/mL			
				Ordered mg dose (1 mg/min) ÷ mg/ml (1.8 mg/mL) = ___ × 60 min/h = mL/h to set on pump					**33**	mL/h × 6 h
	Infusion			Run at **0.5 mg/ min** × 18 h		900 mg/ 500 mL	1.8　mg/mL			
				Ordered mg dose (0.5 mg/min) ÷ mg/mL (1.8 mg/mL) = ___ × 60 min/h = mL/h to set on pump					**17**	mL/h × 18 h
Amrinone	0.75　mg/kg = 48.75　mg			Give mg/kg load over 10 min		300 mg/ 120 mL	2.5　mg/mL		—	
	mg to give ÷ mg/mL = 20　mL				19.5	mL × (60 min/h ÷ 10 min) =			**117**	mL/h × 10 min
	Infusion		0.64		5–10 mcg/ kg/min	300 mg/ 120 mL	2500　mcg/mL		—	
				Take dose you want in mcg ÷ by drug index number = mL/h on pump						
Brevibloc	Infusion		2.56		50–100 mcg/ kg/min	2.5 g/ 250 mL	10,000　mcg/mL		___	mL/h
				Take dose you want in mcg ÷ by drug index number = mL/h on pump						
Cardene	Infusion		—		0.5–10 mg/h	25 mg 250 mL	0.1　mg/mL			
				Ordered mg dose ÷ mg/mL = mL/h to set on pump					___	mL/h
Cardizem	0.25　mg/kg = 16.25　mg			Give mg/kg load over 20 min		50 mg/ 100 mL	0.5　mg/mL		—	
	mg to give ÷ mg/mL = 33　mL				32.5	mL × (60 min/h ÷ 20 min) =			**98**	mL/h
	0.35　mg/kg = 22.75　mg			May repeat loading dose in 15 min			0.5　mg/mL			
	mg to give ÷ mg/mL = 46　mL				45.5	mL × (60 min/h ÷ 20 min) =			**137**	mL/h
	Infusion				5–15 mg/h				—	
				Ordered mg dose ÷ mg/mL = mL/h to set on pump					___	mL/h
Desmopressin	0.3　mcg/kg = 20　mcg			Give dose over 20–30 min			4　mcg/vial			
Dobutamine	Infusion		0.51		2.5–40 mcg/kg/ min	250 mg/ 125 mL	2000　mcg/mL			
				Take dose you want in mcg ÷ by drug index number = mL/h on pump						

(continues)

65 kg (continued)

DRUG	ORDERED AMOUNT		TOTAL DOSE TO GIVE		DRUG INDEX NUMBER	DIRECTIONS	INFUSION RANGE	DRUG MIXTURE	AMOUNT	DRUG/mL	RUN AT	mL/h
Dopamine	Infusion				0.41		1–20 mcg/kg/min	400 mg/250 mL	1600	mcg/mL		
	Take dose you want in mcg ÷ by drug index number = mL/h on pump											
Epinephrine	Infusion		1 mcg/min = 4 mL/h 2 mcg/min = 8 mL/h 3 mcg/min = 11 mL/h 4 mcg/min = 15 mL/h				1–4 mcg/min	4 mg/250 mL	16	mcg/mL		
	Ordered mcg dose/min ÷ mcg/mL × 60 min/h =										___	mL/h
Fenoldapam	Infusion				0.0103		0.01–1.6 mcg/kg/min	10 mg/250 mL	40	mcg/mL		
	Take dose you want in mcg ÷ by drug index number = mL/h on pump											
Heparin	100 u/kg =	6500 u										
	200 u/kg =	13,000 u										
	300 u/kg =	19,500 u										
	400 u/kg =	26,000 u										
Isoproterenol	Infusion						5 mcg/min	1 mg/250 mL	4	mcg/mL		
	Ordered mcg dose/min ÷ mcg/mL × 60 min/h =										**75**	mL/h
Lidocaine	Infusion		1 mg/min = 7.5 mL/h				1–4 mg/min	2 g/250 mL	8	mg/mL	—	
	Ordered mg/min ÷ mg/mL × 60 min/h =										___	mL/h
Nitroglycerin	Infusion		3 mcg/min = 1 mL/h				3–200 mcg/min	50 mg/250 mL	200	mcg/mL	—	
	Ordered mcg/min ÷ mcg/mL × 60 min/h =										___	mL/h
Nitroprusside	Infusion		6.7 mcg/min = 1 mL/h				5–300 mcg/min	100 mg/250 mL	400	mcg/mL	—	
	Ordered mcg/min ÷ mcg/mL × 60 min/h =										___	mL/h
Norepinephrine	Infusion		1 mcg/min = 4 mL/h 2 mcg/min = 8 mL/h 3 mcg/min = 11 mL/h 4 mcg/min = 15 mL/h 5 mcg/min = 19 mL/h				2–20 mcg/min	4 mg/250 mL	16	mcg/mL		
	Ordered mcg dose/min ÷ mcg/mL × 60 min/h =										___	mL/h
Phenylephrine	Infusion		1.3 mcg/min = 1 mL/h				10–200 mcg/min	20 mg/250 mL	80	mcg/mL		
	Ordered mcg/min ÷ mcg/mL × 60 min/h =										___	mL/h
Primacor	0.05 mg/kg =	3.25 mg				Give load over 10 min		40 mg/200 mL	0.2	mg/mL		
	mg to give ÷ mg/mL =	16 mL						16	mL × (60 min/h ÷ 10 min) =		**97.5**	mL/h × 10 min
	Infusion				0.05		0.5 mcg/kg/min	40 mg/200 mL	200	mcg/mL	—	
	Take dose you want in mcg ÷ by drug index number = mL/h on pump											
Trimethaphan	Infusion				—		0.3–6 mg/min	500 mg/500 mL	1	mg/mL	—	
	Ordered mg/min ÷ mg/mL × 60 min/h =										___	mL/h
Vasopressin			0.02 u/min = 3 mL/h 0.04 u/min = 6 mL/h					40 u/100 mL	400	u/mL		

66 kg

DRUG	ORDERED AMOUNT	TOTAL DOSE TO GIVE	DRUG INDEX NUMBER	DIRECTIONS	INFUSION RANGE	DRUG MIXTURE	AMOUNT	DRUG/ mL	RUN AT	mL/h
Aminophylline	5 mg/kg =	**330** mg		Give mg/kg load over 20 min		500 mg/ 250 mL		2 mg/mL		
	mg to give ÷ mg/mL =	**165** mL			**165**	mL × (60 min/h ÷ 20 min) =			**495**	mL/h × 20 min
	Infusion				0.5–1 mg/kg/h	500 mg/ 250 mL		2 mg/mL		
					mg dose ordered × kg ÷ mg/mL =				___	mL/h
Amiodarone	Loading dose			Load **150 mg** over 10 min		900 mg/ 500 mL		1.8 mg/mL	**—**	
				Ordered mg load dose (150 mg) ÷ mg/mL (1.8 mg/mL) = 83 mL to give × (60 min/h ÷ 10 min) = mL/h to set on pump					**500**	mL/h × 83 mL
	Infusion			Run at **1 mg/ min** × 6 h		900 mg/ 500 mL		1.8 mg/mL		
				Ordered mg dose (1 mg/min) ÷ mg/mL (1.8 mg/mL) = ___ × 60 min/h = mL/h to set on pump					**33**	mL/h × 6 h
	Infusion			Run at **0.5 mg/ min** × 18 h		900 mg/ 500 mL		1.8 mg/mL		
				Ordered mg dose (0.5 mg/min) ÷ mg/mL (1.8 mg/mL) = ___ × 60 min/h = mL/h to set on pump					**17**	mL/h × 18 h
Amrinone	0.75 mg/kg =	**49.5** mg		Give mg/kg load over 10 min		300 mg/ 120 mL		2.5 mg/mL	**—**	
	mg to give ÷ mg/mL =	**20** mL			**19.8**	mL × (60 min/h ÷ 10 min) =			**118.8**	mL/h × 10 min
	Infusion		**0.63**		5–10 mcg/ kg/min	300 mg/ 120 mL		2500 mcg/mL	**—**	
				Take dose you want in mcg ÷ by drug index number = mL/h on pump						
Brevibloc	Infusion		**2.52**		50–100 mcg/ kg/min	2.5 g/ 250 mL		10,000 mcg/mL	___	mL/h
				Take dose you want in mcg ÷ by drug index number = mL/h on pump						
Cardene	Infusion		**—**		0.5–10 mg/h	25 mg 250 mL		0.1 mg/mL	**—**	
				Ordered mg dose ÷ mg/mL = mL/h to set on pump					___	mL/h
Cardizem	0.25 mg/kg =	**16.5** mg		Give mg/kg load over 20 min		50 mg/ 100 mL		0.5 mg/mL		
	mg to give ÷ mg/mL =	**33** mL			**33**	mL × (60 min/h ÷ 20 min) =			**99**	mL/h
	0.35 mg/kg =	**23.1** mg		May repeat loading dose in 15 min				0.5 mg/mL	**—**	
	mg to give ÷ mg/mL =	**46** mL			**46.2**	mL × (60 min/h ÷ 20 min) =			**139**	mL/h
	Infusion				5–15 mg/h				**—**	
				Ordered mg dose ÷ mg/mL = mL/h to set on pump					___	mL/h
Desmopressin	0.3 mcg/kg =	**20** mcg		Give dose over 20–30 min				4 mcg/vial		
Dobutamine	Infusion		**0.50**		2.5–40 mcg/kg/ min	250 mg/ 125 mL		2000 mcg/mL		
				Take dose you want in mcg ÷ by drug index number = mL/h on pump						

(continues)

66 kg (continued)

DRUG	ORDERED AMOUNT	TOTAL DOSE TO GIVE		DRUG INDEX NUMBER	DIRECTIONS	INFUSION RANGE	DRUG MIXTURE	AMOUNT	DRUG/mL	RUN AT	mL/h
Dopamine	Infusion			0.40		1–20 mcg/kg/min	400 mg/250 mL	1600	mcg/mL		
	Take dose you want in mcg ÷ by drug index number = mL/h on pump										
Epinephrine	Infusion	1 mcg/min = 4 mL/h 2 mcg/min = 8 mL/h 3 mcg/min = 11 mL/h 4 mcg/min = 15 mL/h				1–4 mcg/min	4 mg/250 mL	16	mcg/mL		
	Ordered mcg dose/min ÷ mcg/mL × 60 min/h =									___	mL/h
Fenoldapam	Infusion			0.0102		0.01–1.6 mcg/kg/min	10 mg/250 mL	40	mcg/mL		
	Take dose you want in mcg ÷ by drug index number = mL/h on pump										
Heparin	100 u/kg = 200 u/kg = 300 u/kg = 400 u/kg =	6600 u 13,200 u 19,800 u 26,400 u									
Isoproterenol	Infusion					5 mcg/min	1 mg/250 mL	4	mcg/mL		
	Ordered mcg dose/min ÷ mcg/mL × 60 min/h =									75	mL/h
Lidocaine	Infusion	1 mg/min = 7.5 mL/h				1–4 mg/min	2 g/250 mL	8	mg/mL	—	
	Ordered mg/min ÷ mg/mL × 60 min/h =									___	mL/h
Nitroglycerin	Infusion	3 mcg/min = 1 mL/h				3–200 mcg/min	50 mg/250 mL	200	mcg/mL	—	
	Ordered mcg/min ÷ mcg/mL × 60 min/h =									___	mL/h
Nitroprusside	Infusion	6.7 mcg/min = 1 mL/h				5–300 mcg/min	100 mg/250 mL	400	mcg/mL	—	
	Ordered mcg/min ÷ mcg/mL × 60 min/h =									___	mL/h
Norepinephrine	Infusion	1 mcg/min = 4 mL/h 2 mcg/min = 8 mL/h 3 mcg/min = 11 mL/h 4 mcg/min = 15 mL/h 5 mcg/min = 19 mL/h				2–20 mcg/min	4 mg/250 mL	16	mcg/mL		
	Ordered mcg dose/min ÷ mcg/mL × 60 min/h =									___	mL/h
Phenylephrine	Infusion	1.3 mcg/min = 1 mL/h				10–200 mcg/min	20 mg/250 mL	80	mcg/mL		
	Ordered mcg/min ÷ mcg/mL × 60 min/h =									___	mL/h
Primacor	0.05 mg/kg =	3.3 mg			Give load over 10 min		40 mg/200 mL	0.2	mg/mL		
	mg to give ÷ mg/mL =	17 mL				17	mL × (60 min/h ÷ 10 min) =			99	mL/h × 10 min
	Infusion			0.05		0.5 mcg/kg/min	40 mg/200 mL	200	mcg/mL	—	
	Take dose you want in mcg ÷ by drug index number = mL/h on pump										
Trimethaphan	Infusion			—		0.3–6 mg/min	500 mg/500 mL	1	mg/mL	—	
	Ordered mg/min ÷ mg/mL × 60 min/h =									___	mL/h
Vasopressin		0.02 u/min = 3 mL/h 0.04 u/min = 6 mL/h					40 u/100 mL	400	u/mL		

67 kg										
DRUG	**ORDERED AMOUNT**	**TOTAL DOSE TO GIVE**		**DRUG INDEX NUMBER**	**DIRECTIONS**	**INFUSION RANGE**	**DRUG MIXTURE**	**AMOUNT**	**DRUG/ mL**	**RUN AT** **mL/h**
Aminophylline	5 mg/kg =	335 mg			Give mg/kg load over 20 min		500 mg/ 250 mL		2 mg/mL	
	mg to give ÷ mg/mL =	168 mL				168	mL × (60 min/h ÷ 20 min) =			502.5 mL/h × 20 min
	Infusion					0.5–1 mg/kg/h	500 mg/ 250 mL		2 mg/mL	
						mg dose ordered × kg ÷ mg/mL =				___ mL/h
Amiodarone	Loading dose				Load **150 mg** over 10 min		900 mg/ 500 mL		1.8 mg/mL	___
					Ordered mg load dose (150 mg) ÷ mg/mL (1.8 mg/mL) = 83 mL to give × (60 min/h ÷ 10 min) = mL/h to set on pump					500 mL/h × 83 mL
	Infusion				Run at **1 mg/ min** × 6 h		900 mg/ 500 mL		1.8 mg/mL	
					Ordered mg dose (1 mg/min) ÷ mg/mL (1.8 mg/mL) = ____ × 60 min/h = mL/h to set on pump					33 mL/h × 6 h
	Infusion				Run at **0.5 mg/ min** × 18 h		900 mg/ 500 mL		1.8 mg/mL	
					Ordered mg dose (0.5 mg/min) ÷ mg/mL (1.8 mg/mL) = ____ × 60 min/h = mL/h to set on pump					17 mL/h × 18 h
Amrinone	0.75 mg/kg =	50.25 mg			Give mg/kg load over 10 min		300 mg/ 120 mL		2.5 mg/mL	___
	mg to give ÷ mg/mL =	20 mL				20.1	mL × (60 min/h ÷ 10 min) =			120.6 mL/h × 10 min
	Infusion			0.62		5–10 mcg/ kg/min	300 mg/ 120 mL	2500	mcg/mL	
					Take dose you want in mcg ÷ by drug index number = mL/h on pump					
Brevibloc	Infusion			2.49		50–100 mcg/ kg/min	2.5 g/ 250 mL	10,000	mcg/mL	___ mL/h
					Take dose you want in mcg ÷ by drug index number = mL/h on pump					
Cardene	Infusion			—		0.5–10 mg/h	25 mg 250 mL		0.1 mg/mL	___
					Ordered mg dose ÷ mg/mL = mL/h to set on pump					___ mL/h
Cardizem	0.25 mg/kg =	16.75 mg			Give mg/kg load over 20 min		50 mg/ 100 mL		0.5 mg/mL	___
	mg to give ÷ mg/mL =	34 mL				33.5	mL × (60 min/h ÷ 20 min) =			101 mL/h
	0.35 mg/kg =	23.45 mg			May repeat loading dose in 15 min				0.5 mg/mL	
	mg to give ÷ mg/mL =	47 mL				46.9	mL × (60 min/h ÷ 20 min) =			141 mL/h
	Infusion					5–15 mg/h				___
					Ordered mg dose ÷ mg/mL = mL/h to set on pump					___ mL/h
Desmopressin	0.3 mcg/kg =	20 mcg			Give dose over 20–30 min				4 mcg/vial	
Dobutamine	Infusion			0.50		2.5–40 mcg/kg/ min	250 mg/ 125 mL	2000	mcg/mL	
					Take dose you want in mcg ÷ by drug index number = mL/h on pump					

(continues)

67 kg (continued)

DRUG	ORDERED AMOUNT	TOTAL DOSE TO GIVE	DRUG INDEX NUMBER	DIRECTIONS	INFUSION RANGE	DRUG MIXTURE	AMOUNT	DRUG/mL	RUN AT	mL/h
Dopamine	Infusion		0.40		1–20 mcg/kg/min	400 mg/250 mL	1600	mcg/mL		
				Take dose you want in mcg ÷ by drug index number = mL/h on pump						
Epinephrine	Infusion	1 mcg/min = 4 mL/h 2 mcg/min = 8 mL/h 3 mcg/min = 11 mL/h 4 mcg/min = 15 mL/h			1–4 mcg/min	4 mg/250 mL	16	mcg/mL		
				Ordered mcg dose/min ÷ mcg/mL × 60 min/h =					___	mL/h
Fenoldapam	Infusion		0.0100		0.01–1.6 mcg/kg/min	10 mg/250 mL	40	mcg/mL		
				Take dose you want in mcg ÷ by drug index number = mL/h on pump						
Heparin	100 u/kg = 6700 u 200 u/kg = 13,400 u 300 u/kg = 20,100 u 400 u/kg = 26,800 u									
Isoproterenol	Infusion				5 mcg/min	1 mg/250 mL	4	mcg/mL		
				Ordered mcg dose/min ÷ mcg/mL × 60 min/h =					75	mL/h
Lidocaine	Infusion	1 mg/min = 7.5 mL/h			1–4 mg/min	2 g/250 mL	8	mg/mL	___	
				Ordered mg/min ÷ mg/mL × 60 min/h =					___	mL/h
Nitroglycerin	Infusion	3 mcg/min = 1 mL/h			3–200 mcg/min	50 mg/250 mL	200	mcg/mL	___	
				Ordered mcg/min ÷ mcg/mL × 60 min/h =					___	mL/h
Nitroprusside	Infusion	6.7 mcg/min = 1 mL/h			5–300 mcg/min	100 mg/250 mL	400	mcg/mL	___	
				Ordered mcg/min ÷ mcg/mL × 60 min/h =					___	mL/h
Norepinephrine	Infusion	1 mcg/min = 4 mL/h 2 mcg/min = 8 mL/h 3 mcg/min = 11 mL/h 4 mcg/min = 15 mL/h 5 mcg/min = 19 mL/h			2–20 mcg/min	4 mg/250 mL	16	mcg/mL		
				Ordered mcg dose/min ÷ mcg/mL × 60 min/h =					___	mL/h
Phenylephrine	Infusion	1.3 mcg/min = 1 mL/h			10–200 mcg/min	20 mg/250 mL	80	mcg/mL		
				Ordered mcg/min ÷ mcg/mL × 60 min/h =					___	mL/h
Primacor	0.05 mg/kg = 3.35 mg			Give load over 10 min		40 mg/200 mL	0.2	mg/mL		
	mg to give ÷ mg/mL = 17 mL					17	mL × (60 min/h ÷ 10 min) =		100.5	mL/h × 10 min
	Infusion		0.05		0.5 mcg/kg/min	40 mg/200 mL	200	mcg/mL	___	
				Take dose you want in mcg ÷ by drug index number = mL/h on pump						
Trimethaphan	Infusion		—		0.3–6 mg/min	500 mg/500 mL	1	mg/mL	___	
				Ordered mg/min ÷ mg/mL × 60 min/h =					___	mL/h
Vasopressin	0.02 u/min = 3 mL/h 0.04 u/min = 6 mL/h					40 u/100 mL	400	u/mL		

63 kg

DRUG	ORDERED AMOUNT	TOTAL DOSE TO GIVE	DRUG INDEX NUMBER	DIRECTIONS	INFUSION RANGE	DRUG MIXTURE	AMOUNT	DRUG/mL	RUN AT	mL/h
Aminophylline	5 mg/kg =	340 mg		Give mg/kg load over 20 min		500 mg/ 250 mL	2 mg/mL			
	mg to give ÷ mg/mL =	170 mL			170	mL × (60 min/h ÷ 20 min) =			510	mL/h × 20 min
	Infusion				0.5–1 mg/kg/h	500 mg/ 250 mL	2 mg/mL			
						mg dose ordered × kg ÷ mg/mL =			___	mL/h
Amiodarone	Loading dose			Load **150 mg** over 10 min		900 mg/ 500 mL	1.8 mg/mL		___	
				Ordered mg load dose (150 mg) ÷ mg/mL (1.8 mg/mL) = 83 mL to give × (60 min/h ÷ 10 min) = mL/h to set on pump					500	mL/h × 83 mL
	Infusion			Run at **1 mg/ min** × 6 h	900 mg/ 500 mL		1.8 mg/mL			
				Ordered mg dose (1 mg/min) ÷ mg/mL (1.8 mg/mL) = _____ × 60 min/h = mL/h to set on pump					33	mL/h × 6 h
	Infusion			Run at **0.5 mg/ min** × 18 h	900 mg/ 500 mL		1.8 mg/mL			
				Ordered mg dose (0.5 mg/min) ÷ mg/mL (1.8 mg/mL) = _____ × 60 min/h = mL/h to set on pump					17	mL/h × 18 h
Amrinone	0.75 mg/kg =	51 mg		Give mg/kg load over 10 min		300 mg/ 120 mL	2.5 mg/mL		___	
	mg to give ÷ mg/mL =	20 mL			20.4	mL × (60 min/h ÷ 10 min) =			122.4	mL/h × 10 min
	Infusion		0.61		5–10 mcg/ kg/min	300 mg/ 120 mL	2500 mcg/mL		___	
				Take dose you want in mcg ÷ by drug index number = mL/h on pump						
Brevibloc	Infusion		2.45		50–100 mcg/ kg/min	2.5 g/ 250 mL	10,000 mcg/mL		___	mL/h
				Take dose you want in mcg ÷ by drug index number = mL/h on pump						
Cardene	Infusion			—	0.5–10 mg/h	25 mg 250 mL	0.1 mg/mL		___	
				Ordered mg dose ÷ mg/mL = mL/h to set on pump					___	mL/h
Cardizem	0.25 mg/kg =	17 mg		Give mg/kg load over 20 min		50 mg/ 100 mL	0.5 mg/mL		___	
	mg to give ÷ mg/mL =	34 mL			34	mL × (60 min/h ÷ 20 min) =			102	mL/h
	0.35 mg/kg =	23.8 mg		May repeat loading dose in 15 min			0.5 mg/mL		___	
	mg to give ÷ mg/mL =	48 mL			47.6	mL × (60 min/h ÷ 20 min) =			143	mL/h
	Infusion				5–15 mg/h				___	
				Ordered mg dose ÷ mg/mL = mL/h to set on pump					___	mL/h
Desmopressin	0.3 mcg/kg =	20 mcg		Give dose over 20–30 min			4 mcg/vial			
Dobutamine	Infusion		0.49		2.5–40 mcg/kg/ min	250 mg/ 125 mL	2000 mcg/mL			
				Take dose you want in mcg ÷ by drug index number = mL/h on pump						

(continues)

68 kg (continued)

DRUG	ORDERED AMOUNT		TOTAL DOSE TO GIVE		DRUG INDEX NUMBER	DIRECTIONS	INFUSION RANGE	DRUG MIXTURE	AMOUNT	DRUG/ mL	RUN AT	mL/h
Dopamine	Infusion				0.39		1–20 mcg/ kg/min	400 mg/ 250 mL	1600	mcg/mL		
	Take dose you want in mcg ÷ by drug index number = mL/h on pump											
Epinephrine	Infusion		1 mcg/min = 4 mL/h 2 mcg/min = 8 mL/h 3 mcg/min = 11 mL/h 4 mcg/min = 15 mL/h				1–4 mcg/min	4 mg/ 250 mL	16	mcg/mL		
			Ordered mcg dose/min ÷ mcg/mL × 60 min/h =								___	mL/h
Fenoldapam	Infusion				0.0099		0.01–1.6 mcg/ kg/min	10 mg/ 250 mL	40	mcg/mL		
	Take dose you want in mcg ÷ by drug index number = mL/h on pump											
Heparin	100 u/kg =	6800 u										
	200 u/kg =	13,600 u										
	300 u/kg =	20,400 u										
	400 u/kg =	27,200 u										
Isoproterenol	Infusion						5 mcg/min	1 mg/ 250 mL	4	mcg/mL		
			Ordered mcg dose/min ÷ mcg/mL × 60 min/h =								75	mL/h
Lidocaine	Infusion		1 mg/min = 7.5 mL/h				1–4 mg/min	2 g/ 250 mL	8	mg/mL	___	
			Ordered mg/min ÷ mg/mL × 60 min/h =								___	mL/h
Nitroglycerin	Infusion		3 mcg/min = 1 mL/h				3–200 mcg/min	50 mg/ 250 mL	200	mcg/mL	___	
			Ordered mcg/min ÷ mcg/mL × 60 min/h =								___	mL/h
Nitroprusside	Infusion		6.7 mcg/min = 1 mL/h				5–300 mcg/min	100 mg/ 250 mL	400	mcg/mL	___	
			Ordered mcg/min ÷ mcg/mL × 60 min/h =								___	mL/h
Norepinephrine	Infusion		1 mcg/min = 4 mL/h 2 mcg/min = 8 mL/h 3 mcg/min = 11 mL/h 4 mcg/min = 15 mL/h 5 mcg/min = 19 mL/h				2–20 mcg/min	4 mg/ 250 mL	16	mcg/mL		
			Ordered mcg dose/min ÷ mcg/mL × 60 min/h =								___	mL/h
Phenylephrine	Infusion		1.3 mcg/min = 1 mL/h				10–200 mcg/min	20 mg/ 250 mL	80	mcg/mL		
			Ordered mcg/min ÷ mcg/mL × 60 min/h =								___	mL/h
Primacor	0.05 mg/kg =	3.4 mg				Give load over 10 min		40 mg/ 200 mL	0.2	mg/mL		
	mg to give ÷ mg/mL =	17 mL					17	mL × (60 min/h ÷ 10 min) =			102	mL/h × 10 min
	Infusion				0.05		0.5 mcg/ kg/min	40 mg/ 200 mL	200	mcg/mL	___	
	Take dose you want in mcg ÷ by drug index number = mL/h on pump											
Trimethaphan	Infusion				—		0.3–6 mg/min	500 mg/ 500 mL	1	mg/mL	___	
			Ordered mg/min ÷ mg/mL × 60 min/h =								___	mL/h
Vasopressin			0.02 u/min = 3 mL/h 0.04 u/min = 6 mL/h					40 u/ 100 mL	400	u/mL		

69 kg

DRUG	ORDERED AMOUNT	TOTAL DOSE TO GIVE	DRUG INDEX NUMBER	DIRECTIONS	INFUSION RANGE	DRUG MIXTURE	AMOUNT	DRUG/ mL	RUN AT	mL/h
Aminophylline	5 mg/kg = 345 mg			Give mg/kg load over 20 min		500 mg/ 250 mL	2 mg/mL		
	mg to give ÷ mg/mL = 173 mL				173	mL × (60 min/h ÷ 20 min) =			517.5	mL/h × 20 min
	Infusion				0.5–1 mg/kg/h	500 mg/ 250 mL	2 mg/mL		
					mg dose ordered × kg ÷ mg/mL =				___	mL/h
Amiodarone	Loading dose			Load **150 mg** over 10 min		900 mg/ 500 mL	1.8 mg/mL	___	
				Ordered mg load dose (150 mg) ÷ mg/mL (1.8 mg/mL) = 83 mL to give × (60 min/h ÷ 10 min) = mL/h to set on pump					500	mL/h × 83 mL
	Infusion			Run at **1 mg/ min** × 6 h	900 mg/ 500 mL		1.8 mg/mL		
				Ordered mg dose (1 mg/min) ÷ mg/mL (1.8 mg/mL) = ____ × 60 min/h = mL/h to set on pump					33	mL/h × 6 h
	Infusion			Run at **0.5 mg/ min** × 18 h	900 mg/ 500 mL		1.8 mg/mL		
				Ordered mg dose (0.5 mg/min) ÷ mg/mL (1.8 mg/mL) = ____ × 60 min/h = mL/h to set on pump					17	mL/h × 18 h
Amrinone	0.75 mg/kg = 51.75 mg			Give mg/kg load over 10 min		300 mg/ 120 mL	2.5 mg/mL	___	
	mg to give ÷ mg/mL = 21 mL				20.7	mL × (60 min/h ÷ 10 min) =			124.2	mL/h × 10 min
	Infusion		0.60		5–10 mcg/ kg/min	300 mg/ 120 mL	2500 mcg/mL	___	
				Take dose you want in mcg ÷ by drug index number = mL/h on pump						
Brevibloc	Infusion		2.41		50–100 mcg/ kg/min	2.5 g/ 250 mL	10,000 mcg/mL	___	mL/h
				Take dose you want in mcg ÷ by drug index number = mL/h on pump						
Cardene	Infusion		—		0.5–10 mg/h	25 mg 250 mL	0.1 mg/mL	___	
				Ordered mg dose ÷ mg/mL = mL/h to set on pump						___ mL/h
Cardizem	0.25 mg/kg = 17.25 mg			Give mg/kg load over 20 min		50 mg/ 100 mL	0.5 mg/mL	___	
	mg to give ÷ mg/mL = 35 mL				34.5	mL × (60 min/h ÷ 20 min) =			104	mL/h
	0.35 mg/kg = 24.15 mg			May repeat loading dose in 15 min			0.5 mg/mL	___	
	mg to give ÷ mg/mL = 48 mL				48.3	mL × (60 min/h ÷ 20 min) =			145	mL/h
	Infusion				5–15 mg/h				___	
				Ordered mg dose ÷ mg/mL = mL/h to set on pump						___ mL/h
Desmopressin	0.3 mcg/kg = 21 mcg			Give dose over 20–30 min			4 mcg/vial		
Dobutamine	Infusion		0.48		2.5–40 mcg/kg/ min	250 mg/ 125 mL	2000 mcg/mL		
				Take dose you want in mcg ÷ by drug index number = mL/h on pump						

(continues)

69 kg (continued)

DRUG	ORDERED AMOUNT	TOTAL DOSE TO GIVE	DRUG INDEX NUMBER	DIRECTIONS	INFUSION RANGE	DRUG MIXTURE	AMOUNT	DRUG/ mL	RUN AT	mL/h
Dopamine	Infusion		0.39		1–20 mcg/ kg/min	400 mg/ 250 mL	1600	mcg/mL		
				Take dose you want in mcg ÷ by drug index number = mL/h on pump						
Epinephrine	Infusion	1 mcg/min = 4 mL/h 2 mcg/min = 8 mL/h 3 mcg/min = 11 mL/h 4 mcg/min = 15 mL/h			1–4 mcg/min	4 mg/ 250 mL	16	mcg/mL		
				Ordered mcg dose/min ÷ mcg/mL × 60 min/h =					___	mL/h
Fenoldapam	Infusion		0.0097		0.01–1.6 mcg/ kg/min	10 mg/ 250 mL	40	mcg/mL		
				Take dose you want in mcg ÷ by drug index number = mL/h on pump						
Heparin	100 u/kg = 6900 u 200 u/kg = 13,800 u 300 u/kg = 20,700 u 400 u/kg = 27,600 u									
Isoproterenol	Infusion				5 mcg/min	1 mg/ 250 mL	4	mcg/mL		
				Ordered mcg dose/min ÷ mcg/mL × 60 min/h =					75	mL/h
Lidocaine	Infusion	1 mg/min = 7.5 mL/h			1–4 mg/min	2 g/ 250 mL	8	mg/mL	___	
				Ordered mg/min ÷ mg/mL × 60 min/h =					___	mL/h
Nitroglycerin	Infusion	3 mcg/min = 1 mL/h			3–200 mcg/min	50 mg/ 250 mL	200	mcg/mL	___	
				Ordered mcg/min ÷ mcg/mL × 60 min/h =					___	mL/h
Nitroprusside	Infusion	6.7 mcg/min = 1 mL/h			5–300 mcg/min	100 mg/ 250 mL	400	mcg/mL	___	
				Ordered mcg/min ÷ mcg/mL × 60 min/h =					___	mL/h
Norepinephrine	Infusion	1 mcg/min = 4 mL/h 2 mcg/min = 8 mL/h 3 mcg/min = 11 mL/h 4 mcg/min = 15 mL/h 5 mcg/min = 19 mL/h			2–20 mcg/min	4 mg/ 250 mL	16	mcg/mL		
				Ordered mcg dose/min ÷ mcg/mL × 60 min/h =					___	mL/h
Phenylephrine	Infusion	1.3 mcg/min = 1 mL/h			10–200 mcg/min	20 mg/ 250 mL	80	mcg/mL		
				Ordered mcg/min ÷ mcg/mL × 60 min/h =					___	mL/h
Primacor	0.05 mg/kg = 3.45 mg			Give load over 10 min		40 mg/ 200 mL	0.2	mg/mL		
	mg to give ÷ mg/mL =	17 mL			17	mL × (60 min/h ÷ 10 min) =			103.5	mL/h × 10 min
	Infusion		0.05		0.5 mcg/ kg/min	40 mg/ 200 mL	200	mcg/mL	___	
				Take dose you want in mcg ÷ by drug index number = mL/h on pump						
Trimethaphan	Infusion			—	0.3–6 mg/min	500 mg/ 500 mL	1	mg/mL	___	
				Ordered mg/min ÷ mg/mL × 60 min/h =					___	mL/h
Vasopressin		0.02 u/min = 3 mL/h 0.04 u/min = 6 mL/h				40 u/ 100 mL	400	u/mL		

70 kg

DRUG	ORDERED AMOUNT	TOTAL DOSE TO GIVE	DRUG INDEX NUMBER	DIRECTIONS	INFUSION RANGE	DRUG MIXTURE	AMOUNT DRUG/mL	RUN AT mL/h
Aminophylline	5 mg/kg =	350 mg		Give mg/kg load over 20 min		500 mg/ 250 mL	2 mg/mL	
	mg to give ÷ mg/mL =	175 mL			175	mL × (60 min/h ÷ 20 min) =		<u>525</u> mL/h × 20 min
		Infusion			0.5–1 mg/kg/h	500 mg/ 250 mL	2 mg/mL	
					mg dose ordered × kg ÷ mg/mL =			___ mL/h
Amiodarone		Loading dose		Load **150 mg** over 10 min		900 mg/ 500 mL	1.8 mg/mL	___
				Ordered mg load dose (150 mg) ÷ mg/mL (1.8 mg/mL) = 83 mL to give × (60 min/h ÷ 10 min) = mL/h to set on pump				<u>500</u> mL/h × 83 mL
		Infusion		Run at **1 mg/ min** × 6 h	900 mg/ 500 mL		1.8 mg/mL	
				Ordered mg dose (1 mg/min) ÷ mg/mL (1.8 mg/mL) = × (60 min/h = mL/h to set on pump				<u>33</u> mL/h × 6 h
		Infusion		Run at **0.5 mg/ min** × 18 h	900 mg/ 500 mL		1.8 mg/mL	
				Ordered mg dose (0.5 mg/min) ÷ mg/mL (1.8 mg/mL) = ____ × 60 min/h = mL/h to set on pump				<u>17</u> mL/h × 18 h
Amrinone	0.75 mg/kg =	52.5 mg		Give mg/kg load over 10 min		300 mg/ 120 mL	2.5 mg/mL	___
	mg to give ÷ mg/mL =	21 mL			21	mL × (60 min/h ÷ 10 min) =		<u>126</u> mL/h × 10 min
		Infusion	0.59		5–10 mcg/ kg/min	300 mg/ 120 mL	2500 mcg/mL	___
				Take dose you want in mcg ÷ by drug index number = mL/h on pump				
Brevibloc		Infusion	2.38		50–100 mcg/ kg/min	2.5 g/ 250 mL	10,000 mcg/mL	___ mL/h
				Take dose you want in mcg ÷ by drug index number = mL/h on pump				
Cardene		Infusion		—	0.5–10 mg/h	25 mg 250 mL	0.1 mg/mL	___
				Ordered mg dose ÷ mg/mL = mL/h to set on pump				___ mL/h
Cardizem	0.25 mg/kg =	17.5 mg		Give mg/kg load over 20 min		50 mg/ 100 mL	0.5 mg/mL	___
	mg to give ÷ mg/mL =	35 mL			35	mL × (60 min/h ÷ 20 min) =		<u>105</u> mL/h
	0.35 mg/kg =	24.5 mg		May repeat loading dose in 15 min			0.5 mg/mL	___
	mg to give ÷ mg/mL =	49 mL			49	mL × (60 min/h ÷ 20 min) =		<u>147</u> mL/h
		Infusion			5–15 mg/h			___
				Ordered mg dose ÷ mg/mL = mL/h to set on pump				___ mL/h
Desmopressin	0.3 mcg/kg =	21 mcg		Give dose over 20–30 min			4 mcg/vial	
Dobutamine		Infusion	0.48		2.5–40 mcg/kg/ min	250 mg/ 125 mL	2000 mcg/mL	
				Take dose you want in mcg ÷ by drug index number = mL/h on pump				

(continues)

70   kg (continued)

DRUG	ORDERED AMOUNT	TOTAL DOSE TO GIVE	DRUG INDEX NUMBER	DIRECTIONS	INFUSION RANGE	DRUG MIXTURE	AMOUNT	DRUG/mL	RUN AT	mL/h
Dopamine	Infusion		0.38		1–20 mcg/kg/min	400 mg/250 mL	1600	mcg/mL		
	Take dose you want in mcg ÷ by drug index number = mL/h on pump									
Epinephrine	Infusion	1 mcg/min = 4 mL/h 2 mcg/min = 8 mL/h 3 mcg/min = 11 mL/h 4 mcg/min = 15 mL/h			1–4 mcg/min	4 mg/250 mL	16	mcg/mL		
		Ordered mcg dose/min ÷ mcg/mL × 60 min/h =							___	mL/h
Fenoldapam	Infusion		0.0096		0.01–1.6 mcg/kg/min	10 mg/250 mL	40	mcg/mL		
		Take dose you want in mcg ÷ by drug index number = mL/h on pump								
Heparin	100 u/kg = 200 u/kg = 300 u/kg = 400 u/kg =	7000 u 14,000 u 21,000 u 28,000 u								
Isoproterenol	Infusion				5 mcg/min	1 mg/250 mL	4	mcg/mL		
		Ordered mcg dose/min ÷ mcg/mL × 60 min/h =							75	mL/h
Lidocaine	Infusion	1 mg/min = 7.5 mL/h			1–4 mg/min	2 g/250 mL	8	mg/mL	___	
		Ordered mg/min ÷ mg/mL × 60 min/h =							___	mL/h
Nitroglycerin	Infusion	3 mcg/min = 1 mL/h			3–200 mcg/min	50 mg/250 mL	200	mcg/mL	___	
		Ordered mcg/min ÷ mcg/mL × 60 min/h =							___	mL/h
Nitroprusside	Infusion	6.7 mcg/min = 1 mL/h			5–300 mcg/min	100 mg/250 mL	400	mcg/mL	___	
		Ordered mcg/min ÷ mcg/mL × 60 min/h =							___	mL/h
Norepinephrine	Infusion	1 mcg/min = 4 mL/h 2 mcg/min = 8 mL/h 3 mcg/min = 11 mL/h 4 mcg/min = 15 mL/h 5 mcg/min = 19 mL/h			2–20 mcg/min	4 mg/250 mL	16	mcg/mL		
		Ordered mcg dose/min ÷ mcg/mL × 60 min/h =							___	mL/h
Phenylephrine	Infusion	1.3 mcg/min = 1 mL/h			10–200 mcg/min	20 mg/250 mL	80	mcg/mL		
		Ordered mcg/min ÷ mcg/mL × 60 min/h =							___	mL/h
Primacor	0.05 mg/kg =	3.5 mg		Give load over 10 min		40 mg/200 mL	0.2	mg/mL		
	mg to give ÷ mg/mL =	18 mL			18	mL × (60 min/h ÷ 10 min) =			105	mL/h × 10 min
	Infusion		0.05		0.5 mcg/kg/min	40 mg/200 mL	200	mcg/mL	___	
		Take dose you want in mcg ÷ by drug index number = mL/h on pump								
Trimethaphan	Infusion		—		0.3–6 mg/min	500 mg/500 mL	1	mg/mL	___	
		Ordered mg/min ÷ mg/mL × 60 min/h =							___	mL/h
Vasopressin		0.02 u/min = 3 mL/h 0.04 u/min = 6 mL/h				40 u/100 mL	400	u/mL		

71 kg

DRUG	ORDERED AMOUNT	TOTAL DOSE TO GIVE	DRUG INDEX NUMBER	DIRECTIONS	INFUSION RANGE	DRUG MIXTURE	AMOUNT DRUG/mL	RUN AT mL/h
Aminophylline	5 mg/kg = **355** mg			Give mg/kg load over 20 min		500 mg/ 250 mL	2 mg/mL	
	mg to give ÷ mg/mL = **178** mL				**178** mL × (60 min/h ÷ 20 min) =			**532.5** mL/h × 20 min
	Infusion				0.5–1 mg/kg/h	500 mg/ 250 mL	2 mg/mL	
				mg dose ordered × kg ÷ mg/mL =				___ mL/h
Amiodarone	Loading dose			Load **150 mg** over 10 min		900 mg/ 500 mL	1.8 mg/mL	___
				Ordered mg load dose (150 mg) ÷ mg/mL (1.8 mg/mL) = 83 mL to give × (60 min/h ÷ 10 min) = mL/h to set on pump				**500** mL/h × 83 mL
	Infusion			Run at **1 mg/ min** × 6 h		900 mg/ 500 mL	1.8 mg/mL	
				Ordered mg dose (1 mg/min) ÷ mg/mL (1.0 mg/mL) = ___ × 60 min/h − mL/h to set on pump				**33** mL/h × 6 h
	Infusion			Run at **0.5 mg/ min** × 18 h		900 mg/ 500 mL	1.8 mg/mL	
				Ordered mg dose (0.5 mg/min) ÷ mg/mL (1.8 mg/mL) = ___ × 60 min/h − mL/h to set on pump				**17** mL/h × 18 h
Amrinone	0.75 mg/kg = **53.25** mg			Give mg/kg load over 10 min		300 mg/ 120 mL	2.5 mg/mL	___
	mg to give ÷ mg/mL = **21** mL				**21.3** mL × (60 min/h ÷ 10 min) =			**127.8** mL/h × 10 min
	Infusion		**0.59**		5–10 mcg/ kg/min	300 mg/ 120 mL	2500 mcg/mL	___
				Take dose you want in mcg ÷ by drug index number = mL/h on pump				
Brevibloc	Infusion		**2.35**		50–100 mcg/ kg/min	2.5 g/ 250 mL	10,000 mcg/mL	___ mL/h
				Take dose you want in mcg ÷ by drug index number = mL/h on pump				
Cardene	Infusion		—		0.5–10 mg/h	25 mg 250 mL	0.1 mg/mL	___
				Ordered mg dose ÷ mg/mL = mL/h to set on pump				___ mL/h
Cardizem	0.25 mg/kg = **17.75** mg			Give mg/kg load over 20 min		50 mg/ 100 mL	0.5 mg/mL	___
	mg to give ÷ mg/mL = **36** mL				**35.5** mL × (60 min/h ÷ 20 min) =			**107** mL/h
	0.35 mg/kg = **24.85** mg			May repeat loading dose in 15 min			0.5 mg/mL	___
	mg to give ÷ mg/mL = **50** mL				**49.7** mL × (60 min/h ÷ 20 min) =			**149** mL/h
	Infusion				5–15 mg/h			___
				Ordered mg dose ÷ mg/mL = mL/h to set on pump				___ mL/h
Desmopressin	0.3 mcg/kg = **21** mcg			Give dose over 20–30 min			4 mcg/vial	
Dobutamine	Infusion		**0.47**		2.5–40 mcg/kg/ min	250 mg/ 125 mL	2000 mcg/mL	
				Take dose you want in mcg ÷ by drug index number = mL/h on pump				

(continues)

71 kg (continued)

DRUG	ORDERED AMOUNT	TOTAL DOSE TO GIVE	DRUG INDEX NUMBER	DIRECTIONS	INFUSION RANGE	DRUG MIXTURE	AMOUNT	DRUG/ mL	RUN AT	mL/h
Dopamine	Infusion		0.38		1–20 mcg/ kg/min	400 mg/ 250 mL	1600	mcg/mL		
	Take dose you want in mcg ÷ by drug index number = mL/h on pump									
Epinephrine	Infusion	1 mcg/min = 4 mL/h 2 mcg/min = 8 mL/h 3 mcg/min = 11 mL/h 4 mcg/min = 15 mL/h			1–4 mcg/min	4 mg/ 250 mL	16	mcg/mL		
		Ordered mcg dose/min ÷ mcg/mL × 60 min/h =								___ mL/h
Fenoldapam	Infusion		0.0094		0.01–1.6 mcg/ kg/min	10 mg/ 250 mL	40	mcg/mL		
	Take dose you want in mcg ÷ by drug index number = mL/h on pump									
Heparin	100 u/kg = 200 u/kg = 300 u/kg = 400 u/kg =	7100 u 14,200 u 21,300 u 28,400 u								
Isoproterenol	Infusion				5 mcg/min	1 mg/ 250 mL	4	mcg/mL		
		Ordered mcg dose/min ÷ mcg/mL × 60 min/h =								**75** mL/h
Lidocaine	Infusion	1 mg/min = 7.5 mL/h			1–4 mg/min	2 g/ 250 mL	8	mg/mL		___
		Ordered mg/min ÷ mg/mL × 60 min/h =								___ mL/h
Nitroglycerin	Infusion	3 mcg/min = 1 mL/h			3–200 mcg/min	50 mg/ 250 mL	200	mcg/mL		___
		Ordered mcg/min ÷ mcg/mL × 60 min/h =								___ mL/h
Nitroprusside	Infusion	6.7 mcg/min = 1 mL/h			5–300 mcg/min	100 mg/ 250 mL	400	mcg/mL		___
		Ordered mcg/min ÷ mcg/mL × 60 min/h =								___ mL/h
Norepinephrine	Infusion	1 mcg/min = 4 mL/h 2 mcg/min = 8 mL/h 3 mcg/min = 11 mL/h 4 mcg/min = 15 mL/h 5 mcg/min = 19 mL/h			2–20 mcg/min	4 mg/ 250 mL	16	mcg/mL		
		Ordered mcg dose/min ÷ mcg/mL × 60 min/h =								___ mL/h
Phenylephrine	Infusion	1.3 mcg/min = 1 mL/h			10–200 mcg/min	20 mg/ 250 mL	80	mcg/mL		
		Ordered mcg/min ÷ mcg/mL × 60 min/h =								___ mL/h
Primacor	0.05 mg/kg =	3.55 mg		Give load over 10 min		40 mg/ 200 mL	0.2	mg/mL		
	mg to give ÷ mg/mL =	18 mL			18	mL × (60 min/h ÷ 10 min) =			**106.5**	mL/h × 10 min
	Infusion		0.05		0.5 mcg/ kg/min	40 mg/ 200 mL	200	mcg/mL		___
	Take dose you want in mcg ÷ by drug index number = mL/h on pump									
Trimethaphan	Infusion		—		0.3–6 mg/min	500 mg/ 500 mL	1	mg/mL		___
		Ordered mg/min ÷ mg/mL × 60 min/h =								___ mL/h
Vasopressin		0.02 u/min = 3 mL/h 0.04 u/min = 6 mL/h				40 u/ 100 mL	400	u/mL		

72 kg										
DRUG	**ORDERED AMOUNT**	**TOTAL DOSE TO GIVE**	**DRUG INDEX NUMBER**	**DIRECTIONS**	**INFUSION RANGE**	**DRUG MIXTURE**	**AMOUNT**	**DRUG/ mL**	**RUN AT**	**mL/h**
Aminophylline	5　mg/kg =	360　mg		Give mg/kg load over 20 min		500 mg/ 250 mL	2　mg/mL			
	mg to give ÷ mg/mL =	180　mL			180	mL × (60 min/h ÷ 20 min) =			**540**	mL/h × 20 min
	Infusion				0.5–1 mg/kg/h	500 mg/ 250 mL	2　mg/mL			
					mg dose ordered × kg ÷ mg/mL =				___	mL/h
Amiodarone	Loading dose			Load **150 mg** over 10 min		900 mg/ 500 mL	1.8　mg/mL		___	
				Ordered mg load dose (150 mg) ÷ mg/mL (1.8 mg/mL) = 83 mL to give × (60 min/h ÷ 10 min) = mL/h to set on pump					**500**	mL/h × 83 mL
	Infusion			Run at **1 mg/ min** × 6 h		900 mg/ 500 mL	1.8　mg/mL			
				Ordered mg dose (1 mg/min) ÷ mg/mL (1.8 mg/mL) = ____ × 60 min/h = mL/h to set on pump					**33**	mL/h × 6 h
	Infusion			Run at **0.5 mg/ min** × 18 h		900 mg/ 500 mL	1.8　mg/mL			
				Ordered mg dose (0.5 mg/min) ÷ mg/mL (1.8 mg/mL) = ____ × 60 min/h = mL/h to set on pump					**17**	mL/h × 18 h
Amrinone	0.75　mg/kg =	54　mg		Give mg/kg load over 10 min		300 mg/ 120 mL	2.5　mg/mL		___	
	mg to give ÷ mg/mL =	22　mL			21.6	mL × (60 min/h ÷ 10 min) =			**129.6**	mL/h × 10 min
	Infusion		0.58		5–10 mcg/ kg/min	300 mg/ 120 mL	2500　mcg/mL		___	
				Take dose you want in mcg ÷ by drug index number = mL/h on pump						
Brevibloc	Infusion		2.31		50–100 mcg/ kg/min	2.5 g/ 250 mL	10,000　mcg/mL		___	mL/h
				Take dose you want in mcg ÷ by drug index number = mL/h on pump						
Cardene	Infusion			—	0.5–10 mg/h	25 mg 250 mL	0.1　mg/mL		___	
				Ordered mg dose ÷ mg/mL = mL/h to set on pump					___	mL/h
Cardizem	0.25　mg/kg =	18　mg		Give mg/kg load over 20 min		50 mg/ 100 mL	0.5　DRUG/mL		___	
	mg to give ÷ mg/mL =	36　mL			36	mL × (60 min/h ÷ 20 min) =			**108**	mL/h
	0.35　mg/kg =	25.2　mg		May repeat loading dose in 15 min			0.5　mg/mL		___	
	mg to give ÷ mg/mL =	50　mL			50.4	mL × (60 min/h ÷ 20 min) =			**151**	mL/h
	Infusion				5–15 mg/h				___	
				Ordered mg dose ÷ mg/mL = mL/h to set on pump					___	mL/h
Desmopressin	0.3　mcg/kg =	22　mcg		Give dose over 20–30 min			4　mcg/vial			
Dobutamine	Infusion		0.46		2.5–40 mcg/kg/ min	250 mg/ 125 mL	2000　mcg/mL			
				Take dose you want in mcg ÷ by drug index number = mL/h on pump						

(continues)

72 kg (continued)

DRUG	ORDERED AMOUNT	TOTAL DOSE TO GIVE	DRUG INDEX NUMBER	DIRECTIONS	INFUSION RANGE	DRUG MIXTURE	AMOUNT	DRUG/ mL	RUN AT	mL/h
Dopamine	Infusion		0.37		1–20 mcg/ kg/min	400 mg/ 250 mL	1600	mcg/mL		
	Take dose you want in mcg ÷ by drug index number = mL/h on pump									
Epinephrine	Infusion	1 mcg/min = 4 mL/h 2 mcg/min = 8 mL/h 3 mcg/min = 11 mL/h 4 mcg/min = 15 mL/h			1–4 mcg/min	4 mg/ 250 mL	16	mcg/mL		
		Ordered mcg dose/min ÷ mcg/mL × 60 min/h =							___	mL/h
Fenoldapam	Infusion		0.0093		0.01–1.6 mcg/ kg/min	10 mg/ 250 mL	40	mcg/mL		
	Take dose you want in mcg ÷ by drug index number = mL/h on pump									
Heparin	100 u/kg = 7200 u 200 u/kg = 14,400 u 300 u/kg = 21,600 u 400 u/kg = 28,800 u									
Isoproterenol	Infusion				5 mcg/min	1 mg/ 250 mL	4	mcg/mL		
		Ordered mcg dose/min ÷ mcg/mL × 60 min/h =							75	mL/h
Lidocaine	Infusion	1 mg/min = 7.5 mL/h			1–4 mg/min	2 g/ 250 mL	8	mg/mL	___	
		Ordered mg/min ÷ mg/mL × 60 min/h =							___	mL/h
Nitroglycerin	Infusion	3 mcg/min = 1 mL/h			3–200 mcg/min	50 mg/ 250 mL	200	mcg/mL	___	
		Ordered mcg/min ÷ mcg/mL × 60 min/h =							___	mL/h
Nitroprusside	Infusion	6.7 mcg/min = 1 mL/h			5–300 mcg/min	100 mg/ 250 mL	400	mcg/mL	___	
		Ordered mcg/min ÷ mcg/mL × 60 min/h =							___	mL/h
Norepinephrine	Infusion	1 mcg/min = 4 mL/h 2 mcg/min = 8 mL/h 3 mcg/min = 11 mL/h 4 mcg/min = 15 mL/h 5 mcg/min = 19 mL/h			2–20 mcg/min	4 mg/ 250 mL	16	mcg/mL		
		Ordered mcg dose/min ÷ mcg/mL × 60 min/h =							___	mL/h
Phenylephrine	Infusion	1.3 mcg/min = 1 mL/h			10–200 mcg/min	20 mg/ 250 mL	80	mcg/mL		
		Ordered mcg/min ÷ mcg/mL × 60 min/h =							___	mL/h
Primacor	0.05 mg/kg = 3.6 mg			Give load over 10 min		40 mg/ 200 mL	0.2	mg/mL		
	mg to give ÷ mg/mL = 18 mL					18	mL × (60 min/h ÷ 10 min) =		108	mL/h × 10 min
	Infusion		0.05		0.5 mcg/ kg/min	40 mg/ 200 mL	200	mcg/mL	___	
	Take dose you want in mcg ÷ by drug index number = mL/h on pump									
Trimethaphan	Infusion		___		0.3–6 mg/min	500 mg/ 500 mL	1	mg/mL	___	
		Ordered mg/min ÷ mg/mL × 60 min/h =							___	mL/h
Vasopressin		0.02 u/min = 3 mL/h 0.04 u/min = 6 mL/h				40 u/ 100 mL	400	u/mL		

73 kg

DRUG	ORDERED AMOUNT	TOTAL DOSE TO GIVE	DRUG INDEX NUMBER	DIRECTIONS	INFUSION RANGE	DRUG MIXTURE	AMOUNT	DRUG/ mL	RUN AT	mL/h
Aminophylline	5 mg/kg =	365 mg		Give mg/kg load over 20 min		500 mg/ 250 mL	2 mg/mL		
	mg to give ÷ mg/mL =	183 mL			183	mL × (60 min/h ÷ 20 min) =			<u>547.5</u>	mL/h × 20 min
	Infusion				0.5–1 mg/kg/h	500 mg/ 250 mL	2 mg/mL		
					mg dose ordered × kg ÷ mg/mL =					___ mL/h
Amiodarone	Loading dose			Load **150 mg** over 10 min		900 mg/ 500 mL	1.8 mg/mL		___
				Ordered mg load dose (150 mg) ÷ mg/mL (1.8 mg/mL) = 83 mL to give × (60 min/h ÷ 10 min) = mL/h to set on pump					<u>500</u>	mL/h × 83 mL
	Infusion			Run at **1 mg/ min)(6 h**		900 mg/ 500 ml	1.8 mg/mL		
				Ordered mg dose (1 mg/min) ÷ mg/mL (1.8 mg/mL) = _____ × 60 min/h = mL/h to set on pump					<u>33</u>	mL/h × 6 h
	Infusion			Run at **0.5 mg/ min × 18 h**		900 mg/ 500 mL	1 8 mg/ml		
				Ordered mg dose (0.5 mg/min) ÷ mg/mL (1.8 mg/mL) = _____ × 60 min/h = mL/h to set on pump					<u>17</u>	mL/h × 18 h
Amrinone	0.75 mg/kg =	54.75 mg		Give mg/kg load over 10 min		300 mg/ 120 mL	2.5 mg/mL		___
	mg to give ÷ mg/mL =	22 mL			21.9	mL × (60 min/h ÷ 10 min) =			<u>131.4</u>	mL/h × 10 min
	Infusion		0.57		5–10 mcg/ kg/min	300 mg/ 120 mL	2500 mcg/mL		___
				Take dose you want in mcg ÷ by drug index number = mL/h on pump						
Brevibloc	Infusion		2.28		50–100 mcg/ kg/min	2.5 g/ 250 mL	10,000 mcg/mL		___ mL/h
				Take dose you want in mcg ÷ by drug index number = mL/h on pump						
Cardene	Infusion		___		0.5–10 mg/h	25 mg 250 mL	0.1 mg/mL		___
				Ordered mg dose ÷ mg/mL = mL/h to set on pump						___ mL/h
Cardizem	0.25 mg/kg =	18.25 mg		Give mg/kg load over 20 min		50 mg/ 100 mL	0.5 mg/mL		___
	mg to give ÷ mg/mL =	37 mL			36.5	mL × (60 min/h ÷ 20 min) =			<u>110</u>	mL/h
	0.35 mg/kg =	25.55 mg		May repeat loading dose in 15 min			0.5 mg/mL		
	mg to give ÷ mg/mL =	51 mL			51.1	mL × (60 min/h ÷ 20 min) =			<u>153</u>	mL/h
	Infusion				5–15 mg/h				___
				Ordered mg dose ÷ mg/mL = mL/h to set on pump						___ mL/h
Desmopressin	0.3 mcg/kg =	22 mcg		Give dose over 20–30 min				4 mcg/vial	
Dobutamine	Infusion		0.46		2.5–40 mcg/kg/ min	250 mg/ 125 mL	2000 mcg/mL		
				Take dose you want in mcg ÷ by drug index number = mL/h on pump						

(continues)

73 kg (continued)

DRUG	ORDERED AMOUNT		TOTAL DOSE TO GIVE		DRUG INDEX NUMBER	DIRECTIONS	INFUSION RANGE	DRUG MIXTURE	AMOUNT	DRUG/mL	RUN AT	mL/h
Dopamine	Infusion				0.37		1–20 mcg/kg/min	400 mg/250 mL	1600	mcg/mL		
	Take dose you want in mcg ÷ by drug index number = mL/h on pump											
Epinephrine	Infusion		1 mcg/min = 4 mL/h 2 mcg/min = 8 mL/h 3 mcg/min = 11 mL/h 4 mcg/min = 15 mL/h				1–4 mcg/min	4 mg/250 mL	16	mcg/mL		
	Ordered mcg dose/min ÷ mcg/mL × 60 min/h =										___	mL/h
Fenoldapam	Infusion				0.0092		0.01–1.6 mcg/kg/min	10 mg/250 mL	40	mcg/mL		
	Take dose you want in mcg ÷ by drug index number = mL/h on pump											
Heparin	100 u/kg =	7300 u										
	200 u/kg =	14,600 u										
	300 u/kg =	21,900 u										
	400 u/kg =	29,200 u										
Isoproterenol	Infusion						5 mcg/min	1 mg/250 mL	4	mcg/mL		
	Ordered mcg dose/min ÷ mcg/mL × 60 min/h =										75	mL/h
Lidocaine	Infusion		1 mg/min = 7.5 mL/h				1–4 mg/min	2 g/250 mL	8	mg/mL	—	
	Ordered mg/min ÷ mg/mL × 60 min/h =										___	mL/h
Nitroglycerin	Infusion		3 mcg/min = 1 mL/h				3–200 mcg/min	50 mg/250 mL	200	mcg/mL	—	
	Ordered mcg/min ÷ mcg/mL × 60 min/h =										___	mL/h
Nitroprusside	Infusion		6.7 mcg/min = 1 mL/h				5–300 mcg/min	100 mg/250 mL	400	mcg/mL	—	
	Ordered mcg/min ÷ mcg/mL × 60 min/h =										___	mL/h
Norepinephrine	Infusion		1 mcg/min = 4 mL/h 2 mcg/min = 8 mL/h 3 mcg/min = 11 mL/h 4 mcg/min = 15 mL/h 5 mcg/min = 19 mL/h				2–20 mcg/min	4 mg/250 mL	16	mcg/mL		
	Ordered mcg dose/min ÷ mcg/mL × 60 min/h =										___	mL/h
Phenylephrine	Infusion		1.3 mcg/min = 1 mL/h				10–200 mcg/min	20 mg/250 mL	80	mcg/mL		
	Ordered mcg/min ÷ mcg/mL × 60 min/h =										___	mL/h
Primacor	0.05 mg/kg =	3.65 mg			Give load over 10 min			40 mg/200 mL	0.2	mg/mL		
	mg to give ÷ mg/mL =	18 mL				18	mL × (60 min/h ÷ 10 min) =				109.5	mL/h × 10 min
	Infusion				0.05		0.5 mcg/kg/min	40 mg/200 mL	200	mcg/mL	—	
	Take dose you want in mcg ÷ by drug index number = mL/h on pump											
Trimethaphan	Infusion		—				0.3–6 mg/min	500 mg/500 mL	1	mg/mL	—	
	Ordered mg/min ÷ mg/mL × 60 min/h =										___	mL/h
Vasopressin			0.02 u/min = 3 mL/h 0.04 u/min = 6 mL/h					40 u/100 mL	400	u/mL		

74 kg

DRUG	ORDERED AMOUNT	TOTAL DOSE TO GIVE	DRUG INDEX NUMBER	DIRECTIONS	INFUSION RANGE	DRUG MIXTURE	AMOUNT DRUG/ mL	RUN AT mL/h
Aminophylline	5 mg/kg =	**370** mg		Give mg/kg load over 20 min		500 mg/ 250 mL	2 mg/mL	
	mg to give ÷ mg/mL =	**185** mL			**185**	mL × (60 min/h ÷ 20 min) =		**555** mL/h × 20 min
	Infusion				0.5–1 mg/kg/h	500 mg/ 250 mL	2 mg/mL	
					mg dose ordered × kg ÷ mg/mL =			___ mL/h
Amiodarone	Loading dose			Load **150 mg** over 10 min		900 mg/ 500 mL	1.8 mg/mL	___
				Ordered mg load dose (150 mg) ÷ mg/mL (1.8 mg/mL) = 83 mL to give × (60 min/h ÷ 10 min) = mL/h to set on pump				**500** mL/h × 83 mL
	Infusion			Run at **1 mg/ min** × 6 h		900 mg/ 500 ml	1.8 mg/mL	
				Ordered mg dose (1 mg/min) ÷ mg/mL (1.8 mg/mL) = ___ × 60 min/h = mL/h to set on pump				**33** mL/h × 6 h
	Infusion			Run at **0.5 mg/ min** × 18 h		900 mg/ 500 mL	1.8 mg/mL	
				Ordered mg dose (0.5 mg/min) ÷ mg/mL (1.8 mg/mL) = ___ × 60 min/h = mL/h to set on pump				**17** mL/h × 18 h
Amrinone	0.75 mg/kg =	**55.5** mg		Give mg/kg load over 10 min		300 mg/ 120 mL	2.5 mg/mL	___
	mg to give ÷ mg/mL =	**22** mL			**22.2**	mL × (60 min/h ÷ 10 min) =		**133.2** mL/h × 10 min
	Infusion		**0.56**		5–10 mcg/ kg/min	300 mg/ 120 mL	2500 mcg/mL	___
				Take dose you want in mcg ÷ by drug index number = mL/h on pump				
Brevibloc	Infusion		**2.25**		50–100 mcg/ kg/min	2.5 g/ 250 mL	10,000 mcg/mL	___ mL/h
				Take dose you want in mcg ÷ by drug index number = mL/h on pump				
Cardene	Infusion		___		0.5–10 mg/h	25 mg 250 mL	0.1 mg/mL	___
				Ordered mg dose ÷ mg/mL = mL/h to set on pump				___ mL/h
Cardizem	0.25 mg/kg =	**18.5** mg		Give mg/kg load over 20 min		50 mg/ 100 mL	0.5 mg/mL	___
	mg to give ÷ mg/mL =	**37** mL			**37**	mL × (60 min/h ÷ 20 min) =		**111** mL/h
	0.35 mg/kg =	**25.9** mg		May repeat loading dose in 15 min			0.5 mg/mL	___
	mg to give ÷ mg/mL =	**52** mL			**51.8**	mL × (60 min/h ÷ 20 min) =		**155** mL/h
	Infusion				5–15 mg/h			___
				Ordered mg dose ÷ mg/mL = mL/h to set on pump				___ mL/h
Desmopressin	0.3 mcg/kg =	**22** mcg		Give dose over 20–30 min			4 mcg/vial	
Dobutamine	Infusion		**0.45**		2.5–40 mcg/kg/ min	250 mg/ 125 mL	2000 mcg/mL	
				Take dose you want in mcg ÷ by drug index number = mL/h on pump				

(continues)

74 kg (continued)

DRUG	ORDERED AMOUNT	TOTAL DOSE TO GIVE	DRUG INDEX NUMBER	DIRECTIONS	INFUSION RANGE	DRUG MIXTURE	AMOUNT	DRUG/ mL	RUN AT	mL/h
Dopamine	Infusion		0.36		1–20 mcg/ kg/min	400 mg/ 250 mL	1600	mcg/mL		
		Take dose you want in mcg ÷ by drug index number = mL/h on pump								
Epinephrine	Infusion	1 mcg/min = 4 mL/h 2 mcg/min = 8 mL/h 3 mcg/min = 11 mL/h 4 mcg/min = 15 mL/h			1–4 mcg/min	4 mg/ 250 mL	16	mcg/mL		
		Ordered mcg dose/min ÷ mcg/mL × 60 min/h =							___	mL/h
Fenoldapam	Infusion		0.0091		0.01–1.6 mcg/ kg/min	10 mg/ 250 mL	40	mcg/mL		
		Take dose you want in mcg ÷ by drug index number = mL/h on pump								
Heparin	100 u/kg = **7400 u** 200 u/kg = **14,800 u** 300 u/kg = **22,200 u** 400 u/kg = **29,600 u**									
Isoproterenol	Infusion				5 mcg/min	1 mg/ 250 mL	4	mcg/mL		
		Ordered mcg dose/min ÷ mcg/mL × 60 min/h =							75	mL/h
Lidocaine	Infusion	1 mg/min = 7.5 mL/h			1–4 mg/min	2 g/ 250 mL	8	mg/mL	___	
		Ordered mg/min ÷ mg/mL × 60 min/h =							___	mL/h
Nitroglycerin	Infusion	3 mcg/min = 1 mL/h			3–200 mcg/min	50 mg/ 250 mL	200	mcg/mL	___	
		Ordered mcg/min ÷ mcg/mL × 60 min/h =							___	mL/h
Nitroprusside	Infusion	6.7 mcg/min = 1 mL/h			5–300 mcg/min	100 mg/ 250 mL	400	mcg/mL	___	
		Ordered mcg/min ÷ mcg/mL × 60 min/h =							___	mL/h
Norepinephrine	Infusion	1 mcg/min = 4 mL/h 2 mcg/min = 8 mL/h 3 mcg/min = 11 mL/h 4 mcg/min = 15 mL/h 5 mcg/min = 19 mL/h			2–20 mcg/min	4 mg/ 250 mL	16	mcg/mL		
		Ordered mcg dose/min ÷ mcg/mL × 60 min/h =							___	mL/h
Phenylephrine	Infusion	1.3 mcg/min = 1 mL/h			10–200 mcg/min	20 mg/ 250 mL	80	mcg/mL		
		Ordered mcg/min ÷ mcg/mL × 60 min/h =							___	mL/h
Primacor	0.05 mg/kg = **3.7 mg**			Give load over 10 min		40 mg/ 200 mL	0.2	mg/mL		
	mg to give ÷ mg/mL =	**19 mL**				19	mL × (60 min/h ÷ 10 min) =		111	mL/h × 10 min
	Infusion		0.05		0.5 mcg/ kg/min	40 mg/ 200 mL	200	mcg/mL	___	
		Take dose you want in mcg ÷ by drug index number = mL/h on pump								
Trimethaphan	Infusion		—		0.3–6 mg/min	500 mg/ 500 mL	1	mg/mL	___	
		Ordered mg/min ÷ mg/mL × 60 min/h =							___	mL/h
Vasopressin		0.02 u/min = 3 mL/h 0.04 u/min = 6 mL/h				40 u/ 100 mL	400	u/mL		

75 kg

DRUG	ORDERED AMOUNT	TOTAL DOSE TO GIVE	DRUG INDEX NUMBER	DIRECTIONS	INFUSION RANGE	DRUG MIXTURE	AMOUNT	DRUG/ mL	RUN AT	mL/h
Aminophylline	5 mg/kg =	375 mg		Give mg/kg load over 20 min		500 mg/ 250 mL	2 mg/mL			
	mg to give ÷ mg/mL =	188 mL			188	mL × (60 min/h ÷ 20 min) =			562.5	mL/h × 20 min
	Infusion				0.5–1 mg/kg/h	500 mg/ 250 mL	2 mg/mL			
					mg dose ordered × kg ÷ mg/mL =					___ mL/h
Amiodarone	Loading dose			Load **150 mg** over 10 min		900 mg/ 500 mL	1.8 mg/mL		___	
				Ordered mg load dose (150 mg) ÷ mg/mL (1.8 mg/mL) = 83 mL to give × (60 min/h ÷ 10 min) = mL/h to set on pump					500	mL/h × 83 mL
	Infusion			Run at **1 mg/ min** × 6 h		900 mg/ 500 mL	1.8 mg/mL			
				Ordered mg dose (1 mg/min) ÷ mg/mL (1.0 mg/mL) = ____ × 60 min/h = mL/h to set on pump					33	mL/h × 6 h
	Infusion			Run at **0.5 mg/ min** × 18 h		900 mg/ 500 mL	1.8 mg/mL			
				Ordered mg dose (0.5 mg/min) ÷ mg/mL (1.8 mg/mL) = ____ × 60 min/h = mL/h to set on pump					17	mL/h × 18 h
Amrinone	0.75 mg/kg =	56.25 mg		Give mg/kg load over 10 min		300 mg/ 120 mL	2.5 mg/mL		___	
	mg to give ÷ mg/mL =	23 mL			22.5	mL × (60 min/h ÷ 10 min) =			135	mL/h × 10 min
	Infusion		0.55		5–10 mcg/ kg/min	300 mg/ 120 mL	2500 mcg/mL		___	
				Take dose you want in mcg ÷ by drug index number = mL/h on pump						
Brevibloc	Infusion		2.22		50–100 mcg/ kg/min	2.5 g/ 250 mL	10,000 mcg/mL		___ mL/h	
				Take dose you want in mcg ÷ by drug index number = mL/h on pump						
Cardene	Infusion		—		0.5–10 mg/h	25 mg 250 mL	0.1 mg/mL		___	
				Ordered mg dose ÷ mg/mL = mL/h to set on pump						___ mL/h
Cardizem	0.25 mg/kg =	18.75 mg		Give mg/kg load over 20 min		50 mg/ 100 mL	0.5 mg/mL		___	
	mg to give ÷ mg/mL =	38 mL			37.5	mL × (60 min/h ÷ 20 min) =			113	mL/h
	0.35 mg/kg =	26.25 mg		May repeat loading dose in 15 min			0.5 mg/mL		___	
	mg to give ÷ mg/mL =	53 mL			52.5	mL × (60 min/h ÷ 20 min) =			158	mL/h
	Infusion				5–15 mg/h				___	
				Ordered mg dose ÷ mg/mL = mL/h to set on pump						___ mL/h
Desmopressin	0.3 mcg/kg =	23 mcg		Give dose over 20–30 min			4 mcg/vial			
Dobutamine	Infusion		0.44		2.5–40 mcg/kg/ min	250 mg/ 125 mL	2000 mcg/mL			
				Take dose you want in mcg ÷ by drug index number = mL/h on pump						

(continues)

75 kg (continued)

DRUG	ORDERED AMOUNT		TOTAL DOSE TO GIVE		DRUG INDEX NUMBER	DIRECTIONS	INFUSION RANGE	DRUG MIXTURE	AMOUNT	DRUG/ mL	RUN AT	mL/h
Dopamine	Infusion				0.36		1–20 mcg/ kg/min	400 mg/ 250 mL	1600	mcg/mL		
	Take dose you want in mcg ÷ by drug index number = mL/h on pump											
Epinephrine	Infusion		1 mcg/min = 4 mL/h 2 mcg/min = 8 mL/h 3 mcg/min = 11 mL/h 4 mcg/min = 15 mL/h				1–4 mcg/min	4 mg/ 250 mL	16	mcg/mL		
	Ordered mcg dose/min ÷ mcg/mL × 60 min/h =										___	mL/h
Fenoldapam	Infusion				0.0089		0.01–1.6 mcg/ kg/min	10 mg/ 250 mL	40	mcg/mL		
	Take dose you want in mcg ÷ by drug index number = mL/h on pump											
Heparin	100 u/kg = 200 u/kg = 300 u/kg = 400 u/kg =		7500 u 15,000 u 22,500 u 30,000 u									
Isoproterenol	Infusion						5 mcg/min	1 mg/ 250 mL	4	mcg/mL		
	Ordered mcg dose/min ÷ mcg/mL × 60 min/h =										75	mL/h
Lidocaine	Infusion		1 mg/min = 7.5 mL/h				1–4 mg/min	2 g/ 250 mL	8	mg/mL	—	
	Ordered mg/min ÷ mg/mL × 60 min/h =										___	mL/h
Nitroglycerin	Infusion		3 mcg/min = 1 mL/h				3–200 mcg/min	50 mg/ 250 mL	200	mcg/mL	—	
	Ordered mcg/min ÷ mcg/mL × 60 min/h =										___	mL/h
Nitroprusside	Infusion		6.7 mcg/min = 1 mL/h				5–300 mcg/min	100 mg/ 250 mL	400	mcg/mL	—	
	Ordered mcg/min ÷ mcg/mL × 60 min/h =										___	mL/h
Norepinephrine	Infusion		1 mcg/min = 4 mL/h 2 mcg/min = 8 mL/h 3 mcg/min = 11 mL/h 4 mcg/min = 15 mL/h 5 mcg/min = 19 mL/h				2–20 mcg/min	4 mg/ 250 mL	16	mcg/mL		
	Ordered mcg dose/min ÷ mcg/mL × 60 min/h =										___	mL/h
Phenylephrine	Infusion		1.3 mcg/min = 1 mL/h				10–200 mcg/min	20 mg/ 250 mL	80	mcg/mL		
	Ordered mcg/min ÷ mcg/mL × 60 min/h =										___	mL/h
Primacor	0.05 mg/kg =		3.75 mg			Give load over 10 min		40 mg/ 200 mL	0.2	mg/mL		
	mg to give ÷ mg/mL =		19 mL				19	mL × (60 min/h ÷ 10 min) =			112.5	mL/h × 10 min
	Infusion				0.04		0.5 mcg/ kg/min	40 mg/ 200 mL	200	mcg/mL	—	
	Take dose you want in mcg ÷ by drug index number = mL/h on pump											
Trimethaphan	Infusion				—		0.3–6 mg/min	500 mg/ 500 mL	1	mg/mL	—	
	Ordered mg/min ÷ mg/mL × 60 min/h =										___	mL/h
Vasopressin			0.02 u/min = 3 mL/h 0.04 u/min = 6 mL/h					40 u/ 100 mL	400	u/mL		

76 kg

DRUG	ORDERED AMOUNT	TOTAL DOSE TO GIVE	DRUG INDEX NUMBER	DIRECTIONS	INFUSION RANGE	DRUG MIXTURE	AMOUNT DRUG/mL	RUN AT mL/h
Aminophylline	5 mg/kg =	380 mg		Give mg/kg load over 20 min		500 mg/250 mL	2 mg/mL	
	mg to give ÷ mg/mL =	190 mL			190	mL × (60 min/h ÷ 20 min) =		570 mL/h × 20 min
	Infusion				0.5–1 mg/kg/h	500 mg/250 mL	2 mg/mL	
					mg dose ordered × kg ÷ mg/mL =			___ mL/h
Amiodarone	Loading dose			Load **150 mg** over 10 min		900 mg/500 mL	1.8 mg/mL	___
				Ordered mg load dose (150 mg) ÷ mg/mL (1.8 mg/mL) = 83 mL to give × (60 min/h ÷ 10 min) = mL/h to set on pump				500 mL/h × 83 mL
	Infusion			Run at **1 mg/min × 6 h**		900 mg/500 mL	1.8 mg/mL	
				Ordered mg dose (1 mg/min) ÷ mg/mL (1.8 mg/mL) = ___ × 60 min/h = mL/h to set on pump				33 mL/h × 6 h
	Infusion			Run at **0.5 mg/min × 18 h**		900 mg/500 mL	1.8 mg/mL	
				Ordered mg dose (0.5 mg/min) ÷ mg/mL (1.8 mg/mL) = ___ × 60 min/h = mL/h to set on pump				17 mL/h × 18 h
Amrinone	0.75 mg/kg =	57 mg		Give mg/kg load over 10 min		300 mg/120 mL	2.5 mg/mL	___
	mg to give ÷ mg/mL =	23 mL			22.8	mL × (60 min/h ÷ 10 min) =		136.8 mL/h × 10 min
	Infusion		0.55		5–10 mcg/kg/min	300 mg/120 mL	2500 mcg/mL	___
	Take dose you want in mcg ÷ by drug index number = mL/h on pump							
Brevibloc	Infusion		2.19		50–100 mcg/kg/min	2.5 g/250 mL	10,000 mcg/mL	___ mL/h
	Take dose you want in mcg ÷ by drug index number = mL/h on pump							
Cardene	Infusion		—		0.5–10 mg/h	25 mg/250 mL	0.1 mg/mL	___
	Ordered mg dose ÷ mg/mL = mL/h to set on pump							___ mL/h
Cardizem	0.25 mg/kg =	19 mg		Give mg/kg load over 20 min		50 mg/100 mL	0.5 mg/mL	___
	mg to give ÷ mg/mL =	38 mL			38	mL × (60 min/h ÷ 20 min) =		114 mL/h
	0.35 mg/kg =	26.6 mg		May repeat loading dose in 15 min			0.5 mg/mL	___
	mg to give ÷ mg/mL =	53 mL			53.2	mL × (60 min/h ÷ 20 min) =		160 mL/h
	Infusion				5–15 mg/h			___
	Ordered mg dose ÷ mg/mL = mL/h to set on pump							___ mL/h
Desmopressin	0.3 mcg/kg =	23 mcg		Give dose over 20–30 min			4 mcg/vial	
Dobutamine	Infusion		0.44		2.5–40 mcg/kg/min	250 mg/125 mL	2000 mcg/mL	
	Take dose you want in mcg ÷ by drug index number = mL/h on pump							

(continues)

76 kg (continued)

DRUG	ORDERED AMOUNT	TOTAL DOSE TO GIVE	DRUG INDEX NUMBER	DIRECTIONS	INFUSION RANGE	DRUG MIXTURE	AMOUNT	DRUG/ mL	RUN AT	mL/h
Dopamine	Infusion		0.35		1–20 mcg/ kg/min	400 mg/ 250 mL	1600	mcg/mL		
			Take dose you want in mcg ÷ by drug index number = mL/h on pump							
Epinephrine	Infusion	1 mcg/min = 4 mL/h 2 mcg/min = 8 mL/h 3 mcg/min = 11 mL/h 4 mcg/min = 15 mL/h			1–4 mcg/min	4 mg/ 250 mL	16	mcg/mL		
			Ordered mcg dose/min ÷ mcg/mL × 60 min/h =						___	mL/h
Fenoldapam	Infusion		0.0088		0.01–1.6 mcg/ kg/min	10 mg/ 250 mL	40	mcg/mL		
			Take dose you want in mcg ÷ by drug index number = mL/h on pump							
Heparin	100 u/kg = 7600 u 200 u/kg = 15,200 u 300 u/kg = 22,800 u 400 u/kg = 30,400 u									
Isoproterenol	Infusion				5 mcg/min	1 mg/ 250 mL	4	mcg/mL		
			Ordered mcg dose/min ÷ mcg/mL × 60 min/h =						75	mL/h
Lidocaine	Infusion	1 mg/min = 7.5 mL/h			1–4 mg/min	2 g/ 250 mL	8	mg/mL	___	
			Ordered mg/min ÷ mg/mL × 60 min/h =						___	mL/h
Nitroglycerin	Infusion	3 mcg/min = 1 mL/h			3–200 mcg/min	50 mg/ 250 mL	200	mcg/mL	___	
			Ordered mcg/min ÷ mcg/mL × 60 min/h =						___	mL/h
Nitroprusside	Infusion	6.7 mcg/min = 1 mL/h			5–300 mcg/min	100 mg/ 250 mL	400	mcg/mL	___	
			Ordered mcg/min ÷ mcg/mL × 60 min/h =						___	mL/h
Norepinephrine	Infusion	1 mcg/min = 4 mL/h 2 mcg/min = 8 mL/h 3 mcg/min = 11 mL/h 4 mcg/min = 15 mL/h 5 mcg/min = 19 mL/h			2–20 mcg/min	4 mg/ 250 mL	16	mcg/mL		
			Ordered mcg dose/min ÷ mcg/mL × 60 min/h =						___	mL/h
Phenylephrine	Infusion	1.3 mcg/min = 1 mL/h			10–200 mcg/min	20 mg/ 250 mL	80	mcg/mL		
			Ordered mcg/min ÷ mcg/mL × 60 min/h =						___	mL/h
Primacor	0.05 mg/kg = 3.8 mg			Give load over 10 min		40 mg/ 200 mL	0.2	mg/mL		
	mg to give ÷ mg/mL = 19 mL					19 mL × (60 min/h ÷ 10 min) =			114	mL/h × 10 min
	Infusion		0.04		0.5 mcg/ kg/min	40 mg/ 200 mL	200	mcg/mL	___	
			Take dose you want in mcg ÷ by drug index number = mL/h on pump							
Trimethaphan	Infusion		—		0.3–6 mg/min	500 mg/ 500 mL	1	mg/mL	___	
			Ordered mg/min ÷ mg/mL × 60 min/h =						___	mL/h
Vasopressin		0.02 u/min = 3 mL/h 0.04 u/min = 6 mL/h				40 u/ 100 mL	400	u/mL		

77 kg

DRUG	ORDERED AMOUNT	TOTAL DOSE TO GIVE	DRUG INDEX NUMBER	DIRECTIONS	INFUSION RANGE	DRUG MIXTURE	AMOUNT DRUG/mL	RUN AT mL/h
Aminophylline	5 mg/kg = **385 mg**			Give mg/kg load over 20 min		500 mg/ 250 mL	2 mg/mL	
	mg to give ÷ mg/mL = **193 mL**				**193**	mL × (60 min/h ÷ 20 min) =		<u>577.5</u> mL/h × 20 min
	Infusion				0.5–1 mg/kg/h	500 mg/ 250 mL	2 mg/mL	
						mg dose ordered × kg ÷ mg/mL =		___ mL/h
Amiodarone	Loading dose			Load **150 mg** over 10 min		900 mg/ 500 mL	1.8 mg/mL	___
				Ordered mg load dose (150 mg) ÷ mg/mL (1.8 mg/mL) = 83 mL to give × (60 min/h ÷ 10 min) = mL/h to set on pump				<u>500</u> mL/h × 83 mL
	Infusion			Run at **1 mg/ min** × 6 h		900 mg/ 500 mL	1.8 mg/mL	
				Ordered mg dose (1 mg/min) ÷ mg/mL (1.0 mg/mL) = ___ × 60 min/h = mL/h to set on pump				<u>33</u> mL/h × 6 h
	Infusion			Run at **0.5 mg/ min** × 18 h		900 mg/ 500 mL	1.8 mg/mL	
				Ordered mg dose (0.5 mg/min) ÷ mg/mL (1.8 mg/mL) = ___ × 60 min/h = mL/h to set on pump				<u>17</u> mL/h × 18 h
Amrinone	0.75 mg/kg = **57.75 mg**			Give mg/kg load over 10 min		300 mg/ 120 mL	2.5 mg/mL	___
	mg to give ÷ mg/mL = **23 mL**				**23.1**	mL × (60 min/h ÷ 10 min) =		<u>138.6</u> mL/h × 10 min
	Infusion		**0.54**		5–10 mcg/ kg/min	300 mg/ 120 mL	2500 mcg/mL	___
				Take dose you want in mcg ÷ by drug index number = mL/h on pump				
Brevibloc	Infusion		**2.16**		50–100 mcg/ kg/min	2.5 g/ 250 mL	10,000 mcg/mL	___ mL/h
				Take dose you want in mcg ÷ by drug index number = mL/h on pump				
Cardene	Infusion		___		0.5–10 mg/h	25 mg 250 mL	0.1 mg/mL	___
				Ordered mg dose ÷ mg/mL = mL/h to set on pump				___ mL/h
Cardizem	0.25 mg/kg = **19.25 mg**			Give mg/kg load over 20 min		50 mg/ 100 mL	0.5 mg/mL	___
	mg to give ÷ mg/mL = **39 mL**				**38.5**	mL × (60 min/h ÷ 20 min) =		**116** mL/h
	0.35 mg/kg = **26.95 mg**			May repeat loading dose in 15 min			0.5 mg/mL	___
	mg to give ÷ mg/mL = **54 mL**				**53.9**	mL × (60 min/h ÷ 20 min) =		**162** mL/h
	Infusion				5–15 mg/h			___
				Ordered mg dose ÷ mg/mL = mL/h to set on pump				___ mL/h
Desmopressin	0.3 mcg/kg = **23 mcg**			Give dose over 20–30 min			4 mcg/vial	
Dobutamine	Infusion		**0.43**		2.5–40 mcg/kg/ min	250 mg/ 125 mL	2000 mcg/mL	
				Take dose you want in mcg ÷ by drug index number = mL/h on pump				

(continues)

77　kg (continued)

DRUG	ORDERED AMOUNT	TOTAL DOSE TO GIVE	DRUG INDEX NUMBER	DIRECTIONS	INFUSION RANGE	DRUG MIXTURE	AMOUNT	DRUG/ mL	RUN AT	mL/h
Dopamine	Infusion		0.35		1–20 mcg/ kg/min	400 mg/ 250 mL	1600	mcg/mL		
	Take dose you want in mcg ÷ by drug index number = mL/h on pump									
Epinephrine	Infusion	1 mcg/min = 4 mL/h 2 mcg/min = 8 mL/h 3 mcg/min = 11 mL/h 4 mcg/min = 15 mL/h			1–4 mcg/min	4 mg/ 250 mL	16	mcg/mL		
		Ordered mcg dose/min ÷ mcg/mL × 60 min/h =							___	mL/h
Fenoldapam	Infusion		0.0087		0.01–1.6 mcg/ kg/min	10 mg/ 250 mL	40	mcg/mL		
	Take dose you want in mcg ÷ by drug index number = mL/h on pump									
Heparin	100　u/kg =	7700　u								
	200　u/kg =	15,400　u								
	300　u/kg =	23,100　u								
	400　u/kg =	30,800　u								
Isoproterenol	Infusion				5 mcg/min	1 mg/ 250 mL	4	mcg/mL		
		Ordered mcg dose/min ÷ mcg/mL × 60 min/h =							**75**	mL/h
Lidocaine	Infusion	1 mg/min = 7.5 mL/h			1–4 mg/min	2 g/ 250 mL	8	mg/mL	___	
		Ordered mg/min ÷ mg/mL × 60 min/h =							___	mL/h
Nitroglycerin	Infusion	3 mcg/min = 1 mL/h			3–200 mcg/min	50 mg/ 250 mL	200	mcg/mL	___	
		Ordered mcg/min ÷ mcg/mL × 60 min/h =							___	mL/h
Nitroprusside	Infusion	6.7 mcg/min = 1 mL/h			5–300 mcg/min	100 mg/ 250 mL	400	mcg/mL	___	
		Ordered mcg/min ÷ mcg/mL × 60 min/h =							___	mL/h
Norepinephrine	Infusion	1 mcg/min = 4 mL/h 2 mcg/min = 8 mL/h 3 mcg/min = 11 mL/h 4 mcg/min = 15 mL/h 5 mcg/min = 19 mL/h			2–20 mcg/min	4 mg/ 250 mL	16	mcg/mL		
		Ordered mcg dose/min ÷ mcg/mL × 60 min/h =							___	mL/h
Phenylephrine	Infusion	1.3 mcg/min = 1 mL/h			10–200 mcg/min	20 mg/ 250 mL	80	mcg/mL		
		Ordered mcg/min ÷ mcg/mL × 60 min/h =							___	mL/h
Primacor	0.05　mg/kg =	3.85　mg		Give load over 10 min		40 mg/ 200 mL	0.2	mg/mL		
	mg to give ÷ mg/mL =	19　mL			19	mL × (60 min/h ÷ 10 min) =			**115.5**	mL/h × 10 min
	Infusion		0.04		0.5 mcg/ kg/min	40 mg/ 200 mL	200	mcg/mL	___	
		Take dose you want in mcg ÷ by drug index number = mL/h on pump								
Trimethaphan	Infusion				0.3–6 mg/min	500 mg/ 500 mL	1	mg/mL	___	
		Ordered mg/min ÷ mg/mL × 60 min/h =							___	mL/h
Vasopressin		0.02 u/min = 3 mL/h 0.04 u/min = 6 mL/h				40 u/ 100 mL	400	u/mL		

78 kg

DRUG	ORDERED AMOUNT	TOTAL DOSE TO GIVE	DRUG INDEX NUMBER	DIRECTIONS	INFUSION RANGE	DRUG MIXTURE	AMOUNT DRUG/mL	RUN AT mL/h
Aminophylline	5 mg/kg =	**390** mg		Give mg/kg load over 20 min		500 mg/ 250 mL	2 mg/mL	
	mg to give ÷ mg/mL =	**195** mL			**195** mL × (60 min/h ÷ 20 min) =			**585** mL/h × 20 min
	\<Infusion\>				0.5–1 mg/kg/h	500 mg/ 250 mL	2 mg/mL	
					mg dose ordered × kg ÷ mg/mL =			___ mL/h
Amiodarone	\<Loading dose\>			Load **150 mg** over 10 min		900 mg/ 500 mL	1.8 mg/mL	—
				Ordered mg load dose (150 mg) ÷ mg/mL (1.8 mg/mL) = 83 mL to give × (60 min/h ÷ 10 min) = mL/h to set on pump				**500** mL/h × 83 mL
	\<Infusion\>			Run at **1 mg/ min** × 6 h		900 mg/ 500 mL	1.8 mg/mL	
				Ordered mg dose (1 mg/min) ÷ mg/mL (1.8 mg/mL) = ___ × 60 min/h = ___ mL/h to set on pump				**33** mL/h × 6 h
	\<Infusion\>			Run at **0.5 mg/ min** × 18 h		900 mg/ 500 mL	1.8 mg/mL	
				Ordered mg dose (0.5 mg/min) ÷ mg/mL (1.8 mg/mL) = ___ × 60 min/h = ___ mL/h to set on pump				**17** mL/h × 18 h
Amrinone	0.75 mg/kg =	**58.5** mg		Give mg/kg load over 10 min		300 mg/ 120 mL	2.5 mg/mL	—
	mg to give ÷ mg/mL =	**23** mL			**23.4** mL × (60 min/h ÷ 10 min) =			**140.4** mL/h × 10 min
	\<Infusion\>		0.53		5–10 mcg/ kg/min	300 mg/ 120 mL	2500 mcg/mL	—
				Take dose you want in mcg ÷ by drug index number = mL/h on pump				
Brevibloc	\<Infusion\>		2.14		50–100 mcg/ kg/min	2.5 g/ 250 mL	10,000 mcg/mL	___ mL/h
				Take dose you want in mcg ÷ by drug index number = mL/h on pump				
Cardene	\<Infusion\>		—		0.5–10 mg/h	25 mg 250 mL	0.1 mg/mL	—
				Ordered mg dose ÷ mg/mL = mL/h to set on pump				___ mL/h
Cardizem	0.25 mg/kg =	**19.5** mg		Give mg/kg load over 20 min		50 mg/ 100 mL	0.5 mg/mL	—
	mg to give ÷ mg/mL =	**39** mL			**39** mL × (60 min/h ÷ 20 min) =			**117** mL/h
	0.35 mg/kg =	**27.3** mg		May repeat loading dose in 15 min			0.5 mg/mL	—
	mg to give ÷ mg/mL =	**55** mL			**54.6** mL × (60 min/h ÷ 20 min) =			**164** mL/h
	\<Infusion\>				5–15 mg/h			—
				Ordered mg dose ÷ mg/mL = mL/h to set on pump				___ mL/h
Desmopressin	0.3 mcg/kg =	**23** mcg		Give dose over 20–30 min			4 mcg/vial	
Dobutamine	\<Infusion\>		0.43		2.5–40 mcg/kg/ min	250 mg/ 125 mL	2000 mcg/mL	
				Take dose you want in mcg ÷ by drug index number = mL/h on pump				

(continues)

78   kg (continued)

DRUG	ORDERED AMOUNT	TOTAL DOSE TO GIVE	DRUG INDEX NUMBER	DIRECTIONS	INFUSION RANGE	DRUG MIXTURE	AMOUNT	DRUG/ mL	RUN AT	mL/h
Dopamine	Infusion		0.34		1–20 mcg/ kg/min	400 mg/ 250 mL	1600	mcg/mL		
	Take dose you want in mcg ÷ by drug index number = mL/h on pump									
Epinephrine	Infusion	1 mcg/min = 4 mL/h 2 mcg/min = 8 mL/h 3 mcg/min = 11 mL/h 4 mcg/min = 15 mL/h			1–4 mcg/min	4 mg/ 250 mL	16	mcg/mL		
	Ordered mcg dose/min ÷ mcg/mL × 60 min/h =								___	mL/h
Fenoldapam	Infusion		0.0086		0.01–1.6 mcg/ kg/min	10 mg/ 250 mL	40	mcg/mL		
	Take dose you want in mcg ÷ by drug index number = mL/h on pump									
Heparin	100 u/kg =	7800 u								
	200 u/kg =	15,600 u								
	300 u/kg =	23,400 u								
	400 u/kg =	31,200 u								
Isoproterenol	Infusion				5 mcg/min	1 mg/ 250 mL	4	mcg/mL		
	Ordered mcg dose/min ÷ mcg/mL × 60 min/h =								**75**	mL/h
Lidocaine	Infusion	1 mg/min = 7.5 mL/h			1–4 mg/min	2 g/ 250 mL	8	mg/mL	___	
	Ordered mg/min ÷ mg/mL × 60 min/h =								___	mL/h
Nitroglycerin	Infusion	3 mcg/min = 1 mL/h			3–200 mcg/min	50 mg/ 250 mL	200	mcg/mL	___	
	Ordered mcg/min ÷ mcg/mL × 60 min/h =								___	mL/h
Nitroprusside	Infusion	6.7 mcg/min = 1 mL/h			5–300 mcg/min	100 mg/ 250 mL	400	mcg/mL	___	
	Ordered mcg/min ÷ mcg/mL × 60 min/h =								___	mL/h
Norepinephrine	Infusion	1 mcg/min = 4 mL/h 2 mcg/min = 8 mL/h 3 mcg/min = 11 mL/h 4 mcg/min = 15 mL/h 5 mcg/min = 19 mL/h			2–20 mcg/min	4 mg/ 250 mL	16	mcg/mL		
	Ordered mcg dose/min ÷ mcg/mL × 60 min/h =								___	mL/h
Phenylephrine	Infusion	1.3 mcg/min = 1 mL/h			10–200 mcg/min	20 mg/ 250 mL	80	mcg/mL		
	Ordered mcg/min ÷ mcg/mL × 60 min/h =								___	mL/h
Primacor	0.05 mg/kg =	3.9 mg		Give load over 10 min		40 mg/ 200 mL	0.2	mg/mL		
	mg to give ÷ mg/mL =	20 mL			20	mL × (60 min/h ÷ 10 min) =			**117**	mL/h × 10 min
	Infusion		0.04		0.5 mcg/ kg/min	40 mg/ 200 mL	200	mcg/mL	___	
	Take dose you want in mcg ÷ by drug index number = mL/h on pump									
Trimethaphan	Infusion		—		0.3–6 mg/min	500 mg/ 500 mL	1	mg/mL	___	
	Ordered mg/min ÷ mg/mL × 60 min/h =								___	mL/h
Vasopressin		0.02 u/min = 3 mL/h 0.04 u/min = 6 mL/h				40 u/ 100 mL	400	u/mL		

79 kg

DRUG	ORDERED AMOUNT	TOTAL DOSE TO GIVE	DRUG INDEX NUMBER	DIRECTIONS	INFUSION RANGE	DRUG MIXTURE	AMOUNT	DRUG/mL	RUN AT	mL/h
Aminophylline	5 mg/kg = 395 mg			Give mg/kg load over 20 min		500 mg/ 250 mL	2 mg/mL			
	mg to give ÷ mg/mL = 198 mL				198	mL × (60 min/h ÷ 20 min) =			592.5	mL/h × 20 min
	Infusion				0.5–1 mg/kg/h	500 mg/ 250 mL	2 mg/mL			
					mg dose ordered × kg ÷ mg/mL =				___	mL/h
Amiodarone	Loading dose			Load **150 mg** over 10 min		900 mg/ 500 mL	1.8 mg/mL		___	
				Ordered mg load dose (150 mg) ÷ mg/mL (1.8 mg/mL) = 83 mL to give × (60 min/h ÷ 10 min) = mL/h to set on pump				500	mL/h × 83 mL	
	Infusion			Run at **1 mg/ min** × 6 h		900 mg/ 500 mL	1.8 mg/mL			
				Ordered mg dose (1 mg/min) ÷ mg/mL (1.8 mg/mL) = ___ × 60 min/h = mL/h to set on pump				33	mL/h × 6 h	
	Infusion			Run at **0.5 mg/ min** × 18 h		900 mg/ 500 mL	1.8 mg/mL			
				Ordered mg dose (0.5 mg/min) ÷ mg/mL (1.8 mg/mL) = ___ × 60 min/h = mL/h to set on pump				17	mL/h × 18 h	
Amrinone	0.75 mg/kg = 59.25 mg			Give mg/kg load over 10 min		300 mg/ 120 mL	2.5 mg/mL		___	
	mg to give ÷ mg/mL = 24 mL				23.7	mL × (60 min/h ÷ 10 min) =			142.2	mL/h × 10 min
	Infusion		0.53		5–10 mcg/ kg/min	300 mg/ 120 mL	2500 mcg/mL		___	
				Take dose you want in mcg ÷ by drug index number = mL/h on pump						
Brevibloc	Infusion		2.11		50–100 mcg/ kg/min	2.5 g/ 250 mL	10,000 mcg/mL		___	mL/h
				Take dose you want in mcg ÷ by drug index number = mL/h on pump						
Cardene	Infusion		___		0.5–10 mg/h	25 mg 250 mL	0.1 mg/mL		___	
				Ordered mg dose ÷ mg/mL = mL/h to set on pump					___	mL/h
Cardizem	0.25 mg/kg = 19.75 mg			Give mg/kg load over 20 min		50 mg/ 100 mL	0.5 mg/mL		___	
	mg to give ÷ mg/mL = 40 mL				39.5	mL × (60 min/h ÷ 20 min) =			119	mL/h
	0.35 mg/kg = 27.65 mg			May repeat loading dose in 15 min			0.5 mg/mL		___	
	mg to give ÷ mg/mL = 55 mL				55.3	mL × (60 min/h ÷ 20 min) =			166	mL/h
	Infusion				5–15 mg/h				___	
				Ordered mg dose ÷ mg/mL = mL/h to set on pump					___	mL/h
Desmopressin	0.3 mcg/kg = 24 mcg			Give dose over 20–30 min			4 mcg/vial			
Dobutamine	Infusion		0.42		2.5–40 mcg/kg/ min	250 mg/ 125 mL	2000 mcg/mL			
				Take dose you want in mcg ÷ by drug index number = mL/h on pump						

(continues)

79 kg (continued)

DRUG	ORDERED AMOUNT	TOTAL DOSE TO GIVE	DRUG INDEX NUMBER	DIRECTIONS	INFUSION RANGE	DRUG MIXTURE	AMOUNT	DRUG/ mL	RUN AT	mL/h
Dopamine	Infusion		0.34		1–20 mcg/ kg/min	400 mg/ 250 mL	1600	mcg/mL		
			Take dose you want in mcg ÷ by drug index number = mL/h on pump							
Epinephrine	Infusion	1 mcg/min = 4 mL/h 2 mcg/min = 8 mL/h 3 mcg/min = 11 mL/h 4 mcg/min = 15 mL/h			1–4 mcg/min	4 mg/ 250 mL	16	mcg/mL		
			Ordered mcg dose/min ÷ mcg/mL × 60 min/h =						___	mL/h
Fenoldapam	Infusion		0.0085		0.01–1.6 mcg/ kg/min	10 mg/ 250 mL	40	mcg/mL		
			Take dose you want in mcg ÷ by drug index number = mL/h on pump							
Heparin	100 u/kg = 7900 u 200 u/kg = 15,800 u 300 u/kg = 23,700 u 400 u/kg = 31,600 u									
Isoproterenol	Infusion				5 mcg/min	1 mg/ 250 mL	4	mcg/mL		
			Ordered mcg dose/min ÷ mcg/mL × 60 min/h =						75	mL/h
Lidocaine	Infusion	1 mg/min = 7.5 mL/h			1–4 mg/min	2 g/ 250 mL	8	mg/mL	___	
			Ordered mg/min ÷ mg/mL × 60 min/h =						___	mL/h
Nitroglycerin	Infusion	3 mcg/min = 1 mL/h			3–200 mcg/min	50 mg/ 250 mL	200	mcg/mL	___	
			Ordered mcg/min ÷ mcg/mL × 60 min/h =						___	mL/h
Nitroprusside	Infusion	6.7 mcg/min = 1 mL/h			5–300 mcg/min	100 mg/ 250 mL	400	mcg/mL	___	
			Ordered mcg/min ÷ mcg/mL × 60 min/h =						___	mL/h
Norepinephrine	Infusion	1 mcg/min = 4 mL/h 2 mcg/min = 8 mL/h 3 mcg/min = 11 mL/h 4 mcg/min = 15 mL/h 5 mcg/min = 19 mL/h			2–20 mcg/min	4 mg/ 250 mL	16	mcg/mL		
			Ordered mcg dose/min ÷ mcg/mL × 60 min/h =						___	mL/h
Phenylephrine	Infusion	1.3 mcg/min = 1 mL/h			10–200 mcg/min	20 mg/ 250 mL	80	mcg/mL		
			Ordered mcg/min ÷ mcg/mL × 60 min/h =						___	mL/h
Primacor	0.05 mg/kg = 3.95 mg			Give load over 10 min		40 mg/ 200 mL	0.2	mg/mL		
	mg to give ÷ mg/mL = 20 mL					20	mL × (60 min/h ÷ 10 min) =		118.5	mL/h × 10 min
	Infusion		0.04		0.5 mcg/ kg/min	40 mg/ 200 mL	200	mcg/mL	___	
			Take dose you want in mcg ÷ by drug index number = mL/h on pump							
Trimethaphan	Infusion		___		0.3–6 mg/min	500 mg/ 500 mL	1	mg/mL	___	
			Ordered mg/min ÷ mg/mL × 60 min/h =						___	mL/h
Vasopressin	0.02 u/min = 3 mL/h 0.04 u/min = 6 mL/h					40 u/ 100 mL	400	u/mL		

80 kg

DRUG	ORDERED AMOUNT	TOTAL DOSE TO GIVE	DRUG INDEX NUMBER	DIRECTIONS	INFUSION RANGE	DRUG MIXTURE	AMOUNT DRUG/mL	RUN AT mL/h
Aminophylline	5 mg/kg = **400** mg			Give mg/kg load over 20 min		500 mg/ 250 mL	2 mg/mL	
	mg to give ÷ mg/mL =	**200** mL				**200**	mL × (60 min/h ÷ 20 min) =	**600** mL/h × 20 min
	Infusion				0.5–1 mg/kg/h	500 mg/ 250 mL	2 mg/mL	
					mg dose ordered × kg ÷ mg/mL =			___ mL/h
Amiodarone	Loading dose			Load **150 mg** over 10 min		900 mg/ 500 mL	1.8 mg/mL	—
				Ordered mg load dose (150 mg) ÷ mg/mL (1.8 mg/mL) = 83 mL to give × (60 min/h ÷ 10 min) = mL/h to set on pump				**500** mL/h × 83 mL
	Infusion			Run at **1 mg/min** × 6 h	900 mg/ 500 mL	1.8 mg/mL	
				Ordered mg dose (1 mg/min) ÷ mg/ml (1.8 mg/mL) = ___ × 60 min/h = mL/h to set on pump				**33** mL/h × 6 h
	Infusion			Run at **0.5 mg/min** × 18 h	900 mg/ 500 mL	1.8 mg/mL	
				Ordered mg dose (0.5 mg/min) ÷ mg/mL (1.8 mg/mL) = ___ × 60 min/h = mL/h to set on pump				**17** mL/h × 18 h
Amrinone	0.75 mg/kg = **60** mg			Give mg/kg load over 10 min		300 mg/ 120 mL	2.5 mg/mL	—
	mg to give ÷ mg/mL =	**24** mL				**24**	mL × (60 min/h ÷ 10 min) =	**144** mL/h × 10 min
	Infusion		0.52		5–10 mcg/ kg/min	300 mg/ 120 mL	2500 mcg/mL	—
				Take dose you want in mcg ÷ by drug index number = mL/h on pump				
Brevibloc	Infusion		2.08		50–100 mcg/ kg/min	2.5 g/ 250 mL	10,000 mcg/mL	___ mL/h
				Take dose you want in mcg ÷ by drug index number = mL/h on pump				
Cardene	Infusion		—		0.5–10 mg/h	25 mg 250 mL	0.1 mg/mL	—
				Ordered mg dose ÷ mg/mL = mL/h to set on pump				___ mL/h
Cardizem	0.25 mg/kg = **20** mg			Give mg/kg load over 20 min		50 mg/ 100 mL	0.5 mg/mL	—
	mg to give ÷ mg/mL =	**40** mL				**40**	mL × (60 min/h ÷ 20 min) =	**120** mL/h
	0.35 mg/kg = **28** mg			May repeat loading dose in 15 min			0.5 mg/mL	—
	mg to give ÷ mg/mL =	**56** mL				**56**	mL × (60 min/h ÷ 20 min) =	**168** mL/h
	Infusion				5–15 mg/h			—
				Ordered mg dose ÷ mg/mL = mL/h to set on pump				___ mL/h
Desmopressin	0.3 mcg/kg = **24** mcg			Give dose over 20–30 min			4 mcg/vial	
Dobutamine	Infusion		0.42		2.5–40 mcg/kg/ min	250 mg/ 125 mL	2000 mcg/mL	
				Take dose you want in mcg ÷ by drug index number = mL/h on pump				

(continues)

80 kg (continued)

DRUG	ORDERED AMOUNT	TOTAL DOSE TO GIVE	DRUG INDEX NUMBER	DIRECTIONS	INFUSION RANGE	DRUG MIXTURE	AMOUNT	DRUG/ mL	RUN AT	mL/h
Dopamine	Infusion		0.33		1–20 mcg/ kg/min	400 mg/ 250 mL	1600	mcg/mL		
	Take dose you want in mcg ÷ by drug index number = mL/h on pump									
Epinephrine	Infusion	1 mcg/min = 4 mL/h 2 mcg/min = 8 mL/h 3 mcg/min = 11 mL/h 4 mcg/min = 15 mL/h			1–4 mcg/min	4 mg/ 250 mL	16	mcg/mL		
	Ordered mcg dose/min ÷ mcg/mL × 60 min/h =								___	mL/h
Fenoldapam	Infusion		0.0084		0.01–1.6 mcg/ kg/min	10 mg/ 250 mL	40	mcg/mL		
	Take dose you want in mcg ÷ by drug index number = mL/h on pump									
Heparin	100 u/kg = 8000 u 200 u/kg = 16,000 u 300 u/kg = 24,000 u 400 u/kg = 32,000 u									
Isoproterenol	Infusion				5 mcg/min	1 mg/ 250 mL	4	mcg/mL		
	Ordered mcg dose/min ÷ mcg/mL × 60 min/h =								75	mL/h
Lidocaine	Infusion	1 mg/min = 7.5 mL/h			1–4 mg/min	2 g/ 250 mL	8	mg/mL	___	
	Ordered mg/min ÷ mg/mL × 60 min/h =								___	mL/h
Nitroglycerin	Infusion	3 mcg/min = 1 mL/h			3–200 mcg/min	50 mg/ 250 mL	200	mcg/mL	___	
	Ordered mcg/min ÷ mcg/mL × 60 min/h =								___	mL/h
Nitroprusside	Infusion	6.7 mcg/min = 1 mL/h			5–300 mcg/min	100 mg/ 250 mL	400	mcg/mL	___	
	Ordered mcg/min ÷ mcg/mL × 60 min/h =								___	mL/h
Norepinephrine	Infusion	1 mcg/min = 4 mL/h 2 mcg/min = 8 mL/h 3 mcg/min = 11 mL/h 4 mcg/min = 15 mL/h 5 mcg/min = 19 mL/h			2–20 mcg/min	4 mg/ 250 mL	16	mcg/mL		
	Ordered mcg dose/min ÷ mcg/mL × 60 min/h =								___	mL/h
Phenylephrine	Infusion	1.3 mcg/min = 1 mL/h			10–200 mcg/min	20 mg/ 250 mL	80	mcg/mL		
	Ordered mcg/min ÷ mcg/mL × 60 min/h =								___	mL/h
Primacor	0.05 mg/kg = 4 mg			Give load over 10 min		40 mg/ 200 mL	0.2	mg/mL		
	mg to give ÷ mg/mL = 20 mL				20 mL × (60 min/h ÷ 10 min) =				120	mL/h × 10 min
	Infusion		0.04		0.5 mcg/ kg/min	40 mg/ 200 mL	200	mcg/mL	___	
	Take dose you want in mcg ÷ by drug index number = mL/h on pump									
Trimethaphan	Infusion		—		0.3–6 mg/min	500 mg/ 500 mL	1	mg/mL	___	
	Ordered mg/min ÷ mg/mL × 60 min/h =								___	mL/h
Vasopressin		0.02 u/min = 3 mL/h 0.04 u/min = 6 mL/h				40 u/ 100 mL	400	u/mL		

81 kg

DRUG	ORDERED AMOUNT	TOTAL DOSE TO GIVE	DRUG INDEX NUMBER	DIRECTIONS	INFUSION RANGE	DRUG MIXTURE	AMOUNT	DRUG/mL	RUN AT	mL/h
Aminophylline	5 mg/kg =	405 mg		Give mg/kg load over 20 min		500 mg/ 250 mL	2	mg/mL		
	mg to give ÷ mg/mL =	203 mL			203	mL × (60 min/h ÷ 20 min) =			607.5	mL/h × 20 min
	Infusion				0.5–1 mg/kg/h	500 mg/ 250 mL	2	mg/mL		
					mg dose ordered × kg ÷ mg/mL =					___ mL/h
Amiodarone	Loading dose			Load **150 mg** over 10 min		900 mg/ 500 mL	1.8	mg/mL		—
	Ordered mg load dose (150 mg) ÷ mg/mL (1.8 mg/mL) = 83 mL to give × (60 min/h ÷ 10 min) = mL/h to set on pump								500	mL/h × 83 mL
	Infusion			Run at **1 mg/ min** × 6 h		900 mg/ 500 mL	1.8	mg/mL		
	Ordered mg dose (1 mg/min) ÷ mg/mL (1.0 mg/mL) = ___ × 60 min/h = mL/h to set on pump								33	mL/h × 6 h
	Infusion			Run at **0.5 mg/ min** × 18 h		900 mg/ 500 mL	1.8	mg/mL		
	Ordered mg dose (0.5 mg/min) ÷ mg/mL (1.8 mg/mL) = ___ × 60 min/h = mL/h to set on pump								17	mL/h × 18 h
Amrinone	0.75 mg/kg =	60.75 mg		Give mg/kg load over 10 min		300 mg/ 120 mL	2.5	mg/mL		
	mg to give ÷ mg/mL =	24 mL			24.3	mL × (60 min/h ÷ 10 min) =			145.8	mL/h × 10 min
	Infusion		0.51		5–10 mcg/ kg/min	300 mg/ 120 mL	2500	mcg/mL		
	Take dose you want in mcg ÷ by drug index number = mL/h on pump									
Brevibloc	Infusion		2.06		50–100 mcg/ kg/min	2.5 g/ 250 mL	10,000	mcg/mL		mL/h
	Take dose you want in mcg ÷ by drug index number = mL/h on pump									
Cardene	Infusion		—		0.5–10 mg/h	25 mg 250 mL	0.1	mg/mL		
	Ordered mg dose ÷ mg/mL = mL/h to set on pump									___ mL/h
Cardizem	0.25 mg/kg =	20.25 mg		Give mg/kg load over 20 min		50 mg/ 100 mL	0.5	mg/mL		
	mg to give ÷ mg/mL =	41 mL			40.5	mL × (60 min/h ÷ 20 min) =			122	mL/h
	0.35 mg/kg =	28.35 mg		May repeat loading dose in 15 min			0.5	mg/mL		
	mg to give ÷ mg/mL =	57 mL			56.7	mL × (60 min/h ÷ 20 min) =			170	mL/h
	Infusion				5–15 mg/h					—
	Ordered mg dose ÷ mg/mL = mL/h to set on pump									___ mL/h
Desmopressin	0.3 mcg/kg =	24 mcg		Give dose over 20–30 min			4	mcg/vial		
Dobutamine	Infusion		0.41		2.5–40 mcg/kg/ min	250 mg/ 125 mL	2000	mcg/mL		
	Take dose you want in mcg ÷ by drug index number = mL/h on pump									

(continues)

81 kg (continued)

DRUG	ORDERED AMOUNT	TOTAL DOSE TO GIVE	DRUG INDEX NUMBER	DIRECTIONS	INFUSION RANGE	DRUG MIXTURE	AMOUNT	DRUG/mL	RUN AT	mL/h
Dopamine	Infusion		0.33		1–20 mcg/kg/min	400 mg/250 mL	1600	mcg/mL		
	Take dose you want in mcg ÷ by drug index number = mL/h on pump									
Epinephrine	Infusion	1 mcg/min = 4 mL/h 2 mcg/min = 8 mL/h 3 mcg/min = 11 mL/h 4 mcg/min = 15 mL/h			1–4 mcg/min	4 mg/250 mL	16	mcg/mL		
	Ordered mcg dose/min ÷ mcg/mL × 60 min/h =								___	mL/h
Fenoldapam	Infusion		0.0083		0.01–1.6 mcg/kg/min	10 mg/250 mL	40	mcg/mL		
	Take dose you want in mcg ÷ by drug index number = mL/h on pump									
Heparin	100 u/kg = 8100 u 200 u/kg = 16,200 u 300 u/kg = 24,300 u 400 u/kg = 32,400 u									
Isoproterenol	Infusion				5 mcg/min	1 mg/250 mL	4	mcg/mL		
	Ordered mcg dose/min ÷ mcg/mL × 60 min/h =								**75**	mL/h
Lidocaine	Infusion	1 mg/min = 7.5 mL/h			1–4 mg/min	2 g/250 mL	8	mg/mL	___	
	Ordered mg/min ÷ mg/mL × 60 min/h =								___	mL/h
Nitroglycerin	Infusion	3 mcg/min = 1 mL/h			3–200 mcg/min	50 mg/250 mL	200	mcg/mL	___	
	Ordered mcg/min ÷ mcg/mL × 60 min/h =								___	mL/h
Nitroprusside	Infusion	6.7 mcg/min = 1 mL/h			5–300 mcg/min	100 mg/250 mL	400	mcg/mL	___	
	Ordered mcg/min ÷ mcg/mL × 60 min/h =								___	mL/h
Norepinephrine	Infusion	1 mcg/min = 4 mL/h 2 mcg/min = 8 mL/h 3 mcg/min = 11 mL/h 4 mcg/min = 15 mL/h 5 mcg/min = 19 mL/h			2–20 mcg/min	4 mg/250 mL	16	mcg/mL		
	Ordered mcg dose/min ÷ mcg/mL × 60 min/h =								___	mL/h
Phenylephrine	Infusion	1.3 mcg/min = 1 mL/h			10–200 mcg/min	20 mg/250 mL	80	mcg/mL		
	Ordered mcg/min ÷ mcg/mL × 60 min/h =								___	mL/h
Primacor	0.05 mg/kg = 4.05 mg			Give load over 10 min		40 mg/200 mL	0.2	mg/mL		
	mg to give ÷ mg/mL = 20 mL				20	mL × (60 min/h ÷ 10 min) =			**121.5**	mL/h × 10 min
	Infusion		0.04		0.5 mcg/kg/min	40 mg/200 mL	200	mcg/mL	___	
	Take dose you want in mcg ÷ by drug index number = mL/h on pump									
Trimethaphan	Infusion	—			0.3–6 mg/min	500 mg/500 mL	1	mg/mL	___	
	Ordered mg/min ÷ mg/mL × 60 min/h =								___	mL/h
Vasopressin		0.02 u/min = 3 mL/h 0.04 u/min = 6 mL/h				40 u/100 mL	400	u/mL		

82 kg

DRUG	ORDERED AMOUNT	TOTAL DOSE TO GIVE	DRUG INDEX NUMBER	DIRECTIONS	INFUSION RANGE	DRUG MIXTURE	AMOUNT	DRUG/mL	RUN AT	mL/h
Aminophylline	5 mg/kg =	410 mg		Give mg/kg load over 20 min		500 mg/250 mL		2 mg/mL		
	mg to give ÷ mg/mL =	205 mL					205	mL × (60 min/h ÷ 20 min) =	**615**	mL/h × 20 min
	Infusion				0.5–1 mg/kg/h	500 mg/250 mL		2 mg/mL		
					mg dose ordered × kg ÷ mg/mL =					___ mL/h
Amiodarone	Loading dose			Load **150 mg** over 10 min		900 mg/500 mL		1.8 mg/mL	—	
				Ordered mg load dose (150 mg) ÷ mg/mL (1.8 mg/mL) = 83 mL to give × (60 min/h ÷ 10 min) = mL/h to set on pump					**500**	mL/h × 83 mL
	Infusion			Run at **1 mg/min** × 6 h		900 mg/500 mL		1.8 mg/mL		
				Ordered mg dose (1 mg/min) ÷ mg/mL (1.8 mg/mL) = _____ × 60 min/h = mL/h to set on pump					**33**	mL/h × 6 h
	Infusion			Run at **0.5 mg/min** × 18 h		900 mg/500 mL		1.8 mg/mL		
				Ordered mg dose (0.5 mg/min) ÷ mg/mL (1.8 mg/mL) = _____ × 60 min/h = mL/h to set on pump					**17**	mL/h × 18 h
Amrinone	0.75 mg/kg =	61.5 mg		Give mg/kg load over 10 min		300 mg/120 mL		2.5 mg/mL	—	
	mg to give ÷ mg/mL =	25 mL					24.6	mL × (60 min/h ÷ 10 min) =	**147.6**	mL/h × 10 min
	Infusion		0.51		5–10 mcg/kg/min	300 mg/120 mL		2500 mcg/mL	—	
				Take dose you want in mcg ÷ by drug index number = mL/h on pump						
Brevibloc	Infusion		2.03		50–100 mcg/kg/min	2.5 g/250 mL		10,000 mcg/mL		___ mL/h
				Take dose you want in mcg ÷ by drug index number = mL/h on pump						
Cardene	Infusion		—		0.5–10 mg/h	25 mg/250 mL		0.1 mg/mL		
				Ordered mg dose ÷ mg/mL = mL/h to set on pump						___ mL/h
Cardizem	0.25 mg/kg =	20.5 mg		Give mg/kg load over 20 min		50 mg/100 mL		0.5 mg/mL	—	
	mg to give ÷ mg/mL =	41 mL					41	mL × (60 min/h ÷ 20 min) =	**123**	mL/h
	0.35 mg/kg =	28.7 mg		May repeat loading dose in 15 min				0.5 mg/mL	—	
	mg to give ÷ mg/mL =	57 mL					57.4	mL × (60 min/h ÷ 20 min) =	**172**	mL/h
	Infusion				5–15 mg/h				—	
				Ordered mg dose ÷ mg/mL = mL/h to set on pump						___ mL/h
Desmopressin	0.3 mcg/kg =	25 mcg		Give dose over 20–30 min				4 mcg/vial		
Dobutamine	Infusion		0.41		2.5–40 mcg/kg/min	250 mg/125 mL		2000 mcg/mL	—	
				Take dose you want in mcg ÷ by drug index number = mL/h on pump						

(continues)

82 kg (continued)

DRUG	ORDERED AMOUNT	TOTAL DOSE TO GIVE	DRUG INDEX NUMBER	DIRECTIONS	INFUSION RANGE	DRUG MIXTURE	AMOUNT	DRUG/mL	RUN AT	mL/h
Dopamine	Infusion		0.33		1–20 mcg/kg/min	400 mg/250 mL	1600	mcg/mL		
		Take dose you want in mcg ÷ by drug index number = mL/h on pump								
Epinephrine	Infusion	1 mcg/min = 4 mL/h 2 mcg/min = 8 mL/h 3 mcg/min = 11 mL/h 4 mcg/min = 15 mL/h			1–4 mcg/min	4 mg/250 mL	16	mcg/mL		
		Ordered mcg dose/min ÷ mcg/mL × 60 min/h = ___ mL/h								
Fenoldapam	Infusion		0.0082		0.01–1.6 mcg/kg/min	10 mg/250 mL	40	mcg/mL		
		Take dose you want in mcg ÷ by drug index number = mL/h on pump								
Heparin	100 u/kg = 8200 u 200 u/kg = 16,400 u 300 u/kg = 24,600 u 400 u/kg = 32,800 u									
Isoproterenol	Infusion				5 mcg/min	1 mg/250 mL	4	mcg/mL		
		Ordered mcg dose/min ÷ mcg/mL × 60 min/h =								75 mL/h
Lidocaine	Infusion	1 mg/min = 7.5 mL/h			1–4 mg/min	2 g/250 mL	8	mg/mL		─
		Ordered mg/min ÷ mg/mL × 60 min/h = ___ mL/h								
Nitroglycerin	Infusion	3 mcg/min = 1 mL/h			3–200 mcg/min	50 mg/250 mL	200	mcg/mL		─
		Ordered mcg/min ÷ mcg/mL × 60 min/h = ___ mL/h								
Nitroprusside	Infusion	6.7 mcg/min = 1 mL/h			5–300 mcg/min	100 mg/250 mL	400	mcg/mL		─
		Ordered mcg/min ÷ mcg/mL × 60 min/h = ___ mL/h								
Norepinephrine	Infusion	1 mcg/min = 4 mL/h 2 mcg/min = 8 mL/h 3 mcg/min = 11 mL/h 4 mcg/min = 15 mL/h 5 mcg/min = 19 mL/h			2–20 mcg/min	4 mg/250 mL	16	mcg/mL		
		Ordered mcg dose/min ÷ mcg/mL × 60 min/h = ___ mL/h								
Phenylephrine	Infusion	1.3 mcg/min = 1 mL/h			10–200 mcg/min	20 mg/250 mL	80	mcg/mL		
		Ordered mcg/min ÷ mcg/mL × 60 min/h = ___ mL/h								
Primacor	0.05 mg/kg = 4.1 mg			Give load over 10 min		40 mg/200 mL	0.2	mg/mL		
	mg to give ÷ mg/mL = 21 mL				21	mL × (60 min/h ÷ 10 min) =			123	mL/h × 10 min
	Infusion		0.04		0.5 mcg/kg/min	40 mg/200 mL	200	mcg/mL		─
		Take dose you want in mcg ÷ by drug index number = mL/h on pump								
Trimethaphan	Infusion		─		0.3–6 mg/min	500 mg/500 mL	1	mg/mL		─
		Ordered mg/min ÷ mg/mL × 60 min/h = ___ mL/h								
Vasopressin		0.02 u/min = 3 mL/h 0.04 u/min = 6 mL/h				40 u/100 mL	400	u/mL		

83 kg								
DRUG	**ORDERED AMOUNT**	**TOTAL DOSE TO GIVE**	**DRUG INDEX NUMBER**	**DIRECTIONS**	**INFUSION RANGE**	**DRUG MIXTURE**	**AMOUNT** / **DRUG/mL**	**RUN AT** / **mL/h**
Aminophylline	5 mg/kg = 415 mg			Give mg/kg load over 20 min		500 mg/ 250 mL	2 mg/mL	
	mg to give ÷ mg/mL = 208 mL				208	mL × (60 min/h ÷ 20 min) =		<u>622.5</u> mL/h × 20 min
	Infusion				0.5–1 mg/kg/h	500 mg/ 250 mL	2 mg/mL	
						mg dose ordered × kg ÷ mg/mL =		___ mL/h
Amiodarone	Loading dose			Load **150 mg** over 10 min		900 mg/ 500 mL	1.8 mg/mL	___
				Ordered mg load dose (150 mg) ÷ mg/mL (1.8 mg/mL) = 83 mL to give × (60 min/h ÷ 10 min) = mL/h to set on pump				<u>500</u> mL/h × 83 mL
	Infusion			Run at **1 mg/ min** × 6 h		900 mg/ 500 mL	1.8 mg/mL	
				Ordered mg dose (1 mg/min) ÷ mg/mL (1.8 mg/mL) = ____ × 60 min/h = mL/h to set on pump				<u>33</u> mL/h × 6 h
	Infusion			Run at **0.5 mg/ min** × 18 h		900 mg/ 500 mL	1.8 mg/mL	
				Ordered mg dose (0.5 mg/min) ÷ mg/mL (1.8 mg/mL) = ____ × 60 min/h = mL/h to set on pump				<u>17</u> mL/h × 18 h
Amrinone	0.75 mg/kg = 62.25 mg			Give mg/kg load over 10 min		300 mg/ 120 mL	2.5 mg/mL	___
	mg to give ÷ mg/mL = 25 mL				24.9	mL × (60 min/h ÷ 10 min) =		<u>149.4</u> mL/h × 10 min
	Infusion		0.50		5–10 mcg/ kg/min	300 mg/ 120 mL	2500 mcg/mL	
				Take dose you want in mcg ÷ by drug index number = mL/h on pump				
Brevibloc	Infusion		2.01		50–100 mcg/ kg/min	2.5 g/ 250 mL	10,000 mcg/mL	___ mL/h
				Take dose you want in mcg ÷ by drug index number = mL/h on pump				
Cardene	Infusion		___		0.5–10 mg/h	25 mg 250 mL	0.1 mg/mL	___
				Ordered mg dose ÷ mg/mL = mL/h to set on pump				___ mL/h
Cardizem	0.25 mg/kg = 20.75 mg			Give mg/kg load over 20 min		50 mg/ 100 mL	0.5 mg/mL	___
	mg to give ÷ mg/mL = 42 mL				41.5	mL × (60 min/h ÷ 20 min) =		<u>125</u> mL/h
	0.35 mg/kg = 29.05 mg			May repeat loading dose in 15 min			0.5 mg/mL	___
	mg to give ÷ mg/mL = 58 mL				58.1	mL × (60 min/h ÷ 20 min) =		<u>174</u> mL/h
	Infusion				5–15 mg/h			___
				Ordered mg dose ÷ mg/mL = mL/h to set on pump				___ mL/h
Desmopressin	0.3 mcg/kg = 25 mcg			Give dose over 20–30 min			4 mcg/vial	
Dobutamine	Infusion		0.40		2.5–40 mcg/kg/ min	250 mg/ 125 mL	2000 mcg/mL	
				Take dose you want in mcg ÷ by drug index number = mL/h on pump				

(continues)

83 kg (continued)

DRUG	ORDERED AMOUNT	TOTAL DOSE TO GIVE	DRUG INDEX NUMBER	DIRECTIONS	INFUSION RANGE	DRUG MIXTURE	AMOUNT	DRUG/mL	RUN AT mL/h
Dopamine	Infusion		0.32		1–20 mcg/kg/min	400 mg/250 mL	1600	mcg/mL	
	Take dose you want in mcg ÷ by drug index number = mL/h on pump								
Epinephrine	Infusion	1 mcg/min = 4 mL/h 2 mcg/min = 8 mL/h 3 mcg/min = 11 mL/h 4 mcg/min = 15 mL/h			1–4 mcg/min	4 mg/250 mL	16	mcg/mL	
		Ordered mcg dose/min ÷ mcg/mL × 60 min/h =							___ mL/h
Fenoldapam	Infusion		0.0081		0.01–1.6 mcg/kg/min	10 mg/250 mL	40	mcg/mL	
	Take dose you want in mcg ÷ by drug index number = mL/h on pump								
Heparin	100 u/kg = 200 u/kg = 300 u/kg = 400 u/kg =	8300 u 16,600 u 24,900 u 33,200 u							
Isoproterenol	Infusion				5 mcg/min	1 mg/250 mL	4	mcg/mL	
		Ordered mcg dose/min ÷ mcg/mL × 60 min/h =							**75** mL/h
Lidocaine	Infusion	1 mg/min = 7.5 mL/h			1–4 mg/min	2 g/250 mL	8	mg/mL	___
		Ordered mg/min ÷ mg/mL × 60 min/h =							___ mL/h
Nitroglycerin	Infusion	3 mcg/min = 1 mL/h			3–200 mcg/min	50 mg/250 mL	200	mcg/mL	___
		Ordered mcg/min ÷ mcg/mL × 60 min/h =							___ mL/h
Nitroprusside	Infusion	6.7 mcg/min = 1 mL/h			5–300 mcg/min	100 mg/250 mL	400	mcg/mL	___
		Ordered mcg/min ÷ mcg/mL × 60 min/h =							___ mL/h
Norepinephrine	Infusion	1 mcg/min = 4 mL/h 2 mcg/min = 8 mL/h 3 mcg/min = 11 mL/h 4 mcg/min = 15 mL/h 5 mcg/min = 19 mL/h			2–20 mcg/min	4 mg/250 mL	16	mcg/mL	
		Ordered mcg dose/min ÷ mcg/mL × 60 min/h =							___ mL/h
Phenylephrine	Infusion	1.3 mcg/min = 1 mL/h			10–200 mcg/min	20 mg/250 mL	80	mcg/mL	
		Ordered mcg/min ÷ mcg/mL × 60 min/h =							___ mL/h
Primacor	0.05 mg/kg =	4.15 mg		Give load over 10 min		40 mg/200 mL	0.2	mg/mL	
	mg to give ÷ mg/mL =	21 mL			21 mL × (60 min/h ÷ 10 min) =				**124.5** mL/h × 10 min
	Infusion		0.04		0.5 mcg/kg/min	40 mg/200 mL	200	mcg/mL	___
	Take dose you want in mcg ÷ by drug index number = mL/h on pump								
Trimethaphan	Infusion		___		0.3–6 mg/min	500 mg/500 mL	1	mg/mL	___
		Ordered mg/min ÷ mg/mL × 60 min/h =							___ mL/h
Vasopressin		0.02 u/min = 3 mL/h 0.04 u/min = 6 mL/h				40 u/100 mL	400	u/mL	

84 kg										
DRUG	**ORDERED AMOUNT**	**TOTAL DOSE TO GIVE**	**DRUG INDEX NUMBER**	**DIRECTIONS**	**INFUSION RANGE**	**DRUG MIXTURE**	**AMOUNT**	**DRUG/ mL**	**RUN AT**	**mL/h**
Aminophylline	5 mg/kg =	420 mg		Give mg/kg load over 20 min		500 mg/ 250 mL	2 mg/mL			
	mg to give ÷ mg/mL =	210 mL			210	mL × (60 min/h ÷ 20 min) =			630	mL/h × 20 min
	Infusion				0.5–1 mg/kg/h	500 mg/ 250 mL	2 mg/mL			
					mg dose ordered × kg ÷ mg/mL =				___	mL/h
Amiodarone	Loading dose			Load **150 mg** over 10 min		900 mg/ 500 mL	1.8 mg/mL		___	
				Ordered mg load dose (150 mg) ÷ mg/mL (1.8 mg/mL) = 83 mL to give × (60 min/h ÷ 10 min) = mL/h to set on pump					500	mL/h × 83 mL
	Infusion			Run at **1 mg/ min** × 6 h		900 mg/ 500 mL	1.8 mg/mL			
				Ordered mg dose (1 mg/min) ÷ mg/mL (1.8 mg/mL) = _____ × 60 min/h = mL/h to set on pump					33	mL/h × 6 h
	Infusion			Run at **0.5 mg/ min** × 18 h		900 mg/ 500 mL	1.8 mg/mL			
				Ordered mg dose (0.5 mg/min) ÷ mg/mL (1.8 mg/mL) = _____ × 60 min/h = mL/h to set on pump					17	mL/h × 18 h
Amrinone	0.75 mg/kg =	63 mg		Give mg/kg load over 10 min		300 mg/ 120 mL	2.5 mg/mL		___	
	mg to give ÷ mg/mL =	25 mL			25.2	mL × (60 min/h ÷ 10 min) =			151.2	mL/h × 10 min
	Infusion		0.50		5–10 mcg/ kg/min	300 mg/ 120 mL	2500 mcg/mL			
				Take dose you want in mcg ÷ by drug index number = mL/h on pump						
Brevibloc	Infusion		1.98		50–100 mcg/ kg/min	2.5 g/ 250 mL	10,000 mcg/mL		___	mL/h
				Take dose you want in mcg ÷ by drug index number = mL/h on pump						
Cardene	Infusion		___		0.5–10 mg/h	25 mg 250 mL	0.1 mg/mL		___	
				Ordered mg dose ÷ mg/mL = mL/h to set on pump					___	mL/h
Cardizem	0.25 mg/kg =	21 mg		Give mg/kg load over 20 min		50 mg/ 100 mL	0.5 mg/mL			
	mg to give ÷ mg/mL =	42 mL			42	mL × (60 min/h ÷ 20 min) =			126	mL/h
	0.35 mg/kg =	29.4 mg		May repeat loading dose in 15 min			0.5 mg/mL		___	
	mg to give ÷ mg/mL =	59 mL			58.8	mL × (60 min/h ÷ 20 min) =			176	mL/h
	Infusion				5–15 mg/h				___	
				Ordered mg dose ÷ mg/mL = mL/h to set on pump					___	mL/h
Desmopressin	0.3 mcg/kg =	25 mcg		Give dose over 20–30 min			4 mcg/vial			
Dobutamine	Infusion		0.40		2.5–40 mcg/kg/ min	250 mg/ 125 mL	2000 mcg/mL			
				Take dose you want in mcg ÷ by drug index number = mL/h on pump						

(continues)

84 kg (continued)

DRUG	ORDERED AMOUNT	TOTAL DOSE TO GIVE	DRUG INDEX NUMBER	DIRECTIONS	INFUSION RANGE	DRUG MIXTURE	AMOUNT	DRUG/mL	RUN AT mL/h
Dopamine	Infusion		0.32		1–20 mcg/kg/min	400 mg/250 mL	1600	mcg/mL	
	Take dose you want in mcg ÷ by drug index number = mL/h on pump								
Epinephrine	Infusion	1 mcg/min = 4 mL/h; 2 mcg/min = 8 mL/h; 3 mcg/min = 11 mL/h; 4 mcg/min = 15 mL/h			1–4 mcg/min	4 mg/250 mL	16	mcg/mL	
	Ordered mcg dose/min ÷ mcg/mL × 60 min/h = ___ mL/h								
Fenoldapam	Infusion		0.0080		0.01–1.6 mcg/kg/min	10 mg/250 mL	40	mcg/mL	
	Take dose you want in mcg ÷ by drug index number = mL/h on pump								
Heparin	100 u/kg = 8400 u; 200 u/kg = 16,800 u; 300 u/kg = 25,200 u; 400 u/kg = 33,600 u								
Isoproterenol	Infusion				5 mcg/min	1 mg/250 mL	4	mcg/mL	
	Ordered mcg dose/min ÷ mcg/mL × 60 min/h =								**75** mL/h
Lidocaine	Infusion	1 mg/min = 7.5 mL/h			1–4 mg/min	2 g/250 mL	8	mg/mL	—
	Ordered mg/min ÷ mg/mL × 60 min/h = ___ mL/h								
Nitroglycerin	Infusion	3 mcg/min = 1 mL/h			3–200 mcg/min	50 mg/250 mL	200	mcg/mL	—
	Ordered mcg/min ÷ mcg/mL × 60 min/h = ___ mL/h								
Nitroprusside	Infusion	6.7 mcg/min = 1 mL/h			5–300 mcg/min	100 mg/250 mL	400	mcg/mL	—
	Ordered mcg/min ÷ mcg/mL × 60 min/h = ___ mL/h								
Norepinephrine	Infusion	1 mcg/min = 4 mL/h; 2 mcg/min = 8 mL/h; 3 mcg/min = 11 mL/h; 4 mcg/min = 15 mL/h; 5 mcg/min = 19 mL/h			2–20 mcg/min	4 mg/250 mL	16	mcg/mL	
	Ordered mcg dose/min ÷ mcg/mL × 60 min/h = ___ mL/h								
Phenylephrine	Infusion	1.3 mcg/min = 1 mL/h			10–200 mcg/min	20 mg/250 mL	80	mcg/mL	
	Ordered mcg/min ÷ mcg/mL × 60 min/h = ___ mL/h								
Primacor	0.05 mg/kg =	4.2 mg		Give load over 10 min		40 mg/200 mL	0.2	mg/mL	
	mg to give ÷ mg/mL =	21 mL			21 mL × (60 min/h ÷ 10 min) =				**126** mL/h × 10 min
	Infusion		0.04		0.5 mcg/kg/min	40 mg/200 mL	200	mcg/mL	—
	Take dose you want in mcg ÷ by drug index number = mL/h on pump								
Trimethaphan	Infusion		—		0.3–6 mg/min	500 mg/500 mL	1	mg/mL	—
	Ordered mg/min ÷ mg/mL × 60 min/h = ___ mL/h								
Vasopressin		0.02 u/min = 3 mL/h; 0.04 u/min = 6 mL/h				40 u/100 mL	400	u/mL	

85 kg

DRUG	ORDERED AMOUNT	TOTAL DOSE TO GIVE	DRUG INDEX NUMBER	DIRECTIONS	INFUSION RANGE	DRUG MIXTURE	AMOUNT	DRUG/mL	RUN AT	mL/h
Aminophylline	5 mg/kg =	425 mg		Give mg/kg load over 20 min		500 mg/ 250 mL	2 mg/mL		
	mg to give ÷ mg/mL =	213 mL			213	mL × (60 min/h ÷ 20 min) =			637.5	mL/h × 20 min
	Infusion				0.5–1 mg/kg/h	500 mg/ 250 mL	2 mg/mL		
					mg dose ordered × kg ÷ mg/mL =				___	mL/h
Amiodarone	Loading dose			Load **150 mg** over 10 min		900 mg/ 500 mL	1.8 mg/mL		___
	Ordered mg load dose (150 mg) ÷ mg/mL (1.8 mg/mL) = 83 mL to give × (60 min/h ÷ 10 min) = mL/h to set on pump								500	mL/h × 83 mL
	Infusion			Run at **1 mg/ min** × 6 h		900 mg/ 500 mL	1.8 mg/mL		
	Ordered mg dose (1 mg/min) ÷ mg/mL (1.8 mg/mL) = _____ × 60 min/h = mL/h to set on pump								33	mL/h × 6 h
	Infusion			Run at **0.5 mg/ min** × 18 h		900 mg/ 500 mL	1.8 mg/mL		
	Ordered mg dose (0.5 mg/min) ÷ mg/mL (1.8 mg/mL) = _____ × 60 min/h = mL/h to set on pump								17	mL/h × 18 h
Amrinone	0.75 mg/kg =	63.75 mg		Give mg/kg load over 10 min		300 mg/ 120 mL	2.5 mg/mL		___
	mg to give ÷ mg/mL =	26 mL			25.5	mL × (60 min/h ÷ 10 min) =			153	mL/h × 10 min
	Infusion		0.49		5–10 mcg/ kg/min	300 mg/ 120 mL	2500 mcg/mL		
	Take dose you want in mcg ÷ by drug index number = mL/h on pump									
Brevibloc	Infusion		1.96		50–100 mcg/ kg/min	2.5 g/ 250 mL	10,000 mcg/mL		___	mL/h
	Take dose you want in mcg ÷ by drug index number = mL/h on pump									
Cardene	Infusion		—		0.5–10 mg/h	25 mg 250 mL	0.1 mg/mL		___
	Ordered mg dose ÷ mg/mL = mL/h to set on pump								___	mL/h
Cardizem	0.25 mg/kg =	21.25 mg		Give mg/kg load over 20 min		50 mg/ 100 mL	0.5 mg/mL		___
	mg to give ÷ mg/mL =	43 mL			42.5	mL × (60 min/h ÷ 20 min) =			128	mL/h
	0.35 mg/kg =	29.75 mg		May repeat loading dose in 15 min			0.5 mg/mL		___
	mg to give ÷ mg/mL =	60 mL			59.5	mL × (60 min/h ÷ 20 min) =			179	mL/h
	Infusion				5–15 mg/h				___
	Ordered mg dose ÷ mg/mL = mL/h to set on pump								___	mL/h
Desmopressin	0.3 mcg/kg =	26 mcg		Give dose over 20–30 min			4 mcg/vial		
Dobutamine	Infusion		0.39		2.5–40 mcg/kg/ min	250 mg/ 125 mL	2000 mcg/mL		
	Take dose you want in mcg ÷ by drug index number = mL/h on pump									

(continues)

85 kg (continued)

DRUG	ORDERED AMOUNT	TOTAL DOSE TO GIVE	DRUG INDEX NUMBER	DIRECTIONS	INFUSION RANGE	DRUG MIXTURE	AMOUNT	DRUG/mL	RUN AT	mL/h
Dopamine	Infusion		0.31		1–20 mcg/kg/min	400 mg/250 mL	1600	mcg/mL		
			Take dose you want in mcg ÷ by drug index number = mL/h on pump							
Epinephrine	Infusion	1 mcg/min = 4 mL/h 2 mcg/min = 8 mL/h 3 mcg/min = 11 mL/h 4 mcg/min = 15 mL/h			1–4 mcg/min	4 mg/250 mL	16	mcg/mL		
				Ordered mcg dose/min ÷ mcg/mL × 60 min/h =					___	mL/h
Fenoldapam	Infusion		0.0079		0.01–1.6 mcg/kg/min	10 mg/250 mL	40	mcg/mL		
			Take dose you want in mcg ÷ by drug index number = mL/h on pump							
Heparin	100 u/kg = 8500 u 200 u/kg = 17,000 u 300 u/kg = 25,500 u 400 u/kg = 34,000 u									
Isoproterenol	Infusion				5 mcg/min	1 mg/250 mL	4	mcg/mL		
				Ordered mcg dose/min ÷ mcg/mL × 60 min/h =					75	mL/h
Lidocaine	Infusion	1 mg/min = 7.5 mL/h			1–4 mg/min	2 g/250 mL	8	mg/mL		___
				Ordered mg/min ÷ mg/mL × 60 min/h =					___	mL/h
Nitroglycerin	Infusion	3 mcg/min = 1 mL/h			3–200 mcg/min	50 mg/250 mL	200	mcg/mL		___
				Ordered mcg/min ÷ mcg/mL × 60 min/h =					___	mL/h
Nitroprusside	Infusion	6.7 mcg/min = 1 mL/h			5–300 mcg/min	100 mg/250 mL	400	mcg/mL		___
				Ordered mcg/min ÷ mcg/mL × 60 min/h =					___	mL/h
Norepinephrine	Infusion	1 mcg/min = 4 mL/h 2 mcg/min = 8 mL/h 3 mcg/min = 11 mL/h 4 mcg/min = 15 mL/h 5 mcg/min = 19 mL/h			2–20 mcg/min	4 mg/250 mL	16	mcg/mL		
				Ordered mcg dose/min ÷ mcg/mL × 60 min/h =					___	mL/h
Phenylephrine	Infusion	1.3 mcg/min = 1 mL/h			10–200 mcg/min	20 mg/250 mL	80	mcg/mL		
				Ordered mcg/min ÷ mcg/mL × 60 min/h =					___	mL/h
Primacor	0.05 mg/kg = 4.25 mg			Give load over 10 min		40 mg/200 mL	0.2	mg/mL		
	mg to give ÷ mg/mL = 21 mL				21	mL × (60 min/h ÷ 10 min) =			127.5	mL/h × 10 min
	Infusion		0.04		0.5 mcg/kg/min	40 mg/200 mL	200	mcg/mL		___
			Take dose you want in mcg ÷ by drug index number = mL/h on pump							
Trimethaphan	Infusion		—		0.3–6 mg/min	500 mg/500 mL	1	mg/mL		___
				Ordered mg/min ÷ mg/mL × 60 min/h =					___	mL/h
Vasopressin		0.02 u/min = 3 mL/h 0.04 u/min = 6 mL/h				40 u/100 mL	400	u/mL		

86 kg

DRUG	ORDERED AMOUNT	TOTAL DOSE TO GIVE	DRUG INDEX NUMBER	DIRECTIONS	INFUSION RANGE	DRUG MIXTURE	AMOUNT DRUG/mL	RUN AT mL/h
Aminophylline	5 mg/kg =	430 mg		Give mg/kg load over 20 min		500 mg/ 250 mL	2 mg/mL	
	mg to give ÷ mg/mL =	215 mL			215	mL × (60 min/h ÷ 20 min) =		645 mL/h × 20 min
	Infusion				0.5–1 mg/kg/h	500 mg/ 250 mL	2 mg/mL	
				mg dose ordered × kg ÷ mg/mL = ___ mL/h				
Amiodarone	Loading dose			Load **150 mg** over 10 min		900 mg/ 500 mL	1.8 mg/mL	—
				Ordered mg load dose (150 mg) ÷ mg/mL (1.8 mg/mL) = 83 mL to give × (60 min/h ÷ 10 min) = mL/h to set on pump				500 mL/h × 83 mL
	Infusion			Run at **1 mg/ min** × 6 h		900 mg/ 500 mL	1.8 mg/mL	
				Ordered mg dose (1 mg/min) ÷ mg/mL (1.8 mg/mL) = ____ × 60 min/h = mL/h to set on pump				33 mL/h × 6 h
	Infusion			Run at **0.5 mg/ min** × 18 h		900 mg/ 500 mL	1.8 mg/mL	
				Ordered mg dose (0.5 mg/min) ÷ mg/mL (1.8 mg/mL) = ____ × 60 min/h = mL/h to set on pump				17 mL/h × 18 h
Amrinone	0.75 mg/kg =	64.5 mg		Give mg/kg load over 10 min		300 mg/ 120 mL	2.5 mg/mL	—
	mg to give ÷ mg/mL =	26 mL			25.8	mL × (60 min/h ÷ 10 min) =		154.8 mL/h × 10 min
	Infusion		0.48		5–10 mcg/ kg/min	300 mg/ 120 mL	2500 mcg/mL	—
				Take dose you want in mcg ÷ by drug index number = mL/h on pump				
Brevibloc	Infusion		1.94		50–100 mcg/ kg/min	2.5 g/ 250 mL	10,000 mcg/mL	___ mL/h
				Take dose you want in mcg ÷ by drug index number = mL/h on pump				
Cardene	Infusion		—		0.5–10 mg/h	25 mg 250 mL	0.1 mg/mL	___
				Ordered mg dose ÷ mg/mL = mL/h to set on pump				___ mL/h
Cardizem	0.25 mg/kg =	21.5 mg		Give mg/kg load over 20 min		50 mg/ 100 mL	0.5 mg/mL	—
	mg to give ÷ mg/mL =	43 mL			43	mL × (60 min/h ÷ 20 min) =		129 mL/h
	0.35 mg/kg =	30.1 mg		May repeat loading dose in 15 min			0.5 mg/mL	—
	mg to give ÷ mg/mL =	60 mL			60.2	mL × (60 min/h ÷ 20 min) =		181 mL/h
					5–15 mg/h			—
	Infusion			Ordered mg dose ÷ mg/mL = mL/h to set on pump				___ mL/h
Desmopressin	0.3 mcg/kg =	26 mcg		Give dose over 20–30 min			4 mcg/vial	
Dobutamine	Infusion		0.39		2.5–40 mcg/kg/ min	250 mg/ 125 mL	2000 mcg/mL	
				Take dose you want in mcg ÷ by drug index number = mL/h on pump				

(continues)

86 kg (continued)

DRUG	ORDERED AMOUNT	TOTAL DOSE TO GIVE	DRUG INDEX NUMBER	DIRECTIONS	INFUSION RANGE	DRUG MIXTURE	AMOUNT	DRUG/mL	RUN AT	mL/h
Dopamine	Infusion		0.31		1–20 mcg/kg/min	400 mg/250 mL	1600	mcg/mL		
	Take dose you want in mcg ÷ by drug index number = mL/h on pump									
Epinephrine	Infusion	1 mcg/min = 4 mL/h 2 mcg/min = 8 mL/h 3 mcg/min = 11 mL/h 4 mcg/min = 15 mL/h			1–4 mcg/min	4 mg/250 mL	16	mcg/mL		
	Ordered mcg dose/min ÷ mcg/mL × 60 min/h =								___	mL/h
Fenoldapam	Infusion		0.0078		0.01–1.6 mcg/kg/min	10 mg/250 mL	40	mcg/mL		
	Take dose you want in mcg ÷ by drug index number = mL/h on pump									
Heparin	100 u/kg =	8600 u								
	200 u/kg =	17,200 u								
	300 u/kg =	25,800 u								
	400 u/kg =	34,400 u								
Isoproterenol	Infusion				5 mcg/min	1 mg/250 mL	4	mcg/mL		
	Ordered mcg dose/min ÷ mcg/mL × 60 min/h =								75	mL/h
Lidocaine	Infusion	1 mg/min = 7.5 mL/h			1–4 mg/min	2 g/250 mL	8	mg/mL	___	
	Ordered mg/min ÷ mg/mL × 60 min/h =								___	mL/h
Nitroglycerin	Infusion	3 mcg/min = 1 mL/h			3–200 mcg/min	50 mg/250 mL	200	mcg/mL		
	Ordered mcg/min ÷ mcg/mL × 60 min/h =								___	mL/h
Nitroprusside	Infusion	6.7 mcg/min = 1 mL/h			5–300 mcg/min	100 mg/250 mL	400	mcg/mL	___	
	Ordered mcg/min ÷ mcg/mL × 60 min/h =								___	mL/h
Norepinephrine	Infusion	1 mcg/min = 4 mL/h 2 mcg/min = 8 mL/h 3 mcg/min = 11 mL/h 4 mcg/min = 15 mL/h 5 mcg/min = 19 mL/h			2–20 mcg/min	4 mg/250 mL	16	mcg/mL		
	Ordered mcg dose/min ÷ mcg/mL × 60 min/h =								___	mL/h
Phenylephrine	Infusion	1.3 mcg/min = 1 mL/h			10–200 mcg/min	20 mg/250 mL	80	mcg/mL		
	Ordered mcg/min ÷ mcg/mL × 60 min/h =								___	mL/h
Primacor	0.05 mg/kg =	4.3 mg		Give load over 10 min		40 mg/200 mL	0.2	mg/mL		
	mg to give ÷ mg/mL =	22 mL				22 mL × (60 min/h ÷ 10 min) =			129	mL/h × 10 min
	Infusion		0.04		0.5 mcg/kg/min	40 mg/200 mL	200	mcg/mL	___	
	Take dose you want in mcg ÷ by drug index number = mL/h on pump									
Trimethaphan	Infusion		—		0.3–6 mg/min	500 mg/500 mL	1	mg/mL	___	
	Ordered mg/min ÷ mg/mL × 60 min/h =								___	mL/h
Vasopressin		0.02 u/min = 3 mL/h 0.04 u/min = 6 mL/h				40 u/100 mL	400	u/mL		

87 kg

DRUG	ORDERED AMOUNT	TOTAL DOSE TO GIVE	DRUG INDEX NUMBER	DIRECTIONS	INFUSION RANGE	DRUG MIXTURE	AMOUNT	DRUG/mL	RUN AT	mL/h
Aminophylline	5 mg/kg = 435 mg			Give mg/kg load over 20 min		500 mg/ 250 mL	2 mg/mL			
	mg to give ÷ mg/mL = 218 mL				218	mL × (60 min/h ÷ 20 min) =			652.5	mL/h × 20 min
	Infusion				0.5–1 mg/kg/h	500 mg/ 250 mL	2 mg/mL			
					mg dose ordered × kg ÷ mg/mL =				___	mL/h
Amiodarone	Loading dose			Load **150 mg** over 10 min		900 mg/ 500 mL	1.8 mg/mL		—	
				Ordered mg load dose (150 mg) ÷ mg/mL (1.8 mg/mL) = 83 mL to give × (60 min/h ÷ 10 min) = mL/h to set on pump					500	mL/h × 83 mL
	Infusion			Run at **1 mg/ min** × 6 h		900 mg/ 500 mL	1.8 mg/mL			
				Ordered mg dose (1 mg/min) ÷ mg/mL (1.8 mg/mL) = ___ × 60 min/h = mL/h to set on pump					33	mL/h × 6 h
	Infusion			Run at **0.5 mg/ min** × 18 h		900 mg/ 500 mL	1.8 mg/mL			
				Ordered mg dose (0.5 mg/min) ÷ mg/mL (1.8 mg/mL) = ___ × 60 min/h = mL/h to set on pump					17	mL/h × 18 h
Amrinone	0.75 mg/kg = 65.25 mg			Give mg/kg load over 10 min		300 mg/ 120 mL	2.5 mg/mL		—	
	mg to give ÷ mg/mL = 26 mL				26.1	mL × (60 min/h ÷ 10 min) =			156.6	mL/h × 10 min
	Infusion		0.48		5–10 mcg/ kg/min	300 mg/ 120 mL	2500 mcg/mL		—	
				Take dose you want in mcg ÷ by drug index number = mL/h on pump						
Brevibloc	Intusion		1.91		50–100 mcg/ kg/min	2.5 g/ 250 mL	10,000 mcg/mL		___	mL/h
				Take dose you want in mcg ÷ by drug index number = mL/h on pump						
Cardene	Infusion		—		0.5–10 mg/h	25 mg 250 mL	0.1 mg/mL		—	
				Ordered mg dose ÷ mg/mL = mL/h to set on pump					___	mL/h
Cardizem	0.25 mg/kg = 21.75 mg			Give mg/kg load over 20 min		50 mg/ 100 mL	0.5 mg/mL		—	
	mg to give ÷ mg/mL = 44 mL				43.5	mL × (60 min/h ÷ 20 min) =			131	mL/h
	0.35 mg/kg = 30.45 mg			May repeat loading dose in 15 min			0.5 mg/mL		—	
	mg to give ÷ mg/mL = 61 mL				60.9	mL × (60 min/h ÷ 20 min) =			183	mL/h
	Infusion				5–15 mg/h				—	
				Ordered mg dose ÷ mg/mL = mL/h to set on pump					___	mL/h
Desmopressin	0.3 mcg/kg = 26 mcg			Give dose over 20–30 min			4 mcg/vial			
Dobutamine	Infusion		0.38		2.5–40 mcg/kg/ min	250 mg/ 125 mL	2000 mcg/mL			
				Take dose you want in mcg ÷ by drug index number = mL/h on pump						

(continues)

87 kg (continued)

DRUG	ORDERED AMOUNT	TOTAL DOSE TO GIVE	DRUG INDEX NUMBER	DIRECTIONS	INFUSION RANGE	DRUG MIXTURE	AMOUNT	DRUG/ mL	RUN AT	mL/h
Dopamine	Infusion		0.31		1–20 mcg/ kg/min	400 mg/ 250 mL	1600	mcg/mL		
	Take dose you want in mcg ÷ by drug index number = mL/h on pump									
Epinephrine	Infusion	1 mcg/min = 4 mL/h 2 mcg/min = 8 mL/h 3 mcg/min = 11 mL/h 4 mcg/min = 15 mL/h			1–4 mcg/min	4 mg/ 250 mL	16	mcg/mL		
	Ordered mcg dose/min ÷ mcg/mL × 60 min/h =								___	mL/h
Fenoldapam	Infusion		0.0077		0.01–1.6 mcg/ kg/min	10 mg/ 250 mL	40	mcg/mL		
	Take dose you want in mcg ÷ by drug index number = mL/h on pump									
Heparin	100 u/kg = 8700 u 200 u/kg = 17,400 u 300 u/kg = 26,100 u 400 u/kg = 34,800 u									
Isoproterenol	Infusion				5 mcg/min	1 mg/ 250 mL	4	mcg/mL		
	Ordered mcg dose/min ÷ mcg/mL × 60 min/h =								75	mL/h
Lidocaine	Infusion	1 mg/min = 7.5 mL/h			1–4 mg/min	2 g/ 250 mL	8	mg/mL	—	
	Ordered mg/min ÷ mg/mL × 60 min/h =								___	mL/h
Nitroglycerin	Infusion	3 mcg/min = 1 mL/h			3–200 mcg/min	50 mg/ 250 mL	200	mcg/mL	—	
	Ordered mcg/min ÷ mcg/mL × 60 min/h =								___	mL/h
Nitroprusside	Infusion	6.7 mcg/min = 1 mL/h			5–300 mcg/min	100 mg/ 250 mL	400	mcg/mL	—	
	Ordered mcg/min ÷ mcg/mL × 60 min/h =								___	mL/h
Norepinephrine	Infusion	1 mcg/min = 4 mL/h 2 mcg/min = 8 mL/h 3 mcg/min = 11 mL/h 4 mcg/min = 15 mL/h 5 mcg/min = 19 mL/h			2–20 mcg/min	4 mg/ 250 mL	16	mcg/mL		
	Ordered mcg dose/min ÷ mcg/mL × 60 min/h =								___	mL/h
Phenylephrine	Infusion	1.3 mcg/min = 1 mL/h			10–200 mcg/min	20 mg/ 250 mL	80	mcg/mL		
	Ordered mcg/min ÷ mcg/mL × 60 min/h =								___	mL/h
Primacor	0.05 mg/kg = 4.35 mg			Give load over 10 min		40 mg/ 200 mL	0.2	mg/mL		
	mg to give ÷ mg/mL = 22 mL				22	mL × (60 min/h ÷ 10 min) =			130.5	mL/h × 10 min
	Infusion		0.04		0.5 mcg/ kg/min	40 mg/ 200 mL	200	mcg/mL	—	
	Take dose you want in mcg ÷ by drug index number = mL/h on pump									
Trimethaphan	Infusion		—		0.3–6 mg/min	500 mg/ 500 mL	1	mg/mL	—	
	Ordered mg/min ÷ mg/mL × 60 min/h =								___	mL/h
Vasopressin		0.02 u/min = 3 mL/h 0.04 u/min = 6 mL/h				40 u/ 100 mL	400	u/mL		

88 kg

DRUG	ORDERED AMOUNT	TOTAL DOSE TO GIVE	DRUG INDEX NUMBER	DIRECTIONS	INFUSION RANGE	DRUG MIXTURE	AMOUNT	DRUG/mL	RUN AT	mL/h
Aminophylline	5 mg/kg = 440 mg			Give mg/kg load over 20 min		500 mg/ 250 mL	2 mg/mL			
	mg to give ÷ mg/mL = 220 mL				220	mL × (60 min/h ÷ 20 min) =			660	mL/h × 20 min
	Infusion				0.5–1 mg/kg/h	500 mg/ 250 mL	2 mg/mL			
					mg dose ordered × kg ÷ mg/mL =				___	mL/h
Amiodarone	Loading dose			Load **150 mg** over 10 min		900 mg/ 500 mL	1.8 mg/mL		___	
				Ordered mg load dose (150 mg) ÷ mg/mL (1.8 mg/mL) = 83 mL to give × (60 min/h ÷ 10 min) = mL/h to set on pump					500	mL/h × 83 mL
	Infusion			Run at **1 mg/ min** × 6 h		900 mg/ 500 mL	1.8 mg/mL			
				Ordered mg dose (1 mg/min) ÷ mg/mL (1.8 mg/mL) = ____ × 60 min/h = mL/h to set on pump					33	mL/h × 6 h
	Infusion			Run at **0.5 mg/ min** × 18 h		900 mg/ 500 mL	1.8 mg/mL			
				Ordered mg dose (0.5 mg/min) ÷ mg/mL (1.8 mg/mL) = ____ × 60 min/h = mL/h to set on pump					17	mL/h × 18 h
Amrinone	0.75 mg/kg = 66 mg			Give mg/kg load over 10 min		300 mg/ 120 mL	2.5 mg/mL		___	
	mg to give ÷ mg/mL = 26 mL				26.4	mL × (60 min/h ÷ 10 min) =			158.4	mL/h × 10 min
	Infusion		0.47		5–10 mcg/ kg/min	300 mg/ 120 mL	2500 mcg/mL		___	
				Take dose you want in mcg ÷ by drug index number = mL/h on pump						
Brevibloc	Infusion		1.89		50–100 mcg/ kg/min	2.5 g/ 250 mL	10,000 mcg/mL		___	mL/h
				Take dose you want in mcg ÷ by drug index number = mL/h on pump						
Cardene	Infusion			—	0.5–10 mg/h	25 mg/ 250 mL	0.1 mg/mL		___	
				Ordered mg dose ÷ mg/mL = mL/h to set on pump					___	mL/h
Cardizem	0.25 mg/kg = 22 mg			Give mg/kg load over 20 min		50 mg/ 100 mL	0.5 mg/mL		___	
	mg to give ÷ mg/mL = 44 mL				44	mL × (60 min/h ÷ 20 min) =			132	mL/h
	0.35 mg/kg = 30.8 mg			May repeat loading dose in 15 min			0.5 mg/mL		___	
	mg to give ÷ mg/mL = 62 mL				61.6	mL × (60 min/h ÷ 20 min) =			185	mL/h
	Infusion				5–15 mg/h				___	
				Ordered mg dose ÷ mg/mL = mL/h to set on pump					___	mL/h
Desmopressin	0.3 mcg/kg = 26 mcg			Give dose over 20–30 min			4 mcg/vial			
Dobutamine	Infusion		0.38		2.5–40 mcg/kg/ min	250 mg/ 125 mL	2000 mcg/mL			
				Take dose you want in mcg ÷ by drug index number = mL/h on pump						

(continues)

88 kg (continued)

DRUG	ORDERED AMOUNT	TOTAL DOSE TO GIVE	DRUG INDEX NUMBER	DIRECTIONS	INFUSION RANGE	DRUG MIXTURE	AMOUNT	DRUG/mL	RUN AT	mL/h
Dopamine	Infusion		0.30		1–20 mcg/kg/min	400 mg/250 mL	1600	mcg/mL		
	Take dose you want in mcg ÷ by drug index number = mL/h on pump									
Epinephrine	Infusion	1 mcg/min = 4 mL/h 2 mcg/min = 8 mL/h 3 mcg/min = 11 mL/h 4 mcg/min = 15 mL/h			1–4 mcg/min	4 mg/250 mL	16	mcg/mL		
	Ordered mcg dose/min ÷ mcg/mL × 60 min/h = ___ mL/h									
Fenoldapam	Infusion		0.0076		0.01–1.6 mcg/kg/min	10 mg/250 mL	40	mcg/mL		
	Take dose you want in mcg ÷ by drug index number = mL/h on pump									
Heparin	100 u/kg = 8800 u 200 u/kg = 17,600 u 300 u/kg = 26,400 u 400 u/kg = 35,200 u									
Isoproterenol	Infusion				5 mcg/min	1 mg/250 mL	4	mcg/mL		
	Ordered mcg dose/min ÷ mcg/mL × 60 min/h = **75** mL/h									
Lidocaine	Infusion	1 mg/min = 7.5 mL/h			1–4 mg/min	2 g/250 mL	8	mg/mL	—	
	Ordered mg/min ÷ mg/mL × 60 min/h = ___ mL/h									
Nitroglycerin	Infusion	3 mcg/min = 1 mL/h			3–200 mcg/min	50 mg/250 mL	200	mcg/mL	—	
	Ordered mcg/min ÷ mcg/mL × 60 min/h = ___ mL/h									
Nitroprusside	Infusion	6.7 mcg/min = 1 mL/h			5–300 mcg/min	100 mg/250 mL	400	mcg/mL	—	
	Ordered mcg/min ÷ mcg/mL × 60 min/h = ___ mL/h									
Norepinephrine	Infusion	1 mcg/min = 4 mL/h 2 mcg/min = 8 mL/h 3 mcg/min = 11 mL/h 4 mcg/min = 15 mL/h 5 mcg/min = 19 mL/h			2–20 mcg/min	4 mg/250 mL	16	mcg/mL		
	Ordered mcg dose/min ÷ mcg/mL × 60 min/h = ___ mL/h									
Phenylephrine	Infusion	1.3 mcg/min = 1 mL/h			10–200 mcg/min	20 mg/250 mL	80	mcg/mL		
	Ordered mcg/min ÷ mcg/mL × 60 min/h = ___ mL/h									
Primacor	0.05 mg/kg = 4.4 mg			Give load over 10 min		40 mg/200 mL	0.2	mg/mL		
	mg to give ÷ mg/mL = 22 mL					22 mL × (60 min/h ÷ 10 min) =		**132**	mL/h × 10 min	
	Infusion		0.04		0.5 mcg/kg/min	40 mg/200 mL	200	mcg/mL	—	
	Take dose you want in mcg ÷ by drug index number = mL/h on pump									
Trimethaphan	Infusion		—		0.3–6 mg/min	500 mg/500 mL	1	mg/mL	—	
	Ordered mg/min ÷ mg/mL × 60 min/h = ___ mL/h									
Vasopressin		0.02 u/min = 3 mL/h 0.04 u/min = 6 mL/h				40 u/100 mL	400	u/mL		

89 kg

DRUG	ORDERED AMOUNT	TOTAL DOSE TO GIVE	DRUG INDEX NUMBER	DIRECTIONS	INFUSION RANGE	DRUG MIXTURE	AMOUNT	DRUG/ mL	RUN AT	mL/h
Aminophylline	5 mg/kg =	445 mg		Give mg/kg load over 20 min		500 mg/ 250 mL	2 mg/mL		
	mg to give ÷ mg/mL =	223 mL				223	mL × (60 min/h ÷ 20 min) =		667.5	mL/h × 20 min
	Infusion				0.5–1 mg/kg/h	500 mg/ 250 mL	2 mg/mL		
					mg dose ordered × kg ÷ mg/mL =				___	mL/h
Amiodarone	Loading dose			Load **150 mg** over 10 min		900 mg/ 500 mL	1.8 mg/mL		___
				Ordered mg load dose (150 mg) ÷ mg/mL (1.8 mg/mL) = 83 mL to give × (60 min/h ÷ 10 min) = mL/h to set on pump					500	mL/h × 83 mL
	Infusion			Run at **1 mg/ min** × 6 h		900 mg/ 500 mL	1.8 mg/mL		
				Ordered mg dose (1 mg/min) ÷ mg/mL (1.8 mg/mL) = _____ × 60 min/h = mL/h to set on pump					33	mL/h × 6 h
	Infusion			Run at **0.5 mg/ min** × 18 h		900 mg/ 500 mL	1.8 mg/mL		
				Ordered mg dose (0.5 mg/min) ÷ mg/mL (1.8 mg/mL) = _____ × 60 min/h = mL/h to set on pump					17	mL/h × 18 h
Amrinone	0.75 mg/kg =	66.75 mg		Give mg/kg load over 10 min		300 mg/ 120 mL	2.5 mg/mL		___
	mg to give ÷ mg/mL =	27 mL				26.7	mL × (60 min/h ÷ 10 min) =		160.2	mL/h × 10 min
	Infusion		0.47		5–10 mcg/ kg/min	300 mg/ 120 mL	2500 mcg/mL		___
				Take dose you want in mcg ÷ by drug index number = mL/h on pump						
Brevibloc	Infusion		1.87		50–100 mcg/ kg/min	2.5 g/ 250 mL	10,000 mcg/mL		___	mL/h
				Take dose you want in mcg ÷ by drug index number = mL/h on pump						
Cardene	Infusion		—		0.5–10 mg/h	25 mg 250 mL	0.1 mg/mL		___
				Ordered mg dose ÷ mg/mL = mL/h to set on pump					___	mL/h
Cardizem	0.25 mg/kg =	22.25 mg		Give mg/kg load over 20 min		50 mg/ 100 mL	0.5 mg/mL		___
	mg to give ÷ mg/mL =	45 mL				44.5	mL × (60 min/h ÷ 20 min) =		134	mL/h
	0.35 mg/kg =	31.15 mg		May repeat loading dose in 15 min			0.5 mg/mL		___
	mg to give ÷ mg/mL =	62 mL				62.3	mL × (60 min/h ÷ 20 min) =		187	mL/h
	Infusion				5–15 mg/h				___
				Ordered mg dose ÷ mg/mL = mL/h to set on pump					___	mL/h
Desmopressin	0.3 mcg/kg =	27 mcg		Give dose over 20–30 min			4 mcg/vial		
Dobutamine	Infusion		0.37		2.5–40 mcg/kg/ min	250 mg/ 125 mL	2000 mcg/mL		
				Take dose you want in mcg ÷ by drug index number = mL/h on pump						

(continues)

89 kg (continued)

DRUG	ORDERED AMOUNT	TOTAL DOSE TO GIVE	DRUG INDEX NUMBER	DIRECTIONS	INFUSION RANGE	DRUG MIXTURE	AMOUNT	DRUG/mL	RUN AT mL/h
Dopamine	Infusion		0.30		1–20 mcg/ kg/min	400 mg/ 250 mL	1600	mcg/mL	
				Take dose you want in mcg ÷ by drug index number = mL/h on pump					
Epinephrine	Infusion	1 mcg/min = 4 mL/h 2 mcg/min = 8 mL/h 3 mcg/min = 11 mL/h 4 mcg/min = 15 mL/h			1–4 mcg/min	4 mg/ 250 mL	16	mcg/mL	
				Ordered mcg dose/min ÷ mcg/mL × 60 min/h =					___ mL/h
Fenoldapam	Infusion		0.0075		0.01–1.6 mcg/ kg/min	10 mg/ 250 mL	40	mcg/mL	
				Take dose you want in mcg ÷ by drug index number = mL/h on pump					
Heparin	100 u/kg = 8900 u 200 u/kg = 17,800 u 300 u/kg = 26,700 u 400 u/kg = 35,600 u								
Isoproterenol	Infusion				5 mcg/min	1 mg/ 250 mL	4	mcg/mL	
				Ordered mcg dose/min ÷ mcg/mL × 60 min/h =					**75** mL/h
Lidocaine	Infusion	1 mg/min = 7.5 mL/h			1–4 mg/min	2 g/ 250 mL	8	mg/mL	___
				Ordered mg/min ÷ mg/mL × 60 min/h =					___ mL/h
Nitroglycerin	Infusion	3 mcg/min = 1 mL/h			3–200 mcg/min	50 mg/ 250 mL	200	mcg/mL	___
				Ordered mcg/min ÷ mcg/mL × 60 min/h =					___ mL/h
Nitroprusside	Infusion	6.7 mcg/min = 1 mL/h			5–300 mcg/min	100 mg/ 250 mL	400	mcg/mL	___
				Ordered mcg/min ÷ mcg/mL × 60 min/h =					___ mL/h
Norepinephrine	Infusion	1 mcg/min = 4 mL/h 2 mcg/min = 8 mL/h 3 mcg/min = 11 mL/h 4 mcg/min = 15 mL/h 5 mcg/min = 19 mL/h			2–20 mcg/min	4 mg/ 250 mL	16	mcg/mL	
				Ordered mcg dose/min ÷ mcg/mL × 60 min/h =					___ mL/h
Phenylephrine	Infusion	1.3 mcg/min = 1 mL/h			10–200 mcg/min	20 mg/ 250 mL	80	mcg/mL	
				Ordered mcg/min ÷ mcg/mL × 60 min/h =					___ mL/h
Primacor	0.05 mg/kg = 4.45 mg			Give load over 10 min		40 mg/ 200 mL	0.2	mg/mL	
	mg to give ÷ mg/mL = 22 mL				**22** mL × (60 min/h ÷ 10 min) =				**133.5** mL/h × 10 min
	Infusion		0.04		0.5 mcg/ kg/min	40 mg/ 200 mL	200	mcg/mL	___
				Take dose you want in mcg ÷ by drug index number = mL/h on pump					
Trimethaphan	Infusion		—		0.3–6 mg/min	500 mg/ 500 mL	1	mg/mL	___
				Ordered mg/min ÷ mg/mL × 60 min/h =					___ mL/h
Vasopressin		0.02 u/min = 3 mL/h 0.04 u/min = 6 mL/h				40 u/ 100 mL	400	u/mL	

90 kg

DRUG	ORDERED AMOUNT	TOTAL DOSE TO GIVE	DRUG INDEX NUMBER	DIRECTIONS	INFUSION RANGE	DRUG MIXTURE	AMOUNT	DRUG/mL	RUN AT	mL/h
Aminophylline	5 mg/kg =	450 mg		Give mg/kg load over 20 min		500 mg/ 250 mL	2 mg/mL			
	mg to give ÷ mg/mL =	225 mL				225 mL × (60 min/h ÷ 20 min) =			**675**	mL/h × 20 min
	Infusion				0.5–1 mg/kg/h	500 mg/ 250 mL	2 mg/mL			
					mg dose ordered × kg ÷ mg/mL =				___	mL/h
Amiodarone	Loading dose			Load **150 mg** over 10 min		900 mg/ 500 mL	1.8 mg/mL		—	
				Ordered mg load dose (150 mg) ÷ mg/mL (1.8 mg/mL) = 83 mL to give × (60 min/h ÷ 10 min) = mL/h to set on pump					**500**	mL/h × 83 mL
	Infusion			Run at **1 mg/ min** × 6 h		900 mg/ 500 mL	1.8 mg/mL			
				Ordered mg dose (1 mg/min) ÷ mg/mL (1.8 mg/mL) = _____ × 60 min/h = mL/h to set on pump					**33**	mL/h × 6 h
	Infusion			Run at **0.5 mg/ min** × 18 h		900 mg/ 500 mL	1.8 mg/mL			
				Ordered mg dose (0.5 mg/min) ÷ mg/mL (1.8 mg/mL) = _____ × 60 min/h = mL/h to set on pump					**17**	mL/h × 18 h
Amrinone	0.75 mg/kg =	67.5 mg		Give mg/kg load over 10 min		300 mg/ 120 mL	2.5 mg/mL		—	
	mg to give ÷ mg/mL =	27 mL				27 mL × (60 min/h ÷ 10 min) =			**162**	mL/h × 10 min
	Infusion		0.46		5–10 mcg/ kg/min	300 mg/ 120 mL	2500 mcg/mL		—	
				Take dose you want in mcg ÷ by drug index number = mL/h on pump						
Brevibloc	Infusion		1.85		50–100 mcg/ kg/min	2.5 g/ 250 mL	10,000 mcg/mL			___ mL/h
				Take dose you want in mcg ÷ by drug index number = mL/h on pump						
Cardene	Infusion		—		0.5–10 mg/h	25 mg 250 mL	0.1 mg/mL		—	
				Ordered mg dose ÷ mg/mL = mL/h to set on pump						___ mL/h
Cardizem	0.25 mg/kg =	22.5 mg		Give mg/kg load over 20 min		50 mg/ 100 mL	0.5 mg/mL		—	
	mg to give ÷ mg/mL =	45 mL				45 mL × (60 min/h ÷ 20 min) =			**135**	mL/h
	0.35 mg/kg =	31.5 mg		May repeat loading dose in 15 min			0.5 mg/mL		—	
	mg to give ÷ mg/mL =	63 mL				63 mL × (60 min/h ÷ 20 min) =			**189**	mL/h
	Infusion				5–15 mg/h				—	
				Ordered mg dose ÷ mg/mL = mL/h to set on pump						___ mL/h
Desmopressin	0.3 mcg/kg =	27 mcg		Give dose over 20–30 min			4 mcg/vial			
Dobutamine	Infusion		0.37		2.5–40 mcg/kg/ min	250 mg/ 125 mL	2000 mcg/mL			
				Take dose you want in mcg ÷ by drug index number = mL/h on pump						

(continues)

90 kg (continued)

DRUG	ORDERED AMOUNT	TOTAL DOSE TO GIVE	DRUG INDEX NUMBER	DIRECTIONS	INFUSION RANGE	DRUG MIXTURE	AMOUNT	DRUG/mL	RUN AT	mL/h
Dopamine	Infusion		0.30		1–20 mcg/kg/min	400 mg/250 mL	1600	mcg/mL		
	Take dose you want in mcg ÷ by drug index number = mL/h on pump									
Epinephrine	Infusion	1 mcg/min = 4 mL/h 2 mcg/min = 8 mL/h 3 mcg/min = 11 mL/h 4 mcg/min = 15 mL/h			1–4 mcg/min	4 mg/250 mL	16	mcg/mL		
	Ordered mcg dose/min ÷ mcg/mL × 60 min/h =								___	mL/h
Fenoldapam	Infusion		0.0074		0.01–1.6 mcg/kg/min	10 mg/250 mL	40	mcg/mL		
	Take dose you want in mcg ÷ by drug index number = mL/h on pump									
Heparin	100 u/kg =	9000 u								
	200 u/kg =	18,000 u								
	300 u/kg =	27,000 u								
	400 u/kg =	36,000 u								
Isoproterenol	Infusion				5 mcg/min	1 mg/250 mL	4	mcg/mL		
	Ordered mcg dose/min ÷ mcg/mL × 60 min/h =								75	mL/h
Lidocaine	Infusion	1 mg/min = 7.5 mL/h			1–4 mg/min	2 g/250 mL	8	mg/mL	___	
	Ordered mg/min ÷ mg/mL × 60 min/h =								___	mL/h
Nitroglycerin	Infusion	3 mcg/min = 1 mL/h			3–200 mcg/min	50 mg/250 mL	200	mcg/mL	___	
	Ordered mcg/min ÷ mcg/mL × 60 min/h =								___	mL/h
Nitroprusside	Infusion	6.7 mcg/min = 1 mL/h			5–300 mcg/min	100 mg/250 mL	400	mcg/mL	___	
	Ordered mcg/min ÷ mcg/mL × 60 min/h =								___	mL/h
Norepinephrine	Infusion	1 mcg/min = 4 mL/h 2 mcg/min = 8 mL/h 3 mcg/min = 11 mL/h 4 mcg/min = 15 mL/h 5 mcg/min = 19 mL/h			2–20 mcg/min	4 mg/250 mL	16	mcg/mL		
	Ordered mcg dose/min ÷ mcg/mL × 60 min/h =								___	mL/h
Phenylephrine	Infusion	1.3 mcg/min = 1 mL/h			10–200 mcg/min	20 mg/250 mL	80	mcg/mL		
	Ordered mcg/min ÷ mcg/mL × 60 min/h =								___	mL/h
Primacor	0.05 mg/kg =	4.5 mg		Give load over 10 min		40 mg/200 mL	0.2	mg/mL		
	mg to give ÷ mg/mL =	23 mL				23 mL × (60 min/h ÷ 10 min) =			135	mL/h × 10 min
	Infusion		0.04		0.5 mcg/kg/min	40 mg/200 mL	200	mcg/mL	___	
	Take dose you want in mcg ÷ by drug index number = mL/h on pump									
Trimethaphan	Infusion		—		0.3–6 mg/min	500 mg/500 mL	1	mg/mL	___	
	Ordered mg/min ÷ mg/mL × 60 min/h =								___	mL/h
Vasopressin		0.02 u/min = 3 mL/h 0.04 u/min = 6 mL/h				40 u/100 mL	400	u/mL		

91 kg

DRUG	ORDERED AMOUNT	TOTAL DOSE TO GIVE	DRUG INDEX NUMBER	DIRECTIONS	INFUSION RANGE	DRUG MIXTURE	AMOUNT	DRUG/ mL	RUN AT	mL/h
Aminophylline	5 mg/kg =	455 mg		Give mg/kg load over 20 min		500 mg/ 250 mL	2 mg/mL			
	mg to give ÷ mg/mL =	228 mL			228	mL × (60 min/h ÷ 20 min) =			**682.5**	mL/h × 20 min
	Infusion				0.5–1 mg/kg/h	500 mg/ 250 mL	2 mg/mL			
						mg dose ordered × kg ÷ mg/mL =			___	mL/h
Amiodarone	Loading dose			Load **150 mg** over 10 min		900 mg/ 500 mL	1.8 mg/mL		___	
				Ordered mg load dose (150 mg) ÷ mg/mL (1.8 mg/mL) = 83 mL to give × (60 min/h ÷ 10 min) = mL/h to set on pump					**500**	mL/h × 83 mL
	Infusion			Run at **1 mg/ min** × 6 h		900 mg/ 500 mL	1.8 mg/mL			
				Ordered mg dose (1 mg/min) ÷ mg/mL (1.8 mg/mL) = _____ × 60 min/h = mL/h to set on pump					**33**	mL/h × 6 h
	Infusion			Run at **0.5 mg/ min** × 18 h		900 mg/ 500 mL	1.8 mg/mL			
				Ordered mg dose (0.5 mg/min) ÷ mg/mL (1.8 mg/mL) = _____ × 60 min/h = mL/h to set on pump					**17**	mL/h × 18 h
Amrinone	0.75 mg/kg =	68.25 mg		Give mg/kg load over 10 min		300 mg/ 120 mL	2.5 mg/mL		___	
	mg to give ÷ mg/mL =	27 mL				27.3	mL × (60 min/h ÷ 10 min) =		**163.8**	mL/h × 10 min
	Infusion		0.46		5–10 mcg/ kg/min	300 mg/ 120 mL	2500 mcg/mL		___	
				Take dose you want in mcg ÷ by drug index number = mL/h on pump						
Brevibloc	Infusion		1.83		50–100 mcg/ kg/min	2.5 g/ 250 mL	10,000 mcg/mL		___	mL/h
				Take dose you want in mcg ÷ by drug index number = mL/h on pump						
Cardene	Infusion		—		0.5–10 mg/h	25 mg 250 mL	0.1 mg/mL		___	
				Ordered mg dose ÷ mg/mL = mL/h to set on pump						mL/h
Cardizem	0.25 mg/kg =	22.75 mg		Give mg/kg load over 20 min		50 mg/ 100 mL	0.5 mg/mL		___	
	mg to give ÷ mg/mL =	46 mL				45.5	mL × (60 min/h ÷ 20 min) =		**137**	mL/h
	0.35 mg/kg =	31.85 mg		May repeat loading dose in 15 min			0.5 mg/mL		___	
	mg to give ÷ mg/mL =	64 mL				63.7	mL × (60 min/h ÷ 20 min) =		**191**	mL/h
	Infusion				5–15 mg/h				___	
				Ordered mg dose ÷ mg/mL = mL/h to set on pump						mL/h
Desmopressin	0.3 mcg/kg =	27 mcg		Give dose over 20–30 min			4 mcg/vial			
Dobutamine	Infusion		0.37		2.5–40 mcg/kg/ min	250 mg/ 125 mL	2000 mcg/mL			
				Take dose you want in mcg ÷ by drug index number = mL/h on pump						

(continues)

91   kg (continued)

DRUG	ORDERED AMOUNT	TOTAL DOSE TO GIVE	DRUG INDEX NUMBER	DIRECTIONS	INFUSION RANGE	DRUG MIXTURE	AMOUNT	DRUG/ mL	RUN AT	mL/h
Dopamine	Infusion		0.29		1–20 mcg/ kg/min	400 mg/ 250 mL	1600	mcg/mL		
	Take dose you want in mcg ÷ by drug index number = mL/h on pump									
Epinephrine	Infusion	1 mcg/min = 4 mL/h 2 mcg/min = 8 mL/h 3 mcg/min = 11 mL/h 4 mcg/min = 15 mL/h			1–4 mcg/min	4 mg/ 250 mL	16	mcg/mL		
		Ordered mcg dose/min ÷ mcg/mL × 60 min/h =							___	mL/h
Fenoldapam	Infusion		0.0074		0.01–1.6 mcg/ kg/min	10 mg/ 250 mL	40	mcg/mL		
	Take dose you want in mcg ÷ by drug index number = mL/h on pump									
Heparin	100 u/kg = 9100 u 200 u/kg = 18,200 u 300 u/kg = 27,300 u 400 u/kg = 36,400 u									
Isoproterenol	Infusion				5 mcg/min	1 mg/ 250 mL	4	mcg/mL		
		Ordered mcg dose/min ÷ mcg/mL × 60 min/h =							75	mL/h
Lidocaine	Infusion	1 mg/min = 7.5 mL/h			1–4 mg/min	2 g/ 250 mL	8	mg/mL	___	
		Ordered mg/min ÷ mg/mL × 60 min/h =							___	mL/h
Nitroglycerin	Infusion	3 mcg/min = 1 mL/h			3–200 mcg/min	50 mg/ 250 mL	200	mcg/mL	___	
		Ordered mcg/min ÷ mcg/mL × 60 min/h =							___	mL/h
Nitroprusside	Infusion	6.7 mcg/min = 1 mL/h			5–300 mcg/min	100 mg/ 250 mL	400	mcg/mL	___	
		Ordered mcg/min ÷ mcg/mL × 60 min/h =							___	mL/h
Norepinephrine	Infusion	1 mcg/min = 4 mL/h 2 mcg/min = 8 mL/h 3 mcg/min = 11 mL/h 4 mcg/min = 15 mL/h 5 mcg/min = 19 mL/h			2–20 mcg/min	4 mg/ 250 mL	16	mcg/mL		
		Ordered mcg dose/min ÷ mcg/mL × 60 min/h =							___	mL/h
Phenylephrine	Infusion	1.3 mcg/min = 1 mL/h			10–200 mcg/min	20 mg/ 250 mL	80	mcg/mL		
		Ordered mcg/min ÷ mcg/mL × 60 min/h =							___	mL/h
Primacor	0.05 mg/kg = 4.55 mg			Give load over 10 min		40 mg/ 200 mL	0.2	mg/mL		
	mg to give ÷ mg/mL = 23 mL				23	mL × (60 min/h ÷ 10 min) =			136.5	mL/h × 10 min
	Infusion		0.04		0.5 mcg/ kg/min	40 mg/ 200 mL	200	mcg/mL	___	
	Take dose you want in mcg ÷ by drug index number = mL/h on pump									
Trimethaphan	Infusion		___		0.3–6 mg/min	500 mg/ 500 mL	1	mg/mL	___	
		Ordered mg/min ÷ mg/mL × 60 min/h =							___	mL/h
Vasopressin		0.02 u/min = 3 mL/h 0.04 u/min = 6 mL/h				40 u/ 100 mL	400	u/mL		

92 kg

DRUG	ORDERED AMOUNT	TOTAL DOSE TO GIVE		DRUG INDEX NUMBER	DIRECTIONS	INFUSION RANGE	DRUG MIXTURE	AMOUNT	DRUG/mL	RUN AT	mL/h
Aminophylline	5 mg/kg =	460	mg		Give mg/kg load over 20 min		500 mg/ 250 mL	2	mg/mL		
	mg to give ÷ mg/mL =	230	mL				230	mL × (60 min/h ÷ 20 min) =		**690**	mL/h × 20 min
	Infusion					0.5–1 mg/kg/h	500 mg/ 250 mL	2	mg/mL		
						mg dose ordered × kg ÷ mg/mL =				___	mL/h
Amiodarone	Loading dose				Load **150 mg** over 10 min		900 mg/ 500 mL	1.8	mg/mL	—	
					Ordered mg load dose (150 mg) ÷ mg/mL (1.8 mg/mL) = 83 mL to give × (60 min/h ÷ 10 min) = mL/h to set on pump					**500**	mL/h × 83 mL
	Infusion				Run at **1 mg/ min** × 6 h		900 mg/ 500 mL	1.8	mg/mL		
					Ordered mg dose (1 mg/min) ÷ mg/mL (1.8 mg/mL) = _____ × 60 min/h = mL/h to set on pump					**33**	mL/h × 6 h
	Infusion				Run at **0.5 mg/ min** × 18 h		900 mg/ 500 mL	1.8	mg/mL		
					Ordered mg dose (0.5 mg/min) ÷ mg/mL (1.8 mg/mL) = _____ × 60 min/h = mL/h to set on pump					**17**	mL/h × 18 h
Amrinone	0.75 mg/kg =	69	mg		Give mg/kg load over 10 min		300 mg/ 120 mL	2.5	mg/mL	—	
	mg to give ÷ mg/mL =	28	mL				27.6	mL × (60 min/h ÷ 10 min) =		**165.6**	mL/h × 10 min
	Infusion			0.45		5–10 mcg/ kg/min	300 mg/ 120 mL	2500	mcg/mL	—	
					Take dose you want in mcg ÷ by drug index number = mL/h on pump						
Brevibloc	Infusion			1.81		50–100 mcg/ kg/min	2.5 g/ 250 mL	10,000	mcg/mL		mL/h
					Take dose you want in mcg ÷ by drug index number = mL/h on pump						
Cardene	Infusion			—		0.5–10 mg/h	25 mg 250 mL	0.1	mg/mL		
					Ordered mg dose ÷ mg/mL = mL/h to set on pump					___	mL/h
Cardizem	0.25 mg/kg =	23	mg		Give mg/kg load over 20 min		50 mg/ 100 mL	0.5	mg/mL		
	mg to give ÷ mg/mL =	46	mL				46	mL × (60 min/h ÷ 20 min) =		**138**	mL/h
	0.35 mg/kg =	32.2	mg		May repeat loading dose in 15 min			0.5	mg/mL		
	mg to give ÷ mg/mL =	64	mL				64.4	mL × (60 min/h ÷ 20 min) =		**193**	mL/h
	Infusion					5–15 mg/h				—	
					Ordered mg dose ÷ mg/mL = mL/h to set on pump					___	mL/h
Desmopressin	0.3 mcg/kg =	28	mcg		Give dose over 20–30 min				4	mcg/vial	
Dobutamine	Infusion			0.36		2.5–40 mcg/kg/ min	250 mg/ 125 mL	2000	mcg/mL		
					Take dose you want in mcg ÷ by drug index number = mL/h on pump						

(continues)

92   kg (continued)

DRUG	ORDERED AMOUNT	TOTAL DOSE TO GIVE	DRUG INDEX NUMBER	DIRECTIONS	INFUSION RANGE	DRUG MIXTURE	AMOUNT	DRUG/ mL	RUN AT	mL/h
Dopamine	Infusion		0.29		1–20 mcg/ kg/min	400 mg/ 250 mL	1600	mcg/mL		
	Take dose you want in mcg ÷ by drug index number = mL/h on pump									
Epinephrine	Infusion	1 mcg/min = 4 mL/h 2 mcg/min = 8 mL/h 3 mcg/min = 11 mL/h 4 mcg/min = 15 mL/h			1–4 mcg/min	4 mg/ 250 mL	16	mcg/mL		
		Ordered mcg dose/min ÷ mcg/mL × 60 min/h =								___ mL/h
Fenoldapam	Infusion		0.0073		0.01–1.6 mcg/ kg/min	10 mg/ 250 mL	40	mcg/mL		
	Take dose you want in mcg ÷ by drug index number = mL/h on pump									
Heparin	100 u/kg = **9200** u 200 u/kg = **18,400** u 300 u/kg = **27,600** u 400 u/kg = **36,800** u									
Isoproterenol	Infusion				5 mcg/min	1 mg/ 250 mL	4	mcg/mL		
		Ordered mcg dose/min ÷ mcg/mL × 60 min/h =							**75** mL/h	
Lidocaine	Infusion	*1 mg/min = 7.5 mL/h*			1–4 mg/min	2 g/ 250 mL	8	mg/mL	—	
		Ordered mg/min ÷ mg/mL × 60 min/h =							___ mL/h	
Nitroglycerin	Infusion	*3 mcg/min = 1 mL/h*			3–200 mcg/min	50 mg/ 250 mL	200	mcg/mL	—	
		Ordered mcg/min ÷ mcg/mL × 60 min/h =							___ mL/h	
Nitroprusside	Infusion	*6.7 mcg/min = 1 mL/h*			5–300 mcg/min	100 mg/ 250 mL	400	mcg/mL	—	
		Ordered mcg/min ÷ mcg/mL × 60 min/h =							___ mL/h	
Norepinephrine	Infusion	1 mcg/min = 4 mL/h 2 mcg/min = 8 mL/h 3 mcg/min = 11 mL/h 4 mcg/min = 15 mL/h 5 mcg/min = 19 mL/h			2–20 mcg/min	4 mg/ 250 mL	16	mcg/mL		
		Ordered mcg dose/min ÷ mcg/mL × 60 min/h =							___ mL/h	
Phenylephrine	Infusion	*1.3 mcg/min = 1 mL/h*			10–200 mcg/min	20 mg/ 250 mL	80	mcg/mL		
		Ordered mcg/min ÷ mcg/mL × 60 min/h =							___ mL/h	
Primacor	0.05 mg/kg = **4.6** mg			Give load over 10 min		40 mg/ 200 mL	0.2	mg/mL		
	mg to give ÷ mg/mL =	**23** mL			**23**	mL × (60 min/h ÷ 10 min) =			**138**	mL/h × 10 min
	Infusion		0.04		0.5 mcg/ kg/min	40 mg/ 200 mL	200	mcg/mL	—	
	Take dose you want in mcg ÷ by drug index number = mL/h on pump									
Trimethaphan	Infusion		—		0.3–6 mg/min	500 mg/ 500 mL	1	mg/mL	—	
		Ordered mg/min ÷ mg/mL × 60 min/h =							___ mL/h	
Vasopressin		0.02 u/min = 3 mL/h 0.04 u/min = 6 mL/h				40 u/ 100 mL	400	u/mL		

93 kg

DRUG	ORDERED AMOUNT	TOTAL DOSE TO GIVE	DRUG INDEX NUMBER	DIRECTIONS	INFUSION RANGE	DRUG MIXTURE	AMOUNT	DRUG/mL	RUN AT	mL/h
Aminophylline	5 mg/kg = **465** mg			Give mg/kg load over 20 min		500 mg/ 250 mL	2 mg/mL			
	mg to give ÷ mg/mL = **233** mL					**233** mL × (60 min/h ÷ 20 min) =			**697.5**	mL/h × 20 min
	Infusion				0.5–1 mg/kg/h	500 mg/ 250 mL	2 mg/mL			
					mg dose ordered × kg ÷ mg/mL = ____ mL/h					
Amiodarone	Loading dose			Load **150 mg** over 10 min		900 mg/ 500 mL	1.8 mg/mL		—	
				Ordered mg load dose (150 mg) ÷ mg/mL (1.8 mg/mL) = 83 mL to give × (60 min/h ÷ 10 min) = mL/h to set on pump					**500**	mL/h × 83 mL
	Infusion			Run at **1 mg/ min** × 6 h		900 mg/ 500 mL	1.8 mg/mL			
				Ordered mg dose (1 mg/min) ÷ mg/mL (1.8 mg/mL) = ____ × 60 min/h = mL/h to set on pump					**33**	mL/h × 6 h
	Infusion			Run at **0.5 mg/ min** × 18 h		900 mg/ 500 mL	1.8 mg/mL			
				Ordered mg dose (0.5 mg/min) ÷ mg/mL (1.8 mg/mL) = ____ × 60 min/h = mL/h to set on pump					**17**	mL/h × 18 h
Amrinone	0.75 mg/kg = **69.75** mg			Give mg/kg load over 10 min		300 mg/ 120 mL	2.5 mg/mL		—	
	mg to give ÷ mg/mL = **28** mL					**27.9** mL × (60 min/h ÷ 10 min) =			**167.4**	mL/h × 10 min
	Infusion		**0.45**		5–10 mcg/ kg/min	300 mg/ 120 mL	2500 mcg/mL		—	
				Take dose you want in mcg ÷ by drug index number = mL/h on pump						
Brevibloc	Infusion		**1.79**		50–100 mcg/ kg/min	2.5 g/ 250 mL	10,000 mcg/mL		____	mL/h
				Take dose you want in mcg ÷ by drug index number = mL/h on pump						
Cardene	Infusion		—		0.5–10 mg/h	25 mg 250 mL	0.1 mg/mL		—	
				Ordered mg dose ÷ mg/mL = mL/h to set on pump					____	mL/h
Cardizem	0.25 mg/kg = **23.25** mg			Give mg/kg load over 20 min		50 mg/ 100 mL	0.5 mg/mL		—	
	mg to give ÷ mg/mL = **47** mL					**46.5** mL × (60 min/h ÷ 20 min) =			**140**	mL/h
	0.35 mg/kg = **32.55** mg			May repeat loading dose in 15 min			0.5 mg/mL		—	
	mg to give ÷ mg/mL = **65** mL					**65.1** mL × (60 min/h ÷ 20 min) =			**195**	mL/h
	Infusion				5–15 mg/h				—	
				Ordered mg dose ÷ mg/mL = mL/h to set on pump					____	mL/h
Desmopressin	0.3 mcg/kg = **28** mcg			Give dose over 20–30 min			4 mcg/vial			
Dobutamine	Infusion		**0.36**		2.5–40 mcg/kg/ min	250 mg/ 125 mL	2000 mcg/mL			
				Take dose you want in mcg ÷ by drug index number = mL/h on pump						

(continues)

93 kg (continued)

DRUG	ORDERED AMOUNT	TOTAL DOSE TO GIVE	DRUG INDEX NUMBER	DIRECTIONS	INFUSION RANGE	DRUG MIXTURE	AMOUNT	DRUG/ mL	RUN AT	mL/h
Dopamine	Infusion		0.29		1–20 mcg/ kg/min	400 mg/ 250 mL	1600	mcg/mL		
	Take dose you want in mcg ÷ by drug index number = mL/h on pump									
Epinephrine	Infusion	1 mcg/min = 4 mL/h 2 mcg/min = 8 mL/h 3 mcg/min = 11 mL/h 4 mcg/min = 15 mL/h			1–4 mcg/min	4 mg/ 250 mL	16	mcg/mL		
		Ordered mcg dose/min ÷ mcg/mL × 60 min/h =							___	mL/h
Fenoldapam	Infusion		0.0072		0.01–1.6 mcg/ kg/min	10 mg/ 250 mL	40	mcg/mL		
		Take dose you want in mcg ÷ by drug index number = mL/h on pump								
Heparin	100 u/kg = 9300 u 200 u/kg = 18,600 u 300 u/kg = 27,900 u 400 u/kg = 37,200 u									
Isoproterenol	Infusion				5 mcg/min	1 mg/ 250 mL	4	mcg/mL		
		Ordered mcg dose/min ÷ mcg/mL × 60 min/h =							75	mL/h
Lidocaine	Infusion	1 mg/min = 7.5 mL/h			1–4 mg/min	2 g/ 250 mL	8	mg/mL	___	
		Ordered mg/min ÷ mg/mL × 60 min/h =							___	mL/h
Nitroglycerin	Infusion	3 mcg/min = 1 mL/h			3–200 mcg/min	50 mg/ 250 mL	200	mcg/mL	___	
		Ordered mcg/min ÷ mcg/mL × 60 min/h =							___	mL/h
Nitroprusside	Infusion	6.7 mcg/min = 1 mL/h			5–300 mcg/min	100 mg/ 250 mL	400	mcg/mL	___	
		Ordered mcg/min ÷ mcg/mL × 60 min/h =							___	mL/h
Norepinephrine	Infusion	1 mcg/min = 4 mL/h 2 mcg/min = 8 mL/h 3 mcg/min = 11 mL/h 4 mcg/min = 15 mL/h 5 mcg/min = 19 mL/h			2–20 mcg/min	4 mg/ 250 mL	16	mcg/mL		
		Ordered mcg dose/min ÷ mcg/mL × 60 min/h =							___	mL/h
Phenylephrine	Infusion	1.3 mcg/min = 1 mL/h			10–200 mcg/min	20 mg/ 250 mL	80	mcg/mL		
		Ordered mcg/min ÷ mcg/mL × 60 min/h =							___	mL/h
Primacor	0.05 mg/kg = 4.65 mg			Give load over 10 min		40 mg/ 200 mL	0.2	mg/mL		
	mg to give ÷ mg/mL = 23 mL					23 mL × (60 min/h ÷ 10 min) =			139.5	mL/h × 10 min
	Infusion		0.04		0.5 mcg/ kg/min	40 mg/ 200 mL	200	mcg/mL	___	
		Take dose you want in mcg ÷ by drug index number = mL/h on pump								
Trimethaphan	Infusion		___		0.3–6 mg/min	500 mg/ 500 mL	1	mg/mL	___	
		Ordered mg/min ÷ mg/mL × 60 min/h =							___	mL/h
Vasopressin		0.02 u/min = 3 mL/h 0.04 u/min = 6 mL/h				40 u/ 100 mL	400	u/mL		

94 kg

DRUG	ORDERED AMOUNT	TOTAL DOSE TO GIVE	DRUG INDEX NUMBER	DIRECTIONS	INFUSION RANGE	DRUG MIXTURE	AMOUNT DRUG/mL	RUN AT mL/h
Aminophylline	5 mg/kg =	470 mg		Give mg/kg load over 20 min		500 mg/ 250 mL	2 mg/mL	
	mg to give ÷ mg/mL =	235 mL			235	mL × (60 min/h ÷ 20 min) =		**705** mL/h × 20 min
	Infusion				0.5–1 mg/kg/h	500 mg/ 250 mL	2 mg/mL	
					mg dose ordered × kg ÷ mg/mL =			___ mL/h
Amiodarone	Loading dose			Load **150 mg** over 10 min		900 mg/ 500 mL	1.8 mg/mL	___
				Ordered mg load dose (150 mg) ÷ mg/mL (1.8 mg/mL) = 83 mL to give × (60 min/h ÷ 10 min) = mL/h to set on pump				**500** mL/h × 83 mL
	Infusion			Run at **1 mg/ min × 6 h**		900 mg/ 500 mL	1.8 mg/mL	
				Ordered mg dose (1 mg/min) ÷ mg/mL (1.8 mg/mL) = _____ × 60 min/h = mL/h to set on pump				**33** mL/h × 6 h
	Infusion			Run at **0.5 mg/ min × 18 h**		900 mg/ 500 mL	1.8 mg/mL	
				Ordered mg dose (0.5 mg/min) ÷ mg/mL (1.8 mg/mL) = _____ × 60 min/h = mL/h to set on pump				**17** mL/h × 18 h
Amrinone	0.75 mg/kg =	70.5 mg		Give mg/kg load over 10 min		300 mg/ 120 mL	2.5 mg/mL	___
	mg to give ÷ mg/mL =	28 mL			28.2	mL × (60 min/h ÷ 10 min) =		**169.2** mL/h × 10 min
	Infusion		0.44		5–10 mcg/ kg/min	300 mg/ 120 mL	2500 mcg/mL	___
				Take dose you want in mcg ÷ by drug index number = mL/h on pump				
Brevibloc	Infusion		1.77		50–100 mcg/ kg/min	2.5 g/ 250 mL	10,000 mcg/mL	___ mL/h
				Take dose you want in mcg ÷ by drug index number = mL/h on pump				
Cardene	Infusion		—		0.5–10 mg/h	25 mg 250 mL	0.1 mg/mL	___
				Ordered mg dose ÷ mg/mL = mL/h to set on pump				___ mL/h
Cardizem	0.25 mg/kg =	23.5 mg		Give mg/kg load over 20 min		50 mg/ 100 mL	0.5 mg/mL	___
	mg to give ÷ mg/mL =	47 mL			47	mL × (60 min/h ÷ 20 min) =		**141** mL/h
	0.35 mg/kg =	32.9 mg		May repeat loading dose in 15 min			0.5 mg/mL	___
	mg to give ÷ mg/mL =	66 mL			65.8	mL × (60 min/h ÷ 20 min) =		**197** mL/h
	Infusion				5–15 mg/h			___
				Ordered mg dose ÷ mg/mL = mL/h to set on pump				___ mL/h
Desmopressin	0.3 mcg/kg =	28 mcg		Give dose over 20–30 min			4 mcg/vial	
Dobutamine	Infusion		0.35		2.5–40 mcg/kg/ min	250 mg/ 125 mL	2000 mcg/mL	
				Take dose you want in mcg ÷ by drug index number = mL/h on pump				

(continues)

94 kg (continued)

DRUG	ORDERED AMOUNT	TOTAL DOSE TO GIVE	DRUG INDEX NUMBER	DIRECTIONS	INFUSION RANGE	DRUG MIXTURE	AMOUNT	DRUG/ mL	RUN AT	mL/h
Dopamine	Infusion		0.28		1–20 mcg/ kg/min	400 mg/ 250 mL	1600	mcg/mL		
			Take dose you want in mcg ÷ by drug index number = mL/h on pump							
Epinephrine	Infusion	1 mcg/min = 4 mL/h 2 mcg/min = 8 mL/h 3 mcg/min = 11 mL/h 4 mcg/min = 15 mL/h			1–4 mcg/min	4 mg/ 250 mL	16	mcg/mL		
				Ordered mcg dose/min ÷ mcg/mL × 60 min/h =					___	mL/h
Fenoldapam	Infusion		0.0071		0.01–1.6 mcg/ kg/min	10 mg/ 250 mL	40	mcg/mL		
			Take dose you want in mcg ÷ by drug index number = mL/h on pump							
Heparin	100 u/kg = 200 u/kg = 300 u/kg = 400 u/kg =	9400 u 18,800 u 28,200 u 37,600 u								
Isoproterenol	Infusion				5 mcg/min	1 mg/ 250 mL	4	mcg/mL		
				Ordered mcg dose/min ÷ mcg/mL × 60 min/h =					75	mL/h
Lidocaine	Infusion	1 mg/min = 7.5 mL/h			1–4 mg/min	2 g/ 250 mL	8	mg/mL	—	
				Ordered mg/min ÷ mg/mL × 60 min/h =					___	mL/h
Nitroglycerin	Infusion	3 mcg/min = 1 mL/h			3–200 mcg/min	50 mg/ 250 mL	200	mcg/mL	—	
				Ordered mcg/min ÷ mcg/mL × 60 min/h =					___	mL/h
Nitroprusside	Infusion	6.7 mcg/min = 1 mL/h			5–300 mcg/min	100 mg/ 250 mL	400	mcg/mL	—	
				Ordered mcg/min ÷ mcg/mL × 60 min/h =					___	mL/h
Norepinephrine	Infusion	1 mcg/min = 4 mL/h 2 mcg/min = 8 mL/h 3 mcg/min = 11 mL/h 4 mcg/min = 15 mL/h 5 mcg/min = 19 mL/h			2–20 mcg/min	4 mg/ 250 mL	16	mcg/mL		
				Ordered mcg dose/min ÷ mcg/mL × 60 min/h =					___	mL/h
Phenylephrine	Infusion	1.3 mcg/min = 1 mL/h			10–200 mcg/min	20 mg/ 250 mL	80	mcg/mL		
				Ordered mcg/min ÷ mcg/mL × 60 min/h =					___	mL/h
Primacor	0.05 mg/kg =	4.7 mg		Give load over 10 min		40 mg/ 200 mL	0.2	mg/mL		
	mg to give ÷ mg/mL =	24 mL			24	mL × (60 min/h ÷ 10 min) =			141	mL/h × 10 min
	Infusion		0.04		0.5 mcg/ kg/min	40 mg/ 200 mL	200	mcg/mL	—	
			Take dose you want in mcg ÷ by drug index number = mL/h on pump							
Trimethaphan	Infusion		—		0.3–6 mg/min	500 mg/ 500 mL	1	mg/mL	—	
				Ordered mg/min ÷ mg/mL × 60 min/h =					___	mL/h
Vasopressin		0.02 u/min = 3 mL/h 0.04 u/min = 6 mL/h				40 u/ 100 mL	400	u/mL		

95 kg

DRUG	ORDERED AMOUNT	TOTAL DOSE TO GIVE	DRUG INDEX NUMBER	DIRECTIONS	INFUSION RANGE	DRUG MIXTURE	AMOUNT	DRUG/ mL	RUN AT	mL/h
Aminophylline	5 mg/kg =	475 mg		Give mg/kg load over 20 min		500 mg/ 250 mL	2 mg/mL		
	mg to give ÷ mg/mL =	238 mL			238	mL × (60 min/h ÷ 20 min) =			712.5	mL/h × 20 min
	Infusion				0.5–1 mg/kg/h	500 mg/ 250 mL	2 mg/mL		
					mg dose ordered × kg ÷ mg/mL =				___	mL/h
Amiodarone	Loading dose			Load **150 mg** over 10 min		900 mg/ 500 mL	1.8 mg/mL	___
				Ordered mg load dose (150 mg) ÷ mg/mL (1.8 mg/mL) = 83 mL to give × (60 min/h ÷ 10 min) = mL/h to set on pump					500	mL/h × 83 mL
	Infusion			Run at **1 mg/ min** × 6 h	900 mg/ 500 ml	1.8 mg/mL		
				Ordered mg dose (1 mg/min) ÷ mg/mL (1.8 mg/mL) = ___ × 60 min/h = mL/h to set on pump					33	mL/h × 6 h
	Infusion			Run at **0.5 mg/ min** × 18 h	900 mg/ 500 mL	1.8 mg/mL		
				Ordered mg dose (0.5 mg/min) ÷ mg/mL (1.8 mg/mL) = ___ × 60 min/h = mL/h to set on pump					17	mL/h × 18 h
Amrinone	0.75 mg/kg =	71.25 mg		Give mg/kg load over 10 min		300 mg/ 120 mL	2.5 mg/mL	___
	mg to give ÷ mg/mL =	29 mL			28.5	mL × (60 min/h ÷ 10 min) =			171	mL/h × 10 min
	Infusion		0.44		5–10 mcg/ kg/min	300 mg/ 120 mL	2500 mcg/mL	___
				Take dose you want in mcg ÷ by drug index number = mL/h on pump				
Brevibloc	Infusion		1.75		50–100 mcg/ kg/min	2.5 g/ 250 mL	10,000 mcg/mL	___	mL/h
				Take dose you want in mcg ÷ by drug index number = mL/h on pump				
Cardene	Infusion		___		0.5–10 mg/h	25 mg 250 mL	0.1 mg/mL	___
				Ordered mg dose ÷ mg/mL = mL/h to set on pump					___	mL/h
Cardizem	0.25 mg/kg =	23.75 mg		Give mg/kg load over 20 min		50 mg/ 100 mL	0.5 mg/mL	___
	mg to give ÷ mg/mL =	48 mL			47.5	mL × (60 min/h ÷ 20 min) =			143	mL/h
	0.35 mg/kg =	33.25 mg		May repeat loading dose in 15 min			0.5 mg/mL		
	mg to give ÷ mg/mL =	67 mL			66.5	mL × (60 min/h ÷ 20 min) =			200	mL/h
	Infusion				5–15 mg/h				___
				Ordered mg dose ÷ mg/mL = mL/h to set on pump					___	mL/h
Desmopressin	0.3 mcg/kg =	29 mcg		Give dose over 20–30 min			4 mcg/vial	
Dobutamine	Infusion		0.35		2.5–40 mcg/kg/ min	250 mg/ 125 mL	2000 mcg/mL	
				Take dose you want in mcg ÷ by drug index number = mL/h on pump				

(continues)

95 kg (continued)

DRUG	ORDERED AMOUNT	TOTAL DOSE TO GIVE	DRUG INDEX NUMBER	DIRECTIONS	INFUSION RANGE	DRUG MIXTURE	AMOUNT	DRUG/mL	RUN AT	mL/h
Dopamine	Infusion		0.28		1–20 mcg/kg/min	400 mg/250 mL	1600	mcg/mL		
				Take dose you want in mcg ÷ by drug index number = mL/h on pump						
Epinephrine	Infusion	1 mcg/min = 4 mL/h 2 mcg/min = 8 mL/h 3 mcg/min = 11 mL/h 4 mcg/min = 15 mL/h			1–4 mcg/min	4 mg/250 mL	16	mcg/mL		
				Ordered mcg dose/min ÷ mcg/mL × 60 min/h =					___	mL/h
Fenoldapam	Infusion		0.0071		0.01–1.6 mcg/kg/min	10 mg/250 mL	40	mcg/mL		
				Take dose you want in mcg ÷ by drug index number = mL/h on pump						
Heparin	100 u/kg =	9500 u								
	200 u/kg =	19,000 u								
	300 u/kg =	28,500 u								
	400 u/kg =	38,000 u								
Isoproterenol	Infusion				5 mcg/min	1 mg/250 mL	4	mcg/mL		
				Ordered mcg dose/min ÷ mcg/mL × 60 min/h =					75	mL/h
Lidocaine	Infusion	1 mg/min = 7.5 mL/h			1–4 mg/min	2 g/250 mL	8	mg/mL	___	
				Ordered mg/min ÷ mg/mL × 60 min/h =					___	mL/h
Nitroglycerin	Infusion	3 mcg/min = 1 mL/h			3–200 mcg/min	50 mg/250 mL	200	mcg/mL	___	
				Ordered mcg/min ÷ mcg/mL × 60 min/h =					___	mL/h
Nitroprusside	Infusion	6.7 mcg/min = 1 mL/h			5–300 mcg/min	100 mg/250 mL	400	mcg/mL	___	
				Ordered mcg/min ÷ mcg/mL × 60 min/h =					___	mL/h
Norepinephrine	Infusion	1 mcg/min = 4 mL/h 2 mcg/min = 8 mL/h 3 mcg/min = 11 mL/h 4 mcg/min = 15 mL/h 5 mcg/min = 19 mL/h			2–20 mcg/min	4 mg/250 mL	16	mcg/mL		
				Ordered mcg dose/min ÷ mcg/mL × 60 min/h =					___	mL/h
Phenylephrine	Infusion	1.3 mcg/min = 1 mL/h			10–200 mcg/min	20 mg/250 mL	80	mcg/mL		
				Ordered mcg/min ÷ mcg/mL × 60 min/h =					___	mL/h
Primacor	0.05 mg/kg =	4.75 mg		Give load over 10 min		40 mg/200 mL	0.2	mg/mL		
	mg to give ÷ mg/mL =	24 mL			24	mL × (60 min/h ÷ 10 min) =			142.5	mL/h × 10 min
	Infusion		0.04		0.5 mcg/kg/min	40 mg/200 mL	200	mcg/mL	___	
				Take dose you want in mcg ÷ by drug index number = mL/h on pump						
Trimethaphan	Infusion		___		0.3–6 mg/min	500 mg/500 mL	1	mg/mL	___	
				Ordered mg/min ÷ mg/mL × 60 min/h =					___	mL/h
Vasopressin		0.02 u/min = 3 mL/h 0.04 u/min = 6 mL/h				40 u/100 mL	400	u/mL		

96 kg

DRUG	ORDERED AMOUNT	TOTAL DOSE TO GIVE	DRUG INDEX NUMBER	DIRECTIONS	INFUSION RANGE	DRUG MIXTURE	AMOUNT	DRUG/ mL	RUN AT	mL/h
Aminophylline	5 mg/kg =	480 mg		Give mg/kg load over 20 min		500 mg/ 250 mL	2 mg/mL		
	mg to give ÷ mg/mL =	240 mL			240	mL × (60 min/h ÷ 20 min) =			<u>720</u>	mL/h × 20 min
	Infusion				0.5–1 mg/kg/h	500 mg/ 250 mL	2 mg/mL		
					mg dose ordered × kg ÷ mg/mL =				___	mL/h
Amiodarone	Loading dose			Load **150 mg** over 10 min		900 mg/ 500 mL	1.8 mg/mL	—
				Ordered mg load dose (150 mg) ÷ mg/mL (1.8 mg/mL) = 83 mL to give × (60 min/h ÷ 10 min) = mL/h to set on pump				<u>500</u>	mL/h × 83 mL
	Infusion			Run at **1 mg/ mln** × 6 h		900 mg/ 500 mL	1.8 mg/mL	
				Ordered mg dose (1 mg/min) ÷ mg/mL (1.8 mg/mL) = _____ × 60 min/h = mL/h to set on pump				<u>33</u>	mL/h × 6 h
	Infusion			Run at **0.5 mg/ min** × 18 h		900 mg/ 500 mL	1.8 mg/mL	
				Ordered mg dose (0.5 mg/min) ÷ mg/mL (1.8 mg/mL) = _____ × 60 min/h = mL/h to set on pump				<u>17</u>	mL/h × 18 h
Amrinone	0.75 mg/kg =	72 mg		Give mg/kg load over 10 min		300 mg/ 120 mL	2.5 mg/mL	—
	mg to give ÷ mg/mL =	29 mL			28.8	mL × (60 min/h ÷ 10 min) =			<u>172.8</u>	mL/h × 10 min
	Infusion		0.43		5–10 mcg/ kg/min	300 mg/ 120 mL	2500 mcg/mL	
				Take dose you want in mcg ÷ by drug index number = mL/h on pump				
Brevibloc	Infusion		1.74		50–100 mcg/ kg/min	2.5 g/ 250 mL	10,000 mcg/mL	___	mL/h
				Take dose you want in mcg ÷ by drug index number = mL/h on pump				
Cardene	Infusion		—		0.5–10 mg/h	25 mg 250 mL	0.1 mg/mL	—
				Ordered mg dose ÷ mg/mL = mL/h to set on pump				___	mL/h
Cardizem	0.25 mg/kg =	24 mg		Give mg/kg load over 20 min		50 mg/ 100 mL	0.5 mg/mL	—
	mg to give ÷ mg/mL =	48 mL			48	mL × (60 min/h ÷ 20 min) =			<u>144</u>	mL/h
	0.35 mg/kg =	33.6 mg		May repeat loading dose in 15 min			0.5 mg/mL	—
	mg to give ÷ mg/mL =	67 mL			67.2	mL × (60 min/h ÷ 20 min) =			<u>202</u>	mL/h
	Infusion				5–15 mg/h				—
				Ordered mg dose ÷ mg/mL = mL/h to set on pump				___	mL/h
Desmopressin	0.3 mcg/kg =	29 mcg		Give dose over 20–30 min			4 mcg/vial	
Dobutamine	Infusion		0.35		2.5–40 mcg/kg/ min	250 mg/ 125 mL	2000 mcg/mL	
				Take dose you want in mcg ÷ by drug index number = mL/h on pump				

(continues)

96 kg (continued)

DRUG	ORDERED AMOUNT	TOTAL DOSE TO GIVE	DRUG INDEX NUMBER	DIRECTIONS	INFUSION RANGE	DRUG MIXTURE	AMOUNT	DRUG/mL	RUN AT	mL/h
Dopamine	Infusion		0.28		1–20 mcg/kg/min	400 mg/250 mL	1600	mcg/mL		
				Take dose you want in mcg ÷ by drug index number = mL/h on pump						
Epinephrine	Infusion	1 mcg/min = 4 mL/h 2 mcg/min = 8 mL/h 3 mcg/min = 11 mL/h 4 mcg/min = 15 mL/h			1–4 mcg/min	4 mg/250 mL	16	mcg/mL		
				Ordered mcg dose/min ÷ mcg/mL × 60 min/h =						___ mL/h
Fenoldapam	Infusion		0.0070		0.01–1.6 mcg/kg/min	10 mg/250 mL	40	mcg/mL		
				Take dose you want in mcg ÷ by drug index number = mL/h on pump						
Heparin	100 u/kg = 9600 u 200 u/kg = 19,200 u 300 u/kg = 28,800 u 400 u/kg = 38,400 u									
Isoproterenol	Infusion				5 mcg/min	1 mg/250 mL	4	mcg/mL		
				Ordered mcg dose/min ÷ mcg/mL × 60 min/h =						75 mL/h
Lidocaine	Infusion	1 mg/min = 7.5 mL/h			1–4 mg/min	2 g/250 mL	8	mg/mL		
				Ordered mg/min ÷ mg/mL × 60 min/h =						___ mL/h
Nitroglycerin	Infusion	3 mcg/min = 1 mL/h			3–200 mcg/min	50 mg/250 mL	200	mcg/mL		
				Ordered mcg/min ÷ mcg/mL × 60 min/h =						___ mL/h
Nitroprusside	Infusion	6.7 mcg/min = 1 mL/h			5–300 mcg/min	100 mg/250 mL	400	mcg/mL		
				Ordered mcg/min ÷ mcg/mL × 60 min/h =						___ mL/h
Norepinephrine	Infusion	1 mcg/min = 4 mL/h 2 mcg/min = 8 mL/h 3 mcg/min = 11 mL/h 4 mcg/min = 15 mL/h 5 mcg/min = 19 mL/h			2–20 mcg/min	4 mg/250 mL	16	mcg/mL		
				Ordered mcg dose/min ÷ mcg/mL × 60 min/h =						___ mL/h
Phenylephrine	Infusion	1.3 mcg/min = 1 mL/h			10–200 mcg/min	20 mg/250 mL	80	mcg/mL		
				Ordered mcg/min ÷ mcg/mL × 60 min/h =						___ mL/h
Primacor	0.05 mg/kg = 4.8 mg			Give load over 10 min		40 mg/200 mL	0.2	mg/mL		
	mg to give ÷ mg/mL =	24 mL			24	mL × (60 min/h ÷ 10 min) =			144	mL/h × 10 min
	Infusion		0.03		0.5 mcg/kg/min	40 mg/200 mL	200	mcg/mL		___
				Take dose you want in mcg ÷ by drug index number = mL/h on pump						
Trimethaphan	Infusion		—		0.3–6 mg/min	500 mg/500 mL	1	mg/mL		___
				Ordered mg/min ÷ mg/mL × 60 min/h =						___ mL/h
Vasopressin		0.02 u/min = 3 mL/h 0.04 u/min = 6 mL/h				40 u/100 mL	400	u/mL		

97 kg

DRUG	ORDERED AMOUNT	TOTAL DOSE TO GIVE	DRUG INDEX NUMBER	DIRECTIONS	INFUSION RANGE	DRUG MIXTURE	AMOUNT	DRUG/mL	RUN AT	mL/h
Aminophylline	5 mg/kg = 485 mg			Give mg/kg load over 20 min		500 mg/ 250 mL	2 mg/mL		
	mg to give ÷ mg/mL = 243 mL				243	mL × (60 min/h ÷ 20 min) =		727.5	mL/h × 20 min
	Infusion				0.5–1 mg/kg/h	500 mg/ 250 mL	2 mg/mL		
				mg dose ordered × kg ÷ mg/mL =			___	mL/h
Amiodarone	Loading dose			Load **150 mg** over 10 min		900 mg/ 500 mL	1.8 mg/mL	___
			Ordered mg load dose (150 mg) ÷ mg/mL (1.8 mg/mL) = 83 mL to give × (60 min/h ÷ 10 min) = mL/h to set on pump				**500**	mL/h × 83 mL
	Infusion			Run at **1 mg/ min** × 6 h	900 mg/ 500 mL	1.8 mg/mL		
			Ordered mg dose (1 mg/min) ÷ mg/mL (1.8 mg/mL) = ____ × 60 min/h = mL/h to set on pump				**33**	mL/h × 6 h
	Infusion			Run at **0.5 mg/ min** × 18 h	900 mg/ 500 mL	1.8 mg/mL		
			Ordered mg dose (0.5 mg/min) ÷ mg/mL (1.8 mg/mL) = ____ × 60 min/h = mL/h to set on pump				**17**	mL/h × 18 h
Amrinone	0.75 mg/kg = 72.75 mg			Give mg/kg load over 10 min		300 mg/ 120 mL	2.5 mg/mL	___
	mg to give ÷ mg/mL = 29 mL				29.1	mL × (60 min/h ÷ 10 min) =		**174.6**	mL/h × 10 min
	Infusion		0.43		5–10 mcg/ kg/min	300 mg/ 120 mL	2500 mcg/mL	___
			Take dose you want in mcg ÷ by drug index number = mL/h on pump					
Brevibloc	Infusion		1.72		50–100 mcg/ kg/min	2.5 g/ 250 mL	10,000 mcg/mL	___ mL/h
			Take dose you want in mcg ÷ by drug index number = mL/h on pump					
Cardene	Infusion		—		0.5–10 mg/h	25 mg 250 mL	0.1 mg/mL	___
			Ordered mg dose ÷ mg/mL = mL/h to set on pump					___ mL/h
Cardizem	0.25 mg/kg = 24.25 mg			Give mg/kg load over 20 min		50 mg/ 100 mL	0.5 mg/mL	___
	mg to give ÷ mg/mL = 49 mL				48.5	mL × (60 min/h ÷ 20 min) =		**146**	mL/h
	0.35 mg/kg = 33.95 mg			May repeat loading dose in 15 min			0.5 mg/mL	___
	mg to give ÷ mg/mL = 68 mL				67.9	mL × (60 min/h ÷ 20 min) =		**204**	mL/h
	Infusion				5–15 mg/h			___
			Ordered mg dose ÷ mg/mL = mL/h to set on pump					___ mL/h
Desmopressin	0.3 mcg/kg = 29 mcg			Give dose over 20–30 min			4 mcg/vial	
Dobutamine	Infusion		0.34		2.5–40 mcg/kg/ min	250 mg/ 125 mL	2000 mcg/mL	
			Take dose you want in mcg ÷ by drug index number = mL/h on pump					

(continues)

97 kg (continued)

DRUG	ORDERED AMOUNT	TOTAL DOSE TO GIVE	DRUG INDEX NUMBER	DIRECTIONS	INFUSION RANGE	DRUG MIXTURE	AMOUNT	DRUG/ mL	RUN AT	mL/h
Dopamine	Infusion		0.28		1–20 mcg/ kg/min	400 mg/ 250 mL	1600	mcg/mL		
	Take dose you want in mcg ÷ by drug index number = mL/h on pump									
Epinephrine	Infusion	1 mcg/min = 4 mL/h 2 mcg/min = 8 mL/h 3 mcg/min = 11 mL/h 4 mcg/min = 15 mL/h			1–4 mcg/min	4 mg/ 250 mL	16	mcg/mL		
	Ordered mcg dose/min ÷ mcg/mL × 60 min/h =									___ mL/h
Fenoldapam	Infusion		0.0069		0.01–1.6 mcg/ kg/min	10 mg/ 250 mL	40	mcg/mL		
	Take dose you want in mcg ÷ by drug index number = mL/h on pump									
Heparin	100 u/kg = 9700 u 200 u/kg = 19,400 u 300 u/kg = 29,100 u 400 u/kg = 38,800 u									
Isoproterenol	Infusion				5 mcg/min	1 mg/ 250 mL	4	mcg/mL		
	Ordered mcg dose/min ÷ mcg/mL × 60 min/h =									75 mL/h
Lidocaine	Infusion	1 mg/min = 7.5 mL/h			1–4 mg/min	2 g/ 250 mL	8	mg/mL		___
	Ordered mg/min ÷ mg/mL × 60 min/h =									___ mL/h
Nitroglycerin	Infusion	3 mcg/min = 1 mL/h			3–200 mcg/min	50 mg/ 250 mL	200	mcg/mL		___
	Ordered mcg/min ÷ mcg/mL × 60 min/h =									___ mL/h
Nitroprusside	Infusion	6.7 mcg/min = 1 mL/h			5–300 mcg/min	100 mg/ 250 mL	400	mcg/mL		___
	Ordered mcg/min ÷ mcg/mL × 60 min/h =									___ mL/h
Norepinephrine	Infusion	1 mcg/min = 4 mL/h 2 mcg/min = 8 mL/h 3 mcg/min = 11 mL/h 4 mcg/min = 15 mL/h 5 mcg/min = 19 mL/h			2–20 mcg/min	4 mg/ 250 mL	16	mcg/mL		
	Ordered mcg dose/min ÷ mcg/mL × 60 min/h =									___ mL/h
Phenylephrine	Infusion	1.3 mcg/min = 1 mL/h			10–200 mcg/min	20 mg/ 250 mL	80	mcg/mL		
	Ordered mcg/min ÷ mcg/mL × 60 min/h =									___ mL/h
Primacor	0.05 mg/kg = 4.85 mg			Give load over 10 min		40 mg/ 200 mL	0.2	mg/mL		
	mg to give ÷ mg/mL = 24 mL				24	mL × (60 min/h ÷ 10 min) =			145.5	mL/h × 10 min
	Infusion		0.03		0.5 mcg/ kg/min	40 mg/ 200 mL	200	mcg/mL		___
	Take dose you want in mcg ÷ by drug index number = mL/h on pump									
Trimethaphan	Infusion		___		0.3–6 mg/min	500 mg/ 500 mL	1	mg/mL		___
	Ordered mg/min ÷ mg/mL × 60 min/h =									___ mL/h
Vasopressin		0.02 u/min = 3 mL/h 0.04 u/min = 6 mL/h				40 u/ 100 mL	400	u/mL		

98 kg

DRUG	ORDERED AMOUNT	TOTAL DOSE TO GIVE	DRUG INDEX NUMBER	DIRECTIONS	INFUSION RANGE	DRUG MIXTURE	AMOUNT / DRUG/mL	RUN AT / mL/h
Aminophylline	5 mg/kg =	490 mg		Give mg/kg load over 20 min		500 mg/ 250 mL	2 mg/mL	
	mg to give ÷ mg/mL =	245 mL			245	mL × (60 min/h ÷ 20 min) =		**735** mL/h × 20 min
	Infusion				0.5–1 mg/kg/h	500 mg/ 250 mL	2 mg/mL	
				mg dose ordered × kg ÷ mg/mL =				___ mL/h
Amiodarone	Loading dose			Load **150 mg** over 10 min		900 mg/ 500 mL	1.8 mg/mL	
				Ordered mg load dose (150 mg) ÷ mg/mL (1.8 mg/mL) = 83 mL to give × (60 min/h ÷ 10 min) = mL/h to set on pump				**500** mL/h × 83 mL
	Infusion			Run at **1 mg/ min** × 6 h		900 mg/ 500 mL	1.8 mg/mL	
				Ordered mg dose (1 mg/min) ÷ mg/mL (1.8 mg/mL) = _____ × 60 min/h = mL/h to set on pump				**33** mL/h × 6 h
	Infusion			Run at **0.5 mg/ min** × 18 h		900 mg/ 500 mL	1.8 mg/mL	
				Ordered mg dose (0.5 mg/min) ÷ mg/mL (1.8 mg/mL) = _____ × 60 min/h = mL/h to set on pump				**17** mL/h × 18 h
Amrinone	0.75 mg/kg =	73.5 mg		Give mg/kg load over 10 min		300 mg/ 120 mL	2.5 mg/mL	___
	mg to give ÷ mg/mL =	29 mL			29.4	mL × (60 min/h ÷ 10 min) =		**176.4** mL/h × 10 min
	Infusion		0.42		5–10 mcg/ kg/min	300 mg/ 120 mL	2500 mcg/mL	___
				Take dose you want in mcg ÷ by drug index number = mL/h on pump				
Brevibloc	Infusion		1.70		50–100 mcg/ kg/min	2.5 g/ 250 mL	10,000 mcg/mL	___ mL/h
				Take dose you want in mcg ÷ by drug index number = mL/h on pump				
Cardene	Infusion	___			0.5–10 mg/h	25 mg 250 mL	0.1 mg/mL	___
				Ordered mg dose ÷ mg/mL = mL/h to set on pump				___ mL/h
Cardizem	0.25 mg/kg =	24.5 mg		Give mg/kg load over 20 min		50 mg/ 100 mL	0.5 mg/mL	___
	mg to give ÷ mg/mL =	49 mL			49	mL × (60 min/h ÷ 20 min) =		**147** mL/h
	0.35 mg/kg =	34.3 mg		May repeat loading dose in 15 min			0.5 mg/mL	___
	mg to give ÷ mg/mL =	69 mL			68.6	mL × (60 min/h ÷ 20 min) =		**206** mL/h
	Infusion				5–15 mg/h			___
				Ordered mg dose ÷ mg/mL = mL/h to set on pump				___ mL/h
Desmopressin	0.3 mcg/kg =	29 mcg		Give dose over 20–30 min			4 mcg/vial	
Dobutamine	Infusion		0.34		2.5–40 mcg/kg/ min	250 mg/ 125 mL	2000 mcg/mL	
				Take dose you want in mcg ÷ by drug index number = mL/h on pump				

(continues)

98 kg (continued)

DRUG	ORDERED AMOUNT	TOTAL DOSE TO GIVE	DRUG INDEX NUMBER	DIRECTIONS	INFUSION RANGE	DRUG MIXTURE	AMOUNT	DRUG/mL	RUN AT	mL/h
Dopamine	Infusion		0.27		1–20 mcg/kg/min	400 mg/250 mL	1600	mcg/mL		
				Take dose you want in mcg ÷ by drug index number = mL/h on pump						
Epinephrine	Infusion	1 mcg/min = 4 mL/h 2 mcg/min = 8 mL/h 3 mcg/min = 11 mL/h 4 mcg/min = 15 mL/h			1–4 mcg/min	4 mg/250 mL	16	mcg/mL		
				Ordered mcg dose/min ÷ mcg/mL × 60 min/h =					___	mL/h
Fenoldapam	Infusion		0.0068		0.01–1.6 mcg/kg/min	10 mg/250 mL	40	mcg/mL		
				Take dose you want in mcg ÷ by drug index number = mL/h on pump						
Heparin	100 u/kg = 9800 u 200 u/kg = 19,600 u 300 u/kg = 29,400 u 400 u/kg = 39,200 u									
Isoproterenol	Infusion				5 mcg/min	1 mg/250 mL	4	mcg/mL		
				Ordered mcg dose/min ÷ mcg/mL × 60 min/h =					75	mL/h
Lidocaine	Infusion	1 mg/min = 7.5 mL/h			1–4 mg/min	2 g/250 mL	8	mg/mL	___	
				Ordered mg/min ÷ mg/mL × 60 min/h =					___	mL/h
Nitroglycerin	Infusion	3 mcg/min = 1 mL/h			3–200 mcg/min	50 mg/250 mL	200	mcg/mL	___	
				Ordered mcg/min ÷ mcg/mL × 60 min/h =					___	mL/h
Nitroprusside	Infusion	6.7 mcg/min = 1 mL/h			5–300 mcg/min	100 mg/250 mL	400	mcg/mL	___	
				Ordered mcg/min ÷ mcg/mL × 60 min/h =					___	mL/h
Norepinephrine	Infusion	1 mcg/min = 4 mL/h 2 mcg/min = 8 mL/h 3 mcg/min = 11 mL/h 4 mcg/min = 15 mL/h 5 mcg/min = 19 mL/h			2–20 mcg/min	4 mg/250 mL	16	mcg/mL		
				Ordered mcg dose/min ÷ mcg/mL × 60 min/h =					___	mL/h
Phenylephrine	Infusion	1.3 mcg/min = 1 mL/h			10–200 mcg/min	20 mg/250 mL	80	mcg/mL		
				Ordered mcg/min ÷ mcg/mL × 60 min/h =					___	mL/h
Primacor	0.05 mg/kg = 4.9 mg			Give load over 10 min		40 mg/200 mL	0.2	mg/mL		
	mg to give ÷ mg/mL =	25 mL		25	mL × (60 min/h ÷ 10 min) =				147	mL/h × 10 min
	Infusion		0.03		0.5 mcg/kg/min	40 mg/200 mL	200	mcg/mL	___	
				Take dose you want in mcg ÷ by drug index number = mL/h on pump						
Trimethaphan	Infusion		—		0.3–6 mg/min	500 mg/500 mL	1	mg/mL	___	
				Ordered mg/min ÷ mg/mL × 60 min/h =					___	mL/h
Vasopressin	0.02 u/min = 3 mL/h 0.04 u/min = 6 mL/h					40 u/100 mL	400	u/mL		

99 kg

DRUG	ORDERED AMOUNT	TOTAL DOSE TO GIVE	DRUG INDEX NUMBER	DIRECTIONS	INFUSION RANGE	DRUG MIXTURE	AMOUNT DRUG/mL	RUN AT mL/h
Aminophylline	5 mg/kg =	495 mg		Give mg/kg load over 20 min		500 mg/ 250 mL	2 mg/mL	
	mg to give ÷ mg/mL =	248 mL			248	mL × (60 min/h ÷ 20 min) =		742.5 mL/h × 20 min
	Infusion				0.5–1 mg/kg/h	500 mg/ 250 mL	2 mg/mL	
					mg dose ordered × kg ÷ mg/mL =			___ mL/h
Amiodarone	Loading dose			Load **150 mg** over 10 min		900 mg/ 500 mL	1.8 mg/mL	—
				Ordered mg load dose (150 mg) ÷ mg/mL (1.8 mg/mL) = 83 mL to give × (60 min/h ÷ 10 min) = mL/h to set on pump				500 mL/h × 83 mL
	Infusion			Run at **1 mg/ min** × 6 h		900 mg/ 500 mL	1.8 mg/mL	
				Ordered mg dose (1 mg/min) ÷ mg/mL (1.8 mg/mL) = _____ × 60 min/h = mL/h to set on pump				33 mL/h × 6 h
	Infusion			Run at **0.5 mg/ min** × 18 h		900 mg/ 500 mL	1.8 mg/mL	
				Ordered mg dose (0.5 mg/min) ÷ mg/mL (1.8 mg/mL) = _____ × 60 min/h = mL/h to set on pump				17 mL/h × 18 h
Amrinone	0.75 mg/kg =	74.25 mg		Give mg/kg load over 10 min		300 mg/ 120 mL	2.5 mg/mL	—
	mg to give ÷ mg/mL =	30 mL			29.7	mL × (60 min/h ÷ 10 min) =		178.2 mL/h × 10 min
	Infusion		0.42		5–10 mcg/ kg/min	300 mg/ 120 mL	2500 mcg/mL	—
				Take dose you want in mcg ÷ by drug index number = mL/h on pump				
Brevibloc	Infusion		1.68		50–100 mcg/ kg/min	2.5 g/ 250 mL	10,000 mcg/mL	___ mL/h
				Take dose you want in mcg ÷ by drug index number = mL/h on pump				
Cardene	Infusion		—		0.5–10 mg/h	25 mg 250 mL	0.1 mg/mL	—
				Ordered mg dose ÷ mg/mL = mL/h to set on pump				___ mL/h
Cardizem	0.25 mg/kg =	24.75 mg		Give mg/kg load over 20 min		50 mg/ 100 mL	0.5 mg/mL	
	mg to give ÷ mg/mL =	50 mL			49.5	mL × (60 min/h ÷ 20 min) =		149 mL/h
	0.35 mg/kg =	34.65 mg		May repeat loading dose in 15 min			0.5 mg/mL	
	mg to give ÷ mg/mL =	69 mL			69.3	mL × (60 min/h ÷ 20 min) =		208 mL/h
	Infusion				5–15 mg/h			—
				Ordered mg dose ÷ mg/mL = mL/h to set on pump				___ mL/h
Desmopressin	0.3 mcg/kg =	30 mcg		Give dose over 20–30 min			4 mcg/vial	
Dobutamine	Infusion		0.34		2.5–40 mcg/kg/ min	250 mg/ 125 mL	2000 mcg/mL	
				Take dose you want in mcg ÷ by drug index number = mL/h on pump				

(continues)

99 kg (continued)

DRUG	ORDERED AMOUNT		TOTAL DOSE TO GIVE		DRUG INDEX NUMBER	DIRECTIONS	INFUSION RANGE	DRUG MIXTURE	AMOUNT	DRUG/ mL	RUN AT	mL/h
Dopamine	Infusion				0.27		1–20 mcg/ kg/min	400 mg/ 250 mL	1600	mcg/mL		
	Take dose you want in mcg ÷ by drug index number = mL/h on pump											
Epinephrine	Infusion		1 mcg/min = 4 mL/h 2 mcg/min = 8 mL/h 3 mcg/min = 11 mL/h 4 mcg/min = 15 mL/h				1–4 mcg/min	4 mg/ 250 mL	16	mcg/mL		
							Ordered mcg dose/min ÷ mcg/mL × 60 min/h =				___	mL/h
Fenoldapam	Infusion				0.0068		0.01–1.6 mcg/ kg/min	10 mg/ 250 mL	40	mcg/mL		
						Take dose you want in mcg ÷ by drug index number = mL/h on pump						
Heparin	100 u/kg =	9900 u										
	200 u/kg =	19,800 u										
	300 u/kg =	29,700 u										
	400 u/kg =	39,600 u										
Isoproterenol	Infusion						5 mcg/min	1 mg/ 250 mL	4	mcg/mL		
							Ordered mcg dose/min ÷ mcg/mL × 60 min/h =				**75**	mL/h
Lidocaine	Infusion		1 mg/min = 7.5 mL/h				1–4 mg/min	2 g/ 250 mL	8	mg/mL	—	
							Ordered mg/min ÷ mg/mL × 60 min/h =				___	mL/h
Nitroglycerin	Infusion		3 mcg/min = 1 mL/h				3–200 mcg/min	50 mg/ 250 mL	200	mcg/mL	—	
							Ordered mcg/min ÷ mcg/mL × 60 min/h =				___	mL/h
Nitroprusside	Infusion		6.7 mcg/min = 1 mL/h				5–300 mcg/min	100 mg/ 250 mL	400	mcg/mL	—	
							Ordered mcg/min ÷ mcg/mL × 60 min/h =				___	mL/h
Norepinephrine	Infusion		1 mcg/min = 4 mL/h 2 mcg/min = 8 mL/h 3 mcg/min = 11 mL/h 4 mcg/min = 15 mL/h 5 mcg/min = 19 mL/h				2–20 mcg/min	4 mg/ 250 mL	16	mcg/mL		
							Ordered mcg dose/min ÷ mcg/mL × 60 min/h =				___	mL/h
Phenylephrine	Infusion		1.3 mcg/min = 1 mL/h				10–200 mcg/min	20 mg/ 250 mL	80	mcg/mL		
							Ordered mcg/min ÷ mcg/mL × 60 min/h =				___	mL/h
Primacor	0.05 mg/kg =	4.95 mg				Give load over 10 min		40 mg/ 200 mL	0.2	mg/mL		
	mg to give ÷ mg/mL =	25 mL					25	mL × (60 min/h ÷ 10 min) =			**148.5**	mL/h × 10 min
	Infusion				0.03		0.5 mcg/ kg/min	40 mg/ 200 mL	200	mcg/mL	—	
						Take dose you want in mcg ÷ by drug index number = mL/h on pump						
Trimethaphan	Infusion		—				0.3–6 mg/min	500 mg/ 500 mL	1	mg/mL	—	
							Ordered mg/min ÷ mg/mL × 60 min/h =				___	mL/h
Vasopressin			0.02 u/min = 3 mL/h 0.04 u/min = 6 mL/h					40 u/ 100 mL	400	u/mL		

100 kg										
DRUG	**ORDERED AMOUNT**	**TOTAL DOSE TO GIVE**	**DRUG INDEX NUMBER**	**DIRECTIONS**	**INFUSION RANGE**	**DRUG MIXTURE**	**AMOUNT**	**DRUG/ mL**	**RUN AT**	**mL/h**
Aminophylline	5 mg/kg =	500 mg		Give mg/kg load over 20 min		500 mg/ 250 mL	2 mg/mL			
	mg to give ÷ mg/mL =	250 mL			250	mL × (60 min/h ÷ 20 min) =			750	mL/h × 20 min
	Infusion				0.5–1 mg/kg/h	500 mg/ 250 mL	2 mg/mL			
					mg dose ordered × kg ÷ mg/mL =					___ mL/h
Amiodarone	Loading dose			Load **150 mg** over 10 min		900 mg/ 500 mL	1.8 mg/mL		—	
				Ordered mg load dose (150 mg) ÷ mg/mL (1.8 mg/mL) = 83 mL to give × (60 min/h ÷ 10 min) = mL/h to set on pump					500	mL/h × 83 mL
	Infusion			Run at **1 mg/ min** × 6 h		900 mg/ 500 mL	1.8 mg/mL			
				Ordered mg dose (1 mg/min) ÷ mg/mL (1.8 mg/mL) = _____ × 60 min/h = mL/h to set on pump					33	mL/h × 6 h
	Infusion			Run at **0.5 mg/ min** × 18 h		900 mg/ 500 mL	1.8 mg/mL			
				Ordered mg dose (0.5 mg/min) ÷ mg/mL (1.8 mg/mL) = _____ × 60 min/h = mL/h to set on pump					17	mL/h × 18 h
Amrinone	0.75 mg/kg =	75 mg		Give mg/kg load over 10 min		300 mg/ 120 mL	2.5 mg/mL		—	
	mg to give ÷ mg/mL =	30 mL			30	mL × (60 min/h ÷ 10 min) =			180	mL/h × 10 min
	Infusion		0.42		5–10 mcg/ kg/min	300 mg/ 120 mL	2500 mcg/mL		—	
				Take dose you want in mcg ÷ by drug index number = mL/h on pump						
Brevibloc	Infusion		1.67		50–100 mcg/ kg/min	2.5 g/ 250 mL	10,000 mcg/mL		___ mL/h	
				Take dose you want in mcg ÷ by drug index number = mL/h on pump						
Cardene	Infusion		—		0.5–10 mg/h	25 mg 250 mL	0.1 mg/mL		___ mL/h	
				Ordered mg dose ÷ mg/mL = mL/h to set on pump						
Cardizem	0.25 mg/kg =	25 mg		Give mg/kg load over 20 min		50 mg/ 100 mL	0.5 mg/mL		—	
	mg to give ÷ mg/mL =	50 mL			50	mL × (60 min/h ÷ 20 min) =			150	mL/h
	0.35 mg/kg =	35 mg		May repeat loading dose in 15 min			0.5 mg/mL		—	
	mg to give ÷ mg/mL =	70 mL			70	mL × (60 min/h ÷ 20 min) =			210	mL/h
	Infusion				5–15 mg/h				—	
				Ordered mg dose ÷ mg/mL = mL/h to set on pump						___ mL/h
Desmopressin	0.3 mcg/kg =	30 mcg		Give dose over 20–30 min			4 mcg/vial			
Dobutamine	Infusion		0.33		2.5–40 mcg/kg/ min	250 mg/ 125 mL	2000 mcg/mL			
				Take dose you want in mcg ÷ by drug index number = mL/h on pump						

(continues)

100 kg (continued)

DRUG	ORDERED AMOUNT	TOTAL DOSE TO GIVE	DRUG INDEX NUMBER	DIRECTIONS	INFUSION RANGE	DRUG MIXTURE	AMOUNT	DRUG/mL	RUN AT	mL/h
Dopamine	Infusion		0.27		1–20 mcg/kg/min	400 mg/250 mL	1600 mcg/mL			
		Take dose you want in mcg ÷ by drug index number = mL/h on pump								
Epinephrine	Infusion	1 mcg/min = 4 mL/h 2 mcg/min = 8 mL/h 3 mcg/min = 11 mL/h 4 mcg/min = 15 mL/h			1–4 mcg/min	4 mg/250 mL	16 mcg/mL			
		Ordered mcg dose/min ÷ mcg/mL × 60 min/h =								___ mL/h
Fenoldapam	Infusion		0.0067		0.01–1.6 mcg/kg/min	10 mg/250 mL	40 mcg/mL			
		Take dose you want in mcg ÷ by drug index number = mL/h on pump								
Heparin	100 u/kg = 10,000 u 200 u/kg = 20,000 u 300 u/kg = 30,000 u 400 u/kg = 40,000 u									
Isoproterenol	Infusion				5 mcg/min	1 mg/250 mL	4 mcg/mL			
		Ordered mcg dose/min ÷ mcg/mL × 60 min/h =								**75** mL/h
Lidocaine	Infusion	1 mg/min = 7.5 mL/h			1–4 mg/min	2 g/250 mL	8 mg/mL			___
		Ordered mg/min ÷ mg/mL × 60 min/h =								___ mL/h
Nitroglycerin	Infusion	3 mcg/min = 1 mL/h			3–200 mcg/min	50 mg/250 mL	200 mcg/mL			___
		Ordered mcg/min ÷ mcg/mL × 60 min/h =								___ mL/h
Nitroprusside	Infusion	6.7 mcg/min = 1 mL/h			5–300 mcg/min	100 mg/250 mL	400 mcg/mL			___
		Ordered mcg/min ÷ mcg/mL × 60 min/h =								___ mL/h
Norepinephrine	Infusion	1 mcg/min = 4 mL/h 2 mcg/min = 8 mL/h 3 mcg/min = 11 mL/h 4 mcg/min = 15 mL/h 5 mcg/min = 19 mL/h			2–20 mcg/min	4 mg/250 mL	16 mcg/mL			
		Ordered mcg dose/min ÷ mcg/mL × 60 min/h =								___ mL/h
Phenylephrine	Infusion	1.3 mcg/min = 1 mL/h			10–200 mcg/min	20 mg/250 mL	80 mcg/mL			
		Ordered mcg/min ÷ mcg/mL × 60 min/h =								___ mL/h
Primacor	0.05 mg/kg = 5 mg			Give load over 10 min		40 mg/200 mL	0.2 mg/mL			
	mg to give ÷ mg/mL = 25 mL					25 mL × (60 min/h ÷ 10 min) =			**150**	mL/h × 10 min
	Infusion		0.03		0.5 mcg/kg/min	40 mg/200 mL	200 mcg/mL			___
		Take dose you want in mcg ÷ by drug index number = mL/h on pump								
Trimethaphan	Infusion	___			0.3–6 mg/min	500 mg/500 mL	1 mg/mL			___
		Ordered mg/min ÷ mg/mL × 60 min/h =								___ mL/h
Vasopressin		0.02 u/min = 3 mL/h 0.04 u/min = 6 mL/h				40 u/100 mL	400 u/mL			

101 kg

DRUG	ORDERED AMOUNT	TOTAL DOSE TO GIVE	DRUG INDEX NUMBER	DIRECTIONS	INFUSION RANGE	DRUG MIXTURE	AMOUNT DRUG/mL	RUN AT mL/h
Aminophylline	5 mg/kg =	**505** mg		Give mg/kg load over 20 min		500 mg/ 250 mL	2 mg/mL	
	mg to give ÷ mg/mL =	**253** mL			253	mL × (60 min/h ÷ 20 min) =		**757.5** mL/h × 20 min
	Infusion				0.5–1 mg/kg/h	500 mg/ 250 mL	2 mg/mL	
						mg dose ordered × kg ÷ mg/mL =		___ mL/h
Amiodarone	Loading dose			Load **150 mg** over 10 min		900 mg/ 500 mL	1.8 mg/mL	___
				Ordered mg load dose (150 mg) ÷ mg/mL (1.8 mg/mL) = 83 mL to give × (60 min/h ÷ 10 min) = mL/h to set on pump				**500** mL/h × 83 mL
	Infusion			Run at **1 mg/ min** × 6 h		900 mg/ 500 mL	1.8 mg/mL	
				Ordered mg dose (1 mg/min) ÷ mg/mL (1.8 mg/mL) = _____ × 60 min/h = mL/h to set on pump				**33** mL/h × 6 h
	Infusion			Run at **0.5 mg/ min** × 18 h		900 mg/ 500 mL	1.8 mg/mL	
				Ordered mg dose (0.5 mg/min) ÷ mg/mL (1.8 mg/mL) = _____ × 60 min/h = mL/h to set on pump				**17** mL/h × 18 h
Amrinone	0.75 mg/kg =	**75.75** mg		Give mg/kg load over 10 min		300 mg/ 120 mL	2.5 mg/mL	___
	mg to give ÷ mg/mL =	**30** mL			30.3	mL × (60 min/h ÷ 10 min) =		**181.8** mL/h × 10 min
	Infusion		0.41		5–10 mcg/ kg/min	300 mg/ 120 mL	2500 mcg/mL	
				Take dose you want in mcg ÷ by drug index number = mL/h on pump				
Brevibloc	Infusion		1.65		50–100 mcg/ kg/min	2.5 g/ 250 mL	10,000 mcg/mL	___ mL/h
				Take dose you want in mcg ÷ by drug index number = mL/h on pump				
Cardene	Infusion		___		0.5–10 mg/h	25 mg 250 mL	0.1 mg/mL	___
				Ordered mg dose ÷ mg/mL = mL/h to set on pump				___ mL/h
Cardizem	0.25 mg/kg =	**25.25** mg		Give mg/kg load over 20 min		50 mg/ 100 mL	0.5 mg/mL	
	mg to give ÷ mg/mL =	**51** mL			50.5	mL × (60 min/h ÷ 20 min) =		**152** mL/h
	0.35 mg/kg =	**35.35** mg		May repeat loading dose in 15 min			0.5 mg/mL	___
	mg to give ÷ mg/mL =	**71** mL			70.7	mL × (60 min/h ÷ 20 min) =		**212** mL/h
	Infusion				5–15 mg/h			___
				Ordered mg dose ÷ mg/mL = mL/h to set on pump				___ mL/h
Desmopressin	0.3 mcg/kg =	**30** mcg		Give dose over 20–30 min			4 mcg/vial	
Dobutamine	Infusion		0.33		2.5–40 mcg/kg/ min	250 mg/ 125 mL	2000 mcg/mL	
				Take dose you want in mcg ÷ by drug index number = mL/h on pump				

(continues)

101 kg (continued)

DRUG	ORDERED AMOUNT	TOTAL DOSE TO GIVE	DRUG INDEX NUMBER	DIRECTIONS	INFUSION RANGE	DRUG MIXTURE	AMOUNT	DRUG/ mL	RUN AT	mL/h
Dopamine	Infusion		0.26		1–20 mcg/ kg/min	400 mg/ 250 mL	1600	mcg/mL		
	Take dose you want in mcg ÷ by drug index number = mL/h on pump									
Epinephrine	Infusion	1 mcg/min = 4 mL/h 2 mcg/min = 8 mL/h 3 mcg/min = 11 mL/h 4 mcg/min = 15 mL/h			1–4 mcg/min	4 mg/ 250 mL	16	mcg/mL		
	Ordered mcg dose/min ÷ mcg/mL × 60 min/h =								___	mL/h
Fenoldapam	Infusion		0.0066		0.01–1.6 mcg/ kg/min	10 mg/ 250 mL	40	mcg/mL		
	Take dose you want in mcg ÷ by drug index number = mL/h on pump									
Heparin	100 u/kg = 10,100 u 200 u/kg = 20,200 u 300 u/kg = 30,300 u 400 u/kg = 40,400 u									
Isoproterenol	Infusion				5 mcg/min	1 mg/ 250 mL	4	mcg/mL		
	Ordered mcg dose/min ÷ mcg/mL × 60 min/h =								75	mL/h
Lidocaine	Infusion	1 mg/min = 7.5 mL/h			1–4 mg/min	2 g/ 250 mL	8	mg/mL	___	
	Ordered mg/min ÷ mg/mL × 60 min/h =								___	mL/h
Nitroglycerin	Infusion	3 mcg/min = 1 mL/h			3–200 mcg/min	50 mg/ 250 mL	200	mcg/mL	___	
	Ordered mcg/min ÷ mcg/mL × 60 min/h =								___	mL/h
Nitroprusside	Infusion	6.7 mcg/min = 1 mL/h			5–300 mcg/min	100 mg/ 250 mL	400	mcg/mL	___	
	Ordered mcg/min ÷ mcg/mL × 60 min/h =								___	mL/h
Norepinephrine	Infusion	1 mcg/min = 4 mL/h 2 mcg/min = 8 mL/h 3 mcg/min = 11 mL/h 4 mcg/min = 15 mL/h 5 mcg/min = 19 mL/h			2–20 mcg/min	4 mg/ 250 mL	16	mcg/mL		
	Ordered mcg dose/min ÷ mcg/mL × 60 min/h =								___	mL/h
Phenylephrine	Infusion	1.3 mcg/min = 1 mL/h			10–200 mcg/min	20 mg/ 250 mL	80	mcg/mL		
	Ordered mcg/min ÷ mcg/mL × 60 min/h =								___	mL/h
Primacor	0.05 mg/kg = 5.05 mg			Give load over 10 min		40 mg/ 200 mL	0.2	mg/mL		
	mg to give ÷ mg/mL =	25 mL					25	mL × (60 min/h ÷ 10 min) =	151.5	mL/h × 10 min
	Infusion		0.03		0.5 mcg/ kg/min	40 mg/ 200 mL	200	mcg/mL	___	
	Take dose you want in mcg ÷ by drug index number = mL/h on pump									
Trimethaphan	Infusion		___		0.3–6 mg/min	500 mg/ 500 mL	1	mg/mL	___	
	Ordered mg/min ÷ mg/mL × 60 min/h =								___	mL/h
Vasopressin		0.02 u/min = 3 mL/h 0.04 u/min = 6 mL/h				40 u/ 100 mL	400	u/mL		

102 kg

DRUG	ORDERED AMOUNT	TOTAL DOSE TO GIVE	DRUG INDEX NUMBER	DIRECTIONS	INFUSION RANGE	DRUG MIXTURE	AMOUNT DRUG/mL	RUN AT mL/h
Aminophylline	5 mg/kg =	510 mg		Give mg/kg load over 20 min		500 mg/ 250 mL	2 mg/mL	
	mg to give ÷ mg/mL =	255 mL			255	mL × (60 min/h ÷ 20 min) =		765 mL/h × 20 min
	Infusion				0.5–1 mg/kg/h	500 mg/ 250 mL	2 mg/mL	
					mg dose ordered × kg ÷ mg/mL =			___ mL/h
Amiodarone	Loading dose			Load **150 mg** over 10 min		900 mg/ 500 mL	1.8 mg/mL	___
				Ordered mg load dose (150 mg) ÷ mg/mL (1.8 mg/mL) = 83 mL to give × (60 min/h ÷ 10 min) = mL/h to set on pump				500 mL/h × 83 mL
	Infusion			Run at **1 mg/ min** × 6 h		900 mg/ 500 mL	1.8 mg/mL	
				Ordered mg dose (1 mg/min) ÷ mg/mL (1.8 mg/mL) = ____ × 60 min/h = mL/h to set on pump				33 mL/h × 6 h
	Infusion			Run at **0.5 mg/ min** × 18 h		900 mg/ 500 mL	1.8 mg/mL	
				Ordered mg dose (0.5 mg/min) ÷ mg/mL (1.8 mg/mL) = ____ × 60 min/h = mL/h to set on pump				17 mL/h × 18 h
Amrinone	0.75 mg/kg =	76.5 mg		Give mg/kg load over 10 min		300 mg/ 120 mL	2.5 mg/mL	___
	mg to give ÷ mg/mL =	31 mL			30.6	mL × (60 min/h ÷ 10 min) =		183.6 mL/h × 10 min
	Infusion		0.41		5–10 mcg/ kg/min	300 mg/ 120 mL	2500 mcg/mL	___
				Take dose you want in mcg ÷ by drug index number = mL/h on pump				
Brevibloc	Infusion		1.63		50–100 mcg/ kg/min	2.5 g/ 250 mL	10,000 mcg/mL	___ mL/h
				Take dose you want in mcg ÷ by drug index number = mL/h on pump				
Cardene	Infusion		—		0.5–10 mg/h	25 mg 250 mL	0.1 mg/mL	___
				Ordered mg dose ÷ mg/mL = mL/h to set on pump				___ mL/h
Cardizem	0.25 mg/kg =	25.5 mg		Give mg/kg load over 20 min		50 mg/ 100 mL	0.5 mg/mL	___
	mg to give ÷ mg/mL =	51 mL			51	mL × (60 min/h ÷ 20 min) =		153 mL/h
	0.35 mg/kg =	35.7 mg		May repeat loading dose in 15 min			0.5 mg/mL	___
	mg to give ÷ mg/mL =	71 mL			71.4	mL × (60 min/h ÷ 20 min) =		214 mL/h
	Infusion				5–15 mg/h			___
				Ordered mg dose ÷ mg/mL = mL/h to set on pump				___ mL/h
Desmopressin	0.3 mcg/kg =	31 mcg		Give dose over 20–30 min			4 mcg/vial	
Dobutamine	Infusion		0.33		2.5–40 mcg/kg/ min	250 mg/ 125 mL	2000 mcg/mL	
				Take dose you want in mcg ÷ by drug index number = mL/h on pump				

(continues)

102 kg (continued)

DRUG	ORDERED AMOUNT	TOTAL DOSE TO GIVE	DRUG INDEX NUMBER	DIRECTIONS	INFUSION RANGE	DRUG MIXTURE	AMOUNT	DRUG/ mL	RUN AT	mL/h
Dopamine	Infusion		0.26		1–20 mcg/ kg/min	400 mg/ 250 mL	1600	mcg/mL		
	Take dose you want in mcg ÷ by drug index number = mL/h on pump									
Epinephrine	Infusion	1 mcg/min = 4 mL/h 2 mcg/min = 8 mL/h 3 mcg/min = 11 mL/h 4 mcg/min = 15 mL/h			1–4 mcg/min	4 mg/ 250 mL	16	mcg/mL		
		Ordered mcg dose/min ÷ mcg/mL × 60 min/h =							___	mL/h
Fenoldapam	Infusion		0.0066		0.01–1.6 mcg/ kg/min	10 mg/ 250 mL	40	mcg/mL		
	Take dose you want in mcg ÷ by drug index number = mL/h on pump									
Heparin	100 u/kg = 10,200 u 200 u/kg = 20,400 u 300 u/kg = 30,600 u 400 u/kg = 40,800 u									
Isoproterenol	Infusion				5 mcg/min	1 mg/ 250 mL	4	mcg/mL		
		Ordered mcg dose/min ÷ mcg/mL × 60 min/h =							75	mL/h
Lidocaine	Infusion	1 mg/min = 7.5 mL/h			1–4 mg/min	2 g/ 250 mL	8	mg/mL	___	
		Ordered mg/min ÷ mg/mL × 60 min/h =							___	mL/h
Nitroglycerin	Infusion	3 mcg/min = 1 mL/h			3–200 mcg/min	50 mg/ 250 mL	200	mcg/mL	___	
		Ordered mcg/min ÷ mcg/mL × 60 min/h =							___	mL/h
Nitroprusside	Infusion	6.7 mcg/min = 1 mL/h			5–300 mcg/min	100 mg/ 250 mL	400	mcg/mL	___	
		Ordered mcg/min ÷ mcg/mL × 60 min/h =							___	mL/h
Norepinephrine	Infusion	1 mcg/min = 4 mL/h 2 mcg/min = 8 mL/h 3 mcg/min = 11 mL/h 4 mcg/min = 15 mL/h 5 mcg/min = 19 mL/h			2–20 mcg/min	4 mg/ 250 mL	16	mcg/mL		
		Ordered mcg dose/min ÷ mcg/mL × 60 min/h =							___	mL/h
Phenylephrine	Infusion	1.3 mcg/min = 1 mL/h			10–200 mcg/min	20 mg/ 250 mL	80	mcg/mL		
		Ordered mcg/min ÷ mcg/mL × 60 min/h =							___	mL/h
Primacor	0.05 mg/kg = 5.1 mg			Give load over 10 min		40 mg/ 200 mL	0.2	mg/mL		
	mg to give ÷ mg/mL = 26 mL				25 mL × (60 min/h ÷ 10 min) =				153	mL/h × 10 min
	Infusion		0.03		0.5 mcg/ kg/min	40 mg/ 200 mL	200	mcg/mL	___	
	Take dose you want in mcg ÷ by drug index number = mL/h on pump									
Trimethaphan	Infusion		—		0.3–6 mg/min	500 mg/ 500 mL	1	mg/mL	___	
		Ordered mg/min ÷ mg/mL × 60 min/h =							___	mL/h
Vasopressin		0.02 u/min = 3 mL/h 0.04 u/min = 6 mL/h				40 u/ 100 mL	400	u/mL		

103 kg								
DRUG	**ORDERED AMOUNT**	**TOTAL DOSE TO GIVE**	**DRUG INDEX NUMBER**	**DIRECTIONS**	**INFUSION RANGE**	**DRUG MIXTURE**	**AMOUNT DRUG/ mL**	**RUN AT mL/h**
Aminophylline	5 mg/kg =	515 mg		Give mg/kg load over 20 min		500 mg/ 250 mL	2 mg/mL	
	mg to give ÷ mg/mL =	258 mL			258	mL × (60 min/h ÷ 20 min) =		<u>772.5</u> mL/h × 20 min
	Infusion				0.5–1 mg/kg/h	500 mg/ 250 mL	2 mg/mL	
					mg dose ordered × kg ÷ mg/mL =			___ mL/h
Amiodarone	Loading dose			Load **150 mg** over 10 min		900 mg/ 500 mL	1.8 mg/mL	—
				Ordered mg load dose (150 mg) ÷ mg/mL (1.8 mg/mL) = 83 mL to give × (60 min/h ÷ 10 min) = mL/h to set on pump				<u>500</u> mL/h × 83 mL
	Infusion			Run at **1 mg/ min** × 6 h		900 mg/ 500 mL	1.8 mg/mL	
				Ordered mg dose (1 mg/min) ÷ mg/mL (1.8 mg/mL) = _____ × 60 min/h = mL/h to set on pump				<u>33</u> mL/h × 6 h
	Infusion			Run at **0.5 mg/ min** × 18 h		900 mg/ 500 mL	1.8 mg/mL	
				Ordered mg dose (0.5 mg/min) ÷ mg/mL (1.8 mg/mL) = _____ × 60 min/h = mL/h to set on pump				<u>17</u> mL/h × 18 h
Amrinone	0.75 mg/kg =	77.25 mg		Give mg/kg load over 10 min		300 mg/ 120 mL	2.5 mg/mL	___
	mg to give ÷ mg/mL =	31 mL			30.9	mL × (60 min/h ÷ 10 min) =		<u>185.4</u> mL/h × 10 min
	Infusion		0.40		5–10 mcg/ kg/min	300 mg/ 120 mL	2500 mcg/mL	___
				Take dose you want in mcg ÷ by drug index number = mL/h on pump				
Brevibloc	Infusion		1.62		50–100 mcg/ kg/min	2.5 g/ 250 mL	10,000 mcg/mL	___ mL/h
				Take dose you want in mcg ÷ by drug index number = mL/h on pump				
Cardene	Infusion		—		0.5–10 mg/h	25 mg 250 mL	0.1 mg/mL	___
				Ordered mg dose ÷ mg/mL = mL/h to set on pump				___ mL/h
Cardizem	0.25 mg/kg =	25.75 mg		Give mg/kg load over 20 min		50 mg/ 100 mL	0.5 mg/mL	___
	mg to give ÷ mg/mL =	52 mL			51.5	mL × (60 min/h ÷ 20 min) =		<u>155</u> mL/h
	0.35 mg/kg =	36.05 mg		May repeat loading dose in 15 min			0.5 mg/mL	___
	mg to give ÷ mg/mL =	72 mL			72.1	mL × (60 min/h ÷ 20 min) =		<u>216</u> mL/h
	Infusion				5–15 mg/h			___
				Ordered mg dose ÷ mg/mL = mL/h to set on pump				___ mL/h
Desmopressin	0.3 mcg/kg =	31 mcg		Give dose over 20–30 min			4 mcg/vial	
Dobutamine	Infusion		0.32		2.5–40 mcg/kg/ min	250 mg/ 125 mL	2000 mcg/mL	
				Take dose you want in mcg ÷ by drug index number = mL/h on pump				

(continues)

103　kg (continued)

DRUG	ORDERED AMOUNT		TOTAL DOSE TO GIVE		DRUG INDEX NUMBER	DIRECTIONS	INFUSION RANGE	DRUG MIXTURE	AMOUNT	DRUG/ mL	RUN AT	mL/h
Dopamine	Infusion				0.26		1–20 mcg/ kg/min	400 mg/ 250 mL	1600	mcg/mL		
	Take dose you want in mcg ÷ by drug index number = mL/h on pump											
Epinephrine	Infusion		1 mcg/min = 4 mL/h 2 mcg/min = 8 mL/h 3 mcg/min = 11 mL/h 4 mcg/min = 15 mL/h				1–4 mcg/min	4 mg/ 250 mL	16	mcg/mL		
						Ordered mcg dose/min ÷ mcg/mL × 60 min/h =						___	mL/h
Fenoldapam	Infusion				0.0065		0.01–1.6 mcg/ kg/min	10 mg/ 250 mL	40	mcg/mL		
	Take dose you want in mcg ÷ by drug index number = mL/h on pump											
Heparin	100　u/kg = 200　u/kg = 300　u/kg = 400　u/kg =		10,300　u 20,600　u 30,900　u 41,200　u										
Isoproterenol	Infusion						5 mcg/min	1 mg/ 250 mL	4	mcg/mL		
						Ordered mcg dose/min ÷ mcg/mL × 60 min/h =						75	mL/h
Lidocaine	Infusion		1 mg/min = 7.5 mL/h				1–4 mg/min	2 g/ 250 mL	8	mg/mL		
						Ordered mg/min ÷ mg/mL × 60 min/h =						___	mL/h
Nitroglycerin	Infusion		3 mcg/min = 1 mL/h				3–200 mcg/min	50 mg/ 250 mL	200	mcg/mL		
						Ordered mcg/min ÷ mcg/mL × 60 min/h =						___	mL/h
Nitroprusside	Infusion		6.7 mcg/min = 1 mL/h				5–300 mcg/min	100 mg/ 250 mL	400	mcg/mL		
						Ordered mcg/min ÷ mcg/mL × 60 min/h =						___	mL/h
Norepinephrine	Infusion		1 mcg/min = 4 mL/h 2 mcg/min = 8 mL/h 3 mcg/min = 11 mL/h 4 mcg/min = 15 mL/h 5 mcg/min = 19 mL/h				2–20 mcg/min	4 mg/ 250 mL	16	mcg/mL		
						Ordered mcg dose/min ÷ mcg/mL × 60 min/h =						___	mL/h
Phenylephrine	Infusion		1.3 mcg/min = 1 mL/h				10–200 mcg/min	20 mg/ 250 mL	80	mcg/mL		
						Ordered mcg/min ÷ mcg/mL × 60 min/h =						___	mL/h
Primacor	0.05　mg/kg =		5.15　mg			Give load over 10 min		40 mg/ 200 mL	0.2	mg/mL		
	mg to give ÷ mg/mL =		26　mL					26 mL × (60 min/h ÷ 10 min) =			154.5	mL/h × 10 min
	Infusion				0.03		0.5 mcg/ kg/min	40 mg/ 200 mL	200	mcg/mL		
	Take dose you want in mcg ÷ by drug index number = mL/h on pump											
Trimethaphan	Infusion				—		0.3–6 mg/min	500 mg/ 500 mL	1	mg/mL		
						Ordered mg/min ÷ mg/mL × 60 min/h =						___	mL/h
Vasopressin			0.02 u/min = 3 mL/h 0.04 u/min = 6 mL/h					40 u/ 100 mL	400	u/mL		

104 kg

DRUG	ORDERED AMOUNT	TOTAL DOSE TO GIVE	DRUG INDEX NUMBER	DIRECTIONS	INFUSION RANGE	DRUG MIXTURE	AMOUNT	DRUG/mL	RUN AT	mL/h
Aminophylline	5 mg/kg =	520 mg		Give mg/kg load over 20 min		500 mg/ 250 mL		2 mg/mL		
	mg to give ÷ mg/mL =	260 mL					260	mL × (60 min/h ÷ 20 min) =	780	mL/h × 20 min
	Infusion				0.5–1 mg/kg/h	500 mg/ 250 mL		2 mg/mL		
						mg dose ordered × kg ÷ mg/mL =				___ mL/h
Amiodarone	Loading dose			Load **150 mg** over 10 min		900 mg/ 500 mL		1.8 mg/mL		—
				Ordered mg load dose (150 mg) ÷ mg/mL (1.8 mg/mL) = 83 mL to give × (60 min/h ÷ 10 min) = mL/h to set on pump					500	mL/h × 83 mL
	Infusion			Run at **1 mg/ min** × 6 h		900 mg/ 500 mL		1.8 mg/mL		
				Ordered mg dose (1 mg/min) ÷ mg/mL (1.8 mg/mL) = ____ × 60 min/h = mL/h to set on pump					33	mL/h × 6 h
	Infusion			Run at **0.5 mg/ min** × 18 h		900 mg/ 500 mL		1.8 mg/mL		
				Ordered mg dose (0.5 mg/min) ÷ mg/mL (1.8 mg/mL) = ____ × 60 min/h = mL/h to set on pump					17	mL/h × 18 h
Amrinone	0.75 mg/kg =	78 mg		Give mg/kg load over 10 min		300 mg/ 120 mL		2.5 mg/mL		—
	mg to give ÷ mg/mL =	31 mL					31.2	mL × (60 min/h ÷ 10 min) =	187.2	mL/h × 10 min
	Infusion		0.40		5–10 mcg/ kg/min	300 mg/ 120 mL		2500 mcg/mL		—
				Take dose you want in mcg ÷ by drug index number = mL/h on pump						
Brevibloc	Infusion		1.60		50–100 mcg/ kg/min	2.5 g/ 250 mL		10,000 mcg/mL		___ mL/h
				Take dose you want in mcg ÷ by drug index number = mL/h on pump						
Cardene	Infusion		—		0.5–10 mg/h	25 mg 250 mL		0.1 mg/mL		—
				Ordered mg dose ÷ mg/mL = mL/h to set on pump						___ mL/h
Cardizem	0.25 mg/kg =	26 mg		Give mg/kg load over 20 min		50 mg/ 100 mL		0.5 mg/mL		—
	mg to give ÷ mg/mL =	52 mL					52	mL × (60 min/h ÷ 20 min) =	156 mL/h	
	0.35 mg/kg =	36.4 mg		May repeat loading dose in 15 min				0.5 mg/mL		—
	mg to give ÷ mg/mL =	73 mL					72.8	mL × (60 min/h ÷ 20 min) =	218 mL/h	
	Infusion				5–15 mg/h					—
				Ordered mg dose ÷ mg/mL = mL/h to set on pump						___ mL/h
Desmopressin	0.3 mcg/kg =	31 mcg		Give dose over 20–30 min				4 mcg/vial		
Dobutamine	Infusion		0.32		2.5–40 mcg/kg/ min	250 mg/ 125 mL		2000 mcg/mL		
				Take dose you want in mcg ÷ by drug index number = mL/h on pump						

(continues)

104 kg (continued)

DRUG	ORDERED AMOUNT	TOTAL DOSE TO GIVE	DRUG INDEX NUMBER	DIRECTIONS	INFUSION RANGE	DRUG MIXTURE	AMOUNT	DRUG/mL	RUN AT	mL/h
Dopamine	Infusion		0.26		1–20 mcg/kg/min	400 mg/250 mL	1600	mcg/mL		
	Take dose you want in mcg ÷ by drug index number = mL/h on pump									
Epinephrine	Infusion	1 mcg/min = 4 mL/h 2 mcg/min = 8 mL/h 3 mcg/min = 11 mL/h 4 mcg/min = 15 mL/h			1–4 mcg/min	4 mg/250 mL	16	mcg/mL		
	Ordered mcg dose/min ÷ mcg/mL × 60 min/h =								___	mL/h
Fenoldapam	Infusion		0.0064		0.01–1.6 mcg/kg/min	10 mg/250 mL	40	mcg/mL		
	Take dose you want in mcg ÷ by drug index number = mL/h on pump									
Heparin	100 u/kg = 10,400 u 200 u/kg = 20,800 u 300 u/kg = 31,200 u 400 u/kg = 41,600 u									
Isoproterenol	Infusion				5 mcg/min	1 mg/250 mL	4	mcg/mL		
	Ordered mcg dose/min ÷ mcg/mL × 60 min/h =								**75**	mL/h
Lidocaine	Infusion	1 mg/min = 7.5 mL/h			1–4 mg/min	2 g/250 mL	8	mg/mL	___	
	Ordered mg/min ÷ mg/mL × 60 min/h =								___	mL/h
Nitroglycerin	Infusion	3 mcg/min = 1 mL/h			3–200 mcg/min	50 mg/250 mL	200	mcg/mL	___	
	Ordered mcg/min ÷ mcg/mL × 60 min/h =								___	mL/h
Nitroprusside	Infusion	6.7 mcg/min = 1 mL/h			5–300 mcg/min	100 mg/250 mL	400	mcg/mL	___	
	Ordered mcg/min ÷ mcg/mL × 60 min/h =								___	mL/h
Norepinephrine	Infusion	1 mcg/min = 4 mL/h 2 mcg/min = 8 mL/h 3 mcg/min = 11 mL/h 4 mcg/min = 15 mL/h 5 mcg/min = 19 mL/h			2–20 mcg/min	4 mg/250 mL	16	mcg/mL		
	Ordered mcg dose/min ÷ mcg/mL × 60 min/h =								___	mL/h
Phenylephrine	Infusion	1.3 mcg/min = 1 mL/h			10–200 mcg/min	20 mg/250 mL	80	mcg/mL		
	Ordered mcg/min ÷ mcg/mL × 60 min/h =								___	mL/h
Primacor	0.05 mg/kg =	5.2 mg		Give load over 10 min		40 mg/200 mL	0.2	mg/mL		
	mg to give ÷ mg/mL =	26 mL			26	mL × (60 min/h ÷ 10 min) =			**156**	mL/h × 10 min
	Infusion		0.03		0.5 mcg/kg/min	40 mg/200 mL	200	mcg/mL	___	
	Take dose you want in mcg ÷ by drug index number = mL/h on pump									
Trimethaphan	Infusion	—			0.3–6 mg/min	500 mg/500 mL	1	mg/mL	___	
	Ordered mg/min ÷ mg/mL × 60 min/h =								___	mL/h
Vasopressin		0.02 u/min = 3 mL/h 0.04 u/min = 6 mL/h				40 u/100 mL	400	u/mL		

105 kg

DRUG	ORDERED AMOUNT	TOTAL DOSE TO GIVE	DRUG INDEX NUMBER	DIRECTIONS	INFUSION RANGE	DRUG MIXTURE	AMOUNT	DRUG/mL	RUN AT	mL/h
Aminophylline	5 mg/kg =	525 mg		Give mg/kg load over 20 min		500 mg/ 250 mL		2 mg/mL		
	mg to give ÷ mg/mL =	263 mL	263			mL × (60 min/h ÷ 20 min) =			787.5	mL/h × 20 min
	Infusion				0.5–1 mg/kg/h	500 mg/ 250 mL		2 mg/mL		
						mg dose ordered × kg ÷ mg/mL =				___ mL/h
Amiodarone	Loading dose			Load **150 mg** over 10 min		900 mg/ 500 mL		1.8 mg/mL	—	
				Ordered mg load dose (150 mg) ÷ mg/mL (1.8 mg/mL) = 83 mL to give × (60 min/h ÷ 10 min) = mL/h to set on pump					500	mL/h × 83 mL
	Infusion			Run at **1 mg/ min** × 6 h		900 mg/ 500 mL		1.8 mg/mL		
				Ordered mg dose (1 mg/min) ÷ mg/mL (1.8 mg/mL) = _____ × 60 min/h = mL/h to set on pump					33	mL/h × 6 h
	Infusion			Run at **0.5 mg/ min** × 18 h		900 mg/ 500 mL		1.8 mg/mL		
				Ordered mg dose (0.5 mg/min) ÷ mg/mL (1.8 mg/mL) = _____ × 60 min/h = mL/h to set on pump					17	mL/h × 18 h
Amrinone	0.75 mg/kg =	78.75 mg		Give mg/kg load over 10 min		300 mg/ 120 mL		2.5 mg/mL	—	
	mg to give ÷ mg/mL =	32 mL				31.5 mL × (60 min/h ÷ 10 min) =			189	mL/h × 10 min
	Infusion		0.40		5–10 mcg/ kg/min	300 mg/ 120 mL		2500 mcg/mL		
				Take dose you want in mcg ÷ by drug index number = mL/h on pump						
Brevibloc	Infusion		1.59		50–100 mcg/ kg/min	2.5 g/ 250 mL		10,000 mcg/mL		___ mL/h
				Take dose you want in mcg ÷ by drug index number = mL/h on pump						
Cardene	Infusion			—	0.5–10 mg/h	25 mg 250 mL		0.1 mg/mL		
				Ordered mg dose ÷ mg/mL = mL/h to set on pump						___ mL/h
Cardizem	0.25 mg/kg =	26.25 mg		Give mg/kg load over 20 min		50 mg/ 100 mL		0.5 mg/mL		
	mg to give ÷ mg/mL =	53 mL				52.5 mL × (60 min/h ÷ 20 min) =			158	mL/h
	0.35 mg/kg =	36.75 mg		May repeat loading dose in 15 min				0.5 mg/mL		
	mg to give ÷ mg/mL =	74 mL				73.5 mL × (60 min/h ÷ 20 min) =			221	mL/h
	Infusion				5–15 mg/h					
				Ordered mg dose ÷ mg/mL = mL/h to set on pump						___ mL/h
Desmopressin	0.3 mcg/kg =	32 mcg		Give dose over 20–30 min				4 mcg/vial		
Dobutamine	Infusion		0.32		2.5–40 mcg/kg/ min	250 mg/ 125 mL		2000 mcg/mL		
				Take dose you want in mcg ÷ by drug index number = mL/h on pump						

(continues)

105 kg (continued)

DRUG	ORDERED AMOUNT	TOTAL DOSE TO GIVE	DRUG INDEX NUMBER	DIRECTIONS	INFUSION RANGE	DRUG MIXTURE	AMOUNT	DRUG/mL	RUN AT	mL/h
Dopamine	Infusion		0.25		1–20 mcg/kg/min	400 mg/250 mL	1600	mcg/mL		
	Take dose you want in mcg ÷ by drug index number = mL/h on pump									
Epinephrine	Infusion	1 mcg/min = 4 mL/h 2 mcg/min = 8 mL/h 3 mcg/min = 11 mL/h 4 mcg/min = 15 mL/h			1–4 mcg/min	4 mg/250 mL	16	mcg/mL		
		Ordered mcg dose/min ÷ mcg/mL × 60 min/h =							___	mL/h
Fenoldapam	Infusion		0.0064		0.01–1.6 mcg/kg/min	10 mg/250 mL	40	mcg/mL		
	Take dose you want in mcg ÷ by drug index number = mL/h on pump									
Heparin	100 u/kg = 10,500 u 200 u/kg = 21,000 u 300 u/kg = 31,500 u 400 u/kg = 42,000 u									
Isoproterenol	Infusion				5 mcg/min	1 mg/250 mL	4	mcg/mL		
		Ordered mcg dose/min ÷ mcg/mL × 60 min/h =							**75**	mL/h
Lidocaine	Infusion	1 mg/min = 7.5 mL/h			1–4 mg/min	2 g/250 mL	8	mg/mL	___	
		Ordered mg/min ÷ mg/mL × 60 min/h =							___	mL/h
Nitroglycerin	Infusion	3 mcg/min = 1 mL/h			3–200 mcg/min	50 mg/250 mL	200	mcg/mL	___	
		Ordered mcg/min ÷ mcg/mL × 60 min/h =							___	mL/h
Nitroprusside	Infusion	6.7 mcg/min = 1 mL/h			5–300 mcg/min	100 mg/250 mL	400	mcg/mL	___	
		Ordered mcg/min ÷ mcg/mL × 60 min/h =							___	mL/h
Norepinephrine	Infusion	1 mcg/min = 4 mL/h 2 mcg/min = 8 mL/h 3 mcg/min = 11 mL/h 4 mcg/min = 15 mL/h 5 mcg/min = 19 mL/h			2–20 mcg/min	4 mg/250 mL	16	mcg/mL		
		Ordered mcg dose/min ÷ mcg/mL × 60 min/h =							___	mL/h
Phenylephrine	Infusion	1.3 mcg/min = 1 mL/h			10–200 mcg/min	20 mg/250 mL	80	mcg/mL	___	
		Ordered mcg/min ÷ mcg/mL × 60 min/h =							___	mL/h
Primacor	0.05 mg/kg = 5.25 mg			Give load over 10 min		40 mg/200 mL	0.2	mg/mL		
	mg to give ÷ mg/mL = 26 mL				26 mL × (60 min/h ÷ 10 min) =				**157.5**	mL/h × 10 min
	Infusion		0.03		0.5 mcg/kg/min	40 mg/200 mL	200	mcg/mL	___	
		Take dose you want in mcg ÷ by drug index number = mL/h on pump								
Trimethaphan	Infusion			___	0.3–6 mg/min	500 mg/500 mL	1	mg/mL	___	
		Ordered mg/min ÷ mg/mL × 60 min/h =							___	mL/h
Vasopressin		0.02 u/min = 3 mL/h 0.04 u/min = 6 mL/h				40 u/100 mL	400	u/mL		

106 kg

DRUG	ORDERED AMOUNT	TOTAL DOSE TO GIVE	DRUG INDEX NUMBER	DIRECTIONS	INFUSION RANGE	DRUG MIXTURE	AMOUNT / DRUG/mL	RUN AT / mL/h
Aminophylline	5 mg/kg =	530 mg		Give mg/kg load over 20 min		500 mg/ 250 mL	2 mg/mL	
	mg to give ÷ mg/mL =	265 mL			265	mL × (60 min/h ÷ 20 min) =		<u>795</u> mL/h × 20 min
	Infusion				0.5–1 mg/kg/h	500 mg/ 250 mL	2 mg/mL	
					mg dose ordered × kg ÷ mg/mL =			___ mL/h
Amiodarone	Loading dose			Load **150 mg** over 10 min		900 mg/ 500 mL	1.8 mg/mL	___
				Ordered mg load dose (150 mg) ÷ mg/mL (1.8 mg/mL) = 83 mL to give × (60 min/h ÷ 10 min) = mL/h to set on pump				<u>500</u> mL/h × 83 mL
	Infusion			Run at **1 mg/ min** × 6 h		900 mg/ 500 mL	1.8 mg/mL	
				Ordered mg dose (1 mg/min) ÷ mg/mL (1.8 mg/mL) = ___ × 60 min/h = mL/h to set on pump				<u>33</u> mL/h × 6 h
	Infusion			Run at **0.5 mg/ min** × 18 h		900 mg/ 500 mL	1.8 mg/mL	
				Ordered mg dose (0.5 mg/min) ÷ mg/mL (1.8 mg/mL) = ___ × 60 min/h = mL/h to set on pump				<u>17</u> mL/h × 18 h
Amrinone	0.75 mg/kg =	79.5 mg		Give mg/kg load over 10 min		300 mg/ 120 mL	2.5 mg/mL	___
	mg to give ÷ mg/mL =	32 mL			31.8	mL × (60 min/h ÷ 10 min) =		<u>190.8</u> mL/h × 10 min
	Infusion		0.39		5–10 mcg/ kg/min	300 mg/ 120 mL	2500 mcg/mL	___
				Take dose you want in mcg ÷ by drug index number = mL/h on pump				
Brevibloc	Infusion		1.57		50–100 mcg/ kg/min	2.5 g/ 250 mL	10,000 mcg/mL	___ mL/h
				Take dose you want in mcg ÷ by drug index number = mL/h on pump				
Cardene	Infusion		___		0.5–10 mg/h	25 mg 250 mL	0.1 mg/mL	___
				Ordered mg dose ÷ mg/mL = mL/h to set on pump				___ mL/h
Cardizem	0.25 mg/kg =	26.5 mg		Give mg/kg load over 20 min		50 mg/ 100 mL	0.5 mg/mL	
	mg to give ÷ mg/mL =	53 mL			53	mL × (60 min/h ÷ 20 min) =		<u>159</u> mL/h
	0.35 mg/kg =	37.1 mg		May repeat loading dose in 15 min			0.5 mg/mL	
	mg to give ÷ mg/mL =	74 mL			74.2	mL × (60 min/h ÷ 20 min) =		<u>223</u> mL/h
	Infusion				5–15 mg/h			___
				Ordered mg dose ÷ mg/mL = mL/h to set on pump				___ mL/h
Desmopressin	0.3 mcg/kg =	32 mcg		Give dose over 20–30 min			4 mcg/vial	
Dobutamine	Infusion		0.31		2.5–40 mcg/kg/ min	250 mg/ 125 mL	2000 mcg/mL	
				Take dose you want in mcg ÷ by drug index number = mL/h on pump				

(continues)

106 kg (continued)

DRUG	ORDERED AMOUNT	TOTAL DOSE TO GIVE	DRUG INDEX NUMBER	DIRECTIONS	INFUSION RANGE	DRUG MIXTURE	AMOUNT	DRUG/mL	RUN AT	mL/h
Dopamine	Infusion		0.25		1–20 mcg/ kg/min	400 mg/ 250 mL	1600	mcg/mL		
						Take dose you want in mcg ÷ by drug index number = mL/h on pump				
Epinephrine	Infusion	1 mcg/min = 4 mL/h 2 mcg/min = 8 mL/h 3 mcg/min = 11 mL/h 4 mcg/min = 15 mL/h			1–4 mcg/min	4 mg/ 250 mL	16	mcg/mL		
					Ordered mcg dose/min ÷ mcg/mL × 60 min/h =				___	mL/h
Fenoldapam	Infusion		0.0063		0.01–1.6 mcg/ kg/min	10 mg/ 250 mL	40	mcg/mL		
						Take dose you want in mcg ÷ by drug index number = mL/h on pump				
Heparin	100 u/kg = 10,600 u 200 u/kg = 21,200 u 300 u/kg = 31,800 u 400 u/kg = 42,400 u									
Isoproterenol	Infusion				5 mcg/min	1 mg/ 250 mL	4	mcg/mL		
					Ordered mcg dose/min ÷ mcg/mL × 60 min/h =				75	mL/h
Lidocaine	Infusion	1 mg/min = 7.5 mL/h			1–4 mg/min	2 g/ 250 mL	8	mg/mL	___	
					Ordered mg/min ÷ mg/mL × 60 min/h =				___	mL/h
Nitroglycerin	Infusion	3 mcg/min = 1 mL/h			3–200 mcg/min	50 mg/ 250 mL	200	mcg/mL	___	
					Ordered mcg/min ÷ mcg/mL × 60 min/h =				___	mL/h
Nitroprusside	Infusion	6.7 mcg/min = 1 mL/h			5–300 mcg/min	100 mg/ 250 mL	400	mcg/mL	___	
					Ordered mcg/min ÷ mcg/mL × 60 min/h =				___	mL/h
Norepinephrine	Infusion	1 mcg/min = 4 mL/h 2 mcg/min = 8 mL/h 3 mcg/min = 11 mL/h 4 mcg/min = 15 mL/h 5 mcg/min = 19 mL/h			2–20 mcg/min	4 mg/ 250 mL	16	mcg/mL		
					Ordered mcg dose/min ÷ mcg/mL × 60 min/h =				___	mL/h
Phenylephrine	Infusion	1.3 mcg/min = 1 mL/h			10–200 mcg/min	20 mg/ 250 mL	80	mcg/mL		
					Ordered mcg/min ÷ mcg/mL × 60 min/h =				___	mL/h
Primacor	0.05 mg/kg = 5.3 mg			Give load over 10 min		40 mg/ 200 mL	0.2	mg/mL		
	mg to give ÷ mg/mL = 27 mL				27 mL × (60 min/h ÷ 10 min) =				159	mL/h × 10 min
	Infusion		0.03		0.5 mcg/ kg/min	40 mg/ 200 mL	200	mcg/mL	___	
					Take dose you want in mcg ÷ by drug index number = mL/h on pump				
Trimethaphan	Infusion			—	0.3–6 mg/min	500 mg/ 500 mL	1	mg/mL	___	
					Ordered mg/min ÷ mg/mL × 60 min/h =				___	mL/h
Vasopressin		0.02 u/min = 3 mL/h 0.04 u/min = 6 mL/h				40 u/ 100 mL	400	u/mL		

107 kg

DRUG	ORDERED AMOUNT	TOTAL DOSE TO GIVE	DRUG INDEX NUMBER	DIRECTIONS	INFUSION RANGE	DRUG MIXTURE	AMOUNT DRUG/mL	RUN AT	mL/h
Aminophylline	5 mg/kg =	**535 mg**		Give mg/kg load over 20 min		500 mg/ 250 mL	2 mg/mL		
	mg to give ÷ mg/mL =	**268 mL**			**268**	mL × (60 min/h ÷ 20 min) =		<u>802.5</u>	mL/h × 20 min
	Infusion				0.5–1 mg/kg/h	500 mg/ 250 mL	2 mg/mL		
						mg dose ordered × kg ÷ mg/mL =		___	mL/h
Amiodarone	Loading dose			Load **150 mg** over 10 min		900 mg/ 500 mL	1.8 mg/mL	___	
				Ordered mg load dose (150 mg) ÷ mg/mL (1.8 mg/mL) = 83 mL to give × (60 min/h ÷ 10 min) = mL/h to set on pump				<u>500</u>	mL/h × 83 mL
	Infusion			Run at **1 mg/ min** × 6 h		900 mg/ 500 mL	1.8 mg/mL		
				Ordered mg dose (1 mg/min) ÷ mg/mL (1.8 mg/mL) = _____ × 60 min/h = mL/h to set on pump				<u>33</u>	mL/h × 6 h
	Infusion			Run at **0.5 mg/ min** × 18 h		900 mg/ 500 mL	1.8 mg/mL		
				Ordered mg dose (0.5 mg/min) ÷ mg/mL (1.8 mg/mL) = _____ × 60 min/h = mL/h to set on pump				<u>17</u>	mL/h × 18 h
Amrinone	0.75 mg/kg =	**80.25 mg**		Give mg/kg load over 10 min		300 mg/ 120 mL	2.5 mg/mL	___	
	mg to give ÷ mg/mL =	**32 mL**			**32.1**	mL × (60 min/h ÷ 10 min) =		<u>192.6</u>	mL/h × 10 min
	Infusion		**0.39**		5–10 mcg/ kg/min	300 mg/ 120 mL	2500 mcg/mL	___	
				Take dose you want in mcg ÷ by drug index number = mL/h on pump					
Brevibloc	Infusion		**1.56**		50–100 mcg/ kg/min	2.5 g/ 250 mL	10,000 mcg/mL	___	mL/h
				Take dose you want in mcg ÷ by drug index number = mL/h on pump					
Cardene	Infusion		—		0.5–10 mg/h	25 mg 250 mL	0.1 mg/mL	___	
				Ordered mg dose ÷ mg/mL = mL/h to set on pump				___	mL/h
Cardizem	0.25 mg/kg =	**26.75 mg**		Give mg/kg load over 20 min		50 mg/ 100 mL	0.5 mg/mL		
	mg to give ÷ mg/mL =	**54 mL**			**53.5**	mL × (60 min/h ÷ 20 min) =		<u>161</u>	mL/h
	0.35 mg/kg =	**37.45 mg**		May repeat loading dose in 15 min			0.5 mg/mL		
	mg to give ÷ mg/mL =	**75 mL**			**74.9**	mL × (60 min/h ÷ 20 min) =		<u>225</u>	mL/h
	Infusion				5–15 mg/h			___	
				Ordered mg dose ÷ mg/mL = mL/h to set on pump				___	mL/h
Desmopressin	0.3 mcg/kg =	**32 mcg**		Give dose over 20–30 min			4 mcg/vial		
Dobutamine	Infusion		**0.31**		2.5–40 mcg/kg/ min	250 mg/ 125 mL	2000 mcg/mL		
				Take dose you want in mcg ÷ by drug index number = mL/h on pump					

(continues)

107 kg (continued)

DRUG	ORDERED AMOUNT	TOTAL DOSE TO GIVE	DRUG INDEX NUMBER	DIRECTIONS	INFUSION RANGE	DRUG MIXTURE	AMOUNT	DRUG/ mL	RUN AT	mL/h
Dopamine	Infusion		0.25		1–20 mcg/ kg/min	400 mg/ 250 mL	1600	mcg/mL		
	Take dose you want in mcg ÷ by drug index number = mL/h on pump									
Epinephrine	Infusion	1 mcg/min = 4 mL/h 2 mcg/min = 8 mL/h 3 mcg/min = 11 mL/h 4 mcg/min = 15 mL/h			1–4 mcg/min	4 mg/ 250 mL	16	mcg/mL		
	Ordered mcg dose/min ÷ mcg/mL × 60 min/h =									___ mL/h
Fenoldapam	Infusion		0.0063		0.01–1.6 mcg/ kg/min	10 mg/ 250 mL	40	mcg/mL		
	Take dose you want in mcg ÷ by drug index number = mL/h on pump									
Heparin	100 u/kg = 10,700 u 200 u/kg = 21,400 u 300 u/kg = 32,100 u 400 u/kg = 42,800 u									
Isoproterenol	Infusion				5 mcg/min	1 mg/ 250 mL	4	mcg/mL		
	Ordered mcg dose/min ÷ mcg/mL × 60 min/h =									**75** mL/h
Lidocaine	Infusion	1 mg/min = 7.5 mL/h			1–4 mg/min	2 g/ 250 mL	8	mg/mL	___	
	Ordered mg/min ÷ mg/mL × 60 min/h =									___ mL/h
Nitroglycerin	Infusion	3 mcg/min = 1 mL/h			3–200 mcg/min	50 mg/ 250 mL	200	mcg/mL	___	
	Ordered mcg/min ÷ mcg/mL × 60 min/h =									___ mL/h
Nitroprusside	Infusion	6.7 mcg/min = 1 mL/h			5–300 mcg/min	100 mg/ 250 mL	400	mcg/mL	___	
	Ordered mcg/min ÷ mcg/mL × 60 min/h =									___ mL/h
Norepinephrine	Infusion	1 mcg/min = 4 mL/h 2 mcg/min = 8 mL/h 3 mcg/min = 11 mL/h 4 mcg/min = 15 mL/h 5 mcg/min = 19 mL/h			2–20 mcg/min	4 mg/ 250 mL	16	mcg/mL		
	Ordered mcg dose/min ÷ mcg/mL × 60 min/h =									___ mL/h
Phenylephrine	Infusion	1.3 mcg/min = 1 mL/h			10–200 mcg/min	20 mg/ 250 mL	80	mcg/mL		
	Ordered mcg/min ÷ mcg/mL × 60 min/h =									___ mL/h
Primacor	0.05 mg/kg = 5.35 mg			Give load over 10 min		40 mg/ 200 mL	0.2	mg/mL		
	mg to give ÷ mg/mL = 27 mL				27	mL × (60 min/h ÷ 10 min) =			**160.5**	mL/h × 10 min
	Infusion		0.03		0.5 mcg/ kg/min	40 mg/ 200 mL	200	mcg/mL	___	
	Take dose you want in mcg ÷ by drug index number = mL/h on pump									
Trimethaphan	Infusion	___			0.3–6 mg/min	500 mg/ 500 mL	1	mg/mL	___	
	Ordered mg/min ÷ mg/mL × 60 min/h =									___ mL/h
Vasopressin		0.02 u/min = 3 mL/h 0.04 u/min = 6 mL/h				40 u/ 100 mL	400	u/mL		

108 kg

DRUG	ORDERED AMOUNT	TOTAL DOSE TO GIVE	DRUG INDEX NUMBER	DIRECTIONS	INFUSION RANGE	DRUG MIXTURE	AMOUNT	DRUG/mL	RUN AT — mL/h
Aminophylline	5 mg/kg =	540 mg		Give mg/kg load over 20 min		500 mg/ 250 mL	2 mg/mL		
	mg to give ÷ mg/mL =	270 mL			270	mL × (60 min/h ÷ 20 min) =			810 mL/h × 20 min
	Infusion				0.5–1 mg/kg/h	500 mg/ 250 mL	2 mg/mL		
						mg dose ordered × kg ÷ mg/mL =			___ mL/h
Amiodarone	Loading dose			Load **150 mg** over 10 min		900 mg/ 500 mL	1.8 mg/mL		___
				Ordered mg load dose (150 mg) ÷ mg/mL (1.8 mg/mL) = 83 mL to give × (60 min/h ÷ 10 min) = mL/h to set on pump					500 mL/h × 83 mL
	Infusion			Run at **1 mg/ min** × 6 h		900 mg/ 500 mL	1.8 mg/mL		
				Ordered mg dose (1 mg/min) ÷ mg/mL (1.8 mg/mL) = _____ × 60 min/h = mL/h to set on pump					33 mL/h × 6 h
	Infusion			Run at **0.5 mg/ min** × 18 h		900 mg/ 500 mL	1.8 mg/mL		
				Ordered mg dose (0.5 mg/min) ÷ mg/mL (1.8 mg/mL) = _____ × 60 min/h = mL/h to set on pump					17 mL/h × 18 h
Amrinone	0.75 mg/kg =	81 mg		Give mg/kg load over 10 min		300 mg/ 120 mL	2.5 mg/mL		___
	mg to give ÷ mg/mL =	32 mL			32.4	mL × (60 min/h ÷ 10 min) =			194.4 mL/h × 10 min
	Infusion		0.39		5–10 mcg/ kg/min	300 mg/ 120 mL	2500 mcg/mL		
				Take dose you want in mcg ÷ by drug index number = mL/h on pump					
Brevibloc	Infusion		1.54		50–100 mcg/ kg/min	2.5 g/ 250 mL	10,000 mcg/mL		___ mL/h
				Take dose you want in mcg ÷ by drug index number = mL/h on pump					
Cardene	Infusion		___		0.5–10 mg/h	25 mg 250 mL	0.1 mg/mL		___
				Ordered mg dose ÷ mg/mL = mL/h to set on pump					___ mL/h
Cardizem	0.25 mg/kg =	27 mg		Give mg/kg load over 20 min		50 mg/ 100 mL	0.5 mg/mL		
	mg to give ÷ mg/mL =	54 mL			54	mL × (60 min/h ÷ 20 min) =			162 mL/h
	0.35 mg/kg =	37.8 mg		May repeat loading dose in 15 min			0.5 mg/mL		
	mg to give ÷ mg/mL =	76 mL			75.6	mL × (60 min/h ÷ 20 min) =			227 mL/h
	Infusion				5–15 mg/h				___
				Ordered mg dose ÷ mg/mL = mL/h to set on pump					___ mL/h
Desmopressin	0.3 mcg/kg =	32 mcg		Give dose over 20–30 min			4 mcg/vial		
Dobutamine	Infusion		0.31		2.5–40 mcg/kg/ min	250 mg/ 125 mL	2000 mcg/mL		
				Take dose you want in mcg ÷ by drug index number = mL/h on pump					

(continues)

108 kg (continued)

DRUG	ORDERED AMOUNT	TOTAL DOSE TO GIVE	DRUG INDEX NUMBER	DIRECTIONS	INFUSION RANGE	DRUG MIXTURE	AMOUNT	DRUG/ mL	RUN AT	mL/h
Dopamine	Infusion		0.25		1–20 mcg/ kg/min	400 mg/ 250 mL	1600	mcg/mL		
		Take dose you want in mcg ÷ by drug index number = mL/h on pump								
Epinephrine	Infusion	1 mcg/min = 4 mL/h 2 mcg/min = 8 mL/h 3 mcg/min = 11 mL/h 4 mcg/min = 15 mL/h			1–4 mcg/min	4 mg/ 250 mL	16	mcg/mL		
		Ordered mcg dose/min ÷ mcg/mL × 60 min/h =							___	mL/h
Fenoldapam	Infusion		0.0062		0.01–1.6 mcg/ kg/min	10 mg/ 250 mL	40	mcg/mL		
		Take dose you want in mcg ÷ by drug index number = mL/h on pump								
Heparin	100 u/kg = **10,800** u 200 u/kg = **21,600** u 300 u/kg = **32,400** u 400 u/kg = **43,200** u									
Isoproterenol	Infusion				5 mcg/min	1 mg/ 250 mL	4	mcg/mL		
		Ordered mcg dose/min ÷ mcg/mL × 60 min/h =							**75**	mL/h
Lidocaine	Infusion	1 mg/min = 7.5 mL/h			1–4 mg/min	2 g/ 250 mL	8	mg/mL	___	
		Ordered mg/min ÷ mg/mL × 60 min/h =							___	mL/h
Nitroglycerin	Infusion	3 mcg/min = 1 mL/h			3–200 mcg/min	50 mg/ 250 mL	200	mcg/mL	___	
		Ordered mcg/min ÷ mcg/mL × 60 min/h =							___	mL/h
Nitroprusside	Infusion	6.7 mcg/min = 1 mL/h			5–300 mcg/min	100 mg/ 250 mL	400	mcg/mL	___	
		Ordered mcg/min ÷ mcg/mL × 60 min/h =							___	mL/h
Norepinephrine	Infusion	1 mcg/min = 4 mL/h 2 mcg/min = 8 mL/h 3 mcg/min = 11 mL/h 4 mcg/min = 15 mL/h 5 mcg/min = 19 mL/h			2–20 mcg/min	4 mg/ 250 mL	16	mcg/mL		
		Ordered mcg dose/min ÷ mcg/mL × 60 min/h =							___	mL/h
Phenylephrine	Infusion	1.3 mcg/min = 1 mL/h			10–200 mcg/min	20 mg/ 250 mL	80	mcg/mL		
		Ordered mcg/min ÷ mcg/mL × 60 min/h =							___	mL/h
Primacor	0.05 mg/kg = **5.4** mg			Give load over 10 min		40 mg/ 200 mL	0.2	mg/mL		
	mg to give ÷ mg/mL = **27** mL				**27** mL × (60 min/h ÷ 10 min) =				**162**	mL/h × 10 min
	Infusion		0.03		0.5 mcg/ kg/min	40 mg/ 200 mL	200	mcg/mL	___	
		Take dose you want in mcg ÷ by drug index number = mL/h on pump								
Trimethaphan	Infusion		—		0.3–6 mg/min	500 mg/ 500 mL	1	mg/mL	___	
		Ordered mg/min ÷ mg/mL × 60 min/h =							___	mL/h
Vasopressin		0.02 u/min = 3 mL/h 0.04 u/min = 6 mL/h				40 u/ 100 mL	400	u/mL		

109 kg

DRUG	ORDERED AMOUNT	TOTAL DOSE TO GIVE	DRUG INDEX NUMBER	DIRECTIONS	INFUSION RANGE	DRUG MIXTURE	AMOUNT	DRUG/ mL	RUN AT	mL/h
Aminophylline	5 mg/kg = **545 mg**			Give mg/kg load over 20 min		500 mg/ 250 mL	2 mg/mL			
	mg to give ÷ mg/mL = **273 mL**					**273** mL × (60 min/h ÷ 20 min) =			**817.5**	mL/h × 20 min
	Infusion				0.5–1 mg/kg/h	500 mg/ 250 mL	2 mg/mL			
					mg dose ordered × kg ÷ mg/mL =				___	mL/h
Amiodarone	Loading dose			Load **150 mg** over 10 min		900 mg/ 500 mL	1.8 mg/mL		—	
				Ordered mg load dose (150 mg) ÷ mg/mL (1.8 mg/mL) = 83 mL to give × (60 min/h ÷ 10 min) = mL/h to set on pump					**500**	mL/h × 83 mL
	Infusion			Run at **1 mg/ min** × 6 h		900 mg/ 500 ml	1.8 mg/mL			
				Ordered mg dose (1 mg/min) ÷ mg/mL (1.8 mg/mL) = _____ × 60 min/h = mL/h to set on pump					**33**	mL/h × 6 h
	Infusion			Run at **0.5 mg/ min** × 18 h		900 mg/ 500 mL	1.8 mg/mL			
				Ordered mg dose (0.5 mg/min) ÷ mg/mL (1.8 mg/mL) = _____ × 60 min/h = mL/h to set on pump					**17**	mL/h × 18 h
Amrinone	0.75 mg/kg = **81.75 mg**			Give mg/kg load over 10 min		300 mg/ 120 mL	2.5 mg/mL		—	
	mg to give ÷ mg/mL = **33 mL**					**32.7** mL × (60 min/h ÷ 10 min) =			**196.2**	mL/h × 10 min
	Infusion		**0.38**		5–10 mcg/ kg/min	300 mg/ 120 mL	2500 mcg/mL		—	
				Take dose you want in mcg ÷ by drug index number = mL/h on pump						
Brevibloc	Infusion		**1.53**		50–100 mcg/ kg/min	2.5 g/ 250 mL	10,000 mcg/mL		___	mL/h
				Take dose you want in mcg ÷ by drug index number = mL/h on pump						
Cardene	Infusion		—		0.5–10 mg/h	25 mg 250 mL	0.1 mg/mL		—	
				Ordered mg dose ÷ mg/mL = mL/h to set on pump					___	mL/h
Cardizem	0.25 mg/kg = **27.25 mg**			Give mg/kg load over 20 min		50 mg/ 100 mL	0.5 mg/mL		—	
	mg to give ÷ mg/mL = **55 mL**					**54.5** mL × (60 min/h ÷ 20 min) =			**164**	mL/h
	0.35 mg/kg = **38.15 mg**			May repeat loading dose in 15 min			0.5 mg/mL		—	
	mg to give ÷ mg/mL = **76 mL**					**76.3** mL × (60 min/h ÷ 20 min) =			**229**	mL/h
	Infusion				5–15 mg/h				—	
				Ordered mg dose ÷ mg/mL = mL/h to set on pump					___	mL/h
Desmopressin	0.3 mcg/kg = **33 mcg**			Give dose over 20–30 min			4 mcg/vial			
Dobutamine	Infusion		**0.31**		2.5–40 mcg/kg/ min	250 mg/ 125 mL	2000 mcg/mL			
				Take dose you want in mcg ÷ by drug index number = mL/h on pump						

(continues)

109 kg (continued)

DRUG	ORDERED AMOUNT	TOTAL DOSE TO GIVE	DRUG INDEX NUMBER	DIRECTIONS	INFUSION RANGE	DRUG MIXTURE	AMOUNT	DRUG/ mL	RUN AT mL/h
Dopamine	Infusion		0.24		1–20 mcg/ kg/min	400 mg/ 250 mL	1600	mcg/mL	
	Take dose you want in mcg ÷ by drug index number = mL/h on pump								
Epinephrine	Infusion	1 mcg/min = 4 mL/h 2 mcg/min = 8 mL/h 3 mcg/min = 11 mL/h 4 mcg/min = 15 mL/h			1–4 mcg/min	4 mg/ 250 mL	16	mcg/mL	
		Ordered mcg dose/min ÷ mcg/mL × 60 min/h =							___ mL/h
Fenoldapam	Infusion		0.0061		0.01–1.6 mcg/ kg/min	10 mg/ 250 mL	40	mcg/mL	
	Take dose you want in mcg ÷ by drug index number = mL/h on pump								
Heparin	100 u/kg = 10,900 u 200 u/kg = 21,800 u 300 u/kg = 32,700 u 400 u/kg = 43,600 u								
Isoproterenol	Infusion				5 mcg/min	1 mg/ 250 mL	4	mcg/mL	
		Ordered mcg dose/min ÷ mcg/mL × 60 min/h =							75 mL/h
Lidocaine	Infusion	1 mg/min = 7.5 mL/h			1–4 mg/min	2 g/ 250 mL	8	mg/mL	___
		Ordered mg/min ÷ mg/mL × 60 min/h =							___ mL/h
Nitroglycerin	Infusion	3 mcg/min = 1 mL/h			3–200 mcg/min	50 mg/ 250 mL	200	mcg/mL	___
		Ordered mcg/min ÷ mcg/mL × 60 min/h =							___ mL/h
Nitroprusside	Infusion	6.7 mcg/min = 1 mL/h			5–300 mcg/min	100 mg/ 250 mL	400	mcg/mL	
		Ordered mcg/min ÷ mcg/mL × 60 min/h =							___ mL/h
Norepinephrine	Infusion	1 mcg/min = 4 mL/h 2 mcg/min = 8 mL/h 3 mcg/min = 11 mL/h 4 mcg/min = 15 mL/h 5 mcg/min = 19 mL/h			2–20 mcg/min	4 mg/ 250 mL	16	mcg/mL	
		Ordered mcg dose/min ÷ mcg/mL × 60 min/h =							___ mL/h
Phenylephrine	Infusion	1.3 mcg/min = 1 mL/h			10–200 mcg/min	20 mg/ 250 mL	80	mcg/mL	
		Ordered mcg/min ÷ mcg/mL × 60 min/h =							___ mL/h
Primacor	0.05 mg/kg = 5.45 mg			Give load over 10 min		40 mg/ 200 mL	0.2	mg/mL	
	mg to give ÷ mg/mL = 27 mL				27	mL × (60 min/h ÷ 10 min) =			163.5 mL/h × 10 min
	Infusion		0.03		0.5 mcg/ kg/min	40 mg/ 200 mL	200	mcg/mL	___
	Take dose you want in mcg ÷ by drug index number = mL/h on pump								
Trimethaphan	Infusion		___		0.3–6 mg/min	500 mg/ 500 mL	1	mg/mL	___
		Ordered mg/min ÷ mg/mL × 60 min/h =							___ mL/h
Vasopressin		0.02 u/min = 3 mL/h 0.04 u/min = 6 mL/h				40 u/ 100 mL	400	u/mL	

110 kg

DRUG	ORDERED AMOUNT	TOTAL DOSE TO GIVE	DRUG INDEX NUMBER	DIRECTIONS	INFUSION RANGE	DRUG MIXTURE	AMOUNT	DRUG/ mL	RUN AT	mL/h
Aminophylline	5 mg/kg = **550 mg**			Give mg/kg load over 20 min		500 mg/ 250 mL		2 mg/mL		
	mg to give ÷ mg/mL = **275 mL**					275	mL × (60 min/h ÷ 20 min) =		**825**	mL/h × 20 min
	Infusion				0.5–1 mg/kg/h	500 mg/ 250 mL		2 mg/mL		
						mg dose ordered × kg ÷ mg/mL =			___	mL/h
Amiodarone	Loading dose			Load **150 mg** over 10 min		900 mg/ 500 mL		1.8 mg/mL		—
				Ordered mg load dose (150 mg) ÷ mg/mL (1.8 mg/mL) = 83 mL to give × (60 min/h ÷ 10 min) = mL/h to set on pump					**500**	mL/h × 83 mL
	Infusion			Run at **1 mg/ min** × 6 h		900 mg/ 500 mL		1.8 mg/mL		
				Ordered mg dose (1 mg/min) ÷ mg/mL (1.8 mg/mL) = ____ × 60 min/h = mL/h to set on pump					**33**	mL/h × 6 h
	Infusion			Run at **0.5 mg/ min** × 18 h		900 mg/ 500 mL		1.8 mg/mL		
				Ordered mg dose (0.5 mg/min) ÷ mg/mL (1.8 mg/mL) = ____ × 60 min/h = mL/h to set on pump					**17**	mL/h × 18 h
Amrinone	0.75 mg/kg = **82.5 mg**			Give mg/kg load over 10 min		300 mg/ 120 mL		2.5 mg/mL		—
	mg to give ÷ mg/mL = **33 mL**					33	mL × (60 min/h ÷ 10 min) =		**198**	mL/h × 10 min
	Infusion		**0.38**		5–10 mcg/ kg/min	300 mg/ 120 mL		2500 mcg/mL		—
				Take dose you want in mcg ÷ by drug index number = mL/h on pump						
Brevibloc	Infusion		**1.51**		50–100 mcg/ kg/min	2.5 g/ 250 mL		10,000 mcg/mL		___ mL/h
				Take dose you want in mcg ÷ by drug index number = mL/h on pump						
Cardene	Infusion		—		0.5–10 mg/h	25 mg 250 mL		0.1 mg/mL		
						Ordered mg dose ÷ mg/mL = mL/h to set on pump				___ mL/h
Cardizem	0.25 mg/kg = **27.5 mg**			Give mg/kg load over 20 min		50 mg/ 100 mL		0.5 mg/mL		
	mg to give ÷ mg/mL = **55 mL**					55	mL × (60 min/h ÷ 20 min) =		**165**	mL/h
	0.35 mg/kg = **38.5 mg**			May repeat loading dose in 15 min				0.5 mg/mL		
	mg to give ÷ mg/mL = **77 mL**					77	mL × (60 min/h ÷ 20 min) =		**231**	mL/h
	Infusion				5–15 mg/h					—
						Ordered mg dose ÷ mg/mL = mL/h to set on pump				___ mL/h
Desmopressin	0.3 mcg/kg = **33 mcg**			Give dose over 20–30 min				4 mcg/vial		
Dobutamine	Infusion		**0.30**		2.5–40 mcg/kg/ min	250 mg/ 125 mL		2000 mcg/mL		
				Take dose you want in mcg ÷ by drug index number = mL/h on pump						

(continues)

110 kg (continued)

DRUG	ORDERED AMOUNT	TOTAL DOSE TO GIVE	DRUG INDEX NUMBER	DIRECTIONS	INFUSION RANGE	DRUG MIXTURE	AMOUNT	DRUG/mL	RUN AT	mL/h
Dopamine	Infusion		0.24		1–20 mcg/kg/min	400 mg/250 mL	1600	mcg/mL		
				Take dose you want in mcg ÷ by drug index number = mL/h on pump						
Epinephrine	Infusion	1 mcg/min = 4 mL/h 2 mcg/min = 8 mL/h 3 mcg/min = 11 mL/h 4 mcg/min = 15 mL/h			1–4 mcg/min	4 mg/250 mL	16	mcg/mL		
				Ordered mcg dose/min ÷ mcg/mL × 60 min/h =					___	mL/h
Fenoldapam	Infusion		0.0061		0.01–1.6 mcg/kg/min	10 mg/250 mL	40	mcg/mL		
				Take dose you want in mcg ÷ by drug index number = mL/h on pump						
Heparin	100 u/kg = 200 u/kg = 300 u/kg = 400 u/kg =	11,000 u 22,000 u 33,000 u 44,000 u								
Isoproterenol	Infusion				5 mcg/min	1 mg/250 mL	4	mcg/mL		
				Ordered mcg dose/min ÷ mcg/mL × 60 min/h =					75	mL/h
Lidocaine	Infusion	1 mg/min = 7.5 mL/h			1–4 mg/min	2 g/250 mL	8	mg/mL	___	
				Ordered mg/min ÷ mg/mL × 60 min/h =					___	mL/h
Nitroglycerin	Infusion	3 mcg/min = 1 mL/h			3–200 mcg/min	50 mg/250 mL	200	mcg/mL	___	
				Ordered mcg/min ÷ mcg/mL × 60 min/h =					___	mL/h
Nitroprusside	Infusion	6.7 mcg/min = 1 mL/h			5–300 mcg/min	100 mg/250 mL	400	mcg/mL	___	
				Ordered mcg/min ÷ mcg/mL × 60 min/h =					___	mL/h
Norepinephrine	Infusion	1 mcg/min = 4 mL/h 2 mcg/min = 8 mL/h 3 mcg/min = 11 mL/h 4 mcg/min = 15 mL/h 5 mcg/min = 19 mL/h			2–20 mcg/min	4 mg/250 mL	16	mcg/mL		
				Ordered mcg dose/min ÷ mcg/mL × 60 min/h =					___	mL/h
Phenylephrine	Infusion	1.3 mcg/min = 1 mL/h			10–200 mcg/min	20 mg/250 mL	80	mcg/mL		
				Ordered mcg/min ÷ mcg/mL × 60 min/h =					___	mL/h
Primacor	0.05 mg/kg =	5.5 mg		Give load over 10 min		40 mg/200 mL	0.2	mg/mL		
	mg to give ÷ mg/mL =	28 mL			28	mL × (60 min/h ÷ 10 min) =			165	mL/h × 10 min
	Infusion		0.03		0.5 mcg/kg/min	40 mg/200 mL	200	mcg/mL	___	
				Take dose you want in mcg ÷ by drug index number = mL/h on pump						
Trimethaphan	Infusion		—		0.3–6 mg/min	500 mg/500 mL	1	mg/mL	___	
				Ordered mg/min ÷ mg/mL × 60 min/h =					___	mL/h
Vasopressin		0.02 u/min = 3 mL/h 0.04 u/min = 6 mL/h				40 u/100 mL	400	u/mL		

111 kg										
DRUG	**ORDERED AMOUNT**	**TOTAL DOSE TO GIVE**	**DRUG INDEX NUMBER**	**DIRECTIONS**	**INFUSION RANGE**	**DRUG MIXTURE**	**AMOUNT**	**DRUG/ mL**	**RUN AT**	**mL/h**
Aminophylline	5 mg/kg = 555 mg			Give mg/kg load over 20 min		500 mg/ 250 mL	2 mg/mL			
	mg to give ÷ mg/mL = 278 mL				278	mL × (60 min/h ÷ 20 min) =			832.5	mL/h × 20 min
	Infusion				0.5–1 mg/kg/h	500 mg/ 250 mL	2 mg/mL			
					mg dose ordered × kg ÷ mg/mL =				___	mL/h
Amiodarone	Loading dose			Load **150 mg** over 10 min		900 mg/ 500 mL	1.8 mg/mL		___	
				Ordered mg load dose (150 mg) ÷ mg/mL (1.8 mg/mL) = 83 mL to give × (60 min/h ÷ 10 min) = mL/h to set on pump					500	mL/h × 83 mL
	Infusion			Run at **1 mg/ min** × 6 h		900 mg/ 500 mL	1.8 mg/mL			
				Ordered mg dose (1 mg/min) ÷ mg/mL (1.8 mg/mL) = ____ × 60 min/h = mL/h to set on pump					33	mL/h × 6 h
	Infusion			Run at **0.5 mg/ min** × 18 h		900 mg/ 500 mL	1.8 mg/mL			
				Ordered mg dose (0.5 mg/min) ÷ mg/mL (1.8 mg/mL) = ____ × 60 min/h = mL/h to set on pump					17	mL/h × 18 h
Amrinone	0.75 mg/kg = 83.25 mg			Give mg/kg load over 10 min		300 mg/ 120 mL	2.5 mg/mL		___	
	mg to give ÷ mg/mL = 33 mL				33.3	mL × (60 min/h ÷ 10 min) =			199.8	mL/h × 10 min
	Infusion		0.37		5–10 mcg/ kg/min	300 mg/ 120 mL	2500 mcg/mL		___	
				Take dose you want in mcg ÷ by drug index number = mL/h on pump						
Brevibloc	Infusion		1.50		50–100 mcg/ kg/min	2.5 g/ 250 mL	10,000 mcg/mL		___	mL/h
				Take dose you want in mcg ÷ by drug index number = mL/h on pump						
Cardene	Infusion		—		0.5–10 mg/h	25 mg 250 mL	0.1 mg/mL		___	
				Ordered mg dose ÷ mg/mL = mL/h to set on pump					___	mL/h
Cardizem	0.25 mg/kg = 27.75 mg			Give mg/kg load over 20 min		50 mg/ 100 mL	0.5 mg/mL		___	
	mg to give ÷ mg/mL = 56 mL				55.5	mL × (60 min/h ÷ 20 min) =			167	mL/h
	0.35 mg/kg = 38.85 mg			May repeat loading dose in 15 min			0.5 mg/mL		___	
	mg to give ÷ mg/mL = 78 mL				77.7	mL × (60 min/h ÷ 20 min) =			233	mL/h
	Infusion				5–15 mg/h				___	
				Ordered mg dose ÷ mg/mL = mL/h to set on pump					___	mL/h
Desmopressin	0.3 mcg/kg = 33 mcg			Give dose over 20–30 min			4 mcg/vial			
Dobutamine	Infusion		0.30		2.5–40 mcg/kg/ min	250 mg/ 125 mL	2000 mcg/mL			
				Take dose you want in mcg ÷ by drug index number = mL/h on pump						

(continues)

111 kg (continued)

DRUG	ORDERED AMOUNT	TOTAL DOSE TO GIVE	DRUG INDEX NUMBER	DIRECTIONS	INFUSION RANGE	DRUG MIXTURE	AMOUNT	DRUG/ mL	RUN AT	mL/h
Dopamine	Infusion		0.24		1–20 mcg/ kg/min	400 mg/ 250 mL	1600	mcg/mL		
	Take dose you want in mcg ÷ by drug index number = mL/h on pump									
Epinephrine	Infusion	1 mcg/min = 4 mL/h 2 mcg/min = 8 mL/h 3 mcg/min = 11 mL/h 4 mcg/min = 15 mL/h			1–4 mcg/min	4 mg/ 250 mL	16	mcg/mL		
		Ordered mcg dose/min ÷ mcg/mL × 60 min/h =							___	mL/h
Fenoldapam	Infusion		0.0060		0.01–1.6 mcg/ kg/min	10 mg/ 250 mL	40	mcg/mL		
	Take dose you want in mcg ÷ by drug index number = mL/h on pump									
Heparin	100 u/kg = **11,100** u 200 u/kg = **22,200** u 300 u/kg = **33,300** u 400 u/kg = **44,400** u									
Isoproterenol	Infusion				5 mcg/min	1 mg/ 250 mL	4	mcg/mL		
	Ordered mcg dose/min ÷ mcg/mL × 60 min/h =								**75**	mL/h
Lidocaine	Infusion	1 mg/min = 7.5 mL/h			1–4 mg/min	2 g/ 250 mL	8	mg/mL	___	
		Ordered mg/min ÷ mg/mL × 60 min/h =							___	mL/h
Nitroglycerin	Infusion	3 mcg/min = 1 mL/h			3–200 mcg/min	50 mg/ 250 mL	200	mcg/mL	___	
		Ordered mcg/min ÷ mcg/mL × 60 min/h =							___	mL/h
Nitroprusside	Infusion	6.7 mcg/min = 1 mL/h			5–300 mcg/min	100 mg/ 250 mL	400	mcg/mL	___	
		Ordered mcg/min ÷ mcg/mL × 60 min/h =							___	mL/h
Norepinephrine	Infusion	1 mcg/min = 4 mL/h 2 mcg/min = 8 mL/h 3 mcg/min = 11 mL/h 4 mcg/min = 15 mL/h 5 mcg/min = 19 mL/h			2–20 mcg/min	4 mg/ 250 mL	16	mcg/mL		
		Ordered mcg dose/min ÷ mcg/mL × 60 min/h =							___	mL/h
Phenylephrine	Infusion	1.3 mcg/min = 1 mL/h			10–200 mcg/min	20 mg/ 250 mL	80	mcg/mL		
		Ordered mcg/min ÷ mcg/mL × 60 min/h =							___	mL/h
Primacor	0.05 mg/kg = **5.55** mg			Give load over 10 min		40 mg/ 200 mL	0.2	mg/mL		
	mg to give ÷ mg/mL = **28** mL						**28** mL × (60 min/h ÷ 10 min) =		**166.5**	mL/h × 10 min
	Infusion		0.03		0.5 mcg/ kg/min	40 mg/ 200 mL	200	mcg/mL	___	
	Take dose you want in mcg ÷ by drug index number = mL/h on pump									
Trimethaphan	Infusion		—		0.3–6 mg/min	500 mg/ 500 mL	1	mg/mL	___	
		Ordered mg/min ÷ mg/mL × 60 min/h =							___	mL/h
Vasopressin		0.02 u/min = 3 mL/h 0.04 u/min = 6 mL/h				40 u/ 100 mL	400	u/mL		

112 kg

DRUG	ORDERED AMOUNT	TOTAL DOSE TO GIVE		DRUG INDEX NUMBER	DIRECTIONS	INFUSION RANGE	DRUG MIXTURE	AMOUNT	DRUG/mL	RUN AT	mL/h
Aminophylline	5 mg/kg =	**560**	**mg**		Give mg/kg load over 20 min		500 mg/ 250 mL	2	mg/mL		
	mg to give ÷ mg/mL =	**280**	**mL**			**280**	mL × (60 min/h ÷ 20 min) =			**840**	mL/h × 20 min
	Infusion					0.5–1 mg/kg/h	500 mg/ 250 mL	2	mg/mL		
							mg dose ordered × kg ÷ mg/mL =			___	mL/h
Amiodarone	Loading dose				Load **150 mg** over 10 min		900 mg/ 500 mL	1.8	mg/mL	—	
					Ordered mg load dose (150 mg) ÷ mg/mL (1.8 mg/mL) = 83 mL to give × (60 min/h ÷ 10 min) = mL/h to set on pump					**500**	mL/h × 83 mL
	Intusion				Run at **1 mg/ min ⟩⟨ 6 h**		900 mg/ 500 mL	1.8	mg/mL		
					Ordered mg dose (1 mg/min) ÷ mg/mL (1.8 mg/mL) = _____ × 60 min/h = mL/h to set on pump					**33**	mL/h × 6 h
	Infusion				Run at **0.5 mg/ min × 18 h**		900 mg/ 500 mL	1.8	mg/mL		
					Ordered mg dose (0.5 mg/min) ÷ mg/mL (1.8 mg/mL) = _____ × 60 min/h = mL/h to set on pump					**17**	mL/h × 18 h
Amrinone	0.75 mg/kg =	**84**	**mg**		Give mg/kg load over 10 min		300 mg/ 120 mL	2.5	mg/mL	—	
	mg to give ÷ mg/mL =	**34**	**mL**			**33.6**	mL × (60 min/h ÷ 10 min) =			**201.6**	mL/h × 10 min
	Infusion			**0.37**		5–10 mcg/ kg/min	300 mg/ 120 mL	2500	mcg/mL	—	
					Take dose you want in mcg ÷ by drug index number = mL/h on pump						
Brevibloc	Infusion			**1.49**		50–100 mcg/ kg/min	2.5 g/ 250 mL	10,000	mcg/mL	___	mL/h
					Take dose you want in mcg ÷ by drug index number = mL/h on pump						
Cardene	Infusion			—		0.5–10 mg/h	25 mg 250 mL	0.1	mg/mL	—	
					Ordered mg dose ÷ mg/mL = mL/h to set on pump					___	mL/h
Cardizem	0.25 mg/kg =	**28**	**mg**		Give mg/kg load over 20 min		50 mg/ 100 mL	0.5	mg/mL	—	
	mg to give ÷ mg/mL =	**56**	**mL**			**56**	mL × (60 min/h ÷ 20 min) =			**168**	mL/h
	0.35 mg/kg =	**39.2**	**mg**		May repeat loading dose in 15 min			0.5	mg/mL	—	
	mg to give ÷ mg/mL =	**78**	**mL**			**78.4**	mL × (60 min/h ÷ 20 min) =			**235**	mL/h
	Infusion					5–15 mg/h				—	
					Ordered mg dose ÷ mg/mL = mL/h to set on pump					___	mL/h
Desmopressin	0.3 mcg/kg =	**34**	**mcg**		Give dose over 20–30 min			4	mcg/vial		
Dobutamine	Infusion			**0.30**		2.5–40 mcg/kg/ min	250 mg/ 125 mL	2000	mcg/mL		
					Take dose you want in mcg ÷ by drug index number = mL/h on pump						

(continues)

112 kg (continued)

DRUG	ORDERED AMOUNT	TOTAL DOSE TO GIVE	DRUG INDEX NUMBER	DIRECTIONS	INFUSION RANGE	DRUG MIXTURE	AMOUNT	DRUG/mL	RUN AT mL/h
Dopamine	Infusion		0.24		1–20 mcg/kg/min	400 mg/250 mL	1600	mcg/mL	
	Take dose you want in mcg ÷ by drug index number = mL/h on pump								
Epinephrine	Infusion	1 mcg/min = 4 mL/h 2 mcg/min = 8 mL/h 3 mcg/min = 11 mL/h 4 mcg/min = 15 mL/h			1–4 mcg/min	4 mg/250 mL	16	mcg/mL	
	Ordered mcg dose/min ÷ mcg/mL × 60 min/h =								___ mL/h
Fenoldapam	Infusion		0.0060		0.01–1.6 mcg/kg/min	10 mg/250 mL	40	mcg/mL	
	Take dose you want in mcg ÷ by drug index number = mL/h on pump								
Heparin	100 u/kg =	11,200 u							
	200 u/kg =	22,400 u							
	300 u/kg =	33,600 u							
	400 u/kg =	44,800 u							
Isoproterenol	Infusion				5 mcg/min	1 mg/250 mL	4	mcg/mL	
	Ordered mcg dose/min ÷ mcg/mL × 60 min/h =								75 mL/h
Lidocaine	Infusion	1 mg/min = 7.5 mL/h			1–4 mg/min	2 g/250 mL	8	mg/mL	—
	Ordered mg/min ÷ mg/mL × 60 min/h =								___ mL/h
Nitroglycerin	Infusion	3 mcg/min = 1 mL/h			3–200 mcg/min	50 mg/250 mL	200	mcg/mL	—
	Ordered mcg/min ÷ mcg/mL × 60 min/h =								___ mL/h
Nitroprusside	Infusion	6.7 mcg/min = 1 mL/h			5–300 mcg/min	100 mg/250 mL	400	mcg/mL	—
	Ordered mcg/min ÷ mcg/mL × 60 min/h =								___ mL/h
Norepinephrine	Infusion	1 mcg/min = 4 mL/h 2 mcg/min = 8 mL/h 3 mcg/min = 11 mL/h 4 mcg/min = 15 mL/h 5 mcg/min = 19 mL/h			2–20 mcg/min	4 mg/250 mL	16	mcg/mL	
	Ordered mcg dose/min ÷ mcg/mL × 60 min/h =								___ mL/h
Phenylephrine	Infusion	1.3 mcg/min = 1 mL/h			10–200 mcg/min	20 mg/250 mL	80	mcg/mL	
	Ordered mcg/min ÷ mcg/mL × 60 min/h =								___ mL/h
Primacor	0.05 mg/kg =	5.6 mg		Give load over 10 min		40 mg/200 mL	0.2	mg/mL	
	mg to give ÷ mg/mL =	28 mL			28 mL × (60 min/h ÷ 10 min) =				168 mL/h × 10 min
	Infusion		0.03		0.5 mcg/kg/min	40 mg/200 mL	200	mcg/mL	—
	Take dose you want in mcg ÷ by drug index number = mL/h on pump								
Trimethaphan	Infusion		—		0.3–6 mg/min	500 mg/500 mL	1	mg/mL	—
	Ordered mg/min ÷ mg/mL × 60 min/h =								___ mL/h
Vasopressin		0.02 u/min = 3 mL/h 0.04 u/min = 6 mL/h				40 u/100 mL	400	u/mL	

113 kg										
DRUG	**ORDERED AMOUNT**	**TOTAL DOSE TO GIVE**	**DRUG INDEX NUMBER**	**DIRECTIONS**	**INFUSION RANGE**	**DRUG MIXTURE**	**AMOUNT**	**DRUG/mL**	**RUN AT**	**mL/h**
Aminophylline	5 mg/kg =	565 mg		Give mg/kg load over 20 min		500 mg/ 250 mL	2 mg/mL			
	mg to give ÷ mg/mL =	283 mL			283	mL × (60 min/h ÷ 20 min) =			847.5	mL/h × 20 min
	Infusion				0.5–1 mg/kg/h	500 mg/ 250 mL	2 mg/mL			
					mg dose ordered × kg ÷ mg/mL =				___	mL/h
Amiodarone	Loading dose			Load **150 mg** over 10 min		900 mg/ 500 mL	1.8 mg/mL		___	
				Ordered mg load dose (150 mg) ÷ mg/mL (1.8 mg/mL) = 83 mL to give × (60 min/h ÷ 10 min) = mL/h to set on pump					500	mL/h × 83 mL
	Infusion			Run at **1 mg/ min** × 6 h		900 mg/ 500 mL	1.8 mg/mL			
				Ordered mg dose (1 mg/min) ÷ mg/mL (1.8 mg/mL) = ___ × 60 min/h = mL/h to set on pump					33	mL/h × 6 h
	Infusion			Run at **0.5 mg/ min** × 18 h		900 mg/ 500 mL	1.8 mg/mL			
				Ordered mg dose (0.5 mg/min) ÷ mg/mL (1.8 mg/mL) = ___ × 60 min/h = mL/h to set on pump					17	mL/h × 18 h
Amrinone	0.75 mg/kg =	84.75 mg		Give mg/kg load over 10 min		300 mg/ 120 mL	2.5 mg/mL		___	
	mg to give ÷ mg/mL =	34 mL			33.9	mL × (60 min/h ÷ 10 min) =			203.4	mL/h × 10 min
	Infusion		0.37		5–10 mcg/ kg/min	300 mg/ 120 mL	2500 mcg/mL		___	
				Take dose you want in mcg ÷ by drug index number = mL/h on pump						
Brevibloc	Infusion		1.47		50–100 mcg/ kg/min	2.5 g/ 250 mL	10,000 mcg/mL		___	mL/h
				Take dose you want in mcg ÷ by drug index number = mL/h on pump						
Cardene	Infusion		—		0.5–10 mg/h	25 mg 250 mL	0.1 mg/mL		___	
				Ordered mg dose ÷ mg/mL = mL/h to set on pump					___	mL/h
Cardizem	0.25 mg/kg =	28.25 mg		Give mg/kg load over 20 min		50 mg/ 100 mL	0.5 mg/mL			
	mg to give ÷ mg/mL =	57 mL			56.5	mL × (60 min/h ÷ 20 min) =			170	mL/h
	0.35 mg/kg =	39.55 mg		May repeat loading dose in 15 min			0.5 mg/mL			
	mg to give ÷ mg/mL =	79 mL			79.1	mL × (60 min/h ÷ 20 min) =			237	mL/h
	Infusion				5–15 mg/h				___	
				Ordered mg dose ÷ mg/mL = mL/h to set on pump					___	mL/h
Desmopressin	0.3 mcg/kg =	34 mcg		Give dose over 20–30 min			4 mcg/vial			
Dobutamine	Infusion		0.29		2.5–40 mcg/kg/ min	250 mg/ 125 mL	2000 mcg/mL			
				Take dose you want in mcg ÷ by drug index number = mL/h on pump						

(continues)

113 kg (continued)

DRUG	ORDERED AMOUNT	TOTAL DOSE TO GIVE		DRUG INDEX NUMBER	DIRECTIONS	INFUSION RANGE	DRUG MIXTURE	AMOUNT	DRUG/ mL	RUN AT	mL/h
Dopamine	Infusion			0.24		1–20 mcg/ kg/min	400 mg/ 250 mL	1600	mcg/mL		
					Take dose you want in mcg ÷ by drug index number = mL/h on pump						
Epinephrine	Infusion	1 mcg/min = 4 mL/h 2 mcg/min = 8 mL/h 3 mcg/min = 11 mL/h 4 mcg/min = 15 mL/h				1–4 mcg/min	4 mg/ 250 mL	16	mcg/mL		
					Ordered mcg dose/min ÷ mcg/mL × 60 min/h =					___	mL/h
Fenoldapam	Infusion			0.0059		0.01–1.6 mcg/ kg/min	10 mg/ 250 mL	40	mcg/mL		
					Take dose you want in mcg ÷ by drug index number = mL/h on pump						
Heparin	100 u/kg = 200 u/kg = 300 u/kg = 400 u/kg =	11,300 u 22,600 u 33,900 u 45,200 u									
Isoproterenol	Infusion					5 mcg/min	1 mg/ 250 mL	4	mcg/mL		
					Ordered mcg dose/min ÷ mcg/mL × 60 min/h =					75	mL/h
Lidocaine	Infusion	1 mg/min = 7.5 mL/h				1–4 mg/min	2 g/ 250 mL	8	mg/mL		
					Ordered mg/min ÷ mg/mL × 60 min/h =					___	mL/h
Nitroglycerin	Infusion	3 mcg/min = 1 mL/h				3–200 mcg/min	50 mg/ 250 mL	200	mcg/mL	___	
					Ordered mcg/min ÷ mcg/mL × 60 min/h =					___	mL/h
Nitroprusside	Infusion	6.7 mcg/min = 1 mL/h				5–300 mcg/min	100 mg/ 250 mL	400	mcg/mL	___	
					Ordered mcg/min ÷ mcg/mL × 60 min/h =					___	mL/h
Norepinephrine	Infusion	1 mcg/min = 4 mL/h 2 mcg/min = 8 mL/h 3 mcg/min = 11 mL/h 4 mcg/min = 15 mL/h 5 mcg/min = 19 mL/h				2–20 mcg/min	4 mg/ 250 mL	16	mcg/mL		
					Ordered mcg dose/min ÷ mcg/mL × 60 min/h =					___	mL/h
Phenylephrine	Infusion	1.3 mcg/min = 1 mL/h				10–200 mcg/min	20 mg/ 250 mL	80	mcg/mL		
					Ordered mcg/min ÷ mcg/mL × 60 min/h =					___	mL/h
Primacor	0.05 mg/kg =	5.65 mg			Give load over 10 min		40 mg/ 200 mL	0.2	mg/mL		
	mg to give ÷ mg/mL =	28 mL				28	mL × (60 min/h ÷ 10 min) =			169.5	mL/h × 10 min
	Infusion			0.03		0.5 mcg/ kg/min	40 mg/ 200 mL	200	mcg/mL	___	
					Take dose you want in mcg ÷ by drug index number = mL/h on pump						
Trimethaphan	Infusion			—		0.3–6 mg/min	500 mg/ 500 mL	1	mg/mL	___	
					Ordered mg/min ÷ mg/mL × 60 min/h =					___	mL/h
Vasopressin		0.02 u/min = 3 mL/h 0.04 u/min = 6 mL/h					40 u/ 100 mL	400	u/mL		

114 kg

DRUG	ORDERED AMOUNT	TOTAL DOSE TO GIVE	DRUG INDEX NUMBER	DIRECTIONS	INFUSION RANGE	DRUG MIXTURE	AMOUNT	DRUG/mL	RUN AT	mL/h
Aminophylline	5 mg/kg = 570 mg			Give mg/kg load over 20 min		500 mg/ 250 mL	2 mg/mL			
	mg to give ÷ mg/mL = 285 mL				285	mL × (60 min/h ÷ 20 min) =			**855**	mL/h × 20 min
	Infusion				0.5–1 mg/kg/h	500 mg/ 250 mL	2 mg/mL			
					mg dose ordered × kg ÷ mg/mL =				___	mL/h
Amiodarone	Loading dose			Load **150 mg** over 10 min		900 mg/ 500 mL	1.8 mg/mL		___	
				Ordered mg load dose (150 mg) ÷ mg/mL (1.8 mg/mL) = 83 mL to give × (60 min/h ÷ 10 min) = mL/h to set on pump					**500**	mL/h × 83 mL
	Infusion			Run at **1 mg/ min** × 6 h		900 mg/ 500 mL	1.8 mg/mL			
				Ordered mg dose (1 mg/min) ÷ mg/mL (1.8 mg/mL) = _____ × 60 min/h = mL/h to set on pump					**33**	mL/h × 6 h
	Infusion			Run at **0.5 mg/ min** × 18 h		900 mg/ 500 mL	1.8 mg/mL			
				Ordered mg dose (0.5 mg/min) ÷ mg/mL (1.8 mg/mL) = _____ × 60 min/h = mL/h to set on pump					**17**	mL/h × 18 h
Amrinone	0.75 mg/kg = 85.5 mg			Give mg/kg load over 10 min		300 mg/ 120 mL	2.5 mg/mL		___	
	mg to give ÷ mg/mL = 34 mL				34.2	mL × (60 min/h ÷ 10 min) =			**205.2**	mL/h × 10 min
	Infusion		0.36		5–10 mcg/ kg/min	300 mg/ 120 mL	2500 mcg/mL		___	
				Take dose you want in mcg ÷ by drug index number = mL/h on pump						
Brevibloc	Infusion		1.46		50–100 mcg/ kg/min	2.5 g/ 250 mL	10,000 mcg/mL		___	mL/h
				Take dose you want in mcg ÷ by drug index number = mL/h on pump						
Cardene	Infusion		—		0.5–10 mg/h	25 mg 250 mL	0.1 mg/mL		___	
				Ordered mg dose ÷ mg/mL = mL/h to set on pump					___	mL/h
Cardizem	0.25 mg/kg = 28.5 mg			Give mg/kg load over 20 min		50 mg/ 100 mL	0.5 mg/mL			
	mg to give ÷ mg/mL = 57 mL				57	mL × (60 min/h ÷ 20 min) =			**171**	mL/h
	0.35 mg/kg = 39.9 mg			May repeat loading dose in 15 min			0.5 mg/mL		___	
	mg to give ÷ mg/mL = 80 mL				79.8	mL × (60 min/h ÷ 20 min) =			**239**	mL/h
	Infusion				5–15 mg/h				___	
				Ordered mg dose ÷ mg/mL = mL/h to set on pump					___	mL/h
Desmopressin	0.3 mcg/kg = 34 mcg			Give dose over 20–30 min			4 mcg/vial			
Dobutamine	Infusion		0.29		2.5–40 mcg/kg/ min	250 mg/ 125 mL	2000 mcg/mL			
				Take dose you want in mcg ÷ by drug index number = mL/h on pump						

(continues)

114 kg (continued)

DRUG	ORDERED AMOUNT		TOTAL DOSE TO GIVE		DRUG INDEX NUMBER	DIRECTIONS	INFUSION RANGE	DRUG MIXTURE	AMOUNT	DRUG/ mL	RUN AT	mL/h
Dopamine	Infusion				0.23		1–20 mcg/ kg/min	400 mg/ 250 mL	1600	mcg/mL		
						Take dose you want in mcg ÷ by drug index number = mL/h on pump						
Epinephrine	Infusion		1 mcg/min = 4 mL/h 2 mcg/min = 8 mL/h 3 mcg/min = 11 mL/h 4 mcg/min = 15 mL/h				1–4 mcg/min	4 mg/ 250 mL	16	mcg/mL		
						Ordered mcg dose/min ÷ mcg/mL × 60 min/h =						___	mL/h
Fenoldapam	Infusion				0.0059		0.01–1.6 mcg/ kg/min	10 mg/ 250 mL	40	mcg/mL		
						Take dose you want in mcg ÷ by drug index number = mL/h on pump						
Heparin	100 u/kg =	11,400 u										
	200 u/kg =	22,800 u										
	300 u/kg =	34,200 u										
	400 u/kg =	45,600 u										
Isoproterenol	Infusion						5 mcg/min	1 mg/ 250 mL	4	mcg/mL		
						Ordered mcg dose/min ÷ mcg/mL × 60 min/h =						75	mL/h
Lidocaine	Infusion		1 mg/min = 7.5 mL/h				1–4 mg/min	2 g/ 250 mL	8	mg/mL	___	
						Ordered mg/min ÷ mg/mL × 60 min/h =						___	mL/h
Nitroglycerin	Infusion		3 mcg/min = 1 mL/h				3–200 mcg/min	50 mg/ 250 mL	200	mcg/mL	___	
						Ordered mcg/min ÷ mcg/mL × 60 min/h =						___	mL/h
Nitroprusside	Infusion		6.7 mcg/min = 1 mL/h				5–300 mcg/min	100 mg/ 250 mL	400	mcg/mL	___	
						Ordered mcg/min ÷ mcg/mL × 60 min/h =						___	mL/h
Norepinephrine	Infusion		1 mcg/min = 4 mL/h 2 mcg/min = 8 mL/h 3 mcg/min = 11 mL/h 4 mcg/min = 15 mL/h 5 mcg/min = 19 mL/h				2–20 mcg/min	4 mg/ 250 mL	16	mcg/mL		
						Ordered mcg dose/min ÷ mcg/mL × 60 min/h =						___	mL/h
Phenylephrine	Infusion		1.3 mcg/min = 1 mL/h				10–200 mcg/min	20 mg/ 250 mL	80	mcg/mL		
						Ordered mcg/min ÷ mcg/mL × 60 min/h =						___	mL/h
Primacor	0.05 mg/kg =	5.7 mg				Give load over 10 min		40 mg/ 200 mL	0.2	mg/mL		
	mg to give ÷ mg/mL =	29 mL					29	mL × (60 min/h ÷ 10 min) =			171	mL/h × 10 min
	Infusion				0.03		0.5 mcg/ kg/min	40 mg/ 200 mL	200	mcg/mL	___	
						Take dose you want in mcg ÷ by drug index number = mL/h on pump						
Trimethaphan	Infusion				___		0.3–6 mg/min	500 mg/ 500 mL	1	mg/mL	___	
						Ordered mg/min ÷ mg/mL × 60 min/h =						___	mL/h
Vasopressin			0.02 u/min = 3 mL/h 0.04 u/min = 6 mL/h					40 u/ 100 mL	400	u/mL		

115   kg

DRUG	ORDERED AMOUNT	TOTAL DOSE TO GIVE	DRUG INDEX NUMBER	DIRECTIONS	INFUSION RANGE	DRUG MIXTURE	AMOUNT	DRUG/mL	RUN AT	mL/h
Aminophylline	5 mg/kg = 575 mg			Give mg/kg load over 20 min		500 mg/ 250 mL	2 mg/mL			
	mg to give ÷ mg/mL = 288 mL				288	mL × (60 min/h ÷ 20 min) =			862.5	mL/h × 20 min
	Infusion				0.5–1 mg/kg/h	500 mg/ 250 mL	2 mg/mL			
						mg dose ordered × kg ÷ mg/mL =				___ mL/h
Amiodarone	Loading dose			Load **150 mg** over 10 min		900 mg/ 500 mL	1.8 mg/mL			—
				Ordered mg load dose (150 mg) ÷ mg/mL (1.8 mg/mL) = 83 mL to give × (60 min/h ÷ 10 min) = mL/h to set on pump					500	mL/h × 83 mL
	Infusion			Run at **1 mg/ min** × 6 h		900 mg/ 500 mL	1.8 mg/mL			
				Ordered mg dose (1 mg/min) ÷ mg/mL (1.8 mg/mL) = ___ × 60 min/h = mL/h to set on pump					33	mL/h × 6 h
	Infusion			Run at **0.5 mg/ min** × 18 h		900 mg/ 500 mL	1.8 mg/mL			
				Ordered mg dose (0.5 mg/min) ÷ mg/mL (1.8 mg/mL) = ___ × 60 min/h = mL/h to set on pump					17	mL/h × 18 h
Amrinone	0.75 mg/kg = 86.25 mg			Give mg/kg load over 10 min		300 mg/ 120 mL	2.5 mg/mL			—
	mg to give ÷ mg/mL = 35 mL				34.5	mL × (60 min/h ÷ 10 min) =			207	mL/h × 10 min
	Infusion		0.36		5–10 mcg/ kg/min	300 mg/ 120 mL	2500 mcg/mL			—
				Take dose you want in mcg ÷ by drug index number = mL/h on pump						
Brevibloc	Infusion		1.45		50–100 mcg/ kg/min	2.5 g/ 250 mL	10,000 mcg/mL			___ mL/h
				Take dose you want in mcg ÷ by drug index number = mL/h on pump						
Cardene	Infusion		—		0.5–10 mg/h	25 mg 250 mL	0.1 mg/mL			—
				Ordered mg dose ÷ mg/mL = mL/h to set on pump						___ mL/h
Cardizem	0.25 mg/kg = 28.75 mg			Give mg/kg load over 20 min		50 mg/ 100 mL	0.5 mg/mL			
	mg to give ÷ mg/mL = 58 mL				57.5	mL × (60 min/h ÷ 20 min) =			173	mL/h
	0.35 mg/kg = 40.25 mg			May repeat loading dose in 15 min			0.5 mg/mL			
	mg to give ÷ mg/mL = 81 mL				80.5	mL × (60 min/h ÷ 20 min) =			242	mL/h
	Infusion				5–15 mg/h					—
				Ordered mg dose ÷ mg/mL = mL/h to set on pump						___ mL/h
Desmopressin	0.3 mcg/kg = 35 mcg			Give dose over 20–30 min			4 mcg/vial			
Dobutamine	Infusion		0.29		2.5–40 mcg/kg/ min	250 mg/ 125 mL	2000 mcg/mL			
				Take dose you want in mcg ÷ by drug index number = mL/h on pump						

(continues)

115 kg (continued)

DRUG	ORDERED AMOUNT	TOTAL DOSE TO GIVE	DRUG INDEX NUMBER	DIRECTIONS	INFUSION RANGE	DRUG MIXTURE	AMOUNT	DRUG/mL	RUN AT	mL/h
Dopamine	Infusion		0.23		1–20 mcg/kg/min	400 mg/250 mL	1600	mcg/mL		
	Take dose you want in mcg ÷ by drug index number = mL/h on pump									
Epinephrine	Infusion	1 mcg/min = 4 mL/h 2 mcg/min = 8 mL/h 3 mcg/min = 11 mL/h 4 mcg/min = 15 mL/h			1–4 mcg/min	4 mg/250 mL	16	mcg/mL		
	Ordered mcg dose/min ÷ mcg/mL × 60 min/h =								___	mL/h
Fenoldapam	Infusion		0.0058		0.01–1.6 mcg/kg/min	10 mg/250 mL	40	mcg/mL		
	Take dose you want in mcg ÷ by drug index number = mL/h on pump									
Heparin	100 u/kg = 11,500 u 200 u/kg = 23,000 u 300 u/kg = 34,500 u 400 u/kg = 46,000 u									
Isoproterenol	Infusion				5 mcg/min	1 mg/250 mL	4	mcg/mL		
	Ordered mcg dose/min ÷ mcg/mL × 60 min/h =								75	mL/h
Lidocaine	Infusion	1 mg/min = 7.5 mL/h			1–4 mg/min	2 g/250 mL	8	mg/mL	___	
	Ordered mg/min ÷ mg/mL × 60 min/h =								___	mL/h
Nitroglycerin	Infusion	3 mcg/min = 1 mL/h			3–200 mcg/min	50 mg/250 mL	200	mcg/mL	___	
	Ordered mcg/min ÷ mcg/mL × 60 min/h =								___	mL/h
Nitroprusside	Infusion	6.7 mcg/min = 1 mL/h			5–300 mcg/min	100 mg/250 mL	400	mcg/mL	___	
	Ordered mcg/min ÷ mcg/mL × 60 min/h =								___	mL/h
Norepinephrine	Infusion	1 mcg/min = 4 mL/h 2 mcg/min = 8 mL/h 3 mcg/min = 11 mL/h 4 mcg/min = 15 mL/h 5 mcg/min = 19 mL/h			2–20 mcg/min	4 mg/250 mL	16	mcg/mL		
	Ordered mcg dose/min ÷ mcg/mL × 60 min/h =								___	mL/h
Phenylephrine	Infusion	1.3 mcg/min = 1 mL/h			10–200 mcg/min	20 mg/250 mL	80	mcg/mL		
	Ordered mcg/min ÷ mcg/mL × 60 min/h =								___	mL/h
Primacor	0.05 mg/kg =	5.75 mg		Give load over 10 min		40 mg/200 mL	0.2	mg/mL		
	mg to give ÷ mg/mL =	29 mL			29	mL × (60 min/h ÷ 10 min) =			172.5	mL/h × 10 min
	Infusion		0.03		0.5 mcg/kg/min	40 mg/200 mL	200	mcg/mL	___	
	Take dose you want in mcg ÷ by drug index number = mL/h on pump									
Trimethaphan	Infusion		—		0.3–6 mg/min	500 mg/500 mL	1	mg/mL	___	
	Ordered mg/min ÷ mg/mL × 60 min/h =								___	mL/h
Vasopressin		0.02 u/min = 3 mL/h 0.04 u/min = 6 mL/h				40 u/100 mL	400	u/mL		

116 kg

DRUG	ORDERED AMOUNT	TOTAL DOSE TO GIVE	DRUG INDEX NUMBER	DIRECTIONS	INFUSION RANGE	DRUG MIXTURE	AMOUNT	DRUG/ mL	RUN AT	mL/h
Aminophylline	5 mg/kg =	580 mg		Give mg/kg load over 20 min		500 mg/ 250 mL	2 mg/mL		
	mg to give ÷ mg/mL =	290 mL			290	mL × (60 min/h ÷ 20 min) =			870	mL/h × 20 min
	Infusion				0.5–1 mg/kg/h	500 mg/ 250 mL	2 mg/mL		
						mg dose ordered × kg ÷ mg/mL =			___	mL/h
Amiodarone	Loading dose			Load **150 mg** over 10 min		900 mg/ 500 mL	1.8 mg/mL	___	
				Ordered mg load dose (150 mg) ÷ mg/mL (1.8 mg/mL) = 83 mL to give × (60 min/h ÷ 10 min) = mL/h to set on pump					500	mL/h × 83 mL
	Infusion			Run at **1 mg/ min** × 6 h		900 mg/ 500 mL	1.8 mg/mL		
				Ordered mg dose (1 mg/min) ÷ mg/mL (1.8 mg/mL) = ____ × 60 min/h = mL/h to set on pump					33	mL/h × 6 h
	Infusion			Run at **0.5 mg/ min** × 18 h		900 mg/ 500 mL	1.8 mg/mL		
				Ordered mg dose (0.5 mg/min) ÷ mg/mL (1.8 mg/mL) = ____ × 60 min/h = mL/h to set on pump					17	mL/h × 18 h
Amrinone	0.75 mg/kg =	87 mg		Give mg/kg load over 10 min		300 mg/ 120 mL	2.5 mg/mL	___	
	mg to give ÷ mg/mL =	35 mL			34.8	mL × (60 min/h ÷ 10 min) =			208.8	mL/h × 10 min
	Infusion		0.36		5–10 mcg/ kg/min	300 mg/ 120 mL	2500 mcg/mL	___	
				Take dose you want in mcg ÷ by drug index number = mL/h on pump						
Brevibloc	Infusion		1.44		50–100 mcg/ kg/min	2.5 g/ 250 mL	10,000 mcg/mL	___	mL/h
				Take dose you want in mcg ÷ by drug index number = mL/h on pump						
Cardene	Infusion		—		0.5–10 mg/h	25 mg 250 mL	0.1 mg/mL	___	
				Ordered mg dose ÷ mg/mL = mL/h to set on pump					___	mL/h
Cardizem	0.25 mg/kg =	29 mg		Give mg/kg load over 20 min		50 mg/ 100 mL	0.5 mg/mL	___	
	mg to give ÷ mg/mL =	58 mL			58	mL × (60 min/h ÷ 20 min) =			174	mL/h
	0.35 mg/kg =	40.6 mg		May repeat loading dose in 15 min			0.5 mg/mL	___	
	mg to give ÷ mg/mL =	81 mL			81.2	mL × (60 min/h ÷ 20 min) =			244	mL/h
	Infusion				5–15 mg/h			___	
				Ordered mg dose ÷ mg/mL = mL/h to set on pump					___	mL/h
Desmopressin	0.3 mcg/kg =	35 mcg		Give dose over 20–30 min			4 mcg/vial		
Dobutamine	Infusion		0.29		2.5–40 mcg/kg/ min	250 mg/ 125 mL	2000 mcg/mL		
				Take dose you want in mcg ÷ by drug index number = mL/h on pump						

(continues)

116 kg (continued)

DRUG	ORDERED AMOUNT	TOTAL DOSE TO GIVE	DRUG INDEX NUMBER	DIRECTIONS	INFUSION RANGE	DRUG MIXTURE	AMOUNT	DRUG/mL	RUN AT mL/h
Dopamine	Infusion		0.23		1–20 mcg/kg/min	400 mg/250 mL	1600	mcg/mL	
	Take dose you want in mcg ÷ by drug index number = mL/h on pump								
Epinephrine	Infusion	1 mcg/min = 4 mL/h 2 mcg/min = 8 mL/h 3 mcg/min = 11 mL/h 4 mcg/min = 15 mL/h			1–4 mcg/min	4 mg/250 mL	16	mcg/mL	
	Ordered mcg dose/min ÷ mcg/mL × 60 min/h = ___ mL/h								
Fenoldapam	Infusion		0.0058		0.01–1.6 mcg/kg/min	10 mg/250 mL	40	mcg/mL	
	Take dose you want in mcg ÷ by drug index number = mL/h on pump								
Heparin	100 u/kg =	11,600 u 200 u/kg = 23,200 u 300 u/kg = 34,800 u 400 u/kg = 46,400 u							
Isoproterenol	Infusion				5 mcg/min	1 mg/250 mL	4	mcg/mL	
	Ordered mcg dose/min ÷ mcg/mL × 60 min/h =								75 mL/h
Lidocaine	Infusion	1 mg/min = 7.5 mL/h			1–4 mg/min	2 g/250 mL	8	mg/mL	—
	Ordered mg/min ÷ mg/mL × 60 min/h = ___ mL/h								
Nitroglycerin	Infusion	3 mcg/min = 1 mL/h			3–200 mcg/min	50 mg/250 mL	200	mcg/mL	—
	Ordered mcg/min ÷ mcg/mL × 60 min/h = ___ mL/h								
Nitroprusside	Infusion	6.7 mcg/min = 1 mL/h			5–300 mcg/min	100 mg/250 mL	400	mcg/mL	—
	Ordered mcg/min ÷ mcg/mL × 60 min/h = ___ mL/h								
Norepinephrine	Infusion	1 mcg/min = 4 mL/h 2 mcg/min = 8 mL/h 3 mcg/min = 11 mL/h 4 mcg/min = 15 mL/h 5 mcg/min = 19 mL/h			2–20 mcg/min	4 mg/250 mL	16	mcg/mL	
	Ordered mcg dose/min ÷ mcg/mL × 60 min/h = ___ mL/h								
Phenylephrine	Infusion	1.3 mcg/min = 1 mL/h			10–200 mcg/min	20 mg/250 mL	80	mcg/mL	
	Ordered mcg/min ÷ mcg/mL × 60 min/h = ___ mL/h								
Primacor	0.05 mg/kg =	5.8 mg		Give load over 10 min		40 mg/200 mL	0.2	mg/mL	
	mg to give ÷ mg/mL =	29 mL			29	mL × (60 min/h ÷ 10 min) =			174 mL/h × 10 min
	Infusion		0.03		0.5 mcg/kg/min	40 mg/200 mL	200	mcg/mL	—
	Take dose you want in mcg ÷ by drug index number = mL/h on pump								
Trimethaphan	Infusion		—		0.3–6 mg/min	500 mg/500 mL	1	mg/mL	—
	Ordered mg/min ÷ mg/mL × 60 min/h = ___ mL/h								
Vasopressin		0.02 u/min = 3 mL/h 0.04 u/min = 6 mL/h				40 u/100 mL	400	u/mL	

117 kg

DRUG	ORDERED AMOUNT	TOTAL DOSE TO GIVE	DRUG INDEX NUMBER	DIRECTIONS	INFUSION RANGE	DRUG MIXTURE	AMOUNT	DRUG/ mL	RUN AT	mL/h
Aminophylline	5 mg/kg =	**585** mg		Give mg/kg load over 20 min		500 mg/ 250 mL	2 mg/mL		
	mg to give ÷ mg/mL =	**293** mL			**293**	mL × (60 min/h ÷ 20 min) =			**877.5**	mL/h × 20 min
	Infusion				0.5–1 mg/kg/h	500 mg/ 250 mL	2 mg/mL		
						mg dose ordered × kg ÷ mg/mL =			___ mL/h	
Amiodarone	Loading dose			Load **150 mg** over 10 min		900 mg/ 500 mL	1.8 mg/mL		___
				Ordered mg load dose (150 mg) ÷ mg/mL (1.8 mg/mL) = 83 mL to give × (60 min/h ÷ 10 min) = mL/h to set on pump					**500**	mL/h × 83 mL
	Infusion			Run at **1 mg/ min** × 6 h		900 mg/ 500 mL	1.8 mg/mL		
				Ordered mg dose (1 mg/min) ÷ mg/mL (1.8 mg/mL) = ___ × 60 min/h = mL/h to set on pump					**33**	mL/h × 6 h
	Infusion			Run at **0.5 mg/ min** × 18 h		900 mg/ 500 mL	1.8 mg/mL		
				Ordered mg dose (0.5 mg/min) ÷ mg/mL (1.8 mg/mL) = ___ × 60 min/h = mL/h to set on pump					**17**	mL/h × 18 h
Amrinone	0.75 mg/kg =	**87.75** mg		Give mg/kg load over 10 min		300 mg/ 120 mL	2.5 mg/mL		___
	mg to give ÷ mg/mL =	**35** mL			**35.1**	mL × (60 min/h ÷ 10 min) =			**210.6**	mL/h × 10 min
	Infusion		**0.36**		5–10 mcg/ kg/min	300 mg/ 120 mL	2500 mcg/mL		___
				Take dose you want in mcg ÷ by drug index number = mL/h on pump						
Brevibloc	Infusion		**1.42**		50–100 mcg/ kg/min	2.5 g/ 250 mL	10,000 mcg/mL		___ mL/h
				Take dose you want in mcg ÷ by drug index number = mL/h on pump						
Cardene	Infusion		—		0.5–10 mg/h	25 mg 250 mL	0.1 mg/mL		___
				Ordered mg dose ÷ mg/mL = mL/h to set on pump						___ mL/h
Cardizem	0.25 mg/kg =	**29.25** mg		Give mg/kg load over 20 min		50 mg/ 100 mL	0.5 mg/mL		
	mg to give ÷ mg/mL =	**59** mL			**58.5**	mL × (60 min/h ÷ 20 min) =			**176** mL/h	
	0.35 mg/kg =	**40.95** mg		May repeat loading dose in 15 min			0.5 mg/mL		___
	mg to give ÷ mg/mL =	**82** mL			**81.9**	mL × (60 min/h ÷ 20 min) =			**246** mL/h	
	Infusion				5–15 mg/h				___
				Ordered mg dose ÷ mg/mL = mL/h to set on pump						___ mL/h
Desmopressin	0.3 mcg/kg =	**35** mcg		Give dose over 20–30 min			4 mcg/vial		
Dobutamine	Infusion		**0.28**		2.5–40 mcg/kg/ min	250 mg/ 125 mL	2000 mcg/mL		
				Take dose you want in mcg ÷ by drug index number = mL/h on pump						

(continues)

117　kg (continued)

DRUG	ORDERED AMOUNT	TOTAL DOSE TO GIVE	DRUG INDEX NUMBER	DIRECTIONS	INFUSION RANGE	DRUG MIXTURE	AMOUNT	DRUG/ mL	RUN AT	mL/h
Dopamine	Infusion		0.23		1–20 mcg/ kg/min	400 mg/ 250 mL	1600	mcg/mL		
			Take dose you want in mcg ÷ by drug index number = mL/h on pump							
Epinephrine	Infusion	1 mcg/min = 4 mL/h 2 mcg/min = 8 mL/h 3 mcg/min = 11 mL/h 4 mcg/min = 15 mL/h			1–4 mcg/min	4 mg/ 250 mL	16	mcg/mL		
			Ordered mcg dose/min ÷ mcg/mL × 60 min/h =						___	mL/h
Fenoldapam	Infusion		0.0057		0.01–1.6 mcg/ kg/min	10 mg/ 250 mL	40	mcg/mL		
			Take dose you want in mcg ÷ by drug index number = mL/h on pump							
Heparin	100 u/kg = 11,700 u 200 u/kg = 23,400 u 300 u/kg = 35,100 u 400 u/kg = 46,800 u									
Isoproterenol	Infusion				5 mcg/min	1 mg/ 250 mL	4	mcg/mL		
			Ordered mcg dose/min ÷ mcg/mL × 60 min/h =						75	mL/h
Lidocaine	Infusion	1 mg/min = 7.5 mL/h			1–4 mg/min	2 g/ 250 mL	8	mg/mL	___	
			Ordered mg/min ÷ mg/mL × 60 min/h =						___	mL/h
Nitroglycerin	Infusion	3 mcg/min = 1 mL/h			3–200 mcg/min	50 mg/ 250 mL	200	mcg/mL	___	
			Ordered mcg/min ÷ mcg/mL × 60 min/h =						___	mL/h
Nitroprusside	Infusion	6.7 mcg/min = 1 mL/h			5–300 mcg/min	100 mg/ 250 mL	400	mcg/mL	___	
			Ordered mcg/min ÷ mcg/mL × 60 min/h =						___	mL/h
Norepinephrine	Infusion	1 mcg/min = 4 mL/h 2 mcg/min = 8 mL/h 3 mcg/min = 11 mL/h 4 mcg/min = 15 mL/h 5 mcg/min = 19 mL/h			2–20 mcg/min	4 mg/ 250 mL	16	mcg/mL		
			Ordered mcg dose/min ÷ mcg/mL × 60 min/h =						___	mL/h
Phenylephrine	Infusion	1.3 mcg/min = 1 mL/h			10–200 mcg/min	20 mg/ 250 mL	80	mcg/mL		
			Ordered mcg/min ÷ mcg/mL × 60 min/h =						___	mL/h
Primacor	0.05 mg/kg = 5.85 mg			Give load over 10 min		40 mg/ 200 mL	0.2	mg/mL		
	mg to give ÷ mg/mL = 29 mL					29	mL × (60 min/h ÷ 10 min) =		175.5	mL/h × 10 min
	Infusion		0.03		0.5 mcg/ kg/min	40 mg/ 200 mL	200	mcg/mL		
			Take dose you want in mcg ÷ by drug index number = mL/h on pump							
Trimethaphan	Infusion		—		0.3–6 mg/min	500 mg/ 500 mL	1	mg/mL	___	
			Ordered mg/min ÷ mg/mL × 60 min/h =						___	mL/h
Vasopressin		0.02 u/min = 3 mL/h 0.04 u/min = 6 mL/h				40 u/ 100 mL	400	u/mL		

118 kg										
DRUG	**ORDERED AMOUNT**	**TOTAL DOSE TO GIVE**	**DRUG INDEX NUMBER**	**DIRECTIONS**	**INFUSION RANGE**	**DRUG MIXTURE**	**AMOUNT**	**DRUG/ mL**	**RUN AT**	**mL/h**
Aminophylline	5 mg/kg = **590 mg**			Give mg/kg load over 20 min		500 mg/ 250 mL		2 mg/mL		
	mg to give ÷ mg/mL = **295 mL**					295	mL × (60 min/h ÷ 20 min) =		**885**	mL/h × 20 min
	Infusion				0.5–1 mg/kg/h	500 mg/ 250 mL		2 mg/mL		
						mg dose ordered × kg ÷ mg/mL =				___ mL/h
Amiodarone	Loading dose			Load **150 mg** over 10 min		900 mg/ 500 mL		1.8 mg/mL		___
				Ordered mg load dose (150 mg) ÷ mg/mL (1.8 mg/mL) = 83 mL to give × (60 min/h ÷ 10 min) = mL/h to set on pump					**500**	mL/h × 83 mL
	Infusion			Run at **1 mg/ min** × 6 h	900 mg/ 500 mL		1.8 mg/mL			
				Ordered mg dose (1 mg/min) ÷ mg/mL (1.8 mg/mL) = ___ × 60 min/h = mL/h to set on pump					**33**	mL/h × 6 h
	Infusion			Run at **0.5 mg/ min** × 18 h	900 mg/ 500 mL		1.8 mg/mL			
				Ordered mg dose (0.5 mg/min) ÷ mg/mL (1.8 mg/mL) = ___ × 60 min/h = mL/h to set on pump					**17**	mL/h × 18 h
Amrinone	0.75 mg/kg = **88.5 mg**			Give mg/kg load over 10 min		300 mg/ 120 mL		2.5 mg/mL		___
	mg to give ÷ mg/mL = **35 mL**					35.4	mL × (60 min/h ÷ 10 min) =		**212.4**	mL/h × 10 min
	Infusion		0.35		5–10 mcg/ kg/min	300 mg/ 120 mL		2500 mcg/mL		___
				Take dose you want in mcg ÷ by drug index number = mL/h on pump						
Brevibloc	Infusion		1.41		50–100 mcg/ kg/min	2.5 g/ 250 mL	10,000	mcg/mL		___ mL/h
				Take dose you want in mcg ÷ by drug index number = mL/h on pump						
Cardene	Infusion		___		0.5–10 mg/h	25 mg 250 mL		0.1 mg/mL		___
				Ordered mg dose ÷ mg/mL = mL/h to set on pump						___ mL/h
Cardizem	0.25 mg/kg = **29.5 mg**			Give mg/kg load over 20 min		50 mg/ 100 mL		0.5 mg/mL		
	mg to give ÷ mg/mL = **59 mL**					59	mL × (60 min/h ÷ 20 min) =		**177**	mL/h
	0.35 mg/kg = **41.3 mg**			May repeat loading dose in 15 min				0.5 mg/mL		___
	mg to give ÷ mg/mL = **83 mL**					82.6	mL × (60 min/h ÷ 20 min) =		**248**	mL/h
	Infusion				5–15 mg/h					___
				Ordered mg dose ÷ mg/mL = mL/h to set on pump						___ mL/h
Desmopressin	0.3 mcg/kg = **35 mcg**			Give dose over 20–30 min				4 mcg/vial		
Dobutamine	Infusion		0.28		2.5–40 mcg/kg/ min	250 mg/ 125 mL	2000	mcg/mL		
				Take dose you want in mcg ÷ by drug index number = mL/h on pump						

(continues)

118 kg (continued)

DRUG	ORDERED AMOUNT	TOTAL DOSE TO GIVE	DRUG INDEX NUMBER	DIRECTIONS	INFUSION RANGE	DRUG MIXTURE	AMOUNT	DRUG/ mL	RUN AT	mL/h
Dopamine	Infusion		0.23		1–20 mcg/ kg/min	400 mg/ 250 mL	1600	mcg/mL		
			Take dose you want in mcg ÷ by drug index number = mL/h on pump							
Epinephrine	Infusion	1 mcg/min = 4 mL/h 2 mcg/min = 8 mL/h 3 mcg/min = 11 mL/h 4 mcg/min = 15 mL/h			1–4 mcg/min	4 mg/ 250 mL	16	mcg/mL		
					Ordered mcg dose/min ÷ mcg/mL × 60 min/h =				___	mL/h
Fenoldapam	Infusion		0.0057		0.01–1.6 mcg/ kg/min	10 mg/ 250 mL	40	mcg/mL		
					Take dose you want in mcg ÷ by drug index number = mL/h on pump					
Heparin	100 u/kg = 11,800 u 200 u/kg = 23,600 u 300 u/kg = 35,400 u 400 u/kg = 47,200 u									
Isoproterenol	Infusion				5 mcg/min	1 mg/ 250 mL	4	mcg/mL		
					Ordered mcg dose/min ÷ mcg/mL × 60 min/h =				75	mL/h
Lidocaine	Infusion	1 mg/min = 7.5 mL/h			1–4 mg/min	2 g/ 250 mL	8	mg/mL	___	
					Ordered mg/min ÷ mg/mL × 60 min/h =				___	mL/h
Nitroglycerin	Infusion	3 mcg/min = 1 mL/h			3–200 mcg/min	50 mg/ 250 mL	200	mcg/mL	___	
					Ordered mcg/min ÷ mcg/mL × 60 min/h =				___	mL/h
Nitroprusside	Infusion	6.7 mcg/min = 1 mL/h			5–300 mcg/min	100 mg/ 250 mL	400	mcg/mL	___	
					Ordered mcg/min ÷ mcg/mL × 60 min/h =				___	mL/h
Norepinephrine	Infusion	1 mcg/min = 4 mL/h 2 mcg/min = 8 mL/h 3 mcg/min = 11 mL/h 4 mcg/min = 15 mL/h 5 mcg/min = 19 mL/h			2–20 mcg/min	4 mg/ 250 mL	16	mcg/mL		
					Ordered mcg dose/min ÷ mcg/mL × 60 min/h =				___	mL/h
Phenylephrine	Infusion	1.3 mcg/min = 1 mL/h			10–200 mcg/min	20 mg/ 250 mL	80	mcg/mL		
					Ordered mcg/min ÷ mcg/mL × 60 min/h =				___	mL/h
Primacor	0.05 mg/kg = 5.9 mg			Give load over 10 min		40 mg/ 200 mL	0.2	mg/mL		
	mg to give ÷ mg/mL = 30 mL				30	mL × (60 min/h ÷ 10 min) =			177	mL/h × 10 min
	Infusion		0.03		0.5 mcg/ kg/min	40 mg/ 200 mL	200	mcg/mL	___	
					Take dose you want in mcg ÷ by drug index number = mL/h on pump					
Trimethaphan	Infusion		—		0.3–6 mg/min	500 mg/ 500 mL	1	mg/mL	___	
					Ordered mg/min ÷ mg/mL × 60 min/h =				___	mL/h
Vasopressin		0.02 u/min = 3 mL/h 0.04 u/min = 6 mL/h				40 u/ 100 mL	400	u/mL		

119 kg

DRUG	ORDERED AMOUNT	TOTAL DOSE TO GIVE		DRUG INDEX NUMBER	DIRECTIONS	INFUSION RANGE	DRUG MIXTURE	AMOUNT	DRUG/mL	RUN AT	mL/h
Aminophylline	5 mg/kg =	**595** mg			Give mg/kg load over 20 min		500 mg/ 250 mL	2 mg/mL			
	mg to give ÷ mg/mL =	**298** mL					**298** mL × (60 min/h ÷ 20 min) =			**892.5**	mL/h × 20 min
	Infusion					0.5–1 mg/kg/h	500 mg/ 250 mL	2 mg/mL			
							mg dose ordered × kg ÷ mg/mL =			___	mL/h
Amiodarone	Loading dose				Load **150 mg** over 10 min		900 mg/ 500 mL	1.8 mg/mL		—	
					Ordered mg load dose (150 mg) ÷ mg/mL (1.8 mg/mL) = 83 mL to give × (60 min/h ÷ 10 min) = mL/h to set on pump					**500**	mL/h × 83 mL
	Infusion				Run at **1 mg/ min** × 6 h		900 mg/ 500 ml	1.8 mg/mL			
					Ordered mg dose (1 mg/min) ÷ mg/mL (1.8 mg/mL) = ___ × 60 min/h = mL/h to set on pump					**33**	mL/h × 6 h
	Infusion				Run at **0.5 mg/ min** × 18 h		900 mg/ 500 mL	1.8 mg/mL			
					Ordered mg dose (0.5 mg/min) ÷ mg/mL (1.8 mg/mL) = ___ × 60 min/h = mL/h to set on pump					**17**	mL/h × 18 h
Amrinone	0.75 mg/kg =	**89.25** mg			Give mg/kg load over 10 min		300 mg/ 120 mL	2.5 mg/mL		—	
	mg to give ÷ mg/mL =	**36** mL					**35.7** mL × (60 min/h ÷ 10 min) =			**214.2**	mL/h × 10 min
	Infusion			0.35		5–10 mcg/ kg/min	300 mg/ 120 mL	2500 mcg/mL		—	
					Take dose you want in mcg ÷ by drug index number = mL/h on pump						
Brevibloc	Infusion			1.40		50–100 mcg/ kg/min	2.5 g/ 250 mL	10,000 mcg/mL		___	mL/h
					Take dose you want in mcg ÷ by drug index number = mL/h on pump						
Cardene	Infusion			—		0.5–10 mg/h	25 mg 250 mL	0.1 mg/mL		—	
					Ordered mg dose ÷ mg/mL = mL/h to set on pump					___	mL/h
Cardizem	0.25 mg/kg =	**29.75** mg			Give mg/kg load over 20 min		50 mg/ 100 mL	0.5 mg/mL		—	
	mg to give ÷ mg/mL =	**60** mL					**59.5** mL × (60 min/h ÷ 20 min) =			**179**	mL/h
	0.35 mg/kg =	**41.65** mg			May repeat loading dose in 15 min			0.5 mg/mL		—	
	mg to give ÷ mg/mL =	**83** mL					**83.3** mL × (60 min/h ÷ 20 min) =			**250**	mL/h
	Infusion					5–15 mg/h				—	
					Ordered mg dose ÷ mg/mL = mL/h to set on pump					___	mL/h
Desmopressin	0.3 mcg/kg =	**36** mcg			Give dose over 20–30 min			4 mcg/vial			
Dobutamine	Infusion			0.28		2.5–40 mcg/kg/ min	250 mg/ 125 mL	2000 mcg/mL			
					Take dose you want in mcg ÷ by drug index number = mL/h on pump						

(continues)

119 kg (continued)

DRUG	ORDERED AMOUNT	TOTAL DOSE TO GIVE	DRUG INDEX NUMBER	DIRECTIONS	INFUSION RANGE	DRUG MIXTURE	AMOUNT	DRUG/mL	RUN AT	mL/h
Dopamine	Infusion		0.22		1–20 mcg/kg/min	400 mg/ 250 mL	1600	mcg/mL		
	Take dose you want in mcg ÷ by drug index number = mL/h on pump									
Epinephrine	Infusion	1 mcg/min = 4 mL/h 2 mcg/min = 8 mL/h 3 mcg/min = 11 mL/h 4 mcg/min = 15 mL/h			1–4 mcg/min	4 mg/ 250 mL	16	mcg/mL		
		Ordered mcg dose/min ÷ mcg/mL × 60 min/h =							___	mL/h
Fenoldapam	Infusion		0.0056		0.01–1.6 mcg/kg/min	10 mg/ 250 mL	40	mcg/mL		
	Take dose you want in mcg ÷ by drug index number = mL/h on pump									
Heparin	100 u/kg = 11,900 u 200 u/kg = 23,800 u 300 u/kg = 35,700 u 400 u/kg = 47,600 u									
Isoproterenol	Infusion				5 mcg/min	1 mg/ 250 mL	4	mcg/mL		
		Ordered mcg dose/min ÷ mcg/mL × 60 min/h =							75	mL/h
Lidocaine	Infusion	1 mg/min = 7.5 mL/h			1–4 mg/min	2 g/ 250 mL	8	mg/mL	___	
		Ordered mg/min ÷ mg/mL × 60 min/h =							___	mL/h
Nitroglycerin	Infusion	3 mcg/min = 1 mL/h			3–200 mcg/min	50 mg/ 250 mL	200	mcg/mL	___	
		Ordered mcg/min ÷ mcg/mL × 60 min/h =							___	mL/h
Nitroprusside	Infusion	6.7 mcg/min = 1 mL/h			5–300 mcg/min	100 mg/ 250 mL	400	mcg/mL	___	
		Ordered mcg/min ÷ mcg/mL × 60 min/h =							___	mL/h
Norepinephrine	Infusion	1 mcg/min = 4 mL/h 2 mcg/min = 8 mL/h 3 mcg/min = 11 mL/h 4 mcg/min = 15 mL/h 5 mcg/min = 19 mL/h			2–20 mcg/min	4 mg/ 250 mL	16	mcg/mL		
		Ordered mcg dose/min ÷ mcg/mL × 60 min/h =							___	mL/h
Phenylephrine	Infusion	1.3 mcg/min = 1 mL/h			10–200 mcg/min	20 mg/ 250 mL	80	mcg/mL		
		Ordered mcg/min ÷ mcg/mL × 60 min/h =							___	mL/h
Primacor	0.05 mg/kg = 5.95 mg			Give load over 10 min		40 mg/ 200 mL	0.2	mg/mL		
	mg to give ÷ mg/mL = 30 mL				30	mL × (60 min/h ÷ 10 min) =			178.5	mL/h × 10 min
	Infusion		0.03		0.5 mcg/kg/min	40 mg/ 200 mL	200	mcg/mL	___	
	Take dose you want in mcg ÷ by drug index number = mL/h on pump									
Trimethaphan	Infusion		—		0.3–6 mg/min	500 mg/ 500 mL	1	mg/mL	___	
		Ordered mg/min ÷ mg/mL × 60 min/h =							___	mL/h
Vasopressin		0.02 u/min = 3 mL/h 0.04 u/min = 6 mL/h				40 u/ 100 mL	400	u/mL		

120 kg

DRUG	ORDERED AMOUNT	TOTAL DOSE TO GIVE	DRUG INDEX NUMBER	DIRECTIONS	INFUSION RANGE	DRUG MIXTURE	AMOUNT	DRUG/mL	RUN AT	mL/h
Aminophylline	5 mg/kg =	600 mg		Give mg/kg load over 20 min		500 mg/ 250 mL	2 mg/mL		
	mg to give ÷ mg/mL =	300 mL			300	mL × (60 min/h ÷ 20 min) =			900	mL/h × 20 min
	Infusion				0.5–1 mg/kg/h	500 mg/ 250 mL	2 mg/mL		
					mg dose ordered × kg ÷ mg/mL =				___	mL/h
Amiodarone	Loading dose			Load **150 mg** over 10 min		900 mg/ 500 mL	1.8 mg/mL		___
				Ordered mg load dose (150 mg) ÷ mg/mL (1.8 mg/mL) = 83 mL to give × (60 min/h ÷ 10 min) = mL/h to set on pump					500	mL/h × 83 mL
	Infusion			Run at **1 mg/ min** × 6 h		900 mg/ 500 mL	1.8 mg/mL		
				Ordered mg dose (1 mg/min) ÷ mg/mL (1.8 mg/mL) = _____ × 60 min/h = mL/h to set on pump					33	mL/h × 6 h
	Infusion			Run at **0.5 mg/ min** × 18 h		900 mg/ 500 mL	1.8 mg/mL		
				Ordered mg dose (0.5 mg/min) ÷ mg/mL (1.8 mg/mL) = _____ × 60 min/h = mL/h to set on pump					17	mL/h × 18 h
Amrinone	0.75 mg/kg =	90 mg		Give mg/kg load over 10 min		300 mg/ 120 mL	2.5 mg/mL		___
	mg to give ÷ mg/mL =	36 mL			36	mL × (60 min/h ÷ 10 min) =			216	mL/h × 10 min
	Infusion		0.35		5–10 mcg/ kg/min	300 mg/ 120 mL	2500 mcg/mL		___
				Take dose you want in mcg ÷ by drug index number = mL/h on pump						
Brevibloc	Infusion		1.39		50–100 mcg/ kg/min	2.5 g/ 250 mL	10,000 mcg/mL		___ mL/h
				Take dose you want in mcg ÷ by drug index number = mL/h on pump						
Cardene	Infusion		___		0.5–10 mg/h	25 mg 250 mL	0.1 mg/mL		___
				Ordered mg dose ÷ mg/mL = mL/h to set on pump						___ mL/h
Cardizem	0.25 mg/kg =	30 mg		Give mg/kg load over 20 min		50 mg/ 100 mL	0.5 mg/mL		
	mg to give ÷ mg/mL =	60 mL			60	mL × (60 min/h ÷ 20 min) =			180	mL/h
	0.35 mg/kg =	42 mg		May repeat loading dose in 15 min			0.5 mg/mL		
	mg to give ÷ mg/mL =	84 mL			84	mL × (60 min/h ÷ 20 min) =			252	mL/h
	Infusion				5–15 mg/h				___
				Ordered mg dose ÷ mg/mL = mL/h to set on pump						___ mL/h
Desmopressin	0.3 mcg/kg =	36 mcg		Give dose over 20–30 min			4 mcg/vial		
Dobutamine	Infusion		0.28		2.5–40 mcg/kg/ min	250 mg/ 125 mL	2000 mcg/mL		
				Take dose you want in mcg ÷ by drug index number = mL/h on pump						

(continues)

120   kg (continued)

DRUG	ORDERED AMOUNT		TOTAL DOSE TO GIVE	DRUG INDEX NUMBER	DIRECTIONS	INFUSION RANGE	DRUG MIXTURE	AMOUNT	DRUG/mL	RUN AT	mL/h
Dopamine	Infusion			0.22		1–20 mcg/kg/min	400 mg/250 mL	1600	mcg/mL		
	Take dose you want in mcg ÷ by drug index number = mL/h on pump										
Epinephrine	Infusion		1 mcg/min = 4 mL/h 2 mcg/min = 8 mL/h 3 mcg/min = 11 mL/h 4 mcg/min = 15 mL/h			1–4 mcg/min	4 mg/250 mL	16	mcg/mL		
	Ordered mcg dose/min ÷ mcg/mL × 60 min/h = ___ mL/h										
Fenoldapam	Infusion			0.0056		0.01–1.6 mcg/kg/min	10 mg/250 mL	40	mcg/mL		
	Take dose you want in mcg ÷ by drug index number = mL/h on pump										
Heparin	100 u/kg =	12,000 u									
	200 u/kg =	24,000 u									
	300 u/kg =	36,000 u									
	400 u/kg =	48,000 u									
Isoproterenol	Infusion					5 mcg/min	1 mg/250 mL	4	mcg/mL		
	Ordered mcg dose/min ÷ mcg/mL × 60 min/h =									75	mL/h
Lidocaine	Infusion		1 mg/min = 7.5 mL/h			1–4 mg/min	2 g/250 mL	8	mg/mL		—
	Ordered mg/min ÷ mg/mL × 60 min/h = ___ mL/h										
Nitroglycerin	Infusion		3 mcg/min = 1 mL/h			3–200 mcg/min	50 mg/250 mL	200	mcg/mL		—
	Ordered mcg/min ÷ mcg/mL × 60 min/h = ___ mL/h										
Nitroprusside	Infusion		6.7 mcg/min = 1 mL/h			5–300 mcg/min	100 mg/250 mL	400	mcg/mL		—
	Ordered mcg/min ÷ mcg/mL × 60 min/h = ___ mL/h										
Norepinephrine	Infusion		1 mcg/min = 4 mL/h 2 mcg/min = 8 mL/h 3 mcg/min = 11 mL/h 4 mcg/min = 15 mL/h 5 mcg/min = 19 mL/h			2–20 mcg/min	4 mg/250 mL	16	mcg/mL		
	Ordered mcg dose/min ÷ mcg/mL × 60 min/h = ___ mL/h										
Phenylephrine	Infusion		1.3 mcg/min = 1 mL/h			10–200 mcg/min	20 mg/250 mL	80	mcg/mL		
	Ordered mcg/min ÷ mcg/mL × 60 min/h = ___ mL/h										
Primacor	0.05 mg/kg =	6 mg			Give load over 10 min		40 mg/200 mL	0.2	mg/mL		
	mg to give ÷ mg/mL =	30 mL					30	mL × (60 min/h ÷ 10 min) =		180	mL/h × 10 min
	Infusion			0.03		0.5 mcg/kg/min	40 mg/200 mL	200	mcg/mL		—
	Take dose you want in mcg ÷ by drug index number = mL/h on pump										
Trimethaphan	Infusion			—		0.3–6 mg/min	500 mg/500 mL	1	mg/mL		—
	Ordered mg/min ÷ mg/mL × 60 min/h = ___ mL/h										
Vasopressin			0.02 u/min = 3 mL/h 0.04 u/min = 6 mL/h				40 u/100 mL	400	u/mL		

121 kg

DRUG	ORDERED AMOUNT	TOTAL DOSE TO GIVE	DRUG INDEX NUMBER	DIRECTIONS	INFUSION RANGE	DRUG MIXTURE	AMOUNT	DRUG/ mL	RUN AT	mL/h
Aminophylline	5 mg/kg =	605 mg		Give mg/kg load over 20 min		500 mg/ 250 mL	2	mg/mL		
		mg to give ÷ mg/mL = 303 mL			303	mL × (60 min/h ÷ 20 min) =			907.5	mL/h × 20 min
		Infusion			0.5–1 mg/kg/h	500 mg/ 250 mL	2	mg/mL		
					mg dose ordered × kg ÷ mg/mL =					___ mL/h
Amiodarone		Loading dose		Load **150 mg** over 10 min		900 mg/ 500 mL	1.8	mg/mL	___	
				Ordered mg load dose (150 mg) ÷ mg/mL (1.8 mg/mL) = 83 mL to give × (60 min/h ÷ 10 min) = mL/h to set on pump					500	mL/h × 83 mL
		Infusion		Run at **1 mg/ min** × 6 h		900 mg/ 500 mL	1.8	mg/mL		
				Ordered mg dose (1 mg/min) ÷ mg/mL (1.8 mg/mL) = _____ × 60 min/h = mL/h to set on pump					33	mL/h × 6 h
		Infusion		Run at **0.5 mg/ min** × 18 h		900 mg/ 500 mL	1.8	mg/mL		
				Ordered mg dose (0.5 mg/min) ÷ mg/mL (1.8 mg/mL) = _____ × 60 min/h = mL/h to set on pump					17	mL/h × 18 h
Amrinone	0.75 mg/kg =	90.75 mg		Give mg/kg load over 10 min		300 mg/ 120 mL	2.5	mg/mL	___	
		mg to give ÷ mg/mL = 36 mL			36.3	mL × (60 min/h ÷ 10 min) =			217.8	mL/h × 10 min
		Infusion	0.34		5–10 mcg/ kg/min	300 mg/ 120 mL	2500	mcg/mL	___	
				Take dose you want in mcg ÷ by drug index number = mL/h on pump						
Brevibloc		Infusion	1.38		50–100 mcg/ kg/min	2.5 g/ 250 mL	10,000	mcg/mL	___	mL/h
				Take dose you want in mcg ÷ by drug index number = mL/h on pump						
Cardene		Infusion	—		0.5–10 mg/h	25 mg 250 mL	0.1	mg/mL	___	
				Ordered mg dose ÷ mg/mL = mL/h to set on pump						___ mL/h
Cardizem	0.25 mg/kg =	30.25 mg		Give mg/kg load over 20 min		50 mg/ 100 mL	0.5	mg/mL	___	
		mg to give ÷ mg/mL = 61 mL			60.5	mL × (60 min/h ÷ 20 min) =			182	mL/h
	0.35 mg/kg =	42.35 mg		May repeat loading dose in 15 min			0.5	mg/mL	___	
		mg to give ÷ mg/mL = 85 mL			84.7	mL × (60 min/h ÷ 20 min) =			254	mL/h
		Infusion			5–15 mg/h				___	
				Ordered mg dose ÷ mg/mL = mL/h to set on pump						___ mL/h
Desmopressin	0.3 mcg/kg =	36 mcg		Give dose over 20–30 min			4	mcg/vial		
Dobutamine		Infusion	0.28		2.5–40 mcg/kg/ min	250 mg/ 125 mL	2000	mcg/mL		
				Take dose you want in mcg ÷ by drug index number = mL/h on pump						

(continues)

121   kg (continued)

DRUG	ORDERED AMOUNT	TOTAL DOSE TO GIVE	DRUG INDEX NUMBER	DIRECTIONS	INFUSION RANGE	DRUG MIXTURE	AMOUNT	DRUG/ mL	RUN AT	mL/h
Dopamine	Infusion		0.22		1–20 mcg/ kg/min	400 mg/ 250 mL	1600	mcg/mL		
		Take dose you want in mcg ÷ by drug index number = mL/h on pump								
Epinephrine	Infusion	1 mcg/min = 4 mL/h 2 mcg/min = 8 mL/h 3 mcg/min = 11 mL/h 4 mcg/min = 15 mL/h			1–4 mcg/min	4 mg/ 250 mL	16	mcg/mL		
		Ordered mcg dose/min ÷ mcg/mL × 60 min/h =								___ mL/h
Fenoldapam	Infusion		0.0055		0.01–1.6 mcg/ kg/min	10 mg/ 250 mL	40	mcg/mL		
	Take dose you want in mcg ÷ by drug index number = mL/h on pump									
Heparin	100 u/kg = 200 u/kg = 300 u/kg = 400 u/kg =	12,100 u 24,200 u 36,300 u 48,400 u								
Isoproterenol	Infusion				5 mcg/min	1 mg/ 250 mL	4	mcg/mL		
	Ordered mcg dose/min ÷ mcg/mL × 60 min/h =									**75** mL/h
Lidocaine	Infusion	1 mg/min = 7.5 mL/h			1–4 mg/min	2 g/ 250 mL	8	mg/mL	___	
		Ordered mg/min ÷ mg/mL × 60 min/h =								___ mL/h
Nitroglycerin	Infusion	3 mcg/min = 1 mL/h			3–200 mcg/min	50 mg/ 250 mL	200	mcg/mL	___	
		Ordered mcg/min ÷ mcg/mL × 60 min/h =								___ mL/h
Nitroprusside	Infusion	6.7 mcg/min = 1 mL/h			5–300 mcg/min	100 mg/ 250 mL	400	mcg/mL	___	
		Ordered mcg/min ÷ mcg/mL × 60 min/h =								___ mL/h
Norepinephrine	Infusion	1 mcg/min = 4 mL/h 2 mcg/min = 8 mL/h 3 mcg/min = 11 mL/h 4 mcg/min = 15 mL/h 5 mcg/min = 19 mL/h			2–20 mcg/min	4 mg/ 250 mL	16	mcg/mL		
		Ordered mcg dose/min ÷ mcg/mL × 60 min/h =								___ mL/h
Phenylephrine	Infusion	1.3 mcg/min = 1 mL/h			10–200 mcg/min	20 mg/ 250 mL	80	mcg/mL		
		Ordered mcg/min ÷ mcg/mL × 60 min/h =								___ mL/h
Primacor	0.05 mg/kg =	6.05 mg		Give load over 10 min		40 mg/ 200 mL	0.2	mg/mL		
	mg to give ÷ mg/mL =	30 mL				30 mL × (60 min/h ÷ 10 min) =				**181.5**	mL/h × 10 min
	Infusion		0.03		0.5 mcg/ kg/min	40 mg/ 200 mL	200	mcg/mL	___	
	Take dose you want in mcg ÷ by drug index number = mL/h on pump									
Trimethaphan	Infusion	___			0.3–6 mg/min	500 mg/ 500 mL	1	mg/mL	___	
		Ordered mg/min ÷ mg/mL × 60 min/h =								___ mL/h
Vasopressin		0.02 u/min = 3 mL/h 0.04 u/min = 6 mL/h				40 u/ 100 mL	400	u/mL		

122 kg

DRUG	ORDERED AMOUNT	TOTAL DOSE TO GIVE	DRUG INDEX NUMBER	DIRECTIONS	INFUSION RANGE	DRUG MIXTURE	AMOUNT	DRUG/mL	RUN AT	mL/h
Aminophylline	5 mg/kg =	**610** mg		Give mg/kg load over 20 min		500 mg/ 250 mL	2	mg/mL		
	mg to give ÷ mg/mL =	**305** mL			**305**	mL × (60 min/h ÷ 20 min) =			**915**	mL/h × 20 min
	Infusion				0.5–1 mg/kg/h	500 mg/ 250 mL	2	mg/mL		
					mg dose ordered × kg ÷ mg/mL =				___	mL/h
Amiodarone	Loading dose			Load **150 mg** over 10 min		900 mg/ 500 mL	1.8	mg/mL	—	
				Ordered mg load dose (150 mg) ÷ mg/mL (1.8 mg/mL) = 83 mL to give × (60 min/h ÷ 10 min) = mL/h to set on pump					**500**	mL/h × 83 mL
	Infusion			Run at **1 mg/ min** × 6 h		900 mg/ 500 mL	1.8	mg/mL		
				Ordered mg dose (1 mg/min) ÷ mg/mL (1.8 mg/mL) = _____ × 60 min/h = mL/h to set on pump					**33**	mL/h × 6 h
	Infusion			Run at **0.5 mg/ min** × 18 h		900 mg/ 500 mL	1.8	mg/mL		
				Ordered mg dose (0.5 mg/min) ÷ mg/mL (1.8 mg/mL) = _____ × 60 min/h = mL/h to set on pump					**17**	mL/h × 18 h
Amrinone	0.75 mg/kg =	**91.5** mg		Give mg/kg load over 10 min		300 mg/ 120 mL	2.5	mg/mL	—	
	mg to give ÷ mg/mL =	**37** mL			**36.6**	mL × (60 min/h ÷ 10 min) =			**219.6**	mL/h × 10 min
	Infusion		**0.34**		5–10 mcg/ kg/min	300 mg/ 120 mL	2500	mcg/mL		
				Take dose you want in mcg ÷ by drug index number = mL/h on pump						
Brevibloc	Infusion		**1.37**		50–100 mcg/ kg/min	2.5 g/ 250 mL	10,000	mcg/mL		mL/h
				Take dose you want in mcg ÷ by drug index number = mL/h on pump						
Cardene	Infusion		—		0.5–10 mg/h	25 mg 250 mL	0.1	mg/mL	—	
				Ordered mg dose ÷ mg/mL = mL/h to set on pump					___	mL/h
Cardizem	0.25 mg/kg =	**30.5** mg		Give mg/kg load over 20 min		50 mg/ 100 mL	0.5	mg/mL	—	
	mg to give ÷ mg/mL =	**61** mL			**61**	mL × (60 min/h ÷ 20 min) =			**183**	mL/h
	0.35 mg/kg =	**42.7** mg		May repeat loading dose in 15 min			0.5	mg/mL	—	
	mg to give ÷ mg/mL =	**85** mL			**85.4**	mL × (60 min/h ÷ 20 min) =			**256**	mL/h
	Infusion				5–15 mg/h				—	
				Ordered mg dose ÷ mg/mL = mL/h to set on pump					___	mL/h
Desmopressin	0.3 mcg/kg =	**37** mcg		Give dose over 20–30 min			4	mcg/vial		
Dobutamine	Infusion		**0.27**		2.5–40 mcg/kg/ min	250 mg/ 125 mL	2000	mcg/mL		
				Take dose you want in mcg ÷ by drug index number = mL/h on pump						

(continues)

122 kg (continued)

DRUG	ORDERED AMOUNT	TOTAL DOSE TO GIVE	DRUG INDEX NUMBER	DIRECTIONS	INFUSION RANGE	DRUG MIXTURE	AMOUNT	DRUG/ mL	RUN AT	mL/h
Dopamine	Infusion		0.22		1–20 mcg/ kg/min	400 mg/ 250 mL	1600	mcg/mL		
			Take dose you want in mcg ÷ by drug index number = mL/h on pump							
Epinephrine	Infusion	1 mcg/min = 4 mL/h 2 mcg/min = 8 mL/h 3 mcg/min = 11 mL/h 4 mcg/min = 15 mL/h			1–4 mcg/min	4 mg/ 250 mL	16	mcg/mL		
				Ordered mcg dose/min ÷ mcg/mL × 60 min/h =					___	mL/h
Fenoldapam	Infusion		0.0055		0.01–1.6 mcg/ kg/min	10 mg/ 250 mL	40	mcg/mL		
			Take dose you want in mcg ÷ by drug index number = mL/h on pump							
Heparin	100 u/kg = 12,200 u 200 u/kg = 24,400 u 300 u/kg = 36,600 u 400 u/kg = 48,800 u									
Isoproterenol	Infusion				5 mcg/min	1 mg/ 250 mL	4	mcg/mL		
				Ordered mcg dose/min ÷ mcg/mL × 60 min/h =					75	mL/h
Lidocaine	Infusion	1 mg/min = 7.5 mL/h			1–4 mg/min	2 g/ 250 mL	8	mg/mL	___	
				Ordered mg/min ÷ mg/mL × 60 min/h =					___	mL/h
Nitroglycerin	Infusion	3 mcg/min = 1 mL/h			3–200 mcg/min	50 mg/ 250 mL	200	mcg/mL	___	
				Ordered mcg/min ÷ mcg/mL × 60 min/h =					___	mL/h
Nitroprusside	Infusion	6.7 mcg/min = 1 mL/h			5–300 mcg/min	100 mg/ 250 mL	400	mcg/mL	___	
				Ordered mcg/min ÷ mcg/mL × 60 min/h =					___	mL/h
Norepinephrine	Infusion	1 mcg/min = 4 mL/h 2 mcg/min = 8 mL/h 3 mcg/min = 11 mL/h 4 mcg/min = 15 mL/h 5 mcg/min = 19 mL/h			2–20 mcg/min	4 mg/ 250 mL	16	mcg/mL		
				Ordered mcg dose/min ÷ mcg/mL × 60 min/h =					___	mL/h
Phenylephrine	Infusion	1.3 mcg/min = 1 mL/h			10–200 mcg/min	20 mg/ 250 mL	80	mcg/mL		
				Ordered mcg/min ÷ mcg/mL × 60 min/h =					___	mL/h
Primacor	0.05 mg/kg = 6.1 mg			Give load over 10 min		40 mg/ 200 mL	0.2	mg/mL		
	mg to give ÷ mg/mL = 31 mL				31	mL × (60 min/h ÷ 10 min) =			183	mL/h × 10 min
	Infusion		0.03		0.5 mcg/ kg/min	40 mg/ 200 mL	200	mcg/mL	___	
			Take dose you want in mcg ÷ by drug index number = mL/h on pump							
Trimethaphan	Infusion		—		0.3–6 mg/min	500 mg/ 500 mL	1	mg/mL	___	
				Ordered mg/min ÷ mg/mL × 60 min/h =					___	mL/h
Vasopressin		0.02 u/min = 3 mL/h 0.04 u/min = 6 mL/h				40 u/ 100 mL	400	u/mL		

123 kg

DRUG	ORDERED AMOUNT	TOTAL DOSE TO GIVE	DRUG INDEX NUMBER	DIRECTIONS	INFUSION RANGE	DRUG MIXTURE	AMOUNT	DRUG/ mL	RUN AT	mL/h
Aminophylline	5 mg/kg =	615 mg		Give mg/kg load over 20 min		500 mg/ 250 mL	2	mg/mL		
	mg to give ÷ mg/mL = 308 mL				308	mL × (60 min/h ÷ 20 min) =			**922.5**	mL/h × 20 min
	Infusion				0.5–1 mg/kg/h	500 mg/ 250 mL	2	mg/mL		
					mg dose ordered × kg ÷ mg/mL =				___	mL/h
Amiodarone	Loading dose			Load **150 mg** over 10 min		900 mg/ 500 mL	1.8	mg/mL	___	
				Ordered mg load dose (150 mg) ÷ mg/mL (1.8 mg/mL) = 83 mL to give × (60 min/h ÷ 10 min) = mL/h to set on pump					**500**	mL/h × 83 mL
	Infusion			Run at **1 mg/ min** × 6 h		900 mg/ 500 mL	1.8	mg/mL		
				Ordered mg dose (1 mg/min) ÷ mg/mL (1.8 mg/mL) = ____ × 60 min/h = mL/h to set on pump					**33**	mL/h × 6 h
	Infusion			Run at **0.5 mg/ min** × 18 h		900 mg/ 500 mL	1.8	mg/mL		
				Ordered mg dose (0.5 mg/min) ÷ mg/mL (1.8 mg/mL) = ____ × 60 min/h = mL/h to set on pump					**17**	mL/h × 18 h
Amrinone	0.75 mg/kg =	92.25 mg		Give mg/kg load over 10 min		300 mg/ 120 mL	2.5	mg/mL	___	
	mg to give ÷ mg/mL = 37 mL				36.9	mL × (60 min/h ÷ 10 min) =			**221.4**	mL/h × 10 min
	Infusion		0.34		5–10 mcg/ kg/min	300 mg/ 120 mL	2500	mcg/mL	___	
				Take dose you want in mcg ÷ by drug index number = mL/h on pump						
Brevibloc	Infusion		1.35		50–100 mcg/ kg/min	2.5 g/ 250 mL	10,000	mcg/mL	___	mL/h
				Take dose you want in mcg ÷ by drug index number = mL/h on pump						
Cardene	Infusion			—	0.5–10 mg/h	25 mg 250 mL	0.1	mg/mL	___	
				Ordered mg dose ÷ mg/mL = mL/h to set on pump					___	mL/h
Cardizem	0.25 mg/kg =	30.75 mg		Give mg/kg load over 20 min		50 mg/ 100 mL	0.5	mg/mL		
	mg to give ÷ mg/mL = 62 mL				61.5	mL × (60 min/h ÷ 20 min) =			**185**	mL/h
	0.35 mg/kg =	43.05 mg		May repeat loading dose in 15 min			0.5	mg/mL		
	mg to give ÷ mg/mL = 86 mL				86.1	mL × (60 min/h ÷ 20 min) =			**258**	mL/h
	Infusion				5–15 mg/h				___	
				Ordered mg dose ÷ mg/mL = mL/h to set on pump					___	mL/h
Desmopressin	0.3 mcg/kg =	37 mcg		Give dose over 20–30 min			4	mcg/vial		
Dobutamine	Infusion		0.27		2.5–40 mcg/kg/ min	250 mg/ 125 mL	2000	mcg/mL		
				Take dose you want in mcg ÷ by drug index number = mL/h on pump						

(continues)

123 kg (continued)

DRUG	ORDERED AMOUNT	TOTAL DOSE TO GIVE	DRUG INDEX NUMBER	DIRECTIONS	INFUSION RANGE	DRUG MIXTURE	AMOUNT	DRUG/ mL	RUN AT	mL/h
Dopamine	Infusion		0.22		1–20 mcg/ kg/min	400 mg/ 250 mL	1600	mcg/mL		
		Take dose you want in mcg ÷ by drug index number = mL/h on pump								
Epinephrine	Infusion	1 mcg/min = 4 mL/h 2 mcg/min = 8 mL/h 3 mcg/min = 11 mL/h 4 mcg/min = 15 mL/h			1–4 mcg/min	4 mg/ 250 mL	16	mcg/mL		
		Ordered mcg dose/min ÷ mcg/mL × 60 min/h =								___ mL/h
Fenoldapam	Infusion		0.0054		0.01–1.6 mcg/ kg/min	10 mg/ 250 mL	40	mcg/mL		
		Take dose you want in mcg ÷ by drug index number = mL/h on pump								
Heparin	100 u/kg = 12,300 u 200 u/kg = 24,600 u 300 u/kg = 36,900 u 400 u/kg = 49,200 u									
Isoproterenol	Infusion				5 mcg/min	1 mg/ 250 mL	4	mcg/mL		
		Ordered mcg dose/min ÷ mcg/mL × 60 min/h =								75 mL/h
Lidocaine	Infusion	1 mg/min = 7.5 mL/h			1–4 mg/min	2 g/ 250 mL	8	mg/mL		___
		Ordered mg/min ÷ mg/mL × 60 min/h =								___ mL/h
Nitroglycerin	Infusion	3 mcg/min = 1 mL/h			3–200 mcg/min	50 mg/ 250 mL	200	mcg/mL		___
		Ordered mcg/min ÷ mcg/mL × 60 min/h =								___ mL/h
Nitroprusside	Infusion	6.7 mcg/min = 1 mL/h			5–300 mcg/min	100 mg/ 250 mL	400	mcg/mL		___
		Ordered mcg/min ÷ mcg/mL × 60 min/h =								___ mL/h
Norepinephrine	Infusion	1 mcg/min = 4 mL/h 2 mcg/min = 8 mL/h 3 mcg/min = 11 mL/h 4 mcg/min = 15 mL/h 5 mcg/min = 19 mL/h			2–20 mcg/min	4 mg/ 250 mL	16	mcg/mL		
		Ordered mcg dose/min ÷ mcg/mL × 60 min/h =								___ mL/h
Phenylephrine	Infusion	1.3 mcg/min = 1 mL/h			10–200 mcg/min	20 mg/ 250 mL	80	mcg/mL		
		Ordered mcg/min ÷ mcg/mL × 60 min/h =								___ mL/h
Primacor	0.05 mg/kg = 6.15 mg			Give load over 10 min		40 mg/ 200 mL	0.2	mg/mL		
	mg to give ÷ mg/mL = 31 mL				31 mL × (60 min/h ÷ 10 min) =				184.5	mL/h × 10 min
	Infusion		0.03		0.5 mcg/ kg/min	40 mg/ 200 mL	200	mcg/mL		___
		Take dose you want in mcg ÷ by drug index number = mL/h on pump								
Trimethaphan	Infusion		—		0.3–6 mg/min	500 mg/ 500 mL	1	mg/mL		___
		Ordered mg/min ÷ mg/mL × 60 min/h =								___ mL/h
Vasopressin		0.02 u/min = 3 mL/h 0.04 u/min = 6 mL/h				40 u/ 100 mL	400	u/mL		

124 kg

DRUG	ORDERED AMOUNT	TOTAL DOSE TO GIVE	DRUG INDEX NUMBER	DIRECTIONS	INFUSION RANGE	DRUG MIXTURE	AMOUNT DRUG/mL	RUN AT mL/h
Aminophylline	5 mg/kg =	620 mg		Give mg/kg load over 20 min		500 mg/ 250 mL	2 mg/mL	
	mg to give ÷ mg/mL =	310 mL			310	mL × (60 min/h ÷ 20 min) =		930 mL/h × 20 min
	Infusion				0.5–1 mg/kg/h	500 mg/ 250 mL	2 mg/mL	
					mg dose ordered × kg ÷ mg/mL =			___ mL/h
Amiodarone	Loading dose			Load **150 mg** over 10 min		900 mg/ 500 mL	1.8 mg/mL	___
				Ordered mg load dose (150 mg) ÷ mg/mL (1.8 mg/mL) = 83 mL to give × (60 min/h ÷ 10 min) = mL/h to set on pump				500 mL/h × 83 mL
	Infusion			Run at **1 mg/ min** × 6 h		900 mg/ 500 mL	1.8 mg/mL	
				Ordered mg dose (1 mg/min) ÷ mg/mL (1.8 mg/mL) = ____ × 60 min/h = mL/h to set on pump				33 mL/h × 6 h
	Infusion			Run at **0.5 mg/ min** × 18 h		900 mg/ 500 mL	1.8 mg/mL	
				Ordered mg dose (0.5 mg/min) ÷ mg/mL (1.8 mg/mL) = ____ × 60 min/h = mL/h to set on pump				17 mL/h × 18 h
Amrinone	0.75 mg/kg =	93 mg		Give mg/kg load over 10 min		300 mg/ 120 mL	2.5 mg/mL	___
	mg to give ÷ mg/mL =	37 mL			37.2	mL × (60 min/h ÷ 10 min) =		223.2 mL/h × 10 min
	Infusion		0.34		5–10 mcg/ kg/min	300 mg/ 120 mL	2500 mcg/mL	
				Take dose you want in mcg ÷ by drug index number = mL/h on pump				
Brevibloc	Infusion		1.34		50–100 mcg/ kg/min	2.5 g/ 250 mL	10,000 mcg/mL	___ mL/h
				Take dose you want in mcg ÷ by drug index number = mL/h on pump				
Cardene	Infusion		___		0.5–10 mg/h	25 mg 250 mL	0.1 mg/mL	___
				Ordered mg dose ÷ mg/mL = mL/h to set on pump				___ mL/h
Cardizem	0.25 mg/kg =	31 mg		Give mg/kg load over 20 min		50 mg/ 100 mL	0.5 mg/mL	___
	mg to give ÷ mg/mL =	62 mL			62	mL × (60 min/h ÷ 20 min) =		186 mL/h
	0.35 mg/kg =	43.4 mg		May repeat loading dose in 15 min			0.5 mg/mL	___
	mg to give ÷ mg/mL =	87 mL			86.8	mL × (60 min/h ÷ 20 min) =		260 mL/h
	Infusion				5–15 mg/h			___
				Ordered mg dose ÷ mg/mL = mL/h to set on pump				___ mL/h
Desmopressin	0.3 mcg/kg =	37 mcg		Give dose over 20–30 min			4 mcg/vial	
Dobutamine	Infusion		0.27		2.5–40 mcg/kg/ min	250 mg/ 125 mL	2000 mcg/mL	
				Take dose you want in mcg ÷ by drug index number = mL/h on pump				

(continues)

124 kg (continued)

DRUG	ORDERED AMOUNT	TOTAL DOSE TO GIVE	DRUG INDEX NUMBER	DIRECTIONS	INFUSION RANGE	DRUG MIXTURE	AMOUNT	DRUG/ mL	RUN AT	mL/h
Dopamine	Infusion		0.22		1–20 mcg/ kg/min	400 mg/ 250 mL	1600	mcg/mL		
	Take dose you want in mcg ÷ by drug index number = mL/h on pump									
Epinephrine	Infusion	1 mcg/min = 4 mL/h 2 mcg/min = 8 mL/h 3 mcg/min = 11 mL/h 4 mcg/min = 15 mL/h			1–4 mcg/min	4 mg/ 250 mL	16	mcg/mL		
		Ordered mcg dose/min ÷ mcg/mL × 60 min/h =								___	mL/h
Fenoldapam	Infusion		0.0054		0.01–1.6 mcg/ kg/min	10 mg/ 250 mL	40	mcg/mL		
	Take dose you want in mcg ÷ by drug index number = mL/h on pump									
Heparin	100 u/kg = **12,400** u 200 u/kg = **24,800** u 300 u/kg = **37,200** u 400 u/kg = **49,600** u									
Isoproterenol	Infusion				5 mcg/min	1 mg/ 250 mL	4	mcg/mL		
		Ordered mcg dose/min ÷ mcg/mL × 60 min/h =								**75**	mL/h
Lidocaine	Infusion	1 mg/min = 7.5 mL/h			1–4 mg/min	2 g/ 250 mL	8	mg/mL	___	
		Ordered mg/min ÷ mg/mL × 60 min/h =								___	mL/h
Nitroglycerin	Infusion	3 mcg/min = 1 mL/h			3–200 mcg/min	50 mg/ 250 mL	200	mcg/mL	___	
		Ordered mcg/min ÷ mcg/mL × 60 min/h =								___	mL/h
Nitroprusside	Infusion	6.7 mcg/min = 1 mL/h			5–300 mcg/min	100 mg/ 250 mL	400	mcg/mL	___	
		Ordered mcg/min ÷ mcg/mL × 60 min/h =								___	mL/h
Norepinephrine	Infusion	1 mcg/min = 4 mL/h 2 mcg/min = 8 mL/h 3 mcg/min = 11 mL/h 4 mcg/min = 15 mL/h 5 mcg/min = 19 mL/h			2–20 mcg/min	4 mg/ 250 mL	16	mcg/mL		
		Ordered mcg dose/min ÷ mcg/mL × 60 min/h =								___	mL/h
Phenylephrine	Infusion	1.3 mcg/min = 1 mL/h			10–200 mcg/min	20 mg/ 250 mL	80	mcg/mL		
		Ordered mcg/min ÷ mcg/mL × 60 min/h =								___	mL/h
Primacor	0.05 mg/kg = **6.2** mg			Give load over 10 min		40 mg/ 200 mL	0.2	mg/mL		
	mg to give ÷ mg/mL = **31** mL				**31** mL × (60 min/h ÷ 10 min) =				**186**	mL/h × 10 min
	Infusion		0.03		0.5 mcg/ kg/min	40 mg/ 200 mL	200	mcg/mL	___	
	Take dose you want in mcg ÷ by drug index number = mL/h on pump									
Trimethaphan	Infusion		___		0.3–6 mg/min	500 mg/ 500 mL	1	mg/mL	___	
		Ordered mg/min ÷ mg/mL × 60 min/h =								___	mL/h
Vasopressin		0.02 u/min = 3 mL/h 0.04 u/min = 6 mL/h				40 u/ 100 mL	400	u/mL		

125 kg

DRUG	ORDERED AMOUNT	TOTAL DOSE TO GIVE	DRUG INDEX NUMBER	DIRECTIONS	INFUSION RANGE	DRUG MIXTURE	AMOUNT	DRUG/mL	RUN AT	mL/h
Aminophylline	5 mg/kg =	625 mg		Give mg/kg load over 20 min		500 mg/ 250 mL	2 mg/mL		
	mg to give ÷ mg/mL =	313 mL			313	mL × (60 min/h ÷ 20 min) =			**937.5**	mL/h × 20 min
	Infusion				0.5–1 mg/kg/h	500 mg/ 250 mL	2 mg/mL		
						mg dose ordered × kg ÷ mg/mL =			___	mL/h
Amiodarone	Loading dose			Load **150 mg** over 10 min		900 mg/ 500 mL	1.8 mg/mL		—
				Ordered mg load dose (150 mg) ÷ mg/mL (1.8 mg/mL) = 83 mL to give × (60 min/h ÷ 10 min) = mL/h to set on pump					**500**	mL/h × 83 mL
	Infusion			Run at **1 mg/ min** × 6 h		900 mg/ 500 mL	1.8 mg/mL		
				Ordered mg dose (1 mg/min) ÷ mg/mL (1.8 mg/mL) = ___ × 60 min/h = mL/h to set on pump					**33**	mL/h × 6 h
	Infusion			Run at **0.5 mg/ min** × 18 h		900 mg/ 500 mL	1.8 mg/mL		
				Ordered mg dose (0.5 mg/min) ÷ mg/mL (1.8 mg/mL) = ___ × 60 min/h = mL/h to set on pump					**17**	mL/h × 18 h
Amrinone	0.75 mg/kg =	93.75 mg		Give mg/kg load over 10 min		300 mg/ 120 mL	2.5 mg/mL		—
	mg to give ÷ mg/mL =	38 mL			37.5	mL × (60 min/h ÷ 10 min) =			**225**	mL/h × 10 min
	Infusion		0.33		5–10 mcg/ kg/min	300 mg/ 120 mL	2500 mcg/mL		—
				Take dose you want in mcg ÷ by drug index number = mL/h on pump						
Brevibloc	Infusion		1.33		50–100 mcg/ kg/min	2.5 g/ 250 mL	10,000 mcg/mL		___ mL/h
				Take dose you want in mcg ÷ by drug index number = mL/h on pump						
Cardene	Infusion		—		0.5–10 mg/h	25 mg 250 mL	0.1 mg/mL		—
				Ordered mg dose ÷ mg/mL = mL/h to set on pump						___ mL/h
Cardizem	0.25 mg/kg =	31.25 mg		Give mg/kg load over 20 min		50 mg/ 100 mL	0.5 mg/mL		—
	mg to give ÷ mg/mL =	63 mL			62.5	mL × (60 min/h ÷ 20 min) =			**188**	mL/h
	0.35 mg/kg =	43.75 mg		May repeat loading dose in 15 min			0.5 mg/mL		
	mg to give ÷ mg/mL =	88 mL			87.5	mL × (60 min/h ÷ 20 min) =			**263**	mL/h
	Infusion				5–15 mg/h				
				Ordered mg dose ÷ mg/mL = mL/h to set on pump						___ mL/h
Desmopressin	0.3 mcg/kg =	38 mcg		Give dose over 20–30 min			4 mcg/vial		
Dobutamine	Infusion		0.27		2.5–40 mcg/kg/ min	250 mg/ 125 mL	2000 mcg/mL		
				Take dose you want in mcg ÷ by drug index number = mL/h on pump						

(continues)

125 kg (continued)

DRUG	ORDERED AMOUNT		TOTAL DOSE TO GIVE		DRUG INDEX NUMBER	DIRECTIONS	INFUSION RANGE	DRUG MIXTURE	AMOUNT	DRUG/ mL	RUN AT	mL/h
Dopamine	Infusion				0.21		1–20 mcg/ kg/min	400 mg/ 250 mL	1600	mcg/mL		
	Take dose you want in mcg ÷ by drug index number = mL/h on pump											
Epinephrine	Infusion		1 mcg/min = 4 mL/h 2 mcg/min = 8 mL/h 3 mcg/min = 11 mL/h 4 mcg/min = 15 mL/h				1–4 mcg/min	4 mg/ 250 mL	16	mcg/mL		
	Ordered mcg dose/min ÷ mcg/mL × 60 min/h =										___	mL/h
Fenoldapam	Infusion				0.0054		0.01–1.6 mcg/ kg/min	10 mg/ 250 mL	40	mcg/mL		
	Take dose you want in mcg ÷ by drug index number = mL/h on pump											
Heparin	100 u/kg =	12,500 u										
	200 u/kg =	25,000 u										
	300 u/kg =	37,500 u										
	400 u/kg =	50,000 u										
Isoproterenol	Infusion						5 mcg/min	1 mg/ 250 mL	4	mcg/mL		
	Ordered mcg dose/min ÷ mcg/mL × 60 min/h =										**75**	mL/h
Lidocaine	Infusion		1 mg/min = 7.5 mL/h				1–4 mg/min	2 g/ 250 mL	8	mg/mL	___	
	Ordered mg/min ÷ mg/mL × 60 min/h =										___	mL/h
Nitroglycerin	Infusion		3 mcg/min = 1 mL/h				3–200 mcg/min	50 mg/ 250 mL	200	mcg/mL		
	Ordered mcg/min ÷ mcg/mL × 60 min/h =										___	mL/h
Nitroprusside	Infusion		6.7 mcg/min = 1 mL/h				5–300 mcg/min	100 mg/ 250 mL	400	mcg/mL		
	Ordered mcg/min ÷ mcg/mL × 60 min/h =										___	mL/h
Norepinephrine	Infusion		1 mcg/min = 4 mL/h 2 mcg/min = 8 mL/h 3 mcg/min = 11 mL/h 4 mcg/min = 15 mL/h 5 mcg/min = 19 mL/h				2–20 mcg/min	4 mg/ 250 mL	16	mcg/mL		
	Ordered mcg dose/min ÷ mcg/mL × 60 min/h =										___	mL/h
Phenylephrine	Infusion		1.3 mcg/min = 1 mL/h				10–200 mcg/min	20 mg/ 250 mL	80	mcg/mL		
	Ordered mcg/min ÷ mcg/mL × 60 min/h =										___	mL/h
Primacor	0.05 mg/kg =	6.25 mg				Give load over 10 min		40 mg/ 200 mL	0.2	mg/mL		
	mg to give ÷ mg/mL =	31 mL					31	mL × (60 min/h ÷ 10 min) =			**187.5**	mL/h × 10 min
	Infusion				0.03		0.5 mcg/ kg/min	40 mg/ 200 mL	200	mcg/mL	___	
	Take dose you want in mcg ÷ by drug index number = mL/h on pump											
Trimethaphan	Infusion				___		0.3–6 mg/min	500 mg/ 500 mL	1	mg/mL	___	
	Ordered mg/min ÷ mg/mL × 60 min/h =										___	mL/h
Vasopressin			0.02 u/min = 3 mL/h 0.04 u/min = 6 mL/h					40 u/ 100 mL	400	u/mL		

126 kg

DRUG	ORDERED AMOUNT	TOTAL DOSE TO GIVE	DRUG INDEX NUMBER	DIRECTIONS	INFUSION RANGE	DRUG MIXTURE	AMOUNT	DRUG/ mL	RUN AT	mL/h
Aminophylline	5 mg/kg =	**630** mg		Give mg/kg load over 20 min		500 mg/ 250 mL	2 mg/mL		
	mg to give ÷ mg/mL =	**315** mL			315	mL × (60 min/h ÷ 20 min) =			**945**	mL/h × 20 min
	Infusion				0.5–1 mg/kg/h	500 mg/ 250 mL	2 mg/mL			
						mg dose ordered × kg ÷ mg/mL =			___	mL/h
Amiodarone	Loading dose			Load **150 mg** over 10 min		900 mg/ 500 mL	1.8 mg/mL		___	
				Ordered mg load dose (150 mg) ÷ mg/mL (1.8 mg/mL) = 83 mL to give × (60 min/h ÷ 10 min) = mL/h to set on pump					**500**	mL/h × 83 mL
	Infusion			Run at **1 mg/ min** × 6 h		900 mg/ 500 mL	1.8 mg/mL			
				Ordered mg dose (1 mg/min) ÷ mg/mL (1.8 mg/mL) = _____ × 60 min/h = mL/h to set on pump					**33**	mL/h × 6 h
	Infusion			Run at **0.5 mg/ min** × 18 h		900 mg/ 500 mL	1.8 mg/mL			
				Ordered mg dose (0.5 mg/min) ÷ mg/mL (1.8 mg/mL) = _____ × 60 min/h = mL/h to set on pump					**17**	mL/h × 18 h
Amrinone	0.75 mg/kg =	**94.5** mg		Give mg/kg load over 10 min		300 mg/ 120 mL	2.5 mg/mL		___	
	mg to give ÷ mg/mL =	**38** mL			37.8	mL × (60 min/h ÷ 10 min) =			**227**	mL/h × 10 min
	Infusion		0.33		5–10 mcg/ kg/min	300 mg/ 120 mL	2500 mcg/mL		___	
				Take dose you want in mcg ÷ by drug index number = mL/h on pump						
Brevibloc	Infusion		1.32		50–100 mcg/ kg/min	2.5 g/ 250 mL	10,000 mcg/mL		___	mL/h
				Take dose you want in mcg ÷ by drug index number = mL/h on pump						
Cardene	Infusion		—		0.5–10 mg/h	25 mg 250 mL	0.1 mg/mL		___	
				Ordered mg dose ÷ mg/mL = mL/h to set on pump					___	mL/h
Cardizem	0.25 mg/kg =	**31.5** mg		Give mg/kg load over 20 min		50 mg/ 100 mL	0.5 mg/mL		
	mg to give ÷ mg/mL =	**63** mL			63	mL × (60 min/h ÷ 20 min) =			**189**	mL/h
	0.35 mg/kg =	**44.1** mg		May repeat loading dose in 15 min			0.5 mg/mL		
	mg to give ÷ mg/mL =	**88** mL			88.2	mL × (60 min/h ÷ 20 min) =			**265**	mL/h
	Infusion				5–15 mg/h				___	
				Ordered mg dose ÷ mg/mL = mL/h to set on pump					___	mL/h
Desmopressin	0.3 mcg/kg =	**38** mcg		Give dose over 20–30 min			4 mcg/vial		
Dobutamine	Infusion		0.26		2.5–40 mcg/kg/ min	250 mg/ 125 mL	2000 mcg/mL		
				Take dose you want in mcg ÷ by drug index number = mL/h on pump						

(continues)

126 kg (continued)

DRUG	ORDERED AMOUNT	TOTAL DOSE TO GIVE	DRUG INDEX NUMBER	DIRECTIONS	INFUSION RANGE	DRUG MIXTURE	AMOUNT	DRUG/mL	RUN AT mL/h
Dopamine	Infusion		0.21		1–20 mcg/kg/min	400 mg/250 mL	1600	mcg/mL	
		Take dose you want in mcg ÷ by drug index number = mL/h on pump							
Epinephrine	Infusion	1 mcg/min = 4 mL/h 2 mcg/min = 8 mL/h 3 mcg/min = 11 mL/h 4 mcg/min = 15 mL/h			1–4 mcg/min	4 mg/250 mL	16	mcg/mL	
		Ordered mcg dose/min ÷ mcg/mL × 60 min/h =							___ mL/h
Fenoldapam	Infusion		0.0053		0.01–1.6 mcg/kg/min	10 mg/250 mL	40	mcg/mL	
		Take dose you want in mcg ÷ by drug index number = mL/h on pump							
Heparin	100 u/kg = 12,600 u 200 u/kg = 25,200 u 300 u/kg = 37,800 u 400 u/kg = 50,400 u								
Isoproterenol	Infusion				5 mcg/min	1 mg/250 mL	4	mcg/mL	
		Ordered mcg dose/min ÷ mcg/mL × 60 min/h =							75 mL/h
Lidocaine	Infusion	1 mg/min = 7.5 mL/h			1–4 mg/min	2 g/250 mL	8	mg/mL	___
		Ordered mg/min ÷ mg/mL × 60 min/h =							___ mL/h
Nitroglycerin	Infusion	3 mcg/min = 1 mL/h			3–200 mcg/min	50 mg/250 mL	200	mcg/mL	___
		Ordered mcg/min ÷ mcg/mL × 60 min/h =							___ mL/h
Nitroprusside	Infusion	6.7 mcg/min = 1 mL/h			5–300 mcg/min	100 mg/250 mL	400	mcg/mL	___
		Ordered mcg/min ÷ mcg/mL × 60 min/h =							___ mL/h
Norepinephrine	Infusion	1 mcg/min = 4 mL/h 2 mcg/min = 8 mL/h 3 mcg/min = 11 mL/h 4 mcg/min = 15 mL/h 5 mcg/min = 19 mL/h			2–20 mcg/min	4 mg/250 mL	16	mcg/mL	
		Ordered mcg dose/min ÷ mcg/mL × 60 min/h =							___ mL/h
Phenylephrine	Infusion	1.3 mcg/min = 1 mL/h			10–200 mcg/min	20 mg/250 mL	80	mcg/mL	
		Ordered mcg/min ÷ mcg/mL × 60 min/h =							___ mL/h
Primacor	0.05 mg/kg =	6.3 mg		Give load over 10 min		40 mg/200 mL	0.2	mg/mL	
	mg to give ÷ mg/mL =	32 mL			32	mL × (60 min/h ÷ 10 min) =			189 mL/h × 10 min
	Infusion		0.03		0.5 mcg/kg/min	40 mg/200 mL	200	mcg/mL	___
		Take dose you want in mcg ÷ by drug index number = mL/h on pump							
Trimethaphan	Infusion		—		0.3–6 mg/min	500 mg/500 mL	1	mg/mL	___
		Ordered mg/min ÷ mg/mL × 60 min/h =							___ mL/h
Vasopressin		0.02 u/min = 3 mL/h 0.04 u/min = 6 mL/h				40 u/100 mL	400	u/mL	

127 kg

DRUG	ORDERED AMOUNT	TOTAL DOSE TO GIVE	DRUG INDEX NUMBER	DIRECTIONS	INFUSION RANGE	DRUG MIXTURE	AMOUNT	DRUG/ mL	RUN AT	mL/h
Aminophylline	5 mg/kg =	635 mg		Give mg/kg load over 20 min		500 mg/ 250 mL	2	mg/mL		
	mg to give ÷ mg/mL =	318 mL			318	mL × (60 min/h ÷ 20 min) =			953	mL/h × 20 min
	Infusion				0.5–1 mg/kg/h	500 mg/ 250 mL	2	mg/mL		
					mg dose ordered × kg ÷ mg/mL =				___	mL/h
Amiodarone	Loading dose			Load **150 mg** over 10 min		900 mg/ 500 mL	1.8	mg/mL	___	
				Ordered mg load dose (150 mg) ÷ mg/mL (1.8 mg/mL) = 83 mL to give × (60 min/h ÷ 10 min) — mL/h to set on pump					500	mL/h × 83 mL
	Infusion			Run at **1 mg/ min** × 6 h		900 mg/ 500 mL	1.8	mg/mL		
				Ordered mg dose (1 mg/min) ÷ mg/mL (1.8 mg/mL) = _____ × 60 min/h = mL/h to set on pump					33	mL/h × 6 h
	Infusion			Run at **0.5 mg/ min** × 18 h		900 mg/ 500 mL	1.8	mg/mL		
				Ordered mg dose (0.5 mg/min) ÷ mg/mL (1.8 mg/mL) = _____ × 60 min/h = mL/h to set on pump					17	mL/h × 18 h
Amrinone	0.75 mg/kg =	95.25 mg		Give mg/kg load over 10 min		300 mg/ 120 mL	2.5	mg/mL	___	
	mg to give ÷ mg/mL =	38 mL			38.1	mL × (60 min/h ÷ 10 min) =			229	mL/h × 10 min
	Infusion		0.33		5–10 mcg/ kg/min	300 mg/ 120 mL	2500	mcg/mL	___	
				Take dose you want in mcg ÷ by drug index number = mL/h on pump						
Brevibloc	Infusion		1.31		50–100 mcg/ kg/min	2.5 g/ 250 mL	10,000	mcg/mL	___	mL/h
				Take dose you want in mcg ÷ by drug index number = mL/h on pump						
Cardene	Infusion		___		0.5–10 mg/h	25 mg 250 mL	0.1	mg/mL	___	
				Ordered mg dose ÷ mg/mL = mL/h to set on pump					___	mL/h
Cardizem	0.25 mg/kg =	31.75 mg		Give mg/kg load over 20 min		50 mg/ 100 mL	0.5	mg/mL		
	mg to give ÷ mg/mL =	64 mL			63.5	mL × (60 min/h ÷ 20 min) =			191	mL/h
	0.35 mg/kg =	44.45 mg		May repeat loading dose in 15 min			0.5	mg/mL	___	
	mg to give ÷ mg/mL =	89 mL			88.9	mL × (60 min/h ÷ 20 min) =			267	mL/h
	Infusion				5–15 mg/h				___	
				Ordered mg dose ÷ mg/mL = mL/h to set on pump					___	mL/h
Desmopressin	0.3 mcg/kg =	38 mcg		Give dose over 20–30 min			4	mcg/vial		
Dobutamine	Infusion		0.26		2.5–40 mcg/kg/ min	250 mg/ 125 mL	2000	mcg/mL		
				Take dose you want in mcg ÷ by drug index number = mL/h on pump						

(continues)

127 kg (continued)

DRUG	ORDERED AMOUNT		TOTAL DOSE TO GIVE		DRUG INDEX NUMBER	DIRECTIONS	INFUSION RANGE	DRUG MIXTURE	AMOUNT	DRUG/mL	RUN AT	mL/h
Dopamine	Infusion				0.21		1–20 mcg/kg/min	400 mg/250 mL	1600	mcg/mL		
	Take dose you want in mcg ÷ by drug index number = mL/h on pump											
Epinephrine	Infusion		1 mcg/min = 4 mL/h 2 mcg/min = 8 mL/h 3 mcg/min = 11 mL/h 4 mcg/min = 15 mL/h				1–4 mcg/min	4 mg/250 mL	16	mcg/mL		
						Ordered mcg dose/min ÷ mcg/mL × 60 min/h =						___	mL/h
Fenoldapam	Infusion				0.0053		0.01–1.6 mcg/kg/min	10 mg/250 mL	40	mcg/mL		
	Take dose you want in mcg ÷ by drug index number = mL/h on pump											
Heparin	100 u/kg =	12,700 u										
	200 u/kg =	25,400 u										
	300 u/kg =	38,100 u										
	400 u/kg =	50,800 u										
Isoproterenol	Infusion						5 mcg/min	1 mg/250 mL	4	mcg/mL		
						Ordered mcg dose/min ÷ mcg/mL × 60 min/h =						75	mL/h
Lidocaine	Infusion		1 mg/min = 7.5 mL/h				1–4 mg/min	2 g/250 mL	8	mg/mL	___	
						Ordered mg/min ÷ mg/mL × 60 min/h =						___	mL/h
Nitroglycerin	Infusion		3 mcg/min = 1 mL/h				3–200 mcg/min	50 mg/250 mL	200	mcg/mL	___	
						Ordered mcg/min ÷ mcg/mL × 60 min/h =						___	mL/h
Nitroprusside	Infusion		6.7 mcg/min = 1 mL/h				5–300 mcg/min	100 mg/250 mL	400	mcg/mL	___	
						Ordered mcg/min ÷ mcg/mL × 60 min/h =						___	mL/h
Norepinephrine	Infusion		1 mcg/min = 4 mL/h 2 mcg/min = 8 mL/h 3 mcg/min = 11 mL/h 4 mcg/min = 15 mL/h 5 mcg/min = 19 mL/h				2–20 mcg/min	4 mg/250 mL	16	mcg/mL		
						Ordered mcg dose/min ÷ mcg/mL × 60 min/h =						___	mL/h
Phenylephrine	Infusion		1.3 mcg/min = 1 mL/h				10–200 mcg/min	20 mg/250 mL	80	mcg/mL		
						Ordered mcg/min ÷ mcg/mL × 60 min/h =						___	mL/h
Primacor	0.05 mg/kg =	6.35 mg				Give load over 10 min		40 mg/200 mL	0.2	mg/mL		
	mg to give ÷ mg/mL =	32 mL						32 mL × (60 min/h ÷ 10 min) =			191	mL/h × 10 min
	Infusion				0.03		0.5 mcg/kg/min	40 mg/200 mL	200	mcg/mL	___	
	Take dose you want in mcg ÷ by drug index number = mL/h on pump											
Trimethaphan	Infusion		___				0.3–6 mg/min	500 mg/500 mL	1	mg/mL	___	
						Ordered mg/min ÷ mg/mL × 60 min/h =						___	mL/h
Vasopressin			0.02 u/min = 3 mL/h 0.04 u/min = 6 mL/h					40 u/100 mL	400	u/mL		

128 kg

DRUG	ORDERED AMOUNT	TOTAL DOSE TO GIVE	DRUG INDEX NUMBER	DIRECTIONS	INFUSION RANGE	DRUG MIXTURE	AMOUNT	DRUG/mL	RUN AT	mL/h
Aminophylline	5 mg/kg = **640 mg**			Give mg/kg load over 20 min		500 mg/ 250 mL	2 mg/mL		
	mg to give ÷ mg/mL = **320 mL**				320	mL × (60 min/h ÷ 20 min) =			**960**	mL/h × 20 min
	Infusion				0.5–1 mg/kg/h	500 mg/ 250 mL	2 mg/mL		
						mg dose ordered × kg ÷ mg/mL =				___ mL/h
Amiodarone	Loading dose			Load **150 mg** over 10 min		900 mg/ 500 mL	1.8 mg/mL		___
				Ordered mg load dose (150 mg) ÷ mg/mL (1.8 mg/mL) = 83 mL to give × (60 min/h ÷ 10 min) = mL/h to set on pump					**500**	mL/h × 83 mL
	Infusion			Run at **1 mg/ min** × 6 h		900 mg/ 500 mL	1.8 mg/mL		
				Ordered mg dose (1 mg/min) ÷ mg/mL (1.8 mg/mL) = ___ × 60 min/h = mL/h to set on pump					**33**	mL/h × 6 h
	Infusion			Run at **0.5 mg/ min** × 18 h		900 mg/ 500 mL	1.8 mg/mL		
				Ordered mg dose (0.5 mg/min) ÷ mg/mL (1.8 mg/mL) = ___ × 60 min/h = mL/h to set on pump					**17**	mL/h × 18 h
Amrinone	0.75 mg/kg = **96 mg**			Give mg/kg load over 10 min		300 mg/ 120 mL	2.5 mg/mL		___
	mg to give ÷ mg/mL = **38 mL**				38.4	mL × (60 min/h ÷ 10 min) =			**230**	mL/h × 10 min
	Infusion		0.33		5–10 mcg/ kg/min	300 mg/ 120 mL	2500 mcg/mL		___
				Take dose you want in mcg ÷ by drug index number = mL/h on pump						
Brevibloc	Infusion		1.30		50–100 mcg/ kg/min	2.5 g/ 250 mL	10,000 mcg/mL		___ mL/h
				Take dose you want in mcg ÷ by drug index number = mL/h on pump						
Cardene	Infusion		___		0.5–10 mg/h	25 mg 250 mL	0.1 mg/mL		___
				Ordered mg dose ÷ mg/mL = mL/h to set on pump						___ mL/h
Cardizem	0.25 mg/kg = **32 mg**			Give mg/kg load over 20 min		50 mg/ 100 mL	0.5 mg/mL		___
	mg to give ÷ mg/mL = **64 mL**				64	mL × (60 min/h ÷ 20 min) =			**192**	mL/h
	0.35 mg/kg = **44.8 mg**			May repeat loading dose in 15 min			0.5 mg/mL		___
	mg to give ÷ mg/mL = **90 mL**				89.6	mL × (60 min/h ÷ 20 min) =			**269**	mL/h
	Infusion				5–15 mg/h				___
				Ordered mg dose ÷ mg/mL = mL/h to set on pump						___ mL/h
Desmopressin	0.3 mcg/kg = **38 mcg**			Give dose over 20–30 min			4 mcg/vial		
Dobutamine	Infusion		0.26		2.5–40 mcg/kg/ min	250 mg/ 125 mL	2000 mcg/mL		
				Take dose you want in mcg ÷ by drug index number = mL/h on pump						

(continues)

128 kg (continued)

DRUG	ORDERED AMOUNT	TOTAL DOSE TO GIVE	DRUG INDEX NUMBER	DIRECTIONS	INFUSION RANGE	DRUG MIXTURE	AMOUNT	DRUG/ mL	RUN AT	mL/h
Dopamine	Infusion		0.21		1–20 mcg/ kg/min	400 mg/ 250 mL	1600	mcg/mL		
	Take dose you want in mcg ÷ by drug index number = mL/h on pump									
Epinephrine	Infusion	1 mcg/min = 4 mL/h 2 mcg/min = 8 mL/h 3 mcg/min = 11 mL/h 4 mcg/min = 15 mL/h			1–4 mcg/min	4 mg/ 250 mL	16	mcg/mL		
		Ordered mcg dose/min ÷ mcg/mL × 60 min/h =								___	mL/h
Fenoldapam	Infusion		0.0052		0.01–1.6 mcg/ kg/min	10 mg/ 250 mL	40	mcg/mL		
	Take dose you want in mcg ÷ by drug index number = mL/h on pump									
Heparin	100 u/kg = 12,800 u 200 u/kg = 25,600 u 300 u/kg = 38,400 u 400 u/kg = 51,200 u									
Isoproterenol	Infusion				5 mcg/min	1 mg/ 250 mL	4	mcg/mL		
		Ordered mcg dose/min ÷ mcg/mL × 60 min/h =								75	mL/h
Lidocaine	Infusion	1 mg/min = 7.5 mL/h			1–4 mg/min	2 g/ 250 mL	8	mg/mL	___	
		Ordered mg/min ÷ mg/mL × 60 min/h =								___	mL/h
Nitroglycerin	Infusion	3 mcg/min = 1 mL/h			3–200 mcg/min	50 mg/ 250 mL	200	mcg/mL	___	
		Ordered mcg/min ÷ mcg/mL × 60 min/h =								___	mL/h
Nitroprusside	Infusion	6.7 mcg/min = 1 mL/h			5–300 mcg/min	100 mg/ 250 mL	400	mcg/mL	___	
		Ordered mcg/min ÷ mcg/mL × 60 min/h =								___	mL/h
Norepinephrine	Infusion	1 mcg/min = 4 mL/h 2 mcg/min = 8 mL/h 3 mcg/min = 11 mL/h 4 mcg/min = 15 mL/h 5 mcg/min = 19 mL/h			2–20 mcg/min	4 mg/ 250 mL	16	mcg/mL		
		Ordered mcg dose/min ÷ mcg/mL × 60 min/h =								___	mL/h
Phenylephrine	Infusion	1.3 mcg/min = 1 mL/h			10–200 mcg/min	20 mg/ 250 mL	80	mcg/mL		
		Ordered mcg/min ÷ mcg/mL × 60 min/h =								___	mL/h
Primacor	0.05 mg/kg = 6.4 mg			Give load over 10 min		40 mg/ 200 mL	0.2	mg/mL		
	mg to give ÷ mg/mL =	32 mL			32	mL × (60 min/h ÷ 10 min) =			192	mL/h × 10 min
	Infusion		0.03		0.5 mcg/ kg/min	40 mg/ 200 mL	200	mcg/mL	___	
	Take dose you want in mcg ÷ by drug index number = mL/h on pump									
Trimethaphan	Infusion	—			0.3–6 mg/min	500 mg/ 500 mL	1	mg/mL	___	
		Ordered mg/min ÷ mg/mL × 60 min/h =								___	mL/h
Vasopressin		0.02 u/min = 3 mL/h 0.04 u/min = 6 mL/h				40 u/ 100 mL	400	u/mL		

129 kg

DRUG	ORDERED AMOUNT	TOTAL DOSE TO GIVE	DRUG INDEX NUMBER	DIRECTIONS	INFUSION RANGE	DRUG MIXTURE	AMOUNT	DRUG/ mL	RUN AT	mL/h
Aminophylline	5 mg/kg =	**645** mg		Give mg/kg load over 20 min		500 mg/ 250 mL	2 mg/mL			
	mg to give ÷ mg/mL =	**323** mL			**323**	mL × (60 min/h ÷ 20 min) =			**968**	mL/h × 20 min
	Infusion				0.5–1 mg/kg/h	500 mg/ 250 mL	2 mg/mL			
						mg dose ordered × kg ÷ mg/mL =			___	mL/h
Amiodarone	Loading dose			Load **150 mg** over 10 min		900 mg/ 500 mL	1.8 mg/mL		___	
				Ordered mg load dose (150 mg) ÷ mg/mL (1.8 mg/mL) = 83 mL to give × (60 min/h ÷ 10 min) = mL/h to set on pump					**500**	mL/h × 83 mL
	Infusion			Run at **1 mg/ min** × 6 h		900 mg/ 500 mL	1.8 mg/mL			
				Ordered mg dose (1 mg/min) ÷ mg/mL (1.8 mg/mL) = ____ × 60 min/h = mL/h to set on pump					**33**	mL/h × 6 h
	Infusion			Run at **0.5 mg/ min** × 18 h		900 mg/ 500 mL	1.8 mg/mL			
				Ordered mg dose (0.5 mg/min) ÷ mg/mL (1.8 mg/mL) = ____ × 60 min/h = mL/h to set on pump					**17**	mL/h × 18 h
Amrinone	0.75 mg/kg =	**96.75** mg		Give mg/kg load over 10 min		300 mg/ 120 mL	2.5 mg/mL		___	
	mg to give ÷ mg/mL =	**39** mL			**38.7**	mL × (60 min/h ÷ 10 min) =			**232**	mL/h × 10 min
	Infusion		**0.32**		5–10 mcg/ kg/min	300 mg/ 120 mL	2500 mcg/mL			
				Take dose you want in mcg ÷ by drug index number = mL/h on pump						
Brevibloc	Infusion		**1.29**		50–100 mcg/ kg/min	2.5 g/ 250 mL	10,000 mcg/mL		___	mL/h
				Take dose you want in mcg ÷ by drug index number = mL/h on pump						
Cardene	Infusion		___		0.5–10 mg/h	25 mg 250 mL	0.1 mg/mL		___	
				Ordered mg dose ÷ mg/mL = mL/h to set on pump					___	mL/h
Cardizem	0.25 mg/kg =	**32.25** mg		Give mg/kg load over 20 min		50 mg/ 100 mL	0.5 mg/mL		___	
	mg to give ÷ mg/mL =	**65** mL			**64.5**	mL × (60 min/h ÷ 20 min) =			**194**	mL/h
	0.35 mg/kg =	**45.15** mg		May repeat loading dose in 15 min			0.5 mg/mL			
	mg to give ÷ mg/mL =	**90** mL			**90.3**	mL × (60 min/h ÷ 20 min) =			**271**	mL/h
	Infusion				5–15 mg/h				___	
				Ordered mg dose ÷ mg/mL = mL/h to set on pump					___	mL/h
Desmopressin	0.3 mcg/kg =	**39** mcg		Give dose over 20–30 min			4 mcg/vial			
Dobutamine	Infusion		**0.26**		2.5–40 mcg/kg/ min	250 mg/ 125 mL	2000 mcg/mL			
				Take dose you want in mcg ÷ by drug index number = mL/h on pump						

(continues)

129 kg (continued)

DRUG	ORDERED AMOUNT	TOTAL DOSE TO GIVE	DRUG INDEX NUMBER	DIRECTIONS	INFUSION RANGE	DRUG MIXTURE	AMOUNT	DRUG/mL	RUN AT	mL/h
Dopamine	Infusion		0.21		1–20 mcg/kg/min	400 mg/250 mL	1600	mcg/mL		
			Take dose you want in mcg ÷ by drug index number = mL/h on pump							
Epinephrine	Infusion	1 mcg/min = 4 mL/h 2 mcg/min = 8 mL/h 3 mcg/min = 11 mL/h 4 mcg/min = 15 mL/h			1–4 mcg/min	4 mg/250 mL	16	mcg/mL		
					Ordered mcg dose/min ÷ mcg/mL × 60 min/h =				___	mL/h
Fenoldapam	Infusion		0.0052		0.01–1.6 mcg/kg/min	10 mg/250 mL	40	mcg/mL		
			Take dose you want in mcg ÷ by drug index number = mL/h on pump							
Heparin	100 u/kg = 12,900 u 200 u/kg = 25,800 u 300 u/kg = 38,700 u 400 u/kg = 51,600 u									
Isoproterenol	Infusion				5 mcg/min	1 mg/250 mL	4	mcg/mL		
					Ordered mcg dose/min ÷ mcg/mL × 60 min/h =				75	mL/h
Lidocaine	Infusion	1 mg/min = 7.5 mL/h			1–4 mg/min	2 g/250 mL	8	mg/mL	___	
					Ordered mg/min ÷ mg/mL × 60 min/h =				___	mL/h
Nitroglycerin	Infusion	3 mcg/min = 1 mL/h			3–200 mcg/min	50 mg/250 mL	200	mcg/mL	___	
					Ordered mcg/min ÷ mcg/mL × 60 min/h =				___	mL/h
Nitroprusside	Infusion	6.7 mcg/min = 1 mL/h			5–300 mcg/min	100 mg/250 mL	400	mcg/mL	___	
					Ordered mcg/min ÷ mcg/mL × 60 min/h =				___	mL/h
Norepinephrine	Infusion	1 mcg/min = 4 mL/h 2 mcg/min = 8 mL/h 3 mcg/min = 11 mL/h 4 mcg/min = 15 mL/h 5 mcg/min = 19 mL/h			2–20 mcg/min	4 mg/250 mL	16	mcg/mL		
					Ordered mcg dose/min ÷ mcg/mL × 60 min/h =				___	mL/h
Phenylephrine	Infusion	1.3 mcg/min = 1 mL/h			10–200 mcg/min	20 mg/250 mL	80	mcg/mL	___	
					Ordered mcg/min ÷ mcg/mL × 60 min/h =				___	mL/h
Primacor	0.05 mg/kg = 6.45 mg			Give load over 10 min		40 mg/200 mL	0.2	mg/mL		
	mg to give ÷ mg/mL = 32 mL					32 mL × (60 min/h ÷ 10 min) =			194	mL/h × 10 min
	Infusion		0.03		0.5 mcg/kg/min	40 mg/200 mL	200	mcg/mL	___	
			Take dose you want in mcg ÷ by drug index number = mL/h on pump							
Trimethaphan	Infusion	—			0.3–6 mg/min	500 mg/500 mL	1	mg/mL	___	
					Ordered mg/min ÷ mg/mL × 60 min/h =				___	mL/h
Vasopressin		0.02 u/min = 3 mL/h 0.04 u/min = 6 mL/h				40 u/100 mL	400	u/mL		

130 kg

DRUG	ORDERED AMOUNT	TOTAL DOSE TO GIVE	DRUG INDEX NUMBER	DIRECTIONS	INFUSION RANGE	DRUG MIXTURE	AMOUNT	DRUG/mL	RUN AT	mL/h
Aminophylline	5 mg/kg =	650 mg		Give mg/kg load over 20 min		500 mg/250 mL		2 mg/mL		
	mg to give ÷ mg/mL =	325 mL			325	mL × (60 min/h ÷ 20 min) =			975	mL/h × 20 min
	Infusion				0.5–1 mg/kg/h	500 mg/250 mL		2 mg/mL		
				mg dose ordered × kg ÷ mg/mL =					___	mL/h
Amiodarone	Loading dose			Load **150 mg** over 10 min		900 mg/500 mL		1.8 mg/mL	___	
				Ordered mg load dose (150 mg) ÷ mg/mL (1.8 mg/mL) = 83 mL to give × (60 min/h ÷ 10 min) = mL/h to set on pump					500	mL/h × 83 mL
	Infusion			Run at **1 mg/min** × 6 h		900 mg/500 mL		1.8 mg/mL		
				Ordered mg dose (1 mg/min) ÷ mg/mL (1.8 mg/mL) = ____ × 60 min/h = mL/h to set on pump					33	mL/h × 6 h
	Infusion			Run at **0.5 mg/min** × 18 h		900 mg/500 mL		1.8 mg/mL		
				Ordered mg dose (0.5 mg/min) ÷ mg/mL (1.8 mg/mL) = ____ × 60 min/h = mL/h to set on pump					17	mL/h × 18 h
Amrinone	0.75 mg/kg =	97.5 mg		Give mg/kg load over 10 min		300 mg/120 mL		2.5 mg/mL	___	
	mg to give ÷ mg/mL =	39 mL			39	mL × (60 min/h ÷ 10 min) =			234	mL/h × 10 min
	Infusion		0.32		5–10 mcg/kg/min	300 mg/120 mL	2500 mcg/mL		___	
				Take dose you want in mcg ÷ by drug index number = mL/h on pump						
Brevibloc	Infusion		1.28		50–100 mcg/kg/min	2.5 g/250 mL	10,000 mcg/mL		___	mL/h
				Take dose you want in mcg ÷ by drug index number = mL/h on pump						
Cardene	Infusion			—	0.5–10 mg/h	25 mg/250 mL		0.1 mg/mL	___	
				Ordered mg dose ÷ mg/mL = mL/h to set on pump					___	mL/h
Cardizem	0.25 mg/kg =	32.5 mg		Give mg/kg load over 20 min		50 mg/100 mL		0.5 drug/mL		
	mg to give ÷ mg/mL =	65 mL			65	mL × (60 min/h ÷ 20 min) =			195	mL/h
	0.35 mg/kg =	45.5 mg		May repeat loading dose in 15 min				0.5 mg/mL		
	mg to give ÷ mg/mL =	91 mL			91	mL × (60 min/h ÷ 20 min) =			273	mL/h
	Infusion				5–15 mg/h				___	
				Ordered mg dose ÷ mg/mL = mL/h to set on pump					___	mL/h
Desmopressin	0.3 mcg/kg =	39 mcg		Give dose over 20–30 min			4 mcg/vial			
Dobutamine	Infusion		0.26		2.5–40 mcg/kg/min	250 mg/125 mL	2000 mcg/mL			
				Take dose you want in mcg ÷ by drug index number = mL/h on pump						

(continues)

130 kg (continued)

DRUG	ORDERED AMOUNT	TOTAL DOSE TO GIVE	DRUG INDEX NUMBER	DIRECTIONS	INFUSION RANGE	DRUG MIXTURE	AMOUNT	DRUG/ mL	RUN AT	mL/h
Dopamine	Infusion		0.21		1–20 mcg/ kg/min	400 mg/ 250 mL	1600	mcg/mL		
				Take dose you want in mcg ÷ by drug index number = mL/h on pump						
Epinephrine	Infusion	1 mcg/min = 4 mL/h 2 mcg/min = 8 mL/h 3 mcg/min = 11 mL/h 4 mcg/min = 15 mL/h			1–4 mcg/min	4 mg/ 250 mL	16	mcg/mL		
		Ordered mcg dose/min ÷ mcg/mL × 60 min/h =							___	mL/h
Fenoldapam	Infusion		0.0052		0.01–1.6 mcg/ kg/min	10 mg/ 250 mL	40	mcg/mL		
		Take dose you want in mcg ÷ by drug index number = mL/h on pump								
Heparin	100 u/kg =	13,000 u 26,000 u 39,000 u 52,000 u								
	200 u/kg =									
	300 u/kg =									
	400 u/kg =									
Isoproterenol	Infusion				5 mcg/min	1 mg/ 250 mL	4	mcg/mL		
		Ordered mcg dose/min ÷ mcg/mL × 60 min/h =							75	mL/h
Lidocaine	Infusion	1 mg/min = 7.5 mL/h			1–4 mg/min	2 g/ 250 mL	8	mg/mL		___
		Ordered mg/min ÷ mg/mL × 60 min/h =							___	mL/h
Nitroglycerin	Infusion	3 mcg/min = 1 mL/h			3–200 mcg/min	50 mg/ 250 mL	200	mcg/mL		___
		Ordered mcg/min ÷ mcg/mL × 60 min/h =							___	mL/h
Nitroprusside	Infusion	6.7 mcg/min = 1 mL/h			5–300 mcg/min	100 mg/ 250 mL	400	mcg/mL		___
		Ordered mcg/min ÷ mcg/mL × 60 min/h =							___	mL/h
Norepinephrine	Infusion	1 mcg/min = 4 mL/h 2 mcg/min = 8 mL/h 3 mcg/min = 11 mL/h 4 mcg/min = 15 mL/h 5 mcg/min = 19 mL/h			2–20 mcg/min	4 mg/ 250 mL	16	mcg/mL		
		Ordered mcg dose/min ÷ mcg/mL × 60 min/h =							___	mL/h
Phenylephrine	Infusion	1.3 mcg/min = 1 mL/h			10–200 mcg/min	20 mg/ 250 mL	80	mcg/mL		
		Ordered mcg/min ÷ mcg/mL × 60 min/h =							___	mL/h
Primacor	0.05 mg/kg =	6.5 mg		Give load over 10 min		40 mg/ 200 mL	0.2	mg/mL		
	mg to give ÷ mg/mL =	33 mL			33	mL × (60 min/h ÷ 10 min) =			195	mL/h × 10 min
	Infusion		0.03		0.5 mcg/ kg/min	40 mg/ 200 mL	200	mcg/mL		___
		Take dose you want in mcg ÷ by drug index number = mL/h on pump								
Trimethaphan	Infusion		—		0.3–6 mg/min	500 mg/ 500 mL	1	mg/mL		___
		Ordered mg/min ÷ mg/mL × 60 min/h =							___	mL/h
Vasopressin		0.02 u/min = 3 mL/h 0.04 u/min = 6 mL/h				40 u/ 100 mL	400	u/mL		

131 kg

DRUG	ORDERED AMOUNT	TOTAL DOSE TO GIVE	DRUG INDEX NUMBER	DIRECTIONS	INFUSION RANGE	DRUG MIXTURE	AMOUNT	DRUG/ mL	RUN AT	mL/h
Aminophylline	5 mg/kg =	655 mg		Give mg/kg load over 20 min		500 mg/ 250 mL	2 mg/mL			
	mg to give ÷ mg/mL =	328 mL			328	mL × (60 min/h ÷ 20 min) =			**983**	mL/h × 20 min
	Infusion				0.5–1 mg/kg/h	500 mg/ 250 mL	2 mg/mL			
					mg dose ordered × kg ÷ mg/mL =				___	mL/h
Amiodarone	Loading dose			Load **150 mg** over 10 min		900 mg/ 500 mL	1.8 mg/mL		—	
				Ordered mg load dose (150 mg) ÷ mg/mL (1.8 mg/mL) = 83 mL to give × (60 min/h ÷ 10 min) = mL/h to set on pump					**500**	mL/h × 83 mL
	Infusion			Run at **1 mg/ min** × 6 h		900 mg/ 500 mL	1.8 mg/mL			
				Ordered mg dose (1 mg/min) ÷ mg/mL (1.8 mg/mL) = _____ × 60 min/h = mL/h to set on pump					**33**	mL/h × 6 h
	Infusion			Run at **0.5 mg/ min** × 18 h		900 mg/ 500 mL	1.8 mg/mL			
				Ordered mg dose (0.5 mg/min) ÷ mg/mL (1.8 mg/mL) = _____ × 60 min/h = mL/h to set on pump					**17**	mL/h × 18 h
Amrinone	0.75 mg/kg =	98.25 mg		Give mg/kg load over 10 min		300 mg/ 120 mL	2.5 mg/mL		—	
	mg to give ÷ mg/mL =	39 mL			39.3	mL × (60 min/h ÷ 10 min) =			**236**	mL/h × 10 min
	Infusion		0.32		5–10 mcg/ kg/min	300 mg/ 120 mL	2500 mcg/mL		—	
				Take dose you want in mcg ÷ by drug index number = mL/h on pump						
Brevibloc	Infusion		1.27		50–100 mcg/ kg/min	2.5 g/ 250 mL	10,000 mcg/mL		___	mL/h
				Take dose you want in mcg ÷ by drug index number = mL/h on pump						
Cardene	Infusion		—		0.5–10 mg/h	25 mg 250 mL	0.1 mg/mL		—	
				Ordered mg dose ÷ mg/mL = mL/h to set on pump					___	mL/h
Cardizem	0.25 mg/kg =	32.75 mg		Give mg/kg load over 20 min		50 mg/ 100 mL	0.5 mg/mL		—	
	mg to give ÷ mg/mL =	66 mL			65.5	mL × (60 min/h ÷ 20 min) =			**197**	mL/h
	0.35 mg/kg =	45.85 mg		May repeat loading dose in 15 min			0.5 mg/mL		—	
	mg to give ÷ mg/mL =	92 mL			91.7	mL × (60 min/h ÷ 20 min) =			**275**	mL/h
	Infusion				5–15 mg/h				—	
				Ordered mg dose ÷ mg/mL = mL/h to set on pump					___	mL/h
Desmopressin	0.3 mcg/kg =	39 mcg		Give dose over 20–30 min			4 mcg/vial			
Dobutamine	Infusion		0.25		2.5–40 mcg/kg/ min	250 mg/ 125 mL	2000 mcg/mL			
				Take dose you want in mcg ÷ by drug index number = mL/h on pump						

(continues)

131   kg (continued)

DRUG	ORDERED AMOUNT	TOTAL DOSE TO GIVE	DRUG INDEX NUMBER	DIRECTIONS	INFUSION RANGE	DRUG MIXTURE	AMOUNT	DRUG/mL	RUN AT	mL/h
Dopamine	Infusion		0.20		1–20 mcg/kg/min	400 mg/250 mL	1600	mcg/mL		
	Take dose you want in mcg ÷ by drug index number = mL/h on pump									
Epinephrine	Infusion	1 mcg/min = 4 mL/h 2 mcg/min = 8 mL/h 3 mcg/min = 11 mL/h 4 mcg/min = 15 mL/h			1–4 mcg/min	4 mg/250 mL	16	mcg/mL		
		Ordered mcg dose/min ÷ mcg/mL × 60 min/h =							___	mL/h
Fenoldapam	Infusion		0.0051		0.01–1.6 mcg/kg/min	10 mg/250 mL	40	mcg/mL		
	Take dose you want in mcg ÷ by drug index number = mL/h on pump									
Heparin	100 u/kg =	13,100 u								
	200 u/kg =	26,200 u								
	300 u/kg =	39,300 u								
	400 u/kg =	52,400 u								
Isoproterenol	Infusion				5 mcg/min	1 mg/250 mL	4	mcg/mL		
		Ordered mcg dose/min ÷ mcg/mL × 60 min/h =							75	mL/h
Lidocaine	Infusion	1 mg/min = 7.5 mL/h			1–4 mg/min	2 g/250 mL	8	mg/mL	___	
		Ordered mg/min ÷ mg/mL × 60 min/h =							___	mL/h
Nitroglycerin	Infusion	3 mcg/min = 1 mL/h			3–200 mcg/min	50 mg/250 mL	200	mcg/mL	___	
		Ordered mcg/min ÷ mcg/mL × 60 min/h =							___	mL/h
Nitroprusside	Infusion	6.7 mcg/min = 1 mL/h			5–300 mcg/min	100 mg/250 mL	400	mcg/mL	___	
		Ordered mcg/min ÷ mcg/mL × 60 min/h =							___	mL/h
Norepinephrine	Infusion	1 mcg/min = 4 mL/h 2 mcg/min = 8 mL/h 3 mcg/min = 11 mL/h 4 mcg/min = 15 mL/h 5 mcg/min = 19 mL/h			2–20 mcg/min	4 mg/250 mL	16	mcg/mL		
		Ordered mcg dose/min ÷ mcg/mL × 60 min/h =							___	mL/h
Phenylephrine	Infusion	1.3 mcg/min = 1 mL/h			10–200 mcg/min	20 mg/250 mL	80	mcg/mL		
		Ordered mcg/min ÷ mcg/mL × 60 min/h =							___	mL/h
Primacor	0.05 mg/kg =	6.55 mg		Give load over 10 min		40 mg/200 mL	0.2	mg/mL		
	mg to give ÷ mg/mL =	33 mL			33 mL × (60 min/h ÷ 10 min) =				197	mL/h × 10 min
	Infusion		0.03		0.5 mcg/kg/min	40 mg/200 mL	200	mcg/mL	___	
	Take dose you want in mcg ÷ by drug index number = mL/h on pump									
Trimethaphan	Infusion	___			0.3–6 mg/min	500 mg/500 mL	1	mg/mL	___	
		Ordered mg/min ÷ mg/mL × 60 min/h =							___	mL/h
Vasopressin		0.02 u/min = 3 mL/h 0.04 u/min = 6 mL/h				40 u/100 mL	400	u/mL		

132 kg

DRUG	ORDERED AMOUNT	TOTAL DOSE TO GIVE	DRUG INDEX NUMBER	DIRECTIONS	INFUSION RANGE	DRUG MIXTURE	AMOUNT	DRUG/mL	RUN AT	mL/h
Aminophylline	5 mg/kg =	660 mg		Give mg/kg load over 20 min		500 mg/ 250 mL	2 mg/mL		
	mg to give ÷ mg/mL =	330 mL				330	mL × (60 min/h ÷ 20 min) =		990	mL/h × 20 min
	Infusion				0.5–1 mg/kg/h	500 mg/ 250 mL	2 mg/mL		
						mg dose ordered × kg ÷ mg/mL =			___ mL/h
Amiodarone	Loading dose			Load **150 mg** over 10 min		900 mg/ 500 mL	1.8 mg/mL	___
				Ordered mg load dose (150 mg) ÷ mg/mL (1.8 mg/mL) = 83 mL to give × (60 min/h ÷ 10 min) = mL/h to set on pump					500	mL/h × 83 mL
	Infusion			Run at **1 mg/ min** × 6 h		900 mg/ 500 mL	1.8 mg/mL		
				Ordered mg dose (1 mg/min) ÷ mg/mL (1.8 mg/mL) = ____ × 60 min/h = mL/h to set on pump					33	mL/h × 6 h
	Infusion			Run at **0.5 mg/ min** × 18 h		900 mg/ 500 mL	1.8 mg/mL		
				Ordered mg dose (0.5 mg/min) ÷ mg/mL (1.8 mg/mL) = ____ × 60 min/h = mL/h to set on pump					17	mL/h × 18 h
Amrinone	0.75 mg/kg =	99 mg		Give mg/kg load over 10 min		300 mg/ 120 mL	2.5 mg/mL	___
	mg to give ÷ mg/mL =	40 mL				39.6	mL × (60 min/h ÷ 10 min) =		238	mL/h × 10 min
	Infusion		0.32		5–10 mcg/ kg/min	300 mg/ 120 mL	2500 mcg/mL	___
				Take dose you want in mcg ÷ by drug index number = mL/h on pump					
Brevibloc	Infusion		1.26		50–100 mcg/ kg/min	2.5 g/ 250 mL	10,000 mcg/mL	___ mL/h
				Take dose you want in mcg ÷ by drug index number = mL/h on pump					
Cardene	Infusion		—		0.5–10 mg/h	25 mg 250 mL	0.1 mg/mL	___
				Ordered mg dose ÷ mg/mL = mL/h to set on pump					___ mL/h
Cardizem	0.25 mg/kg =	33 mg		Give mg/kg load over 20 min		50 mg/ 100 mL	0.5 mg/mL	___
	mg to give ÷ mg/mL =	66 mL				66	mL × (60 min/h ÷ 20 min) =		198	mL/h
	0.35 mg/kg =	46.2 mg		May repeat loading dose in 15 min			0.5 mg/mL	___
	mg to give ÷ mg/mL =	92 mL				92.4	mL × (60 min/h ÷ 20 min) =		277	mL/h
	Infusion				5–15 mg/h				
				Ordered mg dose ÷ mg/mL = mL/h to set on pump					___ mL/h
Desmopressin	0.3 mcg/kg =	40 mcg		Give dose over 20–30 min			4 mcg/vial	
Dobutamine	Infusion		0.25		2.5–40 mcg/kg/ min	250 mg/ 125 mL	2000 mcg/mL	
				Take dose you want in mcg ÷ by drug index number = mL/h on pump					

(continues)

132 kg (continued)

DRUG	ORDERED AMOUNT	TOTAL DOSE TO GIVE	DRUG INDEX NUMBER	DIRECTIONS	INFUSION RANGE	DRUG MIXTURE	AMOUNT	DRUG/ mL	RUN AT	mL/h
Dopamine	Infusion		0.20		1–20 mcg/ kg/min	400 mg/ 250 mL	1600	mcg/mL		
	Take dose you want in mcg ÷ by drug index number = mL/h on pump									
Epinephrine	Infusion	1 mcg/min = 4 mL/h 2 mcg/min = 8 mL/h 3 mcg/min = 11 mL/h 4 mcg/min = 15 mL/h			1–4 mcg/min	4 mg/ 250 mL	16	mcg/mL		
		Ordered mcg dose/min ÷ mcg/mL × 60 min/h =								___	mL/h
Fenoldapam	Infusion		0.0051		0.01–1.6 mcg/ kg/min	10 mg/ 250 mL	40	mcg/mL		
	Take dose you want in mcg ÷ by drug index number = mL/h on pump									
Heparin	100 u/kg = 13,200 u 200 u/kg = 26,400 u 300 u/kg = 39,600 u 400 u/kg = 52,800 u									
Isoproterenol	Infusion				5 mcg/min	1 mg/ 250 mL	4	mcg/mL		
		Ordered mcg dose/min ÷ mcg/mL × 60 min/h =								**75**	mL/h
Lidocaine	Infusion	1 mg/min = 7.5 mL/h			1–4 mg/min	2 g/ 250 mL	8	mg/mL		___
		Ordered mg/min ÷ mg/mL × 60 min/h =								___	mL/h
Nitroglycerin	Infusion	3 mcg/min = 1 mL/h			3–200 mcg/min	50 mg/ 250 mL	200	mcg/mL		___
		Ordered mcg/min ÷ mcg/mL × 60 min/h =								___	mL/h
Nitroprusside	Infusion	6.7 mcg/min = 1 mL/h			5–300 mcg/min	100 mg/ 250 mL	400	mcg/mL		___
		Ordered mcg/min ÷ mcg/mL × 60 min/h =								___	mL/h
Norepinephrine	Infusion	1 mcg/min = 4 mL/h 2 mcg/min = 8 mL/h 3 mcg/min = 11 mL/h 4 mcg/min = 15 mL/h 5 mcg/min = 19 mL/h			2–20 mcg/min	4 mg/ 250 mL	16	mcg/mL		
		Ordered mcg dose/min ÷ mcg/mL × 60 min/h =								___	mL/h
Phenylephrine	Infusion	1.3 mcg/min = 1 mL/h			10–200 mcg/min	20 mg/ 250 mL	80	mcg/mL		
		Ordered mcg/min ÷ mcg/mL × 60 min/h =								___	mL/h
Primacor	0.05 mg/kg = 6.6 mg			Give load over 10 min		40 mg/ 200 mL	0.2	mg/mL		
	mg to give ÷ mg/mL = 33 mL					33	mL × (60 min/h ÷ 10 min) =		**198**	mL/h × 10 min
	Infusion		0.03		0.5 mcg/ kg/min	40 mg/ 200 mL	200	mcg/mL		___
	Take dose you want in mcg ÷ by drug index number = mL/h on pump									
Trimethaphan	Infusion		—		0.3–6 mg/min	500 mg/ 500 mL	1	mg/mL		___
		Ordered mg/min ÷ mg/mL × 60 min/h =								___	mL/h
Vasopressin		0.02 u/min = 3 mL/h 0.04 u/min = 6 mL/h				40 u/ 100 mL	400	u/mL		

133 kg

DRUG	ORDERED AMOUNT	TOTAL DOSE TO GIVE	DRUG INDEX NUMBER	DIRECTIONS	INFUSION RANGE	DRUG MIXTURE	AMOUNT	DRUG/mL	RUN AT / mL/h
Aminophylline	5 mg/kg = 665 mg			Give mg/kg load over 20 min		500 mg/ 250 mL		2 mg/mL	
	mg to give ÷ mg/mL = 333 mL				333	mL × (60 min/h ÷ 20 min) =			998 mL/h × 20 min
	Infusion				0.5–1 mg/kg/h	500 mg/ 250 mL		2 mg/mL	
				mg dose ordered × kg ÷ mg/mL =					___ mL/h
Amiodarone	Loading dose			Load **150 mg** over 10 min		900 mg/ 500 mL		1.8 mg/mL	___
				Ordered mg load dose (150 mg) ÷ mg/mL (1.8 mg/mL) = 83 mL to give × (60 min/h ÷ 10 min) = mL/h to set on pump					500 mL/h × 83 mL
	Infusion			Run at **1 mg/ min** × 6 h		900 mg/ 500 mL		1.8 mg/mL	
				Ordered mg dose (1 mg/min) ÷ mg/mL (1.8 mg/mL) = _____ × 60 min/h = mL/h to set on pump					33 mL/h × 6 h
	Infusion			Run at **0.5 mg/ min** × 18 h		900 mg/ 500 mL		1.8 mg/mL	
				Ordered mg dose (0.5 mg/min) ÷ mg/mL (1.8 mg/mL) = _____ × 60 min/h = mL/h to set on pump					17 mL/h × 18 h
Amrinone	0.75 mg/kg = 99.75 mg			Give mg/kg load over 10 min		300 mg/ 120 mL		2.5 mg/mL	___
	mg to give ÷ mg/mL = 40 mL				39.9	mL × (60 min/h ÷ 10 min) =			239 mL/h × 10 min
	Infusion		0.31		5–10 mcg/ kg/min	300 mg/ 120 mL		2500 mcg/mL	___
				Take dose you want in mcg ÷ by drug index number = mL/h on pump					
Brevibloc	Infusion		1.25		50–100 mcg/ kg/min	2.5 g/ 250 mL		10,000 mcg/mL	___ mL/h
				Take dose you want in mcg ÷ by drug index number = mL/h on pump					
Cardene	Infusion		___		0.5–10 mg/h	25 mg 250 mL		0.1 mg/mL	___
				Ordered mg dose ÷ mg/mL = mL/h to set on pump					___ mL/h
Cardizem	0.25 mg/kg = 33.25 mg			Give mg/kg load over 20 min		50 mg/ 100 mL		0.5 mg/mL	
	mg to give ÷ mg/mL = 67 mL				66.5	mL × (60 min/h ÷ 20 min) =			200 mL/h
	0.35 mg/kg = 46.55 mg			May repeat loading dose in 15 min				0.5 mg/mL	___
	mg to give ÷ mg/mL = 93 mL				93.1	mL × (60 min/h ÷ 20 min) =			279 mL/h
	Infusion				5–15 mg/h				___
				Ordered mg dose ÷ mg/mL = mL/h to set on pump					___ mL/h
Desmopressin	0.3 mcg/kg = 40 mcg			Give dose over 20–30 min				4 mcg/vial	
Dobutamine	Infusion		0.25		2.5–40 mcg/kg/ min	250 mg/ 125 mL		2000 mcg/mL	
				Take dose you want in mcg ÷ by drug index number = mL/h on pump					

(continues)

133 kg (continued)

DRUG	ORDERED AMOUNT	TOTAL DOSE TO GIVE	DRUG INDEX NUMBER	DIRECTIONS	INFUSION RANGE	DRUG MIXTURE	AMOUNT	DRUG/ mL	RUN AT	mL/h
Dopamine	Infusion		**0.20**		1–20 mcg/ kg/min	400 mg/ 250 mL	1600	mcg/mL		
	Take dose you want in mcg ÷ by drug index number = mL/h on pump									
Epinephrine	Infusion	1 mcg/min = 4 mL/h 2 mcg/min = 8 mL/h 3 mcg/min = 11 mL/h 4 mcg/min = 15 mL/h			1–4 mcg/min	4 mg/ 250 mL	16	mcg/mL		
		Ordered mcg dose/min ÷ mcg/mL × 60 min/h = ___ mL/h								
Fenoldapam	Infusion		**0.0050**		0.01–1.6 mcg/ kg/min	10 mg/ 250 mL	40	mcg/mL		
	Take dose you want in mcg ÷ by drug index number = mL/h on pump									
Heparin	100 u/kg = 13,300 u 200 u/kg = 26,600 u 300 u/kg = 39,900 u 400 u/kg = 53,200 u									
Isoproterenol	Infusion				5 mcg/min	1 mg/ 250 mL	4	mcg/mL		
	Ordered mcg dose/min ÷ mcg/mL × 60 min/h =								**75**	mL/h
Lidocaine	Infusion	1 mg/min = 7.5 mL/h			1–4 mg/min	2 g/ 250 mL	8	mg/mL	—	
	Ordered mg/min ÷ mg/mL × 60 min/h = ___ mL/h									
Nitroglycerin	Infusion	3 mcg/min = 1 mL/h			3–200 mcg/min	50 mg/ 250 mL	200	mcg/mL	—	
	Ordered mcg/min ÷ mcg/mL × 60 min/h = ___ mL/h									
Nitroprusside	Infusion	6.7 mcg/min = 1 mL/h			5–300 mcg/min	100 mg/ 250 mL	400	mcg/mL	—	
	Ordered mcg/min ÷ mcg/mL × 60 min/h = ___ mL/h									
Norepinephrine	Infusion	1 mcg/min = 4 mL/h 2 mcg/min = 8 mL/h 3 mcg/min = 11 mL/h 4 mcg/min = 15 mL/h 5 mcg/min = 19 mL/h			2–20 mcg/min	4 mg/ 250 mL	16	mcg/mL		
	Ordered mcg dose/min ÷ mcg/mL × 60 min/h = ___ mL/h									
Phenylephrine	Infusion	1.3 mcg/min = 1 mL/h			10–200 mcg/min	20 mg/ 250 mL	80	mcg/mL		
	Ordered mcg/min ÷ mcg/mL × 60 min/h = ___ mL/h									
Primacor	0.05 mg/kg = 6.65 mg			Give load over 10 min		40 mg/ 200 mL	0.2	mg/mL		
	mg to give ÷ mg/mL = 33 mL				33 mL × (60 min/h ÷ 10 min) =				**200**	mL/h × 10 min
	Infusion		**0.03**		0.5 mcg/ kg/min	40 mg/ 200 mL	200	mcg/mL	—	
	Take dose you want in mcg ÷ by drug index number = mL/h on pump									
Trimethaphan	Infusion		—		0.3–6 mg/min	500 mg/ 500 mL	1	mg/mL	—	
	Ordered mg/min ÷ mg/mL × 60 min/h = ___ mL/h									
Vasopressin		0.02 u/min = 3 mL/h 0.04 u/min = 6 mL/h				40 u/ 100 mL	400	u/mL		

134   kg

DRUG	ORDERED AMOUNT	TOTAL DOSE TO GIVE	DRUG INDEX NUMBER	DIRECTIONS	INFUSION RANGE	DRUG MIXTURE	AMOUNT	DRUG/mL	RUN AT	mL/h
Aminophylline	5 mg/kg =	670 mg		Give mg/kg load over 20 min		500 mg/ 250 mL	2 mg/mL		
	mg to give ÷ mg/mL =	335 mL			335	mL × (60 min/h ÷ 20 min) =			**1005**	mL/h × 20 min
	Infusion				0.5–1 mg/kg/h	500 mg/ 250 mL	2 mg/mL		
					mg dose ordered × kg ÷ mg/mL =					___ mL/h
Amiodarone	Loading dose			Load **150 mg** over 10 min		900 mg/ 500 mL	1.8 mg/mL		—
				Ordered mg load dose (150 mg) ÷ mg/mL (1.8 mg/mL) = 83 mL to give × (60 min/h ÷ 10 min) = mL/h to set on pump					**500**	mL/h × 83 mL
	Infusion			Run at **1 mg/ min** × 6 h		900 mg/ 500 mL	1.8 mg/mL		
				Ordered mg dose (1 mg/min) ÷ mg/mL (1.8 mg/mL) = ___ × 60 min/h = mL/h to set on pump					**33**	mL/h × 6 h
	Infusion			Run at **0.5 mg/ min** × 18 h		900 mg/ 500 mL	1.8 mg/mL		
				Ordered mg dose (0.5 mg/min) ÷ mg/mL (1.8 mg/mL) = ___ × 60 min/h = mL/h to set on pump					**17**	mL/h × 18 h
Amrinone	0.75 mg/kg =	100.5 mg		Give mg/kg load over 10 min		300 mg/ 120 mL	2.5 mg/mL		—
	mg to give ÷ mg/mL =	40 mL			40.2	mL × (60 min/h ÷ 10 min) =			**241**	mL/h × 10 min
	Infusion		0.31		5–10 mcg/ kg/min	300 mg/ 120 mL	2500 mcg/mL		—
				Take dose you want in mcg ÷ by drug index number = mL/h on pump						
Brevibloc	Infusion		1.24		50–100 mcg/ kg/min	2.5 g/ 250 mL	10,000 mcg/mL		___ mL/h
				Take dose you want in mcg ÷ by drug index number = mL/h on pump						
Cardene	Infusion		—		0.5–10 mg/h	25 mg 250 mL	0.1 mg/mL		—
				Ordered mg dose ÷ mg/mL = mL/h to set on pump						___ mL/h
Cardizem	0.25 mg/kg =	33.5 mg		Give mg/kg load over 20 min		50 mg/ 100 mL	0.5 mg/mL		—
	mg to give ÷ mg/mL =	67 mL			67	mL × (60 min/h ÷ 20 min) =			**201**	mL/h
	0.35 mg/kg =	46.9 mg		May repeat loading dose in 15 min			0.5 mg/mL		—
	mg to give ÷ mg/mL =	94 mL			93.8	mL × (60 min/h ÷ 20 min) =			**281**	mL/h
	Infusion				5–15 mg/h				—
				Ordered mg dose ÷ mg/mL = mL/h to set on pump						___ mL/h
Desmopressin	0.3 mcg/kg =	40 mcg		Give dose over 20–30 min			4 mcg/vial		
Dobutamine	Infusion		0.25		2.5–40 mcg/kg/ min	250 mg/ 125 mL	2000 mcg/mL		
				Take dose you want in mcg ÷ by drug index number = mL/h on pump						

(continues)

134 kg (continued)

DRUG	ORDERED AMOUNT	TOTAL DOSE TO GIVE	DRUG INDEX NUMBER	DIRECTIONS	INFUSION RANGE	DRUG MIXTURE	AMOUNT	DRUG/mL	RUN AT	mL/h
Dopamine	Infusion		0.20		1–20 mcg/kg/min	400 mg/250 mL	1600	mcg/mL		
	Take dose you want in mcg ÷ by drug index number = mL/h on pump									
Epinephrine	Infusion	1 mcg/min = 4 mL/h 2 mcg/min = 8 mL/h 3 mcg/min = 11 mL/h 4 mcg/min = 15 mL/h			1–4 mcg/min	4 mg/250 mL	16	mcg/mL		
		Ordered mcg dose/min ÷ mcg/mL × 60 min/h =							___	mL/h
Fenoldapam	Infusion		0.0050		0.01–1.6 mcg/kg/min	10 mg/250 mL	40	mcg/mL		
	Take dose you want in mcg ÷ by drug index number = mL/h on pump									
Heparin	100 u/kg =	13,400 u								
	200 u/kg =	26,800 u								
	300 u/kg =	40,200 u								
	400 u/kg =	53,600 u								
Isoproterenol	Infusion				5 mcg/min	1 mg/250 mL	4	mcg/mL		
		Ordered mcg dose/min ÷ mcg/mL × 60 min/h =							75	mL/h
Lidocaine	Infusion	1 mg/min = 7.5 mL/h			1–4 mg/min	2 g/250 mL	8	mg/mL	___	
		Ordered mg/min ÷ mg/mL × 60 min/h =							___	mL/h
Nitroglycerin	Infusion	3 mcg/min = 1 mL/h			3–200 mcg/min	50 mg/250 mL	200	mcg/mL	___	
		Ordered mcg/min ÷ mcg/mL × 60 min/h =							___	mL/h
Nitroprusside	Infusion	6.7 mcg/min = 1 mL/h			5–300 mcg/min	100 mg/250 mL	400	mcg/mL	___	
		Ordered mcg/min ÷ mcg/mL × 60 min/h =							___	mL/h
Norepinephrine	Infusion	1 mcg/min = 4 mL/h 2 mcg/min = 8 mL/h 3 mcg/min = 11 mL/h 4 mcg/min = 15 mL/h 5 mcg/min = 19 mL/h			2–20 mcg/min	4 mg/250 mL	16	mcg/mL		
		Ordered mcg dose/min ÷ mcg/mL × 60 min/h =							___	mL/h
Phenylephrine	Infusion	1.3 mcg/min = 1 mL/h			10–200 mcg/min	20 mg/250 mL	80	mcg/mL		
		Ordered mcg/min ÷ mcg/mL × 60 min/h =							___	mL/h
Primacor	0.05 mg/kg =	6.7 mg		Give load over 10 min		40 mg/200 mL	0.2	mg/mL		
	mg to give ÷ mg/mL =	34 mL			34	mL × (60 min/h ÷ 10 min) =			201	mL/h × 10 min
	Infusion		0.02		0.5 mcg/kg/min	40 mg/200 mL	200	mcg/mL	___	
	Take dose you want in mcg ÷ by drug index number = mL/h on pump									
Trimethaphan	Infusion		___		0.3–6 mg/min	500 mg/500 mL	1	mg/mL	___	
		Ordered mg/min ÷ mg/mL × 60 min/h =							___	mL/h
Vasopressin		0.02 u/min = 3 mL/h 0.04 u/min = 6 mL/h				40 u/100 mL	400	u/mL		

135 kg

DRUG	ORDERED AMOUNT	TOTAL DOSE TO GIVE	DRUG INDEX NUMBER	DIRECTIONS	INFUSION RANGE	DRUG MIXTURE	AMOUNT	DRUG/ mL	RUN AT	mL/h
Aminophylline	5 mg/kg =	675 mg		Give mg/kg load over 20 min		500 mg/ 250 mL		2 mg/mL		
	mg to give ÷ mg/mL =	338 mL			338	500 mg/ 250 mL	mL × (60 min/h ÷ 20 min) =		1013	mL/h × 20 min
	Infusion				0.5–1 mg/kg/h	500 mg/ 250 mL		2 mg/mL		
						mg dose ordered × kg ÷ mg/mL =			___	mL/h
Amiodarone	Loading dose			Load **150 mg** over 10 min		900 mg/ 500 mL		1.8 mg/mL	—	
				Ordered mg load dose (150 mg) ÷ mg/mL (1.8 mg/mL) = 83 mL to give × (60 min/h ÷ 10 min) = mL/h to set on pump					500	mL/h × 83 mL
	Infusion			Run at **1 mg/ min** × 6 h		900 mg/ 500 mL		1.8 mg/mL		
				Ordered mg dose (1 mg/min) ÷ mg/mL (1.8 mg/mL) = ____ × 60 min/h = mL/h to set on pump					33	mL/h × 6 h
	Infusion			Run at **0.5 mg/ min** × 18 h		900 mg/ 500 mL		1.8 mg/mL		
				Ordered mg dose (0.5 mg/min) ÷ mg/mL (1.8 mg/mL) = ____ × 60 min/h = mL/h to set on pump					17	mL/h × 18 h
Amrinone	0.75 mg/kg =	101.25 mg		Give mg/kg load over 10 min		300 mg/ 120 mL		2.5 mg/mL	—	
	mg to give ÷ mg/mL =	41 mL			40.5		mL × (60 min/h ÷ 10 min) =		243	mL/h × 10 min
	Infusion		0.31		5–10 mcg/ kg/min	300 mg/ 120 mL		2500 mcg/mL	—	
				Take dose you want in mcg ÷ by drug index number = mL/h on pump						
Brevibloc	Infusion		1.23		50–100 mcg/ kg/min	2.5 g/ 250 mL		10,000 mcg/mL	___	mL/h
				Take dose you want in mcg ÷ by drug index number = mL/h on pump						
Cardene	Infusion		—		0.5–10 mg/h	25 mg 250 mL		0.1 mg/mL		
				Ordered mg dose ÷ mg/mL = mL/h to set on pump					___	mL/h
Cardizem	0.25 mg/kg =	33.75 mg		Give mg/kg load over 20 min		50 mg/ 100 mL		0.5 mg/mL	—	
	mg to give ÷ mg/mL =	68 mL			67.5		mL × (60 min/h ÷ 20 min) =		203	mL/h
	0.35 mg/kg =	47.25 mg		May repeat loading dose in 15 min				0.5 mg/mL	—	
	mg to give ÷ mg/mL =	95 mL			94.5		mL × (60 min/h ÷ 20 min) =		284	mL/h
	Infusion				5–15 mg/h				—	
				Ordered mg dose ÷ mg/mL = mL/h to set on pump					___	mL/h
Desmopressin	0.3 mcg/kg =	41 mcg		Give dose over 20–30 min				4 mcg/vial		
Dobutamine	Infusion		0.25		2.5–40 mcg/kg/ min	250 mg/ 125 mL		2000 mcg/mL		
				Take dose you want in mcg ÷ by drug index number = mL/h on pump						

(continues)

135 kg (continued)

DRUG	ORDERED AMOUNT	TOTAL DOSE TO GIVE	DRUG INDEX NUMBER	DIRECTIONS	INFUSION RANGE	DRUG MIXTURE	AMOUNT	DRUG/mL	RUN AT	mL/h
Dopamine	Infusion		0.20		1–20 mcg/kg/min	400 mg/250 mL	1600	mcg/mL		
	Take dose you want in mcg ÷ by drug index number = mL/h on pump									
Epinephrine	Infusion	1 mcg/min = 4 mL/h 2 mcg/min = 8 mL/h 3 mcg/min = 11 mL/h 4 mcg/min = 15 mL/h			1–4 mcg/min	4 mg/250 mL	16	mcg/mL		
	Ordered mcg dose/min ÷ mcg/mL × 60 min/h = ___ mL/h									
Fenoldapam	Infusion		0.0050		0.01–1.6 mcg/kg/min	10 mg/250 mL	40	mcg/mL		
	Take dose you want in mcg ÷ by drug index number = mL/h on pump									
Heparin	100 u/kg = 13,500 u 200 u/kg = 27,000 u 300 u/kg = 40,500 u 400 u/kg = 54,000 u									
Isoproterenol	Infusion				5 mcg/min	1 mg/250 mL	4	mcg/mL		
	Ordered mcg dose/min ÷ mcg/mL × 60 min/h =								**75**	mL/h
Lidocaine	Infusion	1 mg/min = 7.5 mL/h			1–4 mg/min	2 g/250 mL	8	mg/mL	—	
	Ordered mg/min ÷ mg/mL × 60 min/h = ___ mL/h									
Nitroglycerin	Infusion	3 mcg/min = 1 mL/h			3–200 mcg/min	50 mg/250 mL	200	mcg/mL	—	
	Ordered mcg/min ÷ mcg/mL × 60 min/h = ___ mL/h									
Nitroprusside	Infusion	6.7 mcg/min = 1 mL/h			5–300 mcg/min	100 mg/250 mL	400	mcg/mL	—	
	Ordered mcg/min ÷ mcg/mL × 60 min/h = ___ mL/h									
Norepinephrine	Infusion	1 mcg/min = 4 mL/h 2 mcg/min = 8 mL/h 3 mcg/min = 11 mL/h 4 mcg/min = 15 mL/h 5 mcg/min = 19 mL/h			2–20 mcg/min	4 mg/250 mL	16	mcg/mL		
	Ordered mcg dose/min ÷ mcg/mL × 60 min/h = ___ mL/h									
Phenylephrine	Infusion	1.3 mcg/min = 1 mL/h			10–200 mcg/min	20 mg/250 mL	80	mcg/mL	—	
	Ordered mcg/min ÷ mcg/mL × 60 min/h = ___ mL/h									
Primacor	0.05 mg/kg = 6.75 mg			Give load over 10 min		40 mg/200 mL	0.2	mg/mL		
	mg to give ÷ mg/mL = 34 mL				34	mL × (60 min/h ÷ 10 min) =			**203**	mL/h × 10 min
	Infusion		0.02		0.5 mcg/kg/min	40 mg/200 mL	200	mcg/mL	—	
	Take dose you want in mcg ÷ by drug index number = mL/h on pump									
Trimethaphan	Infusion		—		0.3–6 mg/min	500 mg/500 mL	1	mg/mL	—	
	Ordered mg/min ÷ mg/mL × 60 min/h = ___ mL/h									
Vasopressin		0.02 u/min = 3 mL/h 0.04 u/min = 6 mL/h				40 u/100 mL	400	u/mL		

136 kg

DRUG	ORDERED AMOUNT	TOTAL DOSE TO GIVE	DRUG INDEX NUMBER	DIRECTIONS	INFUSION RANGE	DRUG MIXTURE	AMOUNT DRUG/mL	RUN AT mL/h
Aminophylline	5 mg/kg = 680 mg			Give mg/kg load over 20 min		500 mg/ 250 mL	2 mg/mL	
	mg to give ÷ mg/mL = 340 mL				340	mL × (60 min/h ÷ 20 min) =		**1020** mL/h × 20 min
	Infusion				0.5–1 mg/kg/h	500 mg/ 250 mL	2 mg/mL	
					mg dose ordered × kg ÷ mg/mL =			___ mL/h
Amiodarone	Loading dose			Load **150 mg** over 10 min		900 mg/ 500 mL	1.8 mg/mL	___
				Ordered mg load dose (150 mg) ÷ mg/mL (1.8 mg/mL) = 83 mL to give × (60 min/h ÷ 10 min) = mL/h to set on pump				**500** mL/h × 83 mL
	Infusion			Run at **1 mg/ min** × 6 h		900 mg/ 500 mL	1.8 mg/mL	
				Ordered mg dose (1 mg/min) ÷ mg/mL (1.8 mg/mL) = ___ × 60 min/h = mL/h to set on pump				**33** mL/h × 6 h
	Infusion			Run at **0.5 mg/ min** × 18 h		900 mg/ 500 mL	1.8 mg/mL	
				Ordered mg dose (0.5 mg/min) ÷ mg/mL (1.8 mg/mL) = ___ × 60 min/h = mL/h to set on pump				**17** mL/h × 18 h
Amrinone	0.75 mg/kg = 102 mg			Give mg/kg load over 10 min		300 mg/ 120 mL	2.5 mg/mL	___
	mg to give ÷ mg/mL = 41 mL				40.8	mL × (60 min/h ÷ 10 min) =		**245** mL/h × 10 min
	Infusion		0.31		5–10 mcg/ kg/min	300 mg/ 120 mL	2500 mcg/mL	___
				Take dose you want in mcg ÷ by drug index number = mL/h on pump				
Brevibloc	Infusion		1.23		50–100 mcg/ kg/min	2.5 g/ 250 mL	10,000 mcg/mL	___ mL/h
				Take dose you want in mcg ÷ by drug index number = mL/h on pump				
Cardene	Infusion		___		0.5–10 mg/h	25 mg 250 mL	0.1 mg/mL	___
				Ordered mg dose ÷ mg/mL = mL/h to set on pump				___ mL/h
Cardizem	0.25 mg/kg = 34 mg			Give mg/kg load over 20 min		50 mg/ 100 mL	0.5 mg/mL	
	mg to give ÷ mg/mL = 68 mL				68	mL × (60 min/h ÷ 20 min) =		**204** mL/h
	0.35 mg/kg = 47.6 mg			May repeat loading dose in 15 min			0.5 mg/mL	
	mg to give ÷ mg/mL = 95 mL				95.2	mL × (60 min/h ÷ 20 min) =		**286** mL/h
	Infusion				5–15 mg/h			___
				Ordered mg dose ÷ mg/mL = mL/h to set on pump				___ mL/h
Desmopressin	0.3 mcg/kg = 41 mcg			Give dose over 20–30 min			4 mcg/vial	
Dobutamine	Infusion		0.24		2.5–40 mcg/kg/ min	250 mg/ 125 mL	2000 mcg/mL	
				Take dose you want in mcg ÷ by drug index number = mL/h on pump				

(continues)

136 kg (continued)

DRUG	ORDERED AMOUNT	TOTAL DOSE TO GIVE	DRUG INDEX NUMBER	DIRECTIONS	INFUSION RANGE	DRUG MIXTURE	AMOUNT	DRUG/ mL	RUN AT	mL/h
Dopamine	Infusion		0.20		1–20 mcg/ kg/min	400 mg/ 250 mL	1600	mcg/mL		
	— Take dose you want in mcg ÷ by drug index number = mL/h on pump									
Epinephrine	Infusion	1 mcg/min = 4 mL/h 2 mcg/min = 8 mL/h 3 mcg/min = 11 mL/h 4 mcg/min = 15 mL/h			1–4 mcg/min	4 mg/ 250 mL	16	mcg/mL		
	Ordered mcg dose/min ÷ mcg/mL × 60 min/h =									___ mL/h
Fenoldapam	Infusion		0.0049		0.01–1.6 mcg/ kg/min	10 mg/ 250 mL	40	mcg/mL		
	Take dose you want in mcg ÷ by drug index number = mL/h on pump									
Heparin	100 u/kg = 13,600 u 200 u/kg = 27,200 u 300 u/kg = 40,800 u 400 u/kg = 54,400 u									
Isoproterenol	Infusion				5 mcg/min	1 mg/ 250 mL	4	mcg/mL		
	Ordered mcg dose/min ÷ mcg/mL × 60 min/h =									75 mL/h
Lidocaine	Infusion	1 mg/min = 7.5 mL/h			1–4 mg/min	2 g/ 250 mL	8	mg/mL		—
	Ordered mg/min ÷ mg/mL × 60 min/h =									___ mL/h
Nitroglycerin	Infusion	3 mcg/min = 1 mL/h			3–200 mcg/min	50 mg/ 250 mL	200	mcg/mL		—
	Ordered mcg/min ÷ mcg/mL × 60 min/h =									___ mL/h
Nitroprusside	Infusion	6.7 mcg/min = 1 mL/h			5–300 mcg/min	100 mg/ 250 mL	400	mcg/mL		—
	Ordered mcg/min ÷ mcg/mL × 60 min/h =									___ mL/h
Norepinephrine	Infusion	1 mcg/min = 4 mL/h 2 mcg/min = 8 mL/h 3 mcg/min = 11 mL/h 4 mcg/min = 15 mL/h 5 mcg/min = 19 mL/h			2–20 mcg/min	4 mg/ 250 mL	16	mcg/mL		
	Ordered mcg dose/min ÷ mcg/mL × 60 min/h =									___ mL/h
Phenylephrine	Infusion	1.3 mcg/min = 1 mL/h			10–200 mcg/min	20 mg/ 250 mL	80	mcg/mL		
	Ordered mcg/min ÷ mcg/mL × 60 min/h =									___ mL/h
Primacor	0.05 mg/kg = 6.8 mg			Give load over 10 min		40 mg/ 200 mL	0.2	mg/mL		
	mg to give ÷ mg/mL = 34 mL				34 mL × (60 min/h ÷ 10 min) =				204	mL/h × 10 min
	Infusion		0.02		0.5 mcg/ kg/min	40 mg/ 200 mL	200	mcg/mL		—
	Take dose you want in mcg ÷ by drug index number = mL/h on pump									
Trimethaphan	Infusion		—		0.3–6 mg/min	500 mg/ 500 mL	1	mg/mL		—
	Ordered mg/min ÷ mg/mL × 60 min/h =									___ mL/h
Vasopressin		0.02 u/min = 3 mL/h 0.04 u/min = 6 mL/h				40 u/ 100 mL	400	u/mL		

137 kg

DRUG	ORDERED AMOUNT	TOTAL DOSE TO GIVE	DRUG INDEX NUMBER	DIRECTIONS	INFUSION RANGE	DRUG MIXTURE	AMOUNT	DRUG/ mL	RUN AT	mL/h
Aminophylline	5 mg/kg =	685 mg		Give mg/kg load over 20 min		500 mg/ 250 mL	2	mg/mL		
	mg to give ÷ mg/mL =	343 mL			343	mL × (60 min/h ÷ 20 min) =			1028	mL/h × 20 min
	Infusion				0.5–1 mg/kg/h	500 mg/ 250 mL	2	mg/mL		
					mg dose ordered × kg ÷ mg/mL =				___	mL/h
Amiodarone	Loading dose			Load **150 mg** over 10 min		900 mg/ 500 mL	1.8	mg/mL	___	
				Ordered mg load dose (150 mg) ÷ mg/mL (1.8 mg/mL) = 83 mL to give × (60 min/h ÷ 10 min) = mL/h to set on pump					500	mL/h × 83 mL
	Infusion			Run at **1 mg/ min** × 6 h		900 mg/ 500 mL	1.8	mg/mL		
				Ordered mg dose (1 mg/min) ÷ mg/mL (1.8 mg/mL) = _____ × 60 min/h = mL/h to set on pump					33	mL/h × 6 h
	Infusion			Run at **0.5 mg/ min** × 18 h		900 mg/ 500 mL	1.8	mg/mL		
				Ordered mg dose (0.5 mg/min) ÷ mg/mL (1.8 mg/mL) = _____ × 60 min/h = mL/h to set on pump					17	mL/h × 18 h
Amrinone	0.75 mg/kg =	102.75 mg		Give mg/kg load over 10 min		300 mg/ 120 mL	2.5	mg/mL	___	
	mg to give ÷ mg/mL =	41 mL			41.1	mL × (60 min/h ÷ 10 min) =			247	mL/h × 10 min
	Infusion		0.30		5–10 mcg/ kg/min	300 mg/ 120 mL	2500	mcg/mL	___	
				Take dose you want in mcg ÷ by drug index number = mL/h on pump						
Brevibloc	Infusion		1.22		50–100 mcg/ kg/min	2.5 g/ 250 mL	10,000	mcg/mL	___	mL/h
				Take dose you want in mcg ÷ by drug index number = mL/h on pump						
Cardene	Infusion		—		0.5–10 mg/h	25 mg 250 mL	0.1	mg/mL	___	
				Ordered mg dose ÷ mg/mL = mL/h to set on pump					___	mL/h
Cardizem	0.25 mg/kg =	34.25 mg		Give mg/kg load over 20 min		50 mg/ 100 mL	0.5	mg/mL	___	
	mg to give ÷ mg/mL =	69 mL			68.5	mL × (60 min/h ÷ 20 min) =			206	mL/h
	0.35 mg/kg =	47.95 mg		May repeat loading dose in 15 min			0.5	mg/mL		
	mg to give ÷ mg/mL =	96 mL			95.9	mL × (60 min/h ÷ 20 min) =			288	mL/h
	Infusion				5–15 mg/h				___	
				Ordered mg dose ÷ mg/mL = mL/h to set on pump					___	mL/h
Desmopressin	0.3 mcg/kg =	41 mcg		Give dose over 20–30 min			4	mcg/vial		
Dobutamine	Infusion		0.24		2.5–40 mcg/kg/ min	250 mg/ 125 mL	2000	mcg/mL		
				Take dose you want in mcg ÷ by drug index number = mL/h on pump						

(continues)

137   kg (continued)

DRUG	ORDERED AMOUNT		TOTAL DOSE TO GIVE		DRUG INDEX NUMBER	DIRECTIONS	INFUSION RANGE	DRUG MIXTURE	AMOUNT	DRUG/mL	RUN AT	mL/h
Dopamine	Infusion				0.19		1–20 mcg/kg/min	400 mg/250 mL	1600	mcg/mL		
	Take dose you want in mcg ÷ by drug index number = mL/h on pump											
Epinephrine	Infusion		1 mcg/min = 4 mL/h 2 mcg/min = 8 mL/h 3 mcg/min = 11 mL/h 4 mcg/min = 15 mL/h				1–4 mcg/min	4 mg/250 mL	16	mcg/mL		
	Ordered mcg dose/min ÷ mcg/mL × 60 min/h =										___	mL/h
Fenoldapam	Infusion				0.0049		0.01–1.6 mcg/kg/min	10 mg/250 mL	40	mcg/mL		
	Take dose you want in mcg ÷ by drug index number = mL/h on pump											
Heparin	100 u/kg = 200 u/kg = 300 u/kg = 400 u/kg =		13,700 u 27,400 u 41,100 u 54,800 u									
Isoproterenol	Infusion						5 mcg/min	1 mg/250 mL	4	mcg/mL		
	Ordered mcg dose/min ÷ mcg/mL × 60 min/h =										75	mL/h
Lidocaine	Infusion		1 mg/min = 7.5 mL/h				1–4 mg/min	2 g/250 mL	8	mg/mL	___	
	Ordered mg/min ÷ mg/mL × 60 min/h =										___	mL/h
Nitroglycerin	Infusion		3 mcg/min = 1 mL/h				3–200 mcg/min	50 mg/250 mL	200	mcg/mL	___	
	Ordered mcg/min ÷ mcg/mL × 60 min/h =										___	mL/h
Nitroprusside	Infusion		6.7 mcg/min = 1 mL/h				5–300 mcg/min	100 mg/250 mL	400	mcg/mL	___	
	Ordered mcg/min ÷ mcg/mL × 60 min/h =										___	mL/h
Norepinephrine	Infusion		1 mcg/min = 4 mL/h 2 mcg/min = 8 mL/h 3 mcg/min = 11 mL/h 4 mcg/min = 15 mL/h 5 mcg/min = 19 mL/h				2–20 mcg/min	4 mg/250 mL	16	mcg/mL		
	Ordered mcg dose/min ÷ mcg/mL × 60 min/h =										___	mL/h
Phenylephrine	Infusion		1.3 mcg/min = 1 mL/h				10–200 mcg/min	20 mg/250 mL	80	mcg/mL		
	Ordered mcg/min ÷ mcg/mL × 60 min/h =										___	mL/h
Primacor	0.05 mg/kg =		6.85 mg			Give load over 10 min		40 mg/200 mL	0.2	mg/mL		
	mg to give ÷ mg/mL =		34 mL				34	mL × (60 min/h ÷ 10 min) =			206	mL/h × 10 min
	Infusion				0.02		0.5 mcg/kg/min	40 mg/200 mL	200	mcg/mL	___	
	Take dose you want in mcg ÷ by drug index number = mL/h on pump											
Trimethaphan	Infusion				—		0.3–6 mg/min	500 mg/500 mL	1	mg/mL	___	
	Ordered mg/min ÷ mg/mL × 60 min/h =										___	mL/h
Vasopressin			0.02 u/min = 3 mL/h 0.04 u/min = 6 mL/h					40 u/100 mL	400	u/mL		

138 kg

DRUG	ORDERED AMOUNT	TOTAL DOSE TO GIVE	DRUG INDEX NUMBER	DIRECTIONS	INFUSION RANGE	DRUG MIXTURE	AMOUNT	DRUG/ mL	RUN AT	mL/h
Aminophylline	5 mg/kg =	690 mg		Give mg/kg load over 20 min		500 mg/ 250 mL	2 mg/mL			
	mg to give ÷ mg/mL =	345 mL			345	mL × (60 min/h ÷ 20 min) =			**1035**	mL/h × 20 min
	Infusion				0.5–1 mg/kg/h	500 mg/ 250 mL	2 mg/mL			
					mg dose ordered × kg ÷ mg/mL =				___ mL/h	
Amiodarone	Loading dose			Load **150 mg** over 10 min		900 mg/ 500 mL	1.8 mg/mL		___	
				Ordered mg load dose (150 mg) ÷ mg/mL (1.8 mg/mL) = 83 mL to give × (60 min/h ÷ 10 min) = mL/h to set on pump					**500**	mL/h × 83 mL
	Infusion			Run at **1 mg/ min** × 6 h		900 mg/ 500 mL	1.8 mg/mL			
				Ordered mg dose (1 mg/min) ÷ mg/mL (1.8 mg/mL) = _____ × 60 min/h = mL/h to set on pump					**33**	mL/h × 6 h
	Infusion			Run at **0.5 mg/ min** × 18 h		900 mg/ 500 mL	1.8 mg/mL			
				Ordered mg dose (0.5 mg/min) ÷ mg/mL (1.8 mg/mL) = _____ × 60 min/h = mL/h to set on pump					**17**	mL/h × 18 h
Amrinone	0.75 mg/kg =	103.5 mg		Give mg/kg load over 10 min		300 mg/ 120 mL	2.5 mg/mL		___	
	mg to give ÷ mg/mL =	41 mL			41.4	mL × (60 min/h ÷ 10 min) =			**248**	mL/h × 10 min
	Infusion		0.30		5–10 mcg/ kg/min	300 mg/ 120 mL	2500 mcg/mL		___	
				Take dose you want in mcg ÷ by drug index number = mL/h on pump						
Brevibloc	Infusion		1.21		50–100 mcg/ kg/min	2.5 g/ 250 mL	10,000 mcg/mL		___ mL/h	
				Take dose you want in mcg ÷ by drug index number = mL/h on pump						
Cardene	Infusion		—		0.5–10 mg/h	25 mg 250 mL	0.1 mg/mL		___	
				Ordered mg dose ÷ mg/mL = mL/h to set on pump					___ mL/h	
Cardizem	0.25 mg/kg =	34.5 mg		Give mg/kg load over 20 min		50 mg/ 100 mL	0.5 mg/mL			
	mg to give ÷ mg/mL =	69 mL			69	mL × (60 min/h ÷ 20 min) =			**207** mL/h	
	0.35 mg/kg =	48.3 mg		May repeat loading dose in 15 min			0.5 mg/mL		___	
	mg to give ÷ mg/mL =	97 mL			96.6	mL × (60 min/h ÷ 20 min) =			**290** mL/h	
	Infusion				5–15 mg/h				___	
				Ordered mg dose ÷ mg/mL = mL/h to set on pump					___ mL/h	
Desmopressin	0.3 mcg/kg =	41 mcg		Give dose over 20–30 min			4 mcg/vial			
Dobutamine	Infusion		0.24		2.5–40 mcg/kg/ min	250 mg/ 125 mL	2000 mcg/mL			
				Take dose you want in mcg ÷ by drug index number = mL/h on pump						

(continues)

138   kg (continued)

DRUG	ORDERED AMOUNT	TOTAL DOSE TO GIVE	DRUG INDEX NUMBER	DIRECTIONS	INFUSION RANGE	DRUG MIXTURE	AMOUNT	DRUG/ mL	RUN AT	mL/h
Dopamine	Infusion		0.19		1–20 mcg/ kg/min	400 mg/ 250 mL	1600	mcg/mL		
					Take dose you want in mcg ÷ by drug index number = mL/h on pump					
Epinephrine	Infusion	1 mcg/min = 4 mL/h 2 mcg/min = 8 mL/h 3 mcg/min = 11 mL/h 4 mcg/min = 15 mL/h			1–4 mcg/min	4 mg/ 250 mL	16	mcg/mL		
					Ordered mcg dose/min ÷ mcg/mL × 60 min/h =				___	mL/h
Fenoldapam	Infusion		0.0049		0.01–1.6 mcg/ kg/min	10 mg/ 250 mL	40	mcg/mL		
					Take dose you want in mcg ÷ by drug index number = mL/h on pump					
Heparin	100 u/kg = 200 u/kg = 300 u/kg = 400 u/kg =	13,800 u 27,600 u 41,400 u 55,200 u								
Isoproterenol	Infusion				5 mcg/min	1 mg/ 250 mL	4	mcg/mL		
					Ordered mcg dose/min ÷ mcg/mL × 60 min/h =				75	mL/h
Lidocaine	Infusion	1 mg/min = 7.5 mL/h			1–4 mg/min	2 g/ 250 mL	8	mg/mL		___
					Ordered mg/min ÷ mg/mL × 60 min/h =				___	mL/h
Nitroglycerin	Infusion	3 mcg/min = 1 mL/h			3–200 mcg/min	50 mg/ 250 mL	200	mcg/mL		___
					Ordered mcg/min ÷ mcg/mL × 60 min/h =				___	mL/h
Nitroprusside	Infusion	6.7 mcg/min = 1 mL/h			5–300 mcg/min	100 mg/ 250 mL	400	mcg/mL		___
					Ordered mcg/min ÷ mcg/mL × 60 min/h =				___	mL/h
Norepinephrine	Infusion	1 mcg/min = 4 mL/h 2 mcg/min = 8 mL/h 3 mcg/min = 11 mL/h 4 mcg/min = 15 mL/h 5 mcg/min = 19 mL/h			2–20 mcg/min	4 mg/ 250 mL	16	mcg/mL		
					Ordered mcg dose/min ÷ mcg/mL × 60 min/h =				___	mL/h
Phenylephrine	Infusion	1.3 mcg/min = 1 mL/h			10–200 mcg/min	20 mg/ 250 mL	80	mcg/mL		
					Ordered mcg/min ÷ mcg/mL × 60 min/h =				___	mL/h
Primacor	0.05 mg/kg =	6.9 mg		Give load over 10 min		40 mg/ 200 mL	0.2	mg/mL		
	mg to give ÷ mg/mL =	35 mL			35	mL × (60 min/h ÷ 10 min) =			207	mL/h × 10 min
	Infusion		0.02		0.5 mcg/ kg/min	40 mg/ 200 mL	200	mcg/mL		___
					Take dose you want in mcg ÷ by drug index number = mL/h on pump					
Trimethaphan	Infusion		___		0.3–6 mg/min	500 mg/ 500 mL	1	mg/mL		___
					Ordered mg/min ÷ mg/mL × 60 min/h =				___	mL/h
Vasopressin		0.02 u/min = 3 mL/h 0.04 u/min = 6 mL/h				40 u/ 100 mL	400	u/mL		

139 kg

DRUG	ORDERED AMOUNT	TOTAL DOSE TO GIVE	DRUG INDEX NUMBER	DIRECTIONS	INFUSION RANGE	DRUG MIXTURE	AMOUNT	DRUG/mL	RUN AT	mL/h
Aminophylline	5 mg/kg =	695 mg		Give mg/kg load over 20 min		500 mg/ 250 mL	2 mg/mL			
	mg to give ÷ mg/mL =	348 mL			348	mL × (60 min/h ÷ 20 min) =			1043	mL/h × 20 min
	Infusion				0.5–1 mg/kg/h	500 mg/ 250 mL	2 mg/mL			
					mg dose ordered × kg ÷ mg/mL =			___	mL/h	
Amiodarone	Loading dose			Load **150 mg** over 10 min		900 mg/ 500 mL	1.8 mg/mL		___	
				Ordered mg load dose (150 mg) ÷ mg/mL (1.8 mg/mL) = 83 mL to give × (60 min/h ÷ 10 min) = mL/h to set on pump					500	mL/h × 83 mL
	Infusion			Run at **1 mg/ min** × 6 h	900 mg/ 500 mL	1.8 mg/mL				
				Ordered mg dose (1 mg/min) ÷ mg/mL (1.8 mg/mL) = ____ × 60 min/h = mL/h to set on pump					33	mL/h × 6 h
	Infusion			Run at **0.5 mg/ min** × 18 h	900 mg/ 500 mL	1.8 mg/mL				
				Ordered mg dose (0.5 mg/min) ÷ mg/mL (1.8 mg/mL) = ____ × 60 min/h = mL/h to set on pump					17	mL/h × 18 h
Amrinone	0.75 mg/kg =	104.25 mg		Give mg/kg load over 10 min		300 mg/ 120 mL	2.5 mg/mL		___	
	mg to give ÷ mg/mL =	42 mL			41.7	mL × (60 min/h ÷ 10 min) =			250	mL/h × 10 min
	Infusion		0.30		5–10 mcg/ kg/min	300 mg/ 120 mL	2500 mcg/mL		___	
				Take dose you want in mcg ÷ by drug index number = mL/h on pump						
Brevibloc	Infusion		1.20		50–100 mcg/ kg/min	2.5 g/ 250 mL	10,000 mcg/mL		___	mL/h
				Take dose you want in mcg ÷ by drug index number = mL/h on pump						
Cardene	Infusion		—		0.5–10 mg/h	25 mg 250 mL	0.1 mg/mL		___	
				Ordered mg dose ÷ mg/mL = mL/h to set on pump					___	mL/h
Cardizem	0.25 mg/kg =	34.75 mg		Give mg/kg load over 20 min		50 mg/ 100 mL	0.5 DRUG/mL			
	mg to give ÷ mg/mL =	70 mL			69.5	mL × (60 min/h ÷ 20 min) =			209	mL/h
	0.35 mg/kg =	48.65 mg		May repeat loading dose in 15 min			0.5 mg/mL			
	mg to give ÷ mg/mL =	97 mL			97.3	mL × (60 min/h ÷ 20 min) =			292	mL/h
	Infusion				5–15 mg/h				___	
				Ordered mg dose ÷ mg/mL = mL/h to set on pump					___	mL/h
Desmopressin	0.3 mcg/kg =	42 mcg		Give dose over 20–30 min			4 mcg/vial			
Dobutamine	Infusion		0.24		2.5–40 mcg/kg/ min	250 mg/ 125 mL	2000 mcg/mL			
				Take dose you want in mcg ÷ by drug index number = mL/h on pump						

(continues)

139 kg (continued)

DRUG	ORDERED AMOUNT	TOTAL DOSE TO GIVE	DRUG INDEX NUMBER	DIRECTIONS	INFUSION RANGE	DRUG MIXTURE	AMOUNT	DRUG/ mL	RUN AT	mL/h
Dopamine	Infusion		0.19		1–20 mcg/ kg/min	400 mg/ 250 mL	1600	mcg/mL		
				Take dose you want in mcg ÷ by drug index number = mL/h on pump						
Epinephrine	Infusion	1 mcg/min = 4 mL/h 2 mcg/min = 8 mL/h 3 mcg/min = 11 mL/h 4 mcg/min = 15 mL/h			1–4 mcg/min	4 mg/ 250 mL	16	mcg/mL		
					Ordered mcg dose/min ÷ mcg/mL × 60 min/h =				___	mL/h
Fenoldapam	Infusion		0.0048		0.01–1.6 mcg/ kg/min	10 mg/ 250 mL	40	mcg/mL		
					Take dose you want in mcg ÷ by drug index number = mL/h on pump					
Heparin	100 u/kg = 200 u/kg = 300 u/kg = 400 u/kg =	13,900 u 27,800 u 41,700 u 55,600 u								
Isoproterenol	Infusion				5 mcg/min	1 mg/ 250 mL	4	mcg/mL		
					Ordered mcg dose/min ÷ mcg/mL × 60 min/h =				75	mL/h
Lidocaine	Infusion	1 mg/min = 7.5 mL/h			1–4 mg/min	2 g/ 250 mL	8	mg/mL		___
					Ordered mg/min ÷ mg/mL × 60 min/h =				___	mL/h
Nitroglycerin	Infusion	3 mcg/min = 1 mL/h			3–200 mcg/min	50 mg/ 250 mL	200	mcg/mL		___
					Ordered mcg/min ÷ mcg/mL × 60 min/h =				___	mL/h
Nitroprusside	Infusion	6.7 mcg/min = 1 mL/h			5–300 mcg/min	100 mg/ 250 mL	400	mcg/mL		___
					Ordered mcg/min ÷ mcg/mL × 60 min/h =				___	mL/h
Norepinephrine	Infusion	1 mcg/min = 4 mL/h 2 mcg/min = 8 mL/h 3 mcg/min = 11 mL/h 4 mcg/min = 15 mL/h 5 mcg/min = 19 mL/h			2–20 mcg/min	4 mg/ 250 mL	16	mcg/mL		
					Ordered mcg dose/min ÷ mcg/mL × 60 min/h =				___	mL/h
Phenylephrine	Infusion	1.3 mcg/min = 1 mL/h			10–200 mcg/min	20 mg/ 250 mL	80	mcg/mL		___
					Ordered mcg/min ÷ mcg/mL × 60 min/h =				___	mL/h
Primacor	0.05 mg/kg =	6.95 mg		Give load over 10 min		40 mg/ 200 mL	0.2	mg/mL		
	mg to give ÷ mg/mL =	35 mL			35	mL × (60 min/h ÷ 10 min) =			209	mL/h × 10 min
	Infusion		0.02		0.5 mcg/ kg/min	40 mg/ 200 mL	200	mcg/mL		___
					Take dose you want in mcg ÷ by drug index number = mL/h on pump					
Trimethaphan	Infusion		—		0.3–6 mg/min	500 mg/ 500 mL	1	mg/mL		___
					Ordered mg/min ÷ mg/mL × 60 min/h =				___	mL/h
Vasopressin		0.02 u/min = 3 mL/h 0.04 u/min = 6 mL/h				40 u/ 100 mL	400	u/mL		

140 kg

DRUG	ORDERED AMOUNT	TOTAL DOSE TO GIVE	DRUG INDEX NUMBER	DIRECTIONS	INFUSION RANGE	DRUG MIXTURE	AMOUNT	DRUG/ mL	RUN AT	mL/h
Aminophylline	5 mg/kg =	700 mg		Give mg/kg load over 20 min		500 mg/ 250 mL	2	mg/mL		
		mg to give ÷ mg/mL = 350 mL				350	mL × (60 min/h ÷ 20 min) =		**1050**	mL/h × 20 min
		Infusion			0.5–1 mg/kg/h	500 mg/ 250 mL	2	mg/mL		
					mg dose ordered × kg ÷ mg/mL =					___ mL/h
Amiodarone		Loading dose		Load **150 mg** over 10 min		900 mg/ 500 mL	1.8	mg/mL		—
				Ordered mg load dose (150 mg) ÷ mg/mL (1.8 mg/mL) = 83 mL to give × (60 min/h ÷ 10 min) = mL/h to set on pump					**500**	mL/h × 83 mL
		Infusion		Run at **1 mg/ min** × 6 h		900 mg/ 500 mL	1.8	mg/mL		
				Ordered mg dose (1 mg/min) ÷ mg/mL (1.8 mg/mL) = _____ × 60 min/h = mL/h to set on pump					**33**	mL/h × 6 h
		Infusion		Run at **0.5 mg/ min** × 18 h		900 mg/ 500 mL	1.8	mg/mL		
				Ordered mg dose (0.5 mg/min) ÷ mg/mL (1.8 mg/mL) = _____ × 60 min/h = mL/h to set on pump					**17**	mL/h × 18 h
Amrinone	0.75 mg/kg =	105 mg		Give mg/kg load over 10 min		300 mg/ 120 mL	2.5	mg/mL		—
		mg to give ÷ mg/mL = 42 mL				42	mL × (60 min/h ÷ 10 min) =		**252**	mL/h × 10 min
		Infusion	0.30		5–10 mcg/ kg/min	300 mg/ 120 mL	2500	mcg/mL		—
				Take dose you want in mcg ÷ by drug index number = mL/h on pump						
Brevibloc		Infusion	1.19		50–100 mcg/ kg/min	2.5 g/ 250 mL	10,000	mcg/mL		___ mL/h
				Take dose you want in mcg ÷ by drug index number = mL/h on pump						
Cardene		Infusion	—		0.5–10 mg/h	25 mg 250 mL	0.1	mg/mL		—
				Ordered mg dose ÷ mg/mL = mL/h to set on pump						___ mL/h
Cardizem	0.25 mg/kg =	35 mg		Give mg/kg load over 20 min		50 mg/ 100 mL	0.5	DRUG/mL		—
		mg to give ÷ mg/mL = 70 mL				70	mL × (60 min/h ÷ 20 min) =		**210**	mL/h
	0.35 mg/kg =	49 mg		May repeat loading dose in 15 min			0.5	mg/mL		—
		mg to give ÷ mg/mL = 98 mL				98	mL × (60 min/h ÷ 20 min) =		**294**	mL/h
		Infusion			5–15 mg/h					—
				Ordered mg dose ÷ mg/mL = mL/h to set on pump						___ mL/h
Desmopressin	0.3 mcg/kg =	42 mcg		Give dose over 20–30 min			4	mcg/vial		
Dobutamine		Infusion	0.24		2.5–40 mcg/kg/ min	250 mg/ 125 mL	2000	mcg/mL		
				Take dose you want in mcg ÷ by drug index number = mL/h on pump						

(continues)

140 kg (continued)

DRUG	ORDERED AMOUNT	TOTAL DOSE TO GIVE	DRUG INDEX NUMBER	DIRECTIONS	INFUSION RANGE	DRUG MIXTURE	AMOUNT	DRUG/mL	RUN AT	mL/h
Dopamine	Infusion		0.19		1–20 mcg/kg/min	400 mg/250 mL	1600	mcg/mL		
	Take dose you want in mcg ÷ by drug index number = mL/h on pump									
Epinephrine	Infusion	1 mcg/min = 4 mL/h 2 mcg/min = 8 mL/h 3 mcg/min = 11 mL/h 4 mcg/min = 15 mL/h			1–4 mcg/min	4 mg/250 mL	16	mcg/mL		
	Ordered mcg dose/min ÷ mcg/mL × 60 min/h =								___	mL/h
Fenoldapam	Infusion		0.0048		0.01–1.6 mcg/kg/min	10 mg/250 mL	40	mcg/mL		
	Take dose you want in mcg ÷ by drug index number = mL/h on pump									
Heparin	100 u/kg = 14,000 u 200 u/kg = 28,000 u 300 u/kg = 42,000 u 400 u/kg = 56,000 u									
Isoproterenol	Infusion				5 mcg/min	1 mg/250 mL	4	mcg/mL		
	Ordered mcg dose/min ÷ mcg/mL × 60 min/h =								75	mL/h
Lidocaine	Infusion	1 mg/min = 7.5 mL/h			1–4 mg/min	2 g/250 mL	8	mg/mL	___	
	Ordered mg/min ÷ mg/mL × 60 min/h =								___	mL/h
Nitroglycerin	Infusion	3 mcg/min = 1 mL/h			3–200 mcg/min	50 mg/250 mL	200	mcg/mL	___	
	Ordered mcg/min ÷ mcg/mL × 60 min/h =								___	mL/h
Nitroprusside	Infusion	6.7 mcg/min = 1 mL/h			5–300 mcg/min	100 mg/250 mL	400	mcg/mL	___	
	Ordered mcg/min ÷ mcg/mL × 60 min/h =								___	mL/h
Norepinephrine	Infusion	1 mcg/min = 4 mL/h 2 mcg/min = 8 mL/h 3 mcg/min = 11 mL/h 4 mcg/min = 15 mL/h 5 mcg/min = 19 mL/h			2–20 mcg/min	4 mg/250 mL	16	mcg/mL		
	Ordered mcg dose/min ÷ mcg/mL × 60 min/h =								___	mL/h
Phenylephrine	Infusion	1.3 mcg/min = 1 mL/h			10–200 mcg/min	20 mg/250 mL	80	mcg/mL		
	Ordered mcg/min ÷ mcg/mL × 60 min/h =								___	mL/h
Primacor	0.05 mg/kg = 7 mg			Give load over 10 min		40 mg/200 mL	0.2	mg/mL		
	mg to give ÷ mg/mL = 35 mL				35 mL × (60 min/h ÷ 10 min) =				210	mL/h × 10 min
	Infusion		0.02		0.5 mcg/kg/min	40 mg/200 mL	200	mcg/mL	___	
	Take dose you want in mcg ÷ by drug index number = mL/h on pump									
Trimethaphan	Infusion		—		0.3–6 mg/min	500 mg/500 mL	1	mg/mL	___	
	Ordered mg/min ÷ mg/mL × 60 min/h =								___	mL/h
Vasopressin		0.02 u/min = 3 mL/h 0.04 u/min = 6 mL/h				40 u/100 mL	400	u/mL		

141 kg

DRUG	ORDERED AMOUNT	TOTAL DOSE TO GIVE	DRUG INDEX NUMBER	DIRECTIONS	INFUSION RANGE	DRUG MIXTURE	AMOUNT	DRUG/ mL	RUN AT	mL/h
Aminophylline	5 mg/kg = 705 mg			Give mg/kg load over 20 min		500 mg/ 250 mL	2 mg/mL			
	mg to give ÷ mg/mL = 353 mL				353	mL × (60 min/h ÷ 20 min) =			1058	mL/h × 20 min
	Infusion				0.5–1 mg/kg/h	500 mg/ 250 mL	2 mg/mL			
					mg dose ordered × kg ÷ mg/mL =				___	mL/h
Amiodarone	Loading dose			Load **150 mg** over 10 min		900 mg/ 500 mL	1.8 mg/mL		___	
				Ordered mg load dose (150 mg) ÷ mg/mL (1.8 mg/mL) = 83 mL to give × (60 min/h ÷ 10 min) = mL/h to set on pump					500	mL/h × 83 mL
	Infusion			Run at **1 mg/ min** × 6 h		900 mg/ 500 mL	1.8 mg/mL			
				Ordered mg dose (1 mg/min) ÷ mg/mL (1.8 mg/mL) = _____ × 60 min/h = mL/h to set on pump					33	mL/h × 6 h
	Infusion			Run at **0.5 mg/ min** × 18 h		900 mg/ 500 mL	1.8 mg/mL			
				Ordered mg dose (0.5 mg/min) ÷ mg/mL (1.8 mg/mL) = _____ × 60 min/h = mL/h to set on pump					17	mL/h × 18 h
Amrinone	0.75 mg/kg = 105.75 mg			Give mg/kg load over 10 min		300 mg/ 120 mL	2.5 mg/mL		___	
	mg to give ÷ mg/mL = 42 mL				42.3	mL × (60 min/h ÷ 10 min) =			254	mL/h × 10 min
	Infusion		0.30		5–10 mcg/ kg/min	300 mg/ 120 mL	2500 mcg/mL		___	
				Take dose you want in mcg ÷ by drug index number = mL/h on pump						
Brevibloc	Infusion		1.18		50–100 mcg/ kg/min	2.5 g/ 250 mL	10,000 mcg/mL		___	mL/h
				Take dose you want in mcg ÷ by drug index number = mL/h on pump						
Cardene	Infusion		—		0.5–10 mg/h	25 mg 250 mL	0.1 mg/mL		___	
				Ordered mg dose ÷ mg/mL = mL/h to set on pump					___	mL/h
Cardizem	0.25 mg/kg = 35.25 mg			Give mg/kg load over 20 min		50 mg/ 100 mL	0.5 mg/mL		___	
	mg to give ÷ mg/mL = 71 mL				70.5	mL × (60 min/h ÷ 20 min) =			212	mL/h
	0.35 mg/kg = 49.35 mg			May repeat loading dose in 15 min			0.5 mg/mL		___	
	mg to give ÷ mg/mL = 99 mL				98.7	mL × (60 min/h ÷ 20 min) =			296	mL/h
	Infusion				5–15 mg/h				___	
				Ordered mg dose ÷ mg/mL = mL/h to set on pump					___	mL/h
Desmopressin	0.3 mcg/kg = 42 mcg			Give dose over 20–30 min			4 mcg/vial			
Dobutamine	Infusion		0.24		2.5–40 mcg/kg/ min	250 mg/ 125 mL	2000 mcg/mL			
				Take dose you want in mcg ÷ by drug index number = mL/h on pump						

(continues)

141 kg (continued)

DRUG	ORDERED AMOUNT	TOTAL DOSE TO GIVE	DRUG INDEX NUMBER	DIRECTIONS	INFUSION RANGE	DRUG MIXTURE	AMOUNT	DRUG/ mL	RUN AT	mL/h
Dopamine	Infusion		0.19		1–20 mcg/ kg/min	400 mg/ 250 mL	1600	mcg/mL		
			Take dose you want in mcg ÷ by drug index number = mL/h on pump							
Epinephrine	Infusion	1 mcg/min = 4 mL/h 2 mcg/min = 8 mL/h 3 mcg/min = 11 mL/h 4 mcg/min = 15 mL/h			1–4 mcg/min	4 mg/ 250 mL	16	mcg/mL		
				Ordered mcg dose/min ÷ mcg/mL × 60 min/h =					___	mL/h
Fenoldapam	Infusion		0.0048		0.01–1.6 mcg/ kg/min	10 mg/ 250 mL	40	mcg/mL		
			Take dose you want in mcg ÷ by drug index number = mL/h on pump							
Heparin	100 u/kg = 200 u/kg = 300 u/kg = 400 u/kg =	14,100 u 28,200 u 42,300 u 56,400 u								
Isoproterenol	Infusion				5 mcg/min	1 mg/ 250 mL	4	mcg/mL		
				Ordered mcg dose/min ÷ mcg/mL × 60 min/h =					75	mL/h
Lidocaine	Infusion	1 mg/min = 7.5 mL/h			1–4 mg/min	2 g/ 250 mL	8	mg/mL	___	
				Ordered mg/min ÷ mg/mL × 60 min/h =					___	mL/h
Nitroglycerin	Infusion	3 mcg/min = 1 mL/h			3–200 mcg/min	50 mg/ 250 mL	200	mcg/mL	___	
				Ordered mcg/min ÷ mcg/mL × 60 min/h =					___	mL/h
Nitroprusside	Infusion	6.7 mcg/min = 1 mL/h			5–300 mcg/min	100 mg/ 250 mL	400	mcg/mL	___	
				Ordered mcg/min ÷ mcg/mL × 60 min/h =					___	mL/h
Norepinephrine	Infusion	1 mcg/min = 4 mL/h 2 mcg/min = 8 mL/h 3 mcg/min = 11 mL/h 4 mcg/min = 15 mL/h 5 mcg/min = 19 mL/h			2–20 mcg/min	4 mg/ 250 mL	16	mcg/mL		
				Ordered mcg dose/min ÷ mcg/mL × 60 min/h =					___	mL/h
Phenylephrine	Infusion	1.3 mcg/min = 1 mL/h			10–200 mcg/min	20 mg/ 250 mL	80	mcg/mL		
				Ordered mcg/min ÷ mcg/mL × 60 min/h =					___	mL/h
Primacor	0.05 mg/kg =	7.05 mg		Give load over 10 min		40 mg/ 200 mL	0.2	mg/mL		
	mg to give ÷ mg/mL =	35 mL				35	mL × (60 min/h ÷ 10 min) =		212	mL/h × 10 min
	Infusion		0.02		0.5 mcg/ kg/min	40 mg/ 200 mL	200	mcg/mL	___	
			Take dose you want in mcg ÷ by drug index number = mL/h on pump							
Trimethaphan	Infusion		—		0.3–6 mg/min	500 mg/ 500 mL	1	mg/mL	___	
				Ordered mg/min ÷ mg/mL × 60 min/h =					___	mL/h
Vasopressin		0.02 u/min = 3 mL/h 0.04 u/min = 6 mL/h				40 u/ 100 mL	400	u/mL		

142 kg

DRUG	ORDERED AMOUNT	TOTAL DOSE TO GIVE	DRUG INDEX NUMBER	DIRECTIONS	INFUSION RANGE	DRUG MIXTURE	AMOUNT DRUG/mL	RUN AT mL/h
Aminophylline	5 mg/kg =	710 mg		Give mg/kg load over 20 min		500 mg/ 250 mL	2 mg/mL	
	mg to give ÷ mg/mL =	355 mL			355	mL × (60 min/h ÷ 20 min) =		<u>1065</u> mL/h × 20 min
	Infusion				0.5–1 mg/kg/h	500 mg/ 250 mL	2 mg/mL	
				mg dose ordered × kg ÷ mg/mL =				___ mL/h
Amiodarone	Loading dose			Load **150 mg** over 10 min		900 mg/ 500 mL	1.8 mg/mL	___
				Ordered mg load dose (150 mg) ÷ mg/mL (1.8 mg/mL) = 83 mL to give × (60 min/h ÷ 10 min) = mL/h to set on pump				<u>500</u> mL/h × 83 mL
	Infusion			Run at **1 mg/ min** × 6 h		900 mg/ 500 mL	1.8 mg/mL	
				Ordered mg dose (1 mg/min) ÷ mg/mL (1.8 mg/mL) = ____ × 60 min/h = mL/h to set on pump				<u>33</u> mL/h × 6 h
	Infusion			Run at **0.5 mg/ min** × 18 h		900 mg/ 500 mL	1.8 mg/mL	
				Ordered mg dose (0.5 mg/min) ÷ mg/mL (1.8 mg/mL) = ____ × 60 min/h = mL/h to set on pump				<u>17</u> mL/h × 18 h
Amrinone	0.75 mg/kg =	106.5 mg		Give mg/kg load over 10 min		300 mg/ 120 mL	2.5 mg/mL	___
	mg to give ÷ mg/mL =	43 mL			42.6	mL × (60 min/h ÷ 10 min) =		<u>256</u> mL/h × 10 min
	Infusion		0.29		5–10 mcg/ kg/min	300 mg/ 120 mL	2500 mcg/mL	___
				Take dose you want in mcg ÷ by drug index number = mL/h on pump				
Brevibloc	Infusion		1.17		50–100 mcg/ kg/min	2.5 g/ 250 mL	10,000 mcg/mL	___ mL/h
				Take dose you want in mcg ÷ by drug index number = mL/h on pump				
Cardene	Infusion		—		0.5–10 mg/h	25 mg 250 mL	0.1 mg/mL	___
				Ordered mg dose ÷ mg/mL = mL/h to set on pump				___ mL/h
Cardizem	0.25 mg/kg =	35.5 mg		Give mg/kg load over 20 min		50 mg/ 100 mL	0.5 mg/mL	___
	mg to give ÷ mg/mL =	71 mL			71	mL × (60 min/h ÷ 20 min) =		<u>213</u> mL/h
	0.35 mg/kg =	49.7 mg		May repeat loading dose in 15 min			0.5 mg/mL	___
	mg to give ÷ mg/mL =	99 mL			99.4	mL × (60 min/h ÷ 20 min) =		<u>298</u> mL/h
	Infusion				5–15 mg/h			___
				Ordered mg dose ÷ mg/mL = mL/h to set on pump				___ mL/h
Desmopressin	0.3 mcg/kg =	43 mcg		Give dose over 20–30 min			4 mcg/vial	
Dobutamine	Infusion		0.23		2.5–40 mcg/kg/ min	250 mg/ 125 mL	2000 mcg/mL	
				Take dose you want in mcg ÷ by drug index number = mL/h on pump				

(continues)

142 kg (continued)

DRUG	ORDERED AMOUNT	TOTAL DOSE TO GIVE	DRUG INDEX NUMBER	DIRECTIONS	INFUSION RANGE	DRUG MIXTURE	AMOUNT	DRUG/mL	RUN AT	mL/h
Dopamine	Infusion		0.19		1–20 mcg/kg/min	400 mg/250 mL	1600	mcg/mL		
	— Take dose you want in mcg ÷ by drug index number = mL/h on pump									
Epinephrine	Infusion	1 mcg/min = 4 mL/h 2 mcg/min = 8 mL/h 3 mcg/min = 11 mL/h 4 mcg/min = 15 mL/h			1–4 mcg/min	4 mg/250 mL	16	mcg/mL		
	Ordered mcg dose/min ÷ mcg/mL × 60 min/h =								___	mL/h
Fenoldapam	Infusion		0.0047		0.01–1.6 mcg/kg/min	10 mg/250 mL	40	mcg/mL		
	Take dose you want in mcg ÷ by drug index number = mL/h on pump									
Heparin	100 u/kg = 14,200 u 200 u/kg = 28,400 u 300 u/kg = 42,600 u 400 u/kg = 56,800 u									
Isoproterenol	Infusion				5 mcg/min	1 mg/250 mL	4	mcg/mL		
	Ordered mcg dose/min ÷ mcg/mL × 60 min/h =								75	mL/h
Lidocaine	Infusion	1 mg/min = 7.5 mL/h			1–4 mg/min	2 g/250 mL	8	mg/mL	___	
	Ordered mg/min ÷ mg/mL × 60 min/h =								___	mL/h
Nitroglycerin	Infusion	3 mcg/min = 1 mL/h			3–200 mcg/min	50 mg/250 mL	200	mcg/mL	___	
	Ordered mcg/min ÷ mcg/mL × 60 min/h =								___	mL/h
Nitroprusside	Infusion	6.7 mcg/min = 1 mL/h			5–300 mcg/min	100 mg/250 mL	400	mcg/mL	___	
	Ordered mcg/min ÷ mcg/mL × 60 min/h =								___	mL/h
Norepinephrine	Infusion	1 mcg/min = 4 mL/h 2 mcg/min = 8 mL/h 3 mcg/min = 11 mL/h 4 mcg/min = 15 mL/h 5 mcg/min = 19 mL/h			2–20 mcg/min	4 mg/250 mL	16	mcg/mL		
	Ordered mcg dose/min ÷ mcg/mL × 60 min/h =								___	mL/h
Phenylephrine	Infusion	1.3 mcg/min = 1 mL/h			10–200 mcg/min	20 mg/250 mL	80	mcg/mL		
	Ordered mcg/min ÷ mcg/mL × 60 min/h =								___	mL/h
Primacor	0.05 mg/kg = 7.1 mg			Give load over 10 min		40 mg/200 mL	0.2	mg/mL		
	mg to give ÷ mg/mL = 36 mL				36	mL × (60 min/h ÷ 10 min) =			213	mL/h × 10 min
	Infusion		0.02		0.5 mcg/kg/min	40 mg/200 mL	200	mcg/mL	___	
	Take dose you want in mcg ÷ by drug index number = mL/h on pump									
Trimethaphan	Infusion		___		0.3–6 mg/min	500 mg/500 mL	1	mg/mL	___	
	Ordered mg/min ÷ mg/mL × 60 min/h =								___	mL/h
Vasopressin	0.02 u/min = 3 mL/h 0.04 u/min = 6 mL/h					40 u/100 mL	400	u/mL		

143 kg										
DRUG	**ORDERED AMOUNT**	**TOTAL DOSE TO GIVE**	**DRUG INDEX NUMBER**	**DIRECTIONS**	**INFUSION RANGE**	**DRUG MIXTURE**	**AMOUNT**	**DRUG/ mL**	**RUN AT**	**mL/h**
Aminophylline	5 mg/kg =	715 mg		Give mg/kg load over 20 min		500 mg/ 250 mL	2 mg/mL			
	mg to give ÷ mg/mL =	358 mL			358	mL × (60 min/h ÷ 20 min) =			1073	mL/h × 20 min
	Infusion				0.5–1 mg/kg/h	500 mg/ 250 mL	2 mg/mL			
					mg dose ordered × kg ÷ mg/mL =					___ mL/h
Amiodarone	Loading dose			Load **150 mg** over 10 min		900 mg/ 500 mL	1.8 mg/mL			___
				Ordered mg load dose (150 mg) ÷ mg/mL (1.8 mg/mL) = 83 mL to give × (60 min/h ÷ 10 min) = mL/h to set on pump					500	mL/h × 83 mL
	Infusion			Run at **1 mg/ min** × 6 h		900 mg/ 500 mL	1.8 mg/mL			
				Ordered mg dose (1 mg/min) ÷ mg/mL (1.8 mg/mL) = ____ × 60 min/h = mL/h to set on pump					33	mL/h × 6 h
	Infusion			Run at **0.5 mg/ min** × 18 h		900 mg/ 500 mL	1.8 mg/mL			
				Ordered mg dose (0.5 mg/min) ÷ mg/mL (1.8 mg/mL) = ____ × 60 min/h = mL/h to set on pump					17	mL/h × 18 h
Amrinone	0.75 mg/kg =	107.25 mg		Give mg/kg load over 10 min		300 mg/ 120 mL	2.5 mg/mL			___
	mg to give ÷ mg/mL =	43 mL			42.9	mL × (60 min/h ÷ 10 min) =			257	mL/h × 10 min
	Infusion		0.29		5–10 mcg/ kg/min	300 mg/ 120 mL	2500 mcg/mL			
				Take dose you want in mcg ÷ by drug index number = mL/h on pump						
Brevibloc	Infusion		1.17		50–100 mcg/ kg/min	2.5 g/ 250 mL	10,000 mcg/mL			___ mL/h
				Take dose you want in mcg ÷ by drug index number = mL/h on pump						
Cardene	Infusion			—	0.5–10 mg/h	25 mg 250 mL	0.1 mg/mL			___
				Ordered mg dose ÷ mg/mL = mL/h to set on pump						___ mL/h
Cardizem	0.25 mg/kg =	35.75 mg		Give mg/kg load over 20 min		50 mg/ 100 mL	0.5 mg/mL			___
	mg to give ÷ mg/mL =	72 mL			71.5	mL × (60 min/h ÷ 20 min) =			215	mL/h
	0.35 mg/kg =	50.05 mg		May repeat loading dose in 15 min			0.5 mg/mL			___
	mg to give ÷ mg/mL =	100 mL			100.1	mL × (60 min/h ÷ 20 min) =			300	mL/h
	Infusion				5–15 mg/h					___
				Ordered mg dose ÷ mg/mL = mL/h to set on pump						___ mL/h
Desmopressin	0.3 mcg/kg =	43 mcg		Give dose over 20–30 min			4 mcg/vial			
Dobutamine	Infusion		0.23		2.5–40 mcg/kg/ min	250 mg/ 125 mL	2000 mcg/mL			
				Take dose you want in mcg ÷ by drug index number = mL/h on pump						

(continues)

143 kg (continued)

DRUG	ORDERED AMOUNT	TOTAL DOSE TO GIVE	DRUG INDEX NUMBER	DIRECTIONS	INFUSION RANGE	DRUG MIXTURE	AMOUNT	DRUG/mL	RUN AT	mL/h
Dopamine	Infusion		0.19		1–20 mcg/kg/min	400 mg/250 mL	1600 mcg/mL			
		Take dose you want in mcg ÷ by drug index number = mL/h on pump								
Epinephrine	Infusion	1 mcg/min = 4 mL/h 2 mcg/min = 8 mL/h 3 mcg/min = 11 mL/h 4 mcg/min = 15 mL/h			1–4 mcg/min	4 mg/250 mL	16 mcg/mL			
		Ordered mcg dose/min ÷ mcg/mL × 60 min/h =								___ mL/h
Fenoldapam	Infusion		0.0047		0.01–1.6 mcg/kg/min	10 mg/250 mL	40 mcg/mL			
		Take dose you want in mcg ÷ by drug index number = mL/h on pump								
Heparin	100 u/kg = 14,300 u 200 u/kg = 28,600 u 300 u/kg = 42,900 u 400 u/kg = 57,200 u									
Isoproterenol	Infusion				5 mcg/min	1 mg/250 mL	4 mcg/mL			
		Ordered mcg dose/min ÷ mcg/mL × 60 min/h =								75 mL/h
Lidocaine	Infusion	1 mg/min = 7.5 mL/h			1–4 mg/min	2 g/250 mL	8 mg/mL			___
		Ordered mg/min ÷ mg/mL × 60 min/h =								___ mL/h
Nitroglycerin	Infusion	3 mcg/min = 1 mL/h			3–200 mcg/min	50 mg/250 mL	200 mcg/mL			___
		Ordered mcg/min ÷ mcg/mL × 60 min/h =								___ mL/h
Nitroprusside	Infusion	6.7 mcg/min = 1 mL/h			5–300 mcg/min	100 mg/250 mL	400 mcg/mL			___
		Ordered mcg/min ÷ mcg/mL × 60 min/h =								___ mL/h
Norepinephrine	Infusion	1 mcg/min = 4 mL/h 2 mcg/min = 8 mL/h 3 mcg/min = 11 mL/h 4 mcg/min = 15 mL/h 5 mcg/min = 19 mL/h			2–20 mcg/min	4 mg/250 mL	16 mcg/mL			
		Ordered mcg dose/min ÷ mcg/mL × 60 min/h =								___ mL/h
Phenylephrine	Infusion	1.3 mcg/min = 1 mL/h			10–200 mcg/min	20 mg/250 mL	80 mcg/mL			
		Ordered mcg/min ÷ mcg/mL × 60 min/h =								___ mL/h
Primacor	0.05 mg/kg = 7.15 mg			Give load over 10 min		40 mg/200 mL	0.2 mg/mL			
	mg to give ÷ mg/mL = 36 mL					36 mL × (60 min/h ÷ 10 min) =			215	mL/h × 10 min
	Infusion		0.02		0.5 mcg/kg/min	40 mg/200 mL	200 mcg/mL			___
		Take dose you want in mcg ÷ by drug index number = mL/h on pump								
Trimethaphan	Infusion		___		0.3–6 mg/min	500 mg/500 mL	1 mg/mL			___
		Ordered mg/min ÷ mg/mL × 60 min/h =								___ mL/h
Vasopressin		0.02 u/min = 3 mL/h 0.04 u/min = 6 mL/h				40 u/100 mL	400 u/mL			

144 kg

DRUG	ORDERED AMOUNT	TOTAL DOSE TO GIVE	DRUG INDEX NUMBER	DIRECTIONS	INFUSION RANGE	DRUG MIXTURE	AMOUNT	DRUG/ mL	RUN AT	mL/h
Aminophylline	5 mg/kg = 720 mg			Give mg/kg load over 20 min		500 mg/ 250 mL	2 mg/mL			
	mg to give ÷ mg/mL = 360 mL					360 mL × (60 min/h ÷ 20 min) =			1080	mL/h × 20 min
	Infusion				0.5–1 mg/kg/h	500 mg/ 250 mL	2 mg/mL			
					mg dose ordered × kg ÷ mg/mL =				___ mL/h	
Amiodarone	Loading dose			Load **150 mg** over 10 min		900 mg/ 500 mL	1.8 mg/mL		___	
				Ordered mg load dose (150 mg) ÷ mg/mL (1.8 mg/mL) = 83 mL to give × (60 min/h ÷ 10 min) = mL/h to set on pump					**500**	mL/h × 83 mL
	Infusion			Run at **1 mg/ min** × 6 h		900 mg/ 500 mL	1.8 mg/mL			
				Ordered mg dose (1 mg/min) ÷ mg/mL (1.8 mg/mL) = ____ × 60 min/h = mL/h to set on pump					**33**	mL/h × 6 h
	Infusion			Run at **0.5 mg/ min** × 18 h		900 mg/ 500 mL	1.8 mg/mL			
				Ordered mg dose (0.5 mg/min) ÷ mg/mL (1.8 mg/mL) = ____ × 60 min/h = mL/h to set on pump					**17**	mL/h × 18 h
Amrinone	0.75 mg/kg = 108 mg			Give mg/kg load over 10 min		300 mg/ 120 mL	2.5 mg/mL		___	
	mg to give ÷ mg/mL = 43 mL					43.2 mL × (60 min/h ÷ 10 min) =			**259**	mL/h × 10 min
	Infusion		0.29		5–10 mcg/ kg/min	300 mg/ 120 mL	2500 mcg/mL		___	
				Take dose you want in mcg ÷ by drug index number = mL/h on pump						
Brevibloc	Infusion		1.16		50–100 mcg/ kg/min	2.5 g/ 250 mL	10,000 mcg/mL		___	mL/h
				Take dose you want in mcg ÷ by drug index number = mL/h on pump						
Cardene	Infusion		—		0.5–10 mg/h	25 mg 250 mL	0.1 mg/mL		___	
				Ordered mg dose ÷ mg/mL = mL/h to set on pump						___ mL/h
Cardizem	0.25 mg/kg = 36 mg			Give mg/kg load over 20 min		50 mg/ 100 mL	0.5 mg/mL		___	
	mg to give ÷ mg/mL = 72 mL					72 mL × (60 min/h ÷ 20 min) =			**216**	mL/h
	0.35 mg/kg = 50.4 mg			May repeat loading dose in 15 min			0.5 mg/mL		___	
	mg to give ÷ mg/mL = 101 mL					100.8 mL × (60 min/h ÷ 20 min) =			**302**	mL/h
	Infusion				5–15 mg/h				___	
				Ordered mg dose ÷ mg/mL = mL/h to set on pump						___ mL/h
Desmopressin	0.3 mcg/kg = 43 mcg			Give dose over 20–30 min			4 mcg/vial			
Dobutamine	Infusion		0.23		2.5–40 mcg/kg/ min	250 mg/ 125 mL	2000 mcg/mL			
				Take dose you want in mcg ÷ by drug index number = mL/h on pump						

(continues)

144 kg (continued)

DRUG	ORDERED AMOUNT		TOTAL DOSE TO GIVE		DRUG INDEX NUMBER	DIRECTIONS	INFUSION RANGE	DRUG MIXTURE	AMOUNT	DRUG/ mL	RUN AT	mL/h
Dopamine	Infusion				0.19		1–20 mcg/ kg/min	400 mg/ 250 mL	1600	mcg/mL		
	Take dose you want in mcg ÷ by drug index number = mL/h on pump											
Epinephrine	Infusion		1 mcg/min = 4 mL/h 2 mcg/min = 8 mL/h 3 mcg/min = 11 mL/h 4 mcg/min = 15 mL/h				1–4 mcg/min	4 mg/ 250 mL	16	mcg/mL		
			Ordered mcg dose/min ÷ mcg/mL × 60 min/h =								___	mL/h
Fenoldapam	Infusion				0.0047		0.01–1.6 mcg/ kg/min	10 mg/ 250 mL	40	mcg/mL		
	Take dose you want in mcg ÷ by drug index number = mL/h on pump											
Heparin	100 u/kg =	14,400 u										
	200 u/kg =	28,800 u										
	300 u/kg =	43,200 u										
	400 u/kg =	57,600 u										
Isoproterenol	Infusion						5 mcg/min	1 mg/ 250 mL	4	mcg/mL		
	Ordered mcg dose/min ÷ mcg/mL × 60 min/h =										75	mL/h
Lidocaine	Infusion		1 mg/min = 7.5 mL/h				1–4 mg/min	2 g/ 250 mL	8	mg/mL	___	
	Ordered mg/min ÷ mg/mL × 60 min/h =										___	mL/h
Nitroglycerin	Infusion		3 mcg/min = 1 mL/h				3–200 mcg/min	50 mg/ 250 mL	200	mcg/mL	___	
	Ordered mcg/min ÷ mcg/mL × 60 min/h =										___	mL/h
Nitroprusside	Infusion		6.7 mcg/min = 1 mL/h				5–300 mcg/min	100 mg/ 250 mL	400	mcg/mL	___	
	Ordered mcg/min ÷ mcg/mL × 60 min/h =										___	mL/h
Norepinephrine	Infusion		1 mcg/min = 4 mL/h 2 mcg/min = 8 mL/h 3 mcg/min = 11 mL/h 4 mcg/min = 15 mL/h 5 mcg/min = 19 mL/h				2–20 mcg/min	4 mg/ 250 mL	16	mcg/mL		
	Ordered mcg dose/min ÷ mcg/mL × 60 min/h =										___	mL/h
Phenylephrine	Infusion		1.3 mcg/min = 1 mL/h				10–200 mcg/min	20 mg/ 250 mL	80	mcg/mL		
	Ordered mcg/min ÷ mcg/mL × 60 min/h =										___	mL/h
Primacor	0.05 mg/kg =	7.2 mg				Give load over 10 min		40 mg/ 200 mL	0.2	mg/mL		
	mg to give ÷ mg/mL =	36 mL					36	mL × (60 min/h ÷ 10 min) =			216	mL/h × 10 min
	Infusion				0.02		0.5 mcg/ kg/min	40 mg/ 200 mL	200	mcg/mL	___	
	Take dose you want in mcg ÷ by drug index number = mL/h on pump											
Trimethaphan	Infusion				—		0.3–6 mg/min	500 mg/ 500 mL	1	mg/mL	___	
	Ordered mg/min ÷ mg/mL × 60 min/h =										___	mL/h
Vasopressin			0.02 u/min = 3 mL/h 0.04 u/min = 6 mL/h					40 u/ 100 mL	400	u/mL		

145 kg

DRUG	ORDERED AMOUNT	TOTAL DOSE TO GIVE	DRUG INDEX NUMBER	DIRECTIONS	INFUSION RANGE	DRUG MIXTURE	AMOUNT	DRUG/ mL	RUN AT	mL/h
Aminophylline	5 mg/kg =	725 mg		Give mg/kg load over 20 min		500 mg/ 250 mL	2 mg/mL		
	mg to give ÷ mg/mL =	363 mL			363	mL × (60 min/h ÷ 20 min) =			1088	mL/h × 20 min
	Infusion				0.5–1 mg/kg/h	500 mg/ 250 mL	2 mg/mL		
						mg dose ordered × kg ÷ mg/mL =			___	mL/h
Amiodarone	Loading dose			Load **150 mg** over 10 min		900 mg/ 500 mL	1.8 mg/mL		___
				Ordered mg load dose (150 mg) ÷ mg/mL (1.8 mg/mL) = 83 mL to give × (60 min/h ÷ 10 min) = mL/h to set on pump					500	mL/h × 83 mL
	Infusion			Run at **1 mg/ min** × 6 h		900 mg/ 500 mL	1.8 mg/mL		
				Ordered mg dose (1 mg/min) ÷ mg/mL (1.8 mg/mL) = ____ × 60 min/h = mL/h to set on pump					33	mL/h × 6 h
	Infusion			Run at **0.5 mg/ min** × 18 h		900 mg/ 500 mL	1.8 mg/mL		
				Ordered mg dose (0.5 mg/min) ÷ mg/mL (1.8 mg/mL) = ____ × 60 min/h = mL/h to set on pump					17	mL/h × 18 h
Amrinone	0.75 mg/kg =	108.75 mg		Give mg/kg load over 10 min		300 mg/ 120 mL	2.5 mg/mL		___
	mg to give ÷ mg/mL =	44 mL			43.5	mL × (60 min/h ÷ 10 min) =			261	mL/h × 10 min
	Infusion		0.29		5–10 mcg/ kg/min	300 mg/ 120 mL	2500 mcg/mL		___
				Take dose you want in mcg ÷ by drug index number = mL/h on pump					
Breviloc	Infusion		1.15		50–100 mcg/ kg/min	2.5 g/ 250 mL	10,000 mcg/mL		___ mL/h
				Take dose you want in mcg ÷ by drug index number = mL/h on pump					
Cardene	Infusion		—		0.5–10 mg/h	25 mg 250 mL	0.1 mg/mL		___
				Ordered mg dose ÷ mg/mL = mL/h to set on pump					___ mL/h
Cardizem	0.25 mg/kg =	36.25 mg		Give mg/kg load over 20 min		50 mg/ 100 mL	0.5 mg/mL		
	mg to give ÷ mg/mL =	73 mL			72.5	mL × (60 min/h ÷ 20 min) =			218	mL/h
	0.35 mg/kg =	50.75 mg		May repeat loading dose in 15 min			0.5 mg/mL		___
	mg to give ÷ mg/mL =	102 mL			101.5	mL × (60 min/h ÷ 20 min) =			305	mL/h
	Infusion				5–15 mg/h				___
				Ordered mg dose ÷ mg/mL = mL/h to set on pump					___ mL/h
Desmopressin	0.3 mcg/kg =	44 mcg		Give dose over 20–30 min			4 mcg/vial		
Dobutamine	Infusion		0.23		2.5–40 mcg/kg/ min	250 mg/ 125 mL	2000 mcg/mL		
				Take dose you want in mcg ÷ by drug index number = mL/h on pump					

(continues)

145　kg (continued)

DRUG	ORDERED AMOUNT	TOTAL DOSE TO GIVE	DRUG INDEX NUMBER	DIRECTIONS	INFUSION RANGE	DRUG MIXTURE	AMOUNT	DRUG/ mL	RUN AT	mL/h
Dopamine	Infusion		0.18		1–20 mcg/ kg/min	400 mg/ 250 mL	1600	mcg/mL		
	Take dose you want in mcg ÷ by drug index number = mL/h on pump									
Epinephrine	Infusion	1 mcg/min = 4 mL/h 2 mcg/min = 8 mL/h 3 mcg/min = 11 mL/h 4 mcg/min = 15 mL/h			1–4 mcg/min	4 mg/ 250 mL	16	mcg/mL		
					Ordered mcg dose/min ÷ mcg/mL × 60 min/h =				___	mL/h
Fenoldapam	Infusion		0.0046		0.01–1.6 mcg/ kg/min	10 mg/ 250 mL	40	mcg/mL		
					Take dose you want in mcg ÷ by drug index number = mL/h on pump					
Heparin	100　u/kg = 200　u/kg = 300　u/kg = 400　u/kg =	14,500　u 29,000　u 43,500　u 58,000　u								
Isoproterenol	Infusion				5 mcg/min	1 mg/ 250 mL	4	mcg/mL		
					Ordered mcg dose/min ÷ mcg/mL × 60 min/h =				<u>75</u>	mL/h
Lidocaine	Infusion	1 mg/min = 7.5 mL/h			1–4 mg/min	2 g/ 250 mL	8	mg/mL	___	
					Ordered mg/min ÷ mg/mL × 60 min/h =				___	mL/h
Nitroglycerin	Infusion	3 mcg/min = 1 mL/h			3–200 mcg/min	50 mg/ 250 mL	200	mcg/mL		
					Ordered mcg/min ÷ mcg/mL × 60 min/h =				___	mL/h
Nitroprusside	Infusion	6.7 mcg/min = 1 mL/h			5–300 mcg/min	100 mg/ 250 mL	400	mcg/mL		
					Ordered mcg/min ÷ mcg/mL × 60 min/h =				___	mL/h
Norepinephrine	Infusion	1 mcg/min = 4 mL/h 2 mcg/min = 8 mL/h 3 mcg/min = 11 mL/h 4 mcg/min = 15 mL/h 5 mcg/min = 19 mL/h			2–20 mcg/min	4 mg/ 250 mL	16	mcg/mL		
					Ordered mcg dose/min ÷ mcg/mL × 60 min/h =				___	mL/h
Phenylephrine	Infusion	1.3 mcg/min = 1 mL/h			10–200 mcg/min	20 mg/ 250 mL	80	mcg/mL		
					Ordered mcg/min ÷ mcg/mL × 60 min/h =				___	mL/h
Primacor	0.05　mg/kg =	7.25　mg		Give load over 10 min		40 mg/ 200 mL	0.2	mg/mL		
	mg to give ÷ mg/mL =	36　mL			36	mL × (60 min/h ÷ 10 min) =			<u>218</u>	mL/h × 10 min
	Infusion		0.02		0.5 mcg/ kg/min	40 mg/ 200 mL	200	mcg/mL	___	
					Take dose you want in mcg ÷ by drug index number = mL/h on pump					
Trimethaphan	Infusion			—	0.3–6 mg/min	500 mg/ 500 mL	1	mg/mL	___	
					Ordered mg/min ÷ mg/mL × 60 min/h =				___	mL/h
Vasopressin		0.02 u/min = 3 mL/h 0.04 u/min = 6 mL/h				40 u/ 100 mL	400	u/mL		

146　kg

DRUG	ORDERED AMOUNT	TOTAL DOSE TO GIVE	DRUG INDEX NUMBER	DIRECTIONS	INFUSION RANGE	DRUG MIXTURE	AMOUNT　DRUG/mL	RUN AT　mL/h
Aminophylline	5　mg/kg =	730　mg		Give mg/kg load over 20 min		500 mg/ 250 mL	2　mg/mL	
	mg to give ÷ mg/mL =	365　mL			365	mL × (60 min/h ÷ 20 min) =		**1095** mL/h × 20 min
	Infusion				0.5–1 mg/kg/h	500 mg/ 250 mL	2　mg/mL	
					mg dose ordered × kg ÷ mg/mL =			___ mL/h
Amiodarone	Loading dose			Load **150 mg** over 10 min		900 mg/ 500 mL	1.8　mg/mL	___
				Ordered mg load dose (150 mg) ÷ mg/mL (1.8 mg/mL) = 83 mL to give × (60 min/h ÷ 10 min) = mL/h to set on pump				**500** mL/h × 83 mL
	Infusion			Run at **1 mg/ min** × 6 h		900 mg/ 500 mL	1.8　mg/mL	
				Ordered mg dose (1 mg/min) ÷ mg/mL (1.8 mg/mL) = ___ × 60 min/h = mL/h to set on pump				**33** mL/h × 6 h
	Infusion			Run at **0.5 mg/ min** × 18 h		900 mg/ 500 mL	1.8　mg/mL	
				Ordered mg dose (0.5 mg/min) ÷ mg/mL (1.8 mg/mL) = ___ × 60 min/h = mL/h to set on pump				**17** mL/h × 18 h
Amrinone	0.75　mg/kg =	109.5　mg		Give mg/kg load over 10 min		300 mg/ 120 mL	2.5　mg/mL	___
	mg to give ÷ mg/mL =	44　mL			43.8	mL × (60 min/h ÷ 10 min) =		**263** mL/h × 10 min
	Infusion		0.28		5–10 mcg/ kg/min	300 mg/ 120 mL	2500　mcg/mL	___
				Take dose you want in mcg ÷ by drug index number = mL/h on pump				
Brevibloc	Infusion		1.14		50–100 mcg/ kg/min	2.5 g/ 250 mL	10,000　mcg/mL	___ mL/h
				Take dose you want in mcg ÷ by drug index number = mL/h on pump				
Cardene	Infusion		___		0.5–10 mg/h	25 mg 250 mL	0.1　mg/mL	___
				Ordered mg dose ÷ mg/mL = mL/h to set on pump				___ mL/h
Cardizem	0.25　mg/kg =	36.5　mg		Give mg/kg load over 20 min		50 mg/ 100 mL	0.5　mg/mL	
	mg to give ÷ mg/mL =	73　mL			73	mL × (60 min/h ÷ 20 min) =		**219** mL/h
	0.35　mg/kg =	51.1　mg		May repeat loading dose in 15 min			0.5　mg/mL	___
	mg to give ÷ mg/mL =	102　mL			102.2	mL × (60 min/h ÷ 20 min) =		**307** mL/h
	Infusion				5–15 mg/h			___
				Ordered mg dose ÷ mg/mL = mL/h to set on pump				___ mL/h
Desmopressin	0.3　mcg/kg =	44　mcg		Give dose over 20–30 min			4　mcg/vial	
Dobutamine	Infusion		0.23		2.5–40 mcg/kg/ min	250 mg/ 125 mL	2000　mcg/mL	
				Take dose you want in mcg ÷ by drug index number = mL/h on pump				

(continues)

146 kg (continued)

DRUG	ORDERED AMOUNT	TOTAL DOSE TO GIVE	DRUG INDEX NUMBER	DIRECTIONS	INFUSION RANGE	DRUG MIXTURE	AMOUNT	DRUG/mL	RUN AT	mL/h
Dopamine	Infusion		0.18		1–20 mcg/kg/min	400 mg/250 mL	1600	mcg/mL		
	Take dose you want in mcg ÷ by drug index number = mL/h on pump									
Epinephrine	Infusion	1 mcg/min = 4 mL/h 2 mcg/min = 8 mL/h 3 mcg/min = 11 mL/h 4 mcg/min = 15 mL/h			1–4 mcg/min	4 mg/250 mL	16	mcg/mL		
		Ordered mcg dose/min ÷ mcg/mL × 60 min/h =							___	mL/h
Fenoldapam	Infusion		0.0046		0.01–1.6 mcg/kg/min	10 mg/250 mL	40	mcg/mL		
	Take dose you want in mcg ÷ by drug index number = mL/h on pump									
Heparin	100 u/kg = 200 u/kg = 300 u/kg = 400 u/kg =	14,600 u 29,200 u 43,800 u 58,400 u								
Isoproterenol	Infusion				5 mcg/min	1 mg/250 mL	4	mcg/mL		
		Ordered mcg dose/min ÷ mcg/mL × 60 min/h =							75	mL/h
Lidocaine	Infusion	1 mg/min = 7.5 mL/h			1–4 mg/min	2 g/250 mL	8	mg/mL	___	
		Ordered mg/min ÷ mg/mL × 60 min/h =							___	mL/h
Nitroglycerin	Infusion	3 mcg/min = 1 mL/h			3–200 mcg/min	50 mg/250 mL	200	mcg/mL	___	
		Ordered mcg/min ÷ mcg/mL × 60 min/h =							___	mL/h
Nitroprusside	Infusion	6.7 mcg/min = 1 mL/h			5–300 mcg/min	100 mg/250 mL	400	mcg/mL	___	
		Ordered mcg/min ÷ mcg/mL × 60 min/h =							___	mL/h
Norepinephrine	Infusion	1 mcg/min = 4 mL/h 2 mcg/min = 8 mL/h 3 mcg/min = 11 mL/h 4 mcg/min = 15 mL/h 5 mcg/min = 19 mL/h			2–20 mcg/min	4 mg/250 mL	16	mcg/mL		
		Ordered mcg dose/min ÷ mcg/mL × 60 min/h =							___	mL/h
Phenylephrine	Infusion	1.3 mcg/min = 1 mL/h			10–200 mcg/min	20 mg/250 mL	80	mcg/mL		
		Ordered mcg/min ÷ mcg/mL × 60 min/h =							___	mL/h
Primacor	0.05 mg/kg =	7.3 mg		Give load over 10 min		40 mg/200 mL	0.2	mg/mL		
	mg to give ÷ mg/mL =	37 mL			37 mL × (60 min/h ÷ 10 min) =				219	mL/h × 10 min
	Infusion		0.02		0.5 mcg/kg/min	40 mg/200 mL	200	mcg/mL	___	
	Take dose you want in mcg ÷ by drug index number = mL/h on pump									
Trimethaphan	Infusion		—		0.3–6 mg/min	500 mg/500 mL	1	mg/mL	___	
		Ordered mg/min ÷ mg/mL × 60 min/h =							___	mL/h
Vasopressin		0.02 u/min = 3 mL/h 0.04 u/min = 6 mL/h				40 u/100 mL	400	u/mL		

147 kg

DRUG	ORDERED AMOUNT	TOTAL DOSE TO GIVE	DRUG INDEX NUMBER	DIRECTIONS	INFUSION RANGE	DRUG MIXTURE	AMOUNT	DRUG/ mL	RUN AT mL/h
Aminophylline	5 mg/kg =	735 mg		Give mg/kg load over 20 min		500 mg/ 250 mL	2 mg/mL		
	mg to give ÷ mg/mL =	368 mL				**368** mL × (60 min/h ÷ 20 min) =			**1103** mL/h × 20 min
	Infusion				0.5–1 mg/kg/h	500 mg/ 250 mL	2 mg/mL		
					mg dose ordered × kg ÷ mg/mL =				___ mL/h
Amiodarone	Loading dose			Load **150 mg** over 10 min		900 mg/ 500 mL	1.8 mg/mL		___
				Ordered mg load dose (150 mg) ÷ mg/mL (1.8 mg/mL) = 83 mL to give × (60 min/h ÷ 10 min) = mL/h to set on pump					**500** mL/h × 83 mL
	Infusion			Run at **1 mg/ min** × 6 h		900 mg/ 500 mL	1.8 mg/mL		
				Ordered mg dose (1 mg/min) ÷ mg/mL (1.8 mg/mL) = _____ × 60 min/h = mL/h to set on pump					**33** mL/h × 6 h
	Infusion			Run at **0.5 mg/ min** × 18 h		900 mg/ 500 mL	1.8 mg/mL		
				Ordered mg dose (0.5 mg/min) ÷ mg/mL (1.8 mg/mL) = _____ × 60 min/h = mL/h to set on pump					**17** mL/h × 18 h
Amrinone	0.75 mg/kg =	110.25 mg		Give mg/kg load over 10 min		300 mg/ 120 mL	2.5 mg/mL		___
	mg to give ÷ mg/mL =	44 mL				**44.1** mL × (60 min/h ÷ 10 min) =			**265** mL/h × 10 min
	Infusion		**0.28**		5–10 mcg/ kg/min	300 mg/ 120 mL	2500 mcg/mL		___
				Take dose you want in mcg ÷ by drug index number = mL/h on pump					
Brevibloc	Infusion		**1.13**		50–100 mcg/ kg/min	2.5 g/ 250 mL	10,000 mcg/mL		___ mL/h
				Take dose you want in mcg ÷ by drug index number = mL/h on pump					
Cardene	Infusion		___		0.5–10 mg/h	25 mg 250 mL	0.1 mg/mL		___
				Ordered mg dose ÷ mg/mL = mL/h to set on pump					___ mL/h
Cardizem	0.25 mg/kg =	36.75 mg		Give mg/kg load over 20 min		50 mg/ 100 mL	0.5 mg/mL		___
	mg to give ÷ mg/mL =	74 mL				**73.5** mL × (60 min/h ÷ 20 min) =			**221** mL/h
	0.35 mg/kg =	51.45 mg		May repeat loading dose in 15 min			0.5 mg/mL		
	mg to give ÷ mg/mL =	103 mL				**102.9** mL × (60 min/h ÷ 20 min) =			**309** mL/h
	Infusion				5–15 mg/h				___
				Ordered mg dose ÷ mg/mL = mL/h to set on pump					___ mL/h
Desmopressin	0.3 mcg/kg =	44 mcg		Give dose over 20–30 min			4 mcg/vial		
Dobutamine	Infusion		**0.23**		2.5–40 mcg/kg/ min	250 mg/ 125 mL	2000 mcg/mL		
				Take dose you want in mcg ÷ by drug index number = mL/h on pump					

(continues)

147 kg (continued)

DRUG	ORDERED AMOUNT	TOTAL DOSE TO GIVE	DRUG INDEX NUMBER	DIRECTIONS	INFUSION RANGE	DRUG MIXTURE	AMOUNT	DRUG/mL	RUN AT	mL/h
Dopamine	Infusion		0.18		1–20 mcg/kg/min	400 mg/250 mL	1600	mcg/mL		
	Take dose you want in mcg ÷ by drug index number = mL/h on pump									
Epinephrine	Infusion	1 mcg/min = 4 mL/h 2 mcg/min = 8 mL/h 3 mcg/min = 11 mL/h 4 mcg/min = 15 mL/h			1–4 mcg/min	4 mg/250 mL	16	mcg/mL		
	Ordered mcg dose/min ÷ mcg/mL × 60 min/h =								___	mL/h
Fenoldapam	Infusion		0.0046		0.01–1.6 mcg/kg/min	10 mg/250 mL	40	mcg/mL		
	Take dose you want in mcg ÷ by drug index number = mL/h on pump									
Heparin	100 u/kg = 14,700 u 200 u/kg = 29,400 u 300 u/kg = 44,100 u 400 u/kg = 58,800 u									
Isoproterenol	Infusion				5 mcg/min	1 mg/250 mL	4	mcg/mL		
	Ordered mcg dose/min ÷ mcg/mL × 60 min/h =								75	mL/h
Lidocaine	Infusion	1 mg/min = 7.5 mL/h			1–4 mg/min	2 g/250 mL	8	mg/mL	___	
	Ordered mg/min ÷ mg/mL × 60 min/h =								___	mL/h
Nitroglycerin	Infusion	3 mcg/min = 1 mL/h			3–200 mcg/min	50 mg/250 mL	200	mcg/mL	___	
	Ordered mcg/min ÷ mcg/mL × 60 min/h =								___	mL/h
Nitroprusside	Infusion	6.7 mcg/min = 1 mL/h			5–300 mcg/min	100 mg/250 mL	400	mcg/mL	___	
	Ordered mcg/min ÷ mcg/mL × 60 min/h =								___	mL/h
Norepinephrine	Infusion	1 mcg/min = 4 mL/h 2 mcg/min = 8 mL/h 3 mcg/min = 11 mL/h 4 mcg/min = 15 mL/h 5 mcg/min = 19 mL/h			2–20 mcg/min	4 mg/250 mL	16	mcg/mL		
	Ordered mcg dose/min ÷ mcg/mL × 60 min/h =								___	mL/h
Phenylephrine	Infusion	1.3 mcg/min = 1 mL/h			10–200 mcg/min	20 mg/250 mL	80	mcg/mL		
	Ordered mcg/min ÷ mcg/mL × 60 min/h =								___	mL/h
Primacor	0.05 mg/kg =	7.35 mg		Give load over 10 min		40 mg/200 mL		0.2 mg/mL		
	mg to give ÷ mg/mL =	37 mL					37 mL × (60 min/h ÷ 10 min) =		221	mL/h × 10 min
	Infusion		0.02		0.5 mcg/kg/min	40 mg/200 mL	200	mcg/mL	___	
	Take dose you want in mcg ÷ by drug index number = mL/h on pump									
Trimethaphan	Infusion		—		0.3–6 mg/min	500 mg/500 mL	1	mg/mL	___	
	Ordered mg/min ÷ mg/mL × 60 min/h =								___	mL/h
Vasopressin		0.02 u/min = 3 mL/h 0.04 u/min = 6 mL/h				40 u/100 mL	400	u/mL		

148 kg

DRUG	ORDERED AMOUNT	TOTAL DOSE TO GIVE	DRUG INDEX NUMBER	DIRECTIONS	INFUSION RANGE	DRUG MIXTURE	AMOUNT	DRUG/mL	RUN AT	mL/h
Aminophylline	5 mg/kg =	740 mg		Give mg/kg load over 20 min		500 mg/ 250 mL	2	mg/mL		
	mg to give ÷ mg/mL =	370 mL			370	mL × (60 min/h ÷ 20 min) =			1110	mL/h × 20 min
	Infusion				0.5–1 mg/kg/h	500 mg/ 250 mL	2	mg/mL		
				mg dose ordered × kg ÷ mg/mL =					___	mL/h
Amiodarone	Loading dose			Load **150 mg** over 10 min		900 mg/ 500 mL	1.8	mg/mL	___	
				Ordered mg load dose (150 mg) ÷ mg/mL (1.8 mg/mL) = 83 mL to give × (60 min/h ÷ 10 min) = mL/h to set on pump					**500**	mL/h × 83 mL
	Infusion			Run at **1 mg/ min** × 6 h		900 mg/ 500 mL	1.8	mg/mL		
				Ordered mg dose (1 mg/min) ÷ mg/mL (1.8 mg/mL) = ___ × 60 min/h = mL/h to set on pump					**33**	mL/h × 6 h
	Infusion			Run at **0.5 mg/ min** × 18 h		900 mg/ 500 mL	1.8	mg/mL		
				Ordered mg dose (0.5 mg/min) ÷ mg/mL (1.8 mg/mL) = ___ × 60 min/h = mL/h to set on pump					**17**	mL/h × 18 h
Amrinone	0.75 mg/kg =	111 mg		Give mg/kg load over 10 min		300 mg/ 120 mL	2.5	mg/mL	___	
	mg to give ÷ mg/mL =	44 mL			44.4	mL × (60 min/h ÷ 10 min) =			**266**	mL/h × 10 min
	Infusion		**0.28**		5–10 mcg/ kg/min	300 mg/ 120 mL	2500	mcg/mL	___	
				Take dose you want in mcg ÷ by drug index number = mL/h on pump						
Brevibloc	Infusion		**1.13**		50–100 mcg/ kg/min	2.5 g/ 250 mL	10,000	mcg/mL	___	mL/h
				Take dose you want in mcg ÷ by drug index number = mL/h on pump						
Cardene	Infusion			—	0.5–10 mg/h	25 mg 250 mL	0.1	mg/mL	___	
				Ordered mg dose ÷ mg/mL = mL/h to set on pump					___	mL/h
Cardizem	0.25 mg/kg =	37 mg		Give mg/kg load over 20 min		50 mg/ 100 mL	0.5	mg/mL		
	mg to give ÷ mg/mL =	74 mL			74	mL × (60 min/h ÷ 20 min) =			222	mL/h
	0.35 mg/kg =	51.8 mg		May repeat loading dose in 15 min			0.5	mg/mL		
	mg to give ÷ mg/mL =	104 mL			103.6	mL × (60 min/h ÷ 20 min) =			311	mL/h
	Infusion				5–15 mg/h				___	
				Ordered mg dose ÷ mg/mL = mL/h to set on pump					___	mL/h
Desmopressin	0.3 mcg/kg =	44 mcg		Give dose over 20–30 min			4	mcg/vial		
Dobutamine	Infusion		**0.23**		2.5–40 mcg/kg/ min	250 mg/ 125 mL	2000	mcg/mL		
				Take dose you want in mcg ÷ by drug index number = mL/h on pump						

(continues)

148 kg (continued)

DRUG	ORDERED AMOUNT		TOTAL DOSE TO GIVE		DRUG INDEX NUMBER	DIRECTIONS	INFUSION RANGE	DRUG MIXTURE	AMOUNT	DRUG/ mL	RUN AT	mL/h
Dopamine	Infusion				0.18		1–20 mcg/ kg/min	400 mg/ 250 mL	1600	mcg/mL		
	Take dose you want in mcg ÷ by drug index number = mL/h on pump											
Epinephrine	Infusion		1 mcg/min = 4 mL/h 2 mcg/min = 8 mL/h 3 mcg/min = 11 mL/h 4 mcg/min = 15 mL/h				1–4 mcg/min	4 mg/ 250 mL	16	mcg/mL		
	Ordered mcg dose/min ÷ mcg/mL × 60 min/h =										___	mL/h
Fenoldapam	Infusion				0.0045		0.01–1.6 mcg/ kg/min	10 mg/ 250 mL	40	mcg/mL		
	Take dose you want in mcg ÷ by drug index number = mL/h on pump											
Heparin	100 u/kg =	14,800 u										
	200 u/kg =	29,600 u										
	300 u/kg =	44,400 u										
	400 u/kg =	59,200 u										
Isoproterenol	Infusion						5 mcg/min	1 mg/ 250 mL	4	mcg/mL		
	Ordered mcg dose/min ÷ mcg/mL × 60 min/h =										75	mL/h
Lidocaine	Infusion		1 mg/min = 7.5 mL/h				1–4 mg/min	2 g/ 250 mL	8	mg/mL	___	
	Ordered mg/min ÷ mg/mL × 60 min/h =										___	mL/h
Nitroglycerin	Infusion		3 mcg/min = 1 mL/h				3–200 mcg/min	50 mg/ 250 mL	200	mcg/mL	___	
	Ordered mcg/min ÷ mcg/mL × 60 min/h =										___	mL/h
Nitroprusside	Infusion		6.7 mcg/min = 1 mL/h				5–300 mcg/min	100 mg/ 250 mL	400	mcg/mL	___	
	Ordered mcg/min ÷ mcg/mL × 60 min/h =										___	mL/h
Norepinephrine	Infusion		1 mcg/min = 4 mL/h 2 mcg/min = 8 mL/h 3 mcg/min = 11 mL/h 4 mcg/min = 15 mL/h 5 mcg/min = 19 mL/h				2–20 mcg/min	4 mg/ 250 mL	16	mcg/mL		
	Ordered mcg dose/min ÷ mcg/mL × 60 min/h =										___	mL/h
Phenylephrine	Infusion		1.3 mcg/min = 1 mL/h				10–200 mcg/min	20 mg/ 250 mL	80	mcg/mL		
	Ordered mcg/min ÷ mcg/mL × 60 min/h =										___	mL/h
Primacor	0.05 mg/kg =	7.4 mg				Give load over 10 min		40 mg/ 200 mL	0.2	mg/mL		
	mg to give ÷ mg/mL =	37 mL						37 mL × (60 min/h ÷ 10 min) =			222	mL/h × 10 min
	Infusion				0.02		0.5 mcg/ kg/min	40 mg/ 200 mL	200	mcg/mL	___	
	Take dose you want in mcg ÷ by drug index number = mL/h on pump											
Trimethaphan	Infusion		—				0.3–6 mg/min	500 mg/ 500 mL	1	mg/mL	___	
	Ordered mg/min ÷ mg/mL × 60 min/h =										___	mL/h
Vasopressin			0.02 u/min = 3 mL/h 0.04 u/min = 6 mL/h					40 u/ 100 mL	400	u/mL		

149 kg

DRUG	ORDERED AMOUNT	TOTAL DOSE TO GIVE	DRUG INDEX NUMBER	DIRECTIONS	INFUSION RANGE	DRUG MIXTURE	AMOUNT	DRUG/ mL	RUN AT	mL/h
Aminophylline	5 mg/kg = 745 mg			Give mg/kg load over 20 min		500 mg/ 250 mL		2 mg/mL		
	mg to give ÷ mg/mL = 373 mL					373	mL × (60 min/h ÷ 20 min) =		<u>1118</u>	mL/h × 20 min
	Infusion				0.5–1 mg/kg/h	500 mg/ 250 mL		2 mg/mL		
						mg dose ordered × kg ÷ mg/mL =			___	mL/h
Amiodarone	Loading dose			Load **150 mg** over 10 min		900 mg/ 500 mL		1.8 mg/mL	___	
				Ordered mg load dose (150 mg) ÷ mg/mL (1.8 mg/mL) = 83 mL to give × (60 min/h ÷ 10 min) = mL/h to set on pump					<u>500</u>	mL/h × 83 mL
	Infusion			Run at **1 mg/ min** × 6 h		900 mg/ 500 mL		1.8 mg/mL		
				Ordered mg dose (1 mg/min) ÷ mg/mL (1.8 mg/mL) = ____ × 60 min/h = mL/h to set on pump					<u>33</u>	mL/h × 6 h
	Infusion			Run at **0.5 mg/ min** × 18 h		900 mg/ 500 mL		1.8 mg/mL		
				Ordered mg dose (0.5 mg/min) ÷ mg/mL (1.8 mg/mL) = ____ × 60 min/h = mL/h to set on pump					<u>17</u>	mL/h × 18 h
Amrinone	0.75 mg/kg = 111.75 mg			Give mg/kg load over 10 min		300 mg/ 120 mL		2.5 mg/mL		
	mg to give ÷ mg/mL = 45 mL					44.7	mL × (60 min/h ÷ 10 min) =		<u>268</u>	mL/h × 10 min
	Infusion		0.28		5–10 mcg/ kg/min	300 mg/ 120 mL	2500	mcg/mL		
				Take dose you want in mcg ÷ by drug index number = mL/h on pump						
Brevibloc	Infusion		1.12		50–100 mcg/ kg/min	2.5 g/ 250 mL	10,000	mcg/mL		mL/h
				Take dose you want in mcg ÷ by drug index number = mL/h on pump						
Cardene	Infusion		—		0.5–10 mg/h	25 mg 250 mL	0.1	mg/mL		
				Ordered mg dose ÷ mg/mL = mL/h to set on pump						mL/h
Cardizem	0.25 mg/kg = 37.25 mg			Give mg/kg load over 20 min		50 mg/ 100 mL		0.5 mg/mL		
	mg to give ÷ mg/mL = 75 mL					74.5	mL × (60 min/h ÷ 20 min) =		<u>224</u>	mL/h
	0.35 mg/kg = 52.15 mg			May repeat loading dose in 15 min			0.5	mg/mL		
	mg to give ÷ mg/mL = 104 mL					104.3	mL × (60 min/h ÷ 20 min) =		<u>313</u>	mL/h
	Infusion				5–15 mg/h					
				Ordered mg dose ÷ mg/mL = mL/h to set on pump						mL/h
Desmopressin	0.3 mcg/kg = 45 mcg			Give dose over 20–30 min				4 mcg/vial		
Dobutamine	Infusion		0.22		2.5–40 mcg/kg/ min	250 mg/ 125 mL	2000	mcg/mL		
				Take dose you want in mcg ÷ by drug index number = mL/h on pump						

(continues)

149   kg (continued)

DRUG	ORDERED AMOUNT	TOTAL DOSE TO GIVE	DRUG INDEX NUMBER	DIRECTIONS	INFUSION RANGE	DRUG MIXTURE	AMOUNT	DRUG/ mL	RUN AT	mL/h
Dopamine	Infusion		0.18		1–20 mcg/ kg/min	400 mg/ 250 mL	1600	mcg/mL		
	Take dose you want in mcg ÷ by drug index number = mL/h on pump									
Epinephrine	Infusion	1 mcg/min = 4 mL/h 2 mcg/min = 8 mL/h 3 mcg/min = 11 mL/h 4 mcg/min = 15 mL/h			1–4 mcg/min	4 mg/ 250 mL	16	mcg/mL		
		Ordered mcg dose/min ÷ mcg/mL × 60 min/h =								___ mL/h
Fenoldapam	Infusion		0.0045		0.01–1.6 mcg/ kg/min	10 mg/ 250 mL	40	mcg/mL		
	Take dose you want in mcg ÷ by drug index number = mL/h on pump									
Heparin	100 u/kg = 14,900 u 200 u/kg = 29,800 u 300 u/kg = 44,700 u 400 u/kg = 59,600 u									
Isoproterenol	Infusion				5 mcg/min	1 mg/ 250 mL	4	mcg/mL		
		Ordered mcg dose/min ÷ mcg/mL × 60 min/h =								75 mL/h
Lidocaine	Infusion	1 mg/min = 7.5 mL/h			1–4 mg/min	2 g/ 250 mL	8	mg/mL	___	
		Ordered mg/min ÷ mg/mL × 60 min/h =								___ mL/h
Nitroglycerin	Infusion	3 mcg/min = 1 mL/h			3–200 mcg/min	50 mg/ 250 mL	200	mcg/mL	___	
		Ordered mcg/min ÷ mcg/mL × 60 min/h =								___ mL/h
Nitroprusside	Infusion	6.7 mcg/min = 1 mL/h			5–300 mcg/min	100 mg/ 250 mL	400	mcg/mL	___	
		Ordered mcg/min ÷ mcg/mL × 60 min/h =								___ mL/h
Norepinephrine	Infusion	1 mcg/min = 4 mL/h 2 mcg/min = 8 mL/h 3 mcg/min = 11 mL/h 4 mcg/min = 15 mL/h 5 mcg/min = 19 mL/h			2–20 mcg/min	4 mg/ 250 mL	16	mcg/mL		
		Ordered mcg dose/min ÷ mcg/mL × 60 min/h =								___ mL/h
Phenylephrine	Infusion	1.3 mcg/min = 1 mL/h			10–200 mcg/min	20 mg/ 250 mL	80	mcg/mL		
		Ordered mcg/min ÷ mcg/mL × 60 min/h =								___ mL/h
Primacor	0.05 mg/kg = 7.45 mg			Give load over 10 min		40 mg/ 200 mL	0.2	mg/mL		
	mg to give ÷ mg/mL = 37 mL					37 mL × (60 min/h ÷ 10 min) =			224	mL/h × 10 min
	Infusion		0.02		0.5 mcg/ kg/min	40 mg/ 200 mL	200	mcg/mL	___	
	Take dose you want in mcg ÷ by drug index number = mL/h on pump									
Trimethaphan	Infusion			—	0.3–6 mg/min	500 mg/ 500 mL	1	mg/mL	___	
		Ordered mg/min ÷ mg/mL × 60 min/h =								___ mL/h
Vasopressin		0.02 u/min = 3 mL/h 0.04 u/min = 6 mL/h				40 u/ 100 mL	400	u/mL		

150 kg

DRUG	ORDERED AMOUNT	TOTAL DOSE TO GIVE	DRUG INDEX NUMBER	DIRECTIONS	INFUSION RANGE	DRUG MIXTURE	AMOUNT	DRUG/mL	RUN AT	mL/h
Aminophylline	5 mg/kg =	750 mg		Give mg/kg load over 20 min		500 mg/ 250 mL	2 mg/mL		
	mg to give ÷ mg/mL =	375 mL			375	mL × (60 min/h ÷ 20 min) =			1125	mL/h × 20 min
	Infusion				0.5–1 mg/kg/h	500 mg/ 250 mL	2 mg/mL		
					mg dose ordered × kg ÷ mg/mL =					___ mL/h
Amiodarone	Loading dose			Load **150 mg** over 10 min		900 mg/ 500 mL	1.8 mg/mL		___
				Ordered mg load dose (150 mg) ÷ mg/mL (1.8 mg/mL) = 83 mL to give × (60 min/h ÷ 10 min) = mL/h to set on pump					500	mL/h × 83 mL
	Infusion			Run at **1 mg/ min** × 6 h		900 mg/ 500 mL	1.8 mg/mL		
				Ordered mg dose (1 mg/min) ÷ mg/mL (1.8 mg/mL) = ____ × 60 min/h = mL/h to set on pump					33	mL/h × 6 h
	Infusion			Run at **0.5 mg/ min** × 18 h		900 mg/ 500 mL	1.8 mg/mL		
				Ordered mg dose (0.5 mg/min) ÷ mg/mL (1.8 mg/mL) = ____ × 60 min/h = mL/h to set on pump					17	mL/h × 18 h
Amrinone	0.75 mg/kg =	112.5 mg		Give mg/kg load over 10 min		300 mg/ 120 mL	2.5 mg/mL		___
	mg to give ÷ mg/mL =	45 mL			45	mL × (60 min/h ÷ 10 min) =			270	mL/h × 10 min
	Infusion		0.28		5–10 mcg/ kg/min	300 mg/ 120 mL	2500 mcg/mL		___
				Take dose you want in mcg ÷ by drug index number = mL/h on pump						
Brevibloc	Infusion		1.11		50–100 mcg/ kg/min	2.5 g/ 250 mL	10,000 mcg/mL		___ mL/h
				Take dose you want in mcg ÷ by drug index number = mL/h on pump						
Cardene	Infusion		___		0.5–10 mg/h	25 mg 250 mL	0.1 mg/mL		___
				Ordered mg dose ÷ mg/mL = mL/h to set on pump						___ mL/h
Cardizem	0.25 mg/kg =	37.5 mg		Give mg/kg load over 20 min		50 mg/ 100 mL	0.5 mg/mL		___
	mg to give ÷ mg/mL =	75 mL			75	mL × (60 min/h ÷ 20 min) =			225	mL/h
	0.35 mg/kg =	52.5 mg		May repeat loading dose in 15 min			0.5 mg/mL		___
	mg to give ÷ mg/mL =	105 mL			105	mL × (60 min/h ÷ 20 min) =			315	mL/h
	Infusion				5–15 mg/h				___
				Ordered mg dose ÷ mg/mL = mL/h to set on pump						___ mL/h
Desmopressin	0.3 mcg/kg =	45 mcg		Give dose over 20–30 min			4 mcg/vial		
Dobutamine	Infusion		0.22		2.5–40 mcg/kg/ min	250 mg/ 125 mL	2000 mcg/mL		
				Take dose you want in mcg ÷ by drug index number = mL/h on pump						

(continues)

150 kg (continued)

DRUG	ORDERED AMOUNT	TOTAL DOSE TO GIVE	DRUG INDEX NUMBER	DIRECTIONS	INFUSION RANGE	DRUG MIXTURE	AMOUNT	DRUG/ mL	RUN AT	mL/h
Dopamine	Infusion		0.18		1–20 mcg/ kg/min	400 mg/ 250 mL	1600	mcg/mL		
	Take dose you want in mcg ÷ by drug index number = mL/h on pump									
Epinephrine	Infusion	1 mcg/min = 4 mL/h 2 mcg/min = 8 mL/h 3 mcg/min = 11 mL/h 4 mcg/min = 15 mL/h			1–4 mcg/min	4 mg/ 250 mL	16	mcg/mL		
	Ordered mcg dose/min ÷ mcg/mL × 60 min/h = ___ mL/h									
Fenoldapam	Infusion		0.0045		0.01–1.6 mcg/ kg/min	10 mg/ 250 mL	40	mcg/mL		
	Take dose you want in mcg ÷ by drug index number = mL/h on pump									
Heparin	100 u/kg = 15,000 u 200 u/kg = 30,000 u 300 u/kg = 45,000 u 400 u/kg = 60,000 u									
Isoproterenol	Infusion				5 mcg/min	1 mg/ 250 mL	4	mcg/mL		
	Ordered mcg dose/min ÷ mcg/mL × 60 min/h =								75	mL/h
Lidocaine	Infusion	1 mg/min = 7.5 mL/h			1–4 mg/min	2 g/ 250 mL	8	mg/mL		___
	Ordered mg/min ÷ mg/mL × 60 min/h =								___	mL/h
Nitroglycerin	Infusion	3 mcg/min = 1 mL/h			3–200 mcg/min	50 mg/ 250 mL	200	mcg/mL		___
	Ordered mcg/min ÷ mcg/mL × 60 min/h =								___	mL/h
Nitroprusside	Infusion	6.7 mcg/min = 1 mL/h			5–300 mcg/min	100 mg/ 250 mL	400	mcg/mL		___
	Ordered mcg/min ÷ mcg/mL × 60 min/h =								___	mL/h
Norepinephrine	Infusion	1 mcg/min = 4 mL/h 2 mcg/min = 8 mL/h 3 mcg/min = 11 mL/h 4 mcg/min = 15 mL/h 5 mcg/min = 19 mL/h			2–20 mcg/min	4 mg/ 250 mL	16	mcg/mL		
	Ordered mcg dose/min ÷ mcg/mL × 60 min/h =								___	mL/h
Phenylephrine	Infusion	1.3 mcg/min = 1 mL/h			10–200 mcg/min	20 mg/ 250 mL	80	mcg/mL		
	Ordered mcg/min ÷ mcg/mL × 60 min/h =								___	mL/h
Primacor	0.05 mg/kg = 7.5 mg			Give load over 10 min		40 mg/ 200 mL	0.2	mg/mL		
	mg to give ÷ mg/mL = 38 mL				38 mL × (60 min/h ÷ 10 min) =				225	mL/h × 10 min
	Infusion		0.02		0.5 mcg/ kg/min	40 mg/ 200 mL	200	mcg/mL		___
	Take dose you want in mcg ÷ by drug index number = mL/h on pump									
Trimethaphan	Infusion			___	0.3–6 mg/min	500 mg/ 500 mL	1	mg/mL		___
	Ordered mg/min ÷ mg/mL × 60 min/h =								___	mL/h
Vasopressin		0.02 u/min = 3 mL/h 0.04 u/min = 6 mL/h				40 u/ 100 mL	400	u/mL		

151 kg

DRUG	ORDERED AMOUNT	TOTAL DOSE TO GIVE	DRUG INDEX NUMBER	DIRECTIONS	INFUSION RANGE	DRUG MIXTURE	AMOUNT	DRUG/mL	RUN AT	mL/h
Aminophylline	5 mg/kg =	755 mg		Give mg/kg load over 20 min		500 mg/ 250 mL	2 mg/mL		
	mg to give ÷ mg/mL =	378 mL			378	mL × (60 min/h ÷ 20 min) =			1133	mL/h × 20 min
	Infusion				0.5–1 mg/kg/h	500 mg/ 250 mL	2 mg/mL		
					mg dose ordered × kg ÷ mg/mL =				___	mL/h
Amiodarone	Loading dose			Load **150 mg** over 10 min		900 mg/ 500 mL	1.8 mg/mL		___
				Ordered mg load dose (150 mg) ÷ mg/mL (1.8 mg/mL) = 83 mL to give × (60 min/h ÷ 10 min) = mL/h to set on pump					500	mL/h × 83 mL
	Infusion			Run at **1 mg/ min** × 6 h		900 mg/ 500 mL	1.8 mg/mL		
				Ordered mg dose (1 mg/min) ÷ mg/mL (1.8 mg/mL) = ____ × 60 min/h = mL/h to set on pump					33	mL/h × 6 h
	Infusion			Run at **0.5 mg/ min** × 18 h		900 mg/ 500 mL	1.8 mg/mL		
				Ordered mg dose (0.5 mg/min) ÷ mg/mL (1.8 mg/mL) = ____ × 60 min/h = mL/h to set on pump					17	mL/h × 18 h
Amrinone	0.75 mg/kg =	113.25 mg		Give mg/kg load over 10 min		300 mg/ 120 mL	2.5 mg/mL		___
	mg to give ÷ mg/mL =	45 mL			45.3	mL × (60 min/h ÷ 10 min) =			272	mL/h × 10 min
	Infusion		0.28		5–10 mcg/ kg/min	300 mg/ 120 mL	2500 mcg/mL		___
				Take dose you want in mcg ÷ by drug index number = mL/h on pump						
Brevibloc	Infusion		1.10		50–100 mcg/ kg/min	2.5 g/ 250 mL	10,000 mcg/mL		___ mL/h
				Take dose you want in mcg ÷ by drug index number = mL/h on pump						
Cardene	Infusion		___		0.5–10 mg/h	25 mg 250 mL	0.1 mg/mL		___
				Ordered mg dose ÷ mg/mL = mL/h to set on pump						___ mL/h
Cardizem	0.25 mg/kg =	37.75 mg		Give mg/kg load over 20 min		50 mg/ 100 mL	0.5 mg/mL		___
	mg to give ÷ mg/mL =	76 mL			75.5	mL × (60 min/h ÷ 20 min) =			227	mL/h
	0.35 mg/kg =	52.85 mg		May repeat loading dose in 15 min			0.5 mg/mL		
	mg to give ÷ mg/mL =	106 mL			105.7	mL × (60 min/h ÷ 20 min) =			317	mL/h
	Infusion				5–15 mg/h				___
				Ordered mg dose ÷ mg/mL = mL/h to set on pump						___ mL/h
Desmopressin	0.3 mcg/kg =	45 mcg		Give dose over 20–30 min			4 mcg/vial		
Dobutamine	Infusion		0.22		2.5–40 mcg/kg/ min	250 mg/ 125 mL	2000 mcg/mL		
				Take dose you want in mcg ÷ by drug index number = mL/h on pump						

(continues)

151 kg (continued)

DRUG	ORDERED AMOUNT	TOTAL DOSE TO GIVE	DRUG INDEX NUMBER	DIRECTIONS	INFUSION RANGE	DRUG MIXTURE	AMOUNT	DRUG/ mL	RUN AT	mL/h
Dopamine	Infusion		**0.18**		1–20 mcg/ kg/min	400 mg/ 250 mL	1600	mcg/mL		
		Take dose you want in mcg ÷ by drug index number = mL/h on pump								
Epinephrine	Infusion	1 mcg/min = 4 mL/h 2 mcg/min = 8 mL/h 3 mcg/min = 11 mL/h 4 mcg/min = 15 mL/h			1–4 mcg/min	4 mg/ 250 mL	16	mcg/mL		
		Ordered mcg dose/min ÷ mcg/mL × 60 min/h =							___	mL/h
Fenoldapam	Infusion		**0.0044**		0.01–1.6 mcg/ kg/min	10 mg/ 250 mL	40	mcg/mL		
		Take dose you want in mcg ÷ by drug index number = mL/h on pump								
Heparin	100 u/kg = 15,100 u 200 u/kg = 30,200 u 300 u/kg = 45,300 u 400 u/kg = 60,400 u									
Isoproterenol	Infusion				5 mcg/min	1 mg/ 250 mL	4	mcg/mL		
		Ordered mcg dose/min ÷ mcg/mL × 60 min/h =							**75**	mL/h
Lidocaine	Infusion	1 mg/min = 7.5 mL/h			1–4 mg/min	2 g/ 250 mL	8	mg/mL	___	
		Ordered mg/min ÷ mg/mL × 60 min/h =							___	mL/h
Nitroglycerin	Infusion	3 mcg/min = 1 mL/h			3–200 mcg/min	50 mg/ 250 mL	200	mcg/mL	___	
		Ordered mcg/min ÷ mcg/mL × 60 min/h =							___	mL/h
Nitroprusside	Infusion	6.7 mcg/min = 1 mL/h			5–300 mcg/min	100 mg/ 250 mL	400	mcg/mL	___	
		Ordered mcg/min ÷ mcg/mL × 60 min/h =							___	mL/h
Norepinephrine	Infusion	1 mcg/min = 4 mL/h 2 mcg/min = 8 mL/h 3 mcg/min = 11 mL/h 4 mcg/min = 15 mL/h 5 mcg/min = 19 mL/h			2–20 mcg/min	4 mg/ 250 mL	16	mcg/mL		
		Ordered mcg dose/min ÷ mcg/mL × 60 min/h =							___	mL/h
Phenylephrine	Infusion	1.3 mcg/min = 1 mL/h			10–200 mcg/min	20 mg/ 250 mL	80	mcg/mL		
		Ordered mcg/min ÷ mcg/mL × 60 min/h =							___	mL/h
Primacor	0.05 mg/kg = 7.55 mg			Give load over 10 min		40 mg/ 200 mL	0.2	mg/mL		
	mg to give ÷ mg/mL = 38 mL				38	mL × (60 min/h ÷ 10 min) =			**227**	mL/h × 10 min
	Infusion		**0.02**		0.5 mcg/ kg/min	40 mg/ 200 mL	200	mcg/mL	___	
		Take dose you want in mcg ÷ by drug index number = mL/h on pump								
Trimethaphan	Infusion		___		0.3–6 mg/min	500 mg/ 500 mL	1	mg/mL	___	
		Ordered mg/min ÷ mg/mL × 60 min/h =							___	mL/h
Vasopressin		0.02 u/min = 3 mL/h 0.04 u/min = 6 mL/h				40 u/ 100 mL	400	u/mL		

152 kg

DRUG	ORDERED AMOUNT	TOTAL DOSE TO GIVE	DRUG INDEX NUMBER	DIRECTIONS	INFUSION RANGE	DRUG MIXTURE	AMOUNT	DRUG/mL	RUN AT	mL/h
Aminophylline	5 mg/kg = 760 mg			Give mg/kg load over 20 min		500 mg/ 250 mL		2 mg/mL		
	mg to give ÷ mg/mL =	380 mL				380 mL × (60 min/h ÷ 20 min) =			**1140**	mL/h × 20 min
	Infusion				0.5–1 mg/kg/h	500 mg/ 250 mL		2 mg/mL		
					mg dose ordered × kg ÷ mg/mL =					___ mL/h
Amiodarone	Loading dose			Load **150 mg** over 10 min		900 mg/ 500 mL		1.8 mg/mL	___	
				Ordered mg load dose (150 mg) ÷ mg/mL (1.8 mg/mL) = 83 mL to give × (60 min/h ÷ 10 min) = mL/h to set on pump					**500**	mL/h × 83 mL
	Infusion			Run at **1 mg/ min** × 6 h		900 mg/ 500 mL		1.8 mg/mL		
				Ordered mg dose (1 mg/min) ÷ mg/mL (1.8 mg/mL) = ____ × 60 min/h = mL/h to set on pump					**33**	mL/h × 6 h
	Infusion			Run at **0.5 mg/ min** × 18 h		900 mg/ 500 mL		1.8 mg/mL		
				Ordered mg dose (0.5 mg/min) ÷ mg/mL (1.8 mg/mL) = ____ × 60 min/h = mL/h to set on pump					**17**	mL/h × 18 h
Amrinone	0.75 mg/kg = 114 mg			Give mg/kg load over 10 min		300 mg/ 120 mL		2.5 mg/mL	___	
	mg to give ÷ mg/mL =	46 mL				45.6 mL × (60 min/h ÷ 10 min) =			**274**	mL/h × 10 min
	Infusion		0.27		5–10 mcg/ kg/min	300 mg/ 120 mL	2500	mcg/mL	___	
				Take dose you want in mcg ÷ by drug index number = mL/h on pump						
Brevibloc	Infusion		1.10		50–100 mcg/ kg/min	2.5 g/ 250 mL	10,000	mcg/mL	___ mL/h	
				Take dose you want in mcg ÷ by drug index number = mL/h on pump						
Cardene	Infusion		___		0.5–10 mg/h	25 mg 250 mL	0.1	mg/mL	___	
				Ordered mg dose ÷ mg/mL = mL/h to set on pump						___ mL/h
Cardizem	0.25 mg/kg = 38 mg			Give mg/kg load over 20 min		50 mg/ 100 mL		0.5 mg/mL	___	
	mg to give ÷ mg/mL =	76 mL				76 mL × (60 min/h ÷ 20 min) =			**228**	mL/h
	0.35 mg/kg = 53.2 mg			May repeat loading dose in 15 min				0.5 mg/mL	___	
	mg to give ÷ mg/mL =	106 mL				106.4 mL × (60 min/h ÷ 20 min) =			**319**	mL/h
	Infusion				5–15 mg/h				___	
				Ordered mg dose ÷ mg/mL = mL/h to set on pump						___ mL/h
Desmopressin	0.3 mcg/kg = 46 mcg			Give dose over 20–30 min				4 mcg/vial		
Dobutamine	Infusion		0.22		2.5–40 mcg/kg/ min	250 mg/ 125 mL	2000	mcg/mL		
				Take dose you want in mcg ÷ by drug index number = mL/h on pump						

(continues)

152   kg (continued)

DRUG	ORDERED AMOUNT	TOTAL DOSE TO GIVE	DRUG INDEX NUMBER	DIRECTIONS	INFUSION RANGE	DRUG MIXTURE	AMOUNT	DRUG/mL	RUN AT	mL/h
Dopamine	Infusion		0.18		1–20 mcg/kg/min	400 mg/250 mL	1600	mcg/mL		
			Take dose you want in mcg ÷ by drug index number = mL/h on pump							
Epinephrine	Infusion	1 mcg/min = 4 mL/h 2 mcg/min = 8 mL/h 3 mcg/min = 11 mL/h 4 mcg/min = 15 mL/h			1–4 mcg/min	4 mg/250 mL	16	mcg/mL		
				Ordered mcg dose/min ÷ mcg/mL × 60 min/h =					___	mL/h
Fenoldapam	Infusion		0.0044		0.01–1.6 mcg/kg/min	10 mg/250 mL	40	mcg/mL		
			Take dose you want in mcg ÷ by drug index number = mL/h on pump							
Heparin	100 u/kg = 15,200 u 200 u/kg = 30,400 u 300 u/kg = 45,600 u 400 u/kg = 60,800 u									
Isoproterenol	Infusion				5 mcg/min	1 mg/250 mL	4	mcg/mL		
				Ordered mcg dose/min ÷ mcg/mL × 60 min/h =					<u>75</u>	mL/h
Lidocaine	Infusion	1 mg/min = 7.5 mL/h			1–4 mg/min	2 g/250 mL	8	mg/mL		
				Ordered mg/min ÷ mg/mL × 60 min/h =					___	mL/h
Nitroglycerin	Infusion	3 mcg/min = 1 mL/h			3–200 mcg/min	50 mg/250 mL	200	mcg/mL		
				Ordered mcg/min ÷ mcg/mL × 60 min/h =					___	mL/h
Nitroprusside	Infusion	6.7 mcg/min = 1 mL/h			5–300 mcg/min	100 mg/250 mL	400	mcg/mL		
				Ordered mcg/min ÷ mcg/mL × 60 min/h =					___	mL/h
Norepinephrine	Infusion	1 mcg/min = 4 mL/h 2 mcg/min = 8 mL/h 3 mcg/min = 11 mL/h 4 mcg/min = 15 mL/h 5 mcg/min = 19 mL/h			2–20 mcg/min	4 mg/250 mL	16	mcg/mL		
				Ordered mcg dose/min ÷ mcg/mL × 60 min/h =					___	mL/h
Phenylephrine	Infusion	1.3 mcg/min = 1 mL/h			10–200 mcg/min	20 mg/250 mL	80	mcg/mL		
				Ordered mcg/min ÷ mcg/mL × 60 min/h =					___	mL/h
Primacor	0.05 mg/kg = 7.6 mg			Give load over 10 min		40 mg/200 mL	0.2	mg/mL		
	mg to give ÷ mg/mL = 38 mL				38 mL × (60 min/h ÷ 10 min) =				<u>228</u>	mL/h × 10 min
	Infusion		0.02		0.5 mcg/kg/min	40 mg/200 mL	200	mcg/mL	___	
			Take dose you want in mcg ÷ by drug index number = mL/h on pump							
Trimethaphan	Infusion		___		0.3–6 mg/min	500 mg/500 mL	1	mg/mL	___	
				Ordered mg/min ÷ mg/mL × 60 min/h =					___	mL/h
Vasopressin		0.02 u/min = 3 mL/h 0.04 u/min = 6 mL/h				40 u/100 mL	400	u/mL		

153 kg

DRUG	ORDERED AMOUNT	TOTAL DOSE TO GIVE	DRUG INDEX NUMBER	DIRECTIONS	INFUSION RANGE	DRUG MIXTURE	AMOUNT / DRUG/mL	RUN AT / mL/h
Aminophylline	5 mg/kg =	765 mg		Give mg/kg load over 20 min		500 mg/ 250 mL	2 mg/mL	
	mg to give ÷ mg/mL =	383 mL			383	mL × (60 min/h ÷ 20 min) =		**1148** mL/h × 20 min
	Infusion				0.5–1 mg/kg/h	500 mg/ 250 mL	2 mg/mL	
						mg dose ordered × kg ÷ mg/mL =		___ mL/h
Amiodarone	Loading dose			Load **150 mg** over 10 min		900 mg/ 500 mL	1.8 mg/mL	___
				Ordered mg load dose (150 mg) ÷ mg/mL (1.8 mg/mL) = 83 mL to give × (60 min/h ÷ 10 min) = mL/h to set on pump				**500** mL/h × 83 mL
	Infusion			Run at **1 mg/ min** × 6 h		900 mg/ 500 mL	1.8 mg/mL	
				Ordered mg dose (1 mg/min) ÷ mg/mL (1.8 mg/mL) = ____ × 60 min/h = mL/h to set on pump				**33** mL/h × 6 h
	Infusion			Run at **0.5 mg/ min** × 18 h		900 mg/ 500 mL	1.8 mg/mL	
				Ordered mg dose (0.5 mg/min) ÷ mg/mL (1.8 mg/mL) = ____ × 60 min/h = mL/h to set on pump				**17** mL/h × 18 h
Amrinone	0.75 mg/kg =	114.75 mg		Give mg/kg load over 10 min		300 mg/ 120 mL	2.5 mg/mL	___
	mg to give ÷ mg/mL =	46 mL			45.9	mL × (60 min/h ÷ 10 min) =		**275** mL/h × 10 min
	Infusion		0.27		5–10 mcg/ kg/min	300 mg/ 120 mL	2500 mcg/mL	___
				Take dose you want in mcg ÷ by drug index number = mL/h on pump				
Brevibloc	Infusion		1.09		50–100 mcg/ kg/min	2.5 g/ 250 mL	10,000 mcg/mL	___ mL/h
				Take dose you want in mcg ÷ by drug index number = mL/h on pump				
Cardene	Infusion		—		0.5–10 mg/h	25 mg 250 mL	0.1 mg/mL	___
				Ordered mg dose ÷ mg/mL = mL/h to set on pump				___ mL/h
Cardizem	0.25 mg/kg =	38.25 mg		Give mg/kg load over 20 min		50 mg/ 100 mL	0.5 mg/mL	___
	mg to give ÷ mg/mL =	77 mL			76.5	mL × (60 min/h ÷ 20 min) =		**230** mL/h
	0.35 mg/kg =	53.55 mg		May repeat loading dose in 15 min			0.5 mg/mL	___
	mg to give ÷ mg/mL =	107 mL			107.1	mL × (60 min/h ÷ 20 min) =		**321** mL/h
	Infusion				5–15 mg/h			___
				Ordered mg dose ÷ mg/mL = mL/h to set on pump				___ mL/h
Desmopressin	0.3 mcg/kg =	46 mcg		Give dose over 20–30 min			4 mcg/vial	
Dobutamine	Infusion		0.22		2.5–40 mcg/kg/ min	250 mg/ 125 mL	2000 mcg/mL	
				Take dose you want in mcg ÷ by drug index number = mL/h on pump				

(continues)

153 kg (continued)

DRUG	ORDERED AMOUNT		TOTAL DOSE TO GIVE		DRUG INDEX NUMBER	DIRECTIONS	INFUSION RANGE	DRUG MIXTURE	AMOUNT	DRUG/ mL	RUN AT	mL/h
Dopamine	Infusion				0.17		1–20 mcg/ kg/min	400 mg/ 250 mL	1600	mcg/mL		
	Take dose you want in mcg ÷ by drug index number = mL/h on pump											
Epinephrine	Infusion		1 mcg/min = 4 mL/h 2 mcg/min = 8 mL/h 3 mcg/min = 11 mL/h 4 mcg/min = 15 mL/h				1–4 mcg/min	4 mg/ 250 mL	16	mcg/mL		
	Ordered mcg dose/min ÷ mcg/mL × 60 min/h =										___	mL/h
Fenoldapam	Infusion				0.0044		0.01–1.6 mcg/ kg/min	10 mg/ 250 mL	40	mcg/mL		
	Take dose you want in mcg ÷ by drug index number = mL/h on pump											
Heparin	100 u/kg = 200 u/kg = 300 u/kg = 400 u/kg =	15,300 u 30,600 u 45,900 u 61,200 u										
Isoproterenol	Infusion						5 mcg/min	1 mg/ 250 mL	4	mcg/mL		
	Ordered mcg dose/min ÷ mcg/mL × 60 min/h =										75	mL/h
Lidocaine	Infusion		1 mg/min = 7.5 mL/h				1–4 mg/min	2 g/ 250 mL	8	mg/mL	___	
	Ordered mg/min ÷ mg/mL × 60 min/h =										___	mL/h
Nitroglycerin	Infusion		3 mcg/min = 1 mL/h				3–200 mcg/min	50 mg/ 250 mL	200	mcg/mL	___	
	Ordered mcg/min ÷ mcg/mL × 60 min/h =										___	mL/h
Nitroprusside	Infusion		6.7 mcg/min = 1 mL/h				5–300 mcg/min	100 mg/ 250 mL	400	mcg/mL	___	
	Ordered mcg/min ÷ mcg/mL × 60 min/h =										___	mL/h
Norepinephrine	Infusion		1 mcg/min = 4 mL/h 2 mcg/min = 8 mL/h 3 mcg/min = 11 mL/h 4 mcg/min = 15 mL/h 5 mcg/min = 19 mL/h				2–20 mcg/min	4 mg/ 250 mL	16	mcg/mL		
	Ordered mcg dose/min ÷ mcg/mL × 60 min/h =										___	mL/h
Phenylephrine	Infusion		1.3 mcg/min = 1 mL/h				10–200 mcg/min	20 mg/ 250 mL	80	mcg/mL		
	Ordered mcg/min ÷ mcg/mL × 60 min/h =										___	mL/h
Primacor	0.05 mg/kg =	7.65 mg				Give load over 10 min		40 mg/ 200 mL	0.2	mg/mL		
	mg to give ÷ mg/mL =	38 mL					38	mL × (60 min/h ÷ 10 min) =			230	mL/h × 10 min
	Infusion				0.02		0.5 mcg/ kg/min	40 mg/ 200 mL	200	mcg/mL	___	
	Take dose you want in mcg ÷ by drug index number = mL/h on pump											
Trimethaphan	Infusion				___		0.3–6 mg/min	500 mg/ 500 mL	1	mg/mL	___	
	Ordered mg/min ÷ mg/mL × 60 min/h =										___	mL/h
Vasopressin			0.02 u/min = 3 mL/h 0.04 u/min = 6 mL/h					40 u/ 100 mL	400	u/mL		

154 kg

DRUG	ORDERED AMOUNT	TOTAL DOSE TO GIVE	DRUG INDEX NUMBER	DIRECTIONS	INFUSION RANGE	DRUG MIXTURE	AMOUNT	DRUG/mL	RUN AT	mL/h
Aminophylline	5 mg/kg =	770 mg		Give mg/kg load over 20 min		500 mg/250 mL		2 mg/mL		
	mg to give ÷ mg/mL =	385 mL					385	mL × (60 min/h ÷ 20 min) =	**1155**	mL/h × 20 min
	Infusion				0.5–1 mg/kg/h	500 mg/250 mL		2 mg/mL		
						mg dose ordered × kg ÷ mg/mL =				___ mL/h
Amiodarone	Loading dose			Load **150 mg** over 10 min		900 mg/500 mL		1.8 mg/mL		___
				Ordered mg load dose (150 mg) ÷ mg/mL (1.8 mg/mL) = 83 mL to give × (60 min/h ÷ 10 min) = mL/h to set on pump					**500**	mL/h × 83 mL
	Infusion			Run at **1 mg/min** × 6 h		900 mg/500 mL		1.8 mg/mL		
				Ordered mg dose (1 mg/min) ÷ mg/mL (1.8 mg/mL) = ___ × 60 min/h = mL/h to set on pump					**33**	mL/h × 6 h
	Infusion			Run at **0.5 mg/min** × 18 h		900 mg/500 mL		1.8 mg/mL		
				Ordered mg dose (0.5 mg/min) ÷ mg/mL (1.8 mg/mL) = ___ × 60 min/h = mL/h to set on pump					**17**	mL/h × 18 h
Amrinone	0.75 mg/kg =	115.5 mg		Give mg/kg load over 10 min		300 mg/120 mL		2.5 mg/mL		___
	mg to give ÷ mg/mL =	46 mL					46.2	mL × (60 min/h ÷ 10 min) =	**277**	mL/h × 10 min
	Infusion		0.27		5–10 mcg/kg/min	300 mg/120 mL		2500 mcg/mL		___
				Take dose you want in mcg ÷ by drug index number = mL/h on pump						
Brevibloc	Infusion		1.08		50–100 mcg/kg/min	2.5 g/250 mL		10,000 mcg/mL		___ mL/h
				Take dose you want in mcg ÷ by drug index number = mL/h on pump						
Cardene	Infusion		—		0.5–10 mg/h	25 mg/250 mL		0.1 mg/mL		___
				Ordered mg dose ÷ mg/mL = mL/h to set on pump						___ mL/h
Cardizem	0.25 mg/kg =	38.5 mg		Give mg/kg load over 20 min		50 mg/100 mL		0.5 mg/mL		___
	mg to give ÷ mg/mL =	77 mL					77	mL × (60 min/h ÷ 20 min) =	**231** mL/h	
	0.35 mg/kg =	53.9 mg		May repeat loading dose in 15 min				0.5 mg/mL		
	mg to give ÷ mg/mL =	108 mL					107.8	mL × (60 min/h ÷ 20 min) =	**323** mL/h	
	Infusion				5–15 mg/h					___
				Ordered mg dose ÷ mg/mL = mL/h to set on pump						___ mL/h
Desmopressin	0.3 mcg/kg =	46 mcg		Give dose over 20–30 min				4 mcg/vial		
Dobutamine	Infusion		0.22		2.5–40 mcg/kg/min	250 mg/125 mL		2000 mcg/mL		
				Take dose you want in mcg ÷ by drug index number = mL/h on pump						

(continues)

154 kg (continued)

DRUG	ORDERED AMOUNT	TOTAL DOSE TO GIVE	DRUG INDEX NUMBER	DIRECTIONS	INFUSION RANGE	DRUG MIXTURE	AMOUNT	DRUG/ mL	RUN AT	mL/h
Dopamine	Infusion		**0.17**		1–20 mcg/ kg/min	400 mg/ 250 mL	1600	mcg/mL		
				Take dose you want in mcg ÷ by drug index number = mL/h on pump						
Epinephrine	Infusion	1 mcg/min = 4 mL/h 2 mcg/min = 8 mL/h 3 mcg/min = 11 mL/h 4 mcg/min = 15 mL/h			1–4 mcg/min	4 mg/ 250 mL	16	mcg/mL		
					Ordered mcg dose/min ÷ mcg/mL × 60 min/h =				___	mL/h
Fenoldapam	Infusion		**0.0044**		0.01–1.6 mcg/ kg/min	10 mg/ 250 mL	40	mcg/mL		
					Take dose you want in mcg ÷ by drug index number = mL/h on pump					
Heparin	100 u/kg = 15,400 u 200 u/kg = 30,800 u 300 u/kg = 46,200 u 400 u/kg = 61,600 u									
Isoproterenol	Infusion				5 mcg/min	1 mg/ 250 mL	4	mcg/mL		
					Ordered mcg dose/min ÷ mcg/mL × 60 min/h =				**75**	mL/h
Lidocaine	Infusion	1 mg/min = 7.5 mL/h			1–4 mg/min	2 g/ 250 mL	8	mg/mL	___	
					Ordered mg/min ÷ mg/mL × 60 min/h =				___	mL/h
Nitroglycerin	Infusion	3 mcg/min = 1 mL/h			3–200 mcg/min	50 mg/ 250 mL	200	mcg/mL	___	
					Ordered mcg/min ÷ mcg/mL × 60 min/h =				___	mL/h
Nitroprusside	Infusion	6.7 mcg/min = 1 mL/h			5–300 mcg/min	100 mg/ 250 mL	400	mcg/mL	___	
					Ordered mcg/min ÷ mcg/mL × 60 min/h =				___	mL/h
Norepinephrine	Infusion	1 mcg/min = 4 mL/h 2 mcg/min = 8 mL/h 3 mcg/min = 11 mL/h 4 mcg/min = 15 mL/h 5 mcg/min = 19 mL/h			2–20 mcg/min	4 mg/ 250 mL	16	mcg/mL		
					Ordered mcg dose/min ÷ mcg/mL × 60 min/h =				___	mL/h
Phenylephrine	Infusion	1.3 mcg/min = 1 mL/h			10–200 mcg/min	20 mg/ 250 mL	80	mcg/mL		
					Ordered mcg/min ÷ mcg/mL × 60 min/h =				___	mL/h
Primacor	0.05 mg/kg = 7.7 mg			Give load over 10 min		40 mg/ 200 mL	0.2	mg/mL		
	mg to give ÷ mg/mL = 39 mL				39	mL × (60 min/h ÷ 10 min) =			**231**	mL/h × 10 min
	Infusion		**0.02**		0.5 mcg/ kg/min	40 mg/ 200 mL	200	mcg/mL	___	
					Take dose you want in mcg ÷ by drug index number = mL/h on pump					
Trimethaphan	Infusion		___		0.3–6 mg/min	500 mg/ 500 mL	1	mg/mL	___	
					Ordered mg/min ÷ mg/mL × 60 min/h =				___	mL/h
Vasopressin		0.02 u/min = 3 mL/h 0.04 u/min = 6 mL/h				40 u/ 100 mL	400	u/mL		

155 kg

DRUG	ORDERED AMOUNT	TOTAL DOSE TO GIVE	DRUG INDEX NUMBER	DIRECTIONS	INFUSION RANGE	DRUG MIXTURE	AMOUNT DRUG/mL	RUN AT mL/h
Aminophylline	5 mg/kg = 775 mg			Give mg/kg load over 20 min		500 mg/ 250 mL	2 mg/mL	
	mg to give ÷ mg/mL = 388 mL				388	mL × (60 min/h ÷ 20 min) =		**1163** mL/h × 20 min
	Infusion				0.5–1 mg/kg/h	500 mg/ 250 mL	2 mg/mL	
					mg dose ordered × kg ÷ mg/mL =			___ mL/h
Amiodarone	Loading dose			Load **150 mg** over 10 min		900 mg/ 500 mL	1.8 mg/mL	___
				Ordered mg load dose (150 mg) ÷ mg/mL (1.8 mg/mL) = 83 mL to give × (60 min/h ÷ 10 min) = mL/h to set on pump				**500** mL/h × 83 mL
	Infusion			Run at **1 mg/ min** × 6 h		900 mg/ 500 mL	1.8 mg/mL	
				Ordered mg dose (1 mg/min) ÷ mg/mL (1.8 mg/mL) = ___ × 60 min/h = mL/h to set on pump				**33** mL/h × 6 h
	Infusion			Run at **0.5 mg/ min** × 18 h		900 mg/ 500 mL	1.8 mg/mL	
				Ordered mg dose (0.5 mg/min) ÷ mg/mL (1.8 mg/mL) = ___ × 60 min/h = mL/h to set on pump				**17** mL/h × 18 h
Amrinone	0.75 mg/kg = 116.25 mg			Give mg/kg load over 10 min		300 mg/ 120 mL	2.5 mg/mL	
	mg to give ÷ mg/mL = 47 mL				46.5	mL × (60 min/h ÷ 10 min) =		**279** mL/h × 10 min
	Infusion		0.27		5–10 mcg/ kg/min	300 mg/ 120 mL	2500 mcg/mL	___
				Take dose you want in mcg ÷ by drug index number = mL/h on pump				
Brevibloc	Infusion		1.07		50–100 mcg/ kg/min	2.5 g/ 250 mL	10,000 mcg/mL	___ mL/h
				Take dose you want in mcg ÷ by drug index number = mL/h on pump				
Cardene	Infusion		___		0.5–10 mg/h	25 mg 250 mL	0.1 mg/mL	___
				Ordered mg dose ÷ mg/mL = mL/h to set on pump				___ mL/h
Cardizem	0.25 mg/kg = 38.75 mg			Give mg/kg load over 20 min		50 mg/ 100 mL	0.5 mg/mL	___
	mg to give ÷ mg/mL = 78 mL				77.5	mL × (60 min/h ÷ 20 min) =		**233** mL/h
	0.35 mg/kg = 54.25 mg			May repeat loading dose in 15 min			0.5 mg/mL	___
	mg to give ÷ mg/mL = 109 mL				108.5	mL × (60 min/h ÷ 20 min) =		**326** mL/h
	Infusion				5–15 mg/h			___
				Ordered mg dose ÷ mg/mL = mL/h to set on pump				___ mL/h
Desmopressin	0.3 mcg/kg = 47 mcg			Give dose over 20–30 min			4 mcg/vial	
Dobutamine	Infusion		0.21		2.5–40 mcg/kg/ min	250 mg/ 125 mL	2000 mcg/mL	
				Take dose you want in mcg ÷ by drug index number = mL/h on pump				

(continues)

155 kg (continued)

DRUG	ORDERED AMOUNT	TOTAL DOSE TO GIVE	DRUG INDEX NUMBER	DIRECTIONS	INFUSION RANGE	DRUG MIXTURE	AMOUNT	DRUG/ mL	RUN AT	mL/h
Dopamine	Infusion		0.17		1–20 mcg/ kg/min	400 mg/ 250 mL	1600	mcg/mL		
		Take dose you want in mcg ÷ by drug index number = mL/h on pump								
Epinephrine	Infusion	1 mcg/min = 4 mL/h 2 mcg/min = 8 mL/h 3 mcg/min = 11 mL/h 4 mcg/min = 15 mL/h			1–4 mcg/min	4 mg/ 250 mL	16	mcg/mL		
		Ordered mcg dose/min ÷ mcg/mL × 60 min/h =							___	mL/h
Fenoldapam	Infusion		0.0043		0.01–1.6 mcg/ kg/min	10 mg/ 250 mL	40	mcg/mL		
		Take dose you want in mcg ÷ by drug index number = mL/h on pump								
Heparin	100 u/kg = 15,500 u 200 u/kg = 31,000 u 300 u/kg = 46,500 u 400 u/kg = 62,000 u									
Isoproterenol	Infusion				5 mcg/min	1 mg/ 250 mL	4	mcg/mL		
		Ordered mcg dose/min ÷ mcg/mL × 60 min/h =							75	mL/h
Lidocaine	Infusion	1 mg/min = 7.5 mL/h			1–4 mg/min	2 g/ 250 mL	8	mg/mL	___	
		Ordered mg/min ÷ mg/mL × 60 min/h =							___	mL/h
Nitroglycerin	Infusion	3 mcg/min = 1 mL/h			3–200 mcg/min	50 mg/ 250 mL	200	mcg/mL	___	
		Ordered mcg/min ÷ mcg/mL × 60 min/h =							___	mL/h
Nitroprusside	Infusion	6.7 mcg/min = 1 mL/h			5–300 mcg/min	100 mg/ 250 mL	400	mcg/mL	___	
		Ordered mcg/min ÷ mcg/mL × 60 min/h =							___	mL/h
Norepinephrine	Infusion	1 mcg/min = 4 mL/h 2 mcg/min = 8 mL/h 3 mcg/min = 11 mL/h 4 mcg/min = 15 mL/h 5 mcg/min = 19 mL/h			2–20 mcg/min	4 mg/ 250 mL	16	mcg/mL		
		Ordered mcg dose/min ÷ mcg/mL × 60 min/h =							___	mL/h
Phenylephrine	Infusion	1.3 mcg/min = 1 mL/h			10–200 mcg/min	20 mg/ 250 mL	80	mcg/mL		
		Ordered mcg/min ÷ mcg/mL × 60 min/h =							___	mL/h
Primacor	0.05 mg/kg = 7.75 mg			Give load over 10 min		40 mg/ 200 mL	0.2	mg/mL		
	mg to give ÷ mg/mL = 39 mL				39	mL × (60 min/h ÷ 10 min) =			233	mL/h × 10 min
	Infusion		0.02		0.5 mcg/ kg/min	40 mg/ 200 mL	200	mcg/mL	___	
		Take dose you want in mcg ÷ by drug index number = mL/h on pump								
Trimethaphan	Infusion		___		0.3–6 mg/min	500 mg/ 500 mL	1	mg/mL	___	
		Ordered mg/min ÷ mg/mL × 60 min/h =							___	mL/h
Vasopressin	0.02 u/min = 3 mL/h 0.04 u/min = 6 mL/h					40 u/ 100 mL	400	u/mL		

156 kg

DRUG	ORDERED AMOUNT	TOTAL DOSE TO GIVE	DRUG INDEX NUMBER	DIRECTIONS	INFUSION RANGE	DRUG MIXTURE	AMOUNT DRUG/mL	RUN AT mL/h
Aminophylline	5 mg/kg = 780 mg			Give mg/kg load over 20 min		500 mg/ 250 mL	2 mg/mL	
	mg to give ÷ mg/mL = 390 mL				390	mL × (60 min/h ÷ 20 min) =		1170 mL/h × 20 min
	Infusion				0.5–1 mg/kg/h	500 mg/ 250 mL	2 mg/mL	
				mg dose ordered × kg ÷ mg/mL =				___ mL/h
Amiodarone	Loading dose			Load **150 mg** over 10 min		900 mg/ 500 mL	1.8 mg/mL	___
				Ordered mg load dose (150 mg) ÷ mg/mL (1.8 mg/mL) = 83 mL to give × (60 min/h ÷ 10 min) = mL/h to set on pump				500 mL/h × 83 mL
	Infusion			Run at **1 mg/ min** × 6 h		900 mg/ 500 mL	1.8 mg/mL	
				Ordered mg dose (1 mg/min) ÷ mg/mL (1.8 mg/mL) = ___ × 60 min/h = mL/h to set on pump				33 mL/h × 6 h
	Infusion			Run at **0.5 mg/ min** × 18 h		900 mg/ 500 mL	1.8 mg/mL	
				Ordered mg dose (0.5 mg/min) ÷ mg/mL (1.8 mg/mL) = ___ × 60 min/h = mL/h to set on pump				17 mL/h × 18 h
Amrinone	0.75 mg/kg = 117 mg			Give mg/kg load over 10 min		300 mg/ 120 mL	2.5 mg/mL	
	mg to give ÷ mg/mL = 47 mL				46.8	mL × (60 min/h ÷ 10 min) =		281 mL/h × 10 min
	Infusion		0.27		5–10 mcg/ kg/min	300 mg/ 120 mL	2500 mcg/mL	___
				Take dose you want in mcg ÷ by drug index number = mL/h on pump				
Brevibloc	Infusion		1.07		50–100 mcg/ kg/min	2.5 g/ 250 mL	10,000 mcg/mL	___ mL/h
				Take dose you want in mcg ÷ by drug index number = mL/h on pump				
Cardene	Infusion		___		0.5–10 mg/h	25 mg 250 mL	0.1 mg/mL	___
				Ordered mg dose ÷ mg/mL = mL/h to set on pump				___ mL/h
Cardizem	0.25 mg/kg = 39 mg			Give mg/kg load over 20 min		50 mg/ 100 mL	0.5 mg/mL	___
	mg to give ÷ mg/mL = 78 mL				78	mL × (60 min/h ÷ 20 min) =		234 mL/h
	0.35 mg/kg = 54.6 mg			May repeat loading dose in 15 min			0.5 mg/mL	___
	mg to give ÷ mg/mL = 109 mL				109.2	mL × (60 min/h ÷ 20 min) =		328 mL/h
	Infusion				5–15 mg/h			___
				Ordered mg dose ÷ mg/mL = mL/h to set on pump				___ mL/h
Desmopressin	0.3 mcg/kg = 47 mcg			Give dose over 20–30 min			4 mcg/vial	
Dobutamine	Infusion		0.21		2.5–40 mcg/kg/ min	250 mg/ 125 mL	2000 mcg/mL	
				Take dose you want in mcg ÷ by drug index number = mL/h on pump				

(continues)

156 kg (continued)

DRUG	ORDERED AMOUNT	TOTAL DOSE TO GIVE	DRUG INDEX NUMBER	DIRECTIONS	INFUSION RANGE	DRUG MIXTURE	AMOUNT	DRUG/ mL	RUN AT	mL/h
Dopamine	Infusion		0.17		1–20 mcg/ kg/min	400 mg/ 250 mL	1600	mcg/mL		
	Take dose you want in mcg ÷ by drug index number = mL/h on pump									
Epinephrine	Infusion	1 mcg/min = 4 mL/h 2 mcg/min = 8 mL/h 3 mcg/min = 11 mL/h 4 mcg/min = 15 mL/h			1–4 mcg/min	4 mg/ 250 mL	16	mcg/mL		
	Ordered mcg dose/min ÷ mcg/mL × 60 min/h =								___	mL/h
Fenoldapam	Infusion		0.0043		0.01–1.6 mcg/ kg/min	10 mg/ 250 mL	40	mcg/mL		
	Take dose you want in mcg ÷ by drug index number = mL/h on pump									
Heparin	100 u/kg = **15,600** u 200 u/kg = **31,200** u 300 u/kg = **46,800** u 400 u/kg = **62,400** u									
Isoproterenol	Infusion				5 mcg/min	1 mg/ 250 mL	4	mcg/mL		
	Ordered mcg dose/min ÷ mcg/mL × 60 min/h =								**75**	mL/h
Lidocaine	Infusion	1 mg/min = 7.5 mL/h			1–4 mg/min	2 g/ 250 mL	8	mg/mL	___	
	Ordered mg/min ÷ mg/mL × 60 min/h =								___	mL/h
Nitroglycerin	Infusion	3 mcg/min = 1 mL/h			3–200 mcg/min	50 mg/ 250 mL	200	mcg/mL	___	
	Ordered mcg/min ÷ mcg/mL × 60 min/h =								___	mL/h
Nitroprusside	Infusion	6.7 mcg/min = 1 mL/h			5–300 mcg/min	100 mg/ 250 mL	400	mcg/mL	___	
	Ordered mcg/min ÷ mcg/mL × 60 min/h =								___	mL/h
Norepinephrine	Infusion	1 mcg/min = 4 mL/h 2 mcg/min = 8 mL/h 3 mcg/min = 11 mL/h 4 mcg/min = 15 mL/h 5 mcg/min = 19 mL/h			2–20 mcg/min	4 mg/ 250 mL	16	mcg/mL		
	Ordered mcg dose/min ÷ mcg/mL × 60 min/h =								___	mL/h
Phenylephrine	Infusion	1.3 mcg/min = 1 mL/h			10–200 mcg/min	20 mg/ 250 mL	80	mcg/mL		
	Ordered mcg/min ÷ mcg/mL × 60 min/h =								___	mL/h
Primacor	0.05 mg/kg = **7.8** mg			Give load over 10 min		40 mg/ 200 mL	0.2	mg/mL		
	mg to give ÷ mg/mL = **39** mL				39 mL × (60 min/h ÷ 10 min) =				**234**	mL/h × 10 min
	Infusion		0.02		0.5 mcg/ kg/min	40 mg/ 200 mL	200	mcg/mL	___	
	Take dose you want in mcg ÷ by drug index number = mL/h on pump									
Trimethaphan	Infusion	___			0.3–6 mg/min	500 mg/ 500 mL	1	mg/mL	___	
	Ordered mg/min ÷ mg/mL × 60 min/h =								___	mL/h
Vasopressin		0.02 u/min = 3 mL/h 0.04 u/min = 6 mL/h				40 u/ 100 mL	400	u/mL		

157 kg

DRUG	ORDERED AMOUNT	TOTAL DOSE TO GIVE	DRUG INDEX NUMBER	DIRECTIONS	INFUSION RANGE	DRUG MIXTURE	AMOUNT DRUG/mL	RUN AT mL/h
Aminophylline	5 mg/kg =	785 mg		Give mg/kg load over 20 min		500 mg/ 250 mL	2 mg/mL	
	mg to give ÷ mg/mL =	393 mL			393	mL × (60 min/h ÷ 20 min) =		__1178__ mL/h × 20 min
	Infusion				0.5–1 mg/kg/h	500 mg/ 250 mL	2 mg/mL	
						mg dose ordered × kg ÷ mg/mL =		___ mL/h
Amiodarone	Loading dose			Load **150 mg** over 10 min		900 mg/ 500 mL	1.8 mg/mL	___
				Ordered mg load dose (150 mg) ÷ mg/mL (1.8 mg/mL) = 83 mL to give × (60 min/h ÷ 10 min) = mL/h to set on pump				__500__ mL/h × 83 mL
	Infusion			Run at **1 mg/ min** × 6 h		900 mg/ 500 mL	1.8 mg/mL	
				Ordered mg dose (1 mg/min) ÷ mg/mL (1.8 mg/mL) = _____ × 60 min/h = mL/h to set on pump				__33__ mL/h × 6 h
	Infusion			Run at **0.5 mg/ min** × 18 h		900 mg/ 500 mL	1.8 mg/mL	
				Ordered mg dose (0.5 mg/min) ÷ mg/mL (1.8 mg/mL) = _____ × 60 min/h = mL/h to set on pump				__17__ mL/h × 18 h
Amrinone	0.75 mg/kg =	117.75 mg		Give mg/kg load over 10 min		300 mg/ 120 mL	2.5 mg/mL	___
	mg to give ÷ mg/mL =	47 mL			47.1	mL × (60 min/h ÷ 10 min) =		__283__ mL/h × 10 min
	Infusion		0.26		5–10 mcg/ kg/min	300 mg/ 120 mL	2500 mcg/mL	___
				Take dose you want in mcg ÷ by drug index number = mL/h on pump				
Brevibloc	Infusion		1.06		50–100 mcg/ kg/min	2.5 g/ 250 mL	10,000 mcg/mL	___ mL/h
				Take dose you want in mcg ÷ by drug index number = mL/h on pump				
Cardene	Infusion			—	0.5–10 mg/h	25 mg 250 mL	0.1 mg/mL	___
				Ordered mg dose ÷ mg/mL = mL/h to set on pump				___ mL/h
Cardizem	0.25 mg/kg =	39.25 mg		Give mg/kg load over 20 min		50 mg/ 100 mL	0.5 mg/mL	
	mg to give ÷ mg/mL =	79 mL			78.5	mL × (60 min/h ÷ 20 min) =		__236__ mL/h
	0.35 mg/kg =	54.95 mg		May repeat loading dose in 15 min			0.5 mg/mL	___
	mg to give ÷ mg/mL =	110 mL			109.9	mL × (60 min/h ÷ 20 min) =		__330__ mL/h
	Infusion				5–15 mg/h			___
				Ordered mg dose ÷ mg/mL = mL/h to set on pump				___ mL/h
Desmopressin	0.3 mcg/kg =	47 mcg		Give dose over 20–30 min			4 mcg/vial	
Dobutamine	Infusion		0.21		2.5–40 mcg/kg/ min	250 mg/ 125 mL	2000 mcg/mL	
				Take dose you want in mcg ÷ by drug index number = mL/h on pump				

(continues)

157 kg (continued)

DRUG	ORDERED AMOUNT	TOTAL DOSE TO GIVE	DRUG INDEX NUMBER	DIRECTIONS	INFUSION RANGE	DRUG MIXTURE	AMOUNT	DRUG/mL	RUN AT	mL/h
Dopamine	Infusion		0.17		1–20 mcg/kg/min	400 mg/250 mL	1600	mcg/mL		
	Take dose you want in mcg ÷ by drug index number = mL/h on pump									
Epinephrine	Infusion	1 mcg/min = 4 mL/h 2 mcg/min = 8 mL/h 3 mcg/min = 11 mL/h 4 mcg/min = 15 mL/h			1–4 mcg/min	4 mg/250 mL	16	mcg/mL		
	Ordered mcg dose/min ÷ mcg/mL × 60 min/h = ___ mL/h									
Fenoldapam	Infusion		0.0043		0.01–1.6 mcg/kg/min	10 mg/250 mL	40	mcg/mL		
	Take dose you want in mcg ÷ by drug index number = mL/h on pump									
Heparin	100 u/kg = 15,700 u 200 u/kg = 31,400 u 300 u/kg = 47,100 u 400 u/kg = 62,800 u									
Isoproterenol	Infusion				5 mcg/min	1 mg/250 mL	4	mcg/mL		
	Ordered mcg dose/min ÷ mcg/mL × 60 min/h =								75	mL/h
Lidocaine	Infusion	1 mg/min = 7.5 mL/h			1–4 mg/min	2 g/250 mL	8	mg/mL	___	
	Ordered mg/min ÷ mg/mL × 60 min/h = ___ mL/h									
Nitroglycerin	Infusion	3 mcg/min = 1 mL/h			3–200 mcg/min	50 mg/250 mL	200	mcg/mL	___	
	Ordered mcg/min ÷ mcg/mL × 60 min/h = ___ mL/h									
Nitroprusside	Infusion	6.7 mcg/min = 1 mL/h			5–300 mcg/min	100 mg/250 mL	400	mcg/mL	___	
	Ordered mcg/min ÷ mcg/mL × 60 min/h = ___ mL/h									
Norepinephrine	Infusion	1 mcg/min = 4 mL/h 2 mcg/min = 8 mL/h 3 mcg/min = 11 mL/h 4 mcg/min = 15 mL/h 5 mcg/min = 19 mL/h			2–20 mcg/min	4 mg/250 mL	16	mcg/mL		
	Ordered mcg dose/min ÷ mcg/mL × 60 min/h = ___ mL/h									
Phenylephrine	Infusion	1.3 mcg/min = 1 mL/h			10–200 mcg/min	20 mg/250 mL	80	mcg/mL		
	Ordered mcg/min ÷ mcg/mL × 60 min/h = ___ mL/h									
Primacor	0.05 mg/kg = 7.85 mg			Give load over 10 min		40 mg/200 mL	0.2	mg/mL		
	mg to give ÷ mg/mL = 39 mL					39 mL × (60 min/h ÷ 10 min) =			236	mL/h × 10 min
	Infusion		0.02		0.5 mcg/kg/min	40 mg/200 mL	200	mcg/mL	___	
	Take dose you want in mcg ÷ by drug index number = mL/h on pump									
Trimethaphan	Infusion		—		0.3–6 mg/min	500 mg/500 mL	1	mg/mL	___	
	Ordered mg/min ÷ mg/mL × 60 min/h = ___ mL/h									
Vasopressin		0.02 u/min = 3 mL/h 0.04 u/min = 6 mL/h				40 u/100 mL	400	u/mL		

158 kg

DRUG	ORDERED AMOUNT	TOTAL DOSE TO GIVE	DRUG INDEX NUMBER	DIRECTIONS	INFUSION RANGE	DRUG MIXTURE	AMOUNT	DRUG/mL	RUN AT	mL/h
Aminophylline	5 mg/kg = **790 mg**			Give mg/kg load over 20 min		500 mg/ 250 mL	2 mg/mL		
	mg to give ÷ mg/mL = **395 mL**				**395**	mL × (60 min/h ÷ 20 min) =			**1185**	mL/h × 20 min
	Infusion				0.5–1 mg/kg/h	500 mg/ 250 mL	2 mg/mL		
				mg dose ordered × kg ÷ mg/mL =					___	mL/h
Amiodarone	Loading dose			Load **150 mg** over 10 min		900 mg/ 500 mL	1.8 mg/mL		___
				Ordered mg load dose (150 mg) ÷ mg/mL (1.8 mg/mL) = 83 mL to give × (60 min/h ÷ 10 min) = mL/h to set on pump					**500**	mL/h × 83 mL
	Infusion			Run at **1 mg/ min** × 6 h	900 mg/ 500 mL		1.8 mg/mL		
				Ordered mg dose (1 mg/min) ÷ mg/mL (1.8 mg/mL) = ____ × 60 min/h = mL/h to set on pump					**33**	mL/h × 6 h
	Infusion			Run at **0.5 mg/ min** × 18 h	900 mg/ 500 mL		1.8 mg/mL		
				Ordered mg dose (0.5 mg/min) ÷ mg/mL (1.8 mg/mL) = ____ × 60 min/h = mL/h to set on pump					**17**	mL/h × 18 h
Amrinone	0.75 mg/kg = **118.5 mg**			Give mg/kg load over 10 min		300 mg/ 120 mL	2.5 mg/mL		___
	mg to give ÷ mg/mL = **47 mL**				**47.4**	mL × (60 min/h ÷ 10 min) =			**284**	mL/h × 10 min
	Infusion		0.26		5–10 mcg/ kg/min	300 mg/ 120 mL	2500 mcg/mL		___
				Take dose you want in mcg ÷ by drug index number = mL/h on pump					
Brevibloc	Infusion		1.05		50–100 mcg/ kg/min	2.5 g/ 250 mL	10,000 mcg/mL		___ mL/h
				Take dose you want in mcg ÷ by drug index number = mL/h on pump					
Cardene	Infusion		—		0.5–10 mg/h	25 mg 250 mL	0.1 mg/mL		___
				Ordered mg dose ÷ mg/mL = mL/h to set on pump					___	mL/h
Cardizem	0.25 mg/kg = **39.5 mg**			Give mg/kg load over 20 min		50 mg/ 100 mL	0.5 mg/mL		___
	mg to give ÷ mg/mL = **79 mL**				**79**	mL × (60 min/h ÷ 20 min) =			**237**	mL/h
	0.35 mg/kg = **55.3 mg**			May repeat loading dose in 15 min			0.5 mg/mL		___
	mg to give ÷ mg/mL = **111 mL**				**110.6**	mL × (60 min/h ÷ 20 min) =			**332**	mL/h
	Infusion				5–15 mg/h				___
				Ordered mg dose ÷ mg/mL = mL/h to set on pump					___	mL/h
Desmopressin	0.3 mcg/kg = **47 mcg**			Give dose over 20–30 min			4 mcg/vial		
Dobutamine	Infusion		0.21		2.5–40 mcg/kg/ min	250 mg/ 125 mL	2000 mcg/mL		
				Take dose you want in mcg ÷ by drug index number = mL/h on pump					

(continues)

158 kg (continued)

DRUG	ORDERED AMOUNT	TOTAL DOSE TO GIVE	DRUG INDEX NUMBER	DIRECTIONS	INFUSION RANGE	DRUG MIXTURE	AMOUNT	DRUG/mL	RUN AT	mL/h
Dopamine	Infusion		0.17		1–20 mcg/kg/min	400 mg/250 mL	1600	mcg/mL		
	Take dose you want in mcg ÷ by drug index number = mL/h on pump									
Epinephrine	Infusion	1 mcg/min = 4 mL/h 2 mcg/min = 8 mL/h 3 mcg/min = 11 mL/h 4 mcg/min = 15 mL/h			1–4 mcg/min	4 mg/250 mL	16	mcg/mL		
	Ordered mcg dose/min ÷ mcg/mL × 60 min/h =								___	mL/h
Fenoldapam	Infusion		0.0042		0.01–1.6 mcg/kg/min	10 mg/250 mL	40	mcg/mL		
	Take dose you want in mcg ÷ by drug index number = mL/h on pump									
Heparin	100 u/kg = 15,800 u 200 u/kg = 31,600 u 300 u/kg = 47,400 u 400 u/kg = 63,200 u									
Isoproterenol	Infusion				5 mcg/min	1 mg/250 mL	4	mcg/mL		
	Ordered mcg dose/min ÷ mcg/mL × 60 min/h =								75	mL/h
Lidocaine	Infusion	1 mg/min = 7.5 mL/h			1–4 mg/min	2 g/250 mL	8	mg/mL	___	
	Ordered mg/min ÷ mg/mL × 60 min/h =								___	mL/h
Nitroglycerin	Infusion	3 mcg/min = 1 mL/h			3–200 mcg/min	50 mg/250 mL	200	mcg/mL	___	
	Ordered mcg/min ÷ mcg/mL × 60 min/h =								___	mL/h
Nitroprusside	Infusion	6.7 mcg/min = 1 mL/h			5–300 mcg/min	100 mg/250 mL	400	mcg/mL	___	
	Ordered mcg/min ÷ mcg/mL × 60 min/h =								___	mL/h
Norepinephrine	Infusion	1 mcg/min = 4 mL/h 2 mcg/min = 8 mL/h 3 mcg/min = 11 mL/h 4 mcg/min = 15 mL/h 5 mcg/min = 19 mL/h			2–20 mcg/min	4 mg/250 mL	16	mcg/mL		
	Ordered mcg dose/min ÷ mcg/mL × 60 min/h =								___	mL/h
Phenylephrine	Infusion	1.3 mcg/min = 1 mL/h			10–200 mcg/min	20 mg/250 mL	80	mcg/mL		
	Ordered mcg/min ÷ mcg/mL × 60 min/h =								___	mL/h
Primacor	0.05 mg/kg = 7.9 mg			Give load over 10 min		40 mg/200 mL	0.2	mg/mL		
	mg to give ÷ mg/mL = 40 mL					40	mL × (60 min/h ÷ 10 min) =		237	mL/h × 10 min
	Infusion		0.02		0.5 mcg/kg/min	40 mg/200 mL	200	mcg/mL	___	
	Take dose you want in mcg ÷ by drug index number = mL/h on pump									
Trimethaphan	Infusion		—		0.3–6 mg/min	500 mg/500 mL	1	mg/mL	___	
	Ordered mg/min ÷ mg/mL × 60 min/h =								___	mL/h
Vasopressin		0.02 u/min = 3 mL/h 0.04 u/min = 6 mL/h				40 u/100 mL	400	u/mL		

159 kg

DRUG	ORDERED AMOUNT	TOTAL DOSE TO GIVE	DRUG INDEX NUMBER	DIRECTIONS	INFUSION RANGE	DRUG MIXTURE	AMOUNT DRUG/mL	RUN AT mL/h
Aminophylline	5 mg/kg =	795 mg		Give mg/kg load over 20 min		500 mg/ 250 mL	2 mg/mL	
	mg to give ÷ mg/mL =	398 mL			398	mL × (60 min/h ÷ 20 min) =		**1193** mL/h × 20 min
	Infusion				0.5–1 mg/kg/h	500 mg/ 250 mL	2 mg/mL	
					mg dose ordered × kg ÷ mg/mL =			___ mL/h
Amiodarone	Loading dose			Load **150 mg** over 10 min		900 mg/ 500 mL	1.8 mg/mL	___
				Ordered mg load dose (150 mg) ÷ mg/mL (1.8 mg/mL) = 83 mL to give × (60 min/h ÷ 10 min) = mL/h to set on pump				**500** mL/h × 83 mL
	Infusion			Run at **1 mg/ min** × 6 h		900 mg/ 500 mL	1.8 mg/mL	
				Ordered mg dose (1 mg/min) ÷ mg/mL (1.8 mg/mL) = ____ × 60 min/h = mL/h to set on pump				**33** mL/h × 6 h
	Infusion			Run at **0.5 mg/ min** × 18 h		900 mg/ 500 mL	1.8 mg/mL	
				Ordered mg dose (0.5 mg/min) ÷ mg/mL (1.8 mg/mL) = ____ × 60 min/h = mL/h to set on pump				**17** mL/h × 18 h
Amrinone	0.75 mg/kg =	119.25 mg		Give mg/kg load over 10 min		300 mg/ 120 mL	2.5 mg/mL	___
	mg to give ÷ mg/mL =	48 mL			47.7	mL × (60 min/h ÷ 10 min) =		**286** mL/h × 10 min
	Infusion		0.26		5–10 mcg/ kg/min	300 mg/ 120 mL	2500 mcg/mL	___
				Take dose you want in mcg ÷ by drug index number = mL/h on pump				
Brevibloc	Infusion		1.05		50–100 mcg/ kg/min	2.5 g/ 250 mL	10,000 mcg/mL	___ mL/h
				Take dose you want in mcg ÷ by drug index number = mL/h on pump				
Cardene	Infusion			—	0.5–10 mg/h	25 mg 250 mL	0.1 mg/mL	
				Ordered mg dose ÷ mg/mL = mL/h to set on pump				___ mL/h
Cardizem	0.25 mg/kg =	39.75 mg		Give mg/kg load over 20 min		50 mg/ 100 mL	0.5 mg/mL	___
	mg to give ÷ mg/mL =	80 mL			79.5	mL × (60 min/h ÷ 20 min) =		**239** mL/h
	0.35 mg/kg =	55.65 mg		May repeat loading dose in 15 min			0.5 mg/mL	___
	mg to give ÷ mg/mL =	111 mL			111.3	mL × (60 min/h ÷ 20 min) =		**334** mL/h
	Infusion				5–15 mg/h			___
				Ordered mg dose ÷ mg/mL = mL/h to set on pump				___ mL/h
Desmopressin	0.3 mcg/kg =	48 mcg		Give dose over 20–30 min			4 mcg/vial	
Dobutamine	Infusion		0.21		2.5–40 mcg/kg/ min	250 mg/ 125 mL	2000 mcg/mL	
				Take dose you want in mcg ÷ by drug index number = mL/h on pump				

(continues)

159 kg (continued)

DRUG	ORDERED AMOUNT	TOTAL DOSE TO GIVE	DRUG INDEX NUMBER	DIRECTIONS	INFUSION RANGE	DRUG MIXTURE	AMOUNT	DRUG/ mL	RUN AT	mL/h
Dopamine	Infusion		0.17		1–20 mcg/ kg/min	400 mg/ 250 mL	1600	mcg/mL		
	Take dose you want in mcg ÷ by drug index number = mL/h on pump									
Epinephrine	Infusion	1 mcg/min = 4 mL/h 2 mcg/min = 8 mL/h 3 mcg/min = 11 mL/h 4 mcg/min = 15 mL/h			1–4 mcg/min	4 mg/ 250 mL	16	mcg/mL		
	Ordered mcg dose/min ÷ mcg/mL × 60 min/h =								___	mL/h
Fenoldapam	Infusion		0.0042		0.01–1.6 mcg/ kg/min	10 mg/ 250 mL	40	mcg/mL		
	Take dose you want in mcg ÷ by drug index number = mL/h on pump									
Heparin	100 u/kg = 15,900 u 200 u/kg = 31,800 u 300 u/kg = 47,700 u 400 u/kg = 63,600 u									
Isoproterenol	Infusion				5 mcg/min	1 mg/ 250 mL	4	mcg/mL		
	Ordered mcg dose/min ÷ mcg/mL × 60 min/h =								**75**	mL/h
Lidocaine	Infusion	1 mg/min = 7.5 mL/h			1–4 mg/min	2 g/ 250 mL	8	mg/mL		___
	Ordered mg/min ÷ mg/mL × 60 min/h =								___	mL/h
Nitroglycerin	Infusion	3 mcg/min = 1 mL/h			3–200 mcg/min	50 mg/ 250 mL	200	mcg/mL		___
	Ordered mcg/min ÷ mcg/mL × 60 min/h =								___	mL/h
Nitroprusside	Infusion	6.7 mcg/min = 1 mL/h			5–300 mcg/min	100 mg/ 250 mL	400	mcg/mL		___
	Ordered mcg/min ÷ mcg/mL × 60 min/h =								___	mL/h
Norepinephrine	Infusion	1 mcg/min = 4 mL/h 2 mcg/min = 8 mL/h 3 mcg/min = 11 mL/h 4 mcg/min = 15 mL/h 5 mcg/min = 19 mL/h			2–20 mcg/min	4 mg/ 250 mL	16	mcg/mL		
	Ordered mcg dose/min ÷ mcg/mL × 60 min/h =								___	mL/h
Phenylephrine	Infusion	1.3 mcg/min = 1 mL/h			10–200 mcg/min	20 mg/ 250 mL	80	mcg/mL		___
	Ordered mcg/min ÷ mcg/mL × 60 min/h =								___	mL/h
Primacor	0.05 mg/kg = 7.95 mg			Give load over 10 min		40 mg/ 200 mL	0.2	mg/mL		
	mg to give ÷ mg/mL = 40 mL				40 mL × (60 min/h ÷ 10 min) =				**239**	mL/h × 10 min
	Infusion		0.02		0.5 mcg/ kg/min	40 mg/ 200 mL	200	mcg/mL		___
	Take dose you want in mcg ÷ by drug index number = mL/h on pump									
Trimethaphan	Infusion		—		0.3–6 mg/min	500 mg/ 500 mL	1	mg/mL		___
	Ordered mg/min ÷ mg/mL × 60 min/h =								___	mL/h
Vasopressin		0.02 u/min = 3 mL/h 0.04 u/min = 6 mL/h				40 u/ 100 mL	400	u/mL		

160 kg

DRUG	ORDERED AMOUNT	TOTAL DOSE TO GIVE		DRUG INDEX NUMBER	DIRECTIONS	INFUSION RANGE	DRUG MIXTURE	AMOUNT	DRUG/ mL	RUN AT	mL/h
Aminophylline	5 mg/kg =	800	mg		Give mg/kg load over 20 min		500 mg/ 250 mL	2	mg/mL		
	mg to give ÷ mg/mL =	400	mL			400	mL × (60 min/h ÷ 20 min) =			1200	mL/h × 20 min
	Infusion					0.5–1 mg/kg/h	500 mg/ 250 mL	2	mg/mL		
							mg dose ordered × kg ÷ mg/mL =			___	mL/h
Amiodarone	Loading dose				Load **150 mg** over 10 min		900 mg/ 500 mL	1.8	mg/mL	___	
					Ordered mg load dose (150 mg) ÷ mg/mL (1.8 mg/mL) = 83 mL to give × (60 min/h ÷ 10 min) = mL/h to set on pump					500	mL/h × 83 mL
	Infusion				Run at **1 mg/ min** × 6 h		900 mg/ 500 mL	1.8	mg/mL		
					Ordered mg dose (1 mg/min) ÷ mg/mL (1.8 mg/mL) = ____ × 60 min/h = mL/h to set on pump					33	mL/h × 6 h
	Infusion				Run at **0.5 mg/ min** × 18 h		900 mg/ 500 mL	1.8	mg/mL		
					Ordered mg dose (0.5 mg/min) ÷ mg/mL (1.8 mg/mL) = ____ × 60 min/h = mL/h to set on pump					17	mL/h × 18 h
Amrinone	0.75 mg/kg =	120	mg		Give mg/kg load over 10 min		300 mg/ 120 mL	2.5	mg/mL	___	
	mg to give ÷ mg/mL =	48	mL			48	mL × (60 min/h ÷ 10 min) =			288	mL/h × 10 min
	Infusion			0.26		5–10 mcg/ kg/min	300 mg/ 120 mL	2500	mcg/mL	___	
					Take dose you want in mcg ÷ by drug index number = mL/h on pump						
Brevibloc	Infusion			1.04		50–100 mcg/ kg/min	2.5 g/ 250 mL	10,000	mcg/mL	___	mL/h
					Take dose you want in mcg ÷ by drug index number = mL/h on pump						
Cardene	Infusion			___		0.5–10 mg/h	25 mg 250 mL	0.1	mg/mL	___	
					Ordered mg dose ÷ mg/mL = mL/h to set on pump					___	mL/h
Cardizem	0.25 mg/kg =	40	mg		Give mg/kg load over 20 min		50 mg/ 100 mL	0.5	mg/mL		
	mg to give ÷ mg/mL =	80	mL			80	mL × (60 min/h ÷ 20 min) =			240	mL/h
	0.35 mg/kg =	56	mg		May repeat loading dose in 15 min			0.5	mg/mL		
	mg to give ÷ mg/mL =	112	mL			112	mL × (60 min/h ÷ 20 min) =			336	mL/h
	Infusion					5–15 mg/h				___	
					Ordered mg dose ÷ mg/mL = mL/h to set on pump					___	mL/h
Desmopressin	0.3 mcg/kg =	48	mcg		Give dose over 20–30 min			4	mcg/vial		
Dobutamine	Infusion			0.21		2.5–40 mcg/kg/ min	250 mg/ 125 mL	2000	mcg/mL		
					Take dose you want in mcg ÷ by drug index number = mL/h on pump						

(continues)

160 kg (continued)

DRUG	ORDERED AMOUNT	TOTAL DOSE TO GIVE	DRUG INDEX NUMBER	DIRECTIONS	INFUSION RANGE	DRUG MIXTURE	AMOUNT	DRUG/ mL	RUN AT	mL/h
Dopamine	Infusion		0.17		1–20 mcg/ kg/min	400 mg/ 250 mL	1600 mcg/mL			
			Take dose you want in mcg ÷ by drug index number = mL/h on pump							
Epinephrine	Infusion	1 mcg/min = 4 mL/h 2 mcg/min = 8 mL/h 3 mcg/min = 11 mL/h 4 mcg/min = 15 mL/h			1–4 mcg/min	4 mg/ 250 mL	16 mcg/mL			
		Ordered mcg dose/min ÷ mcg/mL × 60 min/h =							___ mL/h	
Fenoldapam	Infusion		0.0042		0.01–1.6 mcg/ kg/min	10 mg/ 250 mL	40 mcg/mL			
			Take dose you want in mcg ÷ by drug index number = mL/h on pump							
Heparin	100 u/kg = 16,000 u 200 u/kg = 32,000 u 300 u/kg = 48,000 u 400 u/kg = 64,000 u									
Isoproterenol	Infusion				5 mcg/min	1 mg/ 250 mL	4 mcg/mL			
		Ordered mcg dose/min ÷ mcg/mL × 60 min/h =							75 mL/h	
Lidocaine	Infusion	1 mg/min = 7.5 mL/h			1–4 mg/min	2 g/ 250 mL	8 mg/mL		—	
		Ordered mg/min ÷ mg/mL × 60 min/h =							___ mL/h	
Nitroglycerin	Infusion	3 mcg/min = 1 mL/h			3–200 mcg/min	50 mg/ 250 mL	200 mcg/mL		—	
		Ordered mcg/min ÷ mcg/mL × 60 min/h =							___ mL/h	
Nitroprusside	Infusion	6.7 mcg/min = 1 mL/h			5–300 mcg/min	100 mg/ 250 mL	400 mcg/mL		—	
		Ordered mcg/min ÷ mcg/mL × 60 min/h =							___ mL/h	
Norepinephrine	Infusion	1 mcg/min = 4 mL/h 2 mcg/min = 8 mL/h 3 mcg/min = 11 mL/h 4 mcg/min = 15 mL/h 5 mcg/min = 19 mL/h			2–20 mcg/min	4 mg/ 250 mL	16 mcg/mL			
		Ordered mcg dose/min ÷ mcg/mL × 60 min/h =							___ mL/h	
Phenylephrine	Infusion	1.3 mcg/min = 1 mL/h			10–200 mcg/min	20 mg/ 250 mL	80 mcg/mL		—	
		Ordered mcg/min ÷ mcg/mL × 60 min/h =							___ mL/h	
Primacor	0.05 mg/kg = 8 mg			Give load over 10 min		40 mg/ 200 mL	0.2 mg/mL			
	mg to give ÷ mg/mL = 40 mL				40 mL × (60 min/h ÷ 10 min) =				240	mL/h × 10 min
	Infusion		0.02		0.5 mcg/ kg/min	40 mg/ 200 mL	200 mcg/mL		—	
			Take dose you want in mcg ÷ by drug index number = mL/h on pump							
Trimethaphan	Infusion		—		0.3–6 mg/min	500 mg/ 500 mL	1 mg/mL		—	
		Ordered mg/min ÷ mg/mL × 60 min/h =							___ mL/h	
Vasopressin		0.02 u/min = 3 mL/h 0.04 u/min = 6 mL/h				40 u/ 100 mL	400 u/mL			

161 kg

DRUG	ORDERED AMOUNT	TOTAL DOSE TO GIVE	DRUG INDEX NUMBER	DIRECTIONS	INFUSION RANGE	DRUG MIXTURE	AMOUNT	DRUG/mL	RUN AT	mL/h
Aminophylline	5 mg/kg =	805 mg		Give mg/kg load over 20 min		500 mg/ 250 mL	2 mg/mL			
	mg to give ÷ mg/mL =	403 mL			403	mL × (60 min/h ÷ 20 min) =			1208	mL/h × 20 min
	Infusion				0.5–1 mg/kg/h	500 mg/ 250 mL	2 mg/mL			
					mg dose ordered × kg ÷ mg/mL =				___	mL/h
Amiodarone	Loading dose			Load **150 mg** over 10 min		900 mg/ 500 mL	1.8 mg/mL		___	
				Ordered mg load dose (150 mg) ÷ mg/mL (1.8 mg/mL) = 83 mL to give × (60 min/h ÷ 10 min) = mL/h to set on pump					500	mL/h × 83 mL
	Infusion			Run at **1 mg/ min** × 6 h		900 mg/ 500 mL	1.8 mg/mL			
				Ordered mg dose (1 mg/min) ÷ mg/mL (1.8 mg/mL) = ___ × 60 min/h = mL/h to set on pump					33	mL/h × 6 h
	Infusion			Run at **0.5 mg/ min** × 18 h		900 mg/ 500 mL	1.8 mg/mL			
				Ordered mg dose (0.5 mg/min) ÷ mg/mL (1.8 mg/mL) = ___ × 60 min/h = mL/h to set on pump					17	mL/h × 18 h
Amrinone	0.75 mg/kg =	120.75 mg		Give mg/kg load over 10 min		300 mg/ 120 mL	2.5 mg/mL		___	
	mg to give ÷ mg/mL =	48 mL			48.3	mL × (60 min/h ÷ 10 min) =			290	mL/h × 10 min
	Infusion		0.26		5–10 mcg/ kg/min	300 mg/ 120 mL	2500 mcg/mL		___	
				Take dose you want in mcg ÷ by drug index number = mL/h on pump						
Brevibloc	Infusion		1.03		50–100 mcg/ kg/min	2.5 g/ 250 mL	10,000 mcg/mL		___	mL/h
				Take dose you want in mcg ÷ by drug index number = mL/h on pump						
Cardene	Infusion		___		0.5–10 mg/h	25 mg 250 mL	0.1 mg/mL		___	
				Ordered mg dose ÷ mg/mL = mL/h to set on pump					___	mL/h
Cardizem	0.25 mg/kg =	40.25 mg		Give mg/kg load over 20 min		50 mg/ 100 mL	0.5 mg/mL		___	
	mg to give ÷ mg/mL =	81 mL			80.5	mL × (60 min/h ÷ 20 min) =			242	mL/h
	0.35 mg/kg =	56.35 mg		May repeat loading dose in 15 min			0.5 mg/mL		___	
	mg to give ÷ mg/mL =	113 mL			112.7	mL × (60 min/h ÷ 20 min) =			338	mL/h
	Infusion				5–15 mg/h				___	
				Ordered mg dose ÷ mg/mL = mL/h to set on pump					___	mL/h
Desmopressin	0.3 mcg/kg =	48 mcg		Give dose over 20–30 min			4 mcg/vial			
Dobutamine	Infusion		0.21		2.5–40 mcg/kg/ min	250 mg/ 125 mL	2000 mcg/mL			
				Take dose you want in mcg ÷ by drug index number = mL/h on pump						

(continues)

161   kg (continued)

DRUG	ORDERED AMOUNT	TOTAL DOSE TO GIVE	DRUG INDEX NUMBER	DIRECTIONS	INFUSION RANGE	DRUG MIXTURE	AMOUNT	DRUG/mL	RUN AT mL/h
Dopamine	Infusion		0.17		1–20 mcg/kg/min	400 mg/250 mL	1600	mcg/mL	
	Take dose you want in mcg ÷ by drug index number = mL/h on pump								
Epinephrine	Infusion	1 mcg/min = 4 mL/h 2 mcg/min = 8 mL/h 3 mcg/min = 11 mL/h 4 mcg/min = 15 mL/h			1–4 mcg/min	4 mg/250 mL	16	mcg/mL	
			Ordered mcg dose/min ÷ mcg/mL × 60 min/h =						___ mL/h
Fenoldapam	Infusion		0.0042		0.01–1.6 mcg/kg/min	10 mg/250 mL	40	mcg/mL	
	Take dose you want in mcg ÷ by drug index number = mL/h on pump								
Heparin	100 u/kg =	16,100 u							
	200 u/kg =	32,200 u							
	300 u/kg =	48,300 u							
	400 u/kg =	64,400 u							
Isoproterenol	Infusion				5 mcg/min	1 mg/250 mL	4	mcg/mL	
			Ordered mcg dose/min ÷ mcg/mL × 60 min/h =						75 mL/h
Lidocaine	Infusion	1 mg/min = 7.5 mL/h			1–4 mg/min	2 g/250 mL	8	mg/mL	___
			Ordered mg/min ÷ mg/mL × 60 min/h =						___ mL/h
Nitroglycerin	Infusion	3 mcg/min = 1 mL/h			3–200 mcg/min	50 mg/250 mL	200	mcg/mL	___
			Ordered mcg/min ÷ mcg/mL × 60 min/h =						___ mL/h
Nitroprusside	Infusion	6.7 mcg/min = 1 mL/h			5–300 mcg/min	100 mg/250 mL	400	mcg/mL	___
			Ordered mcg/min ÷ mcg/mL × 60 min/h =						___ mL/h
Norepinephrine	Infusion	1 mcg/min = 4 mL/h 2 mcg/min = 8 mL/h 3 mcg/min = 11 mL/h 4 mcg/min = 15 mL/h 5 mcg/min = 19 mL/h			2–20 mcg/min	4 mg/250 mL	16	mcg/mL	
			Ordered mcg dose/min ÷ mcg/mL × 60 min/h =						___ mL/h
Phenylephrine	Infusion	1.3 mcg/min = 1 mL/h			10–200 mcg/min	20 mg/250 mL	80	mcg/mL	
			Ordered mcg/min ÷ mcg/mL × 60 min/h =						___ mL/h
Primacor	0.05 mg/kg =	8.05 mg		Give load over 10 min		40 mg/200 mL	0.2	mg/mL	
	mg to give ÷ mg/mL =	40 mL			40 mL × (60 min/h ÷ 10 min) =				242 mL/h × 10 min
	Infusion		0.02		0.5 mcg/kg/min	40 mg/200 mL	200	mcg/mL	___
	Take dose you want in mcg ÷ by drug index number = mL/h on pump								
Trimethaphan	Infusion		___		0.3–6 mg/min	500 mg/500 mL	1	mg/mL	___
			Ordered mg/min ÷ mg/mL × 60 min/h =						___ mL/h
Vasopressin		0.02 u/min = 3 mL/h 0.04 u/min = 6 mL/h				40 u/100 mL	400	u/mL	

162 kg

DRUG	ORDERED AMOUNT	TOTAL DOSE TO GIVE	DRUG INDEX NUMBER	DIRECTIONS	INFUSION RANGE	DRUG MIXTURE	AMOUNT	DRUG/ mL	RUN AT	mL/h
Aminophylline	5 mg/kg =	810 mg		Give mg/kg load over 20 min		500 mg/ 250 mL	2 mg/mL			
	mg to give ÷ mg/mL =	405 mL			405	500 mg/ 250 mL	mL × (60 min/h ÷ 20 min) =		1215	mL/h × 20 min
	Infusion				0.5–1 mg/kg/h	500 mg/ 250 mL	2 mg/mL			
					mg dose ordered × kg ÷ mg/mL =				___	mL/h
Amiodarone	Loading dose			Load **150 mg** over 10 min		900 mg/ 500 mL	1.8 mg/mL		___	
				Ordered mg load dose (150 mg) ÷ mg/mL (1.8 mg/mL) = 83 mL to give × (60 min/h ÷ 10 min) = mL/h to set on pump					500	mL/h × 83 mL
	Infusion			Run at **1 mg/ min** × 6 h		900 mg/ 500 mL	1.8 mg/mL			
				Ordered mg dose (1 mg/min) ÷ mg/mL (1.8 mg/mL) = ____ × 60 min/h = mL/h to set on pump					33	mL/h × 6 h
	Infusion			Run at **0.5 mg/ min** × 18 h		900 mg/ 500 mL	1.8 mg/mL			
				Ordered mg dose (0.5 mg/min) ÷ mg/mL (1.8 mg/mL) = ____ × 60 min/h = mL/h to set on pump					17	mL/h × 18 h
Amrinone	0.75 mg/kg =	121.5 mg		Give mg/kg load over 10 min		300 mg/ 120 mL	2.5 mg/mL		___	
	mg to give ÷ mg/mL =	49 mL			48.6		mL × (60 min/h ÷ 10 min) =		292	mL/h × 10 min
	Infusion		0.26		5–10 mcg/ kg/min	300 mg/ 120 mL	2500 mcg/mL		___	
				Take dose you want in mcg ÷ by drug index number = mL/h on pump						
Brevibloc	Infusion		1.03		50–100 mcg/ kg/min	2.5 g/ 250 mL	10,000 mcg/mL		___	mL/h
				Take dose you want in mcg ÷ by drug index number = mL/h on pump						
Cardene	Infusion		—		0.5–10 mg/h	25 mg 250 mL	0.1 mg/mL		___	
				Ordered mg dose ÷ mg/mL = mL/h to set on pump						mL/h
Cardizem	0.25 mg/kg =	40.5 mg		Give mg/kg load over 20 min		50 mg/ 100 mL	0.5 mg/mL		___	
	mg to give ÷ mg/mL =	81 mL			81		mL × (60 min/h ÷ 20 min) =		243	mL/h
	0.35 mg/kg =	56.7 mg		May repeat loading dose in 15 min			0.5 mg/mL		___	
	mg to give ÷ mg/mL =	113 mL			113.4		mL × (60 min/h ÷ 20 min) =		340	mL/h
	Infusion				5–15 mg/h				___	
				Ordered mg dose ÷ mg/mL = mL/h to set on pump						mL/h
Desmopressin	0.3 mcg/kg =	49 mcg		Give dose over 20–30 min			4 mcg/vial			
Dobutamine	Infusion		0.21		2.5–40 mcg/kg/ min	250 mg/ 125 mL	2000 mcg/mL			
				Take dose you want in mcg ÷ by drug index number = mL/h on pump						

(continues)

162 kg (continued)

DRUG	ORDERED AMOUNT		TOTAL DOSE TO GIVE		DRUG INDEX NUMBER	DIRECTIONS	INFUSION RANGE	DRUG MIXTURE	AMOUNT	DRUG/ mL	RUN AT	mL/h
Dopamine	Infusion				0.16		1–20 mcg/ kg/min	400 mg/ 250 mL	1600	mcg/mL		
					Take dose you want in mcg ÷ by drug index number = mL/h on pump							
Epinephrine	Infusion		1 mcg/min = 4 mL/h 2 mcg/min = 8 mL/h 3 mcg/min = 11 mL/h 4 mcg/min = 15 mL/h				1–4 mcg/min	4 mg/ 250 mL	16	mcg/mL		
					Ordered mcg dose/min ÷ mcg/mL × 60 min/h =						___	mL/h
Fenoldapam	Infusion				0.0041		0.01–1.6 mcg/ kg/min	10 mg/ 250 mL	40	mcg/mL		
					Take dose you want in mcg ÷ by drug index number = mL/h on pump							
Heparin	100 u/kg = 200 u/kg = 300 u/kg = 400 u/kg =		16,200 u 32,400 u 48,600 u 64,800 u									
Isoproterenol	Infusion						5 mcg/min	1 mg/ 250 mL	4	mcg/mL		
					Ordered mcg dose/min ÷ mcg/mL × 60 min/h =						<u>75</u>	mL/h
Lidocaine	Infusion		1 mg/min = 7.5 mL/h				1–4 mg/min	2 g/ 250 mL	8	mg/mL	___	
					Ordered mg/min ÷ mg/mL × 60 min/h =						___	mL/h
Nitroglycerin	Infusion		3 mcg/min = 1 mL/h				3–200 mcg/min	50 mg/ 250 mL	200	mcg/mL	___	
					Ordered mcg/min ÷ mcg/mL × 60 min/h =						___	mL/h
Nitroprusside	Infusion		6.7 mcg/min = 1 mL/h				5–300 mcg/min	100 mg/ 250 mL	400	mcg/mL	___	
					Ordered mcg/min ÷ mcg/mL × 60 min/h =						___	mL/h
Norepinephrine	Infusion		1 mcg/min = 4 mL/h 2 mcg/min = 8 mL/h 3 mcg/min = 11 mL/h 4 mcg/min = 15 mL/h 5 mcg/min = 19 mL/h				2–20 mcg/min	4 mg/ 250 mL	16	mcg/mL		
					Ordered mcg dose/min ÷ mcg/mL × 60 min/h =						___	mL/h
Phenylephrine	Infusion		1.3 mcg/min = 1 mL/h				10–200 mcg/min	20 mg/ 250 mL	80	mcg/mL		
					Ordered mcg/min ÷ mcg/mL × 60 min/h =						___	mL/h
Primacor	0.05 mg/kg =		8.1 mg			Give load over 10 min		40 mg/ 200 mL	0.2	mg/mL		
	mg to give ÷ mg/mL =		41 mL					41	mL × (60 min/h ÷ 10 min) =		<u>243</u>	mL/h × 10 min
	Infusion				0.02		0.5 mcg/ kg/min	40 mg/ 200 mL	200	mcg/mL	___	
					Take dose you want in mcg ÷ by drug index number = mL/h on pump							
Trimethaphan	Infusion				—		0.3–6 mg/min	500 mg/ 500 mL	1	mg/mL	___	
					Ordered mg/min ÷ mg/mL × 60 min/h =						___	mL/h
Vasopressin			0.02 u/min = 3 mL/h 0.04 u/min = 6 mL/h					40 u/ 100 mL	400	u/mL		

163 kg

DRUG	ORDERED AMOUNT	TOTAL DOSE TO GIVE	DRUG INDEX NUMBER	DIRECTIONS	INFUSION RANGE	DRUG MIXTURE	AMOUNT	DRUG/ mL	RUN AT	mL/h
Aminophylline	5 mg/kg =	815 mg		Give mg/kg load over 20 min		500 mg/ 250 mL		2 mg/mL		
		mg to give ÷ mg/mL = 408 mL			408		mL × (60 min/h ÷ 20 min) =		**1223**	mL/h × 20 min
		Infusion			0.5–1 mg/kg/h	500 mg/ 250 mL		2 mg/mL		
							mg dose ordered × kg ÷ mg/mL =			___ mL/h
Amiodarone		Loading dose		Load **150 mg** over 10 min		900 mg/ 500 mL		1.8 mg/mL	___	
				Ordered mg load dose (150 mg) ÷ mg/mL (1.8 mg/mL) = 83 mL to give × (60 min/h ÷ 10 min) = mL/h to set on pump					**500**	mL/h × 83 mL
		Infusion		Run at **1 mg/ min** × 6 h		900 mg/ 500 mL		1.8 mg/mL		
				Ordered mg dose (1 mg/min) ÷ mg/mL (1.8 mg/mL) = ___ × 60 min/h = mL/h to set on pump					**33**	mL/h × 6 h
		Infusion		Run at **0.5 mg/ min** × 18 h		900 mg/ 500 mL		1.8 mg/mL		
				Ordered mg dose (0.5 mg/min) ÷ mg/mL (1.8 mg/mL) = ___ × 60 min/h = mL/h to set on pump					**17**	mL/h × 18 h
Amrinone	0.75 mg/kg =	122.25 mg		Give mg/kg load over 10 min		300 mg/ 120 mL		2.5 mg/mL	___	
		mg to give ÷ mg/mL = 49 mL			48.9		mL × (60 min/h ÷ 10 min) =		**293**	mL/h × 10 min
		Infusion	0.26		5–10 mcg/ kg/min	300 mg/ 120 mL		2500 mcg/mL	___	
				Take dose you want in mcg ÷ by drug index number = mL/h on pump						
Brevibloc		Infusion	1.02		50–100 mcg/ kg/min	2.5 g/ 250 mL		10,000 mcg/mL		___ mL/h
				Take dose you want in mcg ÷ by drug index number = mL/h on pump						
Cardene		Infusion	—		0.5–10 mg/h	25 mg 250 mL		0.1 mg/mL		___
				Ordered mg dose ÷ mg/mL = mL/h to set on pump						___ mL/h
Cardizem	0.25 mg/kg =	40.75 mg		Give mg/kg load over 20 min		50 mg/ 100 mL		0.5 mg/mL	___	
		mg to give ÷ mg/mL = 82 mL			81.5		mL × (60 min/h ÷ 20 min) =		**245** mL/h	
	0.35 mg/kg =	57.05 mg		May repeat loading dose in 15 min				0.5 mg/mL	___	
		mg to give ÷ mg/mL = 114 mL			114.1		mL × (60 min/h ÷ 20 min) =		**342** mL/h	
		Infusion			5–15 mg/h				___	
				Ordered mg dose ÷ mg/mL = mL/h to set on pump						___ mL/h
Desmopressin	0.3 mcg/kg =	49 mcg		Give dose over 20–30 min				4 mcg/vial		
Dobutamine		Infusion	0.20		2.5–40 mcg/kg/ min	250 mg/ 125 mL		2000 mcg/mL		
				Take dose you want in mcg ÷ by drug index number = mL/h on pump						

(continues)

163   kg (continued)

DRUG	ORDERED AMOUNT	TOTAL DOSE TO GIVE	DRUG INDEX NUMBER	DIRECTIONS	INFUSION RANGE	DRUG MIXTURE	AMOUNT	DRUG/mL	RUN AT	mL/h
Dopamine	Infusion		0.16		1–20 mcg/kg/min	400 mg/250 mL	1600 mcg/mL			
		Take dose you want in mcg ÷ by drug index number = mL/h on pump								
Epinephrine	Infusion	1 mcg/min = 4 mL/h 2 mcg/min = 8 mL/h 3 mcg/min = 11 mL/h 4 mcg/min = 15 mL/h			1–4 mcg/min	4 mg/250 mL	16 mcg/mL			
		Ordered mcg dose/min ÷ mcg/mL × 60 min/h =							___	mL/h
Fenoldapam	Infusion		0.0041		0.01–1.6 mcg/kg/min	10 mg/250 mL	40 mcg/mL			
		Take dose you want in mcg ÷ by drug index number = mL/h on pump								
Heparin	100 u/kg = 16,300 u 200 u/kg = 32,600 u 300 u/kg = 48,900 u 400 u/kg = 65,200 u									
Isoproterenol	Infusion				5 mcg/min	1 mg/250 mL	4 mcg/mL			
		Ordered mcg dose/min ÷ mcg/mL × 60 min/h =							<u>75</u>	mL/h
Lidocaine	Infusion	1 mg/min = 7.5 mL/h			1–4 mg/min	2 g/250 mL	8 mg/mL		___	
		Ordered mg/min ÷ mg/mL × 60 min/h =							___	mL/h
Nitroglycerin	Infusion	3 mcg/min = 1 mL/h			3–200 mcg/min	50 mg/250 mL	200 mcg/mL		___	
		Ordered mcg/min ÷ mcg/mL × 60 min/h =							___	mL/h
Nitroprusside	Infusion	6.7 mcg/min = 1 mL/h			5–300 mcg/min	100 mg/250 mL	400 mcg/mL		___	
		Ordered mcg/min ÷ mcg/mL × 60 min/h =							___	mL/h
Norepinephrine	Infusion	1 mcg/min = 4 mL/h 2 mcg/min = 8 mL/h 3 mcg/min = 11 mL/h 4 mcg/min = 15 mL/h 5 mcg/min = 19 mL/h			2–20 mcg/min	4 mg/250 mL	16 mcg/mL			
		Ordered mcg dose/min ÷ mcg/mL × 60 min/h =							___	mL/h
Phenylephrine	Infusion	1.3 mcg/min = 1 mL/h			10–200 mcg/min	20 mg/250 mL	80 mcg/mL		___	
		Ordered mcg/min ÷ mcg/mL × 60 min/h =							___	mL/h
Primacor	0.05 mg/kg = 8.15 mg			Give load over 10 min		40 mg/200 mL	0.2 mg/mL			
	mg to give ÷ mg/mL = 41 mL					41 mL × (60 min/h ÷ 10 min) =			<u>245</u>	mL/h × 10 min
	Infusion		0.02		0.5 mcg/kg/min	40 mg/200 mL	200 mcg/mL		___	
		Take dose you want in mcg ÷ by drug index number = mL/h on pump								
Trimethaphan	Infusion	___			0.3–6 mg/min	500 mg/500 mL	1 mg/mL		___	
		Ordered mg/min ÷ mg/mL × 60 min/h =							___	mL/h
Vasopressin		0.02 u/min = 3 mL/h 0.04 u/min = 6 mL/h				40 u/100 mL	400 u/mL			

164 kg										
DRUG	**ORDERED AMOUNT**	**TOTAL DOSE TO GIVE**	**DRUG INDEX NUMBER**	**DIRECTIONS**	**INFUSION RANGE**	**DRUG MIXTURE**	**AMOUNT**	**DRUG/ mL**	**RUN AT**	**mL/h**
Aminophylline	5 mg/kg =	820 mg		Give mg/kg load over 20 min		500 mg/ 250 mL	2 mg/mL			
	mg to give ÷ mg/mL =	410 mL				410	mL × (60 min/h ÷ 20 min) =		<u>1230</u>	mL/h × 20 min
	Infusion				0.5–1 mg/kg/h	500 mg/ 250 mL	2 mg/mL			
					mg dose ordered × kg ÷ mg/mL =				___	mL/h
Amiodarone	Loading dose			Load **150 mg** over 10 min		900 mg/ 500 mL	1.8 mg/mL		___	
				Ordered mg load dose (150 mg) ÷ mg/mL (1.8 mg/mL) = 83 mL to give × (60 min/h ÷ 10 min) = mL/h to set on pump					<u>500</u>	mL/h × 83 mL
	Infusion			Run at **1 mg/ min** × 6 h		900 mg/ 500 mL	1.8 mg/mL			
				Ordered mg dose (1 mg/min) ÷ mg/mL (1.8 mg/mL) = ___ × 60 min/h = mL/h to set on pump					<u>33</u>	mL/h × 6 h
	Infusion			Run at **0.5 mg/ min** × 18 h		900 mg/ 500 mL	1.8 mg/mL			
				Ordered mg dose (0.5 mg/min) ÷ mg/mL (1.8 mg/mL) = ___ × 60 min/h = mL/h to set on pump					<u>17</u>	mL/h × 18 h
Amrinone	0.75 mg/kg =	123 mg		Give mg/kg load over 10 min		300 mg/ 120 mL	2.5 mg/mL		___	
	mg to give ÷ mg/mL =	49 mL				49.2	mL × (60 min/h ÷ 10 min) =		<u>295</u>	mL/h × 10 min
	Infusion		0.25		5–10 mcg/ kg/min	300 mg/ 120 mL	2500 mcg/mL		___	
				Take dose you want in mcg ÷ by drug index number = mL/h on pump						
Brevibloc	Infusion		1.02		50–100 mcg/ kg/min	2.5 g/ 250 mL	10,000 mcg/mL		___	mL/h
				Take dose you want in mcg ÷ by drug index number = mL/h on pump						
Cardene	Infusion		—		0.5–10 mg/h	25 mg 250 mL	0.1 mg/mL		___	
				Ordered mg dose ÷ mg/mL = mL/h to set on pump					___	mL/h
Cardizem	0.25 mg/kg =	41 mg		Give mg/kg load over 20 min		50 mg/ 100 mL	0.5 mg/mL		___	
	mg to give ÷ mg/mL =	82 mL				82	mL × (60 min/h ÷ 20 min) =		<u>246</u>	mL/h
	0.35 mg/kg =	57.4 mg		May repeat loading dose in 15 min			0.5 mg/mL		___	
	mg to give ÷ mg/mL =	115 mL				114.8	mL × (60 min/h ÷ 20 min) =		<u>344</u>	mL/h
	Infusion				5–15 mg/h				___	
				Ordered mg dose ÷ mg/mL = mL/h to set on pump					___	mL/h
Desmopressin	0.3 mcg/kg =	49 mcg		Give dose over 20–30 min			4 mcg/vial			
Dobutamine	Infusion		0.20		2.5–40 mcg/kg/ min	250 mg/ 125 mL	2000 mcg/mL			
				Take dose you want in mcg ÷ by drug index number = mL/h on pump						

(continues)

164 kg (continued)

DRUG	ORDERED AMOUNT	TOTAL DOSE TO GIVE		DRUG INDEX NUMBER	DIRECTIONS	INFUSION RANGE	DRUG MIXTURE	AMOUNT	DRUG/ mL	RUN AT	mL/h
Dopamine	Infusion			0.16		1–20 mcg/ kg/min	400 mg/ 250 mL	1600	mcg/mL		
	Take dose you want in mcg ÷ by drug index number = mL/h on pump										
Epinephrine	Infusion	1 mcg/min = 4 mL/h 2 mcg/min = 8 mL/h 3 mcg/min = 11 mL/h 4 mcg/min = 15 mL/h				1–4 mcg/min	4 mg/ 250 mL	16	mcg/mL		
	Ordered mcg dose/min ÷ mcg/mL × 60 min/h =									___	mL/h
Fenoldapam	Infusion			0.0041		0.01–1.6 mcg/ kg/min	10 mg/ 250 mL	40	mcg/mL		
	Take dose you want in mcg ÷ by drug index number = mL/h on pump										
Heparin	100 u/kg = 16,400 u 200 u/kg = 32,800 u 300 u/kg = 49,200 u 400 u/kg = 65,600 u										
Isoproterenol	Infusion					5 mcg/min	1 mg/ 250 mL	4	mcg/mL		
	Ordered mcg dose/min ÷ mcg/mL × 60 min/h =									75	mL/h
Lidocaine	Infusion	1 mg/min = 7.5 mL/h				1–4 mg/min	2 g/ 250 mL	8	mg/mL	___	
	Ordered mg/min ÷ mg/mL × 60 min/h =									___	mL/h
Nitroglycerin	Infusion	3 mcg/min = 1 mL/h				3–200 mcg/min	50 mg/ 250 mL	200	mcg/mL	___	
	Ordered mcg/min ÷ mcg/mL × 60 min/h =									___	mL/h
Nitroprusside	Infusion	6.7 mcg/min = 1 mL/h				5–300 mcg/min	100 mg/ 250 mL	400	mcg/mL	___	
	Ordered mcg/min ÷ mcg/mL × 60 min/h =									___	mL/h
Norepinephrine	Infusion	1 mcg/min = 4 mL/h 2 mcg/min = 8 mL/h 3 mcg/min = 11 mL/h 4 mcg/min = 15 mL/h 5 mcg/min = 19 mL/h				2–20 mcg/min	4 mg/ 250 mL	16	mcg/mL		
	Ordered mcg dose/min ÷ mcg/mL × 60 min/h =									___	mL/h
Phenylephrine	Infusion	1.3 mcg/min = 1 mL/h				10–200 mcg/min	20 mg/ 250 mL	80	mcg/mL		
	Ordered mcg/min ÷ mcg/mL × 60 min/h =									___	mL/h
Primacor	0.05 mg/kg = 8.2 mg				Give load over 10 min		40 mg/ 200 mL	0.2	mg/mL		
	mg to give ÷ mg/mL =	41 mL				41	mL × (60 min/h ÷ 10 min) =			246	mL/h × 10 min
	Infusion			0.02		0.5 mcg/ kg/min	40 mg/ 200 mL	200	mcg/mL	___	
	Take dose you want in mcg ÷ by drug index number = mL/h on pump										
Trimethaphan	Infusion			—		0.3–6 mg/min	500 mg/ 500 mL	1	mg/mL	___	
	Ordered mg/min ÷ mg/mL × 60 min/h =									___	mL/h
Vasopressin		0.02 u/min = 3 mL/h 0.04 u/min = 6 mL/h					40 u/ 100 mL	400	u/mL		

165   kg

DRUG	ORDERED AMOUNT	TOTAL DOSE TO GIVE	DRUG INDEX NUMBER	DIRECTIONS	INFUSION RANGE	DRUG MIXTURE	AMOUNT	DRUG/ mL	RUN AT	mL/h
Aminophylline	5 mg/kg =	825 mg		Give mg/kg load over 20 min		500 mg/ 250 mL	2 mg/mL		
	mg to give ÷ mg/mL =	413 mL					413 mL × (60 min/h ÷ 20 min) =			__1238__	mL/h × 20 min
	Infusion				0.5–1 mg/kg/h	500 mg/ 250 mL	2 mg/mL		
					mg dose ordered × kg ÷ mg/mL =			___ mL/h
Amiodarone	Loading dose			Load **150 mg** over 10 min		900 mg/ 500 mL	1.8 mg/mL	__
				Ordered mg load dose (150 mg) ÷ mg/mL (1.8 mg/mL) = 83 mL to give × (60 min/h ÷ 10 min) = mL/h to set on pump				__500__	mL/h × 83 mL
	Infusion			Run at **1 mg/ min × 6 h**		900 mg/ 500 mL	1.8 mg/mL	
				Ordered mg dose (1 mg/min) ÷ mg/mL (1.8 mg/mL) = _____ × 60 min/h = mL/h to set on pump				__33__	mL/h × 6 h
	Infusion			Run at **0.5 mg/ min × 18 h**		900 mg/ 500 mL	1.8 mg/mL	
				Ordered mg dose (0.5 mg/min) ÷ mg/mL (1.8 mg/mL) = _____ × 60 min/h = mL/h to set on pump				__17__	mL/h × 18 h
Amrinone	0.75 mg/kg =	123.75 mg		Give mg/kg load over 10 min		300 mg/ 120 mL	2.5 mg/mL	__
	mg to give ÷ mg/mL =	50 mL					49.5 mL × (60 min/h ÷ 10 min) =			__297__	mL/h × 10 min
	Infusion		0.25		5–10 mcg/ kg/min	300 mg/ 120 mL	2500 mcg/mL	__
				Take dose you want in mcg ÷ by drug index number = mL/h on pump					___
Brevibloc	Infusion		1.01		50–100 mcg/ kg/min	2.5 g/ 250 mL	10,000 mcg/mL	___ mL/h
				Take dose you want in mcg ÷ by drug index number = mL/h on pump
Cardene	Infusion		—		0.5–10 mg/h	25 mg 250 mL	0.1 mg/mL	__
				Ordered mg dose ÷ mg/mL = mL/h to set on pump					___ mL/h
Cardizem	0.25 mg/kg =	41.25 mg		Give mg/kg load over 20 min		50 mg/ 100 mL	0.5 mg/mL	__
	mg to give ÷ mg/mL =	83 mL					82.5 mL × (60 min/h ÷ 20 min) =			__248__	mL/h
	0.35 mg/kg =	57.75 mg		May repeat loading dose in 15 min			0.5 mg/mL	
	mg to give ÷ mg/mL =	116 mL					115.5 mL × (60 min/h ÷ 20 min) =			__347__	mL/h
	Infusion				5–15 mg/h				__
				Ordered mg dose ÷ mg/mL = mL/h to set on pump					___ mL/h
Desmopressin	0.3 mcg/kg =	50 mcg		Give dose over 20–30 min			4 mcg/vial	
Dobutamine	Infusion		0.20		2.5–40 mcg/kg/ min	250 mg/ 125 mL	2000 mcg/mL	
				Take dose you want in mcg ÷ by drug index number = mL/h on pump

(continues)

165 kg (continued)

DRUG	ORDERED AMOUNT	TOTAL DOSE TO GIVE	DRUG INDEX NUMBER	DIRECTIONS	INFUSION RANGE	DRUG MIXTURE	AMOUNT	DRUG/mL	RUN AT	mL/h
Dopamine	Infusion		0.16		1–20 mcg/kg/min	400 mg/250 mL	1600	mcg/mL		
	Take dose you want in mcg ÷ by drug index number = mL/h on pump									
Epinephrine	Infusion	1 mcg/min = 4 mL/h 2 mcg/min = 8 mL/h 3 mcg/min = 11 mL/h 4 mcg/min = 15 mL/h			1–4 mcg/min	4 mg/250 mL	16	mcg/mL		
		Ordered mcg dose/min ÷ mcg/mL × 60 min/h =								___ mL/h
Fenoldapam	Infusion		0.0041		0.01–1.6 mcg/kg/min	10 mg/250 mL	40	mcg/mL		
	Take dose you want in mcg ÷ by drug index number = mL/h on pump									
Heparin	100 u/kg = 16,500 u 200 u/kg = 33,000 u 300 u/kg = 49,500 u 400 u/kg = 66,000 u									
Isoproterenol	Infusion				5 mcg/min	1 mg/250 mL	4	mcg/mL		
		Ordered mcg dose/min ÷ mcg/mL × 60 min/h =								75 mL/h
Lidocaine	Infusion	1 mg/min = 7.5 mL/h			1–4 mg/min	2 g/250 mL	8	mg/mL		—
		Ordered mg/min ÷ mg/mL × 60 min/h =								___ mL/h
Nitroglycerin	Infusion	3 mcg/min = 1 mL/h			3–200 mcg/min	50 mg/250 mL	200	mcg/mL		—
		Ordered mcg/min ÷ mcg/mL × 60 min/h =								___ mL/h
Nitroprusside	Infusion	6.7 mcg/min = 1 mL/h			5–300 mcg/min	100 mg/250 mL	400	mcg/mL		—
		Ordered mcg/min ÷ mcg/mL × 60 min/h =								___ mL/h
Norepinephrine	Infusion	1 mcg/min = 4 mL/h 2 mcg/min = 8 mL/h 3 mcg/min = 11 mL/h 4 mcg/min = 15 mL/h 5 mcg/min = 19 mL/h			2–20 mcg/min	4 mg/250 mL	16	mcg/mL		
		Ordered mcg dose/min ÷ mcg/mL × 60 min/h =								___ mL/h
Phenylephrine	Infusion	1.3 mcg/min = 1 mL/h			10–200 mcg/min	20 mg/250 mL	80	mcg/mL		
		Ordered mcg/min ÷ mcg/mL × 60 min/h =								___ mL/h
Primacor	0.05 mg/kg = 8.25 mg			Give load over 10 min		40 mg/200 mL	0.2	mg/mL		
	mg to give ÷ mg/mL = 41 mL				41	mL × (60 min/h ÷ 10 min) =			248	mL/h × 10 min
	Infusion		0.02		0.5 mcg/kg/min	40 mg/200 mL	200	mcg/mL		—
	Take dose you want in mcg ÷ by drug index number = mL/h on pump									
Trimethaphan	Infusion		—		0.3–6 mg/min	500 mg/500 mL	1	mg/mL		—
		Ordered mg/min ÷ mg/mL × 60 min/h =								___ mL/h
Vasopressin		0.02 u/min = 3 mL/h 0.04 u/min = 6 mL/h				40 u/100 mL	400	u/mL		

Neurovascular Surgery

5

NEUROSURGERY PEARLS

- A preoperative neurologic exam should be done and documented before neurosurgery; especially document *preexisting* deficits and symptoms. Use the Glasgow Coma Scale, do a cranial nerve assessment, note weakness in any extremity, and assess for history of seizures.
- Patients who have been on antiseizure medications or pain medications will be "enzyme induced," meaning their liver CYP 450 system will usually metabolize drugs much faster; be prepared to dose muscle relaxants, narcotics, and other drugs more frequently.
- Check an ABG as soon as possible after induction and intubation to assess the gradient between the $ETCO_2$ and the $PaCO_2$. Guide your ventilation rate based on this information and the surgeon preference for $PaCO_2$.
- Have good IV access in all neurosurgical patients, either peripherally or centrally, to deliver fluids or blood products as needed.
- An arterial line is necessary in most neurosurgical cases.
- Do not use succinylcholine (Anectine) in any patient with increased ICP or increased CBF.

POSTOPERATIVE NAUSEA AND VOMITING

Risk of postoperative nausea and vomiting (PONV) is increased with the following factors:

- Female
- Motion sickness history
- Pediatrics: 6–10 years of age (34% PONV occurrence)
- Pediatrics: 11–14 years of age (35–50% PONV occurrence)
- Nonsmoker
- Anxiety
- Surgery length greater than 45–60 minutes

Surgery Type

- Breast
- Abdominal: endoscopy and laparotomy
- ENT
- Ophthalmic
- *Neurologic*
- Gynecologic

TWO DISEASES COMMONLY ASSOCIATED WITH NEUROSURGERY

Diabetes Insipidus

Several different types of diabetes insipidus (DI) exist, each with a different cause. One common type is associated with patients who have pituitary disease, tumor, or trauma. Called central DI, it is caused by pituitary dysfunction and a deficiency of vasopressin (antidiuretic hormone [ADH]). Signs include the excretion of large amounts of extremely dilute urine, very low urine osmolarity, and high serum sodium. Treatment consists of volume resuscitation, and vasopressin (40 units mixed in 100 mL 0.9% normal saline = 0.4 unit/mL) or DDAVP.

- Vasopressin (ADH): Pitressin
- DDAVP: synthetic desmopressin

Syndrome of Inappropriate Antidiuretic Hormone

Syndrome of inappropriate antidiuretic hormone (SIADH) occurs in patients with central nervous system injury or disease and is characterized by excessive release of antidiuretic hormone from the pituitary gland or other source (vasopressin). Signs include fluid overload and low serum sodium levels. Treatment consists of fluid restriction, sodium loading, and fixing the cause.

BRAIN AND SPINAL CORD ANATOMY BASICS

Brain weight is approximately 1350 to 1500 grams.

Cardiac output to the brain amounts to 15% to 20% of the total cardiac output (750 mL/min).

The brain utilizes 20% of the total body oxygen. The cerebral rate of oxygen consumption ($CMRO_2$) is 3.5 mL per 100 g brain tissue per minute.

The cerebral metabolic rate of glucose consumption (CMRGI) is 5 mg per 100 g brain tissue per minute; this is the basal requirement.

The brain's metabolic demands must be met by adequate delivery of oxygen and glucose. Regular insulin and glucose IV infusions should be titrated to maintain the patient at a normoglycemic level. Hyperglycemia, in the presence of hypoxia, will increase intracellular acidosis. Insulin has a protective effect on ischemic brain tissue by stimulating the sodium–potassium adenosine triphosphatase pump, protecting cell mitochondria, and modulating synaptic transmission between neurons.

Normal CBF is 50 mL per 100 g brain tissue per minute.

- If CBF falls below 20 mL per 100 g brain tissue per minute, it may cause flattened EEG and is associated with cerebral impairment.
- If CBF falls below 6 mL per 100 g brain tissue per minute, it may lead to irreversible damage.

The circle of Willis supplies blood flow to the brain (Figure 5-1):

- 80% supplied by the anterior circulation (internal carotid arteries)
- 20% supplied by the posterior circulation (vertebral arteries)

The circle of Willis allows blood to enter by either internal carotid or vertebral arteries and to be distributed to any part of both cerebral hemispheres. Multiple small branches all arise from the circle and supply the brain parenchyma.

Anterior vessels feed the following structures:

- ACA: midline cerebrum, corpus callosum, and the medial aspect of frontal and parietal lobes
- MCA: lateral surface frontal/parietal/temporal lobes

Posterior vessels feed the following structures through the basilar artery:

- Medulla, brain stem, pons, cerebellum, all occipital lobe, and part of parietal and temporal lobes

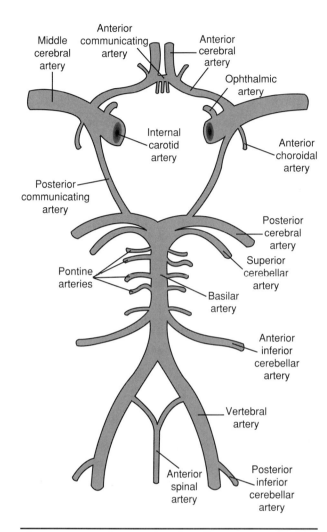

Figure 5-1 *The Circle of Willis*

Dermatomes

Anterior

C4: clavicle

T4–5: nipples

T6–8: xiphoid process

T8: lower ribcage

T10: umbilicus

L1: inguinal ligament

L2–3: knee and below

S2–5: perineal

Posterior

C7: most prominent cervical spinous process

T7: inferior scapular border

L4: superior iliac crest

S2: posterior superior iliac spine

Other

C3–5: supply the diaphragm

C5: supplies the shoulder muscles and the muscle that flex the elbow

C6: extends the wrist back

C7: straightens the elbow

C8: bends the fingers

T1: spreads the fingers

T1–12: supply the chest wall and abdominal muscles

L2: bends the hip

L3: straightens the knee

L4: pulls the foot up

L5: wiggles the toes

S1: pulls the foot down

S3–5: supply the bladder, bowel, and genitals

VENTRICULAR SYSTEM AND CEREBROSPINAL FLUID

The ventricular system is composed of four cavities called ventricles that contain cerebrospinal fluid (CSF). The ventricular system is considered a "communicating system" within the brain.

Intracranial pressure (ICP) is the pressure in the cranium. It results from the presence of the brain tissue, the CSF, and the blood volume in the intracranial blood vessels. ICP is maintained in the normal range through the production and absorption of CSF.

The intracranial compartment can adapt only to a point (contained within a fixed compartment of the skull). When compensatory mechanisms become exhausted, any volume increase in brain tissue (e.g., from an aneurysm, tumor, intracerebral bleed, edema) and/or CSF or intracranial blood vessels will cause the ICP to increase. When the compensatory mechanisms become strained, even a small increase in cerebral blood flow will markedly increase ICP. This can lead to ischemia and then to potential herniation of the brain tissues.

Monroe-Kelly Hypothesis

The Monroe-Kelly hypothesis focuses on the pressure–volume relationship between the CSF, blood, and brain tissue. It states that an increase in the volume of any one of the intracranial contents must be compensated by a decrease in the volume of another. The cranium has three types of intracranial contents:

- Blood (4% of total contents)
- CSF (10%)
- Brain (86%)

The main buffers for any increased volumes in the intracranial vault are (1) a decrease in blood flow (venous) and then, (2) the CSF. If pressure continues to increase, (3) the arterial flow is affected, and last (4) the brain tissue becomes compressed.

Intracranial Pressure

ICP is the supratentorial CSF and brain pressure. The patient must have an intact bony cranium if this pressure is to be measured. The normal range for ICP is 5–15 mm Hg.

Increased ICP

- ICP > 20–25 mm Hg (20 mm Hg can be considered the extreme upper limit of normal ICP): considered an elevated ICP and causes loss of pressure autoregulation.
- ICP levels: sustained > 25–30 mm Hg. These levels are associated with severe neurologic injury and poor outcomes. When ICP is >

30 mm Hg, cerebral blood flow decreases causing ischemia. Ischemia causes brain edema, which further increases the ICP.
- Intracranial hypertension: sustained ICP > 40 mm Hg.
- ICP can be decreased by modulating any of the components within the intracranial compartment (blood, CSF, or brain), or by surgical or pharmacologic techniques. See Chapter 3 for more information.

Increased ICP is associated with the following signs and symptoms in an awake patient: level of consciousness (LOC) changes, blurred or double vision, nausea/vomiting, unilateral pupil dilation, papilledema (optic disc swelling), seizures, and uncoordinated, clumsy movement. Headache and vomiting most frequently occur just after the person wakes up, but decrease during the day.

Signs and symptoms of increased ICP in an anesthetized patient include the following: unilateral papillary dilation, absent brain stem reflexes, decorticate or decerebrate posturing, and Cushing's triad (hypertension, bradycardia, and irregular respirations). Cushing's triad occurs if ICP increases significantly enough to herniate the brain stem. When ICP increases until it is equivalent to arterial pressure, the Cushing reflex acts to elevate blood pressure above ICP.

Risk Factors for ICP Elevation

- *Ischemia:* Can be focal or global. Global changes can cause focal ischemia. Regional ICP symptoms may have a one-sided deviation.
- *Herniation:*

1. Classic: supratentorial pressure gradient causing net movement of structures through the foramen magnum.
2. Transcalvarial: brain tissue extrusion via an opening in the cranial vault.
3. Cingulate: cingulate gyrus herniates over the falx cerebri (arched fold of dura mater which descends vertically between cerebral hemispheres).

4. Uncal: the uncus of the temporal lobe herniates through the incisura of the tentorium cerebelli (an extension of the dura mater; separates the cerebellum from the occipital lobe of the brain).

Cerebrospinal Fluid

Normal values of CSF are as follows:

- pH: 7.3
- pCO_2: 51 mm Hg; metabolically active
- Specific gravity: 1.003–1.008; no blood, no cells, normally looks like water
- Electrolytes:

  Increased: sodium, chloride, and magnesium

  Decreased: potassium, calcium, bicarbonate, and glucose. Calcium is a mediator of ischemic events in the neurological system.

- Pressure: 80–180 mm H_2O

In terms of volume, CSF flow is estimated as follows: 0.35 mL/min = 21 ml/h = 500 mL produced every 24 hours. The static volume of CSF is 120–150 mL (4 oz) in the central nervous system. This volume takes approximately 8 hours to replenish.

CSF is formed in the choroid plexus inside all four ventricles, with 95% being produced in the lateral ventricles. This fluid is formed by active secretion and provides protection, support, nutrition, and chemical regulation for the brain and spinal cord. Its normal composition presupposes an intact blood–brain barrier (BBB).

CSF circulates from the lateral ventricles through interventricular foramen (foramen of Monro) to the third ventricle and, via the aqueduct of Sylvius, to the fourth ventricle (Figure 5-2).

Two lateral ventricles
Largest ventricles of the four;
one lies in each cerebral hemisphere

Aqueduct of Monroe to third ventricle

Third ventricle
Lies in midline between two lateral ventricles;
lies beneath the corpus callosum
and surrounds the thalamus

Aqueduct of Sylvius to fourth ventricle

Fourth ventricle (cerebellum)
Lies in posterior fossa between the inferior brain stem
and the cerebellum; communicates with the subarachnoid
space of the brain and cord

Foramen of Luschka: two lateral apertures
Foramen of Magendie: one median aperture

Cisterna magna, then to the subarachnoid space, arachnoid
villi, and venous sinus

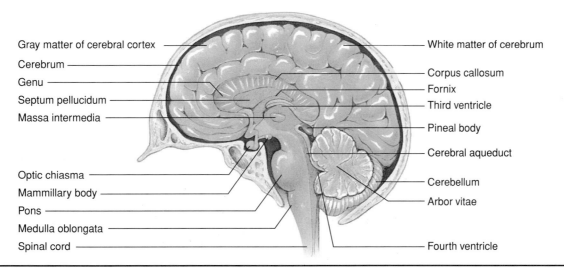

Figure 5-2　*Ventricles of Brain and Interconnections–Lateral View*
Source: Donnersberger, 2010.

It also passes downward to the subarachnoid space, which surrounds the brain and the spinal cord. See Figure 5-3.

Most of the CSF is absorbed via the arachnoid villi (primarily in the superior sagittal sinus) and gradually reabsorbed into veins. Normally, CSF is absorbed as rapidly as it is formed. This process is affected by hydrostatic gradients, so an increased ICP will cause increased absorption.

As a general rule, ICP increases slowly in the presence of a tumor, but more rapidly when bleeding is the cause of the regulation/circulation problems. Symptoms of ICP with growing masses tend to occur after compensatory mechanisms are exhausted. Arterial bleeds are usually from epidural arteries, in which case ICP rises quickly. Venous bleeds are usually subdural, in which case the bleed is usually slow and ICP rises slowly.

The Blood–Brain Barrier

The blood–brain barrier (BBB) refers to a physiologic mechanism that alters the permeability of the cerebral vasculature capillary bed. The cerebral vascular endothelial cells have very tight junctions that limit or allow particles to cross based on their size, ionic charge, degree of protein binding, and lipid solubility in blood. Ionized and large molecules cannot pass through this barrier (i.e., they require facilitated diffusion), while fat-soluble molecules can easily cross (by passive diffusion) the BBB.

Conditions causing alterations in the BBB are closely related to conditions that alter CBF and MAP: dilutional hyponatremia, an acute hypertensive event (affecting autoregulation), high-dose volatile agents, hypercarbia, cerebrovascular vasodilation, tumors, intracerebral bleeding, trauma, infection, hypoxia, or sustained seizure activity. Disease states such as epilepsy, meningitis, multiple sclerosis, and HIV encephalitis can cause BBB disruption. When the BBB is disrupted, fluid movement becomes dependent on hydrostatic pressures instead of osmotic gradients.

Brain Edema and Swelling

Brain edema and swelling may result from four causes:

- Vasogenic: The BBB is disrupted, the junctions are no longer tight, and there is protein

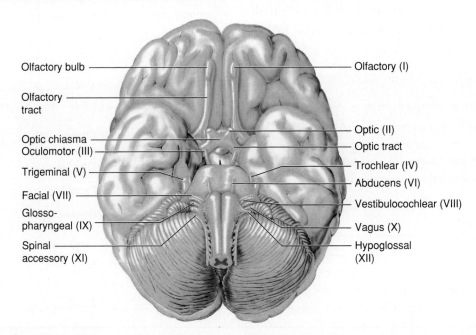

Figure 5-3   *The Cranial Nerves*
Source: Donnersberger, 2010.

movement across the BBB barrier. Vasogenic causes include tumors, hypertension, trauma, and infarctions.

- Cytotoxic: The BBB remains intact. There is an extracellular to intracellular fluid shift. This outcome may occur with pseudo-tumor cerebri, hypoxia, ischemia, and water intoxication (in which there is an acute decrease in osmolality).

- Interstitial: CSF breaks out into the white matter (obstructive hydrocephalus).
- Hyperemic: Vascular volume increases suddenly.

CRANIAL NERVES

Cranial nerves (CN) originate in the base of the brain. They exit from the cranial cavity through various openings in the skull.

CN NUMBER	NAME	ORIGIN	EXIT FROM SKULL	FUNCTION
I	Olfactory	Within the cerebrum, in extensions called olfactory bulbs	Through the cribiform plate of ethmoid bone; terminate in olfactory bulb	Sensory: smell
II	Optic	Ganglion cell in retina	Optic foramen	Sensory: vision; visual acuity and visual fields, circuit for light reflexes
III	Oculomotor	Midbrain	Between the cerebral peduncles	Motor: constriction, movement of eye up, in, and down, elevation of the upper eyelid
IV	Trochlear	Midbrain	Superior orbital fissure	Motor: movement of the eye
V	Trigeminal: sensory has 3 branches, motor has 1 branch	Lateral aspect of pons		Both motor and sensory
	Ophthalmic branch (V$_1$)	Semilunar ganglion	Superior orbital fissure	Sensory: cornea reflex, upper eyelid, nasal, side of nose, forehead, front of scalp
	Maxillary branch (V$_2$)	Semilunar ganglion	Foramen rotundum	Sensory: nose, palate, oral cavity; upper teeth, cheek, lower eyelid

(continues)

CN NUMBER	NAME	ORIGIN	EXIT FROM SKULL	FUNCTION
	Mandibular branch (V_3)	Semilunar ganglion	Foramen ovale	Motor: muscle of mastication (chewing) Sensory: skin over mandible, anterior two-thirds of tongue, floor of mouth
VI	Abducens	Lower margin of pons	Superior orbital fissure	Motor: move eyes laterally
VII	Facial: temporal branch; zygomatic branch; buccal branch; mandibular branch; cervical branch	Lower margin of pons	Through temporal bone to stylomastoid foramen	Motor: muscles of facial expression; close lid, raise and wrinkle brow, smile, puff cheeks Sensory: taste, anterior two-thirds of tongue Parasympathetic: lacrimal, crying, submandibular and sublingual salivary glands (all glands of head except parotid)
VIII	Acoustic			Sensory
	Vestibular (balance)	Lower border of pons	Internal auditory meatus	Sensory: equilibrium
	Cochlear (auditory)	Lower border of pons	Internal auditory meatus	Sensory: hearing; coordinate head and eye movement
IX	Glossopharyngeal	Medulla oblongata	Jugular foramen	Motor: speak, gag, swallowing. Sensory: taste in posterior one-third of tongue; pharynx, tonsils; branch of carotid sinus and carotid body; gag reflex Parasympathetic: parotid gland
X	Vagus	Medulla oblongata	Jugular foramen into the chest and abdomen	Sensory: external meatus, pharynx, larynx, aortic sinus, and

CN NUMBER	NAME	ORIGIN	EXIT FROM SKULL	FUNCTION
				thoracic and abdominal viscera; baro/chemoreceptors Motor: pharynx and larynx, talk/ swallow, lift palate Parasympathetic: thoracic and abdominal viscera (heart, lungs, GI canal)
XI	Spinal accessory (have both cranial and spinal branches)	Medulla oblongata	Jugular foramen	Spinal branch: descends into the neck and supplies motor fibers to the trapezius and sternocleidomastoid muscles, turn and tilt head back, lift shoulders Cranial branch: joins the vagus and carries impulses to the muscles of pharynx and larynx for swallowing and phonation
XII	Hypoglossal	Anterior lateral sulcus on the medulla oblongata	Hypoglossal canal of the tongue	Motor: muscles of (moves) tongue; stick out and push in both sides of cheek; for speaking, chewing, and swallowing

Reflexes

Cranial nerves V–X: trigeminal to vagus
Vagal response (slows heart rate) to traction on extraocular muscle

Cranial nerves IX–X: glossopharyngeal to vagus
Carotid sinus afferent (MAP at least 60 mm Hg or greater) slows heart rate

Cranial nerves X–X: vagus to vagus
Aortic arch afferent (MAP of at least 90 mm Hg or greater): slows heart rate

Baroreceptors

Baroreceptors for low pressure are primarily located at the junction of the vena cava and the right atrium, in the right atrium, and in the pulmonary blood vessels. Baroreceptors for high pressure (arterial) are primarily located in the arch of the aorta and the carotid sinus. These receptors lower the heart rate by affecting the vagal/peripheral vascular tone through sympathetic outflow.

Chemoreceptors: Carotid/Aortic Bodies

Decreased oxygen and increased CO_2 (H^+) excite the vasomotor center. The body responds strongly with an increased heart rate after the blood pressure falls below 80 mm Hg, and breathing is stimulated when the PaO_2 is less than 60 mm Hg.

Atrial/Pulmonary Artery Reflexes

Low pressure stimulates stretch receptors

High pressure stimulates atrial volume receptors

Bainbridge reflex: increased volume causes an increased heart rate

Atrial natriuretic peptide (ANP): powerful vasodilator released by the cells in the atria in response to high blood pressure. ANP acts to reduce the water and sodium (salt) loss, thereby decreasing blood pressure.

Increased volume: afferent arterial dilation of kidney

Hypothalamus: decreases secretion of ADH

Cushing Response

In the Cushing response, increased blood pressure can cause bradycardia. This response may be seen when epinephrine is infiltrated (with a local anesthetic) and a portion enters the blood supply. The bradycardia may become evident first (before the blood pressure cuff can cycle), so the anesthetist can anticipate that the blood pressure will be high.

SNS/PNS Vascular "Tone"

The sympathetic nervous system (SNS) and peripheral nervous system (PNS) affect the basal rates of cardiac activity. Vascular tone is maintained by epinephrine and norepinephrine secretion.

Central Nervous System Control of Heart Rate

Cardio-accelerator function is controlled by the SNS: T1–T4 increases the heart rate by exciting sympathetic neurons to the heart. A neuraxial block at T5 will block out all vascular tone.

Cardio-inhibitory function is controlled by the PNS: CN-10 decreases the heart rate by exciting PNS neurons. This system may produce a profound decrease in heart rate, possibly including asystole.

VASOMOTOR CENTER

Vasoconstriction of the body's vessels is controlled by the medulla (the lower one-third of the pons) and T5–LI (which control venous and arterial tone throughout body and SNS) (Figure 5-4). Vasodilation of the body's vessels is controlled by the lower medulla, which inhibits constriction, thereby causing vasodilation. The sensory area, posterior medulla, and pons all receive CN IX/X signals.

Cerebral Perfusion Pressure

Cerebral perfusion pressure (CPP) measures the amount of blood flow to the brain and is calculated as follows: CPP = MAP − ICP (CVP). *If CVP is used instead of ICP in this equation, it means there is an assumption that there is no obstruction to CSF flow.*

Cerebral perfusion pressure has the following effects on an EEG:

- Normal CPP: 80–90 mm Hg
- CPP < 60 mm Hg: undesirable

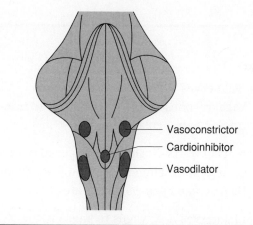

Vasoconstrictor
Cardioinhibitor
Vasodilator

Figure 5-4 *The Vasomotor Center (VMR)*

- CPP = 50 mm Hg: EEG slows
- CPP = 25–40 mm Hg: EEG flattens
- CPP < 20 mm Hg: irreversible damage in normothermic brain

Changes in either MAP or ICP will affect CPP. That is, if MAP remains constant and ICP increases, CPP decreases.

$$MAP = SBP + 2(DBP) \div 3$$

Remember this equation by the "1-2-3 formula": 1 SBP plus 2 DBP, divided by 3.

The MAP goal is 80–100 mm Hg. If MAP is greater than 150 mm Hg, there is autoregulatory breakthrough: The BBB becomes disrupted, causing cerebral edema. (The BBB refers to the cerebrovasculature capillary bed.)

CPP example: MAP 60 − ICP 15 = CPP 45. MAP < 60 mm Hg is undesirable; at MAP < 50, the EEG is slowing.

Transmural Pressure

Transmural pressure (TMP) is calculated as follows:

TMP = MAP − surrounding tissue pressure (ICP)

This is the same formula used to calculate the CPP. *TMP example:* MAP 60 − ICP of 15 = TMP 45.

The TMP calculation is used for aneurysms and determines the amount of pressure across the wall of the aneurysm. The greater the transmural pressure, the more likely the aneurysm is to rupture.

It is very important with aneurysms to keep the pressure gradient tightly controlled with little to no variability. For example, if the ICP decreases, the TMP increases. Similarly, if the MAP increases without a similar rise in ICP, the TMP will also rise, creating a greater likelihood of aneurysm rupture; in this scenario, it would be necessary to lower the MAP accordingly. When placing cranial pins, the MAP is likely to rise if adequate sedation is not achieved. Pentothal or another agent (e.g., propofol, esmolol [Brevibloc]) may be necessary to maintain MAP within an adequate range.

CPP is dependent on MAP when the dura is open.

Cerebral Blood Flow Determinants

See Chapter 3 for more information on altering cerebral blood flow.

Cerebral blood flow (CBF) is determined by three factors:

- I: pressure autoregulation (MAP between 70 and 150 mm Hg)
- II: cerebral oxygen-metabolism flow coupling (CBF and $CMRO_2$)
- III: CO_2 responsiveness (constrict or dilate cerebral vessels)

I: Pressure Autoregulation

Autoregulation refers to the capacity of the cerebral circulation to adjust its resistance to maintain CBF constant over a wide range of the MAP (i.e., between 70 and 150 mm Hg). A mean arterial pressure above or below these values causes the CBF to be pressure dependent disrupting the BBB, making the CBF linearly proportional to the CPP.

Patients who have shifted to the right (e.g., a chronically hypertensive patient in whom autoregulation occurs at higher MAP range) have adapted to higher pressures and will not tolerate hypotension.

Loss of pressure autoregulation may result from the following causes:

- Hypoxia
- Ischemia
- Hypercapnia/hypercarbia
- Trauma
- High-dose volatile agents
- Dilutional hyponatremia
- Acute hypertensive events
- Acute hypotensive events
- Surgery
- Cerebrovascular vasodilation
- Inadvertent dural puncture
- Tumors
- Bleeding into brain tissue

II: Cerebral Oxygen-Metabolism Flow Coupling (CBF and CMRO$_2$)

The goal in neuroanesthesia is to preserve flow coupling:

$$\downarrow CBF = \downarrow CBV = \downarrow ICP = \downarrow CMRO_2$$

CBV control is the most important measure to control ICP elevation.

When CBF and CMRO$_2$ are not matched, the situation is called *uncoupling*. In *unacceptable uncoupling*, cerebral blood flow is less than metabolism. In *acceptable uncoupling*, increased cerebral blood flow is greater than metabolism.

In *luxury perfusion*, supply is greater than demand; thus there is increased CBF with a decreased CMRO$_2$. In a "normal" brain (one that is not hypoxic), this state of luxury perfusion may be desirable, especially during induced hypotension. However, during periods of cerebral ischemia, a circulatory "steal phenomenon" can occur, in which blood flow is increased in normal areas of the brain but not in ischemic areas. In such a case, there is actually a blood flow redistribution away from ischemic areas to normal areas. Volatile agents can create these two states: luxury perfusion in a non-hypoxic brain (not a problem) and the steal phenomenon in a hypoxic brain (a problem).

$$\uparrow CBF = \downarrow CMRO_2: \text{ uncoupled but a "good"}$$
$$\text{uncoupled (luxury perfusion)}$$

Barbiturates also affect CBF and CMRO$_2$, in that both are decreased by use of these medications. In this instance, when barbiturates are given, the CMRO$_2$ is decreased slightly more than CBF, so that metabolic supply exceeds metabolic demand. Barbiturates vasoconstrict cerebral vessels in normal brain areas so that blood flow then becomes redistributed to ischemic areas of the brain. This is called "reverse steal phenomenon" or the "Robin Hood effect" (steal from the rich and give to the poor):

$$\downarrow CBF = \downarrow CMRO_2$$

Factors That Increase Cerebral Blood Flow

Fevers

Decreased hematocrit

Increased PaCO$_2$ (vasodilates): normal vessels dilate but vessels in damaged area don't, leading to intracerebral steal phenomenon

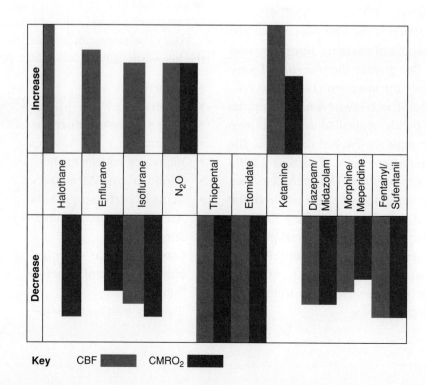

Key   CBF �   CMRO$_2$ ▮

$PaO_2 < 60$ mm Hg

Volatile anesthetics

Ketamine

Vasodilators

Intravenous fluid

Factors That Decrease Cerebral Blood Flow

Hypothermia

Increased hematocrit

Decreased $PaCO_2$ (vasoconstricts): blood diverted to ischemic area

MAP < 70 mm Hg

Barbiturates

Etomidate

Propofol

Benzodiazepines

Lidocaine

III: CO_2 Responsiveness

Increases in $PaCO_2$ lead to dilation of vessels, which increases CBF. Carbon dioxide crosses the BBB without limitation. Thus, when $PaCO_2$ levels are low, pre-capillary areas constrict decreasing flow, thereby decreasing ICP. When $PaCO_2$ levels are elevated, CBF is increased.

A PaO_2 less than 60 mm Hg dilates vessels, which in turn increases CBF.

The vessels dilate with increases in $PaCO_2$ (hypercarbia) or low pH (acidosis) and with decreases in PaO_2 (hypoxia).

CO_2 and flow relationships linear and directly proportional with $PaCO_2$ tensions between 20–80 mm Hg. A patient with a normal CBF has a $PaCO_2$ of 40 mm Hg.

CBF changes ~1–2 mL/100 g brain tissue/min per 1 mm Hg change in $PaCO_2$. Transient effect; CBF and ICP can be acutely decreased when hyperventilating to a lower $PaCO_2$; usually only lasts 6–10 hours.

GLASGOW COMA SCALE

The Glasgow Coma Scale (GCS) measure three factors: eye opening (on a scale of 1–4), motor response (1–6), and verbal response (1–5).

GOALS IN NEUROANESTHESIA

1. Preserve neurons.
2. Preserve flow coupling between CBF and $CMRO_2$.
3. Decrease intracerebral volume by relaxing the brain to provide a better working environment for the surgeon and lower the ICP.

The Glasgow Coma Scale

EYE OPENING		MOTOR RESPONSE		VERBAL RESPONSE	
Spontaneous	4	To verbal command	6	Oriented, converses	5
To speech	3	To pain: localizes	5	Disoriented, converses	4
To pain	2	Flexion withdrawal	4	Inappropriate words	3
No response	1	Flexion abnormal	3	Makes sounds only	2
		Extension	2	No response	1
		No response	1		

Note: Brain injury, mild: 13–15 points
Brain injury, moderate: 9–12 points
Brain injury, severe: < 8 points

4. Decrease brain oxygen consumption ($CMRO_2$).
5. Maintain optimal/normal CPP, but have the ability to reduce CPP rapidly if needed.
6. Avoid abrupt changes in ICP, especially elevations.
7. Avoid seizure activity; seizures increase $CMRO_2$ severely.
8. Provide adequate tissue perfusion to brain and spinal cord so that regional metabolic demand is met.
9. Have a quick and clear wake-up for neurological status assessment.
10. Maintain normal cerebral vasculature response to CO_2.

See Chapter 3 for more information.

Anesthetists must anticipate blood pressure swings and be ready to treat them. Hypertension occurs especially during times of maximum stimulation:

- Laryngoscopy or intubation
- Head pinning
- Skin incision
- When muscle is reflected from the cranium
- When raising a bone flap
- During dural incision

Have propofol 20 mL (200 mg) drawn up and ready to give to the patient during times of high stimulation.

It is rare to see hypertension due to pain when the surgeon is actually working in the brain, as there are no pain receptors in this organ.

Preoperative Measures

Preoperative sedation may be necessary to calm the patient; small doses of a benzodiazepine may be used and are preferred over opiates (which depress respirations). However, the patient should not be allowed to hypoventilate (which increases $PaCO_2$ and vasodilates cerebral arteries, thereby increasing ICP) or receive sedation amounts that affect the neurologic evaluation.

Ideal Induction

It is of crucial importance to keep the ICP and blood pressures as close to normal as possible during induction. Maintaining these values within the patient's normal range can help to prevent an increase in ICP or blood pressure with accompanying stress to the brain.

Induction of anesthesia is best done with drugs that decrease ICP by decreasing $CMRO_2$, CBV, and CBF.

Intraoperative Measures

Be prepared for the possibility of bleeding, either through surgical loss or vascular wall interruption, in any neurosurgical operation. Know the patient's blood bank status (Type and cross or type and screen blood samples received? How many units of blood are available?).

Anesthetic drugs and/or techniques, if improperly used, can worsen an existing intracranial pathology and may produce new damage.

Ideal Maintenance

Ideally, maintenance anesthesia decreases ICP and $CMRO_2$, maintains cerebral regulation, and provides protection from focal ischemia. Muscle relaxants may be required but should not be given if neurophysiologic monitoring is done. Check with surgeon before giving these agents.

Isoflurane in often recommended as the volatile agent of choice for patients with cerebral ischemia. It maintains CBF and reduces $CMRO_2$; thus it can help to protect the brain.

Ideal Emergence

The ability to wake the patient in the immediate postoperative period is essential in neuroanesthesia, whether intracranial or spinal surgery is being performed. It is important to be able to assess the patient's neurologic status as soon as possible after the surgery is completed.

Anesthetic Effects on $CMRO_2$, CBF, CBV, and ICP

Sedation

When sedation is used, watch for hypoventilation: increases in carbon dioxide will increase ICP. Benzodiazepines lower CBF, albeit to a lesser extent than other agents.

IV Anesthetics

Anesthetics that are administered intravenously decrease both $CMRO_2$ and CBF (except ketamine).

- Thiopental (barbiturate) 2–5 mg/kg: decreases CBF, $CMRO_2$, and ICP; potent cerebral vasoconstrictor.
- Propofol 1–3 mg/kg: decreases CBF, $CMRO_2$, and ICP; decreases MAP, which decreases cerebral perfusion pressure); potent cerebral vasoconstrictor.
- Etomidate 0.1–0.4 mg/kg: decreases CBF, $CMRO_2$, and ICP; increases EEG activity; potent cerebral vasoconstrictor.
- Ketamine: generally *increases* $CMRO_2$ and CBF by dilating cerebral vasculature. However, if $PaCO_2$ is *maintain*ed within normal limits in the presence of elevated ICP or cerebral trauma, then ketamine does not adversely alter CBF or ICP.

With the exception of ketamine, all intravenous agents either have little effect or reduce cerebral blood flow.

Opioids

Opioids progressively decrease CBF and $CMRO_2$. They depress respirations, which can increase $PaCO_2$, which in turn increase CBF and ICP.

- Low-dose fentanyl 2–5 mcg/kg
- Sufentanil or alfentanil
- Remifentanil 2–5 mcg/kg, IV, 1–2 minutes before laryngoscopy to help prevent hypertension
- Remifentanil (Ultiva) drip (See Chapter 4 for more information.)

Local Anesthetics

Local anesthetics such as Lidocaine decrease CBF and $CMRO_2$.

Volatile Anesthetics

Volatile anesthetics dilate cerebral vessels (increase CBF) and impair autoregulation in a dose-dependent manner. A MAC greater than 0.6 causes CBF to increase owing to cerebral artery dilation. $CMRO_2$ is decreased with volatile agents.

- Isoflurane is considered the best choice of volatile agent in neurologic procedures, as it maintains CBF and reduces $CMRO_2$.
- CBF can significantly increase with halothane; more than 1 MAC nearly abolishes autoregulation. The relationship can be summarized as follows: halothane $>>$ enflurane $>$ isoflurane $=$ sevoflurane $=$ desflurane; all of these agents increase CBF and decrease $CMRO_2$ (except nitrous oxide)
- Enflurane and isoflurane decrease $CMRO_2$ to the greatest extent.
- Nitrous oxide increases CBF and $CMRO_2$; however, minimal change occurs when this agent is given with other volatile agents.

Hyperventilation can be used to abate the effects of inhalational agents because volatile agents do not abolish CO_2 reactivity completely.

Vasodilators

Vasodilators dilate vessels and may increase CBF in dose-dependent manner. They include nicardipine (Cardene), sodium nitroprusside (SNP), hydralazine (Apresoline), adenosine, and calcium-channel blockers.

Vasoconstrictors

Vasoconstrictors have minimal effects on CBF, within the normal limits of autoregulation.

Depolarizing Muscle Relaxants

Succinylcholine (Anectine) can release histamine. It may be used safely, but a defasiculating dose of a nondepolarizing muscle relaxant (NDMR) should be given first.

Nondepolarizing Muscle Relaxants

NDMRs may not directly affect CBF, but may have important secondary effects (such as histamine-mediated vasodilation) that may increase ICP. Muscle relaxants that *do not* release histamine include vecuronium and cisatricurium. Muscle relaxants that *do* release histamine include rocuronium, atracurium, and pancuronium.

Other Agents

Precedex (Dexmedetomidine) is an alpha$_2$-adrenergic agonist IV drip that helps to maintain stable hemodynamics. See Chapter 10 for more information on this agent.

Anesthetics to Avoid in Patients with Neurological Conditions

Ketamine: increases CBF and increases *or* decreases CMRO$_2$ by dilating the cerebral vasculature

Nitrous oxide: neurotoxic; can increase ICP by increasing CBF and CMRO$_2$

Enflurane: has some positive effects, but also increases the possibility of seizures

Opioids: an increased dose decreases CBF and CMRO$_2$; can cause CO$_2$ to increase due to hypoventilation; can produce seizures

Muscle relaxants that release histamine: atracurium, rocuronium, pancuronium, succinylcholine

Vasoactive Drugs Used in Neurologic Anesthesia

Vasopressors will increase CBF only when MAP is less than 50–60 mm Hg or more than 150–160 mm Hg (assuming an intact BBB).

Vasodilators will induce cerebral vasodilation and, therefore, increase CBF in most cases. Nitroglycerin is one example of a vasodilator to avoid ine patients with neurological conditions.

IV Fluids in Neuroanesthesia

Normal saline solution (NSS) is hyperosmolar, so its administration will help to pull fluid out of the brain tissue. Lactated Ringer's solution may also be used, although it is less osmolar than NSS.

Do not use a dextrose-based solution when administering neuroanesthesia: The body will utilize the glucose, and then only free water will be left, causing edema. In the event of hypoglycemia, small bolus doses of glucose-based solutions can be given.

Patients are usually kept normovolemic during neurosurgery to maintain adequate blood pressure and cardiac output minimizing changes in CBF.

TYPES OF NEUROSURGICAL CASES

- Intracranial-space-occupying lesions
- Intracranial aneurysms
- Vascular: anterior, middle, or posterior

The main consequences of intracranial pathologic conditions are brain tissue hypoxia, acidosis, and edema. In acute brain disorders, cerebral vasoparalysis occurs and coupling between the blood flow and metabolism is impaired (uncoupled). Autoregulation and carbon dioxide reactivity are also disturbed.

Intracranial-Space-Occupying Lesions

Brain Tumors

Slowly expanding tumors cause volume-spatial compensation by compressing the CSF compartment and the blood supply to the brain; they may not always increase ICP. The intracranial compartment can adapt only to a point, after which compensatory mechanisms become exhausted; beyond this point, any increase in tumor size will cause the ICP to increase. When the compensatory mechanisms become strained, even a small increase in cerebral blood flow will markedly increase ICP. This can lead to ischemia and then to herniation of the brain tissues. The primary presenting symptoms indicating the presence of a brain tumor is related to an increased ICP.

In brain tumor cases in which marked cerebral edema is present or the tumor is particularly large, there is a tendency to restrict fluid to reduce brain volume. This practice can cause severe physiological stress that develops due to hypovolemia, hypotension, and possibly ischemia from hypoperfusion. There is only a minimal benefit in brain water reduction (i.e., an 8% decrease in body water produces a 1% decrease in brain fluid volume).

Anesthetic management goals with brain tumors are as follows:

1. Preserve neurons.
2. Preserve stability; control ICP; prevent increases in ICP. Preoperatively, look for midline shifting on head CT or MRI.
3. Control $PaCO_2$.
4. Limit fluids. The patient may be euvolemic to slightly hypovolemic; use normal saline 0.9% for IV fluids. Patients with brain tumors are often hypovolemic and dehydrated; replace obligatory losses slowly. It may be necessary to give additional IV fluids in patients who have undergone angiographic studies because of the diuresis that occurs after someone receives contrast dye.
5. Avoid hypotonic IV fluids such as dextrose 5% in water: The free water goes to the brain, causing edema after body utilizes the glucose.
6. Maintain CPP; prevent decreases in cerebral perfusion and CBF. Only rarely is it necessary to hyperventilate a patient.
7. Ensure normothermia is maintained.
8. Prevent decreases in blood pressure, maintain blood pressure within 20% of baseline. Blood flow and normal blood pressures are needed to maximize blood flow to ischemic areas.
9. Reduce brain bulk to help with retraction.
10. Give corticosteroids if necessary to reduce vasogenic edema surrounding tumors.
11. Protect the patient while in a sitting position from venous air embolism.
12. Provide rapid emergence at the end of the case for neurologic examination purposes.
13. Recognize that the main concerns are hypoxia, hypercapnia, and blood pressure lability.
14. Provide appropriate preoperative treatment for brain tumors: Patients with brain tumors should receive steroids and anticonvulsants for 24–48 hours before surgery.

Other points about treatment of brain tumors follow:

- In adults, the majority of brain tumors are supratentorial (present with seizures, hemiplegia, or aphasia).
- In children, the majority of brain tumors are infratentorial (present with cerebellar dysfunction or brain stem compression).
- The primary symptoms in patients with brain tumors are related to increased ICP—for example, headache and vomiting (not necessarily nausea) in the morning but improving during the day.
- In terms of its pathophysiology, a space-occupying lesion causes cell proliferation, edema, necrosis, and hemorrhage.
- Symptoms are related to infiltration/invasion, compression, and destruction of tissue. Fever, meningeal signs (headache, nuchal rigidity, photophobia), altered level of consciousness, and cranial nerve deficits are all possible.
- Metastasis commonly occurs from tumors of the lung and the breast.
- Vasogenic edema will occur around brain tumors if the BBB altered; brain edema results from interstitial water accumulation.

Supratentorial Masses

The supratentorial region of the brain is the part located above the tentorium cerebelli, which contains the cerebrum. The most common types of tumors in this area are gliomas, meningiomas, and pituitary adenomas.

Supratentorial tumors change intracranial dynamics in predictable ways. Initially, when the lesion is small and slowly expanding, volume-spatial compensation occurs by compression of the CSF compartment and nearby cerebral veins, which prevents increases in ICP. As the lesion grows, compensatory mechanisms become exhausted, and any further increase in tumor mass will cause progressively greater increases in ICP. The intracranial compartment can compensate to a limited extent; up to a point, patients may exhibit minimal neurologic dysfunction despite the presence of a large mass, elevated ICP, and shifts in the position of brain structures.

Significant changes in ICP can occur if the tumor enlarges and develops a central area of hemorrhagic necrotic tissue or a wide border of brain edema (non-autoregulating) around the tumor; such a growing tumor can also increase ICP by blocking the normal flow of cerebrospinal fluid. With this kind of compromised intracranial compliance, small increases in arterial pressure can produce large increases in cerebral blood flow (CBF), which can markedly increase intracranial volume and ICP with its attendant complications.

Significant increases in ICP result in two major deleterious effects on the brain: cerebral ischemia and herniation. The cerebral perfusion pressure (CPP) is determined by the mean arterial pressure (MAP) minus the ICP. If ICP increases to a greater extent than MAP, CPP is reduced. If ICP rises sufficiently, the brain becomes ischemic. Brain herniation can rapidly lead to neurologic deterioration and death. Those elements that can increase cerebral blood volume—such as hypertension, hypercarbia, and hypoxia—are treatable and should be avoided perioperatively.

The goal of neuroanesthetic care for patients with intracranial hypertension is to reduce intracranial volume: Decrease cerebral blood volume means decreased CSF volume. Various maneuvers and pharmacologic agents can be used to reduce brain hypertension.

Infratentorial Masses

The infratentorial region of the brain is the part located below the tentorium cerebelli. It covers the superior surface of the cerebellum, and supports the occipital lobes of the brain. Infratentorial tumors include medulloblastomas, astrocytomas, and ependymomas.

Intracranial Aneurysms

Anesthetic management goals with aneurysm:

1. Preserve neurons.
2. Ensure intravascular volume is appropriate—that is, normovolemia to slightly increased vascular volumes. Avoid the use of hypotonic IV fluids (e.g., dextrose 5% in water): The free water goes to the brain, causing edema after the body has utilized the glucose.
3. Prevent vasospasm, can occur if the aneurysm has already ruptured. Autoregulation is lost in vasospasm, and CBF becomes pressure dependent in vasospastic arteries. Increased MAP and decreasing viscosity can improve CBF.
4. Give calcium-channel blockers, which can help limit vascular smooth muscle contraction, cell ischemia, and platelet aggregation.
5. Maintain normocapnia.
6. Ensure hemodynamics remain stable: Avoid rupture, rebleeding, and vasospasm.
7. Sedate these patients (while watching out for hypoventilation) to decrease the sympathetic response caused by going into the operating room.
8. Watch for venous air embolism, especially if the patient is in a sitting position.

Most neuroanesthesia plans are based on the patient's aneurysm grade, ICP/TMP, CT scan findings, and overall neurological baseline. Patients with Grade I and II aneurysms are generally extubated in the operating room, while patients with higher-grade aneurysms may benefit from longer intubation periods. The goal is a clear wake-up to the patient's previous baseline status or better.

Vasospasm

Vasospasm occurs 30% of the time after subarachnoid hemorrhage from ruptured aneurysm. The incidence of vasospasm reaches its peak approximately 4 to 10 days after rupture.

Signs and symptoms of vasospam include a change in the level of consciousness and focal neurologic deficits. With vasospasm, EKG changes include a prolonged QT interval; ST-segment depression; flat, inverted T waves, premature ventricular contractions; and presence of a U wave.

If a patient is at risk for ischemic neurologic deficits or cerebral infarction caused by vasospasm, the most effective regimen is hypervolemic, hypertensive, and hemodilution therapy (triple-H therapy). Also, treat the patient with nimodipine or nicardipine (calcium-channel blockers) to reduce incidence of vasospasm. Complications with triple-H therapy may include congestive heart failure, myocardial ischemia, dysrhythmias, brain edema, and electrolyte and bleeding abnormalities.

Goals with vasospasm treatment are to maintain CPP, ensure normovolemia, ensure normocapnia, provide tight controls over blood glucose and blood pressure, and preserve neurons.

Vascular Neurosurgery: Anterior, Middle, or Posterior Approaches

Arteriovenous Malformation

Arteriovenous malformations (AVMs) are very similar to aneurysms; they are extremely vascular with the potential for a lot of bleeding. AVMs are characterized by impaired autoregulation because of the direct arterial–venous connection and abnormalities in regional cerebral blood flow. A sudden engorgement in the AVM area can cause focal ischemia as well as global ICP changes.

Treatments include surgical resection, embolization, stereotactic radiosurgery, or a combination of these treatments. Embolization materials include various materials to block the arteries or to obliterate the AVM nidus. Stereotactic radiosurgery involves focused doses of radiation for ablation of AV malformations.

The Spetzler and Martin grading system for AVM is used to predict risk of neurologic impairment. The larger the number, the higher the risk for neurologic impairment:

CRITERION	SCORE
Size of AVM	
< 3 cm	1
3–6 cm	2
> 6 cm	3
Location	
Noneloquent	0
Eloquent (i.e., critical area of brain)	1
Deep Venous Drainage	
Not present	0
Present	1

Anesthetic management goals with vascular neurological conditions (vascular insufficiency) are as follows:

1. Preserve neurons.
2. Maintain normovolemia. If volume replacement is required avoid the use of hypotonic IV fluids (e.g., dextrose 5% in water): The free water goes to the brain, causing edema after the body has utilized the glucose.
3. Maintain normocapnia.
4. Maintain stable hemodynamics, including tight control on blood pressure.
5. Maintain normal cerebral perfusion pressures.

NEUROSURGERY

Neurological Surgical Approaches

- Traditional craniotomy under general anesthesia
- Awake craniotomy
- Neuro-navigation/computer-assisted surgery

Approaches to the Brain

A few of the most common approaches are described here:

- *Burr holes:* a circular, limited opening into the skull through which blood or fluid may be evacuated, instruments inserted, or neural tracts divided. Burr holes can be used to serve

as points that are connected when a bone flap is removed. Burr holes are placed to relieve an increased intracranial pressure; they also allow placement of a ventriculostomy catheter.
  • *Trephination:* larger burr holes.
• *Craniotomy:* opening into the skull.
• *Craniectomy:* excision of cranial bone to permit better exposure, to relieve intracranial pressure, or because it is involved in a disease process.
• *Transsphenoidal:* The sella turcica is located directly above the sphenoid sinus, a relationship that provides direct access to the pituitary gland via the nasal structures. Access is achieved by entering an incision line made under the upper lip and extended over the maxilla into the nasal cavity (rarely used), or an incision on the body septum or at the sphenoid os.

Minimally Invasive Neurologic Procedures

Allergy to contrast dye should be discovered in the preoperative interview. A patient with such an allergy may require preoperative prophylaxis of a steroid and an H_2 blocker.

Endovascular Procedures

An endovascular procedure is a minimally invasive method to treat vascular abnormalities of the brain or spinal cord; this approach does not require a craniotomy. It is performed to clot off or embolize aneurysms, vascular tumors, or arteriovenous malformations, but can also be used to open a stenosed vessel. A small catheter is inserted into an artery or vein, advanced under X-ray or fluoroscopy, to the desired location.

Stereotactic Procedures

A stereotactic procedure is done to obtain a tissue biopsy or treatment of an intracranial lesion; it allows extremely precise localization. Access to the brain gained via a burr hole in the cranium through which a biopsy needle is advanced to the exact spot needed. The head of the bed will be elevated to place head pins and the frame.

Frame-Based Stereotaxy

Local anesthesia with mild sedation can be given for a frame application. Four pins are then used to anchor the frame to the skull. CT, MRI, and angiography studies are used for target localization with the frame in place; markers are applied to the frame to provide reference points during surgery. These patients are usually given sedation anesthesia for their target localization. Access to the patient's airway is restricted with the frame in place; usually fiberoptic intubation is needed for general anesthesia. A key for emergency frame removal should be kept with the patient at all times (while the head in a frame can be extended, the frame may need to be removed for easier access in an emergency intubation). Note: titanium frames must be applied for a patient going through an MRI study.

Frameless Stereotaxy

Instead of a frame providing a reference source, small markers (fiducials) are affixed to the patient's scalp and forehead with adhesive. CT or MRI images of the surgical field are imported into the computer software, while a digitizing camera senses the position of the surgical instruments in space and indicates the position of the instrument on the image displayed on the computer monitor. The fiducials are registered using a probe that is linked to the computer by a camera that detects the probe's position in space. This process marries the position of the head in space with the images in the computer. Surgical instruments incorporating light-emitting diodes (LEDs) are followed by the computer during the operation. The surgeon can navigate through the brain using the computer images linked to the surgical instruments or a microscope. Frameless stereotaxy is thought to be less accurate than a frame-guided system.

Stereotactic Radiosurgery

After application of a frame, focused doses of radiation are used for ablation of small tumors and AV malformations through a closed cranium.

This process is usually done in special leaded surgical suites. Children will need general anesthesia, which is usually initiated before frame placement and continued until after removal of the stereotaxic frame. Cooperative adults may need only sedation.

Functional Neurosurgery

Functional neurosurgery is concerned with the treatment of conditions where the brain and spinal function are abnormal although the anatomy itself is normal. Usually a frame-based procedure is employed in such cases because these techniques depend on absolute precision. Examples of conditions treated by functional neurosurgery include the following:

- *Pallidotomy:* A tiny electrical probe is placed in the globus pallidus, which is then heated to 80°C for 60 seconds, to destroy a small area of brain cells. This approach is used to treat dyskinesias in patients with Parkinson's disease.
- *Thalamotomy:* Precise destruction of the thalamus that controls some involuntary movements.
- Stimulator placement for *chronic pain and movement disorders* such as Parkinson's disease and tremor.
- *Treatment of epilepsy:* either removes or isolates the area of the brain where seizures originate. If the section of this brain tissue is too vital to remove, the surgeon will isolate the area where seizures originate; a series of incisions is made to prevent seizures from spreading to the rest of the brain.

BRAIN AND CRANIUM: INTRACRANIAL NEUROSURGERY

Arteriovenous Malformation: Surgical Resection/Embolization

The vessels feeding the AVM may be surgically clipped and excised, embolized, or stereotactically radiated (such as with gamma knife) with the hope of removing completely, reducing, or clotting the AVM closed. Surgical resection may be indicated for surgically accessible AVMs in noneloquent areas; gamma knife may be becoming a preferred treatment. ("Eloquent" refers to those areas of the brain that deal with the sensory or motor cortex, such as the parts of the brain that control speech, motor functions, and senses.) This technique is used for cerebral/dural AVMs, cavernous malformations, and occult vascular formation and/or malformation.

AVMs are congenital masses of twisted, dilated, arterial-to-venous communication; blood flows directly from the arterial system to the venous system without passing through a capillary system. The direct connection between the arterial and venous systems puts the thin-walled veins (the muscular layers in the vessel walls lack muscle) under significant pressure because there are no capillaries to provide resistance and "slow down" the blood flow. This results in a system of enlarged feeding vessels, the tangled nidus (nest) of the AVM itself, and enlarged draining venous structures. There is a "steal effect" associated with an AVM: A decrease of resistance in the AVM causes a decrease in blood flow in surrounding healthy tissue. Because the blood does not go to the surrounding tissues, but rather is pumped through the shunt and back to the heart without ever delivering its nutrients to the tissues, it can cause progressive neurological deficits from cerebral ischemia, seizures, and headaches.

AVMs can occur anywhere along the spinal cord or in the brain. They vary in size from small to very large lesions occupying a major portion of a cerebral hemisphere. AVMs have a loss of normal vasomotor control.

Operative Procedure

A scalp flap is made and an opening is created into the skull (supratentorial or infratentorial craniotomy) over the AVM site. Feeding vessels (arteries) are exposed, then clipped or coagulated shut.

Once all the feeding vessels have been occluded, the mass is dissected out.

Microsurgical techniques have made total removal of an AVM a reality. Frame-based stereotaxy, frameless stereotaxy, and stereotactic radiosurgery are other approaches to treating AVMs seated deeper in the brain.

Coil occlusion in a neurointerventional lab or stereotactic radiosurgery may have been attempted or even partially successful before the patient is subjected to surgical resection of an AVM. Preoperative embolization may make surgical dissection much easier or unnecessary (many cases are treated completely with embolization).

Anesthetic

General anesthetic (GA), an oral endotracheal tube (OETT), or muscle relaxants may be required; check with the surgeon before providing these measures. If a stereotactic frame has already been applied to the patient's head, fiberoptic intubation is required. An oral RAE tube (a type of pre-formed "U-shaped" endotracheal tube) or reinforced endotracheal tube may be placed to prevent kinking of the tube with movement and positioning of the patient's head.

If the AVM is small, the surgery may be performed under MAC with sedation to allow for continuous neurological evaluation. This technique is rarely used, however.

Positioning

Place the craniotomy site uppermost in the field and parallel to the floor.

If the patient is in the prone position for surgery, special eye care is required. Paper tape is used to close the eyes to prevent corneal drying or abrasions; eye pads are then placed over both eyes to protect them. Eye ointment can be instilled before taping for patients who will remain intubated postoperatively.

If the patient is placed in a prone position and/or head pins are used, maintain general anesthesia until the patient is in the supine position and the head pins have been removed.

Anesthetic Implications

The patient's clinical presentation depends on the size, location, and accessibility of the AVM, as well as the preexisting condition of the patient. Hemorrhage (which occurs in 53% of cases), signaled by acute onset of severe headache, may be described as the worst headache of the patient's life. Other symptoms include headache (34%), progressive neurologic deficit (21%), and seizures. *Hemorrhage is more likely to be caused by small AVM's; seizures are more likely to be caused by large lesions.* In children, seizure is the most common presentation.

Anesthesia Goals for AVM Resection

- Avoid increased venous pressures as well as keep tight blood pressure control. Maintain the CPP approximately 20% lower than the normal level to decrease blood volume and loss. Remember: CPP = MAP − ICP (CVP).
- Hypotensive techniques may be used during resection, with a MAP in the range of 60–65 mm Hg. During dural closing, maintain a minimum MAP of 70 mm Hg.

Preoperative Measures

Do a complete preoperative neurologic assessment and document any deficits.

Preoperative sedation may be necessary to calm the patient; small doses of a benzodiazepine may be used and are preferred for this purpose over opiates (which depress respirations). However, the patient should not be allowed to hypoventilate (hypoventilation increases $PaCO_2$ and vasodilates the cerebral arteries) or have sedation amounts that affect neurologic evaluation.

Type and cross for two units of blood. Blood should be available in the operating room, as extensive blood loss may occur with this surgery.

Monitors and IV Access

- Arterial line placement is required to monitor continuous blood pressure. It also readily permits arterial sampling for blood gases and labs.
- Place two large-bore peripheral IV lines.
- A CVL is needed in case urgent fluid resuscitation is required with extensive blood loss. Use a triple-lumen or Cordis introducer.
- A PA catheter may be needed if the patient has a cardiac history or is hemodynamically unstable.
- The use of EEGs and SSEPs has become common in AVM surgery.
- A ventricular drain may be placed to drain CSF.

IV Vasoactive Agents

- IV pump: nicardipine (Cardene), sodium nitroprusside (SNP), phenylephrine
- Syringe for bolus: phenylephrine, ephedrine, esmolol (Brevibloc), labetalol, metoprolol
- Other drugs to have available: mannitol, furosemide (Lasix), bumetanide (Bumex), lidocaine, atropine, glycopyrrolate (Robinul), calcium-channel blockers (nimodipine, nicardipine), dexamethasone (Decadron), regular insulin, phenytoin (Dilantin), $D_{50}W$

IV Fluids and Volume Requirements

Give normal saline or lactated Ringer's solution to maintain normovolemia, maintenance IVF plus urinary output. Check the patient's urinary output, measuring it every 30 minutes.

Normal saline is more hyperosmolar than lactated Ringer's solution and helps pull fluid out of brain tissue. Colloids, such as albumin or Hextend/Hetastarch, can be given to restore volume deficits and maintain euvolemia. A solution of 6% Hetastarch can cause platelet dysfunction and bleeding; do not give any patient more than 20 mL/kg/day (max 1500 ml in total).

Hypotonic and glucose solutions should be avoided due to their potential for causing increased cerebral metabolism and free water buildup leading to intracerebral edema. Also, do not give D_5W: Once the body utilizes the dextrose, the free water goes to the brain, causing cerebral edema.

Blood Products

Any blood losses should be replaced immediately to keep the patient's hematocrit above 28%. Hypothermia can cause platelet dysfunction.

Pre-induction Measures

- Midazolam 1–2 mg: used to decrease anxiety, produce amnesia
- 100% O_2 by face mask for 3–5 minute
- Lidocaine 1 mg/kg: blunts SNS outflow, which causes hypertension

Induction

Induction of anesthesia must be smooth, with minimal changes in blood pressure occurring. Hypotension can cause ischemic changes in underperfused areas (through the steal phenomenon), whereas hypertension can rupture the aneurysm or worsen the cerebral hypertension (which produces sudden engorgement and hemorrhage). Inhalation, the balance technique, and total intravenous anesthesia (TIVA) have all been used for induction. Low doses of inhaled anesthetics, opioids, and small boluses of propofol or thiopental are used to help with hypertension during the initial surgical stimulation.

Head pinning and intubation can cause hypertension, which may in turn lead to an increase in ICP. Give fentanyl, lidocaine, or beta blockers to blunt the SNS response. Nicardipine or sodium nitroprusside (SNP) IV drips can also be used. Nitroglycerin is usually not preferred in neurosurgery, as it can increase ICP; nicardipine (Cardene) is preferred for blood pressure reduction, particularly during its emergence to ensure tight blood pressure control.

A small dose of a muscle relaxant can also help to avoid coughing and straining. In case of unwanted hypotension, treat the patient with phenylephrine (Neosynephrine), a direct-acting alpha-adrenergic agent.

Induction agent suggestions:

- Thiopental 4 mg/kg: GA induction agent that decreases both $CMRO_2$ and CBF, and has a neuroprotective effect.
- Etomidate: acceptable, but note that it can activate seizure foci.
- Propofol: acceptable, but note that it can produce profound cardiac depression and lead to hypotension.
- Fentanyl 9–10 mcg/kg: analgesia.
- Rocuronium 1 mg/kg: an NDMR that does not release histamine. Vecuronium or pancuronium: both acceptable.

With the stereotactic head frame in place, fiberoptic intubation will be necessary.

Intraoperative Measures/Maintenance

The goal in this setting is to maintain a slightly decreased CPP so as to decrease blood loss during excision of AVM, and to decrease intracranial volume of blood and tissue. Intentional hypotension may be induced before opening of the dura to maintain the TMP/CPP at a constant level, as ICP is now zero; can use i.e.: esmolol (Brevibloc) or nicardipine. Examples of maintenance agents include O_2/air; keep FiO_2 40–50% as long as oxygen saturation is greater than 96%, along with.

- Isoflurane: 0.5 MAC if SSEP used.
- Propofol 75–100 mcg/kg/min infusion; maintain decreased $CMRO_2$ and CBF.
- Rocuronium 0.1–0.2 mg/kg: to TOF 0/4.
- Remifentanil 0.05–0.1 mcg/kg/min: for clear wake-up.
- $PaCO_2$: keep between 30 and 35 mm Hg.

Brain protection strategies may be used such as the use of high-dose barbiturates (2–5 g Pentothal). The use of this technique must be weighed against the possibility of cerebral ischemia; if present, the possible hypotension can compound the ischemia.

Emergence

Titrate IV beta blockers to avoid and manage any hypertension and tachycardia during the patient's emergence from anesthesia. The goal is to achieve a smooth and prompt awakening if possible. The avoidance of hypertension is essential to prevent bleeding or rupture. You may use vasodilators and/or beta blockers—labetalol, metoprolol (Lopressor), esmolol (Brevibloc), hydralazine (Apresoline), nicardipine (Cardene), or sodium nitroprusside (SNP)—to help regulate SBP. It is best to keep the patient's blood pressure within the normal range. If the patient is at risk for hyperemic (increased blood flow to tissues) complications, a mild degree of hypotension may be used.

These patients have increased incidence of postoperative nausea and vomiting, so give antiemetics as necessary to prevent this side effect (see Chapter 4).

Postoperative Measures

Perform a neurologic assessment as soon as the patient can follow commands. The goal is to assess the neurologic status while the patient is still in the operating room. The surgeons would like to evaluate the patient in the immediate postoperative period for complications so they can intervene if needed.

Once the surgery is completed, cover the patient with warmed blankets to prevent shivering. Elevate the head of the bed to approximately 30 degrees.

Complications

Potential complications of this surgery include venous air embolism, cranial nerve injury, intracranial hemorrhage, stroke, cerebral edema, infection, and massive blood loss.

Craniotomy for Brain Tumor

This procedure provides for surgical debulking or removal of a brain tumor. Tumors of the brain can occur anywhere within the head, including, but not limited to, tumors of the skull, meninges, vessels, nerves, and brain itself.

Operative Procedure

The surgical approach and incision depend on the location of the lesion. Tumor resection involves a series of steps: A craniotomy is done and a flap of bone is lifted (a craniotomy *or* a craniectomy may be done); a durotomy is performed; and then the surgeon carefully frees the lesion of interest from the surrounding brain tissue. After removing the specimen, hemostasis is obtained, and the site is closed in reversed order.

If the skull bone cannot be replaced with the bone that has been removed, such as would be the case if the bone were involved in the tumor (for example, in meningiomas or hemangiomas of the skull), or for relieving intracranial pressure, a cranioplasty can be done to cover the defect.

Surgery is sometimes followed by radiation therapy after allowing sufficient time for the wound to heal.

Microsurgical techniques have made total removal of brain tumors a reality. Frame-based stereotaxy, frameless stereotaxy, and stereotactic radiosurgery are other approaches to deeply seated brain tumors.

Anesthetic

General anesthesia, an OETT, and muscle relaxants may be needed; check with surgeon before providing these measures. A pre-formed oral RAE tube or reinforced endotracheal tube may be placed to prevent kinking of the tube with movement and positioning of the patient's head.

The brain tissue is insensate, so the longest part of the surgery requires a lower level of anesthesia. The periods of maximal stimulation include head pinning, scalp incision, cranial opening, and emergence.

Patients undergoing craniotomy require special eye care. Paper tape is used to close the eyes to prevent corneal drying or abrasions; eye pads are then placed over both eyes to protect them. Eye ointment can be instilled before taping for patients who will remain intubated postoperatively. Be aware that patients who have ointment in their eyes will sometimes rub their eyes (to clear their vision postoperatively) and accidentally scratch their eyes or face upon awakening.

Positioning

Patients should have one or both of their arms tucked at the sides. The exact position used depends on the tumor location, though the operative side of the head is always in the uppermost position (the head may be turned laterally). The head of the bed is usually increased 15–30 degrees to ensure venous drainage. The head of the operating table may be turned away at least 90 degrees, if not 180 degrees, from the anesthetist. The patient may be in the supine, lateral, seated, or prone position for craniotomy.

Anesthetic Implications

Patients undergoing craniotomy may be placed in head pins.

Type and cross should be done preoperatively.

The surgeon may need for the ICP to be decreased for help with exposure. See Chapter 3 for more information.

Hypertension after brain tumor dissection is especially detrimental because it increases the chance the patient will bleed into the empty space where the tumor was.

Anesthesia Goals for Craniotomy for Brain Tumor

- Steroids and diuretics may be used to help decrease swelling around a brain tumor.
- Avoid increased venous pressures and maintain tight blood pressure control. Maintain the CPP approximately 20% lower than the normal level to decrease blood volume and loss. Remember: CPP = MAP − ICP (CVP).
- Hypotensive techniques may be used during resection; maintain MAP at 60–65 mm Hg.

During closing, maintain a minimum of 65 mm Hg MAP. The specific pressure depends on the case and the surgeon's preference, but these values are helpful guidelines. Anesthetic care should allow for prompt wake-up for neurologic evaluation at the end of the case.

Preoperative Measures

Perform a complete preoperative neurologic assessment and document any deficits.

Preoperative sedation may be necessary to calm the patient; small doses of a benzodiazepine may be used and are preferred for this purpose over opiates (which depress respirations). The patient should not be allowed to hypoventilate (which increases $PaCO_2$ and vasodilates cerebral arteries) or have sedation amounts that affect neurologic evaluation.

Monitors and IV Access

- Arterial line placement is required to monitor continuous blood pressure. It also readily permits arterial sampling for blood gases and labs.
- Place two large-bore peripheral IV lines.
- All craniotomy patients undergoing tumor resection should have a central line placed.
- CVP may be needed in case urgent fluid resuscitation is required owing to extensive blood loss.
- A PA catheter may be needed if the patient has a cardiac history or is hemodynamically unstable.
- Electrophysiology monitors, EEG, SSEP, BAEP, MEP, and EMG may be used, depending on the site of the tumor and surgeon preference.
- Use a precordial Doppler device to monitor for venous air embolism when the patient is in a sitting position (see Chapter 3).

IV Vasoactive Agents

- IV pump: nicardipine (Cardene), sodium nitroprusside (SNP), phenylephrine
- Syringe for bolus: phenylephrine, ephedrine, esmolol (Brevibloc), labetalol, metoprolol
- Other drugs to have available: mannitol, furosemide (Lasix), bumetanide (Bumex), lidocaine, atropine, glycopyrrolate (Robinul),

calcium-channel blockers (nimodipine, nicardipine), dexamethasone (Decadron), regular insulin, $D_{50}W$, phenytoin (Dilantin)

IV Fluids and Volume Requirements

Use normal saline or lactated Ringer's solution to maintain normovolemia, maintenance IVF plus urinary output. Measure urinary output every 30 minutes.

Normal saline is more hyperosmolar than lactated Ringer's solution and helps pull fluid out of brain tissue. Colloids, such as albumin or Hextend/Hetastarch, can be given to restore volume deficits and maintain euvolemia. A 6% Hetastarch solution can cause platelet dysfunction and bleeding; do not give more 20 mL/kg/day (max 1500 mL total).

Hypotonic and glucose solutions should be avoided owing to their association with increased cerebral metabolism and free water build-up, causing intracerebral edema. Do not give D_5W: Once the body utilizes the dextrose, the free water goes to the brain, causing cerebral edema.

Blood Products

Any blood losses should be replaced immediately to keep HCT at a level greater than 28%. Hypothermia can cause platelet dysfunction.

Pre-induction Measures

- Midazolam 1–2 mg: Used to decrease anxiety and produce amnesia
- 100% O_2 by face mask for 3–5 minutes
- Lidocaine 1 mg/kg: blunts SNS outflow, which causes hypertension

Induction

Induction must be smooth, with minimal changes in blood pressure occurring. Inhalation, the balance technique, and TIVA have all been used for this purpose. Low doses of inhaled anesthetics, opioids, and small boluses of propofol or thiopental are used to help with hypertension during the initial surgical stimulation.

Head pinning and intubation can cause hypertension, which can lead to an increase in ICP. Give fentanyl, lidocaine or beta blockers to blunt the

SNS response. Nicardipine (Cardene) or sodium nitroprusside (SNP) IV drips can also be used.

A small dose of a muscle relaxant can help to avoid coughing and straining.

Treat unwanted hypotension with phenylephrine (Neosynephrine), a direct-acting alpha-adrenergic agent.

Intraoperative Measures/Maintenance
The goal is to maintain a slightly decreased CPP to decrease blood loss during excision of the tumor, and to decrease intracranial volume of blood and tissue for surgical exposure.

Emergence
Titrate IV beta blockers to avoid any hypertensive spike and tachycardia with emergence. The goal is to achieve a smooth and prompt awakening if possible.

Patients undergoing craniotomy have an increased incidence of postoperative nausea and vomiting. Give antiemetics to prevent these side effects (see Chapter 4).

Postoperative Measures
Perform a neurologic assessment as soon as the patient can follow commands. The goal is to assess the neurologic status while the patient is still in the operating room. The surgeons would like to evaluate the patient in the immediate postoperative period for complications so they can intervene if needed.

Once the surgery is completed, cover the patient with warmed blankets to prevent shivering. Elevate the head of the bed to approximately 30 degrees.

Complications
Potential complications include seizures, neurologic deficits, pneumocephalus, venous air embolism, hemorrhage, cerebral edema, cerebrospinal fluid leak, and blood loss.

Craniotomy for Cerebral Embolectomy
This procedure entails the surgical removal of a clot in a cerebral artery. It has largely been abandoned with the increase in endovascular techniques. It may be used when a large embolus cannot be dissolved with intra-arterial thrombolytics or by endovascular approach.

Operative Procedure
A large embolus can occur in the middle cerebral or basilar cerebral arteries. Surgery must take place as soon as possible, with a maximum time limit of 6 hours after the onset of a new neurologic deficit, to decrease the severity of brain injury. In such cases, neurointerventional procedures (e.g., embolectomy, thrombolysis) may have been attempted before the patient comes to the operating room.

A frontal, temporal, or occipital incision and standard craniotomy are done. The involved arterial segment is isolated, temporarily occluded with clips, and opened, removing the blockage. A microscope may be used by the surgeon during this case. The artery is then closed and blood flow reestablished.

Upon opening an occluded vessel, prostaglandins are released. Platelet sequestration, complement activation, and cytokine release occur, which collectively produce oxygen-derived free radicals; metabolic washout causes acidosis and an increased $ETCO_2$. Prepare for hypotension, hypovolemia, and an increase in the potassium level by turning off vasodilators, lightening the anesthetic, and managing volume load (judiciously, so as not to produce volume overload). Mannitol may be given before opening the vessel to decrease the production of thromboxane.

Anesthetic
General endotracheal anesthesia (GETA) is done; muscle relaxants may be needed. Check with surgeon before giving muscle relaxation.

Carefully secure the ETT, as the surgeon will be working around the mouth and face during surgery. A pre-formed oral RAE tube or reinforced endotracheal tube may be placed to prevent kinking of the tube with movement and positioning of the patient's head.

Maintain general anesthesia until the patient is in the supine position and the head pins have been removed (if present).

Positioning
Keep the patient's arms tucked at the sides. The exact position depends on the involved artery's location, but the operative side of the head is always in the uppermost position (the head may be turned laterally). The patient may be in the supine, lateral, sitting, or prone position while undergoing a craniotomy. The head of the bed is usually increased 15–30 degrees to ensure venous drainage. The head of the operating table may be turned away at least 90 degrees, if not 180 degrees, from the anesthetist.

Anesthetic Implications
Patients undergoing craniotomy require special eye care. Paper tape is used to close the eyes to prevent corneal drying or abrasions; eye pads are then placed over both eyes to protect them. Eye ointment may also be instilled before taping for patients who will remain intubated postoperatively.

Anesthesia Goals for Craniotomy for Cerebral Embolectomy

Preoperative Measures

Perform a complete preoperative neurologic assessment and document any deficits. Maintain induced hypertension (via phenylephrine and expanded intravascular volume) to maximize collateral blood flow to the ischemic brain.

Monitors and IV Access
- Arterial line placement is required to monitor continuous blood pressure. It also readily permits arterial sampling for blood gases and labs.
- Place two large-bore peripheral IV lines.
- CVP may be needed in case urgent fluid resuscitation is required owing to extensive blood loss.
- A PA catheter may be needed if the patient has a cardiac history or is hemodynamically unstable.

- Use a precordial Doppler to monitor for venous air embolism while the patient is in a sitting position (see Chapter 3).

IV Vasoactive Agents
- IV pump: nicardipine (Cardene), sodium nitroprusside (SNP), phenylephrine
- Syringe for bolus: phenylephrine, ephedrine, esmolol (Brevibloc), labetalol, metoprolol
- Other drugs to have available: mannitol, furosemide (Lasix), bumetanide (Bumex), lidocaine, atropine, glycopyrrolate (Robinul), calcium-channel blockers (nimodipine, nicardipine), dexamethasone (Decadron), regular insulin, $D_{50}W$

IV Fluids and Volume Requirements

Give normal saline or lactated Ringer's solution to maintain normovolemia, maintenance IVF plus urinary output, and measure urinary output every 30 minutes. Normal saline is more hyperosmolar than lactated Ringer's solution and helps pull fluid out of brain tissue. Colloids, such as albumin or Hextend/Hetastarch, can be given to restore volume deficits and maintain euvolemia. Hetastarch can cause platelet dysfunction and bleeding; do not give more than 20 mL/kg/day (max 1500 mL total).

Hypotonic and glucose solutions should be avoided due to the potential for increased cerebral metabolism and free water build-up, causing intracerebral edema. Don't give D_5W: Once the body utilizes the dextrose, the free water goes to the brain, causing cerebral edema.

Blood Products

Any blood losses should be replaced immediately to keep HCT greater than 28%. Hypothermia can cause platelet dysfunction.

Pre-induction Measures

Preoperative sedation may be necessary to calm the patient; small doses of a benzodiazepine may be used and are preferred for this purpose over opiates (which depress respirations). However, the patient should not be allowed to hypoventilate (which increases $PaCO_2$ and vasodilates cerebral arteries) or have sedation amounts that affect neurologic evaluation.

Induction

Induction should be "slow and controlled"; it must be smooth, with minimal changes in blood pressure. Maintain CPP and MAP to ensure adequate perfusion of brain tissue.

Intraoperative Measures/Maintenance

Maintain the induced hypertension (via phenylephrine and expanded intravascular volume) to maximize collateral blood flow to the ischemic brain.

- Pre-clipping: Decrease blood pressure to approximately 20% of baseline with controlled hypotension. Avoid MAP of less than 80 mm Hg.
- During clipping: Increase blood pressure to 20% to 30% of baseline; phenylephrine (Neosynephrine) is the preferred drug for this purpose.
- Post-clipping: Maintain MAP at 80–100 mm Hg.

Neuroprotective agents are needed because of mechanical retraction of the brain tissue and during arterial segment occlusion (see Chapter 3).

Emergence

Emergence should be "slow and controlled"; it must be smooth with minimal changes in blood pressure. Give prophylactic antiemetics to help patients avoid PONV (see Chapter 4).

Postoperative Measures

Perform a neurologic assessment as soon as the patient can follow commands. The goal is to assess the neurologic status while the patient is still in the operating room. The surgeons would like to evaluate the patient in the immediate postoperative period for complications so they can intervene if needed.

Once the surgery is completed, cover the patient with warmed blankets to prevent shivering. Elevate the head of the bed to approximately 30 degrees.

Complications

Potential complications include stroke and hemorrhage.

Cerebrospinal Fluid Leak Repair

This surgery is performed to repair or stop a CSF leak. A CSF leak may result from head trauma (basilar skull fractures), iatrogenic surgical trauma during endoscopic sinus surgery or transsphenoidal pituitary surgery, benign or malignant tumors, or congenital malformations. CSF usually drains out of the ear canal (otorrhea) or the nose (rhinorrhea). Most leaks involve the anterior cranial fossa from fractures of the ethmoid or sphenoid bones, or the petrous temporal bones in the posterior part of the middle fossa (between the sphenoid and occipital bones).

Operative Procedure

An endoscopic repair can be done that may require placement of a lumbar drain; a bifrontal craniotomy or eyebrow incision approach is done for surgical repair (as well as other approaches such as the middle fossa approach). In surgical repair, a frontal (or bifrontal) bone flap is created, the bone lifted off, and the dura opened. The frontal lobes of the brain are lifted and the defects in the anterior cranial fossa bone are closed with a variety of materials, including fat, bone, cement, or wax. Once the repair is done, the dura is closed and the bone flap replaced. Dural repair may be done by continuous sutures, fascia from the patient's own thigh, fibrin sealants, DuraSeal (synthetic biocompatible hydrogel), or bovine pericardium. Defects in the bone can be repaired with fat, bone, or wax. Once the dura is surgically closed, brain relaxation is no longer needed.

The olfactory tracts may be sacrificed with CSF leak repair, in which case the patient will lose his or her sense of smell.

Anesthetic

General anesthesia and OETT; muscle relaxation not usually needed if the patient's head is placed in tongs. Check with surgeon if relaxation is needed. Many neurosurgeons do not rely on head pinning.

Maintain general anesthesia until the patient is in the supine position and the head pins have been removed.

Positioning

The patient is placed in a supine position, with the arms tucked at sides. The exact position depends on the tumor location, although the operative side of the head is always in the uppermost position (the head may be turned laterally). The head of the bed is usually increased 15–30 degrees to ensure venous drainage. The head of the operating table may be turned away at least 90 degrees, if not 180 degrees, from the anesthetist. The patient's head may be placed in pins for stabilization.

Anesthetic Implications

Neuroprotective agents and brain relaxation are usually necessary to decrease the need for mechanical retraction; these measures may include mannitol, diuretics, or placement of a CSF drain.

Pneumocephalus (presence of air or gas within the cranial cavity) can occur with post-traumatic or spontaneous CSF leak. It is most likely to be attributable to a pressure gradient created during sneezing or nose blowing. See Chapter 3 for more information.

Patients undergoing CSF leak repair require special eye care. Paper tape is used to close the eyes to prevent corneal drying or abrasions; eye pads are then placed over both eyes to protect them. Eye ointment may also be instilled before taping for patients who will remain intubated postoperatively.

Anesthesia Goals for CSF Leak Repair

Preoperative Measures

Perform a complete preoperative neurologic assessment and document any deficits.

Preoperative sedation may be necessary to calm the patient; small doses of a benzodiazepine may be used and are preferred for this purpose over opiates (which depress respirations). The patient should not be allowed to hypoventilate (because it increases $PaCO_2$ and vasodilates cerebral arteries) or have sedation amounts that affect neurologic evaluation.

Monitors and IV Access

- Arterial line placement is required to monitor continuous blood pressure. It also readily permits arterial sampling for blood gases and labs.
- Place at least one large-bore peripheral IV line.
- A CVL may be needed in case urgent fluid resuscitation is required because of extensive blood loss.
- A PA catheter may be needed if the patient has a cardiac history or is hemodynamically unstable.
- A precordial Doppler device may be used for venous air embolism monitoring if the patient is in a sitting position.

IV Vasoactive Agents

- IV pump: nicardipine (Cardene), sodium nitroprusside (SNP), phenylephrine
- Syringe for bolus: phenylephrine, ephedrine, esmolol (Brevibloc), labetalol, metoprolol
- Other drugs to have available: mannitol, furosemide (Lasix), bumetanide (Bumex), lidocaine, atropine, glycopyrrolate (Robinul), calcium-channel blockers (nimodipine, nicardipine), dexamethasone (Decadron), regular insulin, $D_{50}W$

IV Fluids and Volume Requirements

Give normal saline and lactated Ringer's solution to maintain normovolemia, provide maintenance IVF, and measure urinary output every 30 minutes. Normal saline is more hyperosmolar than lactated Ringer's solution and helps pull fluid out of brain tissue. Colloids, such as albumin or Hextend/ Hetastarch, can be given to restore volume deficits and maintain euvolemia. Hetastarch can cause platelet dysfunction and bleeding; do not give more than 20 mL/kg/day (max 1500 mL total).

Hypotonic and glucose solutions should be avoided due to the potential for increased cerebral metabolism and free water build–up, causing intracerebral edema. Don't give D_5W: Once the body utilizes the dextrose, the free water goes to the brain, causing cerebral edema.

Blood Products
Keep HCT at more than 28%.

Induction
Induction should be "slow and controlled"; it must be smooth, with minimal changes in blood pressure occurring. Maintain CPP and MAP so as to provide adequate perfusion of brain tissue.

Intraoperative Measures/Maintenance
The goal is to maintain a slightly decreased CPP to decrease blood loss, and to decrease intracranial volume of blood and tissue for surgical exposure.

Emergence
Emergence should be "slow and controlled"; it must be smooth, with minimal changes in blood pressure to avoid CSF leak. Give prophylactic antiemetics as necessary to help patients avoid PONV (see Chapter 4).

Postoperative Measures
Perform a neurologic assessment as soon as the patient can follow commands. The goal is to assess the neurologic status while the patient is still in the operating room.. The surgeons would like to evaluate the patient in the immediate postoperative period for complications so they can intervene if needed.

Once the surgery is completed, cover the patient with warmed blankets to prevent shivering.

Complications
Potential complications include meningitis, infection, pneumocephalus, continued CSF leak, intracranial hypotension syndrome, hemorrhage, diabetes insipidus, and stroke.

Microvascular Cranial Nerve Decompression
This procedure is performed to treat various disorders of cranial nerves. In particular, it is performed to relieve trigeminal neuralgia (also known as tic douloureux), an extremely painful inflammation or compression of the fifth cranial nerve causing chronic stabbing, lancinating pain (sharp shock-like sensation). An enlarged blood vessel surrounding the trigeminal nerve can also compress against it, injuring the nerve's protective sheath causing paroxysmal, hyperactive functioning. It causes a debilitating pain, often felt around the eye, cheek, lips, gums, or chin on one side of the face; it is elicited by stimulation of affected area by cold, touch, or even sounds.

In addition, this procedure is used to relieve glossopharyngeal neuralgia (a disorder of the ninth cranial nerve—the glossopharyngeal nerve)—that interferes with a patient's ability to taste, can cause chronic pain of tongue and throat and/or unilateral paroxysmal pain of ear and throat, and (similar to tic douloureux), hemifacial spasm, facial nerve disorder, and intractable positional vertigo (by compression of the vestibular nerve).

Operative Procedure
In a retromastoid craniotomy or craniectomy, a slightly curved 2- to 3-inch incision is made behind the affected-side ear; burr holes are made into the cranium; a full craniotomy is done; the dura is opened and the cerebellum is retracted. An opening is enlarged posterior to the transverse and sigmoid sinus to allow access to the cerebellopontine angle. A microscope is used to identify the vessel and dissect the nerve. Shredded Teflon or a small plastic sponge is then placed so as to keep the blood vessel from returning to its position against the nerve, thereby decreasing pain. Occasionally, the nerve is traumatized or a partial section is removed; cutting of the ninth or tenth cranial nerve can cause some vasomotor instability. If cerebral protection is required, see the information in Chapter 3.

Microvascular decompression is a procedure that involves an operating microscope: A small opening is created in the skull behind the ear to visualize and examine the trigeminal nerve at the junction where the trigeminal nerve enters the base of the brain. Any compressive arteries are then repositioned, and a protective pad is placed between the nerve and artery. If the blood vessel pressing on the nerve is a vein, it may be treated in similar fashion or surgically removed.

The addition of an *endoscope* improves visualization of the entire nerve complex and ensures adequate decompression with less retraction.

Anesthetic

General anesthesia, an OETT, and muscle relaxants are usually required; check with the surgeon before giving relaxants.

Some surgeons place the patient in head pins for microvascular nerve decompression. In such a case, maintain general anesthesia until the patient is in the supine position and the head pins have been removed.

A pre-formed oral RAE tube or reinforced endotracheal tube may be placed to prevent kinking of the tube with movement and positioning of the patient's head. This tube should be secured on the side of the mouth opposite from the surgery side.

Positioning

The patient may be placed in a lateral, prone, sitting, or supine position, with the arms tucked at the sides. The exact position depends on the cranial nerve location, but the operative side of the head is always in the uppermost position (the head may be turned laterally). The head of the operating table may be turned away at least 90 degrees, if not 180 degrees, from the anesthetist.

The head of the bed is usually increased 15–30 degrees to ensure venous drainage. See Chapter 2 for more information on cerebral perfusion pressure and transducer levels.

Anesthetic Implications

Type and cross the patient's blood. Although there is usually minimal blood loss with this procedure, massive blood loss is possible secondary to vertebral artery injury.

No muscle relaxation should be given if nerve monitoring is done intraoperatively.

There is a risk of venous air embolism (VAE) if the patient is in a sitting position (see Chapter 3).

Patients undergoing these procedures require special eye care. Paper tape is used to close the eyes to prevent corneal drying or abrasions; eye pads are then placed over both eyes to protect them. Eye ointment may also be instilled before taping for patients who will remain intubated postoperatively.

Anesthesia Goals for Microvascular Cranial Nerve Decompression

Blood pressure is maintained in the normal to slightly lower range during this surgery.

Preoperative Measures

Perform a complete preoperative neurologic assessment and document any deficits.

Preoperative sedation may be necessary to calm the patient; small doses of a benzodiazepine may be used and are preferred for this purpose over opiates (which depress respirations). The patient should not be allowed to hypoventilate (because it increases $PaCO_2$ and vasodilates cerebral arteries) or have sedation amounts that affect neurologic evaluation.

Monitors and IV Access

- Arterial line placement is required to monitor continuous blood pressure. It also readily permits arterial sampling for blood gases and labs.
- Place at least one large-bore peripheral IV line.
- CVP may be needed in case urgent fluid resuscitation is required because of extensive blood loss.
- A PA catheter may be needed if the patient has a cardiac history or is hemodynamically unstable.
- BAEP, facial nerve monitoring, EMG, and/or SSEP may be measured intraoperatively to protect the cranial nerves.

- A precordial Doppler device may be used to monitor for venous air embolism if the patient is in a sitting position (see Chapter 3).

IV Vasoactive Agents

- IV pump: nicardipine (Cardene), sodium nitroprusside (SNP), phenylephrine
- Syringe for bolus: phenylephrine, ephedrine, esmolol (Brevibloc), labetalol, metoprolol
- Other drugs to have available: mannitol, furosemide (Lasix), bumetanide (Bumex), lidocaine, atropine, glycopyrrolate (Robinul), calcium-channel blockers (nimodipine, nicardipine), dexamethasone (Decadron), regular insulin, $D_{50}W$

IV Fluids and Volume Requirements:

Give normal saline or lactated Ringer's solution to maintain normovolemia, provide maintenance IVF, and measure urinary output every 30 minutes. Normal saline is more hyperosmolar than lactated Ringer's solution and helps pull fluid out of brain tissue. Colloids, such as albumin or Hextend/ Hetastarch, can be given to restore volume deficits and maintain euvolemia. Hetastarch can cause platelet dysfunction and bleeding; do not give more than 20 mL/kg/day (max 1500 mL total).

Hypotonic and glucose solutions should be avoided due to the potential for increased cerebral metabolism and free water build-up, causing intra-cerebral edema. Don't give D_5W: Once the body utilizes the dextrose, the free water goes to the brain, causing cerebral edema.

Blood Products

Any blood losses should be replaced immediately to keep HCT higher than 28%. Hypothermia can cause platelet dysfunction.

Intraoperative Measures/Maintenance

The goal is to maintain a slightly decreased CPP so as to decrease blood loss, and to decrease intracranial volume of blood and tissue for surgical exposure. Blood pressure should be maintained in the normal range for the patient.

Emergence

Give prophylactic antiemetics as necessary to help the patient avoid PONV (see Chapter 4).

Postoperative Measures

Perform a neurologic assessment as soon as the patient can follow commands. The goal is to assess the neurologic status while the patient is still in the operating room. The surgeons would like to evaluate the patient in the immediate postoperative period for complications so they can intervene if needed.

Once the surgery is completed, cover the patient with warmed blankets to prevent shivering. Elevate the head of the bed to approximately 30 degrees.

Complications

Potential complications include facial nerve injury, ptosis of facial muscle unilaterally, CSF leak, hemorrhage, and cerebral edema.

Craniopharyngioma

Surgical resection is done to remove a cranio-pharyngioma—a slow-growing, benign epithelial neoplasm of the sellar region. This kind of calcified cystic tumor arises from the region of the pituitary stalk and occupies the (supra) sellar region. It has a benign histology but can behave in a malignant behavior, as craniopharyngiomas have a tendency to invade surrounding structures and recur after what was thought to be total resection. Common presenting symptoms include endocrine dysfunction, vertigo, headache, and mental and visual disturbances.

Operative Procedure

The choice of surgical approach is dictated by the primary location of the tumor and its extension pattern. Some of the common surgical approaches for resection of a craniopharyngioma include the pterional (junction of the greater wing of the sphenoid bone, the temporal, frontal, and parietal bones) approach (Figure 5-5); orbitocranial approaches; the subfrontal, transtemporal, transcallosal (across the top of the head at the coronal suture) approach, which is often preferred for smaller parasellar tumors (as it is less invasive); and the transsphenoidal (above the teeth and below the base of the upper lip at the top of the gum line) approach. At times, a combination of approaches is necessary. For unilateral approaches, the right side is often used with an incision over the frontotemporal region.

Tumor adhesion to surrounding vascular structures and brain (such as the hypothalamus) represents the most common cause of incomplete tumor removal. A subtotal resection with radiation typically gives favorable results, as these tumors are very radiosensitive.

An Ommaya reservoir may be placed to drain the cyst, followed by administration of radiation therapy. The Ommaya reservoir is a small plastic device used to deliver drugs to the brain or spinal cord or to take samples of CSF or drain fluids, depending where the distal tip of the reservoir is placed.

Stereotactic radiotherapy is often used with craniopharyngiomas that could not be completely resected.

Endocrinopathy is common in conjunction with craniopharyngiomas. Permanent diabetes insipidus occurs in 68% to 75% of adults with these tumors and 80% to 93% of children. Replacement of two or more of the anterior pituitary hormones is necessary in 80% to 90% patients. Obesity occurs in 50% of patients. Panhypopituitarism, including

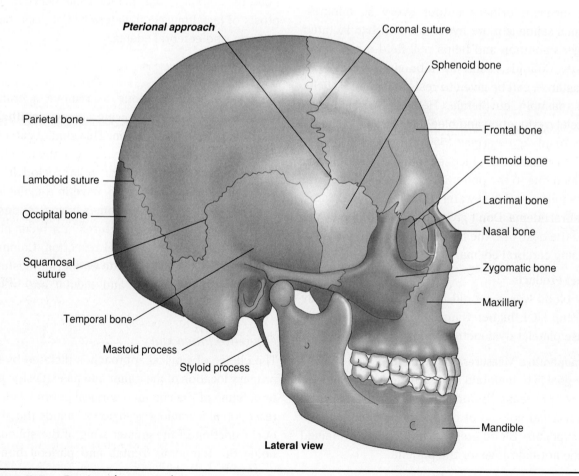

Figure 5-5 *Pterional approach*
Source: Clark, 2005.

hypothyroidism, adrenal insufficiency, and growth hormone deficiency, also occurs frequently. These patients should be referred to an endocrinologist before surgery for appropriate testing and treatment.

Anesthesia Goals for Craniopharyngioma Resection

Assess and monitor for symptoms of diabetes insipidus. These patients may require a continuous intravenous infusion of aqueous vasopression titrated until antidiuresis is established. Perioperative serum sodium levels should be maintained between 130 and 150 mEq/L.

Preoperative Measures

Perform a complete preoperative neurologic assessment and document any deficits. Ophthalmological testing should be done preoperatively to serve as a baseline for postoperative testing.

Have CT scans or MRI scans available in the operating room.

Type and cross the patient's blood, as hemorrhage is a possible complication in this surgery.

Monitors and IV Access

- Arterial line placement is required to monitor continuous blood pressure. It also readily permits arterial sampling for blood gases and labs.
- Place at least two large-bore peripheral IV lines.
- CVP may be needed in case urgent fluid resuscitation is required because of extensive blood loss.
- A PA catheter may be needed if the patient has a cardiac history or is hemodynamically unstable.

IV Vasoactive Agents

- IV pump: nicardipine (Cardene), sodium nitroprusside (SNP), phenylephrine
- Syringe for bolus: phenylephrine, ephedrine, esmolol (Brevibloc), labetalol, metoprolol
- Other drugs to have available: DDAVP/ vasopressin, mannitol, furosemide (Lasix), bumetanide (Bumex), lidocaine, atropine, glycopyrrolate (Robinul), calcium-channel blockers (nimodipine, nicardipine), dexamethasone (Decadron), regular insulin, $D_{50}W$

IV Fluids and Volume Requirements

Normal saline is given and restricted to two-thirds of the calculated maintenance rate. Colloids, such as albumin or Hextend/Hetastarch, can be given to restore volume deficits and blood loss. Hetastarch can cause platelet dysfunction and bleeding; do not give more than 20 mL/kg/day (max 1500 mL total).

Hypotonic and glucose solutions use should be avoided due to the potential for increased cerebral metabolism and free water build-up, causing intracerebral edema. Don't give D_5W: Once the body utilizes the dextrose, the free water goes to the brain, causing cerebral edema.

Blood Products

Any blood losses should be replaced immediately to keep HCT greater than 28%. Hypothermia can cause platelet dysfunction.

Pre-induction Measures

Preoperative sedation may be necessary to calm the patient; small doses of a benzodiazepine may be used and are preferred for this purpose over opiates (which depress respirations). The patient shouldn't be allowed to hypoventilate (because it increases $PaCO_2$ and vasodilates cerebral arteries) or have sedation amounts that affect neurologic evaluation.

Induction

Provide a smooth IV induction; keep MAP within 20% of the patient's baseline.

Intraoperative Measures/Maintenance

The goal is to maintain a slightly decreased CPP to decrease blood loss, and to decrease intracranial volume of blood and tissue for surgical exposure. See Chapter 3 for more information.

Emergence

Give prophylactic antiemetics as necessary to help patients avoid PONV (see Chapter 4).

Postoperative Measures

Once the surgery is completed, cover the patient with warmed blankets to prevent shivering. Elevate the head of the bed to approximately 30 degrees.

Perform a neurologic assessment as soon as the patient can follow commands. The goal is to assess the neurologic status while the patient is still in the operating room. The surgeons would like to evaluate the patient in the immediate postoperative period for complications so they can intervene if needed.

Complications

The olfactory nerve, optic chiasm, optic nerves, and carotid arteries may be injured during this surgery. Hemorrhage and tension pneumocephalus are also possible.

Cranioplasty

Cranioplasty is performed to repair a cranial bone defect. This procedure is done for trauma, fractures, skull/bony tumors, infections, and congenital deformities, and as part of other surgical procedures. It may be used to reduce increased ICP, alleviate pain or seizures from the defect, or for cosmetic reasons.

A cranioplasty is commonly undertaken when a craniectomy has been performed previously, such as in the case of removal of cranial bone if the bone was destroyed/comminuted by trauma or a tumor, or for ICP management. If possible, surgeons will replace the patient's original bone flap if it was removed and stored. It can be stored in a freezer, in a tissue bank, or in the patient's abdominal fat. If the patient's flap is not used, then artificial flaps can be made from autogenous bone grafts (especially in case of infection), titanium mesh, PEEK (poly-ether-ether-ketone), methylmethacrylate, acrylic, mesh, split ribs, and other materials.

Operative Procedure

Local anesthetic with epinephrine is injected in the scalp over the cranial defect to decrease the amount of bleeding, as the scalp tends to be very vascular. The scalp is incised over the defect. The bony defect is excised and smoothed as necessary. If methylmethacrylate is used for reconstruction,

the surgeon molds the material to fit the defect and allows it to harden; bone can also be harvested from the skull, rib, or hip for reconstruction. A craniotome may be used to smooth rough areas.

If an acrylic plate is used to cover the defect, holes are drilled in the periphery of the acrylic plate as well as the defect. The plate is placed over the defect to cover it, and wires are threaded through these holes to secure one to the other.

A drain may be left in the subgaleal space. The skin is then sutured closed.

Anesthetic

General anesthesia is used with an OETT. A pre-formed oral RAE tube or reinforced endotracheal tube may be placed to prevent kinking of the tube with movement and positioning of the patient's head. The head may be placed in head pins. If pins are not placed, muscle relaxation may be needed, check with surgeon before giving relaxation.

Maintain general anesthesia until the patient is in the supine position and the head pins have been removed.

Positioning

The patient may be in a supine, prone, lateral, or sitting position, with arms tucked at the sides. The exact position depends on the tumor location, but the operative side of the head is always in the uppermost position (the head may be turned laterally). The head of the bed is usually increased 15–30 degrees to ensure venous drainage. The head of the operating table may be turned away at least 90 degrees, if not 180 degrees, from the anesthetist.

Anesthetic Implications

Cranioplasty may be done for craniosynostosis. See Chapter 24 for specifics of cranioplasty in the pediatric population

Type and cross the patient's blood.

Patients undergoing cranioplasty require special eye care. Paper tape is used to close the eyes to prevent corneal drying or abrasions; eye pads are then placed over both eyes to protect them. Eye ointment may also be instilled before taping for patients who will remain intubated postoperatively.

Anesthesia Goals for Cranioplasty

Maintain a quiet surgical field. Check with the surgeon before giving muscle relaxants to clarify if nerve monitoring will be needed.

If methylmethacrylate is used, see Chapter 3 for more information.

Patients undergoing cranioplasty may have elevated intracranial pressures and brain relaxation measures may be needed. See Chapter 3 for more information. Lumbar drains are sometimes used for relaxation

Monitor for hemorrhage and maintain a hematocrit greater than 28%. Maintain intravascular volumes with colloids, crystalloids, and/or blood products.

Preoperative Measures

Perform a complete preoperative neurologic assessment and document any deficits.

Preoperative sedation may be necessary to calm the patient; small doses of a benzodiazepine may be used and are preferred for this purpose over opiates (which depress respirations). The patient should not be allowed to hypoventilate (because it increases $PaCO_2$ and vasodilates cerebral arteries) or have sedation amounts that affect neurologic evaluation.

Monitors and IV Access

- Arterial line placement is required to monitor continuous blood pressure. It also readily permits arterial sampling for blood gases and labs.
- Place two large-bore peripheral IV lines.
- CVP may be needed in case urgent fluid resuscitation is required because of extensive blood loss.
- A PA catheter may be needed if the patient has a cardiac history or is hemodynamically unstable.

- Use a precordial Doppler device to monitor for venous air embolism when the patient is in a sitting position (see Chapter 3).

IV Vasoactive Agents

- IV pump: nicardipine (Cardene), sodium nitroprusside (SNP), phenylephrine
- Syringe for bolus: phenylephrine, ephedrine, esmolol (Brevibloc), labetalol, metoprolol
- Other drugs to have available: mannitol, furosemide (Lasix), bumetanide (Bumex), lidocaine, atropine, glycopyrrolate (Robinul), calcium-channel blockers (nimodipine, nicardipine), dexamethasone (Decadron), regular insulin, $D_{50}W$

IV Fluids and Volume Requirements

Give normal saline or lactated Ringer's solution to maintain normovolemia, provide maintenance IVF, and measure urinary output every 30 minutes. Normal saline is more hyperosmolar than lactated Ringer's solution and helps pull fluid out of brain tissue. Colloids, such as albumin or Hextend/Hetastarch, can be given to restore volume deficits and maintain euvolemia. Hetastarch can cause platelet dysfunction and bleeding; do not give more than 20 mL/kg/day (max 1500 mL total).

Hypotonic and glucose solutions should be avoided due to the potential for increased cerebral metabolism and free water build-up, causing intracerebral edema. Don't give D_5W: Once the body utilizes the dextrose, the free water goes to the brain, causing cerebral edema.

Blood Products

Any blood losses should be replaced immediately to keep HCT greater than 28%. Hypothermia can cause platelet dysfunction.

Induction

Use cerebral-protective induction drugs. See Chapter 3 for more information.

Intraoperative Measures/Maintenance

Keep MAP approximately 10% lower than the patient's normal level to help keep bleeding low.

The goal is to maintain a slightly decreased CPP to decrease blood loss, and to decrease intracranial volume of blood and tissue for surgical exposure.

Emergence

Give antiemetics to help patients avoid postoperative nausea and vomiting.

Postoperative Measures

Once the surgery is completed, cover the patient with warmed blankets to prevent shivering. Elevate the head of the bed to approximately 30 degrees.

Perform a neurologic assessment as soon as the patient can follow commands. The goal is to assess the neurologic status while the patient is still in the operating room. The surgeons would like to evaluate the patient in the immediate postoperative period for complications so they can intervene if needed.

Complications

Hemorrhage is a potential complication.

Deep Brain Stimulation: Electrode and Battery Insertion

In deep brain stimulation (DBS), surgical electrodes are inserted into the brain's basal ganglia—the ventral intermedius nucleus in the thalamus—to treat tremors (rhythmic, unintentional, muscle movements of one or more body parts, as with Parkinson's disease) or into the globus pallidus interna or the subthalamic nucleus to treat dystonias (a neurologic movement disorder with sustained muscle contractions or abnormal posture). The electrodes stimulate and inactivate these parts of the brain to stop the tremors or dystonia. Most people with Parkinson's disease will require surgery on both sides of the brain. Indications for this surgery include tremors or dystonia, multiple sclerosis, Parkinson's disease, severe refractory depression, Tourette's syndrome, obsessive–compulsive disorder, and phantom limb pain.

In DBS, electrodes are connected by wires to an impulse generator that is implanted under the skin of the chest, much like a pacemaker battery. Once activated, the generator sends electrical stimulation to targeted areas in the brain, blocking the abnormal nerve signals that cause the tremors. DBS does *not* require destruction of any part of the brain, unlike pallidotomy or thalamotomy. Also, DBS can be programmed on or off using a hand-held magnet or adjusted by a computer that can send radio signals to the device.

Operative Procedure

To start, a stereotactic frame is placed to assist in mapping the target coordinates in an MRI scanner. The patient is then taken to the operating room.

With the stereotactic frame in place, a 14-mm-diameter hole is drilled in the skull, the dura is opened, and a probe is passed down into the deep brain tissues. The electrodes are then inserted. Electrode placement is done under local anesthesia so that the patient can follow commands and give feedback regarding optimal placement. The patient is assessed as different areas are stimulated to monitor for changes or decreases in abnormal movements. Once the correct locations are mapped out, the permanent electrodes are implanted. The pulse generator is calibrated to optimize tremor/dystonia suppression and control side effects.

After the electrodes are successfully placed, the patient is given general anesthesia. An insulated wire is attached to the electrode; it will be tunneled under the skin and subcutaneous tissue from the top of the head, down behind the ear and the side of the neck to the generator.

Subthalamic nucleus stimulation is a new application of the original DBS technique. Stimulation of the subthalamic nucleus has been recognized as the most effective surgical treatment for Parkinson's disease, addressing not only tremors, but also rigidity, slowness of movement, stiffness, and walking concerns. This technique allows patients to slowly reduce their usual medications. The SNS procedure is similar to DBS placement. The operating room may be made dark during the mapping procedure.

Anesthetic

Deep sedation and local anesthesia are necessary for the craniotomy. Lighter sedation is used during electrode testing and placement. Finally, general anesthesia induction is done for tunneling the wire down through the head and neck and pulse generator placement.

Positioning

This procedure is performed with the patient in a supine position.

Anesthetic Implications

Patients will need an arterial line, as this surgery takes an exceedingly long time. Good IV access should be obtained before the drapes go up.

Complications

Potential complications include hemorrhage in the brain, infection, hardware failure, and migration of electrodes.

Evacuation of an Epidural or Subdural Hematoma

An evacuation procedure may be performed to remove a collection of blood that has formed a space-occupying lesion, as a result of an epidural or subdural hematoma. Epidural and subdural hematomas usually have traumatic origins, although they can also occur spontaneously. The majority are supratentorial.

An *epidural hematoma* occurs between the dura of the brain and the skull in a potential space containing mostly arteries. This condition can be deadly because the build-up of blood may increase pressure in the intracranial space and compress delicate brain tissue. The pterion region, which overlies the middle meningeal artery, is exceptionally weak and prone to injury.

In a *subdural hematoma,* blood gathers between the dura and arachnoid mater, in an area containing mostly veins. Unlike with epidural hematomas, subdural bleeding usually results from tears from a shearing force in trauma. Normally, a subdural hematoma is a "venous bleed" in older people who fall; these patients typically exhibit atrophy of the brain and stretching of the veins of the subdural space. This bleeding often separates the dura and the arachnoid layers. Subdural hemorrhages may cause an increase in intracranial pressure, which can cause compression of and damage to the brain tissue. Subdural hematomas may be acute, subacute, or chronic.

An epidural hematoma or even an acute subdural hematoma can have a high mortality rate and is frequently considered a neurosurgical emergency.

Operative Procedure

The skin is incised and reflected, and the cranium is opened. The hematoma is evacuated through a craniotomy (for acute bleeding) or a burr hole (for a chronic hematoma) into the skull. The clot is aspirated to remove the mass and reduce the pressure (a hematoma is a pressure problem, not a volume problem) it puts on the brain.

If an epidural hematoma has occurred, the neurosurgeon not only decompresses the hematoma, but also must stop any further bleeding by ligating or coagulating the injured vessel branches. If there is swelling of the brain tissue, the skull bone may need to be left off (frozen for later use) and the dura closed to protect the brain.

An ICP monitor/ventriculostomy catheter may be placed to monitor ICP levels postoperatively.

Anesthetic

General anesthesia, OETT; muscle relaxation may be needed; check with the surgeon before giving relaxation. Maintain general anesthesia until the patient is in the supine position and the head pins have been removed.

A pre-formed oral RAE tube or reinforced endotracheal tube may be placed to prevent kinking of the tube with movement and positioning of the patient's head.

Positioning

The exact position of the patient depends on hematoma location, but the affected side of the cranium is always placed in the uppermost position (the head may be turned laterally). The patient may be in a supine, lateral, prone, or sitting position, with arms tucked at the sides. The head of the bed is usually increased 15–30 degrees to ensure venous drainage. The head of the operating table may be turned away at least 90 degrees, if not 180 degrees, from the anesthetist.

Anesthetic Implications

These patients may have suffered a traumatic injury and intracranial hypertension may be present with serious neurologic disruption.

Patients undergoing evacuation of an epidural or subdural hematoma require special eye care. Paper tape is used to close the eyes to prevent corneal drying or abrasions; eye pads are then placed over both eyes to protect them. Eye ointment may also be instilled before taping for patients who will remain intubated postoperatively.

See Chapter 2 for more on procedures performed with the patient in a sitting position and cerebral perfusion pressure and transducer levels. See Chapter 3 for information about the potential for embolism.

Anesthesia Goals for Evacuation of Epidural or Subdural Hematoma

The goal is to maintain a slightly decreased CPP to decrease blood loss, and to decrease intracranial volume of blood and tissue for surgical exposure. Patients undergoing hematoma evacuation may have elevated intracranial pressures and brain relaxation measures may be needed (see Chapter 3).

Preoperative Measures

Perform a complete preoperative neurologic assessment and document any deficits.

Preoperative sedation may be necessary to calm the patient; small doses of a benzodiazepine may be used and are preferred for this purpose over opiates (which depress respirations). The patient should not be allowed to hypoventilate (because it increases $PaCO_2$ and vasodilates cerebral arteries) or have sedation amounts that affect neurologic evaluation.

Monitors and IV Access

- Arterial line placement is required to monitor continuous blood pressure. It also readily permits arterial sampling for blood gases and labs.
- Place two large-bore peripheral IV lines.
- CVP may be needed in case urgent fluid resuscitation is required because of extensive blood loss.
- A PA catheter may be needed if the patient has a cardiac history or is hemodynamically unstable.
- Use a precordial Doppler device to monitor for venous air embolism when the patient is placed in a sitting position (see Chapter 3).

IV Vasoactive Agents

- IV pump: nicardipine (Cardene), sodium nitroprusside (SNP), phenylephrine
- Syringe for bolus: phenylephrine, ephedrine, esmolol (Brevibloc), labetalol, metoprolol
- Other drugs to have available: mannitol, furosemide (Lasix), bumetanide (Bumex), lidocaine, atropine, glycopyrrolate (Robinul), calcium-channel blockers (nimodipine, nicardipine), dexamethasone (Decadron), regular insulin, $D_{50}W$

IV Fluids and Volume Requirements

Give normal saline or lactated Ringer's solution to maintain normovolemia, maintenance IVF plus urinary output, and measure urinary output every 30 minutes. Normal saline is more hyperosmolar than lactated Ringer's solution and helps pull fluid out of brain tissue. Colloids, such as albumin or

Hextend/Hetastarch, can be given to restore volume deficits and maintain euvolemia. Hetastarch can cause platelet dysfunction and bleeding; do not give more than 20 mL/kg/day (max 1500 mL total).

Hypotonic and glucose solutions should be avoided due to the potential for increased cerebral metabolism and free water build-up, causing intracerebral edema. Don't give D_5W: Once the body utilizes the dextrose, the free water goes to the brain, causing cerebral edema.

Blood Products
Any blood losses should be replaced immediately to keep HCT greater than 28%. Hypothermia can cause platelet dysfunction.

Pre-induction Measures
Preoperative sedation may be necessary to calm the patient; small doses of a benzodiazepine may be used and are preferred for this purpose over opiates (which depress respirations). The patient should not be allowed to hypoventilate (because it increases $PaCO_2$ and vasodilates cerebral arteries) or have sedation amounts that affect neurologic evaluation.

Induction
Use cerebral-protective induction drugs. See Chapter 3 for more information.

Intraoperative Measures/Maintenance
The goal is to maintain a slightly decreased CPP to decrease blood loss, and to decrease intracranial volume of blood and tissue for surgical exposure.

Emergence
Give prophylactic antiemetics as necessary to help patients avoid PONV (see Chapter 4).

Postoperative Measures
Once the surgery is completed, cover the patient with warmed blankets to prevent shivering. Elevate the head of the bed to approximately 30 degrees.

Perform a neurologic assessment as soon as the patient can follow commands. The goal is to assess the neurologic status while the patient is still in the operating room. The surgeons would like to evaluate the patient in the immediate postoperative period for complications so they can intervene if needed.

Complications
Potential complications include elevated ICP and brain herniation, cranial nerve injury, infection, CSF leak, and neurologic injury.

Hypophysectomy
Hypophysectomy is the excision or destruction of all or a portion of the pituitary gland. It may be performed in case of endocrine disorders, primary tumors of the pituitary, hormonally dependent metastatic breast and prostatic carcinoma, or Cushing's syndrome (elevated levels of cortisol).

The pituitary gland normally sits within the sella turcica at the bottom of the hypothalamus, covered by a dural fold. These tumors are usually found because of the effects of hypersecretion of pituitary hormones or from local symptoms from enlarging lesions. Some pituitary adenomas are hormone-secreting masses that cause side effects; one common side effect of a hypophysectomy is diabetes insipidus, which is treated with vasopressin (Pitressin). Thyroid-stimulating hormone (TSH), follicle-stimulating hormone (FSH), and luteinizing hormones (LH) can be produced by pituitary adenomas as well. Adrenocorticotropic hormone (ACTH) secretion causes Cushing's disease, which in turn leads to hyperaldosteronism, hypertension, hypokalemia, metabolic alkalosis, and congestive heart failure. Growth-stimulating hormone (GSH) can cause gigantism or cretinism that can create airway abnormalities.

Operative Procedure
The approach to the pituitary may be by frontal craniotomy, transsphenoidal approach, or stereotaxic approach.

A *frontal craniotomy* is indicated for large and complex masses and involves a bifrontal incision, opening the skull and lifting the frontal lobe of the brain to expose the pituitary gland. At least 90% of the gland must be removed to achieve the desired results. The total gland (by frontal craniotomy) is removed primarily for the palliative effects on metastatic breast or prostate cancer. *The surgical excision of the pituitary gland in total is a drastic surgery that has largely been abandoned in light of multiple new approaches that can remove the tumor while at least partially preserving the gland.*

There are several approaches to the pituitary that lies directly behind the nose; access is often through the nose or sinuses. Two less invasive and common approaches for hypophysectomy include the transsphenoidal and stereotaxic techniques.

Transsphenoidal hypophysectomy involves a direct approach to the sella turcica. Transsphenoidal tumor resection is done for pituitary tumors that do not have extension outside the sella turcica or growth into the optic nerve. Several approaches can be employed following intubation.

The nasal cavity and gums are infiltrated with local anesthesia containing epinephrine to minimize blood loss. A horizontal incision is made under the upper lip and extended over the maxilla; the surgeon continues through the nasal septum into the nasal cavity. The roof of the sphenoidal sinus is exposed and incised to enter through the floor of the sella turcica.

More recently, many neurosurgeons have chosen go through the nose and through the sphenoid os into the sphenoid sinus. An ENT surgeon may work along with the neurosurgeon: The ENT surgeon creates access to the nasal cavity and closes the wound after the neurosurgeon removes the tumor and repairs the dura.

Fluoroscopy confirms the position of the instruments; care is taken not to penetrate the posterior wall of the sella. Structures at risk include the frontal lobes of the brain, bilateral carotids, and the optic chiasm.

The dura is incised (durotomy), and care is taken not to disturb the gland. Scissors or a knife may be used to sever the stalk. A blunt dissector

frees the remainder of the gland from its dural attachment, and the gland is removed intact. Gelfoam soaked in thrombin can be used to control oozing. A patch of fascia and muscle can be excised (from the patient's thigh) and packed into the empty sella. A segment of previously excised cartilaginous nasal septum is used to seal the muscle plug to the floor of the sella. Nasal packing approximates the nasal mucosa, and the gingival incision is closed with absorbable suture.

Another hypophysectomy approach is *stereotaxic hypophysectomy.* With this technique, the patient's head is secured in a stereotaxic frame (the frame can be placed with local anesthesia). The patient undergoes a CAT scan and vascular angiography so that pituitary mapping can be done. With an integrated system controlled by computers, the patient, with the frame still on, is positioned in surgery. A drill is used to perforate the sphenoid sinus and the floor of the sella turcica. By three-dimensional aiming technique, a cryoprobe is then placed in the sella turcica with pinpoint accuracy and cryodestruction is done. Stereotaxy can be used to direct radiation with extreme precision using a gamma knife. Once the probe is removed, a silicone plug is placed in the sellar opening to prevent cerebrospinal fluid leakage.

Anesthetic

General anesthesia, OETT; muscle relaxants are needed. Carefully secure the endotracheal tube, as the surgeon will be working around the mouth and face during surgery. A pre-formed oral RAE tube or reinforced endotracheal tube may be placed to prevent kinking of the tube with movement and positioning of the patient's head.

Positioning

The patient is positioned supine, with arms tucked at the sides; he or she may be in a beach-chair position, with the head of the bed elevated 30–45 degrees the patient's legs slightly flexed. The head of the operating table may be turned away at least 90 degrees, if not 180 degrees, from the anesthetist.

Anesthetic Implications

Type and cross the patient's blood.

Patients undergoing hypophysectomy require special eye care. Paper tape is used to close the eyes to prevent corneal drying or abrasions; eye pads are then placed over both eyes to protect them. Eye ointment may also be instilled before taping for patients who will remain intubated postoperatively.

Local anesthetic with epinephrine will be infiltrated locally to help decrease bleeding. Monitor the EKG for ST-segment changes or tachycardia.

Hypopituitary function is possible. Prophylactic glucocorticoid administration can be given, consisting of hydrocortisone 100 mg IV once (see Chapter 4).

Monitor urinary output every 30 minutes, checking for increased urinary output that would indicate diabetes insipidus.

The patient will have nasal packing placed by the surgeon at the end of the case. Postoperative oxygen delivery is given by face mask or face tent.

These patients may develop an accumulation of blood in the pharynx and stomach. For this reason, it is necessary to carefully suction the stomach and the oropharynx (by orogastric tube) at the end of the case.

Anesthesia Goals for Hypophysectomy

Preoperative Measures

Perform a complete preoperative neurologic assessment and document any deficits. Labs and tests should include sodium and other electrolytes, CBC, and EKG.

Monitors and IV Access

- Arterial line placement is required to monitor continuous blood pressure. It also readily permits arterial sampling for blood gases and labs.
- Place two large-bore peripheral IV lines.

- CVP may be needed in case urgent fluid resuscitation is required because of extensive blood loss.
- A PA catheter may be needed if the patient has a cardiac history or is hemodynamically unstable.
- Use a precordial Doppler device for venous air embolism monitoring if the patient is placed in a sitting position.
- Visual evoked-potential monitoring may be done if optic nerves are involved.

IV Vasoactive Agents

- IV pump: nicardipine (Cardene), sodium nitroprusside (SNP), phenylephrine
- Syringe for bolus: phenylephrine, ephedrine, esmolol (Brevibloc), labetalol, metoprolol
- Other drugs to have available: DDAVP/vasopressin, mannitol, furosemide (Lasix), bumetanide (Bumex), lidocaine, atropine, glycopyrrolate (Robinul), calcium-channel blockers (nimodipine, nicardipine), dexamethasone (Decadron), regular insulin, $D_{50}W$

IV Fluids and Volume Requirements

Give normal saline or lactated Ringer's solution to maintain normovolemia, maintenance IVF plus urinary output, and measure urinary output every 30 minutes. Normal saline is more hyperosmolar than lactated Ringer's solution and helps pull fluid out of brain tissue. Colloids, such as albumin or Hextend/Hetastarch, can be given to restore volume deficits and maintain euvolemia. Hetastarch can cause platelet dysfunction and bleeding; do not give more than 20 mL/kg/day (max 1500 mL total).

Hypotonic and glucose solutions should be avoided due to the potential for increased cerebral metabolism and free water build-up, causing intracerebral edema. Don't give D_5W: Once the body utilizes the dextrose, the free water goes to the brain, causing cerebral edema.

Blood Products

Keep HCT greater than 28%. Any blood losses should be replaced immediately. Hypothermia can cause platelet dysfunction.

Pre-induction Measures

Preoperative sedation may be necessary to calm the patient; small doses of a benzodiazepine may be used and are preferred for this purpose over opiates (which depress respirations). The patient should not be allowed to hypoventilate (because it increases $PaCO_2$ and vasodilates cerebral arteries) or have sedation amounts that affect neurologic evaluation.

Induction

Use cerebral-protective induction drugs. See Chapter 3 for more information.

Intraoperative Measures/Maintenance

Brain relaxation and cerebral protection may be needed.

Emergence

Give prophylactic antiemetics as necessary to help patients avoid PONV (see Chapter 4). These patients have increased incidence of postoperative nausea and vomiting.

Postoperative Measures

Once the surgery is completed, cover the patient with warmed blankets to prevent shivering. Elevate the head of the bed by approximately 30 degrees.

Perform a neurologic assessment as soon as the patient can follow commands. The goal is to assess the neurologic status while the patient is still in the operating room. The surgeons would like to evaluate the patient in the immediate postoperative period for complications so they can intervene if needed.

Complications

Potential complications include injury to the frontal lobes of the brain, cranial nerves, bilateral carotids, and the optic chiasm with vision loss; diabetes insipidus; sinusitis; CSF leak; epistaxis; meningitis; and hemorrhage.

Craniotomy for Intracranial Aneurysm

Craniotomy for intracranial aneurysm treatment involves opening of the skull to secure a cerebral arterial aneurysm. Intracranial aneurysms occur at major bifurcations on the arteries at the base of the brain in the circle of Willis—commonly in the anterior communicating artery (ACA), posterior communicating artery (PCA), or middle cerebral artery (MCA). The aneurysm may be intact or has already ruptured. The most important surgical considerations include clinical presentation, aneurysm size and location, patient age and neurological status, and medical comorbidities.

Operative Procedure

In these cases, patients have an arterial dilation secondary to muscle weakness in a vessel wall prone to rupture. Generally, a pterional craniotomy is used to approach anterior circulation aneurysms. A subtemporal or a suboccipital exposure is used to approach posterior circulation aneurysms. Intraoperative angiography may be done.

In an open aneurysm repair where the aneurysm has *not* ruptured, keep blood pressure low to prevent rupture of the aneurysm. Temporary clips may be placed on the major feeding vessel to help prevent inadvertent rupture of the aneurysm. While the feeder vessel is clipped, it is important to keep the blood pressure in the normal-high range (increase blood pressure 20% to 30% above baseline) to provide adequate collateral cerebral circulation. Phenylephrine (Neosynephrine) is the preferred vasoactive drug to increase MAP (see Chapter 3).

The most common surgical treatment involves microsurgical clip ligation. Using a microscope, the surgeon identifies the parent vessel feeding the aneurysm; a clip is placed across the aneurysm neck, eliminating the flow of blood into the aneurysm.

Anesthetic

General anesthesia, OETT, and muscle relaxants. Carefully secure the endotracheal tube, as the surgeon will be working around the mouth and face during surgery. A pre-formed oral RAE tube or reinforced endotracheal tube may be placed to prevent kinking of the tube with movement and positioning of the patient's head.

Maintain general anesthesia until the patient is in the supine position and the head pins have been removed.

Positioning

The patient may be positioned supine, sitting, or lateral away from the aneurysm; the head may be placed in Mayfield tongs. The patient's head is turned to the side away from aneurysm. See Chapter 2 for more information on patient positioning.

The exact position depends on the aneurysm location, although the operative side of the head is always in the uppermost position. The head of the bed is usually increased 15–30 degrees to ensure venous drainage. The head of the operating table may be turned away at least 90 degrees, if not 180 degrees, from the anesthetist.

Anesthetic Implications

Consider modest, passive hypothermia (approximately 35°C) for neuroprotection. Avoid hyperthermia.

Muscle relaxation is crucial: Patient movement would be disastrous.

These patients require special eye care. Paper tape is used to close the eyes to prevent corneal drying or abrasions; eye pads are then placed over both eyes to protect them. Eye ointment may also be instilled before taping for patients who will remain intubated postoperatively.

Anesthesia Goals for Craniotomy for Intracranial Aneurysm

"Slow and controlled" induction and emergence are ideal; these anesthesia process must be smooth, with minimal changes in blood pressure occurring. Minimize the transmural pressure gradient (TMP), so as to minimize the stress on the aneurysm and decrease the risk of rupture. Hypotension can cause ischemic changes in underperfused areas, whereas hypertension can rupture the aneurysm or worsen the cerebral hypertension. Avoid stress:

It can increase CMR and increase CBF. Control of blood pressure is crucial for a successful conclusion to a case. Prior to clipping, stability and avoidance of hypertension should be the goals to avoid further bleeding or prevent rupture.

Avoid hyperglycemia, which worsens cerebral ischemia, and hypo-osmolarity, which can increase brain edema.

Preoperative Measures
- Check if the patient has allergies to shellfish or IV iodine, as intraoperative angiography may be done.
- Perform a baseline neurologic assessment. Note the pupil size and reaction to light, presence or absence of vocal/motor deficits, patient's ability to verbalize and understand instructions, ability to follow commands, and Glasgow Coma Scale score. Document these findings.
- Know the location and size of the aneurysm and the patient's ICP. Has there been bleeding from the aneurysm? Have the patient's CT, angiogram films, or MRI results available in the operating room.
- Complete a thorough airway examination to assess ease of intubation.
- Know the patient's baseline cuff blood pressure and keep blood pressures within 20% of normal. Wide swings in blood pressure should be avoided.
- Have a 12-lead EKG report.
- Complete preoperative labs: H&H, platelets, PT/INR/PTT, glucose levels and electrolytes, LFT (hepatic dysfunction can occur after subarachnoid hemorrhage).

Pre-induction Measures
Preoperative sedation may be necessary to calm the patient; small doses of a benzodiazepine may be used and are preferred for this purpose over opiates (which depress respirations). The patient should not be allowed to hypoventilate (because it increases $PaCO_2$ and vasodilates cerebral arteries) or have sedation amounts that affect neurologic evaluation.

Monitors and IV Access
Along with the standard monitoring, make the following preparations:

- Arterial line placement is required to monitor continuous blood pressure. It also readily permits arterial sampling for blood gases and labs (see Chapter 2).
- Place one or two large-bore peripheral IV lines.
- CVP is needed in case urgent fluid resuscitation is required because of extensive blood loss or with VAE precautions.
- A PA catheter may be needed if the patient has a cardiac history or is hemodynamically unstable.
- SSEP, EEG, or BAER (especially with posterior fossa aneurysm resection) may be utilized.
- Use a precordial Doppler device to monitor for venous air embolism while the patient is in a sitting position (see Chapter 3).

IV Vasoactive Agents
- IV pump: nicardipine (Cardene), sodium nitroprusside (SNP), phenylephrine
- Syringe for bolus: phenylephrine, ephedrine, esmolol (Brevibloc), labetalol, metoprolol
- Other drugs to have available: DDAVP, Pitressin, mannitol, furosemide (Lasix), bumetanide (Bumex), lidocaine, atropine, glycopyrrolate (Robinul), calcium-channel blockers (nimodipine, nicardipine), dexamethasone (Decadron), regular insulin, $D_{50}W$

IV Fluids and Volume Requirements
Give normal saline or lactated Ringer's solution to maintain normovolemia, maintenance IVF plus urinary output, and measure urinary output every 30 minutes. Normal saline is more hyperosmolar than lactated Ringer's solution and helps pull fluid out of brain tissue. Colloids, such as albumin or Hextend/Hetastarch, can be given to restore volume deficits and maintain euvolemia. Hetastarch can cause platelet dysfunction and bleeding; do not give more than 20 mL/kg/day (max 1500 mL total).

Hypotonic and glucose solutions should be avoided due to the potential for increased cerebral metabolism and free water build-up, causing intracerebral edema. Don't give D_5W: Once the body utilizes the dextrose, the free water goes to the brain, causing cerebral edema.

Blood Products
Any blood losses should be replaced immediately to keep HCT greater than 28%. Hypothermia can cause platelet dysfunction.

Suggested Induction
- Thiopental 2–5 mg/kg or propofol 1–2 mg/kg for general anesthesia induction; thiopental may also be used for neuroprotection. Provide burst suppression guided by EEG monitoring.
- Succinylcholine (Anectine) 1–2 mg/kg, vecuronium 0.15 mg/kg, rocuronium 1.0 mg/kg, or pancuronium 0.1 mg/kg can be used. Good muscle relaxation is essential.
- Rupture of an aneurysm is often caused by sympathetic surges occurring with intubation and skin incision. Use opioids to facilitate a smooth induction and blunt response to intubation and head pins (if placed). Fentanyl 7–10 mcg/kg and/or Remifentanil 0.5–1 mcg/kg/min can be used. An additional Remifentanil dose of 1 mcg/kg may be administered over 30–60 seconds with application of head pins. The use of opioids, beta blockers, and Stage 3 anesthetics is recommended to avoid spikes in the patient's blood pressure.
- Consider anticonvulsant treatment if not already initiated: Dilantin (phenytoin) 10–15 mg/kg over 30 minutes.

Intraoperative Measures/Maintenance
Maintenance anesthesia is highly individualized. The goal is to preserve adequate cerebral perfusion, control brain tension via CBF and CMR, provide neuroprotection, and control ICP. Be prepared for aneurysm rupture (see Chapter 3).

IV Infusions with Inhaled Agents
- Nitrous oxide 66% with Remifentanil 0.4 mcg/kg/min. *The use of nitrous oxide in cerebral surgery is controversial.*

- Isoflurane at 0.7 (approximately ½ MAC) with Remifentanil 0.25 mcg/kg/min.
- Propofol 100–200 mcg/kg/min with Remifentanil 0.25 mcg/kg/min.
- TIVA (propofol and opioid) or TIVA with 0.5 MAC.
- If evoked-potential monitoring is used, give less than 0.3 MAC or do not use a volatile agent.
- Isoflurane at 1 MAC. *Do not use Enflurane.*

Prior to clipping, decrease MAP to 20% of baseline with controlled hypotension. Avoid a MAP less than 80 mm Hg.

During clipping, increase blood pressure to 20% to 30% of baseline. Phenylephrine (Neosynephrine) is the preferred drug for increasing MAP. A slight blood pressure increases help with collateral circulation.

Post clipping, the MAP should be kept between 80 and 110 mm Hg. Precise control of blood pressure is important; maintain MAP in the normal-high range.

Emergence

Emergence from anesthesia should be smooth and controlled. Short-acting opioids should be used to facilitate a rapid emergence to allow for a full neurological exam as soon as possible following surgery. Beta blocker or arterial dilator titration may be necessary to stabilize the patient's blood pressure and heart rate. When the patient is spontaneously breathing, consider extubating the patient while still on the Remifentanil infusion, and then turn off the infusion.

The head of the bed should be raised by approximately 30 degrees during transport to the ICU. Monitor the patient's heart rate, blood pressure, and pulse oximetry during transport. Prevent shivering.

Blood pressure is lowered during microscopic dissection of the aneurysm. This *controlled hypotension* is utilized to decrease TMP across the aneurysm wall, which reduces the risk of rupture and decreases the potential for bleeding. Also, it allows for better visualization of the anatomy of the aneurysm and perforating vessels. Before controlled hypotension is induced, adequate intravascular volume with optimal viscosity and O_2 delivery should be obtained. In controlled hypotension, keep SBP in the range of 80–90 mm Hg and MAP in the range of 50–65 mm Hg. Any of the following agents may be used to induce hypotension: trimethaphan; propranolol; esmolol (Brevibloc); nicardipine; prostaglandin E_1; direct-acting vasodilating drugs such as sodium nitroprusside, nitroglycerin, or hydralazine (Apresoline); alpha- and beta-adrenergic receptor blockers (e.g., labetalol); Isoflurane. Be aware that controlled hypotension can increase incidence of vasospasm.

Give prophylactic antiemetics as necessary to help patients avoid PONV (see Chapter 4). Retching will dramatically increase the patient's blood pressure.

Postoperative Measures

Once the surgery is completed, cover the patient with warmed blankets to prevent shivering. Elevate the head of the bed by approximately 30 degrees.

Perform a neurologic assessment as soon as the patient can follow commands. The goal is to assess the neurologic status while the patient is still in the operating room. The surgeons would like to evaluate the patient in the immediate postoperative period for complications so they can intervene if needed.

Cerebral Aneurysmal Rupture

Preoperative rupture of cerebral aneurysm may lead to subarachnoid hemorrhage (SAH). In fact, aneurysm rupture into the subarachnoid space is the most common clinical presentation of the presence of an aneurysm. The hallmark sign is eye hemorrhage. While the primary hemorrhage is serious enough, rebleeding is usually more devastating in its effect on the brain tissues.

The *Hunt and Hess clinical grading system* is frequently used to categorize severity of a subarachnoid hemorrhage:

Grade 1 = asymptomatic, or mild headache and slight nuchal rigidity

Grade 2 = cranial nerve palsy, moderate to severe headache, nuchal rigidity

Grade 3 = mild focal deficit, lethargy or confusion

Grade 4 = stupor, moderate to severe hemiparesis, early decerebrate rigidity

Grade 5 = deep coma, decerebrate rigidity, moribund appearance

Knowing the grade helps to give the anesthetist an idea of how the patient will wake up and if he or she can be extubated. Patients with a Grade 4 or 5 SAH will be kept intubated; those with SAHs of other grades may or may not be extubated.

Subarachnoid Hemorrhage Medical Management

The goal is to prevent vasospasm or management of a vasospasm if it occurs. Vasospasm usually occurs 3 to 7 days after SAH occurs. Signs and symptoms include a change in the level of consciousness, worsening neurologic deficits, EKG changes (T-wave inversion and ST-segment changes) due to catecholamine surge.

Treatment consists of giving nimodipine as the first-line treatment. Nimodipine is a calcium-channel blocker and an arterial vasodilator; it is generally given prophylactically when SAH is suspected.

Triple-H (hypervolemic, hypertensive, and hemodilution therapy) treatment is used to improve blood flow to the collateral circulation and reduce ischemia.

Hypervolemia is used to achieve and maintain CVP 10–12, primarily with colloids.

Hypertension is induced in SAH. Take the patient's blood pressure to the highest level ordered, usually MAP 100–120 mm Hg. Higher pressure is needed because cerebral autoregulation is impaired after SAH. Induced hypertension is only done after an aneurysm has been clipped or has already burst; done to help prevent the vessel from going into vasospasm.

Hemodilution is used to bring the patient's hematocrit to 30% (ideal).

Subarachnoid Hemorrhage Surgical Management:

As part of preoperative care, place an arterial line as soon as possible to monitor and control blood pressure. Keep the patient as calm as possible if he or she is still conscious; a clot is sitting at the aneurysm, and a higher blood pressure will blow the clot off.

Hydrocephalus, from increased ICP, may need to be treated with a ventriculostomy to drain the CSF and monitor ICP.

Endovascular coiling in the radiology suite is becoming the preferred method of treating a ruptured aneurysm. This procedure is usually attempted before surgery is done, typically within 72 hours after the SAH occurs. If the aneurysm is coiled, it is not followed by surgery in general, but rather is then considered "treated."

Not all aneurysms can be approached this way. Many factors dictate whether it can be coiled, but the location and size of the aneurysm neck are the main considerations. An aneurysm with a large neck will not hold coils, although many leading centers will now stent a large neck aneurysm and insert coils through the neck stent into the aneurysm, using the stent to hold the coils.

Anesthetic Implications of Subarachnoid Hemorrhage

In patients whose aneurysms have ruptured, treatment must address hemodynamics, blood pressure control, and brain muscle relaxation. Healthcare providers must also address complications of the SAH. To prevent occurrence of rebleeding or ischemic consequences, it may be necessary to provide for early surgery to remove SAH blood so as to prevent tissue irritation, intrathecal thrombolytic treatment to lyse subarachnoid blood, calcium-channel blockers to prevent vasospasm, and anticonvulsant therapy (blood in brain tissue is an irritant and can cause seizures). SAH causes release of norepinephrine from the adrenal medulla, which in turn increases afterload and causes direct myocardial toxicity, leading to subendocardial ischemia; for this reason, healthcare providers should watch for EKG abnormalities.

Once the aneurysm is clipped, initiate triple-H therapy: hypervolemia, hypertension, and hemodilution. According to the literature, triple-H therapy does not provide any benefit if it is initiated before spasm occurs; thus it is generally not used until signs of spasm are seen. Spasm will happen radiographically in 70% of patients, but far fewer actually develop symptoms.

Intraoperative Rupture of Cerebral Aneurysm

If there is a sudden change in the patient's hemodynamics, such as hypertension and tachycardia, suspect aneurysm rupture. If the aneurysm ruptures, decrease MAP to 40–50 mm Hg until the surgeon gains control of the bleeding; temporary compression (2–3 minutes) of bilateral carotid arteries may be necessary to help with control of hemorrhage.

While bleeding is not controlled:

- Decrease MAP to 50 mm Hg.
- Give thiopental or etomidate IVP for cerebral protection.
- Provide blood/fluid resuscitation to maintain MAP at 50 mm Hg.

After control of hemorrhage is achieved, hypertension is needed to perfuse cerebral collateral circulation (CPP and other vital organs). If proximal or distal vessel occlusion is possible, use the following measures to maintain perfusion:

- Thiopental 5–6 mg/kg or etomidate 4–5 mg/kg for cerebral protection
- Blood/fluid resuscitation
- Normotension, to ensure collateral circulation

Postoperative analgesia may consist of Remifentanil 0.1 mcg/kg/min.

Craniotomy for Meningioma

Meningiomas include vascular tumors of the protective covering of the brain, otherwise known as the meninges. They can occur both supratentorially and infratentorially, but occur outside the brain parenchyma (extra-axial). Meningiomas are commonly found at the surface of the brain, either over the convexity or at the skull base.

Commons signs and symptoms of meningiomas include headaches, seizures, mental status changes, paresis, and memory impairment. If an elevated ICP is present, patients may also present with nausea, vomiting, and pupil changes.

Operative Procedure

Staged resection may be done for very large meningiomas. Neurointerventional angiography and embolization may have been used preoperatively to decrease the risk of hemorrhage.

In a craniotomy, the skin is incised and reflected, and the cranium is opened. Meningiomas involve the dura (they are tumors of cap cells), so the dura should be resected and a graft placed. The arterial feeders to the meningioma are clipped/coagulated, and then the surgeon carefully dissects the meningioma away from the brain parenchyma/arachnoid mater. Bleeding is controlled and hemostasis ensured, the cranium is closed, and the skin is sutured or stapled closed.

Anesthetic

Healthcare providers may provide GETA inserting an OETT, and giving short-acting muscle relaxants for intubation and patient positioning. The effects of the muscle relaxant should be gone prior to the need to monitor nerve function in neurophysiologic monitoring.

Carefully secure the endotracheal tube, as the surgeon will be working around the head during surgery. A pre-formed oral RAE tube or reinforced endotracheal tube may be placed to prevent kinking of the tube with movement and positioning of the patient's head.

Maintain general anesthesia until the patient is in the supine position and the head pins have been removed.

Positioning

The patient may be placed in a supine, sitting, or lateral position, with the head in Mayfield tongs or pins; arms are tucked at the sides. The patient's head is turned to the side away from the meningioma; the operative side of the head is in the uppermost position. The head of the bed may be raised 15–30 degrees to ensure venous drainage. The head of the operating table may be turned away at least 90 degrees, if not 180 degrees, from the anesthetist. See Chapter 2 for more on patient positioning and cerebral perfusion pressure and transducer levels.

Anesthetic Implications

Patients undergoing craniotomy require special eye care. Paper tape is used to close the eyes to prevent corneal drying or abrasions; eye pads are then placed over both eyes to protect them. Eye ointment may also be instilled before taping for patients who will remain intubated postoperatively.

Increased ICP can be seen. In such cases, a ventriculostomy may be inserted.

Anesthesia Goals for Craniotomy for Meningioma Resection

Preoperative Measures

Perform a thorough preoperative neurologic assessment and document any deficits. Antiepileptic medications and corticosteroids should have been started before supratentorial meningioma resection begins.

Monitors and IV Access

- Arterial line placement is required to monitor continuous blood pressure. It also readily permits arterial sampling for blood gases and labs.
- Place two large-bore peripheral IV lines.
- CVP may be needed in case urgent fluid resuscitation is required because of extensive blood loss.
- A PA catheter may be needed if the patient has a cardiac history or is hemodynamically unstable.

- VAE monitoring may be necessary, especially if these is bone involvement with meningioma resection (see Chapter 3).

IV Vasoactive Agents

- IV pump: nicardipine (Cardene), sodium nitroprusside (SNP), phenylephrine
- Syringe for bolus: phenylephrine, ephedrine, esmolol (Brevibloc), labetalol, metoprolol
- Other drugs to have available: mannitol, furosemide (Lasix), bumetanide (Bumex), lidocaine, atropine, glycopyrrolate (Robinul), calcium-channel blockers (nimodipine, nicardipine), dexamethasone (Decadron) or other steroids, phenytoin, regular insulin, $D_{50}W$

IV Fluids and Volume Requirements

Give normal saline or lactated Ringer's solution to maintain normovolemia, maintenance IVF plus urinary output, and measure urinary output every 30 minutes. Normal saline is more hyperosmolar than lactated Ringer's solution and helps pull fluid out of brain tissue. Colloids, such as albumin or Hextend/Hetastarch, can be given to restore volume deficits and maintain euvolemia. Hetastarch can cause platelet dysfunction and bleeding; do not give more than 20 mL/kg/day (max 1500 mL total).

Hypotonic and glucose solutions should be avoided due to the potential for increased cerebral metabolism and free water build-up, causing intracerebral edema. Don't give D_5W: Once the body utilizes the dextrose, the free water goes to the brain, causing cerebral edema.

Blood Products

Any blood losses should be replaced immediately to keep HCT greater than 28%. Meningiomas produce a tissue plasminogen activator that leads to significant excessive fibrinolysis and can induce hemorrhage during surgery.

Pre-induction Measures

Preoperative sedation may be necessary to calm the patient; small doses of a benzodiazepine may be used and are preferred for this purpose over opiates (which depress respirations). The patient should not be allowed to hypoventilate (because it increases $PaCO_2$ and vasodilates cerebral arteries) or have sedation amounts that affect neurologic evaluation.

Induction

A "slow and controlled" induction is necessary: It must be smooth, with minimal changes in blood pressure occurring. Maintain CPP and MAP so as to provide adequate perfusion of brain tissue.

Intraoperative Measures/Maintenance

The goal is to maintain a slightly decreased CPP to decrease blood loss, and to decrease intracranial volume of blood and tissue for surgical exposure. See Chapter 3 for more information.

Emergence

Give prophylactic antiemetics as necessary to help patients avoid PONV (see Chapter 4).

Postoperative Measures

Once the surgery is completed, cover the patient with warmed blankets to prevent shivering. Elevate the head of the bed to approximately 30 degrees.

Perform a neurologic assessment as soon as the patient can follow commands. The goal is to assess the neurologic status while the patient is still in the operating room. The surgeons would like to evaluate the patient in the immediate postoperative period for complications so they can intervene if needed.

Complications

Potential complications include hemorrhage, neurologic dysfunction, and infection.

Neurointerventional Procedures (Interventional Neuroradiology)

Neurointerventional techniques are employed to perform endovascular diagnostic and surgical procedures within blood vessels and spinal vertebrae. Multiple types of procedures can be performed through an endovascular approach; access is gained through the blood vessels using very small catheters and wires guided by X-rays.

Neurointerventional procedures may be undertaken to identify the blood supply to a brain tumor, arteriovenous malformations, or aneurysm, usually accompanied by an attempt to inject an AVM with embolizing material, or to open the vessel involved with an embolic stroke. Endovascular treatments are rapidly becoming the preferred option for disorders of the blood vessels of the head and neck, including aneurysms, AVMs, and tumors; they are also the main treatment for pathologies such as carotid–cavernous fistulas.

Neurolytic techniques use a variety of agents to destroy nerves or neural structures: chemicals (glycerol, alcohol, or phenol), heat (radiofrequency coagulation), or cold (cryotherapy). Glycerol is a neurotoxic alcohol solution; it can accidently go into the brain stem or leak into the cerebrospinal fluid or brain tissues if injected.

Operative Procedure

Arterial and venous lines are inserted in one or both femoral vessels for the delivery of contrast agents or treatment modalities such as coils, stents, and retrieval modalities.

Anesthetic

General anesthesia with OETT, and muscle relaxants are typically employed. MAC sedation can sometimes be used.

The choice of anesthetic depends on surgeon preference, anesthetist experience, and patient status. A general anesthetic with muscle relaxation can improve surgical effectiveness and image quality; sedation can allow for continuous neurological assessment. When making this decision, healthcare providers must consider the potential for patient agitation versus the ability to monitor neurologic status. Also, keeping the patient sedated enough to hold still may compromise the airway and the ability to blow off carbon dioxide, leading to hypercapnia (which dilates the brain vessels). If MAC sedation is used, you must have a plan of getting to the head and airway in case such access is needed.

Communication with the radiologist/interventional neurologist is essential.

Positioning

The patient is placed supine, with bilateral arms on egg-crate pads and tucked at sides. After tucking the arms, make sure peripheral IVs and arm arterial lines have a good waveform and blood can be pulled back into the lines.

Neurointerventional surgeries may be exceptionally long procedures, although in experienced hands they may be shorter in duration than craniotomies for identical pathology. Given the potential length of surgery make sure all pressure points are padded carefully and the patient's body and neck are in neutral positions.

Anesthetic Implications

Blood pressure control is of paramount importance. Vasoactive drips as well as syringes of esmolol (Brevibloc), hydralazine (Apresoline), labetalol, Lopressor (metoprolol), phenylephrine (Neosynephrine), and/or ephedrine should be available.

Anesthesia Goals for Neurointerventional Procedures

- Rapid recovery after the procedure is desirable for neurologic evaluation.
- Systemic blood pressures should be controlled by titrating drips and/or bolus medications.
- During deliberate hypertension, the blood pressure is increased by 30% to 40% of the patient's baseline blood pressure. The drug of choice for inducing deliberate hypertension is phenylephrine. It is important to monitor the EKG and ST segments for signs of myocardial ischemia when vasoactive agents are used.
- Drugs to induce hypotension include volatile inhaled agents, propofol, sodium nitroprusside (SNP), nicardipine (Cardene), hydralazine (Apresoline), calcium-channel blockers, beta blockers, and ganglionic blockers. A MAP of

50–60 mm Hg is usually safe for all patients. The cerebral autoregulation lower limit is 50 mm Hg; however, chronic hypertension shifts the autoregulatory curve to the right. Knowing the patient's baseline cuff blood pressure preoperatively is important for this reason.

- Relative normocapnia or modest hypnocapnia should be maintained.
- Patients are anticoagulated with very frequent ACT measurements. Have heparin bolus, heparin drip, and protamine available.

Preoperative Measures

Complete a thorough preoperative neurologic assessment and document any deficits.

Monitors and IV Access

- Arterial line placement is required to monitor continuous blood pressure. It also readily permits arterial sampling for blood gases and labs.
- Place at least two large-bore peripheral IV lines.
- CVL may be needed in case urgent fluid resuscitation is required because of extensive blood loss.
- A PA catheter may be needed if the patient has a cardiac history or is hemodynamically unstable.

IV Vasoactive Agents

- IV pump: nicardipine (Cardene), sodium nitroprusside (SNP), phenylephrine
- Syringe for bolus: phenylephrine, ephedrine, esmolol (Brevibloc), labetalol, metoprolol
- Other drugs to have available: mannitol, furosemide (Lasix), bumetanide (Bumex), lidocaine, atropine, glycopyrrolate (Robinul), calcium-channel blockers (nimodipine, nicardipine), dexamethasone (Decadron), regular insulin, $D_{50}W$
- Heparin bolus, heparin drip, and protamine
- Dexmedetomidine (Precedex)
- Clonidine—an α_2-adrenergic agonist given transdermally or PO

IV Fluids and Volume Requirements

Give normal saline or lactated Ringer's solution to maintain normovolemia, maintenance IVF plus urinary output, and measure urinary output every 30 minutes. Normal saline is more hyperosmolar than lactated Ringer's solution and helps pull fluid out of brain tissue. Colloids, such as albumin or Hextend/Hetastarch, can be given to restore volume deficits and maintain euvolemia. Hetastarch can cause platelet dysfunction and bleeding; do not give more than 20 mL/kg/day (max 1500 mL total).

Hypotonic and glucose solutions should be avoided due to the potential for increased cerebral metabolism and free water build-up, causing intracerebral edema. Don't give D_5W: Once the body utilizes the dextrose, the free water goes to the brain, causing cerebral edema.

Blood Products

Any blood losses should be replaced immediately to keep the HCT more than 28%. Hypothermia can cause platelet dysfunction.

Pre-induction Measures

Preoperative sedation may be necessary to calm the patient; small doses of a benzodiazepine may be used and are preferred for this purpose over opiates (which depress respirations). The patient should not be allowed to hypoventilate (because it increases $PaCO_2$ and vasodilates cerebral arteries) or have sedation amounts that affect neurologic evaluation.

Induction

Ensure smooth IV induction, and maintain blood pressure within 20% of the patient's normal level.

Intraoperative Measures/Maintenance

The goal is to maintain a slightly decreased CPP to decrease blood loss, and to decrease intracranial volume of blood and tissue for surgical exposure. See Chapter 3 for more information.

Emergence

Give prophylactic antiemetics as necessary to help patients avoid PONV (see Chapter 4).

Postoperative Measures

Once the surgery is completed, cover the patient with warmed blankets to prevent shivering. Elevate the head of the bed to approximately 30 degrees.

Perform a neurologic assessment as soon as the patient can follow commands. The goal is to assess the neurologic status while the patient is still in the operating room. The surgeons would like to evaluate the patient in the immediate postoperative period for complications so they can intervene if needed.

POSTERIOR FOSSA SURGERY

The posterior fossa contains the structures below the tentorium cerebelli: cerebellum, fourth ventricle, brain stem, and cranial nerve nuclei (not cranial nerve I or II). It is bordered by the occipital bone posteriorly, the mastoid laterally, the petrous ridge anteriorly, the foramen magnum inferiorly, and the tentorium cerebelli superiorly. Although it is bordered by the occipital bone, the posterior fossa is not the occipital region. The occipital region is supratentorial.

Posterior fossa pathology includes space-occupying lesions that can affect any structure contained within this region:

- Neoplasms: infratentorial tumors; nerve sheath tumors
- Vascular: AVM, basilar artery aneurysm, meningioma
- Cranial nerve syndromes: cranial nerves III–XII dysfunction caused by compression

Posterior fossa pathology can cause injury and dysfunction in the cardiovascular, respiratory, and autonomic nervous systems through changes to the brain stem—namely, the midbrain, upper and lower pons, and medulla oblongata. A decreased level of consciousness may result from changes in the reticular activating system. Cranial nerves or their nuclei can also be damaged. Any abrupt changes in hemodynamics should alert healthcare providers to possible brain stem injury.

Increased ICP from posterior fossa pathology is possible. Symptoms include headache, nausea/vomiting, level of consciousness changes, and papilledema.

Anesthetic management of complex skull base surgical procedures presents unique problems and concerns because of the risks that may influence patient outcome. Knowing the location of the primary skull-based tumor, its proximity to vital structures, and the planned approach can help healthcare providers prepare for neurophysiologic monitoring, recognize the need for blood or intraoperative cerebral protection, and manage the patient's position during surgery.

Postoperative nausea and vomiting are quite common following posterior fossa exploration. Antiemetics should be given to help prevent increased ICP, which can lead to increased bleeding and cerebrospinal fluid leaks.

Cerebral protection strategies are utilized during skull base surgery. See Chapter 3 for more information.

Posterior Fossa Exploration: Craniotomy or Craniectomy

Surgical exploration of the posterior fossa may be necessary to remove a mass. Indications for such surgery include acoustic neuroma (also known as vestibular schwannoma), a benign tumor of cranial nerve VIII, or lesions in the cerebellum (e.g., chiari malformation I and II), fourth ventricle, brain stem, paranasal sinuses, the nasopharynx, cavernous sinus, cerebellopontine angle, jugular foramen, foramen magnum, cranial nerves, or upper cervical spine.

Operative Procedure
The transfacial (transoral, transmandibular, or transmaxillary) approach is rarely used. Suboccipital approaches are often done. The surgeon's preference and the type and location of the tumor will dictate the specific approach used.

The procedure may be unilateral or bilateral. If it is bilateral, the incision may go from the tip of the left mastoid to the tip of the right mastoid. The posterior occipital bone is perforated and removed, the dura mater is opened, and the foramen magnum is exposed.

To gain access to the cerebellum, fourth ventricle, brain stem, and/or cranial nerves, the arch of the atlas (cervical vertebrae 1) must be removed. A ventricular catheter may have been inserted previously; if not, it may be inserted at this time.

The surgeon may request a Valsalva maneuver (closing off the pop-off valve, increasing airway pressures to more than 20–30 mm Hg, and holding these pressures for 10–20 seconds) to check for blood or cerebrospinal fluid leak.

Anesthetic
General anesthesia is used with insertion of an OETT. Muscle relaxation may not be allowed, so check with the surgeon before giving these medications. Preoperative discussions with the surgeon will give details on the planned surgical approach. The airway is shared with the surgeon in a transoral, transmandibular, or transmaxillary approach to the skull base; the patient may require a tracheostomy, which is performed at the beginning of the surgery.

A pre-formed oral RAE tube or reinforced endotracheal tube may be placed to prevent kinking of the tube with movement and positioning of the patient's head.

PEEP and increased airway pressures should be avoided to help prevent an increase in intracranial pressures.

Maintain general anesthesia until the end of the case, when the patient is in the supine position and the head pins have been removed.

Positioning
The patient may be placed in the prone position, with bilateral arms tucked at sides, and the head of the bed elevated 15–30 degrees to facilitate venous drainage; in the sitting position with head immobilization; or in the lateral position. The head may be turned to one side to facilitate surgical exposure. The head of the operating table may be turned away at least 90 degrees, if not 180 degrees, from the anesthetist. See Chapter 2 for more on patient

positioning and cerebral perfusion pressure and transducer levels.

Patient positioning has been found to influence postoperative complication rates with these surgeries. Skull base tumor resections can be extremely long procedures, so meticulous positioning is vital to protect nerves and structures. If the patient's head is to be raised at all, monitoring for venous air embolism is important (see Chapter 3). Venous air embolism is additional concern with any sitting position surgery. A communication between the atmosphere and the venous system can cause air to be drawn into the vascular supply.

When the patient is placed in a sitting position, excessive neck flexion or extension can lead to venous obstruction and quadriplegia from cervical spinal cord compression (see Chapter 2).

Anesthetic

General anesthesia is used with insertion of an OETT; check with the surgeon before giving any muscle relaxants. Avoid nitrous oxide, as it can increase the likelihood of pneumocephalus. Look for cervical subluxation by X-ray and assess for any neurologic changes with head flexion or extension preoperatively.

Secure the OETT on the opposite side of the mouth from the surgeon's approach. A reinforced endotracheal tube or pre-formed RAE tube may be placed to prevent kinking with movement and positioning of the patient's head.

Anesthetic Implications

The tumor may impact on cranial nerve VII (facial nerve), affecting facial sensation; facial paralysis may also be present. Impaired eye movement and difficulty in swallowing and tasting may occur as well. Assess and document for these deficits preoperatively, and check gag, cough, and swallowing ability before extubating the patient.

These patients require special eye care. Paper tape is used to close the eyes to prevent corneal drying or abrasions; eye pads are then placed over both eyes to protect them. Eye ointment may also be instilled before taping for patients who will remain intubated postoperatively.

The vertebral artery and brain stem are accessed by a posterior fossa approach; these structures can be injured by retraction, ischemia, or trauma during surgery. Labile pulse and blood pressures may be observed with any brain stem manipulation. Notify the surgeon if bradycardia or asystole occurs, and have glycopyrrolate (Robinul) and atropine ready for immediate use.

Type and cross the patient's blood. Note, however, that blood transfusion is usually not needed in this surgery.

Anesthesia Goals for Posterior Fossa Exploration

Brain relaxation and cerebral protection are needed. See Chapter 3 for more information.

Preoperative Measures

Perform a complete preoperative neurologic assessment and document any deficits.

Monitors and IV Access

- Arterial line placement is required to monitor continuous blood pressure. It also readily permits arterial sampling for blood gases and labs.
- Place at least two large-bore peripheral IV lines.
- A CVL is needed in case urgent fluid resuscitation is required because of extensive blood loss; it also provides for VAE precaution and treatment. A long-line CVP may be necessary for antecubital versus external jugular versus internal jugular cases. With an antecubital CVP, the basilic vein is the preferred route of access.
- A PA catheter may be needed if the patient has a cardiac history or is hemodynamically unstable.
- Neurological monitoring may include SSEP, BAER, MEP, and/or EMG monitoring, so as to monitor the cranial nerves.
- Transesophageal echocardiography (TEE) may be useful.
- Use a precordial Doppler device for venous air embolism monitoring.

IV Vasoactive Agents

- IV pump: nicardipine (Cardene), sodium nitroprusside (SNP), phenylephrine
- Syringe for bolus: phenylephrine, ephedrine, esmolol (Brevibloc), labetalol, metoprolol
- Other drugs to have available: mannitol, furosemide (Lasix), bumetanide (Bumex), lidocaine, atropine, glycopyrrolate (Robinul), calcium-channel blockers (nimodipine, nicardipine), dexamethasone (Decadron), regular insulin, $D_{50}W$

IV Fluids and Volume Requirements

Give normal saline or lactated Ringer's solution to maintain normovolemia, maintenance IVF plus urinary output, and measure urinary output every 30 minutes. Normal saline is more hyperosmolar than lactated Ringer's solution and helps pull fluid out of brain tissue. Colloids, such as albumin or Hextend/Hetastarch, can be given to restore volume deficits and maintain euvolemia. Hetastarch and Dextran can cause platelet dysfunction and bleeding; do not give more than 20 mL/kg/day (max 1500 mL total).

Hypotonic and glucose solutions should be avoided due to the potential for increased cerebral metabolism and free water build-up, causing intracerebral edema. Don't give D_5W: Once the body utilizes the dextrose, the free water goes to the brain, causing cerebral edema.

Blood Products

Keep HCT greater than 28%. Any blood losses should be replaced immediately.

Pre-induction Measures

Preoperative sedation may be necessary to calm the patient; small doses of a benzodiazepine may be used and are preferred for this purpose over opiates (which depress respirations). The patient should not be allowed to hypoventilate (because it increases $PaCO_2$ and vasodilates cerebral arteries) or have sedation amounts that affect neurologic evaluation.

Induction

Slow, smooth IV induction is necessary to prevent hypertensive episodes. A short-acting muscle relaxant may be needed for intubation and patient positioning; the relaxation should then be reversed if neurophysiologic monitoring is to be done.

Intraoperative Measures/Maintenance

The most stimulating periods during posterior fossa surgery include laryngoscopy, skin incision, dural opening, or cutting/stripping of the membrane covering the bones (periosteal membrane).

Emergence

Provide prophylactic antiemetics to help patients avoid PONV (see Chapter 4).

Postoperative Measures

Perform a neurologic assessment as soon as the patient can follow commands. The goal is to assess the neurologic status while the patient is still in the operating room. The surgeons would like to evaluate the patient in the immediate postoperative period for complications so they can intervene if needed.

Once the surgery is completed, cover the patient with warmed blankets to prevent shivering. Elevate the head of the bed to approximately 30 degrees.

Complications

Potential complications include cranial nerve deficits, especially facial nerve (cranial nerve VII) and auditory nerve (cranial nerve VIII) damage; postoperative CSF leak; and pneumocephalus.

Ventricular Catheter/Shunt Placement for Hydrocephalus

In case of hydrocephalus, insertion of a diversion catheter (called a shunt) may be used to divert cerebrospinal fluid from the ventricular system or subarachnoid space to another absorption space—either the right atrium of the heart (ventriculo-atrial shunt), the pleural cavity (ventriculo-pleural shunt), or the peritoneal cavity (called a ventriculoperitoneal [VP] shunt, where blood reabsorbs the CSF). While carbonic anhydrase inhibitors can temporarily control communicating hydrocephalus, the only definitive treatment is the surgical insertion of a ventricular shunt. A lumbar-peritoneal shunt is a catheter placed into the subarachnoid space in the lumbar spine and tunneled anteriorly to the peritoneal cavity.

A shunt may be placed for treatment of pseudotumor cerebri, benign intracranial hypertension, and obstructive or non-obstructive hydrocephaly; its use is intended to relieve the CSF build-up in the brain and reduce the ICP to normal. Hydrocephalus can be caused by infection, tumor, cyst, congenital defect, or cerebral blood flow abnormalities.

If a ventricular shunt is placed in a child, a revision of the shunt length may be needed as the child grows. This need depends on the child's age and length of the catheter.

Operative Procedure

The shunt can be placed in either lateral ventricle and is most commonly placed from a frontal or parietal approach. In a frontal approach, either the left or right frontal edge of the skull is entered. In the parietal approach, a horseshoe-shaped incision is made several centimeters above and posterior to the ear.

A burr hole is made in the skull, the dura is opened, and a ventricular catheter is passed into the posterior aspect of the lateral ventricle and advanced anterior to the foramen of Munro. Infrequently, air is injected and an X-ray film is taken to confirm catheter placement.

If the distal catheter is to be placed in the peritoneal space, an abdominal incision is made. A small incision is made in the anterior rectus sheath of the abdomen; the peritoneum is grasped and incised. The draining catheter is then tunneled under the skin and subcutaneous tissues from behind the ear, down the neck (the surgeon will sometimes make a small cut along the planned route to help thread the catheter downward) and chest, to the abdominal intraperitoneal reservoir. Tunneling is the most stimulating part of the procedure

If the draining catheter is to end up in the right atrium, the catheter is threaded through the internal jugular vein or placed directly into the atrium or pleural cavity through a thoracotomy.

Shunt Valve

A valve is placed underneath the skin in a subgaleal space created behind the ear, into the pectoral region or the flank. It is attached to both the distal end of the catheter in the ventricle and the proximal end of the drainage shunt. This one-way, pressure-dependent valve regulates the flow of CSF when it becomes increased past a certain preset level. It works at different pressures to avoid excessive drainage of CSF and prevents any flow of CSF back toward the ventricles. When pressure builds, the CSF drains from inside the ventricle down to the right atrium, the pleural cavity, or the peritoneal cavity.

Anesthetic

General anesthesia is done with insertion of with an ETT. Tape the tube carefully, as the patient's head may be moved around during the surgery.

Positioning

The patient is placed in a supine position, with one arm tucked and the other arm extended on an armboard. The head is slightly elevated and turned to one side. The head of the operating table may be turned away at least 90 degrees, if not 180 degrees, from the anesthetist.

The head and the area of the body where the distal shunt/catheter will rest are both exposed, prepped, and ready.

Anesthetic Implications

Patients with hydrocephaly often have other congenital anomalies, so providers should assess the airway very carefully. Have all emergency airway equipment in the room if any question arises about being able to intubate the patient with the first attempt.

These patients are prepped over a large portion of their bodies, so they should be covered with blanket warmers as much as possible. Use fluid warmers as well.

Femoral pulses are bounding in patients with a large shunt.

These patients require special eye care. Paper tape is used to close the eyes to prevent corneal drying or abrasions; eye pads are then placed over both eyes to protect them. Eye ointment may also be instilled before taping for patients who will remain intubated postoperatively.

Anesthesia Goals for Ventriculoperitoneal Shunt Placement

Preoperative Measures

Perform a thorough preoperative neurologic assessment and document any deficits.

Monitors and IV Access

- Arterial line placement is required to monitor continuous blood pressure. It also readily permits arterial sampling for blood gases and labs.
- Place one large-bore peripheral IV line.
- CVL may be needed in case urgent fluid resuscitation is required because of extensive blood loss.
- A PA catheter may be needed if the patient has a cardiac history or is hemodynamically unstable.

IV Vasoactive Agents

- IV pump: nicardipine (Cardene), sodium nitroprusside (SNP), phenylephrine
- Syringe for bolus: phenylephrine, ephedrine, esmolol (Brevibloc), labetalol, metoprolol
- Other drugs to have available: mannitol, furosemide (Lasix), bumetanide (Bumex), lidocaine, atropine, glycopyrrolate (Robinul), calcium-channel blockers (nimodipine, nicardipine), dexamethasone (Decadron), regular insulin, $D_{50}W$

IV Fluids and Volume Requirements

Give normal saline or lactated Ringer's solution to maintain normovolemia, maintenance IVF plus urinary output, and measure urinary output every 30 minutes. Normal saline is more hyperosmolar than lactated Ringer's solution and helps pull fluid out of brain tissue. Colloids, such as albumin or Hextend/Hetastarch, can be given to restore volume deficits and maintain euvolemia. Hetastarch can cause platelet dysfunction and bleeding; do not give more than 20 mL/kg/day (max 1500 mL total).

Hypotonic and glucose solutions should be avoided due to the potential for increased cerebral metabolism and free water build-up, causing intracerebral edema. Don't give D_5W: Once the body utilizes the dextrose, the free water goes to the brain, causing cerebral edema.

Blood Products

Any blood losses should be replaced immediately to keep HCT greater than 28%.

Pre-induction Measures

Preoperative sedation may be necessary to calm the patient; small doses of a benzodiazepine may be used and are preferred for this purpose over opiates (which depress respirations). The patient should not be allowed to hypoventilate (because it increases $PaCO_2$ and vasodilates cerebral arteries) or have sedation amounts that affect neurologic evaluation.

Induction

Slow, smooth IV induction is needed to prevent hypertensive episodes.

Intraoperative Measures/Maintenance

The goal is to maintain a slightly decreased CPP to decrease blood loss, and to decrease intracranial volume of blood and tissue for surgical exposure. See Chapter 3 for more information.

Emergence

Give prophylactic antiemetics as necessary to help patients avoid PONV (see Chapter 4).

Postoperative Measures

Once the surgery is completed, cover the patient with warmed blankets to prevent shivering. Elevate the head of the bed to approximately 30 degrees.

Perform a neurologic assessment as soon as the patient can follow commands. The goal is to assess the neurologic status while the patient is still in the operating room. The surgeons would like to evaluate the patient in the immediate postoperative period for complications so they can intervene if needed.

NEUROPERIPHERAL NERVE SURGERY PEARLS

- See Chapter 3 for more information with these surgeries regarding tourniquet use.
- Assess and document preoperative neurologic deficits.

PERIPHERAL NERVE SURGERY

Peripheral Nerve Repair

The complete or partial anastomosis of a diseased or injured peripheral nerve may be necessary to effect peripheral nerve repair. Injury disrupts a nerve so that it cannot transmit an action potential.

Indications for peripheral nerve repair procedures include trauma, burns, and surgical accidents, especially with excision of malignant tumors. If a significant length of nerve has been damaged, several methods can be employed to achieve tension-free repair. When nerve grafting is necessary, a cutaneous nerve (lateral antebrachial or sural nerve) is used. The operating microscope and nerve stimulator are employed in such procedures.

The peripheral nervous system extends outside the brain and spinal cord. Examples of peripheral nerves include musculocutaneous, radial, median, ulnar, peroneal, tibial, femoral, and intercostal nerves, as well as the brachial, lumbar, and sacral plexus. The purpose of a peripheral nerve is to transmit signals, either from the spinal cord to the periphery, or from the periphery to the spinal cord.

Injured peripheral nerves are very difficult to repair and there is no guarantee of function after a repair is attempted. Even if the patient eventually recovers some of the function served by the particular nerve, healing requires an extensive amount of time. After the nerve is repaired, the axons must regrow into the denervated nerve segment into the muscle. Axon growth occurs at a very slow rate (approximately 1 mm/day), so it may take months, or even years, for the muscle to function again.

After repair of sensory nerves, reinnervation occurs only if the fibers grow to reach their sensory end organs, but mismatch can occur if the sensory fiber reinnervates in a new and different sensory area. Reinnervation can also occur when motor fibers grow to reach their muscle target but may only become partially innervated if the muscle target is a long distance from the site of injury.

Operative Procedure

The operative procedure depends on the nerve that has been damaged. For approximation of nerve ends, primary epineurial nerve suture, and/or secondary nerve repair may be done.

Anesthetic

General and/or local anesthesia may be used. If general anesthesia is given, muscle relaxation is *not* given. Regional anesthesia is not usually provided, as it can make postoperative nerve assessment difficult.

Positioning

Patient positioning depends on which nerve has been damaged.

Anesthetic Implications

A compression tourniquet is used with the pressure setting usually dictated by the surgeon and dependent on whether the tourniquet used on the arm or leg.

The pressure must be released after 2 hours to prevent injury. Chart tourniquet time and setting.

A peripheral IV and blood pressure cuff are placed on the non-operative arm.

SYMPATHECTOMY

Sympathetic pain appears to be the cause of causalgia and reflex sympathetic dystrophy, both complex regional pain syndromes. Symptoms include burning, tingling, shooting, electric-like, lightning-like, pins-and-needles sensations.

The sympathetic nervous system gives rise to complex regional pain syndromes (CRPS), which produce diffuse burning pain and hyperalgesia, usually following injury. This problem is believed to be caused by damage to A-delta and C-nerve fibers, which develop hypersensitivity to circulating nor-epinephrine, pressure, and movement. Central nervous system sensitization that may lead to permanent changes in nerve conduction appears to be involved, but this process is not well understood.

True causalgia follows injury to a major nerve trunk such as the sciatic nerve or its large branches. Reflex sympathetic dystrophy may occur following trauma to the neural structures that accompanies fractures and soft-tissue injuries.

A sympathectomy is the destruction of tissue along one of two sympathetic trunks that lie along either side of the spinal canal; this procedure is undertaken to interrupt neural messages. It involves the division of preganglionic fibers along their segmental origins and resection of corresponding relay ganglia. A sympathectomy can be performed in the cervical, thoracic, or lumbar regions.

Sympathetic denervation can be done endoscopically, by surgical resection, or via laser.

Lumbar Sympathectomy

Lumbar sympathectomy is done in an attempt to increase the local and collateral blood supply to the legs. This procedure can help healing and relieve pain associated with the sympathetic nervous system in the retroperitoneum, pelvis, perineum, and lower extremities. Indications for this surgery include inoperable arterial occlusive disease, reflex sympathetic dystrophy, symptomatic vasospastic disorders, and causalgia; it may also be undertaken as an adjunct to distal revascularization procedures.

Operative Procedure
Lumbar sympathectomy removes the sympathetic nervous system influence in one part of the body. There are two variations:

- *Local with sedation:* After IV sedation, a local anesthetic is injected into the skin at the waist line. Under fluoroscopy, a needle is inserted until the tip is close to the lumbar sympathetic nerves. A chemical blockade of phenol and absolute alcohol is injected. Care must be taken not to inject the solution into a vessel. The procedure can be done unilateral or bilaterally.
- *GA with OETT:* Using a retroperitoneal approach, an oblique incision is made between the ribs and the iliac crest. The lumbar sympathetic chain is located and a chemical blockade is injected.

Anesthetic
Local anesthetic and sedation may be used. Alternatively, GETA is used.

Positioning
The patient is placed in the lateral decubitus with beanbag position.

Anesthetic Implications
Patients may be hypotensive after this procedure.

Upper-Extremity Sympathectomy

Upper-extremity sympathectomy is done in an attempt to increase the local and collateral blood supply to the arm. This procedure can help healing and relieve pain associated with the sympathetic nervous system to the head, neck, and most of the upper extremity.

This type of sympathectomy is undertaken to improve blood flow to the upper arms in the event of arterial vasoconstriction of the arm due to intra-arterial injection of a vasoconstrictor, following frostbite, or to help prevent arterial vasoconstriction after microvascular surgery. It may also be used to relieve pain associated with dystrophies, help with Reynaud's phenomenon, and decrease pain associated with herpes zoster of the head or neck. Upper-extremity sympathectomy can terminate vasomotor control and hyperactive tone of small arteries and arterioles, thereby improving circulation.

This surgery is the procedure of choice to cure hyperhidrosis (excessive sweating) of the hands and/or face, and to stop excessive blushing in the face.

Operative Procedure

Upper-extremity sympathectomy can be done by video-assisted thoracoscopy. Several small incisions are made in the third or fourth intercostal spaces in the axillary area, and thoracic ports are placed to facilitate endoscopic access. The parietal pleura is cut open. The sympathetic nerve is located and collateral branches are dissected. A chest tube is inserted and the chest wall closed.

Anesthetic

General anesthesia with a double-lumen endobronchial tube is used for one-lung ventilation. Avoid nitrous oxide when one-lung ventilation is employed.

Positioning

The patient is placed in the lateral decubitus position.

Anesthetic Implications

Type and cross the patient's blood.
An arterial line is usually placed.
A peripheral IV and blood pressure cuff are placed on the non-operative arm.

Complications

Horner's syndrome can occur after an upper-extremity sympathectomy. Ipsilateral complications may include the following:

- Ptosis (drooping of the upper/lower eyelid and/or face)
- Miosis (pupil constriction)
- Anhydrosis of the neck and face (inability to sweat)
- Enophthalmos (posterior displacement of the globe of the eye)
- Nasal congestion

Pneumothorax is another potential complication.

Ulnar Nerve Transposition (Elbow)

Surgical treatment of ulnar nerve entrapment depends on where the nerve is compressed, it is usually done to relieve an entrapped ulnar nerve; the two most common sites are the elbow and the wrist. Ulnar nerve transposition may involve either decompression in situ or decompression with anterior transposition.

The ulnar nerve travels from under the clavicle to the inside of the upper arm, and then passes through the cubital tunnel at the elbow and toward the little finger. This nerve controls fine movements and large muscles of the forearm that help to make a strong grip. Ulnar nerve compression symptoms include numbness and tingling of half of the ring finger and all of the little finger, and weakening of the grip.

Operative Procedure

In *decompression in situ,* a localized decompression of the nerve is accomplished by incising the Osborne ligament and opening a tunnel beneath the two heads of the flexor carpi ulnaris. A small incision is made beginning at a midpoint between the elbow bone and the medial epicondyle. The incision line is usually extended 6 to 8 cm distally over the flexor carpi ulnaris. This procedure is performed with tourniquet control so as to decrease bleeding. Removal of a portion of the medial epicondyle also removes a compressive area on the ulnar nerve.

Decompression with anterior transposition moves the nerve from its anatomical position and puts it in a location that is more suitable. Transferring the nerve anteriorly effectively lengthens the nerve, decreasing tension on it in flexion. The surgeon will decide where the nerve will end up: either between the muscle and the skin and fat (subcutaneous transposition), within the muscle (intermuscular transposition), or under the muscle (submuscular transposition).

Anesthetic

General and/or local anesthesia may be given. If general anesthesia is given, muscle relaxation is *not* given. Regional anesthesia is not usually employed, as it can make postoperative nerve assessment difficult.

Positioning

The patient is placed in the lateral decubitus position.

Anesthetic Implications

Preoperative and postoperative assessments of arm and hand function should be done and documented. A peripheral IV and blood pressure cuff are placed on the nonoperative arm.

SPINE SURGERY PEARLS

- For any patient being moved into the prone position, make sure the peripheral IV is not placed antecubital, as it will not run when the patient's arms are placed in the "swimmer's position"—elbows flexed, palms down, with shoulders at an angle of less than 90 degrees. Even if the plan is to tuck the patient's arms at the sides, if the patient is too big (wide) it may not be possible to position that way. Keeping the IVs in the forearms or hands is safe with any arm position when the patient is to be prone.

- The prone position, especially if the patient becomes hypotensive, can lead to postoperative vision loss (POVL). This complication is most often associated with long spinal surgery with instrumentation that keeps the patient in the prone position. Raising the head of the bed slightly, preventing any pressure on the eyes or surrounding tissues, maintaining preoperative hematocrit levels, and maintaining a mean arterial pressure greater than 70 mm Hg, normothermia, euglycemia, and urinary output minimum of 0.5 mL/kg/h can help to prevent visual loss in the prone patient. Chart the nose and eyes check at least every 15 minutes on the anesthesia record.

- Secure the endotracheal tube securely before turning the patient in the prone position.

- Patients undergoing spinal surgery have an increased risk for stomach regurgitation due to the extreme position changes. Placing an oral-gastric tube before turning can help to suction out any stomach fluid that may be present.

- An anti-sialagogue (glycopyrrolate or atropine) can be useful in decreasing oral secretions; it can be given in the preoperative area.

- Check with the surgeon as to whether muscle relaxation is to be used at all or if a small amount can be used to turn and settle the patient into the prone position.

- At the beginning of a spine surgery, the surgeon may place a needle at the vertebral level he or she expects to operate on and then take an X-ray to confirm that level. Ventilation should be held while the X-ray is taken.

- Maintaining the blood pressure within 20% of the patient's baseline (with a mean arterial pressure greater than 70 mm Hg) can maintain blood flow while decreasing the risk of bleeding that might affect surgery.

- If the procedure involves opening the dura, the dura will be need to be sutured closed at the end of the case. The surgeon may request a Valsalva maneuver to test the integrity of the sutures. A Valsalva maneuver is performed by turning off ventilated breaths, partially closing the pop-off valve, and squeezing the bag to a sustained pressure of 20–30 mm Hg, which increases the pressure within the intradural space. If cerebrospinal fluid leaks from the suture line, more sutures will be placed to secure the incision line.

- Acute damage to the cervical spine can cause associated spinal cord trauma, leading to a loss of sympathetic tone and subsequently hypotension from vasodilation and bradycardia. Volume load with crystalloid or colloid solutions and/or give an IV vasopressor to treat this problem.

- Cervical fractures may be associated with injuries to the esophagus, airway, and head; severing of vertebral arteries can also occur.

- Multiple techniques for monitoring spinal nerve function may be used during spine surgery. See Chapter 3 for more information.

VERTEBRAE OF THE SPINAL COLUMN, SENSORY LEVELS, AND ASSOCIATED INJURIES

Cervical 1

The C1 (atlas) has no vertebral body. It has a thick anterior arch with two prominent lateral masses and a thin posterior arch.

Cervical 2

The C2 (axis) (also known as the dens or odontoid process) is held in tight approximation to the posterior aspect of the anterior arch of C1 by the transverse ligament, which is the main stabilizing force of the atlanto-axial joint.

Cervical 5 and 6 Vertebrae

The C5 and C6 vertebrae are the source of the most common cervical injuries. C5–6 level spinal injury can lead to:

- Quadriplegia; gross arm movements; diaphragm impaired initially
- Loss of intercostal and abdominal muscles

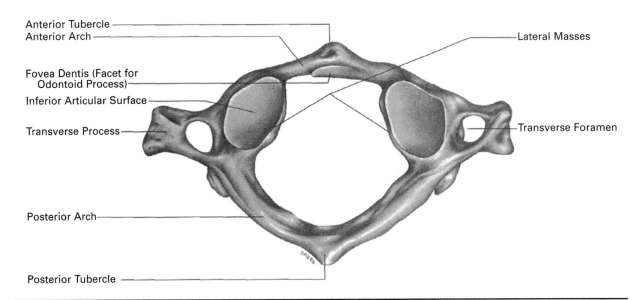

Anterior Tubercle
Anterior Arch
Fovea Dentis (Facet for Odontoid Process)
Inferior Articular Surface
Transverse Process
Posterior Arch
Posterior Tubercle
Lateral Masses
Transverse Foramen

Figure 5-6   *Cervical 1 (atlas)*
Source: Donnersberger, 2010.

- Use of accessory muscles
- No cough
- Paradoxical respiration

Improvement of ventilation may be noted when a patient with a C5–6 injury is in the supine position because the diaphragm works better. Ventilation is improved when the diaphragm is moved cephalad at end-inspiration, causing a decrease in end-expiration volume and allowing for greater excursion on the next inspiration. The upright position worsens ventilation due to the absence of elasticity of abdominal muscles.

Thoracic 1–5 Vertebrae

Injuries to the T1–5 vertebrae may result in paraplegia with diaphragmatic breathing. Such damage may be associated with a rib fracture, aortic tear, or cardiac contusion.

Assessment of Injury and Effect

Lumbar injuries can involve pelvic fracture and retroperitoneal bleeds. Assess the following to determine the damage:

A strong cough can be initiated if injury below *T6*. Quadriplegia is caused by damage to *C2–8* segments.

Paraplegia is caused by damage to *T1–S1* segments.

Perineal damage is caused by damage to *S2–S5* segments

Which anatomical division is how injury levels are defined? *Most caudal segment that has intact motor and sensory function*

A pentaplegic has damage to? *Cranial nerves and accessory muscles*

If the sensory level is at C4, what are you assessing? *Top of acromioclavicular joint*

If the sensory level is at C6, what are you assessing? *Thumb*

If the sensory level is at C7, what are you assessing? *Middle finger*

If the sensory level is at C8, what are you assessing? *Little finger*

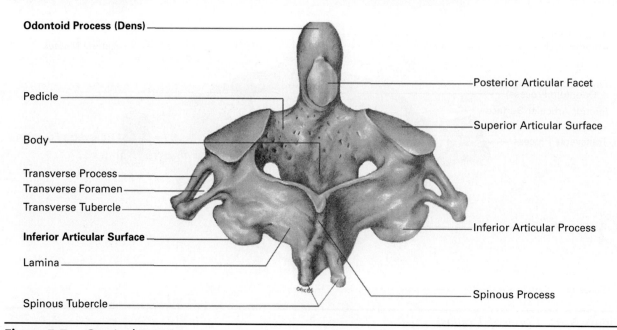

Odontoid Process (Dens)

Pedicle

Body

Transverse Process
Transverse Foramen
Transverse Tubercle

Inferior Articular Surface

Lamina

Spinous Tubercle

Posterior Articular Facet

Superior Articular Surface

Inferior Articular Process

Spinous Process

Figure 5-7 *Cervical 2 (axis)*
Source: Donnersberger, 2010.

If the sensory level is at L1, what are you assessing? *Thigh, groin*

If the sensory level is at T10, what are you assessing? *Naval*

If the sensory level is at L5, what are you assessing? *Foot*

The nerve root for the diaphragm is? *C1–4*

Nerve root for rectal sphincters is? *S2–4*

Foot dorsiflexion nerve root is? *L4–5*

Foot plantar flexion nerve root is? *L5–S1*

Key Definitions

Autograph: bone from own body.

Allograft: bone from cadaver.

Bone morphogenic protein (BMP): used in lieu of autograft/allograft to achieve fusion. BMPs are a group of growth factors and cytokines produced using recombinant DNA technology. They interact with specific receptors on the cell surface and have the ability to induce the formation of bone and cartilage.

Myelopathy: spinal cord compression.

Radiculopathy: nerve root compression.

Vertebrae

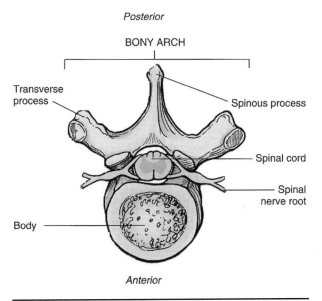

Figure 5-8 *Vertebrae Anatomy*
Source: AAOS, 2004.

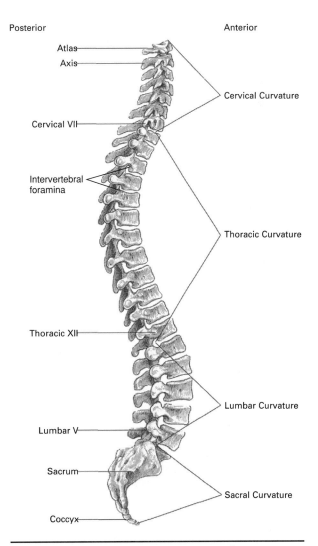

Figure 5-9 *Vertebrae Anatomy (Side View with Differences in Spinous Processes)*
Source: Donnersberger, 2010.

SPINAL SURGERY

Cervical Decompression and Fusion: Anterior Approach

This procedure involves excision of a herniated intervertebral disc with the stabilization of the cervical spine from an anterior approach. It may be undertaken when nerve deficits and pain persist after conservative treatments have been tried; it may also be used to treat a symptomatic nerve root, cord compression, spondylosis, or a herniated disc. Definitive diagnosis may include cervical radiculopathy, cervical myelopathy, degenerative disc disease, and/or cervical trauma including fractures.

Operative Procedure

With the *C1–3 access approach*, the following techniques are used:

- *Transoral*: After soft palate retraction, a midline posterior pharyngeal incision is made; the anterior C1 and C3 vertebrae are exposed. Anterior fixation (arthrodesis) of these vertebrae can be done with plates and screws. Posterior fixation may also be needed and accessed through a posterior cervical midline incision *in the same surgery or at a later date*. The transoral approach is associated with a higher infection rate due to intraoral and pharyngeal contamination, especially when bone grafting is used.

- *Anterior retropharyngeal*: A curved incision is made 2 to 4 cm below the mandible. The facial vein and artery are double-tied and cut. Removal of the submandibular salivary gland aids in better exposure of the cervical spine with less retraction. Anterior cervical decompression, fusion, and plating are done. This approach provides anterior spine exposure equivalent to the transoral approach but without transmucosal contamination. Instrumentation and arthrodesis can be accomplished in conjunction with this approach.

The retropharyngeal approach does have a higher rate of postoperative complications due to tissue swelling—for example, retropharyngeal edema, hematoma, and hemorrhage around the neck structures may lead to airway obstruction and difficulty swallowing. Injury to the mandibular branch of the facial nerve, recurrent laryngeal nerve, and spinal accessory nerve may lead to a motor defect of the sternocleidomastoid and trapezius muscles.

With the *C4–7 access approach,* a transverse incision is made at the level of the cricoid cartilage in a natural skin fold. The carotid sheath and prevertebral muscles are retracted laterally and the trachea and esophagus are retracted medially to expose the anterior spine. The anterior longitudinal ligament is incised, exposing the intervertebral disc. The anterolateral diseased disc is incised and removed piecemeal. The bone graft chips are kept moist until packing of the intervertebral space is complete. Care must be taken to avoid damage to the carotid sheath, vertebral vessels, and recurrent laryngeal nerve. Plates and screws may be used to stabilize the spine. The graft material may be (1) an autograft if performing a corpectomy or discectomy with interbody cage; (2) an allograft for corpectomy or discectomy; or (3) BMP if using an interbody cage or corpectomy. The cervical wound is then closed.

The surgeon usually operates on the right side of the neck due to surgical preference, as most surgeons are right-handed. Also, there is less risk of recurrent laryngeal nerve injury on the right side.

Anesthetic

General anesthesia with insertion of an OETT. A wire-enforced endotracheal tube may be placed to prevent the tube from kinking. Tape the OETT on the side (usually left) away from where surgeon is standing. Muscle relaxants may be needed, but check with the surgeon before giving these medications.

Positioning

Place the patient in a supine position, with the head turned slightly away from the surgical side (the head is usually turned to the left). Both arms may be tucked at the side. A shoulder roll is often used, but make sure the patient's head is not suspended off the table after this roll is placed.

Anesthetic Implications

Careful preoperative assessment of the patient's head flexion and extension range of motion will help to guide your intubation technique. Also check the surgeon's history and physical and preoperative orders to clarify cervical precautions. In-line manual stabilization of the head may be necessary while intubating the patient so as to maintain the head in a neutral position and prevent excessive (or any) extension.

The surgeon may require the anesthetist to apply traction to the patient's head and jaw to extend the neck and separate the cervical vertebrae to place the bone graft. If bone grafting is scheduled, place a warming blanket everywhere else on the lower body.

The surgeon is usually accepting of one tube into the esophagus, either an orogastric tube or an esophageal stethoscope. Be aware that insertion of both tubes may distort the anatomy.

Anesthesia Goals for Cervical Decompression and Fusion, Anterior Approach

Preoperative Measures

Perform a preoperative neurologic exam, and document preexisting abnormalities or deficits.

Type and cross the patient's blood. There is potential for large blood losses if a great vessel is accidentally disrupted.

Monitors and IV Access

- An arterial line may be needed, depending on the patient's age and history.
- Place two large-bore peripheral IV lines.
- SSEPs may be monitored.

Induction

Acute spinal cord compression or damage can result in the loss of sympathetic tone, which causes peripheral vasodilation, hypotension, and bradycardia. Crystalloid or colloid volume load and vasopressors may be required to counteract these effects.

Patients undergoing cervical decompression and fusion require special eye care. Paper tape is used to close the eyes to prevent corneal drying or abrasions; eye pads are then placed over both eyes to protect them. Eye ointment may also be instilled before taping for patients who will remain intubated postoperatively.

Intraoperative Measures/Maintenance

Provide standard maintenance anesthesia.

Emergence

Smooth emergence is important with this surgery. The goal is to avoid coughing, bucking, or nausea/vomiting or retching, thereby minimizing the risk of bleeding, hematoma formation, or suture line disruption from increased head and neck pressures. Have a team member hold gentle pressure over the suture lines if the patient does cough or vomit. Antiemetics should be given to prevent PONV.

The patient may need to remain intubated in the immediate postoperative period, especially if swelling around the airway is a concern. Transport the patient to the ICU with full monitoring.

Postoperative Measures

Perform a neurological exam as soon as the patient is awake.

Complications

Potential complications include great vessel disruption. The trachea, esophagus, and surrounding structures can also be accidentally damaged.

Cervical Decompression and Fusion: Posterior Approach

This procedure involves surgical decompression of cervical neural structures with stabilization of the cervical spine from a posterior approach. It is undertaken when nerve deficits and pain persist even after conservative treatments are applied; it may also be used for treatment of a symptomatic nerve root, cord compression, spondylosis, or herniated disc. Definitive diagnosis may include cervical radiculopathy, cervical myelopathy, degenerative disc disease, and/or cervical trauma including fractures.

Operative Procedure

This type of cervical decompression and fusion relies on a posterior midline cervical incision over the involved vertebrae. Paraspinal muscles are dissected off the spinous process; lamina and bone are removed piecemeal. Wiring, lateral plating, and a pedicle screw plate or rod fixation are inserted; fusion is accomplished with a local bone autograft or BMP. Opening of the dura may be necessary, depending on the extent of the procedure.

Anesthetic

General anesthesia with insertion of an OETT. A wire-enforced endotracheal tube may be placed to prevent the tube from kinking. Muscle relaxants may be needed, but check with the surgeon before giving these medications. Induction is done while the patient is on the stretcher.

Careful preoperative assessment of the patient's head flexion and extension range of motion and history of cervical vertebrae instability will help to guide your intubation technique. In-line manual stabilization of the head (with the patient's head held by a second provider) while intubating the patient or an awake intubation with a fiberoptic scope may be needed to maintain the head in a neutral position and prevent excessive (or any) extension.

Any invasive lines or additional IVs should be placed before turning the patient over to the prone position on the operating room table. Check breath sounds bilaterally after turning the patient prone.

Positioning

Place the patient in a prone position, with the arms in "swimmer's position" and the shoulders at an angle of less than 90 degrees. Perform an eyes and nose check every 15 minutes to confirm no pressure exists on these structures and chart the findings. The head of the bed may be slightly raised to decrease the pressure on the patient's eyes while he or she is in the prone position.

Posterior cervical surgery can also be done with the patient in a sitting (beach-chair) position. A precordial Doppler monitor should be used in such a case, placed to hear the right atrium. A 60-mL syringe must be ready to draw back through a CVP if an "air wheel" is heard on the Doppler monitor.

Monitor the patient for sitting fusion, using an arterial line and a double- or triple-lumen central line.

Head pins are usually applied for a posterior cervical laminectomy when the patient is placed in a sitting position. Have propofol or pentothal available to blunt the sympathetic response to head pin application.

Anesthetic Implications

For surgery in the prone position, following placement of a peripheral IV line (not in the antecubital space), the patient is intubated with an endotracheal tube while still on the stretcher. The patient is then carefully rolled over onto the operating room table into the prone position. Check bilateral breath sounds after turning prone.

Type and cross the patient's blood. Blood for transfusion may need to be made available in the operating room.

A lower-body warming blanket and fluid-warming should be used.

Patients undergoing posterior cervical decompression and fusion require special eye care if they are placed in either a prone or beach-chair position. Paper tape is used to close the eyes to prevent corneal drying or abrasions; eye pads are then placed over both eyes to protect them.

Eye ointment may also be instilled before taping for patients who will remain intubated postoperatively.

A Valsalva maneuver may be requested by the surgeon if the dura needs to be sutured closed at the end of the case.

Cervical Decompression and Fusion: Anterior and Posterior Approaches

This procedure may be required when anterior *and* posterior instability of the cervical spine is present. A transverse incision is usually made; requires rigid fixation of the cervical spine with plating, rods, and screws.

The patient should be placed on a special operating room table that allows the patient to be turned without lifting his or her body on and off the bed. Head fixation is accomplished with pins.

General anesthesia with insertion of an OETT. A wire-enforced endotracheal tube may be placed to prevent the tube from kinking. Muscle relaxation is usually prescribed, but check with the surgeon before giving these medications.

Type and cross the patient's blood. Obtain two units of packed red blood cells, as blood loss can be significant. Cell-saver (autotransfusion) technology may also be used.

Dorsal Root Rhizotomy

Doral root rhizotomy severs problematic nerve roots in the spinal cord. This procedure is most often performed to relieve the symptoms of neuromuscular conditions such as spastic cerebral palsy, multiple sclerosis, or severe back pain. It may also be used to treat spasticity refractory to baclofen (a GABA-receptor agonist muscle relaxant infused into the intrathecal space by a programmable pump or given by mouth)

Operative Procedure

An open laminectomy (removal of lamina) is done; the motor nerve roots are identified and separated from the sensory nerve roots. Electrical stimulation of the nerve fibers identifies the damaged nerves (those producing pain and the source of hypertonia). These damaged nerves are selectively cut, leaving the remaining nerves intact and fully functional.

Anesthetic

General anesthesia with insertion of an OETT. A wire-enforced endotracheal tube may be placed to prevent the tube from kinking. Muscle relaxation is usually not given in dorsal root rhizotomy.

Induction is done while the patient is on the stretcher. Any invasive lines or additional IVs should be placed before turning the patient over to the prone position on the operating room table. Check breath sounds bilaterally after turning the patient prone.

Positioning

The patient is placed in the prone position, with the arms in the "swimmer's position" and the shoulders at an angle of less than 90 degrees. Perform an eyes and nose check every 15 minutes and chart the finding. The head of the bed may be slightly raised to decrease the pressure on the patient's eyes while he or she is in the prone position.

Anesthetic Implications

Following placement of a peripheral IV line (not in the antecubital space), the patient is intubated with an endotracheal tube while still on the stretcher. The patient is then carefully rolled over onto the operating room table into the prone position.

Type and cross the patient's blood, and be aware that blood may need to be available in the operating room. Cell-saver collection is usually done. Have blood tubing with normal saline and an additional IV access for giving blood products readily available.

Patients undergoing dorsal root rhizotomy require special eye care. Paper tape is used to close the eyes to prevent corneal drying or abrasions; eye pads are then placed over both eyes to protect them. Eye ointment may also be instilled before taping for patients who will remain intubated postoperatively.

Foraminotomy

Foraminotomy involves surgical opening of the foramen—that is, a laminectomy with a more lateral opening (see Figure 5-10). This procedure opens and enlarges the neuroforamen (intervertebral foramen), which is the opening at the exit point of the nerve roots. This spinal nerve can develop impingement from a bulging disc, degenerative disc disease, scar tissue, or arthritic changes in the superior facet joint causing radiculopathies.

A foraminotomy does not require an anterior approach and does not require a fusion to preserve motion of the involved vertebral levels. This procedure may be done to decompress several levels.

Operative Procedure

A posterior midline incision is made over the involved vertebrae. Muscles are dissected off the spinous process; lamina and facet joint bone are removed piecemeal. The surgeon will remove the lower edge of the lamina and the inner edge of the inferior and superior facets. The incision is closed in layers.

This procedure can be done endoscopically. No muscles are cut or torn with this approach, and healing occurs much more quickly.

Anesthetic

General anesthesia with insertion of an OETT. A wire-enforced endotracheal tube may be placed to prevent the tube from kinking when the patient is in the prone position. Muscle relaxants may be requested; check with the surgeon before giving these medications.

Positioning

Patients are positioned prone for the posterior cervical, thoracic, or lumbar foraminotomy approach. They are placed supine, with arms tucked at the sides, for the anterior cervical approach.

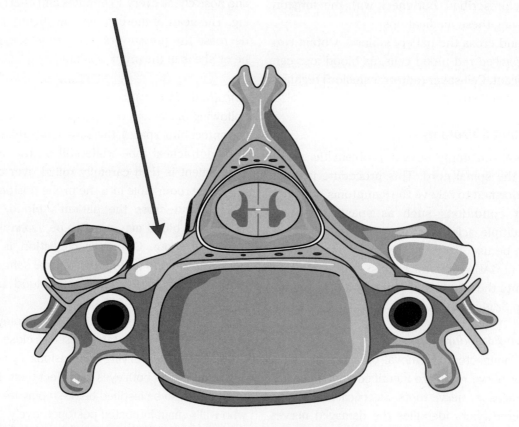

Figure 5-10   *Foraminotomy: Note the Portions of Enlarged Neuroforamen*

Anesthetic Implications

Type and cross the patient's blood, and be aware that blood may need to be available in the operating room. Cell-saver collection is usually done. Have blood tubing with normal saline and an additional IV access readily available for giving blood products.

Patients undergoing foraminotomy require special eye care. Paper tape is used to close the eyes to prevent corneal drying or abrasions; eye pads are then placed over both eyes to protect them. Eye ointment may also be instilled before taping for patients who will remain intubated postoperatively.

Laminectomy with or without Discectomy (Diskectomy)

This variation of laminectomy involves the complete removal of one or more vertebral lamina, usually with the concomitant removal of the spinous process (see Figures 5-11 and 5-12). It is performed to decompress the spinal cord or to access and remove portions of the intervertebral disc. *If instability is created by removing pieces of the vertebrae, a bone graft can be placed.*

A laminectomy may be performed to treat symptomatic nerve root or spinal cord compression from a herniated disc, spinal stenosis, compression fracture, dislocation of vertebrae, or spinal cord tumor or masses (e.g., AVM). The affected areas can be extradural, intradural, extramedullary, or intramedullary, and can occur anywhere along the spinal column; most commonly, they occur in the lumbar region.

The goal of a laminectomy is to relieve pressure on the spinal cord or nerve by widening the spinal canal.

Operative Procedure

A midline incision is made over the spine. The paraspinous muscles and periosteum are reflected. Sponges are packed along the vertebrae. Hemostasis is achieved with bone wax. A large retractor is placed for exposure. Small portions of the laminae overlying the herniated discs are removed with a rongeur; portions of vertebral spines and intervertebral facets may also be excised. The ligamentum flava is incised. Nerve roots are cautiously retracted, exposing the herniated disc; this disc is then removed with a rongeur and curettes. A surgical microscope may be

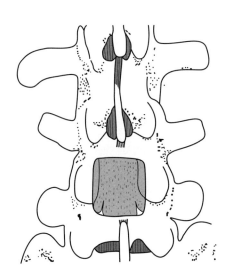

Figure 5-11 *Laminectomy with Spinous Process Removed, Posterior View*

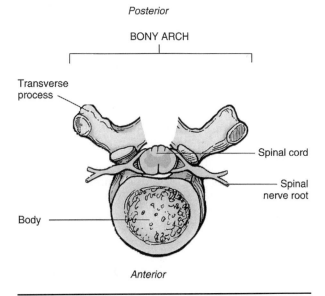

Figure 5-12 *Laminectomy with Spinous Process Removed, Superior View*
Source: AAOS, 2004.

used if a microdiscectomy is done or if a dural tear occurs. The dura is opened only if performing an intradural tumor resection. The wound is irrigated and then closed in layers.

Anesthetic

General anesthesia with insertion of an OETT. A wire-enforced endotracheal tube may be placed to prevent the tube from kinking. Muscle relaxants may be requested; check with the surgeon before giving these medications.

Induction is done while the patient is on the stretcher. Any invasive lines or additional IVs should be placed before turning the patient over to the prone position on the operating room table. Check breath sounds bilaterally after turning the patient prone.

Positioning

Place the patient in the prone position, with the arms in the "swimmer's position" and the shoulders at an angle of less than 90 degrees. Use a modified knee-chest position. Perform an eyes and nose check every 15 minutes to confirm that no pressure are on these structures and chart the findings. The head of the bed may be slightly raised to decrease the pressure on the patient's eyes while he or she is in the prone position.

Anesthetic Implications

Following placement of a peripheral IV line (not in the antecubital space), the patient is intubated with an endotracheal tube while still on the stretcher. The patient is then carefully rolled over onto the operating room table into the prone position.

Type and cross the patient's blood. Blood may need to be available in the operating room.

Patients undergoing laminectomy require special eye care. Paper tape is used to close the eyes to prevent corneal drying or abrasions; eye pads are then placed over both eyes to protect them. Eye ointment may also be instilled before taping for patients who will remain intubated postoperatively.

Check and document the status of the eyes, nose (tip), and chin at least every 15 minutes. Keep the patient's neck in a neutral position.

An upper-body warming blanket can be used.

Monitors

Evoked-potential monitoring may be used.

Laminotomy

Laminotomy involves partial removal of the lamina of the vertebrae (Figure 5-13). The lamina is a thin bony layer covering the spinal canal. This surgery is performed to decompress neural elements, thereby eliminating the pain of a ruptured or herniated intervertebral disc.

Operative Procedure

A midline incision is made over the spine. The paraspinous muscles and periosteum are reflected. A large retractor is placed for exposure. Small portions of the laminae bone are removed with a rongeur. Hemostasis is achieved with bone wax.

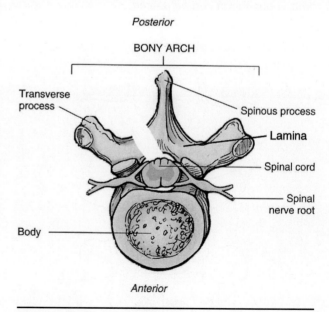

Figure 5-13 *Laminotomy*
Source: AAOS, 2004.

Anesthetic

General anesthesia with insertion of an OETT. A wire-enforced endotracheal tube may be placed to prevent the tube from kinking. Muscle relaxants may be requested; check with surgeon before giving these medications.

Induction is done while the patient is on the stretcher. Any invasive lines or additional IVs should be placed before turning the patient over to the prone position on the operating room table. Check breath sounds bilaterally after turning the patient prone.

Positioning

Place the patient in a prone position, with the arms in the "swimmer's position" and the shoulders at an angle of less than 90 degrees. A modified knee-chest position is used. Perform an eyes and nose check every 15 minutes and chart the findings. The head of the bed may be slightly raised to decrease the pressure on the patient's eyes while he or she is in the prone position.

Anesthetic Implications

Following placement of a peripheral IV line (not in the antecubital space), the patient is intubated with an endotracheal tube while still on the stretcher. The patient is then carefully rolled over onto the operating room table into the prone position.

A type and screen of the patient's blood is usually all that is needed.

Patients undergoing laminotomy require special eye care. Paper tape is used to close the eyes to prevent corneal drying or abrasions; eye pads are then placed over both eyes to protect them. Eye ointment may also be instilled before taping for patients who will remain intubated postoperatively.

Lumbar Discectomy and Microdiscectomy

Removal of an intervertebral disc may be necessary with a herniated or protruding spinal disc into the spinal canal that causes pain and neurologic deficits. A spinal disc is a soft cushion that separates each of the vertebrae of the spine. A herniated disc bulges out from between the vertebrae, compressing the surrounding spinal cord and nerves.

Operative Procedure

Before making an incision, the surgeon will place a spinal needle at the level of the lamina (involved in the surgery) to clarify this position by X-ray. A 1- to 2-inch incision is made over the proposed interspace, and the muscle is retracted laterally. An operating room microscope is used: A small piece of the ligamentum flavum is removed, the nerve root and dura are retracted to expose the disc, and the extruded disc excised. The ligamentum flavum will form a scar over the closing of the surgical incision.

Lumbar discectomy can also be done by endoscopic laser spine surgery through a very small incision in the lower back.

Anesthetic

Multiple methods of anesthesia are used with lumbar discectomy and microdiscectomy.

General anesthesia with insertion of an OETT. A wire-enforced endotracheal tube may be placed to prevent the tube from kinking. Muscle relaxants may be requested; check with the surgeon before giving these medications. Induction is done while the patient is on the stretcher. Any invasive lines are placed before turning the patient over to the prone position on the operating room table. Additional IVs can be placed before or after turning the patient. Check breath sounds bilaterally after turning the patient prone.

Neuraxial anesthesia comprises a spinal or epidural *with sedation* in a cooperative patient. Patients with chronic pain may not be candidates for neuraxial anesthesia.

Positioning

The patient may be placed in the prone position, with the arms in the "swimmer's position" and the shoulders at an angle of less than 90 degrees. Perform an eyes and nose check every 15 minutes and chart the findings. The head of the bed may be slightly raised to decrease the pressure on the patient's eyes while he or she is in the prone position.

With the kneeling position, the patient is placed prone first and then the bed changed into the kneeling position. If the patient is intubated, disconnect the circuit tubing from the endotracheal tube while holding onto the OETT and the patient's head as the patient is moved into the kneeling position (the patient's upper body will move down while the hips are flexed).

Anesthetic Implications

Following placement of a peripheral IV line (not in the antecubital space of the arm), the patient is intubated with an endotracheal tube while still on the stretcher. The patient is then carefully rolled over onto the operating room table into the prone position.

Type and cross the patient's blood. Blood may need to be available in the operating room.

Ventilation may need to be held during X-ray.

Patients undergoing lumbar discectomy and microdiscectomy require special eye care. Paper tape is used to close the eyes to prevent corneal drying or abrasions; eye pads are then placed over both eyes to protect them. Eye ointment may also be instilled before taping for patients who will remain intubated postoperatively.

Lumbar Fusion and Instrumentation: Posterior Approach

The goal with lumbar fusion surgery is to provide stability of the spine and decrease pain by fusing two or more vertebra together to prevent movement. This procedure may be used to treat instability of the lumbar spine from fracture, trauma, infection, degenerative changes, and/or spinal deformity such as scoliosis.

Operative Procedure

Bone graft material is usually obtained from the patient's iliac crest (autograft) or cadaver (allograft) for fusion. BMP can also be used.

Before making an incision, the surgeon may place a spinal needle at the level of the lamina (involved in the surgery) to clarify the vertebrae by X-ray. A 1- to 2-inch incision is made over the proposed vertebrae, and muscle is retracted laterally. The procedure involves removal of the outside layer of the transverse processes and facet joints. Instrumentation refers to metal rods affixed to the vertebrae to internally splint and apply multilevel corrective forces.

Fusion may be done on two or more lumbar vertebrae.

Anesthetic

A wire-enforced endotracheal tube may be placed to prevent the tube from kinking when the patient is in the prone position. Muscle relaxants may be requested; check with the surgeon before giving these medications.

Induction is done while the patient is on the stretcher. Any invasive lines or additional IVs should be placed before turning the patient over to the prone position on the operating room table. Check breath sounds bilaterally after turning the patient prone.

Positioning

Place the patient in the prone position, with the arms in the "swimmer's position" (elbows bent, shoulders less than 90 degrees, palms face down). Perform an eyes and nose check every 15 minutes and chart the findings. The head of the bed may be slightly raised to decrease the pressure on the patient's eyes while he or she is in the prone position.

Anesthetic Implications

Following placement of a peripheral IV line (not in the antecubital space), the patient is intubated with an endotracheal tube while still on the stretcher. The patient is then carefully rolled over onto the operating room table into the prone position.

Type and cross the patient's blood; blood may need to be available in the operating room. Cell-saver collection is usually done. Have blood tubing with normal saline and an additional IV access available for giving blood products.

Assess the patient's neurologic status and document deficits and symptoms preoperatively. Straightening or correcting of spinal abnormalities can cause ischemia to the spinal cord from blood supply compression. Neurophysiologic monitoring (SSEP) can be done to assess for spinal cord ischemia intraoperatively.

A mild hypotensive technique is sometimes used to decrease bleeding.

The surgeon may ask for a Valsalva maneuver to check for a dural tear during surgery. Turn the ventilator off, partially close the ventilator pop-off valve, squeeze ventilator bag to sustain airway pressure at 20 to 30 mm Hg, and count off, indicating you are creating a Valsalva maneuver.

Patients undergoing lumbar fusion require special eye care. Paper tape is used to close the eyes to prevent corneal drying or abrasions; eye pads are then placed over both eyes to protect them. Eye ointment may also be instilled before taping for patients who will remain intubated postoperatively.

Monitors
SSEP neurophysiologic monitoring and MEP monitoring may be used.

Lumbosacral Fusion and Instrumentation: Anterior Approach

Lumbosacral fusion involves removal of degenerative disc(s) and fusion of spine; it also provides for decompression of a cauda equina. This procedure may be performed when nerve deficits and pain persist after conservative treatments; for symptomatic nerve root or cord compression, spondylosis, or a herniated disc; and in case of instability or misalignment of the lumbar spine from fracture, trauma, infection, degenerative changes, or spinal deformity such as scoliosis. Definitive diagnosis may include lumbar radiculopathy, myelopathy, degenerative disc disease, and/or lumbar trauma. The goal is to provide stability of the spine and decrease pain.

Operative Procedure
The anterior approach allows for a limited fusion area but is associated with decreased blood loss. A bone graft, metal implants, bone cement, or a combination of these three, is used to fuse the lumbosacral spine.

In the *transperitoneal* procedure, an incision is made into the lower abdomen with the patient in the supine position. The rectus abdominus fascia is incised and retracted medially or laterally, allowing access to the retroperitoneal space (without violating the peritoneal cavity; there is decreased need for bowel manipulation with less third-space fluid loss and heat loss).

In the *retroperitoneal* procedure, a flank incision is made with the patient in the lateral decubitus position; one or two ribs may be removed to obtain surgical access to the lumbar spine. Risks to this approach include damage to the great vessels of the abdomen, the ureter, and the presacral plexus. The retroperitoneal space can be accessed without entering the peritoneal cavity.

Anesthetic
GETA. A wire-enforced endotracheal tube may be placed to prevent the tube from kinking. Muscle relaxants are usually given but check with the surgeon before giving these medications.

Positioning
The patient may be placed in the either the lateral decubitus position or supine.

Anesthetic Implications

Type and cross the patient's blood; blood may need to be available in the operating room as there is increased blood loss with this surgery. Cell-saver collection is usually done. Have blood tubing with normal saline and multiple large-bore IV access available for giving blood products. Anticipate a large blood loss, and plan on aggressive fluid and blood replacement. These patients usually have large third-space fluid shifts.

There is a greater risk of spinal cord compression and ischemia with the anterior approach, as a larger number of segmental spinal arteries require ligation. SSEP monitoring is very important.

Use aggressive temperature conservation measures.

Anesthesia Goals for Lumbosacral Fusion and Instrumentation Surgery, Anterior Approach

Monitors and IV Access

- Arterial line
- Central venous line if needed
- SSEP neurophysiologic monitoring (possibly)
- A "wake-up" test may also be required.

IV Vasoactive Agents

- IV pump: nitroglycerin, sodium nitroprusside (SNP), phenylephrine
- Syringe for bolus: ephedrine, phenylephrine (Neosynephrine), hydralazine (Apresoline), esmolol (Brevibloc), Lopressor (metoprolol)

IV Fluids and Volume Requirements

Bowel prep may have been given for a transperitoneal approach. These patients tend to present in a very dehydrated state.

Intraoperative Measures/Maintenance

The surgeon may prefer a hypotensive technique to keep blood loss at a minimum. You can use either a labetalol IV bolus or a nitroglycerin or sodium nitroprusside (SNP) drip to maintain a MAP at 60 mm Hg or less.

Spine Reconstruction: Anterior and/or Posterior Approach (Cervical, Thoracic, and/or Transdiaphragmatic for Cervicothoracic Spine Surgery)

Surgery to the cervicothoracic spine may necessitate both anterior and posterior approaches; it can be used to expose the cervical or thoracic spine, or a combination of the two. The cervicothoracic spine involves C6 to T3; the thoracic spine goes from T1 to T12. The transdiaphragmatic spine refers to the three vertebrae above and below the diaphragm.

This surgery is indicated to treat severe instability of the spine from fracture, trauma, infection, degenerative changes, or spinal deformity such as scoliosis.

Operative Procedure

The anterior procedure is usually performed first. It may produce less blood loss because less muscle is dissected. A general surgeon may be called upon to help gain exposure for the neurosurgeon.

Fusion may also be done in reconstructive procedures with bone graft, metal implants, bone cement, or a combination of these three. Bone graft is often taken from the iliac crest.

Cervical surgery is considered the most difficult access in the anterior approach. It may require clavicle or rib resection. Risks associated with this approach include damage to the great vessels at the thoracic outlet, esophagus, left lymphatic duct, brachial plexus, lung parenchyma, and/or trachea.

The patient is placed in the supine position for *cervicothoracic* surgery. Two incisional approaches may be used:

- *Transsternal:* An incision of the anterior sternomastoid border extends to the midline of the sternum. The sternum is divided and retracted to expose the spine.
- *Transclavicular:* A T-shaped incision of the clavicles is made, with the vertical limb extending down the midline of the sternum.

The medial third of the clavicle and manubrium are resected to provide a direct anterior approach.

In *thoracic* surgery, the anterior approach to the upper levels of the thoracic spine is also difficult. Such procedures can potentially cause damage to adjacent structures such as those listed for cervical surgery. *Transthoracic* procedures may require access into the thoracic cavity and will need a collapsed lung on the operative side. In such cases, lateral decubitus positioning is used, a chest tube is usually placed, and the incision lines closed.

In *transdiaphragmatic* surgery, a combined retroperitoneal and transthoracic approach is used to access the thoracic spine. The patient is placed in the lateral decubitus position.

Anesthetic

General anesthesia with insertion of a single-lumen OETT. A wire-enforced endotracheal tube may be placed to prevent the tube from kinking if a single-lumen endotracheal tube is placed. A double-lumen endobronchial tube may be required if thoracic access and partial lung collapse is needed.

Muscle relaxants may be required; check with the surgeon before giving these medications.

Positioning

The patient is placed in the supine or lateral decubitus position with the operative side up; multiple position changes of the patient is usually required. The head of the bed may be slightly raised to decrease the pressure on the patient's eyes while he or she is in the prone position.

Anesthetic Implications

This surgery can be very long in duration. Keeping the patient warm, all body prominences carefully padded, and the body in neutral anatomical alignment is crucial.

The decision whether the patient will be extubated in the operating room or after leaving the operating room depends on the length of the surgery and the amount of IV fluids and blood products given. If there is a lot of facial swelling or third-space fluid shifts, it may be best to wait until the patient is diuresed before attempting extubation.

Patients undergoing spine reconstruction require special eye care if they are placed in the prone position. Paper tape is used to close the eyes to prevent corneal drying or abrasions; eye pads are then placed over both eyes to protect them. Eye ointment may also be instilled before taping for patients who will remain intubated postoperatively.

Anesthesia Goals for Spine Reconstruction

- Maintain hemodynamic stability.
- Type and cross the patient's blood; blood is usually kept on hand in the operating room. Cell-saver collection may also be done.
- There is a potential for massive blood loss if large blood vessels are disrupted.

Monitors and IV Access

- Have multiple large-bore peripheral IV access for crystalloid, colloid, and blood replacement.
- An arterial line is needed due to the potential hemodynamic instability and length of surgical time.
- A CVL may be placed.
- SSEP neurophysiologic monitoring is performed.

For the patient with *scoliosis,* careful preoperative assessment of cardiovascular and pulmonary systems is important, as these systems can also be affected if ribcage deformity is present. Disease states associated with scoliosis include restrictive lung disease, increased pulmonary vascular resistance and pulmonary hypertension, and airway abnormalities. In patients with restrictive lung disease, pulmonary function tests (PFT) will show decreased FRC, decreased VC, decreased TLC, and normal FEV1/FVC. Cardiovascular disease may include congestive heart failure, right ventricular hypertrophy, and cor pulmonale. Patients with scoliosis may also have decreased PaO_2 and an increase in physiologic dead space. These patients are usually hypoxemic (with secondary polycythemia) and hypercapnic.

In any patient with scoliosis, asses the neurologic status and document deficits and symptoms preoperatively. Because the curve of the spine can reach 65 degrees, the stretching of the spinal cord can result in an alteration in the arterial supply, nerves, and muscle from spinal cord compression; this abnormality may cause neurologic deficits that healthcare providers must ascertain preoperatively. In addition, surgical straightening or correcting of spinal abnormalities can cause ischemia to the spinal cord from blood supply compression.

Tumor Resection of the Spine

Tumor resection involves surgical excision of one or more masses of the spine.

Operative Procedure
An incision is made over the spinal section containing the tumor. The surgeon then resects the largest amount of the tumor possible while preserving the spinal nerves. The spine may require support to maintain stability; screws, grafts, and plates may be needed. Hemostasis is achieved and the incision closed.

Anesthetic
General anesthesia with insertion of an OETT. A wire-enforced endotracheal tube may be placed to prevent the tube from kinking if a single-lumen endotracheal tube is used. A double-lumen endobronchial tube may be required if thoracic access and partial lung collapse are needed.

Muscle relaxants may be requested; check with the surgeon before giving these medications.

Induction is done while the patient is on the stretcher. Any invasive lines or additional IVs should be placed before positioning the patient on the operating room table. Check breath sounds bilaterally after turning the patient prone.

Positioning
The patient is placed in the prone position, with the arms in the "swimmer's position" and the shoulders at an angle of less than 90 degrees. Perform an eyes and nose check every 15 minutes and chart the findings. The head of the bed may be slightly raised to decrease the pressure on the patient's eyes while he or she is in the prone position.

Anesthetic Implications
Following placement of a peripheral IV line (not in the antecubital space), the patient is intubated with an endotracheal tube while still on the stretcher. The patient is then carefully rolled over onto the operating room table into the prone position.

This surgery can have a very long duration. Keeping the patient warm, all body prominences carefully padded, and the body in neutral anatomical alignment is crucial.

Have multiple IV access available for crystalloid, colloid, and blood replacement. The length of the surgery and the amount of IV fluids and blood products given will determine whether the patient can be extubated in the operating room or after leaving the operating room. If there is a lot of facial swelling or third-space fluid shifts, it may be best to wait until the patient is diuresed before attempting extubation.

Type and cross the patient's blood; blood is usually kept on hand in the operating room. Large amounts of blood can be lost during these procedures, especially when dealing with metastatic tumors of the spine.

SSEP monitoring may be used.

Patients undergoing tumor resection require special eye care. Paper tape is used to close the eyes to prevent corneal drying or abrasions; eye pads are then placed over both eyes to protect them. Eye ointment may also be instilled before taping for patients who will remain intubated postoperatively.

Craniofacial Surgery

6

CRANIOFACIAL SURGERY PEARLS

- Careful preoperative airway evaluation is imperative in these patients, as they may be difficult to mask-ventilate or intubate due to their injuries or craniofacial abnormalities. Awake fiberoptic intubation may be required. Nasal intubation may be required for surgical access to the upper and lower jaws.
- An endotracheal tube may be in competition with the surgeon for the throat/airway; care is needed so that anesthesia equipment doesn't interfere with the surgeons ability to operate.
- If the frontal sinus or the naso-orbital-ethmoidal (NOE) area is involved or if the patient has isolated fractures, consider inserting an oral endotracheal tube, nasal intubation is not needed.
- If intermaxillary fixation (IMF) is done or arch bars are inserted, a nasal Rae endotracheal tube can be inserted. *Do not nasally intubate the patient if there is a dysjunction at the cranial base* (fracture violation at the cranial base), as with a LeFort III fracture: it is possible to intubate directly into the brain tissue. Also, if there are *nasal, orbital, or zygomatic fractures,* the patient needs to be orally intubated, as an attempt to perform a nasal intubation can violate the cranial vault. These patients will need a surgical airway—that is, a tracheostomy or a submental intubation approach (which goes through the floor of the mouth).
- Because the tissues of the skull and face are quite vascular, maintaining a slight decrease in mean arterial blood pressure (MAP in the range of 60–70 mm Hg) can help to minimize bleeding.

CRANIOFACIAL SURGERY

LeFort Osteotomy

LeFort osteotomy is performed to correct congenital dentofacial abnormalities or establish pre-injury cranial bone relationships with normal height and look of the face. It is indicated to correct maxillary deformities usually caused by motor vehicle accidents, falls, or assault, and/or congenital dentofacial deformities.

Due to the degree of force required to produce facial fractures, these injuries are often associated with other serious eye, intracranial, and/or cervical spine injuries. A combination of LeFort fractures is usually encountered in a patient with facial trauma.

A *LeFort I* fracture consists of horizontal fracture of the maxilla immediately above the teeth and palate, separating the palate from the maxilla (Figure 6-1). It involves a horizontal crack across the maxilla separating the maxilla and teeth from the bone above. Intraoral incisions are made for surgical access and treatment.

A *LeFort II* fracture crosses the nasal bones on the ascending process of the maxilla and lacrimal bone and crosses the medial and inferior orbital rims; it is sometimes called a "pyramidal" fracture (Figure 6-2). The maxilla separates from the face. The LeFort II fracture extends posteriorly to the base of the skull. Brow, coronal, intraoral, and infra-orbital incisions may need to be made for its repair.

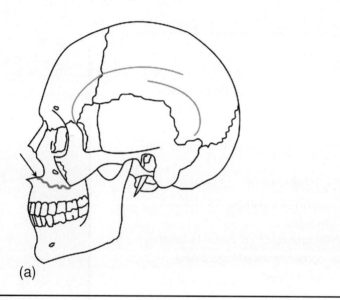

(a)

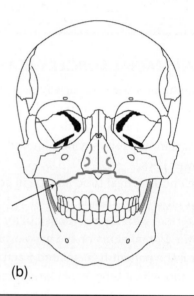

(b)

Figure 6-1   *LeFort I Fracture, (a) Lateral and (b) Anterior Views*

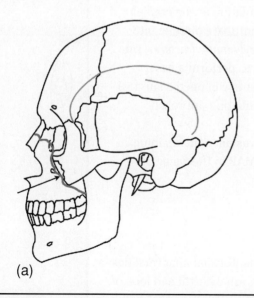

(a)

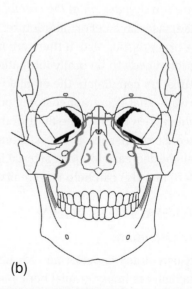

(b)

Figure 6-2   *LeFort II, (a) Lateral and (b) Anterior Views*

With a *LeFort III* fracture, the fracture line traverses the frontal process of the maxilla and the lacrimal bone, extends from the dorsum of the nose and cribiform plate, up along the superior and lateral orbital walls (Figure 6-3). In this suprazygomatic fracture, the facial bones are detached from the anterior cranial base. Such a fracture often involves the posterior plate of the ethmoid. Because of their location, LeFort III fractures are associated with the highest rate of cerebrospinal fluid (CSF) leaks. Brow or coronal incisions may need to be made.

Operative Procedure

The structural buttress of the maxilla must be aligned and stabilized to provide the necessary support and contour to the midface. An osteotomy may be done to one or both jaws to achieve normal occlusion of the teeth and to reestablish the proper maxillomandibular relationships. When trauma and fractures are involved, this proper relationship between the upper and lower jaws can be repaired with intermaxillary fixation (IMF), also known as maxillomandibular fixation. Open reduction and internal fixation is often combined with IMF for maxillomandibular injuries. IMF is established by securing arch bars (either wire or elastic) to the upper and lower dental arches with individual wire ligatures around the teeth.

An iliac or cranial bone graft (autogenic or allogenic) may be necessary to complete any reconstruction.

Anesthetic

Both GETA and muscle relaxants are used. Fiberoptic intubation should be performed if there is any doubt about the ease of intubation. If nasal intubation is required, it should be done with an armored endotracheal tube or RAE tube.

Patients with nasal, orbital, or zygomatic fractures need to be orally intubated, as an attempt to do a nasal intubation can violate the cranial vault. The same applies to inserting a nasogastric tube: If the patient has these facial fractures and a gastric tube is needed, place it orally.

If this procedure is being done for trauma or is considered an emergency procedure, rapid-sequence induction should be done.

Patients may be extubated at the end of the procedure but need to be fully awake to do so. They may need to remain intubated if facial swelling will interfere with normal respiration.

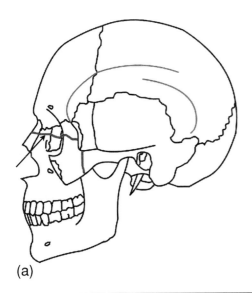

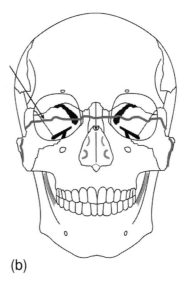

(a)   (b)

Figure 6-3   *LeFort III, (a) Lateral and (b) Anterior Views*

Positioning

The patient is placed supine, with the arms tucked at the sides. The operating table is usually turned at least 90 degrees, if not 180 degrees, away from the anesthetist. The head of the bed is usually increased 15–30 degrees to ensure venous drainage and to decrease swelling.

Anesthetic Implications

CT scanning is the gold standard for detecting facial fractures. It is superior to clinical examination in this respect, and is more than 95% accurate. Have CT films available in the OR.

Depending on the severity of the fracture, a minimum of a type and cross should be available. Blood may need to be available in the operating room.

Positive-pressure ventilation can increase pressure in the nasopharynx and force foreign material or air into the skull.

Use paper tape to secure the patient's eyelids closed; cover the eyes with eye pads and tape them securely unless they are within the surgical field. Eye lubrication may be used to protect the cornea.

As the tissues of the skull and face are quite vascular, maintaining a slight decrease in mean arterial blood pressure (MAP in the range of 60–70 mm Hg) can help to minimize bleeding.

A throat pack may be inserted. Chart its insertion and the point at which it is removed.

The jaw is usually wired shut at the end of the case. If it is, *always* have wire cutters accompany the patient when leaving the OR.

Smooth emergence is important with this surgery. The goal is to avoid coughing, bucking, nausea/vomiting, or retching to prevent increased risk of bleeding, hematoma formation, or suture line disruption from the increased head and neck pressures. Vomiting is especially dangerous if the jaw is wired closed; aggressively treat patients to prevent nausea and vomiting. Check with the surgeon before using Decadron as an antiemetic adjunct, as this agent may retard bone growth.

Reduction of Mandibular Fracture

This procedure is performed for correction of a malocclusion resulting from a fracture of the lower jaw. All lower jaw fractures should be reduced and fixed as soon as possible after the injury. Reduction is indicated for fractures that occur within the occlusion and body of mandible, intermaxillary fixation may suffice.

Operative Procedure

In *closed reduction,* an arch bar is bent to conform to the teeth and the dental arch. Fine wire encircles the necks of each tooth; the wires are then attached to the bars. The maxillary and mandibular arches are placed to effectively reduce the fractures. Small latex bands or wires may be used for intermaxillary fixation.

In *open reduction,* for fractures posterior to the teeth, intermaxillary fixation and open reduction may be necessary. An incision can be made externally (extraorally) to the inferior border of the mandible or internally (intraorally) via a vestibular incision. The fracture site(s) is exposed and the periosteum reflected. Holes may be drilled into the mandible on both sides of the fracture, and plates and screws used to reduce and fix the fracture into optimal alignment.

Anesthetic

Both GETA and muscle relaxants are used. Nasal intubation with an armored tube or RAE tube may be necessary. Patients may be extubated at the end of the procedure but need to be fully awake to do so. They may remain intubated if facial swelling will interfere with normal respiration.

Positioning

The patient is placed in the supine position, with the arms tucked at the sides. The operating table is usually turned at least 90 degrees, if not 180 degrees, away from the anesthetist. The head of the bed is usually increased 15–30 degrees to ensure venous drainage and to decrease swelling.

Anesthetic Implications

Depending on the severity of the fracture, a minimum of a type and cross should be available; blood may need to be available in the operating room.

Use paper tape to secure the patient's eyelids closed. Cover the eyes with eye pads and tape them securely.

Because the tissues of the skull and face are quite vascular, maintaining a slight decrease in mean arterial blood pressure (MAP in the range of 60–70 mm Hg) can help to minimize bleeding.

A throat pack may be inserted. Chart its insertion and the point at which it is removed.

The jaw is usually wired shut. If so, *always* have wire cutters accompany the patient when leaving the OR.

Smooth emergence is important with this surgery. The goal is to avoid coughing, bucking, nausea/vomiting, or retching to prevent increased risk of bleeding, hematoma formation, or suture line disruption from the increased head and neck pressures. Vomiting is especially dangerous if the patient's jaw is wired closed; aggressively treat such patients to prevent nausea and vomiting. Check with the surgeon before using Decadron as an antiemetic adjunct, as it may retard bone growth.

Mandibular Osteotomy

Mandibular osteotomy entails surgical correction of deformities of the mandible (lower jaw) from congenital or accidental causes. Osteotomy refers to cutting of the bone; bone grafting can also be done to correct the deformity. These procedures are done for a retruded (thrust backward) or prognathic (thrust forward) mandible. Because dental malocclusion may be present, orthodontics may be needed. Mandibular osteotomy may also be done to repair mandibular fractures from facial trauma.

Operative Procedure

This surgery is undertaken to advance or retrude the mandible so as to align the jaw and teeth; it is most commonly performed at the ramus area of the mandible (back corner of the lower jaw). Depending on the size of the deformity and surgical preference, an incision may be external or internal and an iliac or cranial bone graft (autogenous or allogenic) may be necessary to complete any reconstruction. Rigid fixation can be done with miniplates and screws. A genioplasty (chin deformity correction) may be done in conjunction with the osteotomy.

Anesthetic

Both GETA and muscle relaxants are used. Nasal intubation is carried out with an armored tube or RAE tube. Patients may be extubated at the end of the procedure but need to be fully awake to do so. They may remain intubated if facial swelling will interfere with normal respiration.

Positioning

The patient is placed in the supine position, with the arms tucked at the sides. The operating table is usually turned at least 90 degrees, if not 180 degrees, away from the anesthetist. The head of the bed is usually increased 15–30 degrees to ensure venous drainage and to decrease swelling.

Anesthetic Implications

Depending on the severity of the fracture, a minimum of a type and cross should be available; blood may need to be available in the operating room if the trauma is severe.

Use paper tape to secure the patient's eyelids closed. Cover the eyes with eye pads and tape them securely.

Because the tissues of the skull and face are quite vascular, maintaining a slight decrease in mean arterial blood pressure (MAP in the range of 60–70 mm Hg) can help to minimize bleeding.

A throat pack may be inserted. Chart its insertion and the point at which it is removed.

The patient's jaw is usually wired shut. If so, *always* have wire cutters accompany the patient when leaving the OR.

Smooth emergence is important with this surgery. The goal is to avoid coughing, bucking, nausea/vomiting, or retching to prevent increased risk of bleeding, hematoma formation, or suture line disruption from the increased head and neck pressures. Vomiting is especially dangerous if the patient's jaw is wired closed; aggressively treat such patients to prevent nausea and vomiting. Check with the surgeon before using Decadron as an antiemetic adjunct, as it may retard bone growth.

Reduction of Maxillary Fractures

Fractures of the maxilla (upper jaw) are more rare than mandibular (lower jaw) fractures. They are often associated with fractures to the nose or other parts of the central face. The maxilla acts as a central support bone in the face, and impact to it can affect bone around the nose and eyes along specific "planes of weakness" in the bone structure. Fractures to the maxilla often cause teeth to fracture as well.

Because the tissues of the skull and face are quite vascular, maintaining a slight decrease in mean arterial blood pressure (MAP in the range of 60–70 mm Hg) can help to minimize bleeding.

A throat pack may be inserted. Chart its insertion and the point at which it is removed.

See the earlier discussion of LeFort fractures for more information.

Open Reduction of Orbital Floor Fractures

Open reduction of orbital floor fractures is intended to restore the integrity and elevation of the thin bone that supports the eye and periorbital tissues. Other facial fractures can occur in combination with orbital floor fractures. A blowout fracture refers to an isolated depressed fracture of the orbital floor, often with the orbital contents protruding into the maxillary sinus. Repair of such injuries should be done promptly.

Operative Procedure

An infraorbital rim incision is made. The periosteum is incised and reflected over the fracture site. The defect can be covered with a synthetic material, autogenous cartilage, or bone.

The globe is rotated (forced duction test) to test the security of the implant and to make certain the inferior rectus muscle is not trapped. An ice pack may be applied after an eye patch placed.

Anesthetic

Both GETA and muscle relaxants are used. Plan to extubate the patient at the end of the case.

Positioning

The patient is placed in a supine position, with the arms tucked at the sides. The operating table is usually turned at least 90 degrees, if not 180 degrees, away from the anesthetist. The head of the bed is usually increased 15–30 degrees to ensure venous drainage and to decrease swelling.

Anesthetic Implications

Use paper tape to secure the non-operative eyelid closed; cover it with an eye pad and tape it securely. This area may also be covered with a plastic occlusive dressing to prevent skin prep liquid from going into the non-operative eye.

Because the tissues of the skull and face are quite vascular, maintaining a slight decrease in mean arterial blood pressure (MAP in the range of 60–70 mm Hg) can help to minimize bleeding.

Smooth emergence is important with this surgery. The goal is to avoid coughing, bucking, nausea/vomiting, or retching to prevent increased risk of bleeding, hematoma formation, or suture line disruption from the increased head and neck pressures. Aggressively treat patients to prevent nausea and vomiting. Check with the surgeon before using Decadron as an antiemetic adjunct, as it may retard bone growth.

Reduction of Zygomatic Fracture

This surgery is performed to correct cheek(s) fracture(s). Closed reduction is used if the treatment is for zygomatic arch fractures. Open reduction and internal fixation are done to treat zygomatico maxillary complex (ZMC) fractures.

Operative Procedure

Small incisions are made in the lateral third of the eyebrow and in the infraorbital region to access the fracture fragments. Intraoral access is often utilized. Wires are passed through holes that have been drilled in the fragments, realigning and maintaining the fragments in alignment.

Anesthetic

Both GETA and muscle relaxants may be needed. Plan to extubate the patient at the end of the case.

Positioning

Place the patient in the supine position, with the arms tucked at the sides. The operating table is usually turned at least 90 degrees, if not 180 degrees, away from the anesthetist. The head of the bed is usually increased 15–30 degrees to ensure venous drainage and to decrease swelling.

Anesthetic Implications

Use paper tape to secure the patient's eyelids closed; cover them with eye pads and tape them securely. Both eyes may be covered with a plastic occlusive dressing to prevent skin prep liquid from going into the eyes.

Because the tissues of the skull and face are quite vascular, maintaining a slight decrease in mean arterial blood pressure (MAP in the range of 60–70 mm Hg) can help to minimize bleeding.

Smooth emergence is important with this surgery. The goal is to avoid coughing, bucking, nausea/vomiting, or retching to prevent increased risk of bleeding, hematoma formation, or suture line disruption from the increased head and neck pressures. Aggressively treat patients to prevent nausea and vomiting. Check with the surgeon before using Decadron as an antiemetic adjunct, as it may retard bone growth.

7

Ophthalmic Surgery

IMPORTANT EYE ANATOMY AND TERMS RELATED TO OPHTHALMIC SURGERY

Aqueous humor: a watery fluid continuously produced by the choroid plexus of the ciliary body. Intraocular pressure is due to a balance of production and drainage of aqueous humor. Secreted in the posterior chamber (behind the iris), this fluid moves forward through the pupil into the anterior chamber, where it is drained through the canal of Schlemm into the blood.

Intraocular pressure (IOP): a measurement of the fluid pressure inside the eye; it measures the balance between the production and drainage of aqueous humor through the trabecular meshwork (in the anterior chamber). Resistance to outflow of aqueous humor maintains IOP within physiologic range.

- Measured by a tonometer, the normal IOP is 12–20 mm Hg in the sitting position and increases slightly in the supine position. The normal eye produces approximately 4 mL of aqueous humor every 24 hours. This fluid circulates around the eye, nourishing the cornea, iris, and lens; it also helps the eye maintain its shape.
- IOP is acutely increased with hypertension, straining, breath holding, vomiting, or straining (e.g., Valsalva maneuver).
- An increase in CVP or blood pressure will cause an increase in IOP.
- An increase in carbon dioxide will cause an increase in IOP.
- Benzodiazepines increase IOP.
- Barbiturates and mannitol decrease IOP.

Conjunctiva: thin transparent tissue covering the sclera (white portion) of the eye.

Choroid: dark-brown vascular coat of the eye between the sclera and the retina.

Palpebral: eyelid.

Pars plana: part of the uvea and choroidea; approximately 4 mm long and located near the iris and the sclera. It is the anterior attachment of the retina.

Periorbita: a fascial sheet that encloses the eyeball and its muscles; it is continuous with the periosteum of the bones forming the orbit.

Retina: light-sensitive layer in the back of the eye; it converts images into electrical impulses and sends these images to the brain along the optic nerve.

Tarsal (Meibomian) gland: sebaceous oil gland that prevents the eyelids from sticking together.

Tarsal plate: inner wall of the eyelids; it provides form and support to the eyelids.

Tenon's capsule: a thin membrane that envelops the eyeball from the optic nerve to the limbus, separating it from the orbital fat and forming a socket in which it moves. Its inner surface is smooth and is separated from the outer surface of the sclera by the lymph space.

Uvea: the middle of the three layers that make up the eye; it includes the iris, ciliary body, pars plana, and choroid.

Vitreous humor: a clear, jelly-like mass that fills the space inside the posterior cavity (rear two-thirds of the eyeball) between the lens and the retina; it contributes to IOP and prevents the eyeball from collapsing. It does not undergo constant replacement.

OPHTHALMIC SURGERY PEARLS

- The head of the bed with ophthalmic surgery patients is always turned away—at least 90 degrees, if not 180 degrees. Have extra length tubing on all monitoring and support equipment.
- Place the IV site in the arm closest to you (after the head of the bed is turned away) for ease in giving medications.
- Placing the EKG pads and leads, a blood pressure cuff, and the nasal cannula oxygen on the patient in the preoperative area as this expedites surgery starting once in the operating room. Just connect the cables

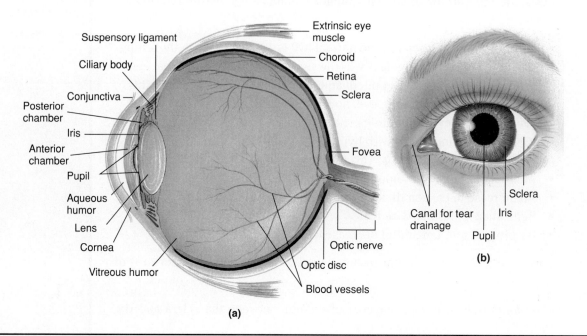

(a)

(b)

Figure 7-1   *Anatomy of the Eye*
Source: Chiras, 2008.

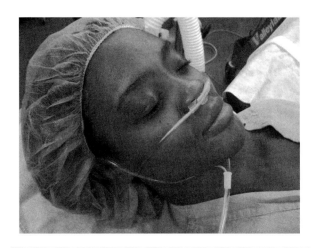

Figure 7-2 *Nasal Cannula Placement for Ophthalmic Surgery*

(still attached to the monitor) to the patient once in the room.

- The nasal cannula can be placed with the tubing (that goes behind the ears) flipped so that no tubing goes near the eye (Figure 7-2).
- Any breach of technique or errors during ophthalmic surgery could lead to partial or complete loss of vision or infection in the operative eye.

ANESTHESIA FOR OPHTHALMIC SURGERY

Anesthesia may require immobility of the globe and lid, anesthesia of the globe and adnexa (appendages of organ—extraocular muscles, eyelids, lacrimal glands), control of IOP, general relaxation of the patient, and prevention of retching, coughing, and BP fluctuation, even after the procedure is finished. The choice of anesthetic depends on the nature of the procedure, the surgeon's and the patient's preference, and the general status and level of anxiety of the patient.

Proper anesthesia is a must for any eye surgery. Ophthalmic surgery is usually performed under MAC anesthesia. It is imperative for the patient to lie still during any eye procedure as to avoid damage or injury to the eye.

Topical anesthesia is the most commonly employed option, with tetracaine (Pontocaine) eye drops or lidocaine gel being instilled into the conjunctival sac. This application may suffice for superficial procedures or may precede administration of local anesthetic. If topical anesthesia is used alone, the patient must be totally oriented and cooperative, as eye movement remains under the control of the patient.

Infiltration anesthesia is the direct injection of a local anesthetic into the surgical site. A form of regional anesthesia, eye blocks involve a block of cranial nerve branches. Lidocaine 2%, tetracaine 0.5%, or longer-acting bupivacaine local anesthetic may be injected into the area for a *retrobulbar block* or a *facial block* to completely immobilize the extraocular muscles, reduce eye lid movement, and minimize pain sensation. A *peribulbar block* is an alternative to the retrobulbar block and offers an effective way to provide anesthesia (Figure 7-3).

For globe immobilization (akinesia of the eyeball) or more involved procedures, a retrobulbar block is performed by injecting the anesthetic agent into the muscle cone behind the globe, which blocks the ciliary ganglion and nerves and cranial nerves (CN) III, IV, and VI. CN IV is not affected totally in a retrobulbar block because it lies outside the muscle cone.

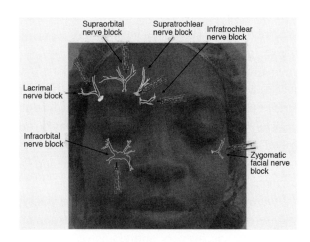

Figure 7-3 *Regional Anesthesia in Ophthalmic Surgery*

- CN III (oculomotor): supplies the levator palpebrae superioris, the superior, medial, and inferior rectus muscles, and the inferior oblique muscles
- CN IV (trochlear): supplies the superior oblique muscle
- CN VI (abducens): supplies the lateral rectus muscle

A retrobulbar block can elicit the oculocardiac reflex transiently. It is performed as follows:

- Local anesthetic (2–5 mL) is injected behind the eye into the cone where the extraocular muscles converge.
- Using a 25-gauge needle, injection is made 0.5 cm medial to the lateral canthus in a supranasal direction, to a depth of 3.5 cm.
- Success will result in anesthesia, akinesia, and an abolished oculocardiac reflex.

If performed incorrectly, this block may result in inadvertent injection into the subarachnoid space that causes a "total spinal." Cardiopulmonary support must be initiated and maintained until the local anesthetic wears off.

A small bolus dose of a hypnotic can be given IV just a minute or two before starting to give regional anesthesia; this helps to stun the patient and prevent movement. Even just 20–50 mg propofol IV can help to keep the patient still, yet able to follow the surgeon's directions.

O'Brien block (into the facial nerve over the condyle of the mandible, inferior to the posterior zygomatic process, to paralyze the orbicularis oculi muscle) and/or *Van Lint block* (paralysis of the orbicularis muscle and facial nerve branches over the periosteum just lateral to the orbital rim) may be performed to provide akinesia of the lids and extraocular muscles (Figure 7-4). Combining the O'Brien and Van Lint blocks ensures complete akinesia.

General anesthesia in ophthalmic surgery is typically employed for children, in case of traumatic eye injuries, and for very apprehensive or uncooperative patients. Care must be taken when placing

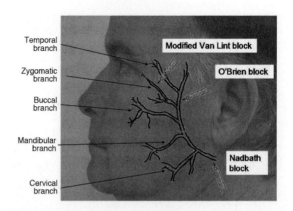

Figure 7-4   *Facial Nerve Blocks*

and holding a face mask over the mouth and the nose so that it does not worsen or cause injury to the eye(s).

Succinylcholine (Anectine) can increase intraocular pressure and should not be used with any eye surgery or where intraocular pressure increases would be detrimental to the patient. Examples include corneal transplants and open globe/penetrating eye injuries.

Do *not* give ketamine if IOP is increased or if the eye is injured, as this drug increases intraocular pressure.

OCULOCARDIAC REFLEX

The *oculocardiac reflex* is a vagally mediated reflex arc that, when stimulated, can cause a decreased output to the sinoatrial node of the heart, leading to reflex bradycardia, junctional rhythm, premature ventricular contractions (PVCs), and possibly sinus arrest. It is associated with ophthalmic surgery, specifically when *traction is applied to extraocular muscles* (especially the medial rectus) and/or there is *compression of the eyeball*. The arc is located between the ophthalmic nerve division of the trigeminal cranial nerve (CN VI) and the vagus nerve (CN X)—the cardiovascular center of the medulla oblongata in the brain stem—of the parasympathetic nervous system.

Treatment of the oculocardiac reflex includes removal of the stimulus; notify the surgeon to release any traction or pressure on the eye. Rarely, an anticholinergic (glycopyrrolate or atropine) will need to be given to increase the heart rate. Give ephedrine if the patient's blood pressure and heart rate drop. In extreme cases, cardiopulmonary resuscitation may be needed. Preoperative treatment may be given: Pretreatment with IV anticholinergics (glycopyrrolate) can be given immediately before surgery.

POSTOPERATIVE NAUSEA AND VOMITING

The following characteristics are associated with increased risk of PONV following ophthalmic surgery:

- Female
- Motion sickness history
- Pediatrics (6–10 years of age): 34% PONV occurrence
- Pediatrics (11–14 years of age): 35–50% PONV occurrence
- Nonsmoker
- Anxiety
- Surgery length greater than 45–60 minutes
- ***Surgery type: Ophthalmic***

OPHTHALMIC SURGERY: EYELIDS

Blepharoptosis Repair

Blepharoptosis repair involves correction of either unilateral or bilateral drooping of the upper eyelid. This defect can be congenital, acquired (neurogenic, myogenic, or aponeurosis defects), traumatic (ocular surgery), and/or mechanical (blepharochalasis—loss of elasticity of the skin of the upper eyelid; enophthalmos—recession of the eyeball within the orbit). Eyelid drooping can be severe enough to obstruct vision. (Also see the discussion of blepharoplasty—eyelid lift in the plastic surgery chapter.)

Operative Procedure

External levator resection or advancement is indicated in patients with moderate to severe ptosis and fair to poor levator function. A traction suture may be placed in the upper lid to permit downward traction. An incision is made from medial canthus to lateral canthus and carried through the orbicularis oculi to the superior border of the eyelid (tarsus). The upper half of the eyelid is exposed. The upper skin edge is grasped, and the orbicularis is separated from the orbital septum. Fat is retracted posteriorly, and the levator aponeurosis is exposed. The excess levator aponeurosis is excised. Lid crease skin sutures are placed.

A surgical alternative to levator advancement of the upper eyelid, used in cases involving severe eyelid drooping from poor levator muscle function, involves lifting the orbicularis oculi muscle flap before attaching to the connective tissue framing the eyelid.

Anesthetic

Local anesthesia eye drops with IV sedation may be used or general anesthesia is used with a laryngeal mask airway (LMA) or oral endotracheal tube (OETT). An oral RAE tube may be needed to keep the endotracheal tube out of the surgical field.

Positioning

The patient is positioned supine, with the operative-side arm tucked and the non-operative-side arm extended on a padded armboard. The bed is usually turned at least 90 degrees, if not 180 degrees, away from the anesthetist. The head of the bed may be raised approximately 20 degrees.

Anesthetic Implications

Give antiemetic treatment for prophylactic avoidance of vomiting and retching.

If the patient is moved from a bed onto the operating room table, have a lift sheet placed under the patient for ease in lifting him or her back onto the stretcher at the end of the case. This prevents the patient from straining during moving, thereby increasing intraocular pressure and possibly disrupting sutures.

Monitor for bradycardia and the oculocardiac reflex.

Canthorrhaphy

Canthorrhaphy involves surgical shortening of the palpebral fissure (the opening between the upper and lower eyelids at the medial or lateral canthus) by suturing the margins of the eyelids either partially or totally to narrow the opening. It is done at either canthus. This procedure is performed to surgically protect the eye when the eyelids cannot adequately protect the cornea and to prevent undue drying of the conjunctival membranes.

Operative Procedure

A corneal shield is placed. The lid margin is split to the canthal angle, and a segment is excised including the lash follicles; the mucosa adjacent is abraded. Sutures approximate the lid margins and are tied over stents. If further support is needed, the canthal tendon is shortened and/or sutured to the adjacent orbital periosteum. For temporary closure, the lateral lid margins are approximated by sutures passed through the lid margins (avoiding the eyelash-bearing surfaces).

Anesthetic

General anesthesia with an LMA or OETT may be needed; an oral RAE tube may be needed to keep the endotracheal tube out of surgical field. Local anesthesia and sedation can be done.

Positioning

The patient is positioned supine, with the operative-side arm tucked and the non-operative-side arm extended on a padded armboard. The bed is usually turned at least 90 degrees, if not 180 degrees, away from the anesthetist. The head of the bed may be raised approximately 20 degrees.

Anesthetic Implications

Give antiemetic treatment for prophylactic avoidance of vomiting and retching.

If the patient is moved from a bed onto the operating room table, have a lift sheet placed under the patient for ease in lifting him or her back onto the stretcher at the end of the case. This prevents the patient from straining during moving.

Monitor for bradycardia and the oculocardiac reflex.

Canthotomy

Canthotomy involves an incision of the canthus (where the upper and lower eyelids meet) of the eye; it may be made at either the medial or lateral canthus. This procedure is indicated when there is an adhesion of the eyelids or when exposure to the globe is inadequate. It is done to open and restore the canthus, and may be performed in tandem with other procedures.

Operative Procedure

After the canthus and the conjunctiva are incised, a hemostat can be clamped over the area for 60 seconds to cause hemostasis. Antibiotic ointment or drops may be instilled and an eye patch applied.

Anesthetic

This procedure is usually performed under local anesthetic eye drops and sedation.

Positioning

The patient is positioned supine, with the affected eye tilted up toward the ceiling; the operative-side arm may be tucked with the non-operative-side arm extended on a padded armboard. The bed is usually turned at least 90 degrees, if not 180 degrees, away from the anesthetist. The head of the bed may be raised approximately 20 degrees.

Anesthetic Implications

Give antiemetic treatment for prophylactic avoidance of vomiting and retching.

If the patient is moved from a bed onto the operating room table, have a lift sheet placed under the patient for ease in lifting him or her back onto the stretcher at the end of the case. This prevents the patient from straining during moving.

Monitor for bradycardia and the oculocardiac reflex.

Excision of Chalazion

Excision of a chalazion involves incision and curettage of a granulomatous swelling of the Meibomian gland(s), caused by hardened oils blocking the gland's duct from draining. Usually occurring on one of the upper eyelids, a chalazion can be a single or multiple swelling; it can subside spontaneously but may also become infected. Chalazions differ from stys in that they are, in and of themselves, painless, and are usually larger than a sty of the eyelid (a sty is a defined abscess caused by a bacterial infection).

Operative Procedure

A *conjunctival approach* is used if the chalazion is pointing through the conjunctiva on the outer edge of the eyelid or to avoid scarring on the upper lid. The lid is everted and the chalazion is incised at right angles to the lid margin; the contents are removed by scraping with a curette.

In the *skin approach*, an incision is made parallel to the lid. The orbicularis oculi muscle is cut, exposing the Meibomian gland. The contents are removed with a curette, and the wound is closed. Antibiotic eye ointment or drops may be instilled and an eye patch placed over the operative eye.

Anesthetic

Usually a local anesthetic injection into the eyelids is employed along with sedation. General anesthesia with a LMA may sometimes be necessary; an oral RAE tube may be needed to keep the endotracheal tube out of the surgical field.

Positioning

The patient is positioned supine, with the operative-side arm tucked and the non-operative-side arm extended on a padded armboard. The bed is usually turned at least 90 degrees, if not 180 degrees, away from the anesthetist. The head of the bed may be raised approximately 20 degrees.

Anesthetic Implications

If general anesthesia is used, tape the nonoperative eyelid closed. Place an eye pad over the eye and cover it with an occlusive clear dressing (Tegaderm) to protect it from cleansing solutions and any movement or grazing of instruments by the surgeon or scrub team as they are working over the face.

Give antiemetic treatment for prophylactic avoidance of vomiting and retching.

If the patient is moved from a bed onto the operating room table, have a lift sheet placed under the patient for ease in lifting him or her back onto the stretcher at the end of the case. This prevents the patient from straining during moving.

Monitor for bradycardia and the oculocardiac reflex.

Correction of Ectropion

This procedure is performed to correct a drooping, and eversion, of the lower eyelid margin.

- *Involutional:* most common type; caused by relaxation of the orbicular muscle; may be part of aging.
- *Congenital:* associated with Down syndrome; result of an elongation of the lower lid.
- *Paralytic:* caused by cranial nerve VII paralysis; the orbicularis oculi has lost its tone.

Operative Procedure

An incision is made in the lower lid margin from the punctum (the hole that drains tears from the eye) to just beyond the lateral canthus. A continued incision is made in the direction of the earlobe. A skin–muscle flap is developed and elevated across the lower lid. A vertical incision is made in the lateral third of the eyelid and angled into the inferior cul-de-sac. The two free edges of the lid are overlapped until tight, and the redundant portion is excised. The two lid edges are approximated. The orbicularis oculi muscle is approximated. The skin is pulled laterally; redundant skin is resected.

The skin is approximated. Antibiotic ophthalmic ointment is instilled and an eye pad placed.

Anesthetic
A local anesthesia injection is required. Rarely, general anesthesia may be used with a LMA; an oral RAE tube may be needed to keep the endotracheal tube out of the surgical field.

Positioning
The patient is positioned supine, with the operative-side arm tucked and the non-operative-side arm extended on a padded armboard. The bed is usually turned at least 90 degrees, if not 180 degrees, away from the anesthetist. The head of the bed may be raised approximately 20 degrees.

Anesthetic Implications
If general anesthesia is used and only one eye is operated on, tape the nonoperative eyelid closed. Place an eye pad over the eye and cover it with an occlusive clear dressing (Tegaderm) to protect it from cleansing solutions and any movement or grazing of instruments by the surgeon or scrub team as they are working over the face.

Give antiemetic treatment for prophylactic avoidance of vomiting and retching

If the patient is moved from a bed onto the operating room table, have a lift sheet placed under the patient for ease in lifting him or her back onto the stretcher at the end of the case. This prevents the patient from straining during moving, thereby increasing intraocular pressure and possibly disrupting sutures.

Monitor for bradycardia and the oculocardiac reflex.

Correction of Entropion
This surgery corrects an inversion (inward rotation) of the lid margins and eyelashes.
- *Congenital:* due to hypertrophy of the marginal and pretarsal orbicularis oculi muscle; causes the eyelid margin to be pushed up and against the globe.

- *Involutional:* most common. Occurs when canthal tendons retain their rigidity but the apposition of the lid to the globe is changed, resulting in the inversion of the eyelid; alternatively, it may occur as a result of weakness of the retractor muscles, causing muscle laxity of the lower lid.
- *Scarring:* burns, trauma.

Operative Procedure
The lower lid is everted. A base-down triangle of skin, orbicularis oculi muscle, and eyelid is excised. The edges are sutured together, and the remaining tissue is excised. In an alternative method, a tarsal strip is created by performing a canthotomy, denuding the area of skin, mucosa, and lashes. The strip is shortened and sutured to the inner aspect of the orbital rim. The skin is closed with sutures or tissue glue. An eye patch and shield are placed over the operative eye at the end of surgery.

A mucosal graft may be needed for repair.

Anesthetic
A local anesthesia injection is usual. General anesthesia with a LMA may be used in children and uncooperative patients; an oral RAE tube may be needed to keep the endotracheal tube out of the surgical field.

Nasal intubation may be needed if a mucosal graft is to be taken from the hard palate.

Positioning
The patient is positioned supine, with the operative-side arm tucked and the non-operative-side arm extended on a padded armboard. The bed is usually turned at least 90 degrees, if not 180 degrees, away from the anesthetist. The head of the bed may be raised approximately 20 degrees.

Anesthetic Implications
If general anesthesia is used and only one eye is operated on, tape the nonoperative eyelid closed.

Place an eye pad over the eye and cover it with an occlusive clear dressing (Tegaderm) to protect it from cleansing solutions and any movement or grazing of instruments by the surgeon or scrub team as they are working over the face.

Give antiemetic treatment for prophylactic avoidance of vomiting and retching.

If the patient is moved from a bed onto the operating room table, have a lift sheet placed under the patient for ease in lifting him or her back onto the stretcher at the end of the case. This prevents the patient from straining during moving, thereby increasing intraocular pressure and possibly disrupting sutures.

Monitor for bradycardia and the oculocardiac reflex.

Eyelid Laceration Repair

This procedure repairs one or more traumatic lacerations of the eyelid(s).

Operative Procedure

If the tear duct (canaliculus) is injured, a special rod may be placed through the lacerated end of the duct. A nonabsorbable suture is used to reapproximate the tear ducts around the rod. First the subcutaneous tissue and then the skin are sutured. An eye patch and shield are placed over the operative eye at the end of surgery.

Anesthetic

Local anesthesia eye drops or infiltration with sedation may be used. General anesthesia may be used with a LMA; an oral RAE tube may be needed to keep the endotracheal tube out of the surgical field.

Positioning

The patient is positioned supine, with the operative-side arm tucked and the non-operative-side arm extended on a padded armboard. The bed is usually turned at least 90 degrees, if not 180 degrees, away from the anesthetist. The head of the bed may be raised approximately 20 degrees.

Anesthetic Implications

If general anesthesia is used and only one eye is operated on, tape the nonoperative eyelid closed. Place an eye pad over the eye and cover it with an occlusive clear dressing (Tegaderm) to protect it from cleansing solutions and any movement or grazing of instruments by the surgeon or scrub team as they are working over the face.

Give antiemetic treatment for prophylactic avoidance of vomiting and retching.

If the patient is moved from a bed onto the operating room table, have a lift sheet placed under the patient for ease in lifting him or her back onto the stretcher at the end of the case. This prevents the patient from straining during moving, thereby increasing intraocular pressure and possibly disrupting sutures.

Monitor for bradycardia and the oculocardiac reflex.

Excision of Eyelid Lesion

Excision of an eyelid lesion may be performed for biopsy and/or cosmetic removal of eyelid lesions.

Operative Procedure

Cosmetically, skin lines are oriented to prevent closure without tension. The lesion is cut away with a pentagon-shaped pattern with a wide enough margin to ensure adequate tumor margins. An incision of the lateral canthus is done to effect closure without undue traction. Sutures are placed through the lid to restore continuity. The connective tissue of the eyelid is closed first, and then the skin is closed with non-absorbable sutures. Topical anesthetic drops may be instilled into the operative eye if the procedure is done with only local anesthesia. An eye patch and shield are placed over the operative eye at the end of surgery.

Anesthetic

This procedure may be performed using local anesthesia with sedation. General anesthesia with a LMA may also be used; an oral RAE tube may be needed to keep the endotracheal tube out of the surgical field.

Positioning

The patient is positioned supine, with the operative-side arm tucked and the nonoperative-side arm extended on a padded armboard. The bed is usually turned at least 90 degrees, if not 180 degrees, away from the anesthetist. The head of the bed may be raised approximately 20 degrees.

Anesthetic Implications

If general anesthesia is used and only one eye is operated on, tape the nonoperative eyelid closed. Place an eye pad over the eye and cover it with an occlusive clear dressing (Tegaderm) to protect it from cleansing solutions and any movement or grazing of instruments by the surgeon or scrub team as they are working over the face.

Give antiemetic treatment for prophylactic avoidance of vomiting and retching.

If the patient is moved from a bed onto the operating room table, have a lift sheet placed under the patient for ease in lifting him or her back onto the stretcher at the end of the case. This prevents the patient from straining during moving, thereby possibly disrupting sutures.

Monitor for bradycardia and the oculocardiac reflex.

Tarsorrhaphy

In tarsorraphy, the upper and lower eyelids are surgically sewn closed, either partially or for the total eyelid. The approximation of the eyelids does not involve just the canthus (see the discussion of canthorrhaphy), but rather the middle section outward.

This surgery is performed on patients who cannot close their eyes fully—for example, in Graves' disease, when the eye is abnormally widened and unable to close, with chronic corneal abrasions, after total globe removal without insertion of a prosthesis, or when the eyelids are abnormally widened as with facial nerve palsy and lower eyelid ptosis. Inability to close the eyes completely may result from either a temporary or permanent widening of the eyelids. As the eyeball moves about under the lid, there is less exposure to the air and the tears help bathe the eye.

Operative Procedure

A corneal shield is placed. The lid margins are approximated by sutures (avoiding the eyelash-bearing surfaces). For a more permanent union, a section of conjunctiva is excised prior to suture placement. For reversal after temporary closure, the tarsorrhaphy is incised and the wound surfaces are sutured to prevent re-adhesion.

Anesthetic

General anesthesia is used with a LMA or OETT; an oral RAE tube may be needed to keep the endotracheal tube out of the surgical field. Local anesthesia and sedation may also be used.

Positioning

The patient is positioned supine, with the operative-side arm tucked and the non-operative-side arm extended on a padded armboard. The bed is usually turned at least 90 degrees, if not 180 degrees, away from the anesthetist. The head of the bed may be raised approximately 20 degrees.

Anesthetic Implications

Give antiemetic treatment for prophylactic avoidance of vomiting and retching.

If the patient is moved from a bed onto the operating room table, have a lift sheet placed under the patient for ease in lifting him or her back onto the stretcher at the end of the case. This prevents the patient from straining during moving, thereby increasing intraocular pressure and possibly disrupting sutures.

Monitor for bradycardia and the oculocardiac reflex.

OPHTHALMIC SURGERY: LACRIMAL GLAND

Dacryocystorhinostomy

Dacryocystorhinostomy is performed to restore the flow of tears from the lacrimal sac into the nose when the nasolacrimal duct is blocked. A "drain" is created between the lacrimal sac and the nasopharynx.

This procedure is indicated to prevent infection or chronic tearing if the nasolacrimal duct is blocked—for example, due to chronic dacryocystitis. Probing or irrigation of the duct is necessary if medical management is unsuccessful.

Operative Procedure

A small incision is made on the side of the nose, starting 1 cm from the medial canthus and moving down to just above the level of the nose wings. The nose may be packed with gauze packing (packing may be soaked in cocaine or phenylephrine) or Gelfoam pledgets to help stop oozing. The lacrimal sac is separated from the bone and retracted as the part of the lacrimal crest is cut and removed to make a connection to the nose. An indwelling silicone tube is inserted into the duct to serve as a stent if probing or irrigation is unsuccessful. Silicone tubing is inserted to prevent the hole from closing and is removed several weeks later. Antibiotic ophthalmic drops may be instilled.

This procedure can be performed endoscopically, where the lacrimal sac can be visualized and an opening is created into the lacrimal sac to facilitate the drainage of tears from within the nasal cavity. Doing this procedure endoscopically avoids the formation of a scar.

Anesthetic

In infants (up to six months of age), probing may be done with a topical anesthetic. The baby is wrapped in a papoose-like wrap. In patients older than six months, general anesthesia may be used.

Positioning

The patient is positioned supine, with the operative-side arm tucked and the nonoperative-side arm extended on a padded armboard. Arms should be secured because the table may be placed in reverse Trendelenburg position; a padded footboard is used. The bed is usually turned at least 90 degrees, if not 180 degrees, away from the anesthetist. The head of the bed may be raised approximately 20 degrees.

Anesthetic Implications

Monitor the heart rate and ST segments on the EKG if local anesthetic with epinephrine is administered during the procedure (the vasoconstrictor may be infiltrated to minimize bleeding). A block of local anesthetic may cause a temporary dilated pupil or medial rectus muscle paralysis.

Give antiemetic treatment for prophylactic avoidance of vomiting and retching for patients older than one year of age.

If general anesthesia is used, a throat pack may be placed (document its insertion and removal time) to prevent blood from draining into the upper airway during surgery.

If general anesthesia is used and only one eye is operated on, tape the nonoperative eyelid closed. Place an eye pad over the eye and cover it with an occlusive clear dressing (Tegaderm) to protect it from cleansing solutions and any movement or grazing of instruments by the surgeon or scrub team as they are working over the face.

Lacrimal Duct Probing

This procedure opens the nasolacrimal duct. It may be performed to prevent acute infection of the lacrimal duct system if conservative management is unsuccessful in alleviating the blockage. If repeated probing is necessary to maintain patency, the placement of an indwelling silicone tube is done. (See the discussion of dacryocystorhinostomy earlier in this section.)

Operative Procedure

A lacrimal dilator is placed into the upper tear ducts; increasing-size probes are placed until the duct is opened. A solution is then irrigated through the tear duct into the nose. Antibiotic ophthalmic drops are instilled at the end of the case.

Anesthetic

A topical local anesthetic is instilled in patients who are six months of age and younger; general anesthesia is usual for children older than six months.

Positioning

The patient is positioned supine, with the operative-side arm tucked and the nonoperative-side arm extended on a padded armboard. The bed is usually turned at least 90 degrees, if not 180 degrees, away from the anesthetist. The head of the bed may be raised approximately 20 degrees.

Anesthetic Implications

Give antiemetic treatment for prophylactic avoidance of vomiting and retching in patients greater than one year of age.

If general anesthesia is used and only one eye is operated on, tape the nonoperative eyelid closed. Place an eye pad over the eye and cover it with an occlusive clear dressing (Tegaderm) to protect it from cleansing solutions and any movement or grazing of instruments by the surgeon or scrub team as they are working over the face.

OPHTHALMIC SURGERY: GLOBE AND ORBIT

Removal of the eye by enucleation or evisceration is done not only to minimize the risk of death from malignant processes, but also to relieve pain and to maintain the well-being of the patient. With any procedure removing the eye, the postoperative appearance should be considered. After removal of the eye, an orbital implant or prosthesis, made from plastic, metal alloy, or glass, can be used to give the area a more natural appearance by restoring volume and providing a stable eye socket. If the extraocular muscles are left, an ocular prosthesis will have enhanced motility and movement, tracking and moving simultaneously with the other eye. The conjunctiva is sewn closed over the implant at the end of the case. Once the conjunctiva is healed and postoperative swelling has subsided, a cupped disc can be formed and placed over the prosthesis, painted and finished to mimic the appearance of the patient's natural eye color. This disc, which is placed in the pocket behind the eyelids, can be removed and cleaned periodically.

Succinylcholine (Anectine) can increase intraocular pressure and should *not* be used with any eye surgery or any other procedure where IOP increases would be detrimental to the patient.

Eye Enucleation

Eye enucleation involves removal of the eyeball and a portion of the optic nerve; the eyelids and the eye socket are not removed. This surgery may be performed in the following circumstances:

- Cancer of the eye: malignant intraocular tumors, melanomas, any other cancers of the eye or orbit
- Severe injury of the eye when the eye cannot be saved or attempts to save the eye have failed
- End-stage glaucoma
- A painful blind eye or for cosmetic reasons with a blind eye
- Congenital cystic eye
- Eye removal for corneal harvesting
- After ocular trauma to prevent sympathetic ophthalmia (inflammation of the eye) from traveling to other eye, which, if untreated, can cause blindness

Operative Procedure

A cut is made separating the conjunctiva and Tenon's capsule from the globe. The superior oblique tendon is grasped with a muscle hook and divided. The inferior oblique muscle is double-clamped with hemostats for hemostasis; the muscle is then cut between the hemostats. All attachments to the globe are separated, permitting the globe to move freely. The conjunctiva, connective tissue, and extraocular muscles are left in place to help in stabilizing an implant. The location of the optic nerve is identified with the nerve being transected and the globe delivered. Hemostasis is achieved. A spherical prosthesis is inserted into Tenon's capsule and the conjunctiva is approximated. An intermarginal suture is placed to produce a mild pressure effect. An antibiotic ointment may be instilled, an eye pad is placed, and a pressure dressing is applied.

Anesthetic

General anesthesia is used with an OETT; an oral RAE tube may be needed to keep the endotracheal tube out of the surgical field. Muscle relaxants may be used. Succinylcholine (Anectine) may be given as the injured eye is being removed.

Positioning

The patient is positioned supine, with the operative-side arm tucked and the nonoperative-side arm extended on a padded armboard. The bed is usually turned at least 90 degrees, if not 180 degrees, away from the anesthetist. The head of the bed may be raised approximately 20 degrees.

Anesthetic Implications

When only one eye is operated on, tape the nonoperative eyelid closed. Place an eye pad over the eye and cover it with an occlusive clear dressing (Tegaderm) to protect it from cleansing solutions and any movement or grazing of instruments by the surgeon or scrub team as they are working over the face.

Give antiemetic treatment for prophylactic avoidance of vomiting and retching

If the patient is moved from a bed onto the operating room table, have a lift sheet placed under the patient for ease in lifting him or her back onto the stretcher at the end of the case. This prevents the patient from straining during moving, thereby increasing intraocular pressure and possibly disrupting sutures.

Monitor for bradycardia and the oculocardiac reflex.

Eye Evisceration

Eye evisceration involves removal of the internal contents of the eye within the scleral shell (white of the eye), while leaving the sclera and extraocular muscles intact. Maintaining the extraocular muscles attached to the scleral shell allows a prosthesis to be moveable after its insertion. This surgery may be performed for the following indications:

- Endophthalmitis unresponsive to antibiotics
- Cancer of the eye: retinoblastoma, melanomas, any other cancers of the eye or orbit
- Severe injury of the eye when the eye cannot be saved or attempts to save the eye have failed
- End-stage glaucoma
- A painful blind eye or for cosmetic reasons with a blind eye
- Congenital cystic eye
- Eye removal for corneal harvesting
- To prevent sympathetic ophthalmia (inflammation of the eye) from traveling to other eye, which, if untreated, can cause blindness

Operative Procedure

A circumferential 360-degree incision across the sclera through to the uvea, separating the conjunctiva and Tenon's capsule from the globe, is made around the eye. An eviscerating spoon is used to separate the entire uvea from the sclera and is removed. Any remaining uvea is removed with gauze rotated within the scleral shell. The shell is irrigated and hemostasis achieved. The posterior surface of the cornea is removed to prevent sensitivity to the patient in the postoperative period. A spherical prosthesis is then inserted. The sclera and the conjunctiva are approximated; antibiotic ointment is instilled and an eye patch applied.

Anesthetic

General anesthesia is used with an OETT; an oral RAE tube may be needed to keep the endotracheal tube out of the surgical field. Muscle relaxants. Succinylcholine (Anectine) may be given as the injured eye is being removed.

Positioning

The patient is positioned supine, with the operative-side arm tucked and the non-operative-side arm extended on a padded armboard. The bed is usually turned at least 90 degrees, if not 180 degrees, away from the anesthetist. The head of the bed may be raised approximately 20 degrees.

Anesthetic Implications

When only one eye is operated on, tape the nonoperative eyelid closed. Place an eye pad over the eye and cover it with an occlusive clear dressing (Tegaderm) to protect it from cleansing solutions and any movement or grazing of instruments by the surgeon or scrub team as they are working over the face.

Give antiemetic treatment for prophylactic avoidance of vomiting and retching.

If the patient is moved from a bed onto the operating room table, have a lift sheet placed under the patient for ease in lifting him or her back onto the stretcher at the end of the case. This prevents the patient from straining during moving, thereby increasing intraocular pressure and possibly disrupting sutures.

Monitor for bradycardia and the oculocardiac reflex.

Eye Exenteration

Eye exenteration is the most radical of the three eye removal procedures. It involves removal of the eye, adnexa (parts attached or adjacent structures in relation to the eyeball—that is, fat, tear glands, muscles), and part of the bony orbit. The amount of the tissues removed beyond the globe depends on the origin and extent of the disease process. The eyelids may also be removed in cases of cutaneous cancers and unrelenting infection. Exenteration is sometimes done together with removal of the maxilla or the upper jaw bone and cheekbone.

This procedure is usually performed for large orbital tumors or extended intraocular tumors, but may also be performed for benign disease such as phycomycosis. Indications for its use are as follows:

- Cancer of the eye: retinoblastoma, melanomas, any other cancers of the eye or orbit

- Severe injury of the eye when the eye cannot be saved or attempts to save the eye have failed
- End-stage glaucoma
- A painful blind eye or for cosmetic reasons with a blind eye
- Congenital cystic eye
- Eye removal for corneal harvesting
- To prevent sympathetic ophthalmia (inflammation of the eye) from traveling to other eye, which, if untreated, can cause blindness

Operative Procedure

- *Subtotal:* excision of eye and epibulbar tissues. Done to remove tumors of the anterior portion of the eye and the conjunctiva.
- *Total:* excision of all tissues within the eye orbit, including the periorbita, with or without removal of the eye lids. Indicated when an intraocular tumor extends into the orbit.
- *Radical:* removal of one or more bony orbital walls in addition to soft tissues and periosteum. Indicated when a malignant sinus tumor invades the orbit or when a malignant skin tumor involves the orbital bones.

If the eyelid is to be preserved, an incision is made circumferentially around the palpebral fissure. The skin is dissected to the orbital rim. The orbicularis muscle may be incised with the cutting blade of an electrosurgical pencil. The periosteum is separated from the orbital rim and walls. The eye and soft tissues within the orbit are removed. The skin is undermined and closed over the lateral orbital rim. A split-thickness skin graft may be used to cover the denuded orbital walls. The orbital cavity is packed with gauze impregnated with antibiotic ointment and a moderate pressure dressing is applied.

After the wound has healed, the cavity may be covered with a black patch or a cosmetic plastic prosthesis.

Anesthetic

General anesthesia is used with an OETT; an oral RAE tube may be needed to keep the endotracheal tube out of the surgical field. Muscle relaxants may be used. Succinylcholine (Anectine) may be given as the injured eye is being removed.

Positioning

The patient is positioned supine, with the operative-side arm tucked and the nonoperative-side arm extended on a padded armboard. The bed is usually turned at least 90 degrees, if not 180 degrees, away from the anesthetist. The head of the bed may be raised approximately 20 degrees.

Anesthetic Implications

Determine if a skin graft is to be used.

When only one eye is operated on, tape the non-operative eyelid closed. Place an eye pad over the eye and cover it with an occlusive clear dressing (Tegaderm) to protect it from cleansing solutions and any movement or grazing of instruments by the surgeon or scrub team as they are working over the face.

Give antiemetic treatment for prophylactic avoidance of vomiting and retching.

If the patient is moved from a bed onto the operating room table, have a lift sheet placed under the patient for ease in lifting him or her back onto the stretcher at the end of the case. This prevents the patient from straining during moving, thereby increasing intraocular pressure and possibly disrupting sutures.

Monitor for bradycardia and the oculocardiac reflex.

Extraction of Intraocular Foreign Body

Foreign bodies within the eye should be removed, if possible, unless they can be tolerated indefinitely and are of no harm to the patient. Particles of iron or copper must be removed to prevent ocular tissue degeneration; metallic foreign bodies must also be removed as their inadvertent dislodgement can have catastrophic effects (e.g., during an MRI owing to magnetic effects). Particles of glass or porcelain can be tolerated and may be better left alone.

Several methods are used to localize intraocular foreign bodies: ultrasonography, coronal CT scan of the orbits, and an electronic metal locator (sterilized and passed over the eye during surgery).

Operative Procedure

If the foreign object (FO) is anterior to the lens zonules, it is removed through an incision into the anterior chamber at the limbus. If it is behind the lens but anterior to the equator, it is removed through the area of the pars plana (part of the uvea and choroid; approximately 4 mm long and located near the iris and the sclera) nearest to the FO. If the FO is lodged posterior to the equator, it is removed through the pars plana by vitrectomy and intraocular forceps to avoid major choroidal hemorrhages from incisions into the posterior wall of the eyeball.

Should any area of the retina be damaged, it should be treated with diathermy, photocoagulation, or endolaser coagulation to prevent retinal detachment.

An eye patch and shield are placed over the operative eye at the end of surgery.

Anesthetic

General anesthesia is used with OETT; an oral RAE tube may be needed to keep the endotracheal tube out of the surgical field. Muscle relaxants may be used. Do *not* use succinylcholine (Anectine). Do *not* use nitrous oxide.

These patients are considered an emergency and to have a full stomach. A rapid-sequence induction should be done. A smooth induction is necessary to maintain hemodynamics and to avoid hypertension and the Valsalva maneuver (both of which increase intraocular pressure). Regional anesthesia is contraindicated.

An increase in intraocular pressure during the time when the patient's own eye is open (e.g., because of coughing, vomiting, movement, straining, breath holding) can cause the intraocular contents to be expelled.

Positioning

The patient is positioned supine, with the operative-side arm tucked and the nonoperative-side arm extended on a padded armboard. The bed is usually turned at least 90 degrees, if not 180 degrees, away from the anesthetist. The head of the bed may be raised approximately 20 degrees.

Anesthetic Implications

Give antiemetic treatment for prophylactic avoidance of vomiting and retching.

When only one eye is operated on, tape the nonoperative eyelid closed. Place an eye pad over the eye and cover it with an occlusive clear dressing (Tegaderm) to protect it from cleansing solutions and any movement or grazing of instruments by the surgeon or scrub team as they are working over the face.

If the patient is moved from a bed onto the operating room table, have a lift sheet placed under the patient for ease in lifting him or her back onto the stretcher at the end of the case. This prevents the patient from straining during moving, thereby increasing intraocular pressure and possibly disrupting sutures.

Monitor for bradycardia and the oculocardiac reflex.

Orbit Fracture Repair

Orbit fractures are usually caused by mid-facial, blunt trauma (usually not penetrating), such as from a motor vehicle collision, industrial accident, sports trauma, or assault. Fractures vary in their displacement and type of fracture; likewise, the injury severity ranges from small minimally displaced fractures of an isolated wall that require no surgical intervention to major disruption of the orbit. Discerning which orbital wall is fractured is important because of the possible associated damage in surrounding structures. This determination will help to diagnose injury to the soft tissues, neurovascular structures, and the globe. The surgical approach is dependent on this information.

Operative Procedure

The goal of orbital reconstruction is to achieve normal bony projection by reduction, replacement of lost bone, and/or fixation of comminuted bone; to release or resuspend any entrapped orbital soft tissue; and to replace normal orbital volume. This surgery may be done transcutaneously or by transconjunctival or endoscopic (transmaxillary or transnasal) approaches.

Complex multiple-wall orbit fractures or fractures that extend laterally to the infraorbital nerve must be repaired using an open approach because of the greater risk of postoperative paresthesias. Additional incisions may be required to provide adequate exposure along with periosteal elevation, to adequately expose the fracture, and to ensure anatomic alignment. During an open approach (either transcutaneous or transconjunctival), excessive pressure or retraction should be avoided on the globe and surrounding nerves. Extreme care is required around the sides or back of the eye to prevent injury to the surrounding sinuses and ethmoidal blood vessels. With these approaches, dissection is carried down to the periosteum to expose the orbital rim where the limits of the fracture can be assessed. Herniated or entrapped orbital soft tissue is reduced and repositioned. Once the soft tissues are repositioned, an orbital implant may be placed to completely cover the bony defect, preventing any further movement of the soft tissue. Implants are chosen based on surgeon and institutional preference, and all have their own advantages and disadvantages. Implants can be autogenous (patient's own cartilage, bone, fascia), allogenic dura, or artificial materials (e.g., Teflon, silicon, titanium); such implants are used to rebuild the orbital walls and facial skeleton. A skeletal fracture may also need plates to rigidly affix a fracture. Conjunctiva or skin is then closed with absorbable sutures.

Orbital floor, orbital roof, and medial wall fractures are the best candidates for an endoscopic endonasal approach. However, an additional septoplasty may be needed to obtain an adequate view of these structures. When obtaining patient consent for surgery, the surgeon must discuss with the patient the possibility of switching to an open approach if the endoscopic approach fails.

The transmaxillary endoscopic approach offers excellent visualization of the entire orbital floor. A safe and efficacious procedure, it eliminates any postoperative eyelid complications. With this approach, a 1- to 2-inch incision under the lip at the top of the upper gum (sublabial) is made over the canine fossa to expose the maxillary sinus; a hole (antrostomy) is made and enlarged to just below the infraorbital foramen and lateral to the nasomaxillary support, thus avoiding injury to nerves and dental roots.

In orbital floor fractures (trapdoor fractures), a malleable retractor can be passed through the maxillary sinus antrostomy and used to reduce the orbital contents. In medial blow-out fractures, a circumferential dissection is made first and, after the margins are defined, a small dissection is made on the orbital side of the defect to allow placement of the implant.

Anesthetic

General anesthesia with an OETT; an oral RAE tube may be needed to keep the endotracheal tube out of the surgical field. Muscle relaxants may be used. Do *not* use succinylcholine (Anectine). An increase in intraocular pressure during the time when the patient's own eye is open (e.g., because of coughing, vomiting, movement, straining, breath holding) can cause the intraocular contents to be expelled.

If this procedure is done as an emergency case, the patient should be considered to have a full stomach and a rapid-sequence induction should be done. A smooth induction is necessary to maintain hemodynamics and to avoid hypertension and the Valsalva maneuver (both of which increase intraocular pressure). Regional anesthesia is contraindicated.

Positioning

The patient is positioned supine, with the operative-side arm tucked and the nonoperative-side arm extended on a padded armboard. The bed is usually turned at least 90 degrees, if not 180 degrees, away from the anesthetist. The head of the bed may be raised approximately 20 degrees.

Anesthetic Implications

Most patients who require orbit fracture repair present with a history of blunt trauma and, therefore, must be assessed and managed for potential airway difficulty, cervical neck injury, and hemodynamic instability. The patient may have had head and neck CT scans assessing bone fractures and soft-tissue injuries, and possibly MRI studies to assess for bleeding in the sheath of the optic nerve. Severe head injury should have been ruled out before the patient arrives in the OR. Imaging study films should be present in the operating room before beginning surgery.

Patients should be told to avoid blowing their nose and performing Valsalva maneuvers to limit intraorbital subcutaneous emphysema and possible cerebrospinal fluid leaks.

Intraoperatively, analgesia and antiemetics are given for prophylactic avoidance of pain and vomiting and retching. The use of steroids (Decadron 0.25 mg/kg IV) has been suggested to augment antiemetics and to decrease soft-tissue edema.

When only one eye is operated on, tape the nonoperative eyelid closed. Place an eye pad over the eye and cover it with an occlusive clear dressing (Tegaderm) to protect it from cleansing solutions and any movement or grazing of instruments by the surgeon or scrub team as they are working over the face.

If the patient is moved from a bed onto the operating room table, have a lift sheet placed under the patient for ease in lifting him or her back onto the stretcher at the end of the case. This prevents the patient from straining during moving, thereby increasing intraocular pressure and possibly disrupting sutures.

Recording the patient's visual acuity when the patient has regained consciousness is prudent. Maintaining the patient in a head-up position may be useful in decreasing postoperative edema.

Monitor for bradycardia and the oculocardiac reflex.

Ruptured Globe Repair

Repair of a ruptured globe is undertaken when the integrity of the eye's outer membranes is disrupted. Such a procedure is indicated for any full-thickness injury to the cornea, the sclera, or both by blunt or penetrating trauma. These conditions are major ophthalmic emergencies that always require surgical intervention. The goal is to replace extruded intraocular contents, to remove any foreign body, and to close the defect.

A CT scan (axial and coronal views of the brain) is the most sensitive imaging study to visualize the anatomy of the eye and the orbit to detect eye rupture and optic nerve injury. An MRI is useful in identifying soft-tissue injuries but cannot be done if a metallic foreign body is suspected to be present in any wound. Ultrasound of the eye cannot be done due to the risks of applying direct pressure on or around the globe.

Early recognition of a ruptured globe, along with identification of injury to surrounding structures, especially the eye orbit, is crucial to maximizing the functional outcome. A ruptured globe will allow aqueous humor to escape the anterior chamber, which will result in a flat-appearing eye, air bubbles under the cornea, or an asymmetric pupil secondary to the iris protruding through the corneal defect. Posterior eye injuries may require a complete opening of the conjunctiva to allow assessment.

Operative Procedure

An eye speculum is placed to provide exposure. The eye is examined and the laceration(s) identified. Scissors and forceps can be used to dissect the conjunctiva away from the wound. Any prolapsed tissue is brought back into its normal position. Nylon sutures are used to close any scleral or corneal lacerations. A puncture is made into the anterior chamber, and a balanced salt solution is injected to fill the chamber. The wound is checked—it should be water-tight. A Vicryl suture is used to close the conjunctival tear. An antibiotic and steroid injection is instilled under the conjunctiva; in grossly contaminated eye wounds, intravitreal antibiotic prophylaxis may be given. The eye speculum is removed; a soft dressing is then placed and covered with a rigid eye shield.

In some cases, the eye may be determined to be unrepairable and need to be enucleated.

Anesthetic

General anesthesia with an OETT; an oral RAE tube may be needed to keep the endotracheal tube out of the surgical field. Muscle relaxants may be used. Do *not* use succinylcholine (Anectine). Do *not* use nitrous oxide.

These patients are considered an emergency and to have a full stomach. A rapid-sequence induction should be done. A smooth induction is necessary to maintain hemodynamics and to avoid hypertension and the Valsalva maneuver (both of which increase intraocular pressure). Regional anesthesia is contraindicated.

An increase in intraocular pressure during the time when the patient's own eye is open (e.g., because of coughing, vomiting, movement, straining, breath holding) can cause the intraocular contents to be expelled.

Positioning

The patient is positioned supine, with the operative-side arm tucked and the non-operative-side arm extended on a padded armboard. The bed is usually turned at least 90 degrees, if not 180 degrees, away from the anesthetist. The head of the bed may be raised approximately 20 degrees.

Anesthetic Implications

Most patients requiring ruptured globe repair present with a history of blunt trauma and, therefore, must be assessed and managed for potential airway difficulty, cervical neck injury, and hemodynamic instability. The patient may have had head and neck CT scans assessing bone fractures and soft-tissue injuries, and possibly MRI studies to assess for bleeding in the sheath of the optic nerve. Severe head injury should have been ruled out before the patient arrives in the OR. Imaging study films should be present in the operating room before beginning surgery.

When only one eye is operated on, tape the nonoperative eyelid closed. Place an eye pad over the eye and cover it with an occlusive clear dressing (Tegaderm) to protect it from cleansing solutions and any movement or grazing of instruments by the surgeon or scrub team as they are working over the face.

Give antiemetic treatment for prophylactic avoidance of vomiting and retching. Give analgesics to prevent the patient from attempting the Valsalva maneuver.

Avoid all pressure on or around the eye. If there is an impaled object, do not attempt to remove it or touch it in any way.

If the patient is moved from a bed onto the operating room table, have a lift sheet placed under the patient for ease in lifting him or her back onto the stretcher at the end of the case. This prevents the patient from straining during moving, thereby increasing intraocular pressure and possibly disrupting sutures.

Monitor for bradycardia and the oculocardiac reflex.

Although the globe's position within the orbit protects it from injury in many situations, damage to the posterior segment of the eye is associated with a very high frequency of permanent visual loss.

Correction of Strabismus

This procedure is undertaken to align the eyes' visual axes. It is performed when medical treatment (patching, glasses, eye exercises) fails to align the visual axes of the eyes. Surgical alignment cannot guarantee complete restoration.

Operative Procedure

Lateral rectus resection involves shortening of this extraocular muscle. An eye speculum is inserted; an incision is made in the conjunctiva at the limbus to expose the lateral rectus muscle. The eye is then retracted medially as far as possible. Two traction sutures are placed in the conjunctiva, and it is freed from underlying tissue. A muscle hook is passed under the muscle insertion site. The amount of muscle to be resected is measured with a caliper. A muscle clamp is clamped over the muscle and the measured portion is excised. The end of the muscle is reattached to the original point of insertion. The conjunctiva is then closed, antibiotic ophthalmic ointment may be instilled, and an eye pad is applied.

Medial rectus recession is the lengthening of this extraocular muscle by detaching it from its original insertion and reattaching it more posteriorly on the sclera. An eye speculum is inserted. An incision is made in the conjunctiva at the limbus, and it is freed from underlying tissue. The distance from the original point of insertion to the new one is measured with a caliper. Two absorbable sutures are placed in the eye of the muscle. A straight mosquito hemostat is clamped across the muscle to compress small blood vessels and discourage oozing. The hemostat is removed once hemostasis has occurred; a muscle hook is passed under the muscle to lift it, and the muscle is incised. The muscle is reattached at the new point of insertion farther back on the globe with the previously placed sutures. The conjunctiva is then closed.

Anesthetic

General anesthesia is used with or without a retrobulbar injection. An oral RAE tube may be needed to keep the endotracheal tube out of the surgical field.

Positioning

The patient is positioned supine, with the operative-side arm tucked and the nonoperative-side arm extended on a padded armboard. The bed is usually turned at least 90 degrees, if not 180 degrees, away from the anesthetist. The head of the bed may be raised approximately 20 degrees.

Anesthetic Implications

Give antiemetic treatment for prophylactic avoidance of vomiting and retching.

If only one eye is operated on, tape the nonoperative eyelid closed. Place an eye pad over the eye and cover it with an occlusive clear dressing (Tegaderm) to protect it from cleansing solutions and any movement or grazing of instruments by the surgeon or scrub team as they are working over the face.

If the patient is moved from a bed onto the operating room table, have a lift sheet placed under the patient for ease in lifting him or her back onto the stretcher at the end of the case. This prevents the patient from straining during moving, thereby increasing intraocular pressure and possibly disrupting sutures.

The oculocardiac reflex is seen in strabismus surgery especially because of work done to the medial rectus. Monitor all patients undergoing this procedure for bradycardia and asystole.

OPHTHALMIC SURGERY: CONJUNCTIVA

Excision of Pterygium

Excision of a pterygium is defined as removal of a growth of tissue that extends from the conjunctiva onto the superficial cornea. A pterygium is a benign growth of the conjunctiva, usually found on the medial aspect of the eye. It is thought to be associated with exposure to ultraviolet light, dust, wind, sand, and low humidity, and is caused by a degeneration of collagen and fibrovascular proliferation.

A pterygium can be excised if it interferes with the person's vision, if the growth becomes inflamed and does not respond to topical medications, or for cosmetic reasons. The only definitive treatment is surgical removal.

Operative Procedure

An eye speculum is inserted. One side of the pterygium is dissected from the cornea and undermined toward the sclera. A suture is passed under the main portion of the pterygium; with the surgeon using a sawing motion, it is stripped from the cornea as the suture is moved from one end of the growth to the other. Hemostasis is achieved with cautery.

A conjunctival autograft can be taken from the inside of the patient's upper eyelid and used to replace the bare sclera that has been removed with pterygium excision. This graft is fixated with sutures or adhesive.

Amniotic membrane transplantation, where the source material is taken from the innermost layer of the human placenta, has been used in place of a conjunctival graft. Use of an amniotic membrane graft facilitates epithelialization and has anti-inflammatory properties as well. Like the conjunctival autograft, it is fixated with sutures or adhesive. An eye patch and shield are placed over the operative eye at the end of surgery.

Anesthetic

Topical local anesthesia eye drops or subconjunctival anesthesia is applied with IV sedation; a retrobulbar block is also done.

Positioning

The patient is positioned supine, with the operative-side arm tucked and the nonoperative-side arm extended on a padded armboard. The bed is usually turned at least 90 degrees, if not 180 degrees, away from the anesthetist. The head of the bed may be raised approximately 20 degrees.

Anesthetic Implications

Give antiemetic treatment for prophylactic avoidance of vomiting and retching.

If only one eye is operated on, tape the nonoperative eyelid closed. Place an eye pad over the eye and cover it with an occlusive clear dressing (Tegaderm) to protect it from cleansing solutions and any movement or grazing of instruments by the surgeon or scrub team as they are working over the face.

If the patient is moved from a bed onto the operating room table, have a lift sheet placed under the patient for ease in lifting him or her back onto the stretcher at the end of the case. This prevents the patient from straining during moving, thereby increasing intraocular pressure and possibly disrupting sutures.

Monitor for bradycardia and the oculocardiac reflex.

OPHTHALMIC SURGERY: CORNEA

Repair of Corneal Lacerations

A corneal laceration is either a partial- or full-thickness injury to the cornea. A partial-thickness injury does not violate the globe of the eye. A full-thickness injury causes a ruptured globe (see the earlier discussion of ruptured globe repair).

Operative Procedure

An eye speculum is placed to provide exposure. The eye is examined and the laceration(s) identified. Scissors and forceps can be used to dissect the conjunctiva away from the wound. Any prolapsed tissue is brought back into its normal position. Nylon sutures are used to close any scleral or corneal laceration. Vicryl sutures are used to close the conjunctival tear. An antibiotic and steroid injection is instilled under the conjunctiva. The eye speculum is removed, a soft dressing is placed, and the eye is covered with a rigid eye shield.

Anesthetic

General anesthesia is used with insertion of an OETT; an oral RAE tube may be needed to keep the endotracheal tube out of the surgical field.

These patients are considered an emergency and to have a full stomach. A rapid-sequence induction should be done. A smooth induction is necessary to maintain hemodynamics and to avoid hypertension and the Valsalva maneuver (both of which increase intraocular pressure). Regional anesthesia is contraindicated.

Positioning

The patient is positioned supine, with the operative-side arm tucked and the nonoperative-side arm extended on a padded armboard. The bed is usually turned at least 90 degrees, if not 180 degrees, away from the anesthetist. The head of the bed may be raised approximately 20 degrees.

Anesthetic Implications

The patient's eye will be intensely painful and tearing profusely.

If only one eye is operated on, tape the nonoperative eyelid closed. Place an eye pad over the eye and cover it with an occlusive clear dressing (Tegaderm) to protect it from cleansing solutions and any movement or grazing of instruments by the surgeon or scrub team as they are working over the face.

Give antiemetic treatment for prophylactic avoidance of vomiting and retching.

If the patient is moved from a bed onto the operating room table, have a lift sheet placed under the patient for ease in lifting him or her back onto the stretcher at the end of the case. This prevents the patient from straining during moving, thereby increasing intraocular pressure and possibly disrupting sutures.

Monitor for bradycardia and the oculocardiac reflex.

OPHTHALMIC SURGERY: TRANSPLANTATION

Corneal Transplant: Keratoplasty

In keratoplasty (also known as corneal grafting or penetrating keratoplasty), a diseased opaque host cornea is replaced with a donated clear cornea.

A corneal transplant is indicated in case of opacification of the cornea due to injury, disease, or old age; the goal is to improve vision and restore corneal integrity. The retina and optic nerve must be functioning properly to do a corneal transplant.

Indications for corneal transplantation include the following:

- *Optical:* to improve visual acuity by replacing the opaque host tissue with clear healthy donor tissue.
- *Reconstructive:* to restore corneal anatomy and integrity in patients with stromal thinning, or to reconstruct the anatomy of the eye after corneal perforation.
- *Therapeutic:* to remove inflamed corneal tissue unresponsive to treatment consisting of antibiotic or antiviral agents.
- *Cosmetic:* to improve the appearance of patients with corneal scars.

Operative Procedure

Lamellar keratoplasty and endothelial keratoplasty are newer procedures that are undertaken when only certain layers of the cornea need transplantation. They can sometimes be performed with local anesthesia with sedation. An eye patch and shield are placed over the operative eye at the end of the case.

- In *lamellar* keratoplasty, a partial thickness of the cornea is replaced.
- In *penetrating* keratoplasty, a full thickness of the cornea is replaced. This surgery is often preformed as an emergency procedure.
- *Total* keratoplasty provides for replacement of the entire cornea.

With the *donor cornea*, the donor tissue graft comes from a cadaver with no known diseases that might affect the donated cornea. The donor cornea is placed with the epithelial side down on a moistened gauze pad, and fluid is placed on the endothelial surface to prevent it from drying out.

Preparation of the *host cornea* proceeds as follows: An eye speculum is placed to keep the lids open; lubrication is placed on the eye to prevent it from drying out. A metal ring may be stitched to the sclera, which will provide a base for a trephine (a surgical instrument with a cylindrical blade). The trephine is then used to cut a circular graft (a "button") from the donor cornea. A second trephine and scissors are used to remove the diseased cornea. The donor button is brought into the surgical field and maneuvered into place with forceps. Once in place, the surgeon fastens the cornea to the eye with sutures, first at 12 o'clock, then 3 o'clock, then 6 o'clock, and finally 9 o'clock; the cornea is then secured around the circle. Before the last suture is tied, the surgeon reforms the anterior chamber to a normal depth with a sterile balanced salt solution, testing for water-tightness by placing a dye on the exterior wound. With the metal ring removed, antibiotic ointment is placed and the eye is patched.

Anesthetic

General anesthesia is used with insertion of an OETT; an oral RAE tube may be needed to keep the endotracheal tube out of the surgical field. A retrobulbar injection may be done intraoperatively for postoperative pain control. Do *not* use succinylcholine (Anectine). Do *not* use nitrous oxide. An increase in intraocular pressure during the time when the patient's own cornea has been removed and the eye is "open" (e.g., because of coughing, vomiting, movement, straining, breath holding) can cause the intraocular contents to be expelled.

Positioning

The patient is positioned supine, with the operative-side arm tucked and the nonoperative-side arm extended on a padded armboard. The bed is usually turned at least 90 degrees, if not 180 degrees, away from the anesthetist. The head of the bed may be raised approximately 20 degrees.

Anesthetic Implications

Give antiemetic treatment for prophylactic avoidance of vomiting and retching.

If only one eye is operated on, tape the nonoperative eyelid closed. Place an eye pad over the eye and cover it with an occlusive clear dressing (Tegaderm) to protect it from cleansing solutions and any movement or grazing of instruments by the surgeon or scrub team as they are working over the face.

If the patient is moved from a bed onto the operating room table, have a lift sheet placed under the patient for ease in lifting him or her back onto the stretcher at the end of the case. This prevents the patient from straining during moving, thereby increasing intraocular pressure and possibly disrupting sutures.

Monitor for bradycardia and the oculocardiac reflex.

Strict aseptic precautions are needed with IV insertion, invasive monitoring, drug administration, airway management, and blood sampling.

OPHTHALMIC SURGERY: GLAUCOMA

Iridectomy

Iridectomy (also known as corectomy) involves surgical removal of the iris. During a surgical iridectomy, if the patient has a high intraocular pressure and the globe is opened, it greatly increases the risk of suprachoroidal hemorrhage and possibly content expulsion. "Surgical removal" iridectomy has been replaced with a much safer procedure: the Nd:YAG laser iridotomy (see the discussion of laser iridotomy later in this chapter).

Iridectomy may be performed to treat narrow-angle or angle-closure glaucoma, to treat iris melanoma, as part of cataract surgery in a glaucoma patient, to repair posterior capsular tears with vitreous loss, for anterior chamber intraocular lens implantation, and to relieve increased intraocular pressure.

Operative Procedure

- *Antiphlogistic iridectomy:* surgical removal of part of the iris to reduce intraocular pressure in inflammatory conditions of the eye.
- *Basal iridectomy:* an iridectomy that includes the root of the iris.
- *Optical iridectomy:* surgical removal of part of the iris to enlarge the existing pupil or to form an artificial pupil.
- *Peripheral iridectomy:* surgical removal of a portion of the iris in the region of its root, leaving the pupillary margin and sphincter pupillae muscle intact. This procedure is used in the treatment of glaucoma.
- *Preliminary iridectomy:* surgical removal of part of the iris preceding cataract extraction.
- *Sector iridectomy* (also known as a *complete iridectomy* or *total iridectomy*): surgical removal of a complete radial section of the iris extending from the pupillary margin to the root of the iris. A *key-hole pupil* is left by the removal of a wedge-shaped section of iris.
- *Stenopeic iridectomy:* surgical removal of a narrow slit or a minute portion of the iris, leaving the sphincter pupillae muscle intact.
- *Therapeutic iridectomy:* surgical removal of a portion of the iris for the cure or prevention of an ocular disease.

An eye patch and/or shield are placed over the operative eye at the end of surgery.

Anesthetic

Local anesthesia eye drops and infiltration with sedation are used. Do *not* give succinylcholine (Anectine). Do *not* use nitrous oxide. An increase in intraocular pressure during the time when the patient's own eye is open (e.g., because of coughing, vomiting, movement, straining, breath holding) can cause the intraocular contents to be expelled.

Positioning

The patient is positioned supine, with the operative-side arm tucked and the nonoperative-side arm extended on a padded armboard. The bed is usually turned at least 90 degrees, if not 180 degrees, away from the anesthetist. The head of the bed may be raised approximately 20 degrees.

Anesthetic Implications

Give antiemetic treatment for prophylactic avoidance of vomiting and retching.

If only one eye is operated on, tape the nonoperative eyelid closed. Place an eye pad over the eye and cover it with an occlusive clear dressing (Tegaderm) to protect it from cleansing solutions and any movement or grazing of instruments by the surgeon or scrub team as they are working over the face.

If the patient is moved from a bed onto the operating room table, have a lift sheet placed under the patient for ease in lifting him or her back onto the stretcher at the end of the case. This prevents the patient from straining during moving, thereby increasing intraocular pressure and possibly disrupting sutures.

Monitor for bradycardia and the oculocardiac reflex.

Trabeculectomy

Trabeculectomy (filtration surgery) involves drainage of the anterior chamber of the eye to reduce intraocular pressure; it employs a partial-thickness scleral flap. Normally, aqueous humor drains through a network of canals known as the trabecular meshwork; the fluid then flows from the meshwork into the bloodstream through a small structure called Schlemm's canal.

Trabeculectomy is performed to treat primary glaucoma when an iridectomy is considered inadequate; it may also be used in cases involving infantile glaucoma or in secondary glaucoma to relieve intraocular pressure. Glaucoma is a progressive optic neuropathy associated with increased intraocular pressure.

Operative Procedure

A piece of tissue is removed at the point in the eye where the iris and the sclera meet. This creates an opening that allows aqueous humor to drain out of the eye, bypassing the clogged drainage canals (trabecular meshwork) through which most of the fluid of the inner eye empties from the anterior space to the subconjunctival space. This new opening is partially covered with a flap of tissue from the sclera and the conjunctiva. As the aqueous humor drains through the new opening, the tissue over the opening rises to form a little blister on the conjunctiva called a bleb; the fluid is absorbed from this bleb. The surgeon may treat the wound bed with a chemotherapeutic agent to help prevent scarring of the bleb by inhibiting fibroblast proliferation. The scleral flap is sutured loosely and the conjunctiva is closed in a watertight fashion at the end of the procedure. An eye patch and shield are placed over the operative eye at the end of surgery.

Anesthetic

Usually, anesthesia consists of a retrobulbar block with local anesthetic injection or Tenon's capsule block. If general anesthesia is used, an oral RAE tube may be needed to keep the endotracheal tube out of the surgical field. Do *not* give succinylcholine (Anectine). Do *not* use nitrous oxide. An increase in intraocular pressure during the time when the patient's own cornea has been removed and the eye is "open" (e.g., because of coughing, vomiting, movement, straining, breath holding) can cause the intraocular contents to be expelled.

Positioning

The patient is positioned supine, with the operative-side arm tucked and the nonoperative-side arm extended on a padded armboard. The bed is usually turned at least 90 degrees, if not 180 degrees, away from the anesthetist. The head of the bed may be raised approximately 20 degrees.

Anesthetic Implications

Give antiemetic treatment for prophylactic avoidance of vomiting and retching.

If only one eye is operated on, tape the nonoperative eyelid closed. Place an eye pad over the eye and cover it with an occlusive clear dressing (Tegaderm) to protect it from cleansing solutions and any movement or grazing of instruments by the surgeon or scrub team as they are working over the face.

If the patient is moved from a bed onto the operating room table, have a lift sheet placed under the patient for ease in lifting him or her back onto the stretcher at the end of the case. This prevents the patient from straining during moving, thereby increasing intraocular pressure and possibly disrupting sutures.

Monitor for bradycardia and the oculocardiac reflex.

OPHTHALMIC SURGERY: LENS

Cataract Extraction with Intraocular Lens Implant

This procedure involves removal of an opaque ocular lens (cataract) of the eye and the placement of a synthetic intraocular lens implant (IOL). Opacification is primarily caused by aging but can be due to trauma or metabolic changes of the crystalline lens fibers. Surgery is indicated if loss of vision is significant. Advances in cataract surgery have led to the use of multifocal and accommodating lens implants, allowing patients to see better than ever before.

Operative Procedure

Local anesthetic drops may be instilled. A lid speculum is placed to hold the upper and lower lids open. The lens to be implanted may be a foldable lens made of acrylic or silicone, which is placed through a small incision, or a polymethylmethacrylate (PMMA) lens, which is placed through a larger incision. The lens is inserted into the capsular bag in the posterior chamber, and the corneal incision is closed. Using a foldable IOL requires few or no stitches placed and provides for a shorter recovery time. An eye patch and shield are placed over the operative eye at the end of the case.

The *intracapsular method* provides for removal of the opaque lens with its intact capsule; this technique is rarely used today. An iridotomy is performed as the cornea is retracted by suture traction. A medication is instilled into the anterior chamber to dissolve the zonules suspending the lens. A cryoprobe is usually applied to the cataract and the lens, and they are removed by gentle pressure. The corneal incision is then closed, the traction sutures removed, and the conjunctival flap approximated. Ophthalmic ointment is instilled and an eye pad applied.

In the *extracapsular method*, a large (usually 10–12 mm) incision is made in the cornea or sclera; the anterior lens is opened (capsulectomy) and the opaque lens cortex is removed by irrigation and manual expression, leaving the posterior capsule in situ. Because the posterior capsule is left intact, an extracapsular intraocular lens may be placed in the posterior chamber behind the iris. Although a larger incision and stitches are required, this method may be required if the patient has very hard cataracts or if phacoemulsification is too difficult.

In *phacoemulsification*, the anterior lens capsule is excised, the lens nucleus is prolapsed into the anterior chamber, and an ultrasonic probe is inserted into the capsule. The contents of the lens capsule are fragmented with ultrasonic energy as the lens material is emulsified; it is simultaneously irrigated and aspirated. After emulsification of the hard central lens nucleus, a probe is used to suction out the softer outer lens cortex. The posterior capsule is left intact to provide support. Aspirated fluids are replaced with a balanced salt solution, thereby maintaining the anterior chamber. An artificial lens is then implanted into the remaining lens capsule after the cataract is removed. Phacoemulsification leaves a smaller wound.

Anesthetic

IV sedation and topical anesthesia eye drops is the usual anesthetic. General anesthesia with insertion of an OETT may be used in extreme instances; an oral RAE tube may be needed to keep the endotracheal tube out of the surgical field. If general anesthesia is used, do *not* give succinylcholine (Anectine). Do *not* use nitrous oxide. An increase in intraocular pressure during the time when the patient's own eye is open (e.g., because of coughing, vomiting, movement, straining, breath holding) can cause the intraocular contents to be expelled.

Positioning

The patient is positioned supine, with the operative-side arm tucked and the nonoperative-side arm extended on a padded armboard. The bed is usually turned at least 90 degrees, if not 180 degrees, away from the anesthetist. The head of the bed may be raised approximately 20 degrees.

Anesthetic Implications

Give antiemetic treatment for prophylactic avoidance of vomiting and retching.

If only one eye is operated on, tape the nonoperative eyelid closed. Place an eye pad over the eye and cover it with an occlusive clear dressing (Tegaderm) to protect it from cleansing solutions and any movement or grazing of instruments by the surgeon or scrub team as they are working over the face.

If the patient is moved from a bed onto the operating room table, have a lift sheet placed under the patient for ease in lifting him or her back onto the stretcher at the end of the case. This prevents the patient from straining during moving, thereby increasing intraocular pressure and possibly disrupting sutures.

The oculocardiac reflex is often seen in cataract extraction surgery. Monitor all patients undergoing this procedure for bradycardia and asystole.

OPHTHALMIC SURGERY: RETINA

The ultimate goal of retinal surgery is the preservation and/or recovery of vision through the restoration of normal retina anatomy.

Repair of Retinal Detachment: Scleral Buckling

Retinal detachment repair is undertaken to place and secure the retina to its normal position. The retina is a transparent tissue that allows a person to see the images that are focused on it by the cornea and the lens. Retinal detachment is a potentially blinding condition where the light-sensitive lining in the back of the eye peels loose and floats freely within the interior of the eye. It can be caused by trauma, advanced diabetes, an inflammatory disorder, or a condition called posterior vitreous detachment. In other cases, it occurs spontaneously due to changes in the consistency or volume of the vitreous humor. Retinal detachment is associated with a tear or hole in the retina through which eye fluids may leak.

Most detachment repair operations are urgent. A detached retina lacks oxygen, which causes cells in the area to die. This can lead to blindness.

Operative Procedure

If the retina has just started to separate, a procedure called a pneumatic retinopexy can be done in the ophthalmologist's office. A gas bubble is injected into the eye; the patient is then placed in the prone position to allow the bubble to float up against the hole in the retina, pushing it back into place. This bubble also allows fluid to be pumped out from beneath the retina. The bubble remains in place for about a week to help flatten the retina, until a seal forms between the retina and the wall of the eye. The eye gradually absorbs the gas bubble.

If the retina has just started to separate or a hole is found before a detachment occurs, the physician can also use a laser or a freezing probe (cropexy) to permanently seal the hole. A variation of this surgery uses a large bubble of silicone oil instead of a gas bubble to close and flatten the retina. The vitreous humor is removed to create space for the silicone oil to be injected. Because the silicone oil cannot be absorbed, a second procedure may be needed to remove the oil after the retinal detachment has healed. Silicone oil is used instead of gas in patients who may have trouble staying in a specified position (not supine), for young children, or to make recovery easier for older adults.

A larger retinal detachment requires surgery, either in a hospital or at an outpatient surgery center. For some complex detachments, multiple procedures may be done during the same operation.

The scleral buckle method involves suturing a piece of rubber to the sclera, which bends the wall of the eye inward so that it meets the hole in the retina. This procedure uses very small instruments inside the eye to pull the retina forward.

Additional steps to reattach the retina may include a membranectomy to remove scar tissue, use of photocoagulation or a laser to bond the retina back against the wall of the eye, and scleral buckling to create a support for the reattached retina.

An eye patch and shield are placed over the operative eye at the end of surgery.

Anesthetic

Anesthesia options include topical local anesthesia eye drops and sedation with MAC. General anesthesia and an OETT may be necessary; an oral RAE tube may be needed to keep the endotracheal tube out of the surgical field. If general anesthesia is used, do *not* give succinylcholine (Anectine). Do *not* use nitrous oxide. Regional anesthesia is contraindicated.

These patients may be considered an emergency and to have a full stomach. A rapid-sequence induction should be done. A smooth induction is necessary to maintain hemodynamics and to avoid hypertension and the Valsalva maneuver (both of which increase intraocular pressure). An increase in intraocular pressure during the time when the

patient's own eye is open (e.g., because of coughing, vomiting, movement, straining, breath holding) can cause the intraocular contents to be expelled.

Positioning

The patient is positioned supine, with the operative-side arm tucked and the nonoperative-side arm extended on a padded armboard. The bed is usually turned at least 90 degrees, if not 180 degrees, away from the anesthetist.

The patient may need to be placed in the prone position if a "gas–fluid" exchange is done for a large retinal tear.

Anesthetic Implications

Give antiemetic treatment for prophylactic avoidance of vomiting and retching.

If only one eye is operated on, tape the nonoperative eyelid closed. Place an eye pad over the eye and cover it with an occlusive clear dressing (Tegaderm) to protect it from cleansing solutions and any movement or grazing of instruments by the surgeon or scrub team as they are working over the face.

If the patient is moved from a bed onto the operating room table, have a lift sheet placed under the patient for ease in lifting him or her back onto the stretcher at the end of the case. This prevents the patient from straining during moving, thereby increasing intraocular pressure and possibly disrupting sutures.

The oculocardiac reflex is often seen in retinal detachment repair. Monitor all patients undergoing this procedure for bradycardia and asystole.

OPHTHALMIC SURGERY: VITREOUS

Vitrectomy: Anterior and Posterior Approaches

In a vitrectomy, the surgeon removes some or all of the vitreous humor from the inside the eye. The vitreous humor makes up two-thirds of the volume of the eye. In an *anterior vitrectomy*, small portions of the vitreous humor are removed from the front of the eye. These portions are usually tangled in an intraocular lens or other structures. A *Posterior vitrectomy* is accomplished in the deeper part of the eye to remove some or all of the vitreous humor.

"Floaters" are deposits in the normally clear vitreous fluid of various size and shape that can obstruct vision; a vitrectomy may be performed to remove them. This procedure is also used in cases involving retinal detachment, endophthalmitis, and foreign body removal. In some cases, vitreous hemorrhage from injuries or diabetic retinopathy forms free-bleeding blood vessels within the eye and a vitrectomy is needed to clear the bloody gel. The vitreous is replaced as the eye secretes aqueous and nutritive fluids.

Operative Procedure

This procedure is performed through a microscope, using special lenses designed to provide a clear image of the retina at the back of the eye. Several tiny incisions are made on the sclera. Microsurgical instruments are inserted through the incisions to illuminate the inside of the eye and to cut and remove the vitreous. In addition, the surgeon may seal blood vessels or inject a gas or silicone oil bubble into the eye to maintain the retina's position. A balanced salt solution is injected to replace the vitreous removed during the surgery. An eye patch and shield are placed over the operative eye at the end of surgery.

Anesthetic

A vitrectomy is usually done with general anesthesia and an OETT; an oral RAE tube may be needed to keep the endotracheal tube out of the surgical field. If general anesthesia is used, do *not* give succinylcholine (Anectine). Do *not* use nitrous oxide. This procedure may also be done with a regional block and sedation.

An increase in intraocular pressure during the time when the patient's own eye is open (e.g., because of coughing, vomiting, movement, straining, breath holding) can cause the intraocular contents to be expelled.

Positioning

The patient is positioned supine, with the operative-side arm tucked and the nonoperative-side arm extended on a padded armboard. The operating table is placed in a slight reverse Trendelenburg position. The bed is usually turned at least 90 degrees, if not 180 degrees, away from the anesthetist.

Anesthetic Implications

Give antiemetic treatment for prophylactic avoidance of vomiting and retching.

If the patient is moved from a bed onto the operating room table, have a lift sheet placed under the patient for ease in lifting him or her back onto the stretcher at the end of the case. This prevents the patient from straining during moving, thereby increasing intraocular pressure and possibly disrupting sutures.

If only one eye is operated on, tape the nonoperative eyelid closed. Place an eye pad over the eye and cover it with an occlusive clear dressing (Tegaderm) to protect it from cleansing solutions and any movement or grazing of instruments by the surgeon or scrub team as they are working over the face.

Monitor for bradycardia and the oculocardiac reflex.

LASER THERAPY AND PHOTOCOAGULATION

Laser surgery carries a variety of risks, including a temporary, usually short-term increase in eye pressure, a temporary inflammation of the eye, and the increased risk of developing cataracts. If cautery or laser is used, airway fire is also a risk. See Chapter 1 for more information on these safety concerns.

Laser Cyclophotocoagulation

Laser cyclophotocoagulation is used to destroy the ciliary body—that is, the part of the eye that makes aqueous fluid. This procedure is necessary in severe cases of glaucoma that have not improved with medical treatment.

Operative Procedure
A laser beam is used to destroy the ciliary body.

Anesthetic
Anesthesia consists of a retrobulbar block and sedation. Patients usually do not feel any pain with these procedures, although some report a slight stinging. Do *not* give succinylcholine (Anectine). Do *not* use nitrous oxide. An increase in intraocular pressure during the time when the patient's own eye is open (e.g., because of coughing, vomiting, movement) can cause the intraocular contents to be expelled.

Positioning
The patient is positioned supine, with the operative-side arm tucked and the nonoperative-side arm extended on a padded armboard. The bed is usually turned at least 90 degrees, if not 180 degrees, away from the anesthetist. The head of the bed may be raised approximately 20 degrees.

Anesthetic Implications
Give antiemetic treatment for prophylactic avoidance of vomiting and retching.

If the patient is moved from a bed onto the operating room table, have a lift sheet placed under the patient for ease in lifting him or her back onto the stretcher at the end of the case. This prevents the patient from straining during moving, thereby increasing intraocular pressure and possibly disrupting sutures.

If only one eye is operated on, tape the nonoperative eyelid closed. Place an eye pad over the eye and cover it with an occlusive clear dressing (Tegaderm) to protect it from cleansing solutions and any movement or grazing of instruments by the surgeon or scrub team as they are working over the face.

Monitor for bradycardia and the oculocardiac reflex.

Complications
Potential complications from this procedure include bleeding from the laser site, inflammation of the eye, and pain.

Laser Iridotomy

In laser iridotomy, a tiny hole is created in the iris with an Nd:YAG laser. A laser iridotomy is considered a much safer procedure than a surgical iridectomy. It may be used to treat narrow-angle or angle-closure glaucoma; to treat iris melanoma, in conjunction with cataract surgery in a glaucoma patient, to repair posterior capsular tears with vitreous loss, for anterior chamber intraocular lens implantation, and to relieve increased intraocular pressure.

Operative Procedure
The laser iridotomy creates a hole in the iris, letting the pressure in front of the iris become the same as the pressure behind the iris. This allows the iris to move away from the junction of the iris and the cornea, opening a passageway for the aqueous fluid to leave the eye.

The aqueous fluid is continuously produced by the ciliary body, which is located behind the iris (Figure 7-1). The aqueous fluid enters the eye through the ciliary body and flows between the iris and lens through the pupil. The fluid passes out of the eye through a tissue called the trabecular meshwork, which is at the drainage angle (at the junction of the cornea and the iris). As the aqueous fluid passes through the eye, it supplies the lens and cornea with nutrients and carries away waste products. This thin, watery fluid nourishes the cornea and the lens with nutrients, carries away waste products, and fills the space in the anterior chamber.

Anesthetic
Laser iridotomy is usually performed in the physician's office with topical local anesthetic eye drops.

Laser Photocoagulation

With laser photocoagulation, a fine-point laser light ray is used to cauterize abnormal blood vessels that grow beneath the retina. This procedure is used to treat a number of eye conditions but is not considered a cure; rather, it is a treatment employed to delay deterioration of the patient's eyesight.

Laser photocoagulation is undertaken to treat proliferative diabetic retinopathy, macular edema, or the "wet" form of macular degeneration. Macular degeneration is a deterioration of the macula (the central area of the retina in the back of the eye that is responsible for fine, detailed central vision) that takes two forms: wet and dry. Macular degeneration is one of the leading causes of blindness.

Operative Procedure

Dilating eye drops are instilled; the laser light seals the vessels from further leaking. The laser may be either a focal beam (to seal vessels in a small place in the retina) or a scatter beam (to seal vessels over a larger area). This procedure does not restore lost vision, but rather slows its deterioration.

Anesthetic

Laser photocoagulation is usually an office-based procedure, but may sometimes be done in the operating room, especially when combined with a vitrectomy. Local anesthetic eye drops are instilled. Some permanent vision loss from the photocoagulation is possible, though this loss is considered smaller than the vision loss from the disease. If general anesthesia must be used, do *not* give succinylcholine (Anectine). Do *not* use nitrous oxide. An increase in intraocular pressure during the time when the patient's own eye is open (e.g., because of coughing, vomiting, movement, straining, breath holding) can cause the intraocular contents to be expelled.

Positioning

The patient is positioned supine, with the operative-side arm tucked and the nonoperative-side arm extended on a padded armboard. The bed is usually turned at least 90 degrees, if not 180 degrees, away from the anesthetist. The head of the bed may be raised approximately 20 degrees.

Anesthetic Implications

Give antiemetic treatment for prophylactic avoidance of vomiting and retching.

If the patient is moved from a bed onto the operating room table, have a lift sheet placed under the patient for ease in lifting him or her back onto the stretcher at the end of the case. This prevents the patient from straining during moving, thereby increasing intraocular pressure and possibly disrupting sutures.

Laser Photodynamic Therapy

Laser photodynamic therapy destroys abnormal blood vessels in the retina. It is used in cases involving the "wet" form of macular degeneration.

Operative Procedure

Visudyne is injected into the patient's arm. This drug is activated as it passes through the retinal blood vessels by a nonthermal laser light beam, in the process destroying abnormal blood vessels in the retina.

Anesthetic

This procedure is virtually painless and is usually done in the physician's office.

Positioning

The patient is placed upright, in semi-Fowler's position. The bed is usually turned at least 90 degrees, if not 180 degrees, away from the anesthetist.

Anesthetic Implications

A topical local anesthetic is used, as this procedure is typically performed on an in-office basis.

If only one eye is operated on, tape the nonoperative eyelid closed. Place an eye pad over the eye and cover it with an occlusive clear dressing (Tegaderm) to protect it from cleansing solutions and any movement or grazing of instruments by the surgeon or scrub team as they are working over the face.

Laser Trabeculoplasty

Laser trabeculoplasty improves the drainage of aqueous humor by creating laser holes in the outflow pathways of the eye. This procedure is used for severe glaucoma, to relieve intraocular pressure.

Operative Procedure

A laser is used to make 50 to 100 tiny burn holes in the trabecular outflow pathway to improve aqueous humor drainage from the eye. The benefit of the treatment may last for several years, but it is not a cure.

Normally, aqueous humor drains through a network of canals known as the trabecular meshwork. The fluid then flows from the meshwork into the bloodstream through a small structure called Schlemm's canal.

Anesthetic

Anesthesia consists of topical local anesthetic eye drops.

Positioning

The patient is placed upright, in a semi-Fowler's position. The bed is usually turned at least 90 degrees, if not 180 degrees, away from the anesthetist.

Anesthetic Implications

Laser trabeculoplasty is usually performed in the physician's office under topical anesthesia.

If only one eye is operated on, tape the nonoperative eyelid closed. Place an eye pad over the eye and cover it with an occlusive clear dressing (Tegaderm) to protect it from cleansing solutions and any movement or grazing of instruments by the surgeon or scrub team as they are working over the face.

REFRACTIVE EYE SURGERY

Refractive eye surgery includes any eye surgery done to improve the refractive state of the eye and decrease or eliminate dependency on glasses or contact lenses. Such procedures include various methods of surgical remodeling of the cornea or cataract surgery. Successful refractive eye surgery can reduce or cure common vision disorders such as myopia, hyperopia, and astigmatism.

Radial Keratotomy

Radial keratotomy (RK), also known as refractive keratoplasty, is a refractive surgical procedure to correct myopia (near-sightedness).

Operative Procedure

Incisions are made deep into the cornea with a precision-calibrated diamond knife. Numerous radial incisions are made that extend from the pupil to the periphery of the cornea in a pattern like the spokes of a wheel. Antibiotic ointment and an eye patch may be applied at the end of the case.

Anesthetic

Anesthesia consists of topical local anesthetic eye drops with mild sedation.

Positioning

The patient is positioned supine, with the operative-side arm tucked and the nonoperative-side arm extended on a padded armboard. Patient cooperation is important as the patient will be asked to focus his or her gaze straight ahead during the surgery. The bed is usually turned at least 90 degrees, if not 180 degrees, away from the anesthetist. The head of the bed may be raised approximately 20 degrees.

Anesthetic Implications

Monitor for bradycardia and the oculocardiac reflex.

Laser-Assisted In Situ Keratomileusis (LASIK)

LASIK is a type of refractive laser eye surgery that changes the dynamics of the cornea to correct myopia, hyperopia, and astigmatism in patients who prefer an alternative to wearing corrective eyeglasses or contact lenses. Keratomileusis is a form of keratoplasty in which a slice of the patient's cornea is removed, shaped to the desired curvature, and then sutured back on the remaining cornea to correct the optical error.

Operative Procedure

After instillation of local anesthetic drops, a corneal suction ring is applied to the eye to immobilize the eye. A corneal flap is then cut, maintaining a hinge on one end of the flap; a metal blade or an IntraLASIK laser then creates a series of tiny, closely arranged bubbles within the cornea. This flap is folded back, and a laser is used to remodel the corneal stroma (the middle section of the cornea) by vaporizing tissue in a finely controlled manner. Even with a corneal suction ring, the eye can still move slightly; current lasers have an eye-tracking system that can follow the patient's eye position and redirect laser impulses. After the surgeon finishes the laser work, the flap site is checked for air bubbles and debris and is repositioned normally. The flap site will heal on its own.

Anesthetic

Anesthesia consists of sedation with MAC, plus local anesthetic eye drops.

Positioning

The patient is positioned supine, with the operative-side arm tucked and the nonoperative-side arm extended on a padded armboard. The bed is usually turned at least 90 degrees, if not 180 degrees, away from the anesthetist. The head of the bed may be raised approximately 20 degrees.

Anesthetic Implications

Preoperatively, let the patient know that the procedure can cause small blood vessels to burst, resulting in a subconjunctival hemorrhage; this type of hemorrhage is harmless and should resolve in 1 to 2 weeks. Intraoperatively, the patient can find the suction ring or lid speculum uncomfortable.

Monitor for bradycardia and the oculocardiac reflex.

EAR SURGERY PEARLS

- Do not use nitrous oxide in ear surgery.
- A laryngeal mask airway (LMA) can be used in ear surgery, as it is less stimulating than an oral endotracheal tube (OETT) and is associated with decreased coughing.
- The facial nerve may be monitored during ear surgery; check with the surgeon before giving muscle relaxation agents. The facial nerve travels through a bony canal in the temporal bone before passing into the middle ear just above the stapes.
- A postauricular incision is made behind the ear in the natural fold, from the upper ear to the tip of the mastoid process, to expose the mastoid process and the internal auditory meatus.
- The middle fossa can be approached by an incision made above the ear at the upper level of the zygomatic arch.

POSTOPERATIVE NAUSEA AND VOMITING

The following characteristics are associated with increased risk of PONV following ear surgery:

- Female
- Motion sickness history
- Pediatrics (6–10 years of age): 34% PONV occurrence
- Pediatrics (11–14 years of age): 35–50% PONV occurrence
- Nonsmoker
- Anxiety
- Surgery length greater than 45–60 minutes
- ***Surgery type: ENT***

EAR SURGERY

Removal of Acoustic Neuroma (Vestibular Schwannoma)

This procedure entails the surgical removal of a fibroid tumor of the acoustic cranial nerve (CN VIII). It is indicated as treatment for nonmalignant tumors of the eighth cranial nerve (auditory) that arise from the Schwann cells of the vestibular nerve. These masses can present as intracranial, brain stem, or cerebellopontine-angle tumors. Affected patients may present with progressive, unilateral hearing loss, facial sensory disturbances, headaches, and/or dizziness.

The facial nerve, acoustic nerve, and superior and inferior vestibular nerves all course through the internal auditory canal. While some procedures may make a strong effort to preserve the acoustic and facial nerves, because the tumor often splays out the nerves, it may not be possible to preserve them.

Operative Procedure

Surgical removal of the tumor is the preferred option because it prevents potentially fatal complications of tumor growth. Surgical approaches to acoustic neuroma include the following options:

- *Translabyrinthine approach.* The surgeon removes the mastoid bone and bone of the inner ear for access to the ear canal and tumor. This approach is not appropriate for very large tumors. It is used if the patient's hearing is already minimal, as hearing loss is total and inevitable with this procedure. The translabyrinthine approach makes no attempt to preserve hearing but may protect the facial nerve.
- *Middle fossa approach.* An incision is made 1 to 2 inches behind the back of the ear into the scalp and temporalis muscle. A bone flap is removed from the temporal bone to expose the middle fossa dura. A microscope is used when elevating the dura and cauterizing any bleeding. This approach is appropriate when there is a good chance that hearing may be preserved.
- *Retrosigmoid or suboccipital approach.* A retromastoid incision is made, and retraction

of the cerebellum is necessary. This approach is used with both small and large tumors. It is appropriate when there is a good chance that hearing may be preserved. Headaches are common after this approach.

A portion of the facial nerve may need to be removed. It may be necessary to sew the facial nerve ends together or to insert a nerve graft. A piece of nerve is used for the nerve graft. Graft material from fat, fascia, or muscle may be harvested to pack the mastoid cavity.

This surgery requires both an otologist and a neurosurgeon.

A pressure dressing is applied over the incision and ear. Elastic wrap is used to hold the dressing against the outer ear and skull.

Anesthetic

General endotracheal anesthesia (GETA) is done. Facial nerve monitoring is almost always done during this surgery. No paralytics are used if nerve monitoring is done. Do *not* give nitrous oxide.

Positioning

The patient is placed in the lateral decubitus position.

Anesthetic Implications

An acoustic neuroma may need to be removed from both the middle and posterior fossa. Stereotactic radiotherapy may have been attempted previously and proved unsuccessful in reducing the tumor effects.

An arterial line is needed for this procedure.

Patients undergoing this procedure require special eye care. Paper tape is used to close the eyes to prevent corneal drying or abrasions; eye pads are then placed over both eyes to protect them.

IV *steroids* can be given to help decrease swelling unless otherwise contraindicated. Patients are usually started on steroids preoperatively.

Smooth emergence from anesthesia is important with this surgery. The goal is to avoid coughing, bucking, or nausea/vomiting or retching so as to prevent increased risk of bleeding, hematoma formation, or suture line disruption from the increased head and neck pressures.

Complications

Potential complications include stroke; injury to the cerebellum, pons, or temporal lobe of the brain; CSF leak; meningitis; facial muscle weakness; imbalance and dizziness; and death.

Cochlear Implantation

Cochlear implantation involves surgical implantation of an electronic device that does not amplify sound, but rather bypasses damaged portions of the ear to directly stimulate functioning of the eighth cranial nerve (auditory) inside the cochlea (auditory portion of the inner ear) with an electric field. This device helps to provide a sense of sound for a patient who is profoundly deaf. While the resulting hearing is different from "normal" hearing, the implant gives recipients sound discrimination fine enough to understand speech in quiet environments.

External components (which sit behind the ear) of the cochlear implant include a microphone/receiver, a speech processor, and a radiofrequency transmitter (primary coil or antenna). The external component receives the sound, converts the sound into an electric signal, and sends this signal to the internal cochlear component. The internal component is a secondary coil implanted in the temporal bone; it receives signals from the speech processor, converts them into electric signals, and sends them to the brain. The brain interprets these signals as sound.

Operative Procedure

An incision is made behind the mastoid bone, and the skin and muscle are elevated. A circular depression is made into the temporal bone to place the receiver (i.e., the external component). A mastoidectomy is done so that an intracochlear electrode can be passed into the cochlea. Next, a small piece of temporalis fascia is used to secure the electrode in place, and the incisions are closed. A pressure dressing is applied over the incision and ear; elastic wrap is used to hold the dressing against the outer ear and skull.

Anesthetic

General anesthesia and endotracheal intubation. Facial nerve monitoring is almost always done during this surgery; no paralytics are given when nerve monitoring is done. Do *not* give nitrous oxide.

Positioning

The patient is positioned supine, with the head turned away from the operative side. Tuck the patient's ipsilateral arm.

Anesthetic Implications

These patients require special eye care. Paper tape is used to close the eyes to prevent corneal drying or abrasions; eye pads are then placed over both eyes to protect them.

IV *steroids* can be given to help decrease swelling unless otherwise contraindicated.

Smooth emergence from anesthesia is important with this surgery. The goal is to avoid coughing, bucking, or nausea/vomiting or retching so as to prevent increased risk of bleeding, hematoma formation, or suture line disruption from the increased head and neck pressures.

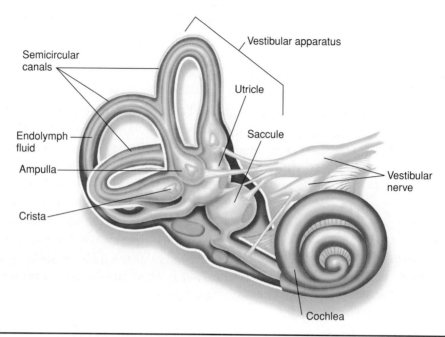

Figure 8-1 *Anatomy of the Inner Ear and Cochlea*
Source: Chiras, 2008.

Facial Nerve Decompression

Facial nerve decompression relieves an area of facial nerve compression. The patient with facial nerve compression may present with Bell's palsy, which is characterized by decreased tearing with unilateral faceptosis and inability to close the eye on the affected side. Increased tearing can occur if the eye becomes irritated

Operative Procedure

In the *transmastoid approach*, the surgeon removes the mastoid bone and may remove the incus to obtain access to the facial canal. The bone over the compressed section of nerve is carefully removed. The facial nerve sheath is incised and the nerve decompressed.

In the *middle fossa approach*, an incision is made 1 to 2 inches behind the back of the ear into the scalp and temporalis muscle. A bone flap is removed from the temporal bone to expose the middle fossa dura. A microscope is used when elevating the dura and cauterizing any bleeding. The facial nerve sheath is identified and opened, and the nerve is decompressed. The bone flap is replaced into the hole, after which the temporalis muscle and the skin are sutured closed.

A pressure dressing is placed over the operative ear. Elastic wrap is used to hold the dressing against the outer ear and skull.

Anesthetic

Facial nerve monitoring may be done during this surgery, but may not be needed if the facial nerve is already nonfunctional. Check with the surgeon before giving paralytics. Do *not* give nitrous oxide. GETA is done.

Positioning

Place the patient supine, with the head turned away from the operative side. Alternatively, the patient may be placed in the lateral decubitus position. The arm on the operative ear side is padded and tucked at the side; the non-operative-side arm may be extended on a padded armboard and positioned with the shoulder bent at an angle less than 90 degrees.

Anesthetic Implications

These patients require special eye care. Paper tape is used to close the eyes to prevent corneal drying or abrasions; eye pads are then placed over both eyes to protect them.

IV *steroids* can be given to help decrease swelling unless otherwise contraindicated.

Smooth emergence from anesthesia is important with this surgery. The goal is to avoid coughing, bucking, or nausea/vomiting or retching so as to prevent increased risk of bleeding, hematoma formation, or suture line disruption from the increased head and neck pressures.

Labyrinthectomy

The labyrinthectomy surgical procedure destroys the labyrinth of the middle ear. The labyrinth is a system of passages in the inner ear that includes the cochlea (hearing) and the vestibule (sense of balance, position, and movement). A labyrinthectomy is undertaken to control episodic vertigo and disequilibrium, such as occur with severe vertigo or Ménière's disease. See also the discussion of vestibular neurectomy later in this chapter

Operative Procedure

This procedure provides for a complete unilateral vestibular ablation.

- *Chemical labyrinthectomy:* injection of intratympanic aminoglycoside or gentamicin to destroy the balance receptors in the labyrinth. The use of this outpatient procedure is growing rapidly.
- *Selective vestibular neurectomy (SVN):* procedure in which the surgeon cuts the vestibular nerve, stopping faulty signals from traveling from the inner ear to the brain. It is done by a transmastoid approach.
- *Labyrinthectomy:* removal of the membranous labyrinth of the inner ear.

If a transmastoid approach is used, a pressure dressing is applied over the incision and ear.

Elastic wrap is used to hold the dressing against the outer ear and skull.

Anesthetic

GETA with oral endotracheal tube insertion. Facial nerve monitoring may be done during this surgery. Check with the surgeon before giving paralytics. Do *not* give nitrous oxide.

Positioning

The patient is placed supine, with the head turned away from the operative side. Alternatively, the patient may be placed in the lateral decubitus position. The arm on the operative ear side is padded and tucked at the side; the non-operative-side arm may be extended on a padded armboard and positioned with the shoulder bent at an angle less than 90 degrees.

Anesthetic Implications

These patients require special eye care. Paper tape is used to close the eyes to prevent corneal drying or abrasions; eye pads are then placed over both eyes to protect them.

IV *steroids* can be given to help decrease swelling unless otherwise contraindicated.

Smooth emergence from anesthesia is important with this surgery. The goal is to avoid coughing, bucking, or nausea/vomiting or retching so as to prevent increased risk of bleeding, hematoma formation, or suture line disruption from the increased head and neck pressures.

Mastoidectomy

Mastoidectomy, which involves removal of bony partitions, is undertaken to remove infected mastoid air cells within the mastoid bone or as an approach for labyrinthectomy, transmastoid surgery, or translabyrinthine surgery. Infected bone cells may result from middle ear infections, an inflammatory disease of the middle ear, cholesteatoma (cyst-like mass in the mastoid), or mastoiditis. The air cells are connected to the upper part of the mastoid, which is in turn connected to the middle ear. As a consequence, infections and inflammation of the middle ear can readily spread to the mastoid bone. When antibiotics cannot clear this infection, it may be necessary to remove the infected air cells via surgery. A mastoidectomy is also performed sometimes to repair paralyzed facial nerves.

Operative Procedure

Three types of procedures are used to perform a mastoidectomy.

Simple mastoidectomy entails removal of the diseased mastoid air cells only. An incision is made behind the ear, exposing the cortex. The mastoid cells are then removed with a burr, but the ossicles, eardrum, and ear canal are left intact. A drain is placed and the incision is closed. A myringotomy may also be performed.

Modified radical mastoidectomy involves removal of the mastoid air cells, part of the ossicular chain, and the posterior external auditory canal wall. The posterior and superior walls of the auditory canal are resected, combining the middle ear, the attic, and the mastoid cavity into a single space. Drills and burrs are employed; care is taken to avoid injury to the facial nerve and canal skin. A tympanomeatal flap is created and draped over the ossicles to partially line the mastoid cavity. The incision is closed. This type of mastoidectomy leaves the patient able to hear.

Radical mastoidectomy excises the mastoid air cells and tympanic membrane, along with the malleus, incus, and stapes (ossicular chain) and mucoperiosteal lining. A strip of temporalis muscle or an absorbable sponge may be used to fill the cavity. The wound is packed, and a pressure dressing is applied over the incision and ear. Elastic wrap is used to hold the dressing against the outer ear and skull.

Anesthetic

GETA and a LMA or endotracheal tube are required. Facial nerve monitoring is usually done during this surgery. Check with the surgeon before giving paralytics. Do *not* give nitrous oxide.

Positioning

The patient is positioned supine, with the affected ear up. The arm on the operative ear side is padded and tucked at the side; the nonoperative-side arm may be extended on a padded armboard and positioned with the shoulder bent at an angle less than 90 degrees.

Anesthetic Implications

These patients require special eye care. Paper tape is used to close the eyes to prevent corneal drying or abrasions; eye pads are then placed over both eyes to protect them.

IV *steroids* can be given to help decrease swelling unless otherwise contraindicated.

Smooth emergence from anesthesia is important with this surgery. The goal is to avoid coughing, bucking, or nausea/vomiting or retching so as to prevent increased risk of bleeding, hematoma formation, or suture line disruption from the increased head and neck pressures.

Myringotomy

In myringotomy, an incision is made into the tympanic membrane to remove fluid accumulation or drain pus from the middle ear. This procedure becomes necessary when the eustachian tube is either partially or completely blocked and unable to perform this function. It is used in cases of acute and chronic otitis media that have not responded to antibiotic therapy or are repeated problems; such indications can occur in both children and adults.

Operative Procedure

A speculum is inserted into the ear canal. A small incision is made in the pars tensa of the tympanic membrane, and fluid or pus is suctioned out. A culture may be done. Ear drops are instilled, and a cotton ball is placed in the ear canal.

A carbon dioxide laser-assisted myringotomy can be done. With this approach, the laser is used to create a precise hole in the tympanic membrane.

In *myringotomy with tube placement (tympanostomy)*, a tube made from polyethylene is implanted unilaterally or bilaterally to equalize pressure and facilitate drainage of the middle ear. The tube prevents the incision from closing and decreases the number of ear infections by helping the middle ear to drain.

Anesthetic

General anesthesia may be used with children and uncooperative adults. Mask ventilation with volatile inhaled agents is usually adequate for the brief microsurgical procedure. Do not give nitrous oxide.

A topical anesthetic may be adequate for a cooperative adult.

Positioning

The patient is placed supine, with the head turned so that the operative ear is upward. The arm on the operative ear side is padded and tucked at the side; the nonoperative-side arm may be extended on a padded armboard and positioned with the shoulder bent at an angle less than 90 degrees.

Anesthetic Implications

Paper tape is used to close the eyes to prevent corneal drying or abrasions.

A peripheral IV is usually not started for these cases. If it is, IV steroids can be given to help decrease swelling unless otherwise contraindicated.

Ossicular Chain Reconstruction

The ossicular chain is the small bones of the middle ear (the bones of hearing: malleus, incus, and stapes); they transmit sound from the tympanic membrane to the oval window. Long-standing perforations of this membrane can have severe consequences, including infection and erosion of the bones of hearing, which disrupt the bony chain of the middle ear. Reconstructive procedures of the ossicular chain seek to repair this damage, using microinstrumentation.

Operative Procedure

Entering the ear through the external ear canal, the surgeon checks the ossicular bone chain to see if these bones are mobile and functioning. If they are not, ossicular reconstruction may be necessary.

After injecting the area with local anesthesia with epinephrine, an incision is made in the external ear canal; alternatively, a postauricular incision can be done to access the middle ear. The goal of ossicular chain reconstruction is to reestablish the connection between an intact tympanic membrane and the oval window. This can be done with a variety of techniques and materials, both homograft and allograft.

Removed ossicles may be reshaped and replaced. If the ossicles are diseased beyond repair, they may be replaced with a total ossicular replacement prosthesis (TORP).

If the external meatus is entered, the tympanic membrane is closed, usually with a temporalis fascia graft (taken from the fascia over the temporal bone).

The external ear canal is packed with a moistened packing. A pressure dressing is applied over the ear. Elastic wrap is used to hold the dressing against the outer ear and skull.

Anesthetic

GETA and an LMA or endotracheal tube is required. Facial nerve monitoring may be done during this surgery. Check with the surgeon before giving paralytics. Do *not* give nitrous oxide.

Positioning

The patient is positioned supine, with the head turned away from the operative side. Alternatively, the patient may be placed in the lateral decubitus position. If the patient is supine, the arm on the operative ear side is padded and tucked at the side; the non-operative-side arm may be extended on a padded armboard and positioned with the shoulder bent at an angle less than 90 degrees.

Anesthetic Implications

Closely monitor the EKG if local anesthesia with epinephrine is injected.

These patients require special eye care. Paper tape is used to close the eyes to prevent corneal drying or abrasions; eye pads are then placed over both eyes to protect them.

IV *steroids* can be given to help decrease swelling unless otherwise contraindicated.

Smooth emergence from anesthesia is important with this surgery. The goal is to avoid coughing, bucking, or nausea/vomiting or retching so as to prevent increased risk of bleeding, hematoma formation, or suture line disruption from the increased head and neck pressures.

Stapedectomy

In a stapedectomy, the stapes bone of the middle ear is removed. (The stapes is one of the three bones in the ossicular chain that transmit sound.) A prosthesis may be inserted to restore ossicular continuity and alleviate conductive hearing loss. This procedure is performed in cases involving otosclerosis (overgrowth of bone around the stapes).

Operative Procedure

In this microsurgical procedure, the surgeon enters through the external ear canal. Local anesthesia with epinephrine is infiltrated to help with pain control and decrease bleeding. An incision is made into the ear canal near the tympanic membrane. The membrane is lifted, allowing the surgeon to see into the middle ear; the stapes is pressed in an attempt to move it to confirm otosclerosis. If the stapes footplate is fixed, then the stapes is separated from the incus (anvil). A laser or a microsurgical instrument is used to remove the arch of the stapes bone, and the stapes remnant is removed from the ear. An artificial stapes prosthesis is gently inserted and attached to the incus. A piece of fat or other tissue may be taken from a small incision behind the ear lobe and used to seal the hole in the window and space around the prosthesis.

A cotton ball is inserted into the external auditory canal at the end of the case.

Anesthetic

Local anesthesia with IV sedation may be used with a cooperative adult; otherwise, GETA may be required. Do *not* give nitrous oxide. Facial nerve monitoring may be done during this surgery. Check with the surgeon before giving paralytics.

Positioning

The patient is positioned supine, with the head turned away from the operative side. Alternatively, the patient may be placed in the lateral decubitus position. If the patient is supine, the arm on the operative ear side is padded and tucked at the side; the non-operative-side arm may be extended on a padded armboard and positioned with the shoulder bent at an angle less than 90 degrees.

Anesthetic Implications

Closely monitor the EKG if local anesthesia with epinephrine is injected.

These patients require special eye care. Paper tape is used to close the eyes to prevent corneal drying or abrasions; eye pads are then placed over both eyes to protect them.

IV *steroids* can be given to help decrease swelling unless otherwise contraindicated.

The surgeon may require a rapid wake-up at the end of the case so that a hearing test can be done.

Smooth emergence from anesthesia is important with this surgery. The goal is to avoid coughing, bucking, or nausea/vomiting or retching so as to prevent increased risk of bleeding, hematoma formation, or suture line disruption from the increased head and neck pressures.

Tympanoplasty

Tympanoplasty is the reconstruction or repair of the tympanic membrane (ear drum); it can also refer to reconstructive procedures of the ossicular chain in the middle ear (discussed earlier in this chapter).

This surgery is performed in cases in which hearing loss results from a perforated eardrum, trauma, and chronic otitis media.

Operative Procedure

Before tympanoplasty is required, the surgeon may debride the edge of the perforation (after instilling Xylocaine drops) with a sharp instrument, stimulating the membrane to heal and the eardrum to close. If this measure is unsuccessful, a patch of very thin paper-like substance is placed onto the outer surface of the eardrum, creating a matrix to allow the membrane to close.

Perforations do not always heal with these approaches, however. If a tympanoplasty becomes necessary, a microsurgical approach is employed. Local anesthetic with epinephrine is injected into the external auditory canal to decrease pain and bleeding. Tissue is taken either from the back of the ear or from the small cartilaginous lobe of skin in front of the ear (called the tragus). The tissues are thinned and dried. The graft is then inserted underneath the remaining eardrum remnant. An absorbable Gelfoam sponge is placed under the eardrum to allow for support of the graft. The graft and the remaining eardrum remnant are then replaced into their normal position.

Anesthetic

Anesthesia may consist of either local anesthesia with sedation or GETA with a LMA or endotracheal tube. Do *not* give nitrous oxide. Facial nerve monitoring may be done during this surgery. Check with the surgeon before giving paralytics.

Positioning

The patient is positioned supine, with the operative ear up; the head is placed on a soft headrest. The arm on the operative ear side is padded and tucked at the side; the nonoperative-side arm may be extended on a padded armboard and positioned with the shoulder bent at an angle less than 90 degrees.

Anesthetic Implications

The patient may have been on decongestants or antihistamines to dry the ear following perforation.

The patient's hair must be secured out of the way on the operative side.

Closely monitor the EKG if local anesthesia with epinephrine is injected.

These patients require special eye care. Paper tape is used to close the eyes to prevent corneal drying or abrasions; eye pads are then placed over both eyes to protect them.

IV *steroids* can be given to help decrease swelling unless otherwise contraindicated.

Smooth emergence from anesthesia is important with this surgery. The goal is to avoid coughing, bucking, or nausea/vomiting or retching so as to prevent increased risk of bleeding, hematoma formation, or suture line disruption from the increased head and neck pressures.

Tympanostomy (Myringotomy Tubes)

Tympanostomy involves placement of pressure equalization tube(s) through the tympanic membrane. See the discussion of myringotomy earlier in this chapter.

Vestibular Neurectomy

Vestibular neurectomy involves surgical cutting of the vestibular portion of cranial nerve VIII (auditory nerve), but leaves the cochlear portion of this nerve intact. This procedure may be performed if the patient has severe vertigo but hearing is intact. See the discussion of labyrinthectomy earlier in this chapter.

Sinus and Rhinologic Surgery

9

SINUS AND RHINOLOGIC SURGERY PEARLS

- Offer the surgeon an oral gastric tube at the end of any sinus/rhinologic surgery so he or she can suction out the stomach (for any blood) at the end of the case.
- A laryngeal mask airway (LMA) may be used in sinus surgeries to the decrease risk of coughing and bucking.
- Sinus/rhinologic surgery may require the intubation technique and airway management to be different from standard practice, as anesthesia equipment may be in competition with the surgeon for the throat and airway.
- Because the tissues of the face and sinus are quite vascular, maintaining a slight decrease in mean arterial blood pressure (MAP of approximately 60–70 mm Hg) can help to minimize bleeding.
- A local anesthetic with epinephrine may be injected or applied to the nasal mucosa to decrease swelling. The patient should be questioned regarding a history of cocaine use as it can cause drug interactions (especially vasoactive interactions) if epinephrine is given with the local anesthetic. If the patient has used cocaine (or its equivalent), healthcare providers may want to decrease the amount of epinephrine given.
- Gauze saturated with a local anesthetic with epinephrine (LA with epi) may be placed intranasally (or infiltrated) by the surgeon to decrease mucosal size and to prevent bleeding. Watch for an increase in heart rate or blood pressure or ST-segment changes on the EKG when epinephrine is introduced into the nare(s). In Cushing's response, the blood pressure goes so high that the heart rate decreases.
- A throat pack is usually placed if general anesthesia is used; document its insertion and removal times. Suction the back of the throat gently with a soft suction catheter before extubating the patient.
- Use of a humidified oxygen face tent mask at the end of the case helps to oxygenate the patient if he or she is mouth breathing and does not apply pressure to facial structures.

- Smooth emergence from anesthesia is important with sinus/rhinologic surgery. The goal is to avoid coughing, bucking, or nausea/vomiting or retching so as to prevent increased risk of bleeding, hematoma formation, or suture line disruption from the increased head and neck pressures. Antiemetics should be given.
- Sinus surgery complications include possible injury to the optic nerve, the sphenopalatine artery, the ethmoid arteries, and the skull base.
- A nasal endoscope is used to visualize the sinuses to avoid cutting the patient's skin.

These endoscopes come in varying angles of vision from 0 to 120 degrees. There are four sinuses dealt with by endoscope: the frontal sinus with frontal recess dissection; the maxillary sinus in cases involving uncinectomy and antrostomy; the anterior and posterior ethmoid sinus, which requires careful dissection to the skull base and orbital lamina; and the sphenoid sinus, which is managed via a sphenoidotomy.

- No blood thinners should be given to these patients preoperatively. Postoperatively, watch for excessive swallowing due to bleeding.

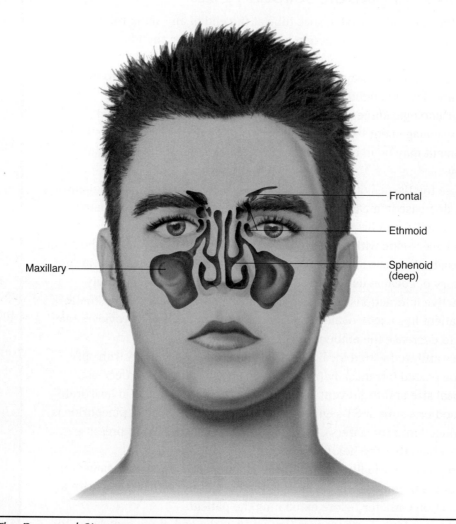

Maxillary

Frontal

Ethmoid

Sphenoid (deep)

Figure 9-1 *The Paranasal Sinuses*
Source: AAOS, 2004.

POSTOPERATIVE NAUSEA AND VOMITING

The following characteristics are associated with increased risk of PONV following sinus/rhinology surgery:

- Female
- Motion sickness history
- Pediatrics (6–10 years of age): 34% PONV occurrence
- Pediatrics (11–14 years of age): 35–50% PONV occurrence
- Nonsmoker
- Anxiety
- Surgery length greater than 45–60 minutes
- ***Surgery type: ENT***

SINUS SURGERY

Intranasal Antrostomy

Intranasal antrostomy makes a surgical opening in the maxillary sinus. At the same time, the natural opening of the sinus into the nasal cavity is often enlarged to improve drainage of normal secretions and reduce the chance of recurrent sinus disease. This surgery may be performed to treat a blocked or chronically infected maxillary sinus; to remove the sinus's diseased lining; to remove polyps, cysts, or foreign bodies; to clean the sinus; to biopsy a tumor; or to gain access to the ethmoid sinus.

Operative Procedure

Local anesthetic with epinephrine is infiltrated to help decrease bleeding and swelling of nasal tissues.

In *intranasal antrostomy*, the nasoantral wall is fenestrated and the opening is enlarged. The inferior nasal wall is removed down to the level of the floor of the nasal cavity. Diseased mucosa is excised. The sinus is irrigated and suctioned and the cavity is inspected. Intranasal packing is done for hemostasis. A mustache dressing is placed under the nose.

A *Caldwell-Luc procedure* is performed if the maxillary disease appears irreversible. A small cut is made between the upper lip and gum (by the canine fossa), and a tiny piece of bone is removed from the anterior wall of the maxillary sinus. The surgeon creates an opening into the antrum of the maxillary sinus through the fossa to allow for evacuation of diseased sinus and scar tissue under direct vision when an intranasal antrostomy alone is not adequate to completely drain the area.

Anesthetic

General endotracheal anesthesia (GETA) and an LMA may be used in sinus surgeries to decrease the risk of coughing and bucking. If an endotracheal tube is placed, an oral RAE tube may be placed to minimize intrusion into the surgical field.

Positioning

The patient is positioned supine, with the arm on the affected side padded and tucked. The nonoperative-side arm can be extended on a padded armboard. Reverse Trendelenburg position of 10–20 degrees is used.

Anesthetic Implications

Tape both eyelids closed. Place eye pads over both eyes and cover them with occlusive clear dressings (Tegaderm) to protect them from cleansing solutions and any movement or grazing of instruments by the surgeon or scrub team as they are working over the face.

A local anesthetic and epinephrine solution may be infiltrated to decrease swelling to prevent bleeding. Watch for an increase in heart rate or blood pressure or EKG changes.

An orogastric tube should be placed after induction and maintained until the end of the case so that any blood or gastric juices can be suctioned out before the patient is extubated.

A throat pack is usually placed if general anesthesia is used; document its insertion and removal times. Suction the back of the throat gently with a soft suction catheter before extubating the patient.

Because the tissues of the face and sinus are quite vascular, maintaining a slight decrease in mean arterial blood pressure (60–70 mm Hg) can help to minimize bleeding.

Smooth emergence from anesthesia is important with this surgery. The goal is to avoid coughing, bucking, or nausea/vomiting and retching so as to prevent increased risk of bleeding, hematoma formation, or suture line disruption from the increased head and neck pressures.

Steroids may be given to decrease tissue swelling and as an antiemetic adjunct unless otherwise contraindicated.

Facial swelling is a common side effect, tending to migrate down the neck.

Use of a humidified oxygen face tent mask at the end of the case helps to oxygenate the patient when he or she is mouth breathing (nose packed) and does not apply pressure to facial structures.

Endoscopic Sinus Surgery (Functional Endoscopic Sinus Surgery)

Endoscopic sinus surgery, also known as functional endoscopic sinus surgery (FESS), involves endoscopic examination of the nasal and paranasal sinuses. It is used in cases of sinusitis and nasal polyposis, including fungal sinusitis. Endoscopy permits the diagnosis to be confirmed by direct visualization. This approach also permits the removal of tissue in the ethmoid sinus, septoplasty, turbinate reduction, partial or total resection of the middle turbinate, and radical procedures such as total sphenoethmoidectomy. Biopsies, cultures, irrigation, and suctioning can also be done as part of this procedure. Endoscopic sinus surgery is indicated in infection, chronic sinus disease, polyps, and benign or malignant tumors.

Operative Procedure
Gauze saturated with a local anesthetic with epinephrine (LA with epi) is placed intranasally and/or infiltrated by the surgeon to help with perioperative discomfort and to decrease risk of bleeding at the start of the surgery.

The endoscope is inserted through each nostril, where the surgeon may inject LA with epi into the ethmoidal prechambers bilaterally so that they can be examined. The procedure performed depends entirely on the pathology encountered. Diseased tissue is excised as necessary with a microdebrider—it has a tiny, curved rotating tip that helps the surgeon to move it in several different directions.

Ethmoidectomy (discussed later in this chapter) and, infrequently, total sphenoethmoidectomy may be performed as part of endoscopic sinus surgery. Nasal packing soaked with LA with epi is placed with strings coming out from the nares to be secured at the end of the case.

Anesthetic
General anesthesia with an OETT may be used; an oral Rae tube may also be requested by the surgeon. An LMA can be used in sinus surgeries to decrease the risk of coughing and bucking. Muscle relaxation may be given to prevent patient movement. MAC with IV sedation and local anesthesia may be employed, albeit only rarely.

Positioning
The patient is placed supine, with a shoulder roll to slightly extend the head with a slight reverse Trendelenburg position of 10–30 degrees. The head of the bed is usually turned at least 90 degrees, if not 180 degrees, away from the anesthetist.

Anesthetic Implications
Tape both eyelids closed. Place eye pads over both eyes and cover them with occlusive clear dressings (Tegaderm) to protect them from cleansing solutions and any movement or grazing of instruments by the surgeon or scrub team as they are working over the face.

Watch for an increase in heart rate or blood pressure or ST-segment changes on the EKG when LA and epinephrine are introduced into the nare(s).

An orogastric tube should be placed after induction and maintained until the end of the case so that any blood or gastric juices can be suctioned out before the patient is extubated.

A throat pack is usually placed if general anesthesia is used; document its insertion and removal times. Suction the back of the throat gently with a soft suction catheter before extubating the patient.

Smooth emergence from anesthesia is important with this surgery. The goal is to avoid coughing, bucking, or nausea/vomiting or retching so as to prevent increased risk of bleeding or hematoma formation from the increased head and neck pressures. Antiemetics should be given.

Steroids may be given to decrease tissue swelling and as an antiemetic adjunct unless otherwise contraindicated.

Because the tissues of the face and sinus are quite vascular, maintaining a slight decrease in mean arterial blood pressure (60–70 mm Hg) can help to minimize bleeding.

Use of a humidified oxygen face tent mask at the end of the case helps to oxygenate the patient when he or she is mouth breathing (nose is packed) and does not apply pressure to facial structures.

Complications

Potential complications of endoscopic sinus surgery include injury to the optic nerve, the sphenopalatine artery, the ethmoid arteries, and the skull base.

Ethmoidectomy

Ethmoidectomy removes the walls separating individual sinus air cells of the ethmoid sinus(es); this opens up the small partition between the cells so that they form one common cavity. This procedure is performed to drain infected mucus and remove inflamed tissues. Depending on how much sinus disease is present, it may involve opening just the front (anterior) portion of the ethmoid; alternatively, in a total ethmoidectomy, both the anterior and posterior portions of the sinus are cleaned out surgically

Located between the eyes, the ethmoid sinuses have a variable number (range of 5 to more than 15) of eggshell-thin bony chambers (much like a honeycomb-like structure), which are divided into anterior and posterior regions. The posterior cells are associated with several important structures—the eye orbit, optic nerve, and sphenoid sinus. The ethmoid sinuses are key to treating most sinus infections because all of the other sinuses drain through or next to them.

Operative Procedure

This procedure is done endoscopically. See the discussion of endoscopic sinus surgery earlier in this section for more information.

Frontal Sinus Drainage

Drainage of the frontal sinus is accomplished by enlarging the frontal sinus outflow tract. This procedure is undertaken for chronic infection not responsive to antibiotics or antihistamines and for any spreading acute infections. The infection is usually drained internally. If it is drained externally, in rare cases it may involve obliteration of the sinus cavity.

Operative Procedure

In *internal* drainage procedures, which are performed endoscopically, balloon or angled-forceps are used to open the natural frontal sinus opening.

In *external* drainage procedures, an incision is made along the inferior margin of the eyebrow to the anterolateral aspect of the nasal bone. The periosteum is reflected. The lacrimal crest is identified. The ethmoid sinus is entered; the frontal sinus is then likewise entered after bone is rongeured, removing the floor of the sinus. Diseased mucous membrane is excised using curettes and pituitary forceps. A nasofrontal passage is made by removing a portion of the middle turbinate. Drains are placed to maintain the passage. The external wound is closed and a dressing is applied.

Anesthetic

General anesthesia is used with an OETT or LMA; an LMA may be used in sinus surgeries to decrease risk of coughing and bucking.

Positioning

The patient is positioned supine, with a shoulder roll to slightly extend the head. The operative-side arm is padded and tucked. The nonoperative-side arm can be extended on an armboard.

Anesthetic Implications

Tape both eyelids closed. Place eye pads over both eyes and cover them with occlusive clear dressings (Tegaderm) to protect them from cleansing solutions and any movement or grazing of instruments by the surgeon or scrub team as they are working over the face.

An orogastric tube should be placed after induction and maintained until the end of the case so that any blood or gastric juices can be suctioned out before the patient is extubated.

A throat pack is usually placed if general anesthesia is used; document its insertion and removal times. Suction the back of the throat gently with a soft suction catheter before extubating the patient.

Smooth emergence from anesthesia is important with this surgery. The goal is to avoid coughing, bucking, or nausea/vomiting or retching so as to prevent increased risk of bleeding, hematoma formation, or suture line disruption from the increased head and neck pressures. Antiemetics should be given.

Steroids may be given to decrease tissue swelling and as an antiemetic adjunct unless otherwise contraindicated.

Because the tissues of the face and sinus are quite vascular, maintaining a slight decrease in mean arterial blood pressure (60–70 mm Hg) can help to minimize bleeding.

Use of a humidified oxygen face tent mask at the end of the case helps to oxygenate the patient when he or she is mouth breathing (nose packed) and does not apply pressure to facial structures.

Maxillectomy: Partial or Total

Maxillectomy involves partial or total surgical excision of the maxilla. This procedure is done to treat neoplastic disease of the maxilla. The maxilla bone forms the upper jaw, the front part of the roof of the mouth, the sidewalls of the nasal cavity, and part of the floor of the eye sockets. It helps shape the tissues around the eyeball, nose, and hard palate. The surgical goal of the maxillectomy is to safely remove all of the tumor and preserve function.

Operative Procedure

A *partial maxillectomy* leaves one or more of the bony walls in place. It involves making a cut inside the mouth under the upper lip; no scar is left on the face. Only part of the maxilla is removed.

Extended or radical maxillectomy is an extensive procedure that is undertaken if the cancer has spread into all the walls as well as into nearby structures. An incision is made along the nasofacial groove and ala, exposing the face of the maxilla, from the eyebrow or the eyelids down to (or through) the upper lip at the midline. The front of the gum is split, going back to the junction of the soft and hard palates; there the incision is directed laterally toward the posterior margin of the alveolar ridge (teeth). An intraoral Caldwell-Luc incision is made and connected to the previously described incision (called a Weber-Ferguson procedure). The orbital contents are retracted downward and laterally to expose the medial wall of the eye orbit. An external ethmoidectomy is done, which involves removing all of the maxilla.

Both of these approaches leave an opening in the roof of the mouth. A dental obturator is fitted immediately after resection by the surgeon; a split-thickness skin graft may also be done.

Anesthetic

General anesthesia with endotracheal intubation is done. The choice of nasal or oral intubation is based on surgeon preference; muscle relaxation is given. Use a smaller, reinforced OETT if the surgeon requests oral intubation, to facilitate surgical exposure and to prevent kinking of the tube during surgical manipulation inside the mouth.

Positioning

The patient is placed supine, in a reverse Trendelenburg position of 20–30 degrees.

Anesthetic Implications

The surgeon will dictate eye protection based on personal preference and surgical method.

Type and cross-match the patient's blood and have 2 units of packed cells available. Moderate to severe blood loss is possible with this procedure.

An orogastric tube should be placed after induction and maintained until the end of the case so that any blood or gastric juices can be suctioned out before the patient is extubated.

A throat pack is usually placed as general anesthesia is used; document its insertion and removal times. Suction the back of the throat gently with a soft suction catheter before extubating the patient.

Smooth emergence from anesthesia is important with this surgery. The goal is to avoid coughing, bucking, or nausea/vomiting or retching so as to prevent increased risk of bleeding, hematoma formation, or suture line disruption from the increased head and neck pressures. Antiemetics should be given.

Steroids may be given to decrease tissue swelling and as an antiemetic adjunct unless otherwise contraindicated.

Because the tissues of the face and sinus are quite vascular, maintaining a slight decrease in mean arterial blood pressure (60–70 mm Hg) can help to minimize bleeding.

Use of a humidified oxygen face tent mask at the end of the case helps to oxygenate the patient if he or she is mouth breathing and does not apply pressure to facial structures.

Complications

Potential complications include transection of the maxillary artery, bleeding, infection, cheek numbness, lip weakness, watery eyes, and double vision.

Nasal Polypectomy

Nasal polypectomy is the excision of a hypertrophic area of the nasal mucosa resulting from a chronic edematous inflammatory process due to chronic allergies or sinusitis. Nasal polyps are usually located in the middle meatus; they may occur singly or in numbers. These polyps may grow large enough to obstruct the entire nasopharynx.

Operative Procedure

If a debrider is not used, each polyp is individually encircled with the wire of a nasal polyp snare, grasped with forceps, and amputated.

Debriders are now more commonly used. The debrider is inserted into the sinus; it has a suction unit that pulls the polyp into the device. A rotating blade transects the polyp.

The nasal cavity is packed with petrolatum-impregnated gauze.

If a choanal polyp (extends from the maxillary sinus into the nose—a very large polyp) is removed, the procedure is done under GA. A snare wire is passed through the nasal cavity into the nasopharynx; the polyp may be grasped by forceps in the oropharynx, and the polyp is amputated. Alternatively, a debrider may be used.

Anesthetic

General anesthesia is used with an OETT or LMA. An LMA may be used in sinus surgeries to decrease the risk of coughing and bucking with a choanal polyp. Local anesthesia with epinephrine may also be used.

Positioning

The patient is positioned supine, with a shoulder roll. The operative-side arm is padded and tucked. The nonoperative-side arm can be extended on an armboard. The is placed in a reverse Trendelenburg position of 10–20 degrees.

Anesthetic Implications

When a local anesthetic and epinephrine solution is infiltrated to decrease swelling and to prevent bleeding, watch for an increase in heart rate or blood pressure or EKG changes.

Tape both eyelids closed. Place eye pads over both eyes and cover them with occlusive clear dressings (Tegaderm) to protect them from cleansing solutions and any movement or grazing of instruments by the surgeon or scrub team as they are working over the face.

An orogastric tube should be placed after induction and maintained until the end of the case so that any blood or gastric juices can be suctioned out before the patient is extubated.

A throat pack is usually placed if general anesthesia is used; document its insertion and removal times. Suction the back of the throat gently with a soft suction catheter before extubating the patient.

Smooth emergence from anesthesia is important with this surgery. The goal is to avoid coughing, bucking, or nausea/vomiting or retching so as to prevent increased risk of bleeding or hematoma formation from the increased head and neck pressures. Antiemetics should be given.

Steroids may be given to decrease tissue swelling and as an antiemetic adjunct unless otherwise contraindicated.

Because the tissues of the face and sinus are quite vascular, maintaining a slight decrease in mean arterial blood pressure (60–70 mm Hg) can help to minimize bleeding.

Use of a humidified oxygen face tent mask at the end of the case helps to oxygenate the patient when he or she is mouth breathing (nose packed) and does not apply pressure to facial structures.

Sphenoidotomy

In sphenoidotomy, an opening into the anterior wall of the sphenoid sinus is made by endoscopic approach through the nasal cavity. The sphenoid sinus is bordered superiorly by the brain and pituitary gland, laterally by the optic nerves and the carotid artery, and anteriorly by the ethmoid sinuses. The sphenoid sinuses can become inflamed and require widening of the drainage canals. The surgeon may use a stereotactic system (see the stereotactic procedures discussed in Chapter 5) to help identify landmarks during surgery. The ethmoid sinuses may be entered first to facilitate access to the sphenoid sinuses.

Operative Procedure

This procedure is done endoscopically. See the discussion of functional endoscopic sinus surgery earlier in this section for more information.

Turbinectomy (Coblation of Turbinates)

Turbinectomy involves surgical removal of a turbinate bone and/or mucous membrane. A turbinate is an extension of the ethmoid bone along the side wall of the nose. The turbinates are the main source of heat exchange, air filtering, humidification, and airflow sensation of the nose; their integrity and function are crucial for maintaining sinus health. The turbinates do not grow back, so removing too much of the bone can lead to a condition called "empty nose syndrome" where heat and moisturization of the nose is no longer possible.

One or more turbinates may become enlarged due to infection or trauma. In such a case, they can block breathing and drainage of the sinuses.

Operative Procedure

The most common method of turbinectomy is manual resection of the bone and extra mucosal tissue with surgical scissors. Alternatively, a microdebrider or coblater probe may be inserted into the inferior turbinate through a small incision.

See the discussion of functional endoscopic sinus surgery earlier in this section for more information on anesthetic, position, and anesthetic implications of turbinectomy.

RHINOLOGIC SURGERY

Treatment of Epistaxis

Treatment of epistaxis is undertaken to stop a severe nosebleed. Nosebleeds can occur from trauma, inherited diseases, or nasal tumors; they may also occur spontaneously due to dry mucous membranes; use of anticoagulants, aspirin, or NSAIDs; allergies; hypertension; or alcohol abuse. In addition, they can result from sinus surgery.

Operative Procedure

Nasal packing options include gauze impregnated with petroleum jelly placed against the bleeding site with forceps; Oxycel cotton with Bacitracin (which dissolves and does not have to be removed); tampon-like packing that expands after it is placed against a bleeding site; and a balloon inflation catheter. If bleeding cannot be stopped with packing alone, endovascular techniques may be used:

- *Cauterization:* electrocauterization (with a "Bovie") or silver nitrate sticks can be used. This procedure is done in one nostril at a time to avoid septal perforation.
- *Ligation of vessels:* sphenopalatine and ethmoid vessels.
- *Angiographic embolization:* involves the sphenopalatine vessels.

Anesthetic

GETA is used with a cuffed endotracheal tube for pediatric patients or for more invasive procedures in adults to prevent blood from dripping down the back of the throat and into the lungs and to prevent oxygen from "blowing" back into the airway during cauterization.

Positioning

The patient is placed supine, with a shoulder roll, in a reverse Trendelenburg position of 10–20 degrees.

Anesthetic Implications

Tape both eyelids closed. Place eye pads over both eyes and cover them with occlusive clear dressings (Tegaderm) to protect them from cleansing solutions and any movement or grazing of instruments by the surgeon or scrub team as they are working over the face.

An orogastric tube should be placed after induction and maintained until the end of the case so that any blood or gastric juices can be suctioned out before the patient is extubated.

A throat pack is usually placed if general anesthesia is used; document its insertion and removal times. Suction the back of the throat gently with a soft suction catheter before extubating the patient.

Decrease FiO_2 as tolerated if cauterization used anywhere in the patient's airway.

Smooth emergence from anesthesia is important with this surgery. The goal is to avoid coughing, bucking, or nausea/vomiting/retching so as to prevent increased risk of bleeding or hematoma formation from the increased head and neck pressures. Antiemetics should be given.

Steroids may be given to decrease tissue swelling and as an antiemetic adjunct unless otherwise contraindicated.

Because the tissues of the face and sinus are quite vascular, maintaining a slight decrease in mean arterial blood pressure (60–70 mm Hg) can help to minimize bleeding.

Use of a humidified oxygen face tent mask at the end of the case helps to oxygenate the patient when he or she is mouth breathing (nose packed) and does not apply pressure to facial structures.

Repair of Nasal Fracture

Surgical repair of a fracture of the paired nasal bones or cartilage may be required in trauma cases. Application of a large force in any direction to the nose can cause comminution of the nasal bones.

Operative Procedure

- *Closed reduction:* can be performed by digital and instrumental manipulation.
- *Open reduction:* done when the fracture is severe or when interosseous wire fixation of bone fragments is necessary.

Anesthetic

- Closed reduction: local anesthetic topically to nasal mucosa with IV sedation.
- Open reduction: GETA with cuffed endotracheal tube, to prevent blood from dripping down the back of the throat and into the lungs. Rapid-sequence induction should be done due to blood in the stomach. Gauze saturated with a local anesthetic with epinephrine (LA with epi) is placed intranasally and/or infiltrated by the surgeon to help with perioperative discomfort and to decrease risk of bleeding.

Positioning

The patient is placed supine, in a reverse Trendelenburg position of 10–30 degrees.

Anesthetic Implications

Tape both eyelids closed. Place eye pads over both eyes and cover them with occlusive clear dressings (Tegaderm) to protect them from cleansing solutions and any movement or grazing of instruments by the surgeon or scrub team as they are working over the face.

An orogastric tube should be placed after induction and maintained until the end of the case so that any blood or gastric juices can be suctioned out before the patient is extubated.

A local anesthetic and epinephrine solution may be infiltrated to decrease swelling to prevent bleeding. Watch for an increase in heart rate or blood pressure or EKG changes.

A throat pack is usually placed if general anesthesia is used; document its insertion and removal times. Suction the back of the throat gently with a soft suction catheter before extubating the patient.

Because the tissues of the skull and face are quite vascular, maintaining a slight decrease in mean arterial blood pressure (60–70 mm Hg) can help to minimize bleeding.

Other injuries that are commonly associated with nasal fractures include midface injuries involving the frontal, ethmoid, and lacrimal bones, as well as fractures of the naso-orbital ethmoid bones, orbital wall, cribriform plate, frontal sinus, and maxillary LeFort I, II, and III.

Steroids may be given to decrease tissue swelling and as an antiemetic adjunct unless otherwise contraindicated.

Smooth emergence from anesthesia is important with this surgery. The goal is to avoid coughing, bucking, or nausea/vomiting and retching so as to prevent increased risk of bleeding or hematoma formation from the increased head and neck pressures. Antiemetics should be given.

Use of a humidified oxygen face tent mask at the end of the case helps to oxygenate the patient when he or she is mouth breathing (nose packed) and does not apply pressure to facial structures.

Nasoseptoplasty: Submucous Resection of Septum

In nasoseptoplasty, also known as submucous resection of the septum (SMR), a portion of the cartilaginous or osseous nasal septum beneath flaps of the mucous membrane, perichondrium, and/or periosteum is excised. This procedure is undertaken to repair or reconstruct a deviated septum so as to alleviate chronic sinus symptoms or correct a nasal airway obstruction. It is also used as part of a treatment plan to treat obstructive sleep apnea.

Operative Procedure

Usually, local anesthesia with epinephrine (LA with epi) is infiltrated into the septum. Incisions are made intranasally, mucosal flaps are raised, and the bony and cartilaginous portions of the septum are either removed or fractured back into the midline. Septal flaps are replaced and sutured, and nasal packing is placed. A mustache dressing is put under the nose to collect drainage.

Anesthetic
GETA with oral endotracheal tube; an LMA may be used to decrease the risk of coughing and bucking.

Positioning
The patient is placed in a reverse Trendelenburg position of 10–20 degrees.

Anesthetic Implications
Tape both eyelids closed. Place eye pads over both eyes and cover them with occlusive clear dressings (Tegaderm) to protect them from cleansing solutions and any movement or grazing of instruments by the surgeon or scrub team as they are working over the face.

An orogastric tube should be placed after induction and maintained until the end of the case so that any blood or gastric juices can be suctioned out before the patient is extubated.

A throat pack is usually placed if general anesthesia is used; document its insertion and removal times. Suction the back of the throat gently with a soft suction catheter before extubating the patient.

A local anesthetic and epinephrine solution may be infiltrated to decrease swelling to prevent bleeding. Watch for an increase in heart rate or blood pressure or EKG changes.

Because the tissues of the face and sinuses are quite vascular, maintaining a slight decrease in mean arterial blood pressure (60–70 mm Hg) can help to minimize bleeding.

Smooth emergence from anesthesia is important with this surgery. The goal is to avoid coughing, bucking, or nausea/vomiting and retching so as to prevent increased risk of bleeding or hematoma formation from the increased head and neck pressures. Antiemetics should be given.

Steroids may be given to decrease tissue swelling and as an antiemetic adjunct unless otherwise contraindicated.

Use of a humidified oxygen face tent mask at the end of the case helps to oxygenate the patient when he or she is mouth breathing (nose packed) and does not apply pressure to facial structures.

Mouth Surgery

10

MOUTH SURGERY PEARLS

- If any procedure uses laser or electrocautery, see Chapter 1 on safety concerns for more information.
- Mouth surgery is in competition with surgeon for the patient's throat and airway. Good communication with the surgeon is essential.

MOUTH SURGERY

Operative Dentistry: Periodontics, Endodontics, and Dentoalveolar Procedures

Operative dentistry is performed to provide dental extractions and/or restoration to a patient who cannot tolerate dental care in an office or clinic setting. It may be performed for the following clinical indications: dental caries, dental fractures/trauma, necrotic teeth, oral—facial abscess/cellulitis, periodontitis, impacted wisdom teeth, supernumerary (extra) teeth, ectopically erupted teeth, severe dental crowding/malalignment, teeth in the line of a mandibular fracture or maxillary alveolar fracture, teeth with associated cysts/tumors, retained primary teeth, and missing teeth. Subjective indications for this surgery include severe situational anxiety, mental retardation, physical disability, or medical compromise precluding dental treatment in a typical office or clinic setting.

Operative Procedure

The operative procedure may include dental examination, dental radiographs, dental hygiene, gingival flap curettage, gingivectomy, dental restorations, root canal treatment, dental implants, dental extractions, and alveoplasty.

Root canal treatment, gingival flap curettage, gingivectomy, dental implant placement, dental extractions, and alveoplasty are all procedures that could necessitate the use of electrocautery. If cautery is used, airway fire is a risk (see Chapter 1 on safety concerns).

Anesthetic

Anesthesia usually consists of inhalational induction with a mask if no IV is already present: one example: nitrous oxide 70%, oxygen 30%, and sevoflurane at 8%. Once the patient is in stage III anesthesia, a peripheral IV is started. Once the IV is placed, the FiO_2 can be turned to 100%.

There are two schools of thought on preparing the nasal passage for nasotracheal intubation. The first approach calls for instilling Neosynephrine nose drops into both nares and then passing a lubricated red-rubber obturator, in increasing size, into the nare you plan to intubate. This technique helps to decrease mucosa size and chance of bleeding. One of the risks of this method is the repeated removal of the face mask and interruption of the continuous levels of inhaled agent. There is an increased risk of laryngospasm and light anesthesia with this repeated removal of the mask. The benefit of this method is that preparing the mucosa for intubation provides for potentially less mucosal damage and, therefore, less bleeding.

The alternative is to not prepare the nasal passage and to simply insert the lubricated nasotracheal tube down through the nose. If there is any mucosal irritation or bleeding, the nasotracheal tube itself will tamponade the mucosal bleeding. The benefit of this method is that it does not require repeatedly removing the face mask away, so it maintains the inhaled anesthetic at a constant level and is associated with a lower incidence of laryngospasm. The risk is that damage to the mucosa can occur and bleeding may not tamponade, allowing blood to drip into the back of the throat and into the stomach or lungs.

To perform *nasal intubation,* with careful pressure insert the appropriate-size nasal RAE endotracheal tube (ETT) through the nare to the back of the throat. With a laryngoscope blade, open the mouth, looking at the back of the throat for the distal tip of the nasotracheal tube; gently insert the tube so that it can be reached with Magill forceps inserted into the mouth. With the Magill forceps, grasp the distal end of the ETT, guiding it through the cords. Check for chest excursion, positive $ETCO_2$, and bilateral breath sounds. The nasotracheal RAE tube is positioned with the tube length (external to the nose) coming up over the forehead. A "flex extender" can be placed to the proximal end of the Naso-Rae to extend the circuit tubing up out of the surgeon's way. A piece of foam or folded gauze may be placed on the patient's forehead under the flex extender to prevent pressure on the skin. Tape the nasal ETT securely at the end of the nare and upper jaw to help prevent tube movement. One recommended practice is to wrap a surgical towel around the patient's head and over the patient's taped and padded eyes, then tape it closed, to secure the tubes inside.

Some surgeons prefer *oral intubation* even with dental surgery. The ETT can be secured over at one side of the mouth while the surgeon operates on the opposite side; that is, the ETT can be moved over to the right side of the mouth so the surgeon can operate on the left side of the mouth, and vice versa. There is a higher risk of damage to the ETT when this method is used, so care should be taken to place the ETT as lateral as possible to avoid inadvertent puncture or tearing of the ETT by the surgeon. Look for positive $ETCO_2$, chest excursion, and listen for bilateral breath sounds each time the ETT is repositioned.

Positioning

The patient is positioned supine, with a shoulder roll used to extend the head. Arms are placed at the patient's sides, with the arm on the operating side tucked. The head of the bed may be moved 90 degrees away from the anesthetist.

Anesthetic Implications

Tape and place eye pads to protect the patient's eyes. The dentist will stand at the head of the bed to work with instruments moved over the face.

There is a potential for blood to drip down from the nose or the mouth into the back of the throat and into the stomach. Antiemetic prophylaxis is needed. A weight-based dose of a steroid (e.g., Decadron) is also very effective, and also helps with postoperative inflammation.

A throat pack should always be inserted; chart its insertion and removal times. It is vital to make sure the throat pack is removed by the surgeon at the end of the case. A throat pack can help prevent blood from dripping down the back of the throat. It also will prevent dental restorative debris, tooth fragments, or bacteria-laden calculus (tartar) from lodging in the throat or potentially being aspirated upon awakening.

A local anesthetic solution, often containing epinephrine, may be infiltrated to assist in diminishing postoperative pain. It also functions as a local hemostatic agent. Watch for an increase in heart rate or blood pressure or EKG changes.

An antisialogogue (scopolamine, robinul) or antihistamines (trimethobenzamide [Tigan]; diphenhydramine [Benadry]) can also be given to decrease oral secretions.

Maintenance anesthesia may consist of a volatile inhaled agent mixed with either air or nitrous oxide. As no muscle relaxation is needed with dental surgery, it is acceptable to get the patient back breathing and then give a narcotic based on his or her respiratory rate and vital signs.

At the end of the case, either the surgeon or the anesthetist may place an orogastric tube to suction any blood out of the stomach. A soft, flexible plastic catheter should be used to suction out the oropharynx prior to extubation; avoid hitting the gums or mucosa to prevent bleeding.

Glossectomy: Partial or Total

Glossectomy involves the surgical removal of all or part of the tongue. It is used in cases of tongue cancer that does not respond to other treatments. Tongue cancer is treated aggressively because it can spread very rapidly to surrounding lymph nodes. A glossectomy can be done in combination with a neck dissection (modified or radical) or a mandibulectomy (see the discussion of marginal resection of the mandible with glossectomy later in this chapter).

Operative Procedure

Partial glossectomy is a relatively simple operation. If the cancer to be excised is small, a hole is created, excising the cancerous tissue. The hole is commonly repaired by sewing the tongue closed. If a larger specimen is taken, a small graft (commonly a piece of skin and blood vessels taken from the inner wrist—a radial forearm free flap) is inserted into the hole, with the vessels from the skin flap anastomosed to the tongue vessels. The goal with any partial glossectomy is to maintain as much mobility of the tongue as possible. Speech and swallowing abilities are usually maintained if at least one-third of the tongue remains.

Depending on the extent of the resection and the location of the lesion, a tracheostomy may be done in combination with the glossectomy.

Complete glossectomy is rarely performed but if it is done, a laryngectomy is performed at the same time (or done before) because of the risk of future aspiration difficulties. This surgery results in enormous difficulty in swallowing and talking. A prosthesis may be inserted but it is done only for cosmetic reasons as it is incapable of movement and cannot assist in speech or eating.

Marginal resection of the mandible may also be performed in conjunction with glossectomy. Lymph channels drain the tongue and floor of the mouth into the cervical lymph nodes; thus tumor cells may extend directly into the periosteum and cortex of the mandible, necessitating removal of part of the mandible bone. A much larger and wider tissue excision may be necessary depending on the spread of the cancer or tissue margins taken. Wire is used to reconstruct and stabilize the remaining mandible.

Anesthetic

General anesthesia is used, and nasotracheal intubation is usually done (depending on the site of the lesion); muscle relaxation is needed. Oral intubation may be requested by the surgeon depending on the site of the lesion and surgical approach. Use care with laryngoscope blade so as to not tear or cause bleeding to any mouth lesion.

Local anesthetic *without* epinephrine may be infiltrated by the surgeon to help numb the remaining tongue in a partial glossectomy or the tongue stump with total glossectomy.

Positioning

The patient is positioned supine, with bilateral arms padded and tucked at the patient's side. The head of the table may be turned away at least 90 degrees, if not 180 degrees, from the anesthetist.

Anesthetic Implications

Type and cross-matching of the patient's blood may be needed.

Tape and place eye pads to protect the patient's eyes, as the surgeon will be operating around the face.

Diligent preoperative assessment of the airway is imperative; have emergency airway equipment available. Awake oral or nasal fiberoptic intubation may be required. Use extra care when oral intubation is needed, so as to not dislodge the tumor or cause bleeding during intubation.

An antisialogogue (scopolamine, robinul) or antihistamines (trimethobenzamide [Tigan]; diphenhydramine [Benadryl]) can be given to decrease oral secretions.

A nasogastric tube or feeding tube should be placed during surgery for a complete or large-excision glossectomy so that nutrition can be given postoperatively.

A throat pack should always be inserted; chart its insertion and removal times. It is vital to make sure that the throat pack is removed by the surgeon at the end of the case. A throat pack can help prevent blood from dripping down the back of the patient's throat.

There is a potential for blood to drip down from the mouth into the back of the throat and into the stomach and/or lungs. Antiemetic prophylaxis is needed. A weight-based dose of an IV steroid (e.g., Decadron) is also very effective, and also helps with postoperative inflammation unless otherwise contraindicated. Give this agent just after induction and intubation.

Because the tissues of the mouth are quite vascular, maintaining a slight decrease in mean arterial blood pressure (MAP of approximately 60–70 mm Hg) can help to minimize bleeding.

Look for airway swelling, and assess whether the patient will tolerate extubation before removing the tube. Deflate the ETT cuff and listen for air moving around the tube; you can listen with a stethoscope at the patient's neck or mouth.

A soft, flexible plastic catheter should be used to suction out the oropharynx prior to extubation. Avoid hitting the suture line or surrounding tissues to prevent bleeding.

Smooth emergence from anesthesia is important with this surgery. The goal is to avoid coughing, bucking, or nausea/vomiting or retching so as to prevent increased risk of bleeding, hematoma formation, or suture line disruption from the increased head and neck pressures.

If a tracheostomy is performed, have the obturator go with the patient when leaving the operating room.

Report the size and make of the tracheostomy tube to the recovery nurse.

Humidified oxygen should be given once the patient is in the recovery room.

Excision of Oral Cavity Lesions

Surgical removal of a single or multiple soft-tissue lesions on the lips, gingiva, oral mucous membranes, hard or soft palate, tongue, or floor of the mouth is the goal of this procedure. It may also involve surgical removal of intraosseous lesions of the maxilla or mandible. These surgeries are undertaken to remove acute or chronic benign or malignant neoplasms; they may also be performed when ulcerative, reactive, or inflammatory lesions not healing with traditional methods require biopsy, to establish their diagnosis or to effect surgical excision. Squamous cell carcinoma is the most common primary oral cavity malignant process. Bone may need to be taken; metastases to cervical nodes may be found.

Operative Procedure

The operative procedure depends on the type of lesion and tissue involved. An intra-oral incision is made. These procedures can also frequently necessitate the use of a laser or electrocautery (see Chapter 1 on safety concerns with these techniques). A total or partial surgical resection may take place. A split-thickness skin graft can also be done to cover the defect. Cervical lymph nodes may be biopsied and removed.

Anesthetic

General anesthesia and nasotracheal intubation are typically used; muscle relaxation is needed. Oral intubation may be requested by the surgeon depending on the site of the lesion and surgical approach. Use care when manipulating the laryngoscope blade so as to not tear or cause bleeding to any mouth lesion.

Extubation can be of particular concern with mentally challenged or cognitively impaired patients.

Positioning

The patient is placed supine, in a reverse Trendelenburg position of 30 degrees.

Anesthetic Implications

Tape the eyelids closed and place eye pads to protect the patient's eyes, as the surgeon will be operating around the face.

An antisialogogue (scopolamine, robinul) or antihistamines (trimethobenzamide [Tigan]; diphenhydramine [Benadryl]) can be given to decrease oral secretions.

Infectious lesions can and do occur in the oral cavity. When lesions such as condylomas are being excised, a laser or electrocautery is often used. An appropriate filtration mask should be worn by all surgical, nursing, and anesthesia staff in the room to prevent possible inhalation of infectious material when these types of lesions are being excised.

Type and cross-matching of the patient's blood may be needed. Preparations should be made for unanticipated complications when resecting osseous lesions—most notably, surgical dissection into an intraosseous arteriovenous malformation that could result in massive bleeding.

Because the tissues of the mouth are quite vascular, maintaining a slight decrease in mean arterial blood pressure (60–70 mm Hg) can help to minimize bleeding.

A throat pack should always be inserted; chart its insertion and removal times. It is vital to make sure the throat pack is removed by the surgeon at the end of the case. A throat pack can help prevent blood from dripping down the back of the patient's throat.

There is a potential for blood to drip down from the mouth into the back of the throat and into the stomach and/or the lungs. Antiemetic prophylaxis is needed. A weight-based dose of a steroid (e.g., Decadron) is very effective, and helps with postoperative inflammation.

At the end of the case, either the surgeon or the anesthetist should place an orogastric tube to suction any blood out of the stomach. A soft, flexible plastic catheter should be used to suction out the oropharynx prior to extubation; avoid hitting the suture line or surrounding tissues to prevent bleeding.

Smooth emergence from anesthesia is important with this surgery. The goal is to avoid coughing, bucking, or nausea/vomiting or retching so as to prevent increased risk of bleeding, hematoma formation, or suture line disruption from the increased head and neck pressures.

Oral gauze packing may be placed postoperatively, depending on the procedure performed, to aid in hemostasis. These materials should be secured to the patient's cheek(s) with umbilical tape to prevent them from potentially being swallowed or aspirated. The umbilical tape also allows for easy access and removal should the patient not tolerate them upon awakening.

Humidified oxygen should be given once the patient is in the recovery room.

Uvulopalatopharyngoplasty

Uvulopalatopharyngoplasty (UPPP) is a surgical procedure to remove redundant tissue and relieve obstruction in the upper airway. Indications for this procedure include obstructive sleep apnea and snoring. A tonsillectomy and adenoidectomy may be done at the same time.

Operative Procedure

The surgeon cuts away a portion of the soft palate, including the tonsils and uvula, which shortens the tissue, thereby preventing its collapse during sleep. A portion of the pharynx and adenoids may also be removed. The mucosa is closed with absorbable sutures. The goal is to reduce the amount of soft-tissue palate, widen the airway, and make breathing easier.

Laser-assisted uvulopalatopharyngoplasty (LA-UPPP) is also done. If any procedure uses laser or electrocautery, see Chapter 1 on safety concerns for more information.

Anesthetic

General anesthesia and nasal intubation with a nasal RAE tube are required; muscle relaxants are usually not necessary. IV steroids can be given if there is no contraindication to their use.

Preoperative oxygenation should be done for a minute or two longer than normal, as patients undergoing this procedure may be chronically hypoxic from obstructive sleep apnea.

To prevent airway fires, use caution with oxygen during this procedure. Good communication with the surgeon is essential, especially as the trachea is to be entered and bleeding is to be cauterized. Decrease FiO_2 to 30% before cauterization starts.

Positioning

The patient should be positioned supine, with a shoulder roll and one arm tucked at the side. The head of the bed can be elevated 30 degrees.

Anesthetic Implications

Occasionally patients with severe obstruction or added risk due to obesity may require a temporary tracheotomy. Postoperative airway obstruction and difficulties are possible in all patients who undergo UPPP.

Tape the eyelids closed and place eye pads to protect the patient's eyes, as the surgeon will be operating around the face.

Heavily sedated patients may also have airway obstruction. For this reason, give minimal sedation preoperatively.

An antisialogogue (scopolamine, robinul) or antihistamines (trimethobenzamide [Tigan]; diphenhydramine [Benadry]) can be given to decrease oral secretions.

A throat pack should always be inserted; chart its insertion and removal times. It is vital to make sure the throat pack is removed by the surgeon at the end of the case. A throat pack can help prevent blood from dripping down the back of the patient's throat.

There is a potential for blood to drip down from the mouth into the back of the throat and into the stomach and/or the lungs. Antiemetic prophylaxis is needed. A weight-based dose of a steroid (e.g., Decadron) is very effective, and also helps with postoperative inflammation.

Because the tissues of the mouth are quite vascular, maintaining a slight decrease in mean arterial blood pressure (60–70 mm Hg) can help to minimize bleeding.

At the end of the case, either the surgeon or the anesthetist should place an orogastric tube to suction any blood out of the stomach. A soft, flexible plastic catheter should be used to suction out the oropharynx prior to extubation; avoid hitting the suture line or surrounding tissues to prevent bleeding.

Smooth emergence from anesthesia is important with this surgery. The goal is to avoid coughing, bucking, or nausea/vomiting or retching so as to prevent increased risk of bleeding, hematoma formation, or suture line disruption from the increased head and neck pressures.

Humidified oxygen should be given once the patient is in the recovery room.

ENDOCRINE SURGERY PEARLS

- The endocrine system is composed of many organs, each of which secretes specific hormones to regulate many body systems. There are several glands that signal each other in a specific sequence, this is referred to as an axis. An example of an axis is the hypothalamus–pituitary axis.

  While there are many organs known specifically as endocrine organs (pituitary, thyroid, pancreas, etc.), there are other organs that also secrete endocrine hormones. One example is the kidney, which secretes endocrine hormones such as renin and erythropoietin.

- Diseases of the endocrine system are classified as primary, secondary, or tertiary. Primary endocrine disease inhibits the endocrine gland itself (i.e., thyroid). Secondary endocrine disease is indicative of a problem with the pituitary gland. Tertiary endocrine disease is associated with dysfunction of the hypothalamus.
- Feedback loops are very important in the stimulation or inhibition of hormone release. A few examples include TRH–TSH–T3/T4 and renin–angiotensin–aldosterone.

ENDOCRINE DISORDERS

Hyperparathyroidism

Signs and symptoms of hyperparathyroidism (characterized by increased calcium levels) may include hypertension, pancreatitis, hyperchloremic metabolic acidosis, muscle weakness, fatigue, renal stones, and renal and cardiac abnormalities including ventricular dysrhythmias. EKG changes can include a shortened QT segment and a prolonged PR interval. Hypercalcemia can cause nausea, vomiting, and polyuria; patients with chronic hypercalcemia may be hypovolemic and/or anorexic.

Avoid hypoventilation (acidosis increases serum calcium levels). Hypercalcemic crisis is treated by hydration with 0.9% normal saline IV at a rate of 200–300 mL/h to correct intravascular volume contraction and aid renal excretion of calcium. To decrease calcium levels, hyperventilate the patient and possibly initiate diuresis with a loop diuretic (furosemide). Loop diuretics inhibit renal absorption of calcium. Patients in renal failure may need dialysis if they cannot tolerate fluid resuscitation. Patients may already be on calcitonin, which helps to retard bone loss. Mithramycin may be prescribed to inhibit parathyroid hormone activity; bisphosphonates are used to inhibit osteoclast activity.

Digoxin potentiates arrhythmia in the setting of hypercalcemia.

Hypoparathyroidism

Hypoparathyroidism (characterized by decreased calcium levels) is most commonly caused by damage to parathyroids during surgery. Its signs and symptoms include neuromuscular irritability, laryngospasm, stridor, Chvostek's sign (muscle spasm of face when the facial nerve is tapped at the angle of the jaw), and Trousseau's sign (carpal spasm with BP cuff inflation greater than systolic BP for 3 minutes). Hypoalbuminemia, defined as an albumin level less than 3.5 g/dL, is also present. EKG changes can include a prolonged QT segment. Hypocalcemia can potentiate a response to neuromuscular blocking agents; vigilance with peripheral nerve monitoring is needed.

Avoid alkalosis with hyperventilation or sodium bicarbonate, as it further decreases serum calcium levels. Treat this disorder with calcium chloride and vitamin D.

Hyperthyroidism

Hyperthyroid (Graves' disease) symptoms include muscle weakness, hyperactive reflexes, exophthalmos, sinus tachycardia, atrial fibrillation, dehydration, diarrhea, heat intolerance, and weight loss due to metabolic derangements. Do not allow the patient's temperature to get too warm.

Patients with large goiters or abnormal airway anatomy may be especially vulnerable to airway compromise with preoperative sedation.

However, increased stress and anxiety can lead to thyrotoxicosis. Sedate these individuals carefully.

Sodium thiopental has antithyroid activity properties and is the induction agent of choice in hyperthyroid patients. Avoid anesthetic agents that stimulate the sympathetic nervous system (SNS) or sympathomimetics, such as ketamine, pancuronium, atropine, robinul, and ephedrine. Agents should ideally blunt the SNS response.

Cardiac function should be closely monitored in hyperthyroidism cases; these patients commonly have atrial fibrillation and premature ventricular contractions. Hyperthyroid patients also tend to have an increased resting heart rate, stroke volume, and cardiac output. A beta blocker may need to be given if the patient has hypertension or tachycardia.

The increased basal metabolic rate associated with hyperthyroid states can mean that these patients will desaturate faster with any interruption in oxygen delivery (e.g., during intubation).

Give an antithyroid medication to block further synthesis of any thyroid hormones and to inhibit peripheral conversion of T_4 to T_3. High-dose propyl thiouracil is preferred because of its early onset of action.

Hyperthyroid patients with exophthalmos (bulging eyes) require special eye care.

Paper tape is used to close the eyes to prevent corneal drying or abrasions; eye pads are then placed over both eyes to protect them. Eye ointment can be instilled before taping for patients who will remain intubated postoperatively. Patients who have ointment in their eyes will sometimes rub their eyes (to clear their vision postoperatively) and can accidentally scratch their eyes or face.

Thyroid Storm

While a rare occurrence, thyroid storm (also known as thyrotoxic crisis or thyrotoxicosis) usually occurs several hours after surgery but can be a sudden development in the operating room. An acute, life-threatening medical emergency, this hypermetabolic state is induced by excessive release of the T_3/T_4 thyroid hormones. It is brought on by an exaggerated peripheral response to high levels of circulating thyroid hormone.

Signs and symptoms include fever greater than 38.5°C, marked tachycardia, atrial fibrillation, ventricular arrhythmias, shock, sudden and profound cardiovascular collapse, and congestive heart failure, hypertension followed by hypotension, seizures, and mental status changes evolving from irritability to coma.

Treatment includes the following measures:

- Provide 100% FiO_2. If the patient is intubated, increase the minute ventilation to control carbon dioxide excess.
- Hydrate the patient: Dextrose solutions are the preferred intravenous fluids to cope with continuously high metabolic demand
- Treat any cardiac arrhythmia. Cardioversion is ineffective.
- Give corticosteroids to block peripheral conversion of T_4 to T_3 (thyroid hormones).
- Apply ice packs and cooling blankets. Give cold IV fluids.
- Beta blockers—such as propranolol or esmolol (Brevibloc), labetalol, and metoprolol) —may be given to minimize sympathomimetic symptoms, decrease hypertension, and slow the heart rate to less than 100 beats per minute.
- Give iodides: potassium iodide, Lugol's solution, or thioamide (propylthiouracil) to block the release of thyroid hormones.
- Aspirin is contraindicated because it binds with protein, and the T_3/T_4 hormones bind with protein. Giving aspirin tears T_3/T_4 from the protein and puts it into the bloodstream.

Differential diagnoses for thyroid storm include malignant hyperthermia, pheochromocytoma, and neuroleptic malignant syndrome. Thyroid storm is *not* associated with muscle rigidity, respiratory acidosis, lactic acidosis, or an increase in creatinine kinase.

Hypothyroidism

Hypothyroidism symptoms include lethargy, dehydration, bradycardia, decreased cardiac function, hypoactive reflexes, intolerance to cold, depression, constipation, and weight gain. Cardiac function should be closely monitored. Patients with this condition also have decreased respiratory responsiveness to hypoxia and hypercarbia.

Ketamine is the induction agent of choice in patients with severe hypothyroidism because they usually have slower heart rates and decreased contractility, stroke volume, and cardiac output. MAC requirements are less than noted with a euthyroid patient. Hypothyroid patients may be slow to recover from general anesthesia. Pain control may be achieved with a nonopioid agent, such as ketorolac (an injectable NSAID). Hypothyroid patients are sensitive to muscle relaxation and all anesthetics; give less of all of these drugs in such cases.

Hyperthyroid patients usually have delayed gastric emptying and need a rapid-sequence induction.

Monitor the patient's temperature and do not allow the patient to get cold.

These patients are usually on Synthroid (levo-thyroxine) preoperatively and should take their medication before surgery. They should be euthyroid preoperatively. Their thyroid-stimulating hormone (TSH) levels should be normal preoperatively.

Myxedema Coma

Severe hypothyroidism in adults may occasionally lead to myxedema coma. This life-threatening emergency is characterized by signs that include a decreased level of consciousness, cardiomegaly, pleural effusions, peripheral edema, and hyponatremia with syndrome of inappropriate antidiuretic hormone (SIADH). Sedation can precipitate myxedema coma in hypothyroid patients. Treat this condition with thyroid replacement, administration of cortisol, and correction of metabolic abnormalities.

Cretinism

Severe hypothyroidism in neonates may lead to cretinism, which is characterized by severe mental retardation.

ENDOCRINE SURGERY

Endocrine surgeries include procedures related to the adrenal glands, parathyroids, pheochromocytomas, and thyroid.

Adrenalectomy

Adrenalectomy involves excision of one or both adrenal glands. This procedure is performed to excise primary benign or malignant tumors of the adrenals, to treat primary hyperaldosteronism, to modify an endocrine-dependent tumor (seen in breast or prostate cancers), and to treat a pheochromocytoma (discussed later in this chapter).

Operative Procedure
With the *posterior* approach, an incision is made from the lower ribs to the posterior iliac crest. The left adrenal vein is divided from the renal vein, and the right adrenal vein is divided from the inferior vena cava. If the pleura is entered, a drain may be inserted.

With the *anterior* approach, an upper abdominal longitudinal incision is made. The retroperitoneal space is entered on the right after reflecting the duodenum, and on the left through the lesser sac.

Adrenalectomy is usually done using a laparoscopic approach at centers experienced with such surgeries. The open approach is reserved for larger masses, local or vascular invasion, lymphadenopathy, or metastasis.

Anesthetic
General endotracheal anesthesia (GETA) is given with insertion of an oral endotracheal tube (OETT); muscle relaxants are given. The patient may need rapid-sequence induction if he or she is obese as a result of Cushing's syndrome.

Monitors and IV Access
An arterial line and a central line may be needed. At least two large-bore peripheral IVs should be available.

IV Fluids and Volume Requirements
Euvolemia is recommended.

Positioning
The patient is positioned lateral or prone for a posterior approach for unilateral adrenalectomy; supine for an anterior approach for a bilateral adrenalectomy. Careful positioning and padding are necessary, as these patients are usually quite sick.

Anesthetic Implications
Corticosteroid replacement must be given throughout the entire perioperative period if the operative indication for adrenalectomy is Cushing's syndrome or if bilateral adrenalectomy has been performed. Have hydrocortisone available. If bilateral adrenalectomy is expected, pretreatment with glucocorticoids (hydrocortisone, cortisone, prednisone, methylprednisolone, betamethasone, or dexamethasone [Decadron]) and mineralocorticoids (aldosterone, progesterone) is necessary.

Assess sodium, potassium, and glucose levels preoperatively.

Type and cross-match the patient's blood, as blood loss may be considerable with this procedure. The spleen, pancreas, and liver may be manipulated for retraction during the surgery, and; injury to these organs may cause enormous blood loss.

Parathyroidectomy

Parathyroidectomy involves removal of one or more of the four parathyroid glands (located behind the thyroid gland). Parathyroid glands control serum calcium and bone calcium levels. This procedure is indicated to excise adenomas, carcinomas, and hyperplasia.

Serum calcium levels are important in muscle and nerve function, and a low calcium level can cause painful muscle spasms (tetany). There is currently no replacement medication for parathyroid hormone, so treatment usually consists of calcium and vitamin D supplements.

Hyperparathyroidism causes excessive secretion of parathyroid hormone with resulting hypercalcemia.

Operative Procedure

Blunt and sharp dissection is conducted to expose the thyroid, followed by identification of the four parathyroid glands, which are located behind the thyroid gland. A sternotomy is rarely needed unless not all of the parathyroid glands are localized in the neck.

Parathyroid reimplantation is done in the setting of total parathyroid removal due to hyperplasia of all the glands; it is not attempted if only one parathyroid gland has been removed. Parathyroids generally are not reimplanted in the neck; if they grow too big, they are more difficult to remove. With reimplantation, multiple pieces of one parathyroid gland are placed in the muscle (not fat) of the forearm; muscle has a good blood supply. The small pieces of parathyroid gland are chopped up to release the capsule around it so there is a better chance of cells touching the blood supply and growing. This reimplanted gland should then be able to maintain adequate calcium levels in the blood. If elevated calcium levels reoccur, some of previously implanted gland may be removed. A drain may be inserted before closing the neck incision.

Anesthetic

General anesthesia is given with insertion of an OETT; an armored ETT may be useful. An awake fiberoptic intubation may be needed if the normal airway anatomy is affected by a large gland and/or tracheal compression or deviation. This surgery may be performed under cervical block and IV sedation.

Succinylcholine (Anectine) may be given with rapid-sequence induction. Nitrous oxide may also be given. Regional anesthesia is not contraindicated.

If general anesthesia is given, check with the surgeon regarding the use of muscle paralytics and nerve monitoring. A NIM EMG endotracheal tube (ETT) may be used to facilitate electromyography (EMG) monitoring of the intrinsic laryngeal musculature during surgery; muscle relaxants are not used if nerve monitoring is performed. This kind of ETT monitors manipulation of the recurrent laryngeal nerve by evaluating EMG signals from the intrinsic laryngeal musculature. It is equipped with audible alarms and provides a visual interpretation of EMG signals. Intrinsic wires of the NIM ETT should be in direct contact with the vocal cords; a blue stripe in the tube should also be positioned right between the cords. A grounding wire is usually pierced through the skin of the patient's shoulder or arm. The NIM EMG ETT is available in whole sizes only: sizes 6, 7, and 8 mm.

If muscle relaxants are used, avoid histamine-releasing paralytics. Note that the action of muscle relaxants may be altered by a low or high calcium level in these patients.

Positioning

The patient is positioned supine, with a shoulder roll to extend the head and neck. The patient's head should not hang freely. Bilateral arms may be tucked. For gland reimplantation, the operative arm will remain on a padded armboard and is not tucked.

Anesthetic Implications

Be very careful with preoperative sedation if the patient's airway is compromised in any way.

A local anesthetic with epinephrine is usually injected into the patient's neck before the incision is made. Monitor the EKG for increased heart rate or ST-segment changes.

Surgical exploration of the parathyroid takes place around highly vascular structures and vessels and around the airway; manipulation of these tissues can cause bleeding, edema, and swelling. Extra monitoring is needed when extubating the patient and in the immediate postoperative period. To look for laryngeal edema, occlude the endotracheal tube, put the cuff down, and listen for patient ventilation around the ETT.

An iPTH (intact parathyroid hormone) lab should be drawn minutes after taking the gland(s) out of the patient's neck. Parathyroid hormone (PTH) levels will drop in 10 minutes, and lab results should be available in 30 minutes.

IV access should be available so that large volumes of fluid or blood product replacement can be given if needed. A large-bore IV "med-lock" may be placed in the nonoperative arm preoperatively to provide for easier blood-draw access for labs.

A frozen section may be used to confirm removal of parathyroid tissue.

Complications

Potential complications of parathyroidectomy include pneumothorax, failure to correct hypercalcemia, hematoma, phrenic nerve injury, superior laryngeal nerve injury (manifested as voice changes; hoarseness is usually not appreciated until a week after surgery), and recurrent laryngeal nerve injury (unilateral: hoarseness; bilateral: aphonia and patient may need reintubation). Even small blood collections can lead to devastating tracheal compression and usually need to be re-explored in the operating room.

Postoperative Measures

Assess for hypocalcemia in the postoperative period, evidenced by laryngeal stridor, tingling in the fingers or lips, and Chvostek's or Trousseau's sign.

Pheochromocytoma

A pheochromocytoma tumor (typically found on the adrenals) may be removed through surgical resection. Some patients may have bilateral tumors, one on each adrenal gland.

A pheochromocytoma is a rare, highly vascular, neuroendocrine tumor, originating in the chromaffin cells, usually found in the adrenal medulla (90% of the time) or in an extra-adrenal location. Extra-adrenal sites include any organ along the paravertebral sympathetic chain from the skull to the pelvis, although most tumors are found below the diaphragm. Such tumors can also be found in the ureters and bladder.

Although these tumors most often arise spontaneously, some are associated with neurofibromatosis and "MEN syndromes." Multiple endocrine neoplasm (MEN) syndromes are conditions that cause overactivity in certain endocrine glands and are associated with tumors of the pancreas, thyroid, adrenal, and pituitary glands. Three major types are identified:

- MEN 1: parathyroid, pancreatic, and pituitary tumors
- MEN 2a: medullary thyroid and parathyroid tumors, and pheochromocytomas
- MEN 2b: medullary thyroid cancer, pheochromocytoma, and neuromas

Pheochromocytoma tumors secrete excessive catecholamines—usually norepinephrine (70%) and epinephrine (30%). Catecholamine secretion may be stimulated by tumor manipulation, postural changes, exertion or anxiety, trauma, pain, and use of sympathomimetics, phenothiazines, Reglan, histamine, or glucagon.

Patients with pheochromocytomas have paroxysmal signs and symptoms of sympathetic nervous system hyperactivity, including diaphoresis, tachycardia, headache, severe hypertension, palpitations, anxiety, elevated blood glucose levels (i.e., catecholamine-stimulated inhibition of glucose uptake), and cardiomyopathy. If these tumors are not removed, patients can die from congestive heart failure, myocardial infarction, and intracerebral hemorrhage.

Operative Procedure

Removal of a pheochromocytoma can be done by laparotomy or laparoscopy. If the procedure is done laterally, the retroperitoneum is entered by the lower ribs.

Anesthetic

General anesthesia is given with insertion of an OETT; muscle relaxants are given. Isoflurane, enflurane, desflurane, sevoflurane (volatile agents); vecuronium and rocuronium (muscle relaxants); and fentanyl (opioid) are all acceptable drugs to use in a patient with a pheochromocytoma.

Drugs to avoid in patients with pheochromocytomas include histamine releasers (e.g., morphine, atracurium), vagolytics and sympathomimetics (e.g., atropine, pancuronium, succinylcholine [Anectine]), ketamine, cocaine, and indirect catechol stimulators (e.g., droperidol, metoclopramide, and ephedrine).

Have vasoactive medications drawn up or in line as an infusion and ready to give at any time, including nitroglycerin, sodium nitroprusside (SNP), beta blockers, and phenylephrine (Neo-Synephrine).

Positioning

The patient may be placed in either the supine or the lateral position.

Anesthetic Implications

Do not allow the sympathetic nervous system (SNS) to be stimulated if at all possible. Sedate the patient before any stimulation occurs.

Start alpha blockade 7 to 10 days preoperatively using a nonspecific and irreversible alpha antagonist; this measure helps to decrease the possibility of severe intraoperative hypertension. The following agents may be used:

- Phentolamine (Regitine): 5 mg for adults, 1 mg for pediatrics; IV. This agent's half-life is 19 minutes (short acting).
- Prazosin (Minipress): 1 mg BID or TID; PO. This agent's half-life is 2–3 hours (moderate action).
- Phenoxybenzamine (Dibenzyline): 40–400 mg/day; PO. This agent's half-life is 24 hours (long acting). A noncompetitive alpha and alpha$_2$ antagonist, dibenzylline is the drug of choice for alpha blockade. Ideally, it should be started several weeks before surgery takes place.

Initiate a "pure" beta blocker only after adequate alpha blockade has been provided in the presence of a pheochromocytoma if the patient is persistently tachycardic. If beta blockade is started prematurely, unopposed alpha stimulation could precipitate a hypertensive crisis. Some authorities recommend that an alpha:beta blocker (e.g., labetalol; 1:7 alpha:beta ratio when given IV) be given to slow the heart rate.

Critical times of sympathetic hyperactivity are during tracheal intubation and during tumor manipulation. Intubation and surgical manipulation of the tumor can cause a massive release of catecholamines; in this event, be prepared with vasodilators to control hypertension. Patients undergoing surgical resection of pheochromocytomas can have severe paroxysmal or sustained hypertension. Blood pressure goals are SBP less than 160 mm Hg and DBP less than 95 mm Hg.

Once the adrenal vein has been ligated, thereby removing the major source of circulating catecholamines, profound hypotension can occur because of very low sympathetic activity and dehydration. The patient may need a vasopressor infusion for emergence from anesthesia and during the immediate postoperative period; phenylephrine (Neo-Synephrine) is an acceptable option for this purpose.

Type and cross-match the patient's blood, as blood loss may be considerable during this procedure.

Patients with pheochromocytomas are often volume depleted. Preoperatively, the patient should be encouraged to take in increased salt amounts; isotonic saline IV fluids are given once the patient is admitted into the hospital. IV volume resuscitation may be necessary intraoperatively.

Treat cardiac arrhythmias, which are common, and control blood glucose levels.

If a bilateral adrenalectomy is expected, pretreat with a glucocorticoid and mineralocorticoid. See Chapter 4 for more information on these steroids.

Preoperative Measures
Obtain a preoperative 12-lead EKG; an echocardiogram may also be needed.

Monitors and IV Access
- An arterial line is required; BP must be monitored during induction and intubation.
- CVP is commonly placed.
- At least two large-bore peripheral IV lines should be available if no central line is placed.
- A pulmonary artery catheter may be needed.
- TEE is helpful.

The following drugs may be required:

- IV vasoactive agents: IV pump: nitroglycerin, sodium nitroprusside (SNP), and phenylephrine; dopamine; norepinephrine; epinephrine
- Syringe for bolus: ephedrine, phenylephrine, esmolol (Brevibloc), labetalol, metoprolol; phentolamine (Regitine) is used for hypertensive emergencies
- Other drugs: glucose, regular insulin

Induction
Don't stimulate the SNS if at all possible. Sedate the patient before any stimulation is attempted.

Use of succinylcholine (Anectine) is usually avoided.

Maintenance
Isoflurane is the volatile anesthetic agent that is least sensitive to catecholamines.

Thyroidectomy: Subtotal or Total (Neck Approach)

Thyroidectomy involves removal of all or part of the thyroid gland. It is performed to correct either a benign or malignant process affecting the thyroid gland.

Operative Procedure

An incision is made above the sternal notch. Blunt and sharp dissection is performed to expose the thyroid gland. Care should be taken to avoid injury to the recurrent and superior laryngeal nerves and the parathyroid glands. A drain may be inserted before the incision is closed.

Anesthetic

General anesthesia is given with insertion of an OETT; an armored ETT may be useful. An awake fiberoptic intubation may be needed if the normal airway anatomy is affected by a large gland and/or tracheal compression or deviation. Be very careful with preoperative sedation if the patient's airway is compromised in any way.

This procedure may also be done under a bilateral deep cervical plexus block and IV sedation.

If general anesthesia is given, check with the surgeon regarding muscle paralytics and nerve monitoring. A NIM (Nerve Integrity Monitor) EMG endotracheal tube may be used to facilitate EMG monitoring of the intrinsic laryngeal musculature during surgery. This kind of ETT monitors manipulation of the recurrent laryngeal nerve by evaluating EMG signals from the intrinsic laryngeal musculature. It is equipped with audible alarms and provides a visual interpretation of EMG signals. Intrinsic wires of the NIM ETT should be in direct contact with the vocal cords; a blue stripe in the tube should also be positioned right between the cords. A grounding wire is usually pierced through the skin of the patient's shoulder or arm. The NIM EMG ETT is available in whole sizes only: sizes 6, 7, and 8 mm.

Muscle relaxants are not used if nerve monitoring is performed. If muscle relaxants are used, avoid histamine-releasing paralytics.

A local anesthetic with epinephrine is usually injected into the patient's neck before the incision is made. Monitor the EKG for increased heart rate and ST-segment changes.

If the patient has hyperthyroidism, have beta blockers available in case of hypertension and tachycardia or any SNS response.

Succinylcholine (Anectine) may be given with rapid-sequence induction. Nitrous oxide may be given. Regional anesthesia is not contraindicated.

Positioning

The patient is positioned supine, with a shoulder roll to extend the neck. The head should not hang. Bilateral arms should be placed on padding and tucked at the patient's sides.

Anesthetic Implications

The thyroid gland is very vascular, so there is a risk of significant blood loss with this procedure. Have at least one 18-gauge or larger peripheral IV available in case blood products need to be given. Type and cross-match the patient's blood. Check for adequate IV drip flow after arms are tucked

These patients should be euthyroid preoperatively, with a resting heart rate of 85 beats/min or less, and stable cardiovascular status and vital signs. It is important to assess for thyrotoxicosis preoperatively, as this imbalance correlates with intraoperative risk and morbidity. Thyroid-stimulating hormone (TSH) levels should be normal preoperatively.

Patients with thyroid disease (both hypothyroid and hyperthyroid) are dehydrated and need volume repletion.

Place a warming/cooling blanket on the patient. Let the patient passively cool if possible; active cooling may be required in the event of thyroid storm.

Surgical stimulation around the trachea can cause the patient to cough and buck. If muscle relaxants are not used, the patient's anesthetic level must be kept a little deeper with vasopressors given to support the blood pressure if needed. Along with a volatile agent, a propofol infusion can be given to help smooth the anesthetic effect.

A frozen section may be done to confirm cancer before removing the entire gland.

Surgical exploration of the thyroid is done around the airway; manipulation of these tissues can cause edema or swelling. Extra monitoring is needed when extubating the patient and in the immediate postoperative period. To look for laryngeal edema, occlude the endotracheal tube, put the cuff down, and listen for patient ventilation around the ETT.

Postoperative Measures

Assess for hypocalcemia in the postoperative period, evidenced by laryngeal stridor, tingling in the fingers or lips, and Chvostek's or Trousseau's sign.

Complications

Potential complications of thyroidectomy include pneumothorax, hematoma, and phrenic nerve injury. Even small blood collections can lead to devastating upper airway edema.

Signs of hypothyroidism and hypoparathyroidism can also develop. Hypocalcemia signs include stridor, laryngospasm, and vocal cord tetanus.

Bilateral injury to the recurrent laryngeal nerves (RLN) can lead to vocal cord paresis and stridor. Unilateral injury to the RLN can cause hoarseness. Superior laryngeal nerve injury may be manifested as voice changes.

Coughing on emergence from anesthesia or vomiting in the immediate postoperative period can cause stress on the suture line and cause bleeding. The trachea is at risk for compression due to hematoma and usually needs to be re-explored in the operating room in these circumstances.

Thyroidectomy: Substernal or Intrathoracic

This type of thyroidectomy involves removal of a thyroid gland with a pronounced downward prolongation of the lower pole or poles; these elements may extend below the level of the manubrial notch. *Most thyroid glands that have a substernal or intrathoracic component can be removed through a neck incision.*

Downward growth from the lower pole of thyroid tissue comes from a single or multiple nodules. The term *substernal* may be used to describe thyroid gland extension above the level of the sternal notch and the term *intrathoracic* to describe extension below the notch. As the nodule grows larger and moves lower through the thoracic strait, symptoms can range from minimal to severe; the difficulty and risk of the surgery also increase with prolongation. Because of its fixed position in the thorax, any swelling or any further growth of the thyroid can result in compression of surrounding structures, leading to swallowing difficulties, breathing difficulties with tracheal compression, superior vena cava compression, transient hoarseness, permanent vocal cord paralysis, or unilateral phrenic nerve paralysis.

Operative Procedure

A median sternotomy and right-sided thoracotomy are viable approaches. This procedure can be done with video-assisted thoracotomy.

Anesthetic

General anesthesia is given with insertion of an OETT. Check with the surgeon regarding nerve monitoring and use of muscle relaxants.

Positioning

The patient is positioned supine, with a shoulder roll to extend the neck. The head should not hang. Bilateral arms are padded and tucked at the patient's sides.

Anesthetic Implications

These patients may have tracheal deviation and may be difficult to intubate. CT or MRI may be needed preoperatively to discern difficult airway anatomy.

There is increased morbidity and mortality associated with this surgery.

See the section on subtotal and total thyroidectomy for thyroid disease information.

Neck and Laryngologic Surgery

12

NECK AND LARYNGOLOGIC SURGERY PEARLS

- If any procedure uses laser or electrocautery, see Chapter 1 on safety concerns for more information.
- Neck and laryngologic surgery is in competition with the anesthetist for the patient's throat and airway.
- Narcotics and premedication measures must avoid airway compromise. Many patients undergoing these types of surgeries may have an airway with abnormal anatomy and be considered a "difficult airway."
- With oral cavity and pharynx surgery, a cuffed tube is needed to prevent volatile gas from blowing into the surgeon's face and contaminating the OR, to prevent oxygen from blowing back up where contact with the cautery or laser can cause a fire, and to prevent blood from going into lungs.
- Because the tissues of the neck and larynx are quite vascular, maintaining a slight decrease in mean arterial blood pressure (MAP of approximately 60–70 mm Hg) can help to minimize bleeding.
- Smooth emergence from anesthesia is important with this surgery. The goal is to avoid coughing, bucking, or nausea/vomiting or retching so as to prevent increased risk of bleeding, hematoma formation, or suture line disruption from the increased chest, neck, and head pressures. Antiemetics should be given (see Chapter 4). Have a team member hold gentle pressure over suture lines if patient does cough or vomit.
- Muscle relaxation is important to avoid bucking during any "scope" procedure.
- Muscle relaxation is imperative if laser surgery of the airway is done, to prevent patient movement or movement of the larynx (so the glottis does not move and stays open).
- Muscle relaxation may or may not be given based on the surgeon's preference and the need for intraoperative nerve monitoring.
- Warmed, humidified gases may be used perioperatively to prevent drying of secretions and mucous plugs.

- These patients may require a different setup from a nasal cannula or face mask postoperatively to avoid placing pressure on tissues of the neck and lower face.
- Surgical manipulation around carotid baroreceptors may cause bradycardia. Notify the surgeon, as he or she may want to infiltrate the area with lidocaine. Atropine IV may be needed.
- Steroids can be given to decrease airway swelling (if there are no contraindications) and as an antiemetic adjunct.
- An antisialagogue (scopolamine, robinul) or antihistamines (trimethobenzamide [Tigan]; diphenhydramine [Benadryl]) can be given to decrease oral secretions.
- Position the patient so that his or her shoulders are at the break of the table, so that the head can be flexed or extended for surgical access.

POSTOPERATIVE NAUSEA AND VOMITING

The following characteristics are associated with increased risk of PONV following neck and laryngologic surgery:

- Female
- Motion sickness history
- Pediatrics (6–10 years of age): 34% PONV occurrence
- Pediatrics (11–14 years of age): 35–50% PONV occurrence
- Nonsmoker
- Anxiety
- Surgery length greater than 45–60 minutes
- *Surgery type: ENT*

TRACHEOSTOMY CONSIDERATIONS

A Passy-Muir valve allows a tracheostomy cannula opening to be closed off so that air can travel upward through the glottis normally, enabling the patient to vocalize. If this valve is on the trachea, the trachea cuff must be deflated or the patient will be unable to breathe. With the cuff inflated,

air cannot travel upward, past the closed-off tracheostomy hole, through the glottis; instead, it becomes trapped in the lung. The valve must be removed prior to anesthesia.

The patient with a tracheostomy who is to receive general anesthesia should have the tracheostomy cuff inflated during surgery.

A patient with a laryngectomy stoma (without an internal cannula) can have oxygen supplementation with a pediatric anesthesia face mask placed over the stoma in their neck. Even a volatile inhaled induction can be given this way. The face mask will prevent gases from leaking out, and as soon as the patient is asleep without lash reflexes, a reinforced endotracheal tube can be placed into the trachea, the balloon inflated, and ventilation initiated.

NECK AND LARYNGOLOGIC SURGERY

Laryngoscopy

Laryngoscopy is an endoscopic examination of the pharynx, hypopharynx, and larynx. It is done to diagnose problems with these structures, biopsy a lesion, remove a foreign body, or treat laryngeal lesions.

Operative Procedure

A soft-plastic dental protector is placed on the upper teeth to prevent damage; use of a microscope facilitates visualization. The patient's head is tilted back and the laryngoscope is inserted by the surgeon. Mirrors can be used to visualize inaccessible areas; stainless steel mirrors are used to reflect a laser beam. Suction is used to clear smoke from tissue evaporation.

Laryngoscopy is often combined with other "scope" procedures.

Anesthetic

General anesthesia is given; a small-diameter oral endotracheal tube (OETT) is inserted; there must be enough room in the trachea to accommodate both the laryngoscope and the ETT. Muscle relaxation is given if a laser is used.

Jet ventilation can be given during a laryngoscopy with a Hunsaker tube or tracheal cannula. The Hunsaker tube allows airway control and appropriate visualization of laryngeal anatomy; it is laser safe, provides subglottic jet ventilation, and allows for the continuous monitoring of end-expiratory and peak airway pressures, as well as periodic sampling of ETCO$_2$ levels.

Topical anesthesia may be used in an awake patient. In such a case, the patient sits up for administration of the local anesthetic and is then placed supine for the procedure.

Positioning

The patient is positioned supine, with a shoulder roll to extend the head. The head of the bed is moved at least 90 degrees, if not 180 degrees, away from the anesthetist.

Anesthetic Implications

These patients may present with "difficult airways," so a thorough preoperative airway assessment must be done. Have emergency airway equipment available.

Airway fire is a risk if cauterization is used. Decrease FiO$_2$ to 30%, have good communication with the surgeon, and be aware of safety concerns (see Chapter 1).

These patients require special eye care. Paper tape is used to close the eyes to prevent corneal drying or abrasions; eye pads are then placed over both eyes to protect them. Eye ointment can be instilled before taping for patients who will remain intubated postoperatively. Goggles should be worn by both patient and caregivers when a laser is used.

Special face masks should be donned if a laser is used to vaporize a lesion, to prevent breathing in airborne contaminants.

IV *steroids* can be given to help decrease swelling unless otherwise contraindicated.

Antisialagogues can be given to decrease secretions.

At the end of the case, suction the back of the throat with a soft suction catheter to prevent further irritation to the tissues.

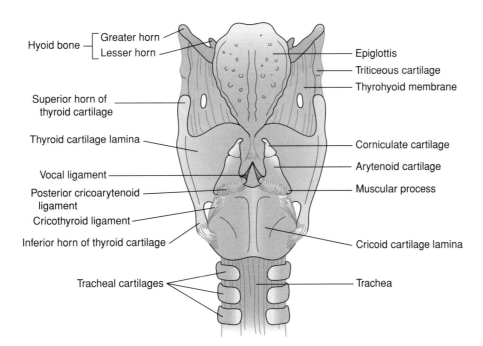

Figure 12-1   *Larynx*

Source: Adapted from Anson, B. J., & McVay, C. B. (1971). Surgical Anatomy. *Philadelphia: W. B. Saunders.*

Laryngectomy: Supraglottic, Hemilaryngectomy (Partial), and Total

Laryngectomy involves partial or complete removal of the larynx. The procedure may be done in combination with a radical neck dissection. It is primarily performed to treat malignancy of the laryngeal muscles or cartilage, usually involving squamous cell carcinoma. It may also be done to remedy intractable aspiration of food or fluid into the lungs.

Operative Procedure

One type of incision is made above the suprasternal notch, consisting of a vertical incision from the hyoid bone to the clavicle. Another type of incision is a "U-shaped" incision, where the lowest part is several finger-breadths above the suprasternal notch. Either incision exposes the hyoid bone to the clavicle.

Supraglottic Laryngectomy

Surgical exposure is from the hyoid bone to the clavicle. This procedure involves removal of larynx from the false cords (which sit just above the true vocal cords) and the epiglottis, to the base of the tongue; it leaves the true vocal cords intact. A temporary tracheostomy is required until swelling resolves.

Hemilaryngectomy (Partial)

Surgical exposure is from the hyoid bone to the clavicle. This procedure involves removal of a unilateral true and false vocal cord. The larynx is usually transected just above the hyoid bone. A temporary tracheostomy is required until swelling resolves.

Total Laryngectomy

If the tracheostomy is done at the beginning of the procedure or is already present, an anode ETT is placed into the tracheostomy hole and the patient is ventilated. The reinforced anode ETT is sutured to the skin to prevent it from becoming dislodged during surgery. Some surgeons require the patient be intubated normally and a tracheostomy is not formed until the end of the procedure.

If the patient has a tracheostomy, surgical exposure is from the hyoid bone to the clavicle. This approach is used when both cords, transglottic lesions, or laryngeal cartilage are involved. It may also necessitate removal of the posterior third of the tongue or the vallecula. The thyroid gland is resected away from the trachea unless it is to be removed with the larynx. The larynx is transected between the hyoid bone and the trachea; the trachea is brought out to skin and sutured into a permanent tracheal stoma. A tracheostomy tube is required until the tracheal stoma heals.

If the patient has been intubated through the mouth, the strap muscles and the isthmus of the thyroid gland are divided. At the surgeon's direction, the endotracheal tube is pulled back to prevent the ETT cuff from being punctured as the trachea is incised and entered between tracheal rings 2 and 3. After entering the trachea safely, the surgeon will ask for the ETT to be advanced into the distal trachea to maintain oxygenation while the surgery continues. Confirmation of adequate oxygenation is confirmed with $ETCO_2$ levels, chest movement, and pulse oximetry.

The superior cornu of the thyroid cartilage and hyoid bone are freed from the strap and supraglottic muscles. A portion of the thyroid may also need to be excised. The posterior aspect of the cricoid cartilage is entered, and dissection continues to the base of the tongue. With traction on the epiglottis and the severed end of the trachea, dissection is completed. The pharynx is closed. A tracheostomy is performed to ensure airway continuity; the tracheostomy stoma is matured to the surrounding skin and a tracheostomy tube is placed. The wound flaps are approximated over a drain. A moderate-pressure dressing is placed.

This procedure may be done in combination with neck dissection and pharyngectomy with flap reconstruction.

Anesthetic

General anesthesia is given with insertion of an OETT; muscle relaxants are usually essential. Check with the surgeon before giving any muscle relaxants; he or she may not want these agents to be given if nerve stimulation will be monitored.

Positioning

The patient is positioned supine, with a shoulder roll to slightly extend head. Arms are tucked at the sides, and a slight reverse Trendelenburg position is used. The head of the bed may be moved at least 90 degrees, if not 180 degrees, away from the anesthetist.

Anesthetic Implications

Type and cross-match the patient's blood before surgery starts. While drastic blood loss is not common with laryngectomy, these patients may already be anemic and the potential blood loss may be close to 1000 mL.

These patients may have already received radiation, laser surgery, and chemotherapy as treatment for advanced lesions. They may have affected tracheal anatomy, making intubation difficult. Diligent preoperative assessment of the airway is imperative; have emergency airway equipment available.

These patients are often smokers and also may have a history of alcohol abuse. Chronic obstructive pulmonary disease, chronic bronchitis, and impaired respiratory function are typical findings. Preoperative baseline arterial blood gases, pulmonary function tests, and oxygen saturation levels will be helpful in preparing for laryngectomy. With possible liver dysfunction, it is also important to have preoperative hematocrit, PT/INR/PTT, hepatic function tests, glucose, and BUN and creatinine levels.

Antisialagogues may be given to decrease secretions.

These patients require special eye care. Paper tape is used to close the eyes to prevent corneal drying or abrasions; eye pads are then placed over both eyes to protect them. Eye ointment can be instilled before taping for patients who will remain intubated postoperatively.

Ask the surgeon about placing an esophageal stethoscope with the orogastric tube placed during surgery. Some surgeons like having something in the esophagus so they can feel where the esophagus is; others do not want the esophageal distortion.

Airway fire is a risk if cauterization ("Bovie") is used. To prevent airway fires, use caution when providing oxygen during this procedure. Good communication with the surgeon is essential, especially as the trachea is to be entered and bleeding is to be cauterized. Decrease FiO_2 to 30% before cauterization is to start. See Chapter 1 on safety concerns for more information.

Because the tissues of the trachea and neck are quite vascular, maintaining a slight decrease in mean arterial blood pressure (60–70 mm Hg) can help to minimize bleeding.

IV *steroids* can be given to help decrease swelling unless otherwise contraindicated.

Have a tracheostomy flex tube extension available to facilitate connecting the ventilator circuit tubing to the tracheostomy tube.

A cuffed tracheostomy tube is inserted into the tracheal stoma during surgery and left there until the edema subsides. For a total laryngectomy, it is then replaced with a laryngectomy tube.

Smooth emergence from anesthesia is important with this surgery. The goal is to avoid coughing, bucking, or nausea/vomiting or retching so as to prevent increased risk of bleeding, hematoma formation, or suture line disruption from the increased head and neck pressures. Have a team member hold gentle pressure over the suture lines if patient does cough or vomit.

At the end of the case, suction the back of the throat to clear any secretions.

Note the tracheostomy manufacturer and size, and report this information during hand-off of the patient to another unit. The obturator for the tracheostomy tube must accompany the patient out of the operating room; it will be needed to replace the tracheostomy if it becomes dislodged. This device may be taped to the head of the bed or the front of the chart in case of tracheostomy dislodgement.

A tracheostomy oxygen collar is needed during transport of the patient to the recovery room or ICU; healthcare providers there will add humidified oxygen.

Monitors and IV Access

An arterial line may be needed. Two large-bore peripheral IVs should be placed.

IV Fluids and Volume Requirements

Patients may be given normal saline or lactated Ringer's solution as IVF. Keep the patient in a normovolemia to slightly dry state.

Complications

Potential complications include hemorrhage, subcutaneous air in tissues and pleural spaces, and pneumothorax.

Modified Neck Dissection

In modified neck dissection, the surgeon excises cervical lymph-node-bearing tissue in the anterior and posterior neck. This procedure is used to treat malignancy of the head and neck region.

Operative Procedure

One or two horizontal neck incisions are made for complete cervical lymph node removal. Although not often done anymore, a vertical incision can be made in the lateral neck from the mandible to the clavicle. The sternocleidomastoid, internal jugular vein, and select cranial nerves may or may not be removed. A tracheostomy may be necessary due to throat and face swelling. Suction drains are inserted and flaps closed. A moderate-pressure dressing is applied.

A neck dissection is usually done in combination with other surgeries. Modified neck dissection is not as extensive as a radical neck dissection.

Anesthetic

Cervical deep or superficial blocks are applied for postoperative pain control. General endotracheal anesthesia (GETA) and possibly muscle relaxants are used during the procedure. The surgeon will occasionally want to monitor nerve stimulation, so check with the surgeon before giving any nondepolarizing muscle relaxants.

Positioning

Place the patient supine, with the head turned away from the surgical site, in a slight reverse Trendelenburg position. The head of the bed may be moved at least 90 degrees, if not 180 degrees, away from the anesthetist.

Anesthetic Implications

These patients may have affected tracheal anatomy with limited head and neck mobility, making intubation difficult. Diligent preoperative assessment of the airway is imperative; have emergency airway equipment available. Some cases may require awake fiberoptic intubation.

Patients may have already received radiation treatment and, therefore, have friable tissues. Special caution must be used during intubation and throat suctioning.

Neck dissection has the potential for a large blood loss owing to the risk to the jugular vein or carotid artery. For this reason, all patients' blood should be typed and cross-matched, and 2 units of packed cells made available in the OR.

These patients require special eye care. Paper tape is used to close the eyes to prevent corneal drying or abrasions; eye pads are then placed over both eyes to protect them. Eye ointment can be instilled before taping for patients who will remain intubated postoperatively.

A nasogastric tube should be placed during surgery.

Because the tissues of the trachea and neck are quite vascular, maintaining a slight decrease in mean arterial blood pressure (60–70 mm Hg) can help to minimize bleeding.

IV *steroids* can be given to help decrease swelling and as an adjunct with antiemetics unless otherwise contraindicated.

Smooth emergence from anesthesia is important with this surgery. The goal is to avoid coughing, bucking, or nausea/vomiting or retching so as to prevent increased risk of bleeding, hematoma formation, or suture line disruption from the increased head and neck pressures. Have a team member hold gentle pressure over the suture lines if the patient does cough or vomit.

At the end of the case, suction the back of the throat with a soft suction catheter to prevent further irritation to the tissues.

Monitors and IV Access

An arterial line may be needed if the patient has a cardiovascular history—which most of these patients have. Two large-bore peripheral IVs should be placed.

IV Fluids and Volume Requirements

Patients may be given normal saline or lactated Ringer's solution as IVF. Keep the patient in a normovolemia to slightly dry state.

Complications

Potential complications include accidental entry into the trachea, carotid artery, jugular vein, or pleura, which can become disastrous. Damage to nerves is also possible, including the brachial plexus, facial nerve, phrenic or vagus nerve, cranial nerve XI (accessory), XII (hypoglossal), and lingual nerve.

Radical Neck Dissection

Radical neck dissection involves complete excision of cervical lymph-node-bearing tissue and adjacent muscular, nerve, and vascular structures if a local tumor extends into surrounding tissue—including the sternocleidomastoid (SCM) muscle, internal jugular veins, and cranial nerve XI (accessory). This procedure is performed in cases of malignancy of the head and neck region. It may be done alone or in conjunction with primary tumor resection of any cancer sites (e.g., larynx, pharynx, tongue, parotid gland) whose lymphatics drain into the cervical lymph nodes. A temporal bone resection may be done if the tumor extends into the ear canal or middle ear.

Operative Procedure

An incision is made in the lateral neck, usually from beneath the jaw to the supraclavicular region; the submental region is exposed and skin flaps are mobilized. The external jugular vein is severed; the deep cervical fascial and the sternoclavicular origins of the SCM muscle are divided. Fatty tissues bearing lymph nodes are dissected; the insertion of the SCM is divided, as is the lower pole of the parotid gland. The facial artery and vein, the submandibular gland, and the proximal end of the internal jugular vein are all divided from under the jaw. The tissue bloc is then excised. Suction drains are inserted and the flaps are closed. A moderate-pressure dressing is applied.

A tracheostomy may be performed with this resection. Radical neck dissection also may be done in conjunction with a laryngectomy.

For a more involved dissection, the outer cortex of the mandible may be exposed and cut. The lower lip may be transected if this procedure is combined with a cheek flap to expose the oral cavity.

Anesthetic

General anesthesia is given with insertion of an OETT; muscle relaxants may be given if a nerve stimulator is not used. Check with the surgeon before giving muscle relaxants. Deep or superficial cervical blocks may be applied for postoperative pain control.

The type of induction may need to be altered depending on the patient's condition.

Secure the OETT to the opposite side of the mouth from the surgical side.

Positioning

The patient is positioned supine, with the arms tucked at the sides. A shoulder roll may be placed to slightly extend the head. The patient's head will be turned away from the operative side. The table is usually turned at least 90 degrees, if not 180 degrees, away from the anesthetist. A slight reverse Trendelenburg position to 30 degrees is often done.

Anesthetic Implications

Because normal airway anatomy may be altered in these patients, a diligent preoperative assessment of the airway is imperative. These patients may have affected tracheal anatomy with limited head and neck mobility, making intubation difficult. Some cases may require an awake fiberoptic intubation. Emergency airway equipment should be immediately available.

Radical neck dissection has the potential for large blood loss owing to the risk to the jugular vein or carotid artery. For this reason, all patients' blood should be typed and cross-matched, and 2 units of packed cells should be made available in the OR.

Injury to the facial nerve (CN VII) is a potential complication. Preoperative and postoperative assessment and documentation of having the patient move his or her face, pout, purse the lips, close the eyes, and wrinkle the nose can assess for damage to CN VII.

These patients require special eye care. Paper tape is used to close the eyes to prevent corneal drying or abrasions; eye pads are then placed over both eyes to protect them. Eye ointment can be instilled before taping for patients who will remain intubated postoperatively.

A nasogastric tube should be placed during surgery.

Special care is needed with a right radical neck dissection, as sympathetic outflow through the right stellate ganglion can be interrupted. This interruption can cause EKG changes, ranging from a prolonged QT interval to cardiac arrest. This complication occurs only with surgery on the right side.

There is a risk of venous air embolism with this procedure. See Chapter 3 for more information.

The surgeon makes every effort to preserve the function of the thoracic duct but must sacrifice both cranial nerve XI (accessory: motor to trapezius and SCM), and cranial nerve XII (hypoglossal: motor to tongue) in a radical neck dissection.

Surgical manipulation around the carotid artery can cause hypotension and cardiac dysrhythmias, especially bradycardia. Monitor and notify the surgeon if this cardiac complication occurs. Local anesthetic infiltration in this area may be needed.

Because the tissues of the trachea and neck are quite vascular, maintaining a slight decrease in mean arterial blood pressure (60–70 mm Hg) can help to minimize bleeding.

IV *steroids* can be given to help decrease swelling unless otherwise contraindicated.

At the end of the case, suction the back of the throat with a soft suction catheter to prevent further irritation to the tissues.

Smooth emergence from anesthesia is important with this surgery. The goal is to avoid coughing, bucking, or nausea/vomiting or retching so as to prevent increased risk of bleeding, hematoma formation, or suture line disruption from the increased head and neck pressures. Have a team member hold gentle pressure over the suture lines if the patient does cough or vomit.

Monitors

An arterial line may be necessary; it is especially helpful for securing samples for serial ABGs and labs.

A central venous line may be necessary but is placed in the arm (brachial) or groin (femoral) vein, or opposite neck.

IV Fluids and Volume Requirements

Maintain patients at normovolemia to a slightly dry state.

Complications

Potential complications include accidental entry into the trachea, carotid artery, or pleura (pneumothorax), which can become disastrous. Injury to the brachial plexus, phrenic, and vagus nerves must be avoided. Diaphragmatic paralysis can develop if the phrenic nerve is injured, affecting the patient's ability to breathe effectively postoperatively. The surgeon must maintain good control of the resected ends of the jugular vein; if control is lost, major blood loss is possible.

Panendoscopy

Panendoscopy may include examination of the pharynx, larynx, hypopharynx, trachea and right and left main bronchus, and digestive tract. It includes a rigid bronchoscopy, pharyngoscopy, laryngoscopy, and rigid/flexible esophagoscopy.

Operative Procedure

If multiple procedures are done at once, a rigid bronchoscopy is performed before intubating the patient. After intubation (a small-caliber OETT should be inserted and secured on the left side of the mouth [if the surgeon is right-handed) and taped to the lower lip), a pharyngoscopy and laryngoscopy are done and/or then a rigid esophagoscopy is performed.

Anesthetic Implications

These patients require special eye care. Paper tape is used to close the eyes to prevent corneal drying or abrasions; eye pads are then placed over both eyes to protect them. Eye ointment can be instilled before taping for patients who will remain intubated postoperatively.

IV *steroids* can be given to help decrease swelling unless otherwise contraindicated.

At the end of the case, suction the back of the throat with a soft suction catheter to prevent further irritation to the tissues.

Parotidectomy: Superficial, Total, and Radical

Parotidectomy involves excision of the parotid gland, the largest salivary gland. This salivary gland is located just in front of and below the ear.

This procedure is performed in case of benign (inflammatory) disease or malignant tumors, chronic infection, or obstruction of the salivary outflow tract causing chronic engorgement of the parotid gland. A radical neck dissection may be needed if a malignant tumor is found.

Operative Procedure

- *Superficial:* removes the entire parotid gland lateral to the facial nerve to protect the nerve.
- *Total:* removes a tumor or infections of the parotid gland medial to facial nerve to protect the nerve.
- *Radical:* resection of the parotid gland and the facial nerve. A nerve graft may be done using the great auricular nerve or the superficial branches of the cervical plexus (microsurgical technique). A radical dissection is done for malignant disease of the parotid gland.

An incision is started around the front of the ear and continues down the side of the jaw and then anteriorly toward the hyoid bone (periauricular incision). The fascia is incised, with careful identification and exposure of the facial nerve (a nerve stimulator may be needed). For benign disease, the superficial portion of the parotid gland is resected; resection of the deeper portions may be necessary for malignant disease. A drain is usually inserted and the wound closed.

Anesthetic

General anesthesia is given and insertion of an OETT is usual; securely tape the endotracheal tube to the opposite side of the mouth from the surgical side. Check with the surgeon whether facial nerve monitoring is to be performed during the surgery and if muscle relaxants are to be given.

Nasal intubation may be warranted for total or radical surgery to allow the mandible to be moved forward for better exposure to the deep lobe of the parotid gland.

Positioning

The patient is placed supine, with the affected side of the face in the uppermost position, in a slight reverse Trendelenburg position. The head of the bed may be moved at least 90 degrees, if not 180 degrees, away from the anesthetist.

Anesthetic Implications

These patients may have affected tracheal anatomy, making intubation difficult. Diligent preoperative assessment of the airway is imperative; have emergency airway equipment available.

All five branches of the facial nerve run directly through the parotid gland, dividing the superficial portion from the deeper portion of the gland. Every effort should be made to salvage this cranial nerve. Preoperative and postoperative assessment and documentation of having the patient move his or her face, pout, purse the lips, close the eyes, and wrinkle the nose can assess for damage.

These patients require special eye care. Paper tape is used to close the eyes to prevent corneal drying or abrasions; eye pads are then placed over both eyes to protect them. Eye ointment can be instilled before taping for patients who will remain intubated postoperatively.

A frozen section may be collected to determine malignancy. A locally invasive malignancy may require resection of the facial nerve, mandible, or skull base.

Because the tissues of the trachea and neck are quite vascular, maintaining a slightly decreased mean arterial blood pressure (60–70 mm Hg) can help to minimize bleeding.

IV *steroids* can be given to help decrease swelling unless otherwise contraindicated.

Smooth emergence from anesthesia is important with this surgery. The goal is to avoid coughing, bucking, or nausea/vomiting or retching so as to prevent increased risk of bleeding, hematoma formation, or suture line disruption from the increased head and neck pressures. Have a team member hold gentle pressure over the suture lines if the patient does cough or vomit.

At the end of the case, suction the back of the throat with a soft suction catheter to prevent further irritation to the tissues.

Submandibular Gland Excision

Excision of the submandibular (submaxillary) gland is usually done for benign disease such as chronic inflammation, a submaxillary salivary stone blockage, or salivary duct stricture. A malignant tumor is less often encountered.

Operative Procedure

A transverse incision is made over the gland parallel to the mandible, usually in a naturally occurring fold in the neck. The anterior facial vein is divided and the fascial envelope about the gland is incised. The gland is dissected free from the surrounding tissues and removed, the facial artery is ligated, and the Wharton's duct is ligated and divided. A drain is inserted and the wound closed and dressed.

Anesthetic

General anesthesia is given with insertion of an OETT; secure the OETT to the opposite side of the mouth from the surgical side. Muscle relaxants may be needed. Check with the surgeon before giving any nondepolarizing muscle relaxants; the surgeon may not want these agents used if facial nerve stimulation monitoring is necessary. An LMA is not used, as it may distort throat tissue.

Positioning

The patient is placed supine, with the head turned with the affected side up, in a slight reverse Trendelenburg position. A shoulder roll is placed to extend the head slightly. The head of the bed may be moved at least 90 degrees, if not 180 degrees, away from the anesthetist.

Anesthetic Implications

These patients may have affected tracheal anatomy, making intubation difficult. Diligent preoperative assessment of the airway is imperative; have emergency airway equipment available.

These patients require special eye care. Paper tape is used to close the eyes to prevent corneal drying or abrasions; eye pads are then placed over both eyes to protect them.

IV *steroids* can be given to help decrease swelling unless otherwise contraindicated.

As the surgery progresses, deeper layers of tissue and muscle are accessed; this is very stimulating. Anesthesia should be deepened during this time.

Nerve damage to the facial nerve (mandibular branch), the lingual nerve (carries fibers from the facial nerve and return taste from anterior two-thirds of the tongue), and hypoglossal nerve is possible. Preoperative and postoperative assessment and documentation of having the patient move his or her face, pout, purse the lips, close the eyes, wrinkle the nose, and demonstrate tongue movement and taste can assess for damage.

Because the tissues of the trachea and neck are quite vascular, maintaining a slightly decreased mean arterial blood pressure (60–70 mm Hg) can help to minimize bleeding.

A frozen section may be taken to determine malignancy. If malignancy is found, a radical neck dissection may be done. The surgical consent form should list all possible surgeries.

Smooth emergence from anesthesia is important with this surgery. The goal is to avoid coughing, bucking, or nausea/vomiting or retching so as to prevent increased risk of bleeding, hematoma formation, or suture line disruption from the increased head and neck pressures.

At the end of the case, suction the back of the throat with a soft suction catheter to prevent further irritation to the tissues.

Thyroglossal Duct Cyst Resection

Thyroglossal duct cyst resection involves excision of a cyst and duct in the midline of the neck, including a portion of the hyoid bone, to correct a congenital defect. The hyoid bone extends from the base of the tongue to the thyroid gland, connected by a tract called the thyroglossal duct. An embryologic remnant, it usually disappears once the thyroid reaches its final position in the neck. Sometimes, however, the duct can leave cavities called cysts along the tract; these cysts can fill with fluid or mucus and can become infected. Very enlarged cysts can causes difficulty swallowing or obstruct breathing passages. Occasionally a cyst will form a tract to the skin, allowing drainage of fluid or mucus externally.

Operative Procedure

An incision is made between the hyoid bone and the thyroid cartilage. Sharp and blunt dissection is used to excise the along with the mid-portion of the hyoid bone; the latter material is removed to prevent recurrence.

Anesthetic

General anesthesia is given with insertion of an OETT; muscle relaxants may also be given. Check with the surgeon before giving any nondepolarizing muscle relaxants, as the surgeon may not want these agents used if nerve stimulation monitoring will occur. Secure the OETT to the opposite side of the mouth from the surgical side.

Positioning

The patient is placed supine, with a shoulder roll to extend the neck, in a slight reverse Trendelenburg position. The head of the bed may be moved at least 90 degrees, if not 180 degrees, away from the anesthetist.

Anesthetic Implications

These patients may have affected tracheal anatomy, making intubation difficult. Diligent preoperative assessment of the airway is imperative; have emergency airway equipment available.

These patients require special eye care. Paper tape is used to close the eyes to prevent corneal drying or abrasions; eye pads are then placed over both eyes to protect them. Eye ointment can be instilled before taping for patients who will remain intubated postoperatively.

IV *steroids* can be given to help decrease swelling unless otherwise contraindicated.

Injection of a methylene blue solution directly into the tract may be needed to identify the thyroglossal duct.

Because the tissues of the trachea and neck are quite vascular, maintaining a slight decrease in mean arterial blood pressure (60–70 mm Hg) can help to minimize bleeding.

Smooth emergence from anesthesia is important with this surgery. The goal is to avoid coughing, bucking, or nausea/vomiting or retching so as to prevent increased risk of bleeding, hematoma formation, or suture line disruption from the increased head and neck pressures.

At the end of the case, suction the back of the throat with a soft suction catheter to prevent further irritation to the tissues.

Tracheostomy

In tracheostomy, an opening is made into the trachea with the insertion of a cannula to facilitate breathing. This procedure may be done emergently or electively to maintain an airway, for prolonged ventilatory support with respiratory insufficiency, or in combination with another procedure.

Operative Procedure

A transverse or longitudinal incision is made over the first and second tracheal rings, approximately 2 fingerbreadths above the suprasternal notch. The strap muscles are divided in the midline, the thyroid isthmus is divided, and the tracheal rings are exposed. An incision is made into the trachea, and an inferiorly based tracheal flap is fashioned, usually at the second or third ring. Stay-sutures may be used to mark the stoma and for retraction. The tracheostomy tube is placed. The ventilator tubing is then attached to the tracheostomy tube. Once $ETCO_2$ is confirmed and the patient's oxygen saturation is acceptable, the surgeon will direct complete removal of the endotracheal tube. The outer flange of the tracheostomy tube is held in place with sutures and umbilical tapes tied around the patient's neck. A split gauze dressing is applied around the bottom part of the tracheostomy cannula and around the wound.

- For *elective tracheostomy* where the patient is not intubated, local anesthetic is injected into the skin and neck tissue over the site and the tracheostomy is done.
- For *emergency tracheostomy*, a "slash and trach" approach is used.

Anesthetic

General anesthesia is given and an OETT with a cuff (to prevent oxygen and volatile agents from leaking out) is inserted. Selection of a reinforced endotracheal tube can help to prevent compression of the ETT during surgical manipulation of the surrounding structures. Have several sizes of reinforced tubes available.

A local anesthetic and epinephrine solution may be infiltrated to decrease swelling to prevent bleeding. Watch for an increase in heart rate or blood pressure or EKG changes.

Muscle relaxants used to prevent coughing and bucking with tracheal manipulation.

Positioning

The patient is positioned supine, with a shoulder roll to extend the head slightly. Bilateral arms are padded and tucked at the patient's side. A slight reverse Trendelenburg position of 20–30 degrees is used. The head of the bed may be moved at least 90 degrees, if not 180 degrees, away from the anesthetist.

Anesthetic Implications

For *elective tracheostomy when the patient is not already intubated,* diligent preoperative assessment of the airway is imperative. Have emergency airway equipment available, as these patients may have affected tracheal anatomy, making intubation difficult.

For *elective tracheostomy with the patient already intubated,* before the patient is draped, make sure the pilot balloon is up toward the forehead and can be reached by the anesthetist, that the orogastric or nasogastric tube is separate and securely taped away from the ETT, and that the tape securing the ETT is away from the back of the neck and the sides of the head. Maintain the tape around the ETT and on the skin for several inches to avoid the ETT becoming dislodged before the tracheostomy is formed. Once the sterile drapes are place, make sure you can reach all necessary parts of the ETT and pilot balloon for later withdrawal.

As the surgeon is placing the tracheostomy, he or she will direct us to slowly withdraw the ETT, stopping when the distal end of the ETT is just above the tracheostomy site. Hand-ventilation may be needed during this time; it may also be necessary to turn off the inhaled agent to prevent it from blowing out into the surgeon's face. When the surgeon has the tracheostomy with the inner cannula placed in the trachea, he or she will indicate when to disconnect the circuit tubing from the ETT. Have an extension ("flex-extender"—corrugated tubing that is attached proximally to the distal right-angled elbow of the circuit tubing and distally to the tracheostomy) tubing ready to attach; hand this tubing to the surgeon from underneath the drape. Once the circuit is attached to the tracheostomy, attempt to hand-ventilate the patient. Look for the $ETCO_2$ waveform, and monitor oxygen saturations. Occasionally the surgeon will have difficulties with the tracheostomy and will need for the ETT to be reinserted. Do not withdraw the ETT completely out of the mouth until directed to do so. The drapes are usually then taken down, and the tracheostomy is sutured into place to secure it.

Airway fire is a risk if cauterization ("Bovie") is used. This procedure requires clear communication between the anesthesia provider and the surgeon, especially after the trachea has been entered by the surgeon. To prevent airway fires, use caution when administering oxygen during this procedure. Decreasing the FiO_2 levels to 30% while the surgeon is entering the airway is necessary to help prevent an airway fire. If the patient's oxygen saturation drops during this period, let the surgeon know. It may be necessary to interrupt the surgery and increase the FiO_2 to get the oxygen saturation up before decreasing the FiO_2 again to restart the surgery.

Patients presenting for tracheostomy may be quite debilitated with pulmonary and cardiac diseases. They may also have already undergone chemotherapy or radiation therapy and have friable tissues that bleed easily.

These patients require special eye care. Paper tape is used to close the eyes to prevent corneal drying or abrasions; eye pads are then placed over both eyes to protect them. Eye ointment can be instilled before taping for patients who will remain intubated postoperatively.

A nasogastric tube should be placed during surgery.

Because the tissues of the trachea and neck are quite vascular, maintaining a slightly decreased mean arterial blood pressure (60–70 mm Hg) can help to minimize bleeding.

IV *steroids* can be given to help decrease swelling unless otherwise contraindicated.

At the end of the case, suction the back of the throat to clear away secretions.

Smooth emergence from anesthesia is important with this surgery. The goal is to avoid coughing, bucking, or nausea/vomiting or retching so as to prevent increased risk of bleeding, hematoma formation, or suture line disruption from the increased head and neck pressures.

Note the tracheostomy manufacturer and size, and report this information during hand-off of the patient to another unit. The obturator for the tracheostomy tube must accompany the patient out of the operating room; it will be needed to replace the tracheostomy if it becomes dislodged. This device may be taped to the head of the bed or the front of the chart in case of tracheostomy dislodgement.

A humidified tracheostomy collar is applied at the end of the case.

If a patient has a tracheostomy (not a total laryngectomy), the patient can be reintubated through the mouth with a laryngoscope.

Complications

Potential complications of a tracheostomy include pneumothorax, hemorrhage, and aspiration of blood.

13

BREAST SURGERY PEARLS

- Monitor the amount of local anesthetic used and alert the surgeon if nearing the maximum amount allowed.
- A paravertebral block regional anesthetic (multiple-level block) may be used for some breast surgeries. Regional anesthesia is associated with less postoperative nausea and vomiting and less postoperative pain.
- The operating table can be tilted to allow the operative breast to be centered in the surgical field.
- Immediate breast reconstruction may be performed at the time of the mastectomy. A prosthesis, a myocutaneous flap, or a combination of the two may be employed. When the temporary prosthesis is used, a muscular pocket is created into which a tissue expander balloon is inserted (to be incrementally inflated postoperatively) to create the appropriate size of cavity for insertion of a permanent prosthesis.
- Preoperative evaluation of the cardiac and pulmonary systems should be done if the patient has already undergone radiation or chemotherapy treatments.
- If a mastectomy is to follow a breast biopsy, the patient is re-prepped and re-draped; the surgical team is re-gowned and gloved.
- The *BRCA* gene has a known relationship with breast cancer; it is used as a DNA-based genetic test for this disease.

POSTOPERATIVE NAUSEA AND VOMITING

The following characteristics are associated with increased risk of PONV following breast surgery:

- Female
- Motion sickness history
- Pediatrics (6–10 years of age): 34% PONV occurrence
- Pediatrics (11–14 years of age): 35–50% PONV occurrence
- Nonsmoker
- Anxiety

- Surgery length greater than 45–60 minutes
- ***Surgery type: Breast***

BREAST SURGERY

Axillary Node Dissection (Lymphadenectomy)

Lymphadenectomy may be done alone or in conjunction with a mastectomy if the sentinel lymph node is positive for cancer. In this procedure, an incision is made into the axilla. Vessels and lymph channels are ligated; lymph nodes are dissected free from their surrounding tissues and removed. Pathologic exam of the nodes allows for staging of the disease; follow-up treatment is planned based on these results.

See the discussion of sentinel lymph node mapping later in this chapter for more information.

Open Breast Biopsy

Open breast biopsy involves excision of a breast lesion and its margins to determine the nature of a lesion.

Operative Procedure

An incision is usually made over the lesion; the lesion, along with margins of healthy tissue, are dissected free and removed. For centrally located lesions, a circumareolar incision is usually done to prevent more obvious scarring. A frozen section can be performed on the specimen immediately, if indicated. Subcuticular tissue is approximated after hemostasis is achieved. A drain may be inserted; the incision line is closed in layers.

Anesthetic

Sedation with local anesthetic is usual; general endotracheal anesthesia (GETA) and a laryngeal mask airway (LMA) may be needed. A local anesthetic and epinephrine solution may be infiltrated to decrease swelling, to prevent bleeding, and to help with postoperative pain. If epinephrine is used with local anesthetic, monitor the EKG for ST-segment changes and heart rate.

Positioning

The patient is positioned supine, with the arm on the affected side extended on a padded armboard and the shoulder at an angle less than 90 degrees. The operative side of the upper body should be at the edge of the table. A folded pad may be placed under the operative area to facilitate surgical exposure.

Anesthetic Implications

The blood pressure cuff and the peripheral IV should both be placed on the nonoperative-side arm.

Smooth emergence from anesthesia is important with this surgery. The goal is to avoid coughing, bucking, or nausea/vomiting or retching so as to prevent increased risk of bleeding, hematoma formation, or suture line disruption from the increased chest pressures. Have a team member hold gentle pressure over the suture lines if the patient does cough or vomit.

The risk of postoperative nausea and vomiting is increased in any breast surgery, so antiemetics should be given.

If a mastectomy is to follow a breast biopsy, the patient is re-prepped and re-draped; the surgical team also changes gowns and gloves. The surgical consent form should include all procedures, both planned and possible.

Breast Biopsy with Needle (Wire) Localization

The patient is taken to the radiology department, where needles are inserted into the breast under imaging techniques to localize the lesion. The wires are left in place and the patient is brought to surgery for the biopsy. The surgeon makes the skin incision as close to these wires as possible. The breast tissue surrounding the wires is removed en bloc and sent to pathology.

Care should be taken to avoid dislodging or hitting these wires. A drinking cup can be placed (and taped) over the wires to avoid touching or moving them.

Lumpectomy (Segmental Resection)

Lumpectomy is a type of partial mastectomy that involves excision of a breast tumor with appropriate tumor-free margins. It is done to excise only one tumor with normal breast tissue margins, where the tumor is between 2.5 and 5 centimeters in size. This procedure may be performed in combination with an axillary node dissection.

Operative Procedure

The incision is usually made over the lesion; the lesion, along with margins of healthy tissue, are dissected free and removed. For centrally located lesions, a circumareolar incision may be done to prevent more obvious scarring. A frozen section can be performed on the specimen immediately, if indicated. Subcuticular tissue is approximated. A drain may be inserted; the incision line is closed in layers after hemostasis is obtained.

Anesthetic

IV sedation and local anesthesia are usual. In some cases, GETA may be necessary due to the extent of the surgery or because of patient preference.

Positioning

The patient is positioned supine, with the arm on the affected side extended on a padded armboard and the shoulder at an angle of less than 90 degrees. The operative side of the upper body should be at the edge of the table. A folded pad may be placed under the operative area to facilitate surgical exposure.

Anesthetic Implications

The blood pressure cuff and the peripheral IV should both be placed on the nonoperative-side arm.

The risk of postoperative nausea and vomiting is increased in any breast surgery, so antiemetics should be given.

If a mastectomy is to follow a lumpectomy, the patient is re-prepped and re-draped; the surgical team also changes gowns and gloves.

Simple Mastectomy

In a simple mastectomy, the entire breast (usually with nipple) is removed. This procedure may be done in a patient with ductal carcinoma in situ that has no lymph node involvement or in a patient with a more involved lesion who is a poor surgical risk.

Operative Procedure

A transverse elliptical incision is usually made over the involved breast. Breast tissue is separated from the pectoral fascia on the chest wall and the subcutaneous tissue at the skin; skin flaps are developed. Hemostasis is achieved during dissection. A drain is inserted and the incised skin edges are brought together with sutures and staples.

Anesthetic

GETA with OETT or LMA are used. Muscle relaxants are usually not required.

Positioning

The patient is positioned supine, with the arm on the affected side extended on a padded armboard and the shoulder at an angle less than 90 degrees. The operative side of the upper body should be at the edge of the table. A folded pad may be placed under the operative area to facilitate surgical exposure.

Anesthetic Implications

The blood pressure cuff and the peripheral IV should both be placed on the nonoperative-side arm.

Smooth emergence from anesthesia is important with this surgery. The goal is to avoid coughing, bucking, or nausea/vomiting or retching so as to prevent increased risk of bleeding, hematoma formation, or suture line disruption from the increased chest pressures. Have a team member hold gentle pressure over the suture lines if the patient does cough or vomit.

The risk of postoperative nausea and vomiting is increased in any breast surgery, so antiemetics should be given.

A bulky pressure dressing and a surgical bra are applied at the end of the case.

The affected arm may be draped into the surgical field.

Immediate breast reconstruction may be performed at the time of the mastectomy. A breast prosthesis, a myocutaneous flap, or a combination of the two may be employed for breast reconstruction. When a prosthesis is used, a muscular pocket is created into which a tissue expander balloon is inserted (to be incrementally inflated postoperatively) to create the appropriate size of cavity for insertion of a permanent prosthesis.

Subcutaneous Mastectomy

Subcutaneous mastectomy removes all tissue of one breast, but leaves the overlying skin and nipple intact. This procedure is appropriate for small, centrally located, noninvasive lesions, including those associated with chronic cystic mastitis, gynecomastia; and patients with a strong family history of breast cancer (prophylactic removal).

Operative Procedure

The incision is usually made in the inframammary fold. If the breast is small, a circumareolar incision may be used. Breast tissue is separated from the pectoral fascia on the chest wall and the subcutaneous tissue at the skin. Hemostasis is achieved with dissection. A drain is inserted and the incision closed.

Anesthetic

GETA with an OETT or LMA are used. Muscle relaxation is not usually required.

Positioning

The patient is positioned supine, with the arm on the affected side extended on a padded armboard and the shoulder at an angle less than 90 degrees. The operative side of the upper body should be at the edge of the table. A folded pad may be placed under the operative area to facilitate surgical exposure.

Anesthetic Implications

The blood pressure cuff and the peripheral IV should both be placed on the nonoperative-side arm.

Smooth emergence from anesthesia is important with this surgery. The goal is to avoid coughing, bucking, or nausea/vomiting or retching so as to prevent increased risk of bleeding, hematoma formation, or suture line disruption from the increased chest pressures. Have a team member hold gentle pressure over the suture lines if the patient does cough or vomit.

The risk of postoperative nausea and vomiting is increased in any breast surgery, so antiemetics should be given.

A light pressure dressing and a surgical bra are applied at the end of the case.

Immediate breast reconstruction may be performed at the time of the mastectomy. A breast prosthesis, a myocutaneous flap, or a combination of the two may be employed for breast reconstruction. When a prosthesis is used, a muscular pocket is created into which a tissue expander balloon is inserted (to be incrementally inflated postoperatively) to create appropriate size of cavity for insertion of a permanent prosthesis.

Modified Radical Mastectomy

Modified radical mastectomy removes the breast, nipple, and all axillary lymph nodes. The muscles and adjacent tissues are not removed with the modified mastectomy. This procedure is used when the patient has a breast mass with cancer spread to the axillary lymph nodes.

Operative Procedure

Usually a transverse elliptical incision is done. Skin flaps are developed; the breast tissue and fascia are dissected free from the underlying pectoral muscle. The underlying pectoral muscles (major and minor) are not removed.

The axillary contents are dissected free from vascular and nervous structures and removed. Hemostasis is achieved. Care is taken to avoid injury to the nerve supply to various muscles. Drainage tube(s) are placed, and the incision line is closed in layers.

Anesthetic

Anesthesia consists of GETA. Check with the surgeon before giving muscle relaxation.

Positioning

The patient is positioned supine, with the arm on the affected side extended on a padded armboard and the shoulder at an angle less than 90 degrees; the operative arm can be suspended over the patient's head with the elbow flexed. The operative side of the upper body should be at the edge of the table. A folded pad may be placed under the operative area to facilitate surgical exposure.

Anesthetic Implications

Preoperative evaluation of the cardiac and pulmonary systems should be done if the patient has already undergone radiation or chemotherapy treatments.

The blood pressure cuff and the peripheral IV should both be placed on the nonoperative-side arm.

Type and cross-match the patient's blood preoperatively, as there is a potential for blood loss with this procedure.

Smooth emergence from anesthesia is important with this surgery. The goal is to avoid coughing, bucking, or nausea/vomiting or retching so as to prevent increased risk of bleeding, hematoma formation, or suture line disruption from the increased chest pressures. Have a team member hold gentle pressure over the suture lines if the patient does cough or vomit.

The risk of postoperative nausea and vomiting is increased in any breast surgery, so antiemetics should be given.

A bulky pressure dressing and a surgical bra are applied at the end of the case.

Radiation treatment to the remaining breast will be done after surgery.

Immediate breast reconstruction may be performed at the time of the mastectomy. A breast prosthesis, a myocutaneous flap, or a combination of the two may be employed for breast reconstruction. When a prosthesis is used, a muscular pocket is created into which a tissue expander balloon is inserted (to be incrementally inflated postoperatively) to create the appropriate size of cavity for insertion of a permanent prosthesis.

Complications

A pneumothorax is a possible complication with deep breast tissue excision.

Radical Mastectomy

Radical mastectomy involves removal of the entire breast, pectoralis muscles, axillary lymph nodes, fat, fascia, and adjacent tissues. It is performed in patients with malignant lesions of the breast.

Operative Procedure

A large oblique or transverse elliptical incision is made, and the entire breast, pectoralis muscles, axillary lymph nodes, fat, fascia, and adjacent tissues are removed. Resection of the ribs and sternum may also be effected. Drains are placed; a skin graft may be required to close the wound.

Anesthetic

General anesthesia is given with insertion of an oral endotracheal tube. Check with the surgeon before giving nondepolarizing muscle relaxants.

Positioning

The patient is positioned supine, with the arm on the affected side on a padded armboard and the shoulder at an angle less than 90 degrees; the operative arm can be suspended over the patient's head with the elbow flexed. A folded pad may be placed under the operative area to facilitate surgical exposure.

Anesthetic Implications

Preoperative evaluation of the cardiac and pulmonary systems should be done if the patient has already undergone radiation or chemotherapy treatments.

The blood pressure cuff and the peripheral IV should both be placed on the nonoperative-side arm.

Type and cross-match the patient's blood pre-operatively, as there is a potential for blood loss with this procedure.

Smooth emergence from anesthesia is important with this surgery. The goal is to avoid coughing, bucking, or nausea/vomiting or retching so as to prevent increased risk of bleeding, hematoma formation, or suture line disruption from the increased chest pressures. Have a team member hold gentle pressure over the suture lines if the patient does cough or vomit.

The risk of postoperative nausea and vomiting is increased in any breast surgery, so antiemetics should be given.

A bulky pressure dressing and a surgical bra are applied at the end of the case.

Immediate breast reconstruction may be performed at the time of the mastectomy. A breast prosthesis, a myocutaneous flap, or a combination of the two may be employed for breast reconstruction. When a prosthesis is used, a muscular pocket is created into which a tissue expander balloon is inserted (to be incrementally inflated postoperatively) to create the appropriate size of cavity for insertion of a permanent prosthesis.

Complications

A pneumothorax is a possible complication with deep breast tissue excision.

Sentinel Lymph Node Biopsy (Lymph Node Mapping)

Sentinel lymph node (SLN) biopsy is a method of determining whether cancer has metastasized beyond the primary breast tumor and into the lymph system (where it can spread to other areas in the body). This procedure allows the surgeon to identify and remove the first nodes that drain the lymphatics from a breast cancer. These lymph nodes are located behind and lateral to the pectoralis minor muscle.

Breast cancer has a marked tendency to metastasize early to the first drainage lymphatic nodes, which usually lie in the axilla. (The SLN may not be the "lowest" lymph node; it is usually located in the axilla, but may be found outside the axilla, such as in the internal mammary chain.) In lymph node mapping, the lymphatic flow carries dye or a radioactive tracer as it drains to the lymph nodes in the armpit and creates a "map" of the nodes, showing which nodes to remove. Sentinel lymph node mapping pinpoints the node that is the most likely to receive the first drainage from the tumor and, therefore, the most likely to contain cancer. If the sentinel node is free from tumor cells, it indicates that the local lymph nodes are negative and a full node dissection is not needed. If the sentinel node is positive for cancer, an axillary node dissection is needed. The mapping procedure is done in conjunction with the SLN biopsy or dissection.

Lymph node mapping allows surgeons to avoid removal of excess nodes in node-negative patients with a positive, small breast cancer. Axillary node status remains the best single predictor of disease outcome in patients with breast cancer and the best guide in selecting the appropriate adjuvant therapy.

Several agents can be used to identify the sentinel node as part of lymph node mapping. Because accuracy in locating the sentinel node is increased by 10% to 15% if both radioactive and dye tracers are used together, this combination is generally employed. The different particulate markers include the following options.

Isosulfan Blue Dye (Lymphazurin 1%)

After injecting the isosulfan blue dye into the tumor (multiple sites) or around the biopsy cavity, the breast is massaged and the axilla is incised 3 to 7 minutes later. The sentinel nodes will be stained; they are identified and excised. After injection of isosulfan dye, allergic reactions can occur, including anaphylactic shock. A transient drop in the pulse oximeter reading occurs, and the patient usually has blue or green urine for approximately 24 hours while the dye is excreted by the kidneys.

Isosulfan is considered to be the most effective dye in lymph node mapping. It is taken up quickly by the lymphatic vessels, with very little diffusion to surrounding tissues.

Technetium

A nuclear isomer, technetium can be injected into the tumor cavity. Technetium has very low radioactivity and, therefore, is safe to handle. It can be injected anywhere from 30 minutes to 24 hours before surgery. A hand-held Geiger probe is used to locate the "hot spot"—the area where the most radioactivity is located. The surgeon uses a sterile marker to mark this area; the area is then prepped and draped for excision.

Methylene Blue Dye 1%

Methylene blue dye 1%, 5 mL, may also be injected intraparenchymally around the tumor mass. The breast is then massaged for 5 minutes. Exposure of the axilla is obtained through an incision; the blue lymphatic channels are identified and carefully followed to a blue-stained sentinel lymph node.

Indigo Carmine

Indigo carmine (also known as India ink) works like methylene blue.

Operative Procedure

A small incision is made over the axilla. The surgeon looks for the node with the blue dye or scans with a special gamma probe to find the node with the highest tracer count—this is the sentinel node (or first filtering lymph node). A biopsy is taken and sent to pathology (frozen section). The surgeon must wait for the pathologist to report on the results before either closing the axilla or removing more lymph nodes. If the sentinel node is cancer free, there is a very high probability that cancer has not spread to any other node. If cancer cells are present in the sentinel node, it is likely that other nodes in the lymph system also contain cancer cells and should be excised.

Anesthetic

General anesthesia is given with insertion of either an OETT or LMA. Muscle relaxants may be contraindicated.

Positioning

The patient is positioned supine, with the operative arm abducted away from the body and laid on armboards or a side table per surgeon requirement. The operative arm can be suspended over the patient's head with the elbow flexed.

Anesthetic Implications

The blood pressure cuff and the peripheral IV should both be placed on the nonoperative-side arm.

The surgeon may want nerve function monitoring, check with the surgeon before giving muscle relaxation.

Be aware of possible allergic reactions, and watch for anaphylactic shock with isosulfan blue injections.

Let the patient know preoperatively that their urine may have a blue or green color for several days postoperatively depending on the dye used.

Along with other preoperative lab tests, liver function tests are performed before sentinel node mapping and dissection.

The surgical consent form should list all possible surgeries that may be done if the sentinel node comes back positive.

Smooth emergence from anesthesia is important with this surgery. The goal is to avoid coughing, bucking, or nausea/vomiting or retching so as to prevent increased risk of bleeding, hematoma formation, or suture line disruption from the increased chest pressures. Have a team member hold gentle pressure over the suture lines if the patient does cough or vomit.

The risk of postoperative nausea and vomiting is increased in any breast surgery, so antiemetics should be given.

SLN biopsy should not be done on patients who have already received chemotherapy, as it can cause tissue changes that alter normal lymph flow.

Complications

Potential complications of SLN biopsy include allergic reaction to the isosulfan dye (if used) and sensory or motor nerve damage.

RECONSTRUCTION OF THE BREAST

"Flaps" created for other parts of the body are also covered in the plastic surgery chapter.

Breast reconstruction may be done either immediately after mastectomy or at a later date.

Breast Reconstruction Using Latissimus Dorsi Myocutaneous Flaps

A latissimus dorsi myocutaneous (LDM) flap may be used to enhance breast symmetry during breast reconstruction. Such breast reconstruction occurs after breast tissue excision, usually due to cancer. A natural-appearing breast offers the patient a sense of wholeness and normalcy and eliminates the need for an external prosthesis.

The LDM flap technique is typically useful if the contralateral breast is small. If the nonoperative breast is significantly larger, a breast implant is usually placed between the latissimus and pectoralis muscles to increase the volume of the reconstructed graft.

The latissimus dorsi muscle is a flat muscle measuring 20 by 40 cm. It extends from the posterior axilla to the midline of the back and down to the posterior portion of the iliac crest.

Operative Procedure

Dissection is carried out under the LDM muscle to separate it from its deep tissues with the patient in the lateral position. The LDM muscle with overlying skin is cut away as a pedicle graft from the back, tunneled through the axilla, and brought to the anterior chest for breast creation; the back wound is then closed. The patient is turned supine, the LDM is brought out through the anterior chest wall, and the graft is rotated and placed on the mastectomy site. A drain is inserted and the incision is closed.

Anesthetic

Anesthesia consists of GETA with muscle relaxation.

Positioning

The patient is placed in the lateral decubitus position for LDM flap harvest, then supine. Reverse Trendelenburg position is also used.

Anesthetic Implications

The blood pressure cuff and the peripheral IV should both be placed on the nonoperative arm or in the lower extremities if either arm cannot be used.

Type and cross-match the patient's blood preoperatively. Moderate blood loss is possible with this surgery, and the patient may require a blood transfusion during the procedure.

Maintain a stable BP (MAP > 70 mm Hg) for continued perfusion of the flap tissue. Avoid the use of vasopressors.

A Doppler may be used to check for flap pulses. Postoperatively, monitor for hematoma formation, flap color, capillary refill, and temperature to assess for vascular constriction/vasospasm.

Keep patients warm and well hydrated to optimize graft perfusion.

IV fluorescin dye may be given to determine the viability of the flap with breast reconstruction. Skin fluorescence correlates with flap survival.

Smooth emergence from anesthesia is important with this surgery. The goal is to avoid coughing, bucking, or nausea/vomiting or retching so as to prevent increased risk of bleeding, hematoma formation, or suture line disruption from the increased chest pressures. Have a team member hold gentle pressure over the suture lines if the patient does cough or vomit.

The risk of postoperative nausea and vomiting is increased in any breast surgery, so antiemetics should be given.

A bulky pressure dressing and a surgical bra are applied at the end of the case.

Breast reconstruction may be performed either at the time of the mastectomy (if the patient has not undergone chemotherapy or radiation) or at a later date.

The surgeon will mark the skin while the patient is in an upright position in the preoperative area.

Complications

There is a higher incidence of flap loss in patients who are obese, smokers, and diabetics, and in those patients who have had prior abdominal surgery

Breast Reconstruction Using Transverse Rectus Abdominis Myocutaneous Flaps: Pedicle or Free TRAM Graft

A transverse rectus abdominus myocutaneous (TRAM) flap is created to replace an area of lost tissue. This procedure is usually done to replace missing breast tissue and to enhance breast symmetry during breast reconstruction after breast tissue excision, usually due for cancer. A natural-appearing breast offers the patient a sense of wholeness and normalcy and eliminates the need for an external prosthesis.

Bilateral breast reconstruction can be done during the same surgery. The patient must have adequate lower abdominal tissue to use this technique.

A TRAM flap is created with an ellipse of abdominal skin, adipose tissue, connective tissue, and the anterior rectus abdominus muscle. Either a pedicle flap or a free flap procedure may be used.

The rectus abdominus muscle is located in the lower abdomen.

Operative Procedure

The incision starts at the ellipse of abdominal skin and subcutaneous tissue on the abdomen.

With a *pedicle TRAM flap,* an ellipse of skin and abdominal wall subcutaneous fat, along with a portion of the anterior rectus abdominus muscle, is partially separated from the posterior rectus muscle. The proximal portion *remains attached* to the rectus abdominus muscle, which provides the blood supply (the superior epigastric and deep inferior epigastric arteries branch to myocutaneous perforators) to the flap. The loosened distal flap is then tunneled under the upper abdominal skin and passed to the mastectomy site at the chest. The flap is rotated and placed into position; it may be either ipsilateral or contralateral to the breast to be reconstructed.

With a *free (microsurgical) TRAM flap,* the flap is cut into the abdominal skin and fat just like the pedicle flap. However, the ellipse of abdominal skin, subcutaneous tissue, and anterior rectus abdominus muscle flap is *separated completely* and removed from the abdomen; it is then brought into the mastectomy wound. An operating microscope is used to suture the vessels of the flap to the recipient vessels, using either the thoracodorsal arteries or internal mammary veins.

A mesh prosthesis can be used to reconstruct an abdominal wall donor site defect as well as for additional adjacent tissue mobilization.

Drains are placed in the chest and abdominal wounds, and the incision lines are closed.

IV fluorescin dye may be used to determine the viability of the flap with breast reconstruction. Skin fluorescence correlates with flap survival.

Breast reconstruction may be performed either at the time of the mastectomy (if the patient has not undergone chemotherapy or radiation) or at a later date.

Anesthetic

GETA and muscle relaxation are used. Nitrous oxide may need to be avoided in this procedure, given that it can distend the abdomen, making abdominal closure more difficult.

Positioning

The patient is positioned supine, with the arm on the affected side extended on a padded armboard and the shoulder at an angle less than 90 degrees. The surgeon may request flexing the table during abdominal wall closure.

Anesthetic Implications

The surgeon will mark the skin while the patient is in an upright position in the preoperative area.

Maintain stable BP (MAP > 70 mm Hg) for continued perfusion of the flap tissue. Avoid the use of vasopressors.

Keep patients warm and well hydrated to optimize graft perfusion.

Type and cross-match the patient's blood preoperatively. Moderate blood loss is possible with this surgery, and the patient may require a blood transfusion during the procedure.

The blood pressure cuff and the peripheral IV should both be placed on the nonoperative-side arm, or in the lower extremities if either arm cannot be used.

Smooth emergence from anesthesia is important with this surgery. The goal is to avoid coughing, bucking, or nausea/vomiting or retching so as to prevent increased risk of bleeding, hematoma formation, or suture line disruption from the increased chest pressures. Have a team member hold gentle pressure over the suture lines if the patient does cough or vomit.

The risk of postoperative nausea and vomiting is increased in any breast surgery, so antiemetics should be given.

A bulky pressure dressing and a surgical bra are applied at the end of the case.

A Doppler may be used to check for flap pulses. Postoperatively, monitor for hematoma formation, flap color, capillary refill, and temperature to assess for vascular constriction/vasospasm.

Breast reconstruction may be performed either at the time of the mastectomy (if the patient has not undergone chemotherapy or radiation) or at a later date.

Complications

There is a higher incidence of flap loss in patients who are obese, smokers, or diabetics, and in those patients who have had prior abdominal surgery.

Nipple Reconstruction

Surgical reconstruction of the nipple is done to improve the cosmetic results after the nipple is removed. A natural-appearing breast offers the patient a sense of wholeness and normalcy.

After optimal symmetry between the breasts has been achieved, the nipple areola reconstruction can be performed. The type of nipple reconstruction depends on the quality of tissue on the reconstructed breast and whether a surrounding graft is needed.

Operative Procedure

In some cases, the nipple is recreated from skin taken as a local flap on the reconstructed breast. Multiple techniques are available, such as the "skate," "C-V," and "star" flap. The goal with any technique is to create a nipple mound using adjacent tissue.

Alternatively, the nipple may be recreated from a skin graft taken from another body location. For example, a graft may be taken from the inner thigh, the abdominal scar from a flap reconstruction, the buttock crease, or a waist tissue flap to construct the nipple mound. Skin from these areas of the body has a natural tendency to heal darker when it is grafted. Areola grafts are performed in the operating room.

The use of dermis, fat grafts, or fillers may be necessary to improve nipple projection.

Nipple tattooing is done months after all other reconstruction is done. This multistep procedure uses colored dye to add a natural-looking nipple;

it can also make scarring less obvious. Tattooing can be done in the physician's office, as most patients have very little sensation in the reconstructed nipple postoperatively.

Patients may also choose the nonsurgical option of tattooing without reconstruction. In this case, color pigmentation simulates the nipple areola without the contour of an actual nipple.

Anesthetic

GETA and insertion of an OETT or a LMA are necessary during nipple reconstruction surgery.

Positioning

The patient is positioned supine, with bilateral arms on padded armboards and the shoulders at an angle less than 90 degrees.

Anesthetic Implications

The surgeon will mark the skin while the patient is in an upright position in the preoperative area. He or she will compare the nonoperative breast and the surgical breast to determine nipple positioning.

The blood pressure cuff and the peripheral IV should both be placed on the nonoperative-side arm.

Make sure to have an extra-long length of ventilator circuit tubing to accommodate putting the patient's head up in high-Fowler's position. This positioning may be used to check position of the nipple in a more natural, dropped position.

Smooth emergence from anesthesia is important with this surgery. The goal is to avoid coughing, bucking, or nausea/vomiting or retching so as to prevent increased risk of bleeding, hematoma formation, or suture line disruption from the increased chest pressures. Have a team member hold gentle pressure over the suture lines if the patient does cough or vomit.

The risk of postoperative nausea and vomiting is increased in any breast surgery, so antiemetics should be given.

Tissue Expanders

An inflatable silicone balloon may be placed in the chest following breast surgery and in some other areas of the body to slowly and serially expand the surrounding tissue and skin. This technique takes advantage of the skin's ability to accommodate a slowly enlarging mass by increasing its surface area, thereby enabling the skin to accommodate a permanent implant. The goal is for the patient's breasts to be symmetrical bilaterally.

Tissue expanders are commonly used with breast reconstruction (as described earlier in this chapter) but can also be inserted to repair or replace tissue areas such in the scalp, face, neck, hands, arms, and legs. Expanders are placed when there is not enough skin to accommodate a permanent implant.

Operative Procedure

In breast reconstruction, a tissue expander is surgically placed underneath the pectoralis major muscle and a part of the serratus anterior muscle, usually at the junction of the lesion and the area of the proposed expansion. The incision made is one-third the length of the expander. The filling port can be externalized for ease in filling; alternatively, it may be placed under the skin (much like a port-a-cath, a catheter connects the reservoir to the balloon). Under sterile technique, a small amount of saline is instilled or injected into the filling port during surgery. Drains are placed; the incision lines are closed.

The balloon is incrementally inflated postoperatively. The amount instilled into the expander depends on the patient's comfort, skin tension, and blanching of the overlying skin. Usually 50–100 mL of saline is injected into the implant every 1 to 2 weeks. It can take 2 to 3 months to inflate the balloon fully.

Anesthetic

Anesthesia consists of GETA with insertion of an OETT or an LMA.

Positioning
The patient is positioned supine, with bilateral arms placed on padded armboards and the shoulders at an angle less than 90 degrees.

Anesthetic Implications
The blood pressure cuff and the peripheral IV should both be placed on the nonoperative-side arm, or on one of the legs if an arm cannot be used

Smooth emergence from anesthesia is important with this surgery. The goal is to avoid coughing, bucking, or nausea/vomiting or retching so as to prevent increased risk of bleeding, hematoma formation, or suture line disruption from the increased chest pressures. Have a team member hold gentle pressure over the suture lines if the patient does cough or vomit.

The risk of postoperative nausea and vomiting is increased in any breast surgery, so antiemetics should be given.

A bulky pressure dressing and a surgical bra are applied at the end of the case.

The expander is surgically removed after the tissue is expanded.

Complications
Potential complications include infection, rupture, and exposure.

Thoracic Surgery

14

THORACIC SURGERY PEARLS

- Operative sites within the thorax include the heart, esophagus, and lungs, and somatically innervated structures such as the ribs, superficial chest wall, and breast. When patients undergo thoracic surgery, preexisting diseases of these organs or prior medical treatment (e.g., radiation) is common. These factors contribute to postoperative morbidity through a variety of mechanisms such as decreased pulmonary reserve.

- *Chest wall disorders:* benign and malignant tumors of the ribs, sternum, and muscles of the chest wall; bony defects of the chest wall such as pectus excavatum and pectus carinatum; thoracic outlet syndrome, reflex sympathetic dystrophy, ankylosing spondylitis (chronic inflammatory arthritis), lung hernia, and the need for stabilization of the chest after trauma.

- *Pleural disorders:* pleural effusion, pleurisy, empyema, pneumothorax, hemothorax, and tumors of the pleura.

- *Pulmonary disorders:* lung cancer, lung metastasis, pulmonary nodules, carcinoid tumors, hamartomas (benign tumor-like malformation in the tissue of its origin), emphysema, alveolar proteinosis, giant bullas disease, spontaneous pneumothorax, hemangioma, bronchopleural fistulas, and infections.

- *Tracheal/bronchial disorders:* tumors and strictures of the trachea including those involving the subglottic larynx or carina, extrinsic tracheal compression, tracheal malacia, sarcoidosis, Wegener's granulomatosis, tracheostomy, bronchial stenosis, and bronchiectasis.

- *Mediastinal disorders:* mediastinal tumors and cysts, thymoma, teratoma, neurogenic tumors, germ cell tumors, mediastinitis, chronic fibrosing mediastinitis, and mediastinal lymphadenopathy. The mediastinum is the anatomic region between the lungs that contains all the principal organs of the chest except for the lungs—that is, the heart, trachea, esophagus, trachea, and thoracic duct. It extends from the sternum to the vertebral column and laterally to the mediastinal pleurae.

- *Disorders of the diaphragm:* eventration (disorder in which all or part of the diaphragmatic muscle is replaced by fibroelastic tissue), hiatal hernia, and phrenic nerve paralysis.
- *Esophageal disorders:* See Chapter 16 on abdominal and gastrointestinal surgery.

Source: Adapted from http://www.surgery.usc.edu/foregut/index.html.

ANESTHESIA FOR THORACIC SURGERIES: KEY POINTS

- One of the main problems with thoracic surgery patients is hypothermia. The mediastinum is very vascular, and heat loss occurs when the chest is opened.
- The main goal related to anesthesia is to provide optimal conditions for surgery of intrathoracic structures while maintaining oxygenation and hemodynamic stability.
- Inhalational agents relax smooth muscle of the airways and depress airway reflexes.
- The use of an anticholinergic for its anti-sialagogue effect reduces the secretions created with airway manipulation.
- The goal may be to have an awake, comfortable, and extubated patient at the end of surgery. Advantages of prompt extubation include avoiding the potentially disruptive effects of higher airway pressures on fresh suture lines.
- There is always a potential for a significant alteration in oxygenation and ventilation with intrathoracic procedures. Monitoring should include pulse oximetry, capnography, arterial blood gas (ABG) sampling, airway pressure measurements, and expiratory tidal volumes. When possible, the use of a ventilator with pressure-control ventilation and pressure support is advantageous to limit peak airway pressures and facilitate emergence from anesthesia.
- EKG changes may be noted during thoracic surgery. Specifically, tachydysrhythmias may be triggered by mechanical stimulation during intrathoracic procedures. Bradycardia from vagal nerve stimulation is also frequently elicited during chest wall dissection.
- Arterial line placement is needed to monitor continuous blood pressure and readily permits arterial sampling for blood gases. With a patient in the lateral position, placing the arterial line on the dependent arm not only improves stability of the site, but also ensures that any compression of that arm will be manifested as a flattened arterial waveform.
- In terms of IV fluids, a slightly dry to an extremely conservative fluid regimen is needed to help decrease the risk of pulmonary edema associated with standard crystalloid solutions.
- Thoracic surgeries are usually quite painful. Placing an epidural catheter preoperatively for postoperative pain control is quite effective. When the epidural catheter is placed, a test dose is given to confirm placement but neither local anesthesia nor narcotics are given at that time to avoid the vasodilatation from the sympathectomy response that occurs with these agents (causing hypothermia and hypotension). Instead, drugs are given through the epidural when the patient is waking up from surgery. It is best to place the catheter preoperatively so that third-space fluid shifts and edema do not make insertion of the catheter more difficult. A urethral catheter should be placed whenever an epidural catheter has been placed, as these patients have more difficulty voiding.
- An epidural increases the patient's fluid requirements and risk of hypothermia. An epidural catheter helps with postoperative pain control and assists the patient to be able to take deep breaths and cough effectively.
- For any thoracic procedure using laser or electrocautery, see Chapter 1 on safety concerns for more information.

- Monitoring central venous pressure (CVP), if available, may aid in fluid management.
- One-lung ventilation allows for the collapse of the operative lung, which facilitates exposure for the surgeon. See Chapter 3 for more information on use of a double-lumen endobronchial tube (DLEBT).

THORACIC ENDOSCOPY

Flexible Bronchoscopy

Flexible bronchoscopy includes endoscopic visualization of the trachea, main bronchi and their openings, and most of the segmental bronchi with a flexible scope. It is used for diagnosis, biopsy, tumor staging, removal of a foreign object, and aspiration of secretions in these areas. The flexible scope allows more peripheral subdivisions to be inspected (more than a rigid scope); a disadvantage is that foreign objects or thick mucus cannot be removed through the lumen. The flexile scope is also used to aid in placement of an ETT/DLEBT and to confirm or reposition endotracheal/DLEBT and/or tracheostomy tubes.

Operative Procedure

Place the largest oral endotracheal tube (OETT) so that a flexible bronchoscope can be inserted through it, but a small enough OETT that the patient can ventilate *around* it (the fiberoptic scope may occlude the inside of the tube). A pediatric fiberoptic scope may be needed if the endotracheal tube is too small to accommodate the adult scope. The flexible scope is placed through a T-piece diaphragm adaptor placed at the end of the endotracheal tube.

Anesthetic

General endotracheal anesthesia (GETA) is used. In some cases, the procedure may be carried out with only local anesthesia to abolish the gag reflex or hemodynamic changes and increase patient comfort. Topical local anesthesia (LA) consists of anesthesia to the mouth, oropharynx, or base of tongue.

Methods include lidocaine gel/nebulizer, lidocaine 2% Cetacaine spray, and use of Krause forceps with local anesthetic soaked gauze/Q-tips placed into the piriform recess (lateral to the aryepiglottic folds—they are deep recesses on either side of the larynx).

Airway block consists of a translaryngeal/transtracheal block to the vagus nerve (CN X) with Lidocaine 1%, 2%, or 4%, 3–4 mL, with or without epinephrine. When epinephrine is used in conjunction with local anesthetic infiltration, monitor the EKG for tachycardia or ST-segment changes.

Positioning

The patient is placed in a sitting position with awake flexible bronchoscopy; or supine when general anesthesia is used. The head of the operating table may be turned away at least 90 degrees, if not 180 degrees, from the anesthetist.

Anesthetic Implications

Glycopyrrolate, given as an antisialagogue preoperatively, can be used to decrease airway/oral secretions.

Flexible fiberoptic scope sizes range from 3.5 mm (pediatric) to 6.0 mm (adult). If the scope is to be passed through an endotracheal tube, a valve port can be placed at the end of the ETT with a right-angle side port for circuit placement. This arrangement allows the flexible scope to be passed through the valve, forming a tight seal around the scope while maintaining circuit integrity and the ability to ventilate with full tidal volumes, giving volatile agents if desired.

Rigid Bronchoscopy

Rigid bronchoscopy provides for endoscopic visualization of the trachea, main bronchi, and their openings with a rigid scope. Using this technique, a foreign body can be removed, washings and biopsy samples can be obtained, and tumor staging can be performed.

Rigid bronchoscopy is preferred when airway patency is paramount, as with airways occluded with foreign material (e.g., blood, foreign body, aspiration of particulate matter, or tumor). Suctioning ability is better with a rigid scope than with a flexible scope. It is also easier to manipulate and grasp foreign bodies during rigid bronchoscopy, and increased choices of types and sizes of forceps available with the rigid scope. Also, the rigid scope can be passed distal to a strictured segment of the airway (tumor, granuloma) and provides better access for laser equipment and for stent placement (tracheal or tracheobronchial). Disadvantages of using a rigid scope include increased potential risk for damage to soft tissue and inability of the rigid scope to visualize the deeper peripheral subdivisions of the bronchioles.

Operative Procedure

After general anesthesia and muscle relaxants have been given (without inserting an endotracheal tube), the head of the bed is turned 90 degrees to the surgeon. The surgeon immediately introduces a well-lubricated straight steel bronchoscope into the mouth, lifting the epiglottis and passing the scope into the trachea. Once the scope is in the trachea, the anesthesia circuit tubing is attached to the bronchoscope adaptor and the patient ventilated. A telescope is advanced through the bronchoscope and then into the bronchi. Further instrumentation may then be inserted, such as a laser for removal of tracheal papillomas or forceps for retrieval of a foreign body.

Anesthetic

General anesthesia; muscle relaxation may also be used. Once the anesthesia circuit tubing is attached to the bronchoscope adaptor, oxygen and a volatile agent can be given with manual ventilation (hand-bagging), although it may be difficult to achieve normal tidal volumes due to the leaking of gases around the narrow diameter of the bronchoscope.

For general anesthesia, instead of using a volatile inhaled agent—which can blow up into the surgeon's face—a total intravenous anesthetic (TIVA) with remifentanil and propofol infusions and a BIS monitor can be used. If volatile inhaled agents are used, keep the percentage lower to prevent "gassing" the surgeon.

In some cases, local anesthesia can be given to diminish hemodynamic changes from the stimulation. Topical local anesthesia (LA) consists of anesthesia to the mouth, oropharynx, or base of tongue. Methods include lidocaine gel/nebulizer, lidocaine 2% 2–4 mL infiltrated each side, Cetacaine spray, and use of Krause forceps with local anesthetic soaked gauze/Q-tips placed into the piriform recess (lateral to the aryepiglottic folds—they are deep recesses on either side of the larynx).

Airway block consists of a translaryngeal/transtracheal block to the vagus nerve (CN X) with lidocaine 1%, 2%, or 4%, 3–4 mL, with or without epinephrine. When epinephrine is used in conjunction with local anesthetic infiltration, monitor the EKG for tachycardia or ST-segment changes.

Positioning

The patient is placed in a sitting position when topical anesthesia is used; positioned supine for induction and the procedure. A shoulder roll is placed to help extend the head and align the airway axis to aid in nontraumatic insertion of the rigid scope. Position the patient so that his or her shoulders are at the break of the table, allowing the head to be flexed or extended for surgical access. Arms should be padded and tucked at the sides bilaterally.

Anesthetic Implications

Four techniques for oxygenation and carbon dioxide elimination are used with the rigid scope:

- *Spontaneous ventilation* with or without an endotracheal tube in place. This technique is rarely used unless forced breaths risk displacement of a foreign object.

- *Apneic oxygenation*, which requires the surgeon to work in between withdrawal of the rigid bronchoscope and mask ventilations. Alert the surgeon to a predetermined drop in the oxygen saturation percent. The surgeon will then withdraw the scope and allow mask ventilation to bring the saturation back up to 100%. After a time of higher saturations, the surgeon can then reinsert the rigid scope and continue working until decreased oxygenation saturations, again, requires scope removal and manual mask ventilation.
- *Positive-pressure ventilation.* The circuit is attached to a side port on the rigid bronchoscope with oxygen given by manual ventilation. Excessive leaking of gases through the glottis and around the scope can be controlled by packing the posterior pharynx.
- *Jet ventilation.* The jet must be pointed straight into the trachea; ventilation can be assessed by chest rise, pulse oximetry, and ABGs.

A rubber tooth guard should be placed over the patient's upper teeth by the surgeon to protect against damage from the rigid scope.

This procedure can be quite stimulating to the patient. If the patient coughs with the rigid scope in the trachea, soft-tissue damage may occur. Muscle relaxation will prevent this complication.

If the laser is used to remove tracheal papillomas, a special facemask for all caregivers in the room should be used as aerosolized papillomas can be inhaled by any person in the room.

Prevent airway fires by inserting a fire-resistant ETT. Filling the ETT balloon with saline can help to put out any fire or spark that is started. Alternatively, the balloon can be filled with a mix of saline and methylene blue to indicate if the balloon's patency has been compromised at any time during the surgery. Keep the FiO_2 as low as possible. If the patient's saturation falls, notify the surgeon, who can stop the laser. Increase the FiO_2 settings and manually ventilate the patient to increase the saturation level. The surgeon can begin to use the laser again when the FiO_2 returns to 30%. Avoid using nitrous oxide, as this gas is also highly combustible. Keep a bottle of sterile water nearby to use in case of a fire. See Chapter 1 on safety concerns for more information.

Glycopyrrolate, given as an antisialagogue preoperatively, can be used to decrease airway and oral secretions.

Mediastinoscopy

Mediastinoscopy involves endoscopic visualization of the mediastinum, including the tracheobronchial junction, bronchi, aortic arch, and regional lymph nodes. It is performed to assess for suspected intrathoracic malignancy; for biopsy; for tumor staging to determine the resectability of lung cancers; and for evaluation of lymph nodes in the superior mediastinum and the paratracheal areas.

Mediastinal masses are classified as anterior, middle, or posterior, based on their relationship to the heart. Anterior mediastinal masses can cause distal airway obstructions; patients with these tumors are often unable to lie flat and anesthesia must be induced in a partially sitting position. Middle mediastinal masses are approached through a posterolateral thoracotomy or thoracoscopically. Posterior mediastinal masses may cause Horner's syndrome when excised.

Operative Procedure

A small incision is made at the level of the suprasternal notch. The surgeon clears a path into the mediastinum manually before placing the mediastinoscope into the incision. Important structures lying within the mediastinum include the heart and its major vessels, the lymph nodes, the trachea, the esophagus, and the thymus. Through the mediastinoscope, instruments are inserted to perform the biopsy. Note the following variations depending on the approach used:

- *Cervical mediastinoscopy:* An incision is made approximately one fingerbreadth above the suprasternal notch. The scope is passed anteriorly to the trachea; the lymph nodes are visually assessed and a biopsy completed.
- *Anterior mediastinoscopy and mediastinotomy* (also known as a Chamberlain procedure): An incision is made into the second intercostal space to the left of the sternum. It may be necessary to remove the cartilage. Lymph node assessment and dissection in the subaortic and periaortic regions are then completed.

After the biopsy is sent to pathology, the surgeon may elect to close the incision and get the results of the biopsy at a later time, or he or she may decide to wait for the pathology report prior to closing. In the latter situation, the surgeon will likely continue on to pulmonary resection if a malignancy is found.

Anesthetic
General anesthesia is given with insertion of a single-lumen endotracheal tube. Adequate muscle relaxation is imperative to prevent coughing and movement by the patient, which may lead to vascular trauma if the mediastinoscope in place.

Mask induction with 100% FiO_2 and a volatile agent while the patient is in a sitting position may be the induction of choice with a patient who has a mediastinal tumor. In individuals with a significant mediastinal mass, supine positioning may result in compression of the airway and the heart by the tumor. Ketamine and narcotic-based induction can be used to avoid cardiovascular compromise.

A left radial arterial line should be used to accurately monitor the blood pressure during mediastinoscopy. The pulse oximeter may be placed on the patient's right hand to monitor possible compression of the right innominate artery. Inadvertent compression of the innominate artery will decrease blood flow to the right arm, resulting in a poor pulse oximetry waveform. As compression continues, the decreasing saturation levels will alert the anesthetist to ask the surgeon to reposition the scope. The left radial arterial line blood pressures will remain accurate.

Positioning
The patient is positioned supine, with a neck roll and head and neck extension to aid in surgical

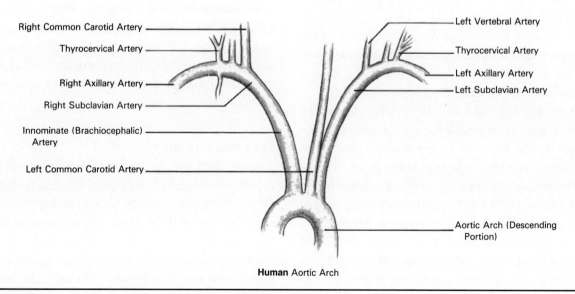

Right Common Carotid Artery

Thyrocervical Artery

Right Axillary Artery

Right Subclavian Artery

Innominate (Brachiocephalic) Artery

Left Common Carotid Artery

Left Vertebral Artery

Thyrocervical Artery

Left Axillary Artery

Left Subclavian Artery

Aortic Arch (Descending Portion)

Human Aortic Arch

Figure 14-1 *Important Anatomy in Mediastinoscopy*
Chiras, 2008

access and visualization. Position the patient so that his or her shoulders are at the break of the table, allowing the head to be flexed or extended more easily.

Anesthetic Implications

Mediastinal biopsies can be sent for frozen section and immediately evaluated by a pathologist. This allows the surgeon to make a decision whether to proceed with a thoracotomy or thoracoscopy.

Enlarged lymph nodes or tumors may compress the trachea and surrounding structures, creating the potential for severe respiratory or cardiovascular compromise with supine positioning and/or induction of general anesthesia.

The innominate artery crosses from left to right within the mediastinum. It can be compressed by the scope, leading to decreased blood flow to the right cerebral hemisphere and the right upper extremity.

If a superior vena caval syndrome is present, it is important to have IV access in a lower extremity.

Preoperative evaluation is crucial—specifically examining for airway obstruction (stridor, wheezing, cyanosis, atelectasis, pneumonia) and signs and symptoms of respiratory compromise during position changes such as supine or lateral. CT scans of the chest are invaluable in assessing the mediastinum.

Complications

Multiple complications may occur secondary to the mediastinoscopy. Important structures lying within the mediastinum—including the heart and its major vessels, the lymph nodes, the trachea, the esophagus, and the thymus—may be injured.

- Excessive hemorrhage from vascular trauma from the procedure may necessitate blood transfusion. For this reason, the patient's blood should, at a minimum, be typed and screened prior to surgery. Due to the small incision and the limited visibility through

the mediastinoscope, if bleeding should occur, the surgeon may have difficulty getting it under control.

- If the innominate artery is compressed, cerebral ischemia may occur. To prevent this complication, the anesthesia provider must notify the surgeon immediately of a loss of pulsatile flow in the right arm arterial line or the pulse oximeter.
- Vagally mediated reflex bradycardia may occur secondary to compression of the trachea or great vessels. If this problem arises, the surgeon should be notified immediately and the anesthesia provider should determine whether discontinuing the compression is sufficient to return the patient's heart rate to normal or whether pharmacologic support is needed.
- Recurrent laryngeal nerve damage and phrenic nerve injury may occur due to surgical manipulation. Careful assessment of the airway and the patient's ability to protect the airway should be completed prior to extubation.
- Pneumothorax may be seen postoperatively and may require chest tube placement.

Thoracoscopy

Thoracoscopy consists of endoscopic visualization of the pleural spaces. It is performed for tumor staging. This procedure is indicated when noninvasive or minimally invasive diagnostic procedures have not yielded sufficient information or in patients with reduced pulmonary function such that the risk of formal thoracotomy is too great. Thoracoscopy, which may be performed with a video-assisted system (see the discussion of video-assisted thoracoscopic surgery later in this chapter), permits inspection of the entire hemithorax.

Operative Procedure

A small incision is made at the fourth to seventh intercostal space midaxillary to the posterior axillary line, and an initial entry port is established. A telescope attached to a camera is inserted. Two or three additional ports are placed according to the location of the lesion. Endoscopic instruments are deployed to retract, dissect, ligate, excise, and suture the tissues. Specimens are removed in a specimen bag to prevent seeding of malignant cells or infectious materials. Larger specimens may require extension of the small incision or the creation of an additional, larger incision for removal. A chest tube may be inserted and connected to a sealed drainage unit. Chest tubes are often placed through one of the endoscopic ports created for surgical exposure.

Anesthetic

General anesthesia is given with insertion of a double-lumen ETT for one-lung ventilation; muscle relaxants are used as well. An epidural or patient-controlled analgesia may facilitate postoperative pain management.

Positioning

The patient is placed in the lateral decubitus position with the affected side up.

Anesthetic Implications

Always be prepared for the potential to convert to an open thoracotomy procedure.

The patient's X-rays, CT scans, MRIs, PET scans, and other images should be available in the OR. The patient may have been asked to bring them in from home.

Type and cross-match the patient's blood. Ensure that blood products are readily available.

Contraindications to a thoracoscopy include lesions in close proximity to the great vessels and patients who cannot tolerate single-lung ventilation.

Monitors and IV Access

An arterial line; placed in a dependent upper extremity.

Complications

Risks of this procedure include hemorrhage, air embolism, diaphragmatic injury, and injury to adjacent organs.

Thoracic Sympathectomy

Thoracic sympathectomy involves cauterization, ultrasound dissection, excision, or clamping of a sympathetic chain within the chest cavity, most commonly at T2, T3, or T4. This procedure may be performed to treat Raynaud's phenomenon or hyperhydrosis (excessive hand or facial sweating or facial blushing not relieved by more conservative measures, such as Drysol, Drionic, or Botox).

Operative Procedure

One to three small incisions (less than ½ inch) are made under the armpit, and a gas is insufflated through the incision into the chest cavity. Endoscopic equipment is inserted, and the sympathetic chain is located along the head of the rib. The sympathetic chain is clamped, excised, dissected, and/or cauterized. The procedure is then repeated on the opposite side.

Anesthetic

General anesthesia is given with insertion of either a double-lumen ETT or single endotracheal tube, depending on surgeon preference. An epidural or patient-controlled analgesia may facilitate postoperative pain management.

Positioning

The patient is placed in a supine or lateral decubitus position, depending on surgeon preference.

Anesthetic Implications

If a single-lumen tube is used, peak airway pressures will likely increase, requiring pressure-control ventilation.

Horner syndrome (ptosis, miosis, enophthalmos, and anhydrosis) or decreasing heart rate and/or blood pressure are possible complications.

Other potential complications include excessive bleeding, infection, or injury to surrounding organs. Pneumothorax can occur and may require placement of a chest tube.

LUNG SURGERY

Excision of Blebs and Bullae

Lung resection may be used to remove blebs or bullae that could potentially lead to spontaneous pneumothorax.

These problems may be an incidental or a concomitant finding, especially in patients with COPD or as the cause of spontaneous pneumothorax.

Operative Procedure

Excision of blebs and bullae is commonly performed as a video-assisted thoracoscopic surgery (VATS). During this procedure, blebs or bullae are isolated and resected.

Anesthetic

General anesthesia is given with insertion of a double-lumen endotracheal tube; muscle relaxants are given. An epidural or patient-controlled analgesia may facilitate postoperative pain management.

Positioning

The patient is placed in the lateral decubitus position.

Anesthetic Implications

Avoid nitrous oxide, as it may increase the size of bullae. Positive-pressure ventilation may rupture bullae with subsequent development of a tension pneumothorax. Pressure-control ventilation may aid the anesthesia provider in providing the lowest possible pressure while maintaining adequate oxygenation and ventilation. A bronchopleurocutaneous fistula may result, with subsequent loss of ability to ventilate the patient.

Bronchoplastic Resection

Bronchoplastic resection involves removal of lung tissue along with a segment of a major bronchus affected by tumor. This surgery is performed to treat major bronchi cancer, involving either the three lobes of the right lung or the two lobes of the left lung.

Operative Procedure

Access obtained through a posterolateral or lateral incision. The surgeon requires intraluminal access to the ipsilateral main stem bronchus. Removal of a portion of the bronchus entails transient disruption of the airway. The surgeon must reattach the proximal to the distal bronchial margins during nonoperative one-lung ventilation.

Anesthetic

General anesthesia is given with insertion of a double-lumen endobronchial tube; muscle relaxants are given. An epidural or patient-controlled analgesia may facilitate postoperative pain management.

Positioning

The patient may be placed in either a supine or a lateral position.

Anesthetic Implications

Sterile ventilator tubing is required for sleeve resection.

Temperature loss is common with an open-chest procedure. Upper- and lower-body warming blankets are needed as well as fluid warmers. The ambient temperature in the room may also need to be warmed.

There is a potential for a large amount of blood loss, so the patient's blood should be type and cross-matched prior to surgery. Blood may need to be available in the OR.

Bronchopleural Fistula

A bronchopleural fistula is a fistula found between the pleural space and the bronchial tree. It may develop following adult respiratory distress syndrome (ARDS), pneumonia, lung abscesses, tuberculosis (TB), chemotherapy or radiotherapy for lung cancer, or previous lung resection surgery including, but not limited to, pneumonectomy, lobectomy, bullectomy, or lung volume reduction.

Symptoms include dyspnea, subcutaneous emphysema, contralateral deviation of the trachea, expectoration of purulent material, persistent air leak, and purulent drainage from the chest tube. Diagnosis is confirmed by bronchoscopy.

Small fistulas may spontaneously resolve with conservative therapy (e.g., antibiotics, nutrition, chest tube). Fistulas involving larger bronchi require surgical intervention.

Operative Procedure

The bronchopleural fistula approached through an open thoracotomy. Surgical options include the following:

- Decortication if the lung if surrounded by a thick purulent layer
- Revision of a bronchial stump
- Closure of the fistula with a muscle flap from the intercostal space
- Thoracoplasty, often in combination with a pedicled muscle flap over the bronchial stump
- Bronchoscopic application of fibrin glue, sealant, or coils to seal the fistula

A staged closure may be necessary for complicated bronchopleural fistulas.

Anesthetic

General anesthesia is given with placement of a double-lumen ETT (DLEBT) via rapid-sequence induction or intubation in a spontaneously breathing patient. Muscle relaxants are given. Use of a DLEBT is essential to isolate one lung from the other. An epidural or patient-controlled analgesia may facilitate postoperative pain management.

Positioning

The patient is placed in a lateral decubitus position.

Anesthetic Implications

Prevention of spillage of purulent contents into the unaffected lung is of greatest importance when planning induction of anesthesia. Rapid-sequence induction aids in minimizing the time between induction and lung isolation. Placement of a double-lumen ETT in the spontaneously ventilating patient can prevent aspiration of gastric contents in patients with a bronchopleuroenteric fistula.

Regardless of the method of induction, the affected lung should be isolated immediately following ETT placement, and the head of the bed should be raised to decrease the potential for contamination of the healthy lung. Application of positive-pressure ventilation may suggest apparent inadequate ventilation secondary to the loss of tidal volume through the fistula. If a chest tube is not in place or if it malfunctions, accumulation of air in the pleural space may lead to pneumothorax.

Independent lung ventilation with two ventilators is sometimes used to treat each lung separately. High-frequency jet ventilation has also been used.

These patients usually have one or more chest tubes placed before coming to surgery.

Temperature loss is common with an open-chest procedure. Upper- and lower-body warming blankets are needed as well as fluid warmers. The ambient temperature in the room may also need to be warmed.

Bronchopulmonary Lavage

In bronchopulmonary lavage, either unilateral lung lavage of the tracheobronchial tree or sequential lavage of both lungs is performed. This procedure is used to treat alveolar proteinosis, a disease characterized by accumulation of a substance rich in lipids in the alveoli, which prevents gas exchange at the alveolar level. It is also performed to treat severe bronchitis or asthma.

Operative Procedure

This procedure is performed by instilling warm isotonic saline into one lung at a time while oxygenating the other lung with 100% FiO_2. The lung can accommodate approximately 700 mL to 1.0 L of fluid. Vigorous chest percussion is performed throughout the instillation of fluid; the lavage fluid is then passively drained. Placing the patient in the Trendelenburg position may facilitate drainage. This procedure is repeated until the drainage decreases in turbidity and is nearly clear. When the lavage is complete, the affected lung is thoroughly suctioned and ventilation reestablished.

Anesthetic

General anesthesia is given with insertion of a double-lumen ETT; muscle relaxants are given. The trachea should be intubated with the largest double-lumen ETT that can be positioned correctly. Placement of the ETT should be confirmed by bronchoscopy.

Positioning

Patient positioning depends on surgeon preference. Lavage of the nondependent lung may improve oxygenation by decreasing blood flow to the nonventilated lung; however, this position increases the risk of displacement of the ETT, which may result in spillage from the nondependent lung to the dependent lung. Lavage of the dependent lung decreases the likelihood of spillage, but may lead to hypoxia secondary to shunted blood flow. The supine position may balance the risk of hypoxia and aspiration/spillage.

Anesthetic Implications

These patients are often seriously ill and in severe respiratory insufficiency when coming for pulmonary lavage.

Ensuring proper placement of the DLEBT and carefully securing it in place are the two most important aspects of anesthesia in bronchopulmonary lavage. Failure to adequately isolate the lungs can result in a severe loss of compliance and acute arterial desaturation. Signs and symptoms of leakage include appearance of bubbles in the lavage fluid, rales or rhonchi in the ventilated lung, arterial desaturation, and discrepancies between the volume of fluid instilled and the volume of fluid drained. If leakage should occur, the lavage should be stopped immediately, the lung should be drained, and the position of the ETT confirmed.

Prior to isolation of the lung to be lavaged, the patient should be administered 100% FiO_2 to denitrogenate the lung. Failure to denitrogenate the lung prior to lavage may result in nitrogen pockets that limit the effectiveness of the procedure. When ventilation is reestablished to the lung after lavage, the lung will exhibit decreased compliance and will require larger than normal tidal volumes (15–20 mL/kg).

Patients typically remain hemodynamically stable during the bronchopulmonary lavage procedure, although decreased left ventricular filling and right heart strain resulting in decreased BP may occur. PVR increases with the instillation of fluid into the lung and decreases with fluid drainage.

Anesthesia Goals for Bronchopulmonary Lavage

Preoperative Measures

V/Q scans are usually done preoperatively to characterize the distribution of the impairment. The lung with the least perfusion is lavaged first if sequential lavage is anticipated.

Induction

Correct placement of the ETT is of paramount importance. The ETT should be carefully secured once placement has been verified.

Maintenance

Maintain ETT placement and monitor for signs and symptoms of leakage.

Emergence

Ensure lung compliance has returned sufficiently to allow the patient to adequately oxygenate/ventilate.

Postoperative Measures

A chest X-ray should be taken within an hour of the completion of lavage for comparison with the pre-lavage examination.

Decortication (Pleural Stripping)

Decortication consists of the stripping of a restrictive membrane on the visceral pleura that interferes with respiration. The pleural space is the potential space between the visceral and parietal layers of the pleurae. This space usually contains a small amount of fluid, which serves as a lubricant to allow the pleurae to slide over each other as the lungs expand and contract with respiration.

Chronic empyema, clotted hemothorax, tuberculosis, and other types of pleural inflammation, either infectious or noninfectious, may lead to large effusions that decrease pulmonary function. The collection of empyema or blood in the pleural space can lead to the formation of a fibrin layer on the pleura. As the fibrin layer (also called a peel) matures, the underlying lung becomes trapped. Surgical intervention may be necessary to remove the fibrin layer, thereby allowing the lung to reexpand and help with infection management.

Operative Procedure

The surgical approach can be either thoracoscopy or thoracotomy, although access by thoracoscopy may be limited. Thus, a thoracotomy may be required for definitive treatment.

In an open approach, a posterolateral thoracotomy incision is made. A rib resection may be necessary for adequate exposure. The fibrous membrane is then peeled away from the visceral pleura. Chest tubes are inserted and connected to a sealed drainage system.

Occasionally, an additional procedure, known as *pleurodesis,* is necessary to prevent reaccumulation of the effusion. During pleurodesis, a chemical agent is introduced into the pleural space that causes formation of adhesions and destruction of the pleural space. Agents used for chemical pleurodesis include tetracycline, talc, and bleomycin. Alternatively, mechanical pleurodesis can be done by the surgeon by scraping an abrasive surface, such as sterile gauze, against the pleura.

Anesthetic

General anesthesia is given, a double-lumen endobronchial tube is needed for one-lung ventilation. Muscle relaxants are given. An epidural or patient-controlled analgesia may facilitate postoperative pain management.

Positioning

The patient is placed lateral decubitus, with the affected lung in the nondependent position.

Anesthetic Implications

The most common anesthetic issues are hypovolemia and hypotension due to bleeding and sepsis, along with postoperative pain related to the decortication and pleurodesis. See "Anesthesia for Thoracic Surgeries: Key Points" earlier in this chapter for more information.

Positive-pressure ventilation following decortications may facilitate the breakdown of residual fibrous deposits, further allowing for lung expansion.

A posterolateral incision can affect the patient's efforts to cough postoperatively.

Temperature loss is common with an open-chest procedure. Upper- and lower-body warming blankets are needed as well as fluid warmers. The ambient temperature in the room may also need to be warmed.

Monitors

An arterial line is inserted for these cases.

Drainage of Empyema

Empyemas not responding to conservative treatment (e.g., intercostal chest tube drainage, antibiotics) require surgical drainage of the infected fluid.

The pleural space is the potential space between the visceral (lung) and parietal (chest wall) layers of the pleurae. This space usually contains a small amount of fluid that serves as a lubricant to allow the pleurae to slide over each other as the lungs expand and contract with respiration.

An empyema consists of infected pleural fluid; it may occur secondary to infectious processes such as pneumonia, tuberculosis, or a lung abscess, or after thoracic surgery, thoracic trauma, or needle puncture of the pleural space. The pus and fibrin deposits resulting from the infection cover the surface of the lung and chest, which leads to loculations (divided into smaller compartments) and pleural thickening. These changes, in turn, may cause partial collapse of the lung and impair ventilation. If the empyema is left untreated, the lung may become entrapped, allowing the pus to erode into the airways and potentially creating a bronchopleural fistula.

Operative Procedure

Drainage of an empyema is performed by either VATS or lateral thoracotomy (with or without rib resection and decortication).

In a *VATS* procedure, a small incision (½ inch) is made in the chest wall and a telescope is inserted into the pleural space. One or two additional incisions are made to allow insertion of additional instruments, and the pus, fluid, and debris are evacuated from the chest.

In a *thoracotomy,* a 5- to 6-inch incision is made into the intercostal space; the infected fluid is removed and sent for analysis. The pleura is carefully removed from the lung and chest wall and the lung reexpanded.

Chest tubes are usually placed through the incisions at the end of the case to facilitate further drainage postoperatively.

Anesthetic

General anesthesia is given with insertion of a double-lumen endotracheal tube; short-acting muscle relaxants are given. An epidural or patient-controlled analgesia may facilitate postoperative pain management. See "Anesthesia for Thoracic Surgeries: Key Points" earlier in this chapter for more information.

Positioning

The patient is placed in a lateral decubitus position, with the affected lung in the nondependent position.

Anesthetic Implications

The most common anesthetic issues are hypovolemia and hypotension due to bleeding and sepsis. If decortication is planned, epidural placement may facilitate the treatment of postoperative pain.

Temperature loss is common with an open-chest procedure. Upper- and lower-body warming blankets are needed as well as fluid warmers. The ambient temperature in the room may also need to be warmed.

Monitors

Arterial line placement can facilitate careful blood pressure monitoring as well as allow for regular arterial blood gases monitoring, which can indicate the patient's oxygenation/ventilation.

Lobectomy

Lobectomy is excision of one or more lobes of the lung. See the discussion of wedge resection later in this chapter for more information.

This surgery may be performed when a lesion is limited to a specific lobe. The most common indications for pulmonary resection are bronchogenic carcinoma (small cell, large cell, squamous cell, and adenocarcinoma), carcinoid tumors, infectious lung abscesses (bacterial, fungal, myobacterial), vascular disease, congenital abnormalities, and trauma.

Operative Procedure

Lobectomy may be performed via either a thoracotomy or during a VATS procedure. A posterolateral incision is made, and the muscles and ribs of the chest are retracted. The visceral pleura is dissected free from the hilus; the pulmonary artery and vein of the diseased lobe are ligated and divided. The bronchus is then transsected and the stump is sutured closed. The surgeon may test for air leaks by filling the chest with warm saline and observing for bubbles while the anesthesia provider performs a Valsalva maneuver (see information regarding Valsalva in "Anesthetic Implications"). At the end of the case, chest tubes are inserted and connected to a sealed drainage unit.

Anesthetic

General anesthesia is given with insertion of a double-lumen endotracheal tube for one-lung ventilation; muscle relaxants are given. An epidural or patient-controlled analgesia may facilitate postoperative pain management.

Positioning

The patient is placed in a lateral decubitus position, with the affected lung in the nondependent position.

Anesthetic Implications

Patients in whom pulmonary resection is necessary have a high prevalence of significant coexisting cardiac and pulmonary diseases. Following resection, acute respiratory insufficiency is the most serious complication. Partial airway obstruction and aspiration from an incompetent glottis can be seen postoperatively. Major causes of death include respiratory failure, pneumonia, pulmonary embolism, and myocardial infarction.

When resecting the left upper lobe of the lung, the risk of significant hemorrhage is high, owing to accidental injury of the anterior pulmonary arteries. For this reason, the patients' blood should be typed and cross-matched prior to transport to the OR. There is

also risk of injury to the recurrent laryngeal nerve, causing ipsilateral vocal cord paralysis.

Resection of the left upper lobe of the lung is an indication for a right-sided endobronchial tube. In such a case, the right lung will be the inflated/ventilated lung.

The surgeon may ask for a pressure stress test of the resection suture line. Close off the pop-off valve and inflate the lung to 35–40 mm Hg of peak pressure, essentially creating Valsalva pressure. The surgeon will then check the suture line for bubbling air leaks. If the surgeon fills the chest cavity with warm fluids to assist with verification of the suture line, careful monitoring of the patient's cardiac status to avoid arrhythmias and hypotension is necessary.

Temperature loss is common with an open-chest procedure. Upper- and lower-body warming blankets are needed as well as fluid warmers. The ambient temperature in the room may also need to be warmed.

Lung Biopsy

Lung biopsy involves removal of a small piece of lung tissue, which can then be examined microscopically. A lung biopsy is performed to diagnose certain lung conditions, including lung cancer, pulmonary fibrosis, sarcoidosis, and pneumonia, or to evaluate abnormalities seen on other tests (e.g., chest X-ray or CT scan).

Operative Procedure

Four techniques for biopsy are commonly used:

- *Bronchoscopy.* This method may be used if an infectious disease is suspected, if the abnormal lung tissue is located in the bronchi, or before trying more invasive techniques, such as the needle biopsy.
- *Needle biopsy.* With this technique, a needle is inserted into the chest wall and aspirated to remove the lung tissue. This method is most often used if the abnormal lung tissue is

located next to the chest wall. A CT scan, ultrasound, or fluoroscopy is used to guide the needle to the abnormal tissue.

- *Open biopsy.* With this technique, a small incision is made between the ribs and a small sample of lung tissue is removed. This method is often used after other methods of getting a biopsy have failed, if they are not feasible, or when a larger piece of tissue is needed for diagnosis.
- *VATS.* A small incision is made in the chest wall, through which a telescope is passed to visualize the abnormal tissue. Additional small incisions may be made to allow passage of instruments into the chest cavity to remove the tissue.

Anesthetic
- Bronchoscopy: airway topicalization, sedation, or GETA
- Needle biopsy: local anesthesia
- Open biopsy/VATS: GETA, double-lumen endotracheal tube, muscle relaxation

An epidural or patient-controlled IV analgesia may facilitate postoperative pain management in an open biopsy or VATS procedure.

Positioning
For bronchoscopy and needle biopsy, the patient will most likely remain in the supine position. For open biopsy or VATS, the patient will be placed in the lateral decubitus position with the affected lung in the nondependent position following induction.

Anesthetic Implications
One or two large-bore peripheral IVs are needed.

Complications
During this procedure, patients are at risk for pneumothorax requiring chest tube placement, bleeding, bronchospasm, and arrhythmias.

Lung Volume Reduction Surgery (Reduction Pneumoplasty)

Lung volume reduction surgery (LVRS) involves reduction of the size of the lungs in patients with severe emphysema by removing approximately 30% of the most diseased lung tissue, allowing the healthier lung tissue to perform more optimally. This procedure is performed to improve the quality of life for individuals with severe emphysema. It is *not* a cure for emphysema, but may be considered as an alternative to lung transplantation in this patient population. Additionally, this procedure may allow the diaphragm to return to its normal shape and allow the patient's breathing to normalize. LVRS is usually not done bilaterally.

Operative Procedure
One-lung ventilation is required. This procedure can be done with an open thoracotomy or VATS procedure.

In an *open thoracotomy,* through a median sternotomy, the diseased portions of the operative lung are resected surgically by thermal laser. Usually 20% to 30% of lung tissue is removed. Multiple materials can be used to support or strengthen the staple line of the lung; bovine pericardium is a popular choice, but Gortex and other materials may be used.

In a *VATS approach,* port incisions are made; instrumentation is inserted to facilitate manipulation of the lung. Forceps grasp the portion of the lung to be resected and a stapler is used to close 30% of lung. Bovine pericardium often used to support the staple line of the lung, but other materials may be used.

The surgeon may request that anesthesia personnel hand-ventilate the patient's lungs and hold pressure at 20 cm Hg to test for staple line leaks. The pleura and chest wall are closed in a normal fashion. One or two chest tubes are commonly placed at the end of the procedure, as prolonged air leaks are a common side effect of LVRS. The chest tube is attached to suction so that pleural cavity pressures do not disrupt the suture lines of the lung.

If bilateral lungs require LVRS, the reductions are almost always done in two separate procedures.

Anesthetic

General anesthesia is given with insertion of a double-lumen endotracheal tube; muscle relaxants are given. An epidural or patient-controlled analgesia may facilitate postoperative pain management.

Positioning

Place the patient lateral decubitus, with the operative lung in the nondependent position.

Anesthetic Implications

The goal is to have these patients emerge from anesthesia immediately after surgery, with extubation occurring as soon as possible, preferably in the operating room.

Temperature loss is common with an open-chest procedure. Upper- and lower-body warming blankets are needed as well as fluid warmers. The ambient temperature in the room may also need to be warmed.

Monitors and IV Access

Arterial line placement can facilitate careful blood pressure monitoring as well as allow for regular arterial blood gases monitoring, which can indicate the patient's oxygenation and ventilation.

Complications

Complications of LVRS may include pneumonia, bleeding, stroke, and myocardial infarction.

Pneumonectomy

Pneumonectomy consists of removal of one of the lungs. Lung removal may be necessitated by bronchogenic carcinoma, extensive unilateral tuberculosis, some benign tumors, bronchiectasis, or multiple lung abscesses. Pneumonectomy is usually performed for centrally located lesions that cannot be adequately resected by lobectomy. These patients will have had pulmonary function tests (PFTs) to determine if they will be able to remain oxygenated when one entire lung is removed.

Operative Procedure

In an *open* procedure, a posterolateral thoracotomy is made and the mediastinal pleura is dissected free. The bronchus, pulmonary artery, and superior and inferior pulmonary veins are isolated. The pulmonary artery and veins are ligated. The bronchial stump is clamped, transsected, and sutured closed. Lymph-node tissue is excised.

Pneumonectomy can also be done using a video-assisted thoracoscopic approach (VATS). Three ports are inserted and a submammary incision is made. A grasper is used to seize and retract the lung. Major vessels are dissected, divided, and stapled. The main stem bronchus is exposed, peribronchial nodes are removed, and the bronchus is stapled and divided. The superior pulmonary vein is divided, periaortic nodes excised, and the specimen removed through the incision.

A chest tube may or may not be inserted to create a slightly negative pressure in the affected pleural space to stabilize the mediastinum, but suction is *not* applied to the system. A chest tube may not be placed, however, as fluid typically "fills up" the empty hemithorax after lung removal.

Anesthetic

General anesthesia is given with insertion of a double-lumen endobronchial tube; muscle relaxants are given. If the left lung is to be removed, a right-sided double-lumen endobronchial tube must be used. Thoracic epidurals are typically placed for postoperative pain management. See "Anesthesia for Thoracic Surgeries: Key Points" earlier in this chapter for more information.

Positioning

The patient is placed lateral decubitus, with the affected side in the nondependent position.

Anesthetic Implications

The surgeon may ask for a pressure stress test of the pneumonectomy suture line. Close off the pop-off valve and inflate the lung to 20–30 mm Hg of peak pressure, essentially creating Valsalva pressure. The surgeon will check the suture line for bubbling air leaks. Alternatively, the surgeon may test for air leaks by filling the chest with warm saline and observing for bubbles when the anesthesia provider administers positive-pressure ventilation. If the surgeon does instill warm fluids into the chest cavity, careful monitoring of the patient's cardiac status to avoid arrhythmias and hypotension is necessary.

Temperature loss is common with an open-chest procedure. Upper- and lower-body warming blankets are needed as well as fluid warmers. The ambient temperature in the room may also need to be warmed.

Monitors and IV Access

An arterial line should be placed in the dependent upper extremity, either prior to induction or immediately after induction/intubation.

A central line with central venous pressure monitoring is advantageous in monitoring fluid volume status. Also, a central line and/or large-bore IV will allow for easy transfusion of blood products if the vasculature is inadvertently compromised.

IV Fluids and Volume Requirements

Careful fluid management is required as these patients are at increased risk for adult respiratory distress syndrome (ARDS). Patients should be kept vascularly "dry" both throughout the procedure and into the postoperative recovery area. Blood loss is ideally replaced with colloids (e.g., packed red blood cells) rather than crystalloids.

Complications

Injury to the vagus nerve is possible. Manifestations of vagus nerve injury may include bradycardia, hypotension, respiratory compromise, and gastroparesis.

Pneumonectomy is associated with a greater risk of complications than lobectomy, including pulmonary hypertension and right heart failure, pulmonary edema, dysrhythmias, and cardiac herniation into the pleural space. A greater incidence of complications is observed with removal of the right lung (55% of the total lung capacity). When the right lung is removed, the lymphatic system is disturbed and fluid can build up in the chest.

Cardiac herniation—a rare complication—manifests rapidly due to compression of the superior and inferior vena cava with an acute decrease in systemic venous return, causing severe hypotension with the potential for cardiac arrest. This problem is most likely to occur in the immediate postoperative period. The risk of cardiac herniation increases if the patient is placed in the lateral position with the postoperative side down.

Pneumonectomy with Extrapleural Resection

In this variation of pneumonectomy, radical pulmonary resection is done along with removal of the parietal and visceral pleura, mediastinal pleura, the pericardium, and the diaphragm. This procedure is used to treat malignant pleural mesothelioma.

Operative Procedure

A posterolateral thoracotomy incision is made, typically in the fifth intercostal space. During extrapleural dissection, care is taken to avoid entering into the pleural cavity to avoid spillage of malignant cells into the operative field. The superior component of the dissection is done first, with care being taken to avoid injury to the internal mammary artery and vein. Medial resection occurs from -the apex of the lung to the azygos vein. The mediastinal pleura is then dissected free from the superior vena cava and the azygos vein. The pericardium at the level of the azygos vein is opened to determine myocardial involvement, if any. If no myocardial involvement is found, the pericardiotomy is extended. Intrapericardially, the pulmonary artery and the superior and inferior vena cava and superior and inferior pulmonary veins are dissected free.

The diaphragm is excised starting anteriorly and working posteriorly. After the diaphragm dissection is completed, a complete mediastinal lymphadenectomy is completed and the thoracic duct (AKA left lymphatic duct, the largest lymphatic conduit in the body) is ligated to prevent postoperative chylothorax (lymphatic fluid [chyle] collects in the pleural cavity that can cause a type of pleural effusion). The right pulmonary artery and the superior and inferior pulmonary veins are ligated. The specimen is then retracted anteriorly, and the main stem bronchus is stapled and the specimen removed.

Prior to closure, a tissue flap is used to cover the bronchial stump and the pericardium and diaphragm are reconstructed, often with synthetic materials. Chest tubes are inserted at the end of the case.

Anesthetic
General anesthesia is given with insertion of a double-lumen endotracheal tube; muscle relaxants are given. A thoracic epidural is typically provided for postoperative pain management. See "Anesthesia for Thoracic Surgeries: Key Points" earlier in this chapter for more information.

Positioning
The patient is placed lateral decubitus, with the affected side in the nondependent position.

Anesthetic Implications
Placement of a nasogastric tube during induction can facilitate surgical palpation of the esophagus during dissection. After dissection is complete, the surgeon may request administration of IV steroids.

This procedure has a large potential for massive blood loss, especially if compromise occurs to the pulmonary artery, superior or inferior vena cava, superior or inferior pulmonary veins or the aorta (with a left pneumonectomy). For this reason, blood typing and cross-matching should be done prior to surgery.

Any atrial arrhythmias noted perioperatively should be treated aggressively to prevent cardiac dysfunction. This procedure is associated with high morbidity and mortality.

Temperature loss is common with an open-chest procedure. Upper- and lower-body warming blankets are needed as well as fluid warmers. The ambient temperature in the room may also need to be warmed.

Monitors and IV Access
An arterial line should be placed in the dependent upper extremity, either prior to induction or immediately after induction/intubation.

A central line with central venous pressure monitoring can facilitate monitoring of the patient's fluid volume status. Also, a central line and/or large-bore IV will allow for easy transfusion of blood products if the vasculature is inadvertently compromised.

IV Fluids and Volume Requirements
A negative fluid balance (dry intravascularly) should be maintained postoperatively to prevent post-pneumonectomy pulmonary edema.

Complications
Complications associated with this procedure are similar to those for pneumonectomy without extrapleural resection. Specific to this surgical population, however, is the risk for postoperative hypotension after the patient is placed in the supine position, due to the reconstruction of the pericardium. If the hypotension is uncorrectable, the patient may be experiencing a pericardial patch that is too tight or cardiac herniation secondary to dehiscence of the pericardial patch. In such a case, the patient should be placed in the lateral position and taken to the OR.

Segmental Resection
Segmental resection involves excision of anatomic subdivisions of the pulmonary lobes that contain diseased lung tissue, with ligation of segmental branches of the pulmonary artery and vein. This

procedure is performed to treat bronchiectasis, cysts or blebs, benign or metastatic tumors, and tuberculosis.

The individual lobes of the lung can be divided primarily by the anatomy of the blood supply. The limited resection involved in segmental resection is associated with decreased morbidity due to lung tissue conservation.

Operative Procedure

A posterolateral incision is made over the affected lung, and the segmental pulmonary vein and segmental branches of the pulmonary artery are ligated. The segmental bronchus is isolated and transsected, and the bronchial stump is sutured or stapled closed. The suture line is tested for air leaks (see the discussion of lobectomy earlier in this chapter). Chest tubes are inserted at the end of the case and connected to a sealed drainage unit.

Limited resections may be performed via a thoracotomy or video-assisted thoracoscopy (VATS).

Anesthetic

General anesthesia is given with insertion of a double-lumen endotracheal tube; muscle relaxants are given. An epidural or patient-controlled analgesia may facilitate postoperative pain management.

Positioning

The patient is placed lateral decubitus, with the affected side in the nondependent position.

Anesthetic Implications

X-ray films should be available in the operating room prior to the start of the case.

The patient's blood should be typed and screened, with two units of blood cross-matched and made available in the OR prior to starting the case. Hemorrhage is possible due to the increased vascularity associated with malignancy or inflammation.

Patient difficulty with postoperative coughing and deep breathing may increase secondary to pain from the incision site. Consideration to preoperative placement of a thoracic epidural for pain management may

facilitate pulmonary toileting postoperatively. See "Anesthesia for Thoracic Surgeries: Key Points" earlier in this chapter for more information.

The surgeon may ask for a pressure stress test of the pneumonectomy suture line. Close off the pop-off valve and inflate the lung to 20–30 mm Hg of peak pressure, essentially creating Valsalva pressure. The surgeon will check the suture line for bubbling air leaks. Alternatively, the surgeon may test for air leaks by filling the chest with warm saline and observing for bubbles when the anesthesia provider administers positive-pressure ventilation. If the surgeon does instill warm fluids into the chest cavity, careful monitoring of the patient's cardiac status to avoid arrhythmias and hypotension is necessary.

Temperature loss is common with an open-chest procedure. Upper- and lower-body warming blankets are needed as well as fluid warmers. The ambient temperature in the room may also need to be warmed.

Monitors and IV Access

Arterial line placement can facilitate careful blood pressure monitoring as well as allow for regular arterial blood gases monitoring, which can indicate the patient's oxygenation/ventilation status. Placement of the arterial line in the dependent arm not only improves stability of the site, but also ensures that any compression of that arm will be manifested as a flattened arterial waveform.

Wedge Resection

Wedge resection involves excision of a small wedge-shaped portion of the lung periphery containing a well-circumscribed lesion. This procedure is used to remove a contained pulmonary lesion for diagnostic or therapeutic purposes—for example, a primary benign or malignant lesion, metastatic malignant lesions, a localized infectious lesion, and bullae.

Operative Procedure

Depending on the location of the lesion and the level of exposure, a full or "mini" posterolateral thoracotomy may be performed. Clamps are placed outside the margins of the lesion and the peripheral lung tissue is excised. The lung tissue held in the clamps is sutured, and the suture line is tested for air leaks. Chest tubes are inserted at the end of the case and connected to a sealed drainage unit.

Limited resections can be performed via a thoracotomy or video-assisted thoracoscopy (VATS).

When wedge resection is done under *thoracoscopy,* a port is inserted at the fifth or sixth intercostal space (ICS), then at the fourth or fifth ICS anterior axillary line, and at the seventh or eighth ICS midaxillary line. A grasper is used to grab the affected site, and a staple line is placed to give a clear margin from the lesion. A second or third staple line completes the wedge. The specimen is retrieved in a specimen bag. The suture line is then tested for air leaks, and a chest tube is inserted at the end of the case and connected to a sealed drainage system.

A *median sternotomy incision* may be used in a patient with marginal lung function, as this approach helps the patient return to normal pulmonary function more quickly.

Anesthetic

General anesthesia is given with insertion of a double-lumen endotracheal tube; muscle relaxants are given. Resection of the left upper lobe of the lung is an indication for a right-sided endobronchial tube; the right lung will be the inflated/ventilated lung. Preoperative placement of a thoracic epidural aids in postoperative pain control and facilitates deep breathing and effective coughing. See "Anesthesia for Thoracic Surgeries: Key Points" earlier in this chapter for more information.

Positioning

The patient is placed lateral decubitus, with the affected side in the nondependent position.

Anesthetic Implications

Patients who undergo pulmonary resection have a high prevalence of significant coexisting cardiac and pulmonary diseases. Following resection, acute respiratory insufficiency is the most serious complication in this population. Partial airway obstruction and aspiration from an incompetent glottis may be seen postoperatively. Major causes of death in such cases include respiratory failure, pneumonia, pulmonary embolism, and myocardial infarction.

The surgeon may ask for a pressure stress test of the pneumonectomy suture line. Close off the pop-off valve and inflate the lung to 20–30 mm Hg of peak pressure, essentially creating Valsalva pressure. The surgeon will check the suture line for bubbling air leaks. Alternatively, the surgeon may test for air leaks by filling the chest with warm saline and observing for bubbles when the anesthesia provider administers positive-pressure ventilation. If the surgeon does instill warm fluids into the chest cavity, careful monitoring of the patient's cardiac status to avoid arrhythmias and hypotension is necessary.

The patient's blood should be typed and screened, with two units of blood cross-matched and made available in the OR prior to starting the case.

Temperature loss is common with an open-chest procedure. Upper- and lower-body warming blankets are needed as well as fluid warmers. The ambient temperature in the room may also need to be warmed.

Monitors and IV Access

Arterial line placement can facilitate careful blood pressure monitoring as well as allow for regular arterial blood gases monitoring, which can indicate the patient's oxygenation/ventilation status. Placement of the arterial line in the dependent arm not only improves stability of the site, but also ensures that any compression of that arm will be manifested as a flattened arterial waveform.

Complications

Following resection of the left upper lobe of the lung, the risk of significant hemorrhage is high secondary to accidental injury of the anterior pulmonary arteries.

Wedge resection is also associated with a risk of damage to the recurrent laryngeal nerve, resulting in ipsilateral vocal cord paralysis. Careful assessment of the airway and the patient's ability to protect the airway should be completed prior to extubation.

Thoracostomy (Chest Tube)

Placement of a chest tube is a short-term method of providing drainage of air or fluid from the pleural space. Chest tube thoracostomy (commonly referred to as "putting in a chest tube") involves placing a hollow plastic tube between the ribs and into the chest to drain fluid or air from around the lungs. The tube is often hooked up to suction to help with drainage. Drainage may be necessary due to large or recurrent pleural effusions, pneumothorax, empyema, or hemothorax.

Operative Procedure

A 2-cm skin incision is made at the fourth intercostal space for pneumothorax or at the fifth or sixth intercostal space for fluid drainage. The intercostal soft tissue down to the pleura is bluntly dissected, and the pleura is perforated. A thoracostomy tube is inserted through the tract and directed inferoposteriorly for effusions or apically for pneumothorax. The thoracostomy tube is sutured to the chest wall, and a sterile dressing with petroleum gauze is placed over the insertion site to seal the wound. Finally, the thoracostomy tube is connected to a sealed drainage system.

Anesthetic

Commonly, chest tube placement occurs at the end of a thoracic procedure. If a thoracostomy tube is to be inserted without concurrent procedures, local anesthesia with or without monitored anesthesia care should be provided.

Positioning

If the thoracostomy tube is placed in the operating room following thoracic surgery, the tube may be inserted while the patient is in the lateral decubitus position. If the thoracostomy tube is inserted without concurrent procedure, the patient will be in the supine position, with or without placement of a positioning device to tilt the patient so that the operative side is in the nondependent position.

Anesthetic Implications

One peripheral IV is usually all that is needed.

Complications

Potential complications of thoracostomy tube placement include malpositioning of the tube; clotting, kinking or dislodgement of the tube; infection; and pulmonary or diaphragmatic laceration.

Thoracotomy

In a thoracotomy, an incision is made into the chest wall to allow visualization into the chest cavity. Thoracotomy allows for examination of the lungs, removal of part or all of a lung, removal of a rib or ribs, or examination, treatment, or removal of any organs in the chest cavity. In addition to the lungs, a thoracotomy incision provides access to the heart, esophagus, diaphragm, and a portion of the aorta.

Lung cancer is the most common reason for thoracotomy, as this procedure allows for both biopsies and resections.

An emergency thoracotomy may be performed on a patient in extremis following chest injury. In this case, a thoracotomy is used to access the chest cavity to control injury-related bleeding from the heart, to initiate cardiac compressions, or to relieve pressure on the heart from cardiac tamponade

Chest wall resection may be required for the management of benign or malignant thoracic diseases. When the disease process is limited to the pleura, chest resection with parietal pleurectomy may be adequate. For disease processes that are not confined, pulmonary resection as well as removal of involved intercostal muscles and ribs may be necessary. If ribs must be resected, they can be disarticulated from the vertebral column.

Operative Procedure

A thoracotomy may be performed in a variety of ways. An *axillary* thoracotomy is made on the patient's side underneath the arm. A *posterolateral* thoracotomy is a slanted incision traversing from the patient's back to the patient's side. Finally, an *anterolateral* thoracotomy is made under the patient's breast. The type of thoracotomy depends on the reason for the surgery.

When possible, the incision is made through the intercostal space so as to preserve nerves, muscle, and bone. Typical thoracotomy incisions range in length from 5 to 10 inches.

Anesthetic

General anesthesia is given with insertion of a double-lumen endotracheal tube; muscle relaxants are given. An epidural or patient-controlled analgesia may facilitate postoperative pain management.

Positioning

The patient is placed lateral decubitus, with the affected side in the nondependent position.

Anesthetic Implications

A thoracotomy may affect the patient's efforts to cough and deep breath postoperatively. Preoperative placement of a thoracic epidural for pain control may facilitate pulmonary toileting following surgery.

The patient's blood should be typed and screened, with two units of blood cross-matched and made available in the OR prior to starting the case.

Bradycardia from vagal nerve stimulation can be elicited during chest wall dissection.

Temperature loss is common with an open-chest procedure. Upper- and lower-body warming blankets are needed as well as fluid warmers. The ambient temperature in the room may also need to be warmed.

Monitors and IV Access

An arterial line is typically placed in the dependent arm to promote stability of the line and to allow for monitoring of compression of the arteries in the dependent arm. If the procedure is expected to be prolonged in duration or involve large fluid shifts, placement of a central line to transducer central venous pressure is beneficial for determining the patient's fluid status.

Complications

Thoracotomy is associated with a significant risk of bleeding or hemorrhage secondary to accidental injury of the major vascular structures in the chest cavity.

Video-Assisted Thoracoscopic Surgery

Video-assisted thoracoscopic surgery (VATS) involves endoscopic visualization of the pleural space(s) with the ability to provide a video feed in the OR and record the surgery and its findings. This approach allows for visualization and inspection of the entire hemothorax.

VATS is used for the diagnosis and treatment of numerous pleural and intrapleural conditions, including diseases of the pleura, mediastinum, pericardium, esophagus, lungs, and thoracic trauma. Tissue sampling, drainage of fluid collections, and surgical resections can all be performed via a VATS procedure. This procedure is also indicated when noninvasive or minimally invasive diagnostic procedures have not yielded sufficient information and for treatment of patients with reduced pulmonary function for whom the risks associated with thoracotomy are too great. In patients with severe cardiopulmonary disease, the VATS procedure may be better tolerated than an open thoracotomy.

Operative Procedure

The first thoroscopic port is established at the level of the fourth to seventh intercostal space, in the midaxillary to posterior axillary line. A telescope is inserted into this port and used to visualize the chest cavity during placement of additional ports. Two or three other ports are placed based on the location of the lesion. Endoscopic instruments are deployed through the ports to retract, dissect, ligate, excise, and suture the tissues. Limited exposure can be accomplished without spreading the ribs. Specimens are removed in a specimen bag to prevent seeding of malignant cells or infectious materials. Larger specimens are removed through a larger incision. At the end of the procedure, a chest tube may be inserted and connected to a sealed drainage unit.

Anesthetic

General anesthesia is given with insertion of a double-lumen endotracheal tube; muscle relaxants are given. An epidural or patient-controlled analgesia may facilitate postoperative pain management.

A very limited procedure may be done under local anesthesia and sedation with or without regional blockade.

Positioning

The patient is placed lateral decubitus, with the affected side in the nondependent position.

Anesthetic Implications

The patient's X-rays (or CT, PET scans, MRI, or other images) should be available in the OR prior to the start of surgery.

Approximately 35% of VATS procedures require conversion to open thoracotomy. The anesthesia provider must be prepared to adjust the anesthetic plan at any time.

The patient's blood should be typed and screened, and two units of blood cross-matched and made available in the OR prior to surgery.

Contraindications to VATS include lesions in close proximity to the great vessels and patients who cannot tolerate one-lung ventilation.

Monitors

An arterial line is typically placed in the dependent arm to promote stability of the line and to allow for monitoring of compression of the arteries in the dependent arm in the lateral decubitus position.

Complications

Potential complications with a VATS procedure include hemorrhage, air embolism, diaphragmatic injury, and injury to adjacent organs.

THORACIC SURGERY

Mediastinal Anatomy

Functionally, the mediastinum is divided into the anterior, middle, and posterior divisions based on their relationship to the heart. Defects usually develop in only one division. Further, mediastinal diseases fall into three major categories: masses, infections, and pneumomediastinum.

- *Anterior:* lymphomas, lymphangiomas, teratomas, thymomas, and thymic cysts. These lesions may present as compression of pulmonary or vascular structures (e.g., superior vena caval syndrome, cardiac tamponade, and lung compression and distal airway obstructions).
- *Middle:* bronchogenic cysts (usually next to the trachea or main stem bronchi at the level of the carina and potentially able to produce sudden, life-threatening airway obstruction), granulomas, and lymphomas. These masses are approached through a posterolateral thoracotomy or thoracoscopically.
- *Posterior:* enteric cysts and tumors of neurogenic origin (neuroblastoma, ganglioneuroma, neurofibroma). Posterior mediastinal masses may cause Horner's syndrome when excised.

Preoperative evaluation is crucial to successfully anesthetizing and managing the airway of patients with mediastinal pathology. The anesthetists should carefully note any signs of airway obstruction (e.g., stridor, wheezing, cyanosis, atelectasis, pneumonia) and signs of respiratory distress or compromise during position changes. CT scans of the chest are invaluable in assessing the mediastinum and should be carefully examined prior to initiating anesthesia.

Sympathetic tone is diminished with anesthesia and may cause cardiovascular decompensation. Ketamine and narcotic-based induction can be used to avoid cardiovascular compromise in patients at risk.

Patients at risk for airway compromise (due to compression or shifting of the airway by the mediastinal pathology) may benefit from mask induction with 100% FiO_2 and a volatile agent while in a sitting position. When the patient is in this position, the mass is unable to compress the airway. Use of muscle relaxants during induction with these patients should be determined on a case-by-case basis based on each patient's pathology and risk of relaxed tissues leading to further airway compromise.

Mediastinal Tumor Excision: Open Approach

This procedure involves removal of a benign or malignant anterior mediastinal mass or thymoma. If left in place, these tumors or thymomas may spread to the heart or begin to compress the spinal cord.

Operative Procedure

Traditional resection requires a median sternotomy so that the surgeon can access the anterior mediastinum. An alternative technique involves use of a VATS procedure, although this approach is limited by tumor location and size and the structures around the mass or thymoma. The mass may need to be dissected away from major nerves, arteries, the heart, and the airway, regardless of the surgical approach. At the end of the procedure, a chest tube is inserted and connected to a sealed drainage unit.

Anesthetic

General anesthesia is given with insertion of a single-lumen endotracheal tube; muscle relaxants are given. An epidural may be beneficial for postoperative pain control.

Positioning

The patient is positioned supine, with bilateral arms padded and tucked at the sides.

Anesthetic Implications

Prior to induction, the anesthesia provider must carefully examine the patient's airway for any risk of compromise after induction/muscle relaxation and for any tracheal deviation. Careful communication with the surgeon as to the likelihood of airway compromise with induction should be discussed prior to taking the patient to the operating room. If a significant risk for airway compromise is likely, a predetermined plan of action should be identified prior to entry into the OR, including, but not limited to, awake fiberoptic intubation and elective tracheostomy.

Multiple anatomic structures are at risk for trauma during mediastinal excision surgery, including the innominate vein and artery, the right atrium, the esophagus, and the spinal cord. Due to the increased risk of bleeding, the patient's blood should be typed and screened, and cross-matched blood should be immediately available.

Temperature loss is common with an open-chest procedure. Upper- and lower-body warming blankets are needed as well as fluid warmers. The ambient temperature in the room may also need to be warmed.

Monitors and IV Access

Two large-bore intravenous lines should be placed prior to incision. An arterial line should be placed to facilitate careful blood pressure monitoring as well as allow for regular arterial blood gases monitoring, which will indicate the patient's oxygenation and ventilation. Depending upon the patient's comorbid conditions and stability at the time of surgery, a central line may be beneficial.

Thymectomy

Thymectomy is the removal of the thymus gland. This procedure is undertaken to remove benign or malignant tumors of the thymus gland, or to alleviate the symptoms of myasthenia gravis.

Operative Procedure

The most common approach is usually a full or partial midline sternotomy to access the thymus gland, which is located just below the sternum. An alternative approach is a transverse cervical neck incision, although it is used much less commonly.

The mediastinal fat pad is incised and the thymus gland is dissected away from the underlying pericardium and mediastinal pleura. Vascular attachments, such as the internal mammary arteries and the innominate vein, are ligated. If either pleural space is entered, a chest tube is inserted and connected to a sealed drainage system. Sternal wires are used to close the chest.

Thymectomy may also be done by video-assisted thoracoscopic surgery. In such a case, the patient should be intubated with a double-lumen endobronchial tube for the VATS procedure.

Anesthetic

General anesthesia is given with insertion of a single-lumen endotracheal tube (for open procedure); muscle relaxants are given.

Positioning

The patient is placed in a supine position for an open procedure. Discuss with the surgeon whether the patient's arms should be tucked at his or her sides with armboards, as in cardiac surgery, or whether the arms should be extended less than 90 degrees on armboards.

Anesthetic Implications

When a thymectomy is done to treat myasthenia gravis, the possibility of respiratory compromise must be anticipated. Careful assessment of the airway prior to extubation at the end of the case is paramount, as residual weakness may require prolonged intubation. Additionally, the phrenic nerve is at increased risk for intraoperative damage due to its close proximity to the surgical site. Careful titration of anticholinesterase therapy in the postoperative period may aid in minimizing patient weakness and support earlier extubation.

Patients with myasthenia gravis are particularly sensitive to nondepolarizing muscle relaxants. In general, *long-acting* nondepolarizing medications are not used in these patients, and nondepolarizers of *moderate duration* are given in smaller than normal dosages. Conversely, patients with myasthenia gravis are more likely to show resistance to depolarizing agents, including succinylcholine (Anectine). In this population, the dose of succinylcholine for rapid-sequence intubation is typically 1.5–2 mg/kg body weight.

Because this surgery is done in close proximity to the great vessels, the patient's blood should be type and screened, with cross-matched blood made available in the OR prior to the start of the surgery.

Temperature loss is common with an open-chest procedure. Upper- and lower-body warming blankets are needed as well as fluid warmers. The ambient temperature in the room may also need to be warmed.

Tracheal Tumor Resection

In tracheal tumor resection, a portion of the trachea that is diseased (stenosis) or contains tumor growth is removed.

Operative Procedure

A rigid bronchoscope is passed immediately into the airway after induction to assess the trachea. An incision is made over the neck, and the diseased segment of the trachea is separated away from the healthy trachea. An armored endotracheal tube is inserted by the surgeon into the distal end of the trachea, and a sterile anesthesia circuit is connected to the armored tube to provide for oxygenation and ventilation of the patient. The diseased tracheal segment is then removed and the posterior walls of the remaining healthy trachea are anastomosed.

The anesthesia provider will then insert an oral endotracheal tube, with the assistance of the surgeon, across the suture line into the lower portion of the trachea. The anterior trachea is then anastomosed over the endotracheal tube. Flexing the head sharply forward will assist with the tracheal closure. After the neck is closed, a large retention stitch is placed between the patient's chin and chest, to hold the head in this flexed position and minimize strain in the anastomosis.

Anesthetic
General anesthesia is given with insertion of a single-lumen endotracheal tube; muscle relaxants are given.

Positioning
The patient is placed in a supine position, with bilateral arms tucked at the patient's sides. The head of the operating table may be turned away at least 90 degrees, if not 180 degrees, from the anesthetist.

Anesthetic Implications
Have different sizes of armored endotracheal tubes available (maintain sterile packaging for surgeon use) as well as a sterile anesthesia circuit.

Careful communication between the anesthesia provider and the surgeon is necessary both prior to induction and during induction. The two providers should jointly decide how induction will be accomplished and how the patency of the airway will be maintained until the rigid bronchoscope is in place.

The operating room table is often repositioned or angled away from the anesthesia provider during these cases to allow for increased operative space. The position of the bed should allow for optimal surgical exposure while still allowing the anesthesia provider the ability to place the oral endotracheal tube midway through the surgery.

Temperature loss is common with an open-chest procedure. Upper- and lower-body warming blankets are needed as well as fluid warmers. The ambient temperature in the room may also need to be warmed.

Extubation at the conclusion of the procedure is ideal, as removal of the endotracheal tube limits potential internal irritation to the tracheal anastomosis. However, careful airway assessment to determine readiness for extubation is needed. Reintubation must be done with a flexible fiberoptic approach while maintaining the patient's head and neck in the flexed position.

TRANSPLANTATION
Lung Transplant Recipient
This procedure involves the surgical placement of one or two donated cadaveric lungs after removal of the patient's diseased native lung(s).

When retrieving cadaveric lungs for transplant, the surgeon removes the donor lung with the greatest possible length of main pulmonary artery and bronchus. Lung ischemia time is measured from the time of removal to reperfusion in the recipient. A maximum ischemic time of 4 to 8 hours is essential to limit reperfusion injury.

Unilateral lung transplantation is done for end-stage pulmonary disease, idiopathic pulmonary fibrosis, sarcoidosis, Eisenmenger's syndrome, bronchiolitis obliterans, primary pulmonary hypertension, and eosinophilic granuloma of the lung.

Bilateral lung transplantation is done for severe infection, bronchiectasis (irreversible dilatation of part of the bronchial tree, often from necrotizing bacterial infections), and cystic fibrosis. It is especially indicated for cystic fibrosis patients because of the risk of infectious contamination of the transplanted lung by the native lung.

Operative Procedure
In *single lung transplant,* a transverse thoracotomy is made on the side of the diseased lung. The patient is placed in the lateral position.

In *bilateral lung transplant,* a large clamshell thoracotomy is made across the chest and the patient's native lung is dissected free and removed. Each lung is sequentially removed before introducing each donor lung for anastomosis.

The donated lung is then placed in the recipient's chest and the artery and vein are anastomosed. The lung is then perfused while the bronchial anastomosis is being done. A flap of omentum from the intestine can be excised and wrapped around the bronchial anastomosis for support.

Anesthetic

General anesthesia is given with insertion of a double-lumen endotracheal tube. The choice of a left- or right-sided double-lumen ETT is based on surgeon preference. Fiberoptic bronchoscopy is used to verify correct placement of the tube.

All lung transplant patients are considered "full stomach" cases and require rapid-sequence intubation secondary to their regular preoperative administration of oral immunosuppressants and the emergency nature of procedure.

Positioning

For bilateral lung transplant, the patient is placed in the supine position, with bilateral arms secured above the head (forearms crossed). For unilateral lung transplant, the patient is placed in the lateral position, with the operative lung in the upward position.

Anesthetic Implications

Preoperative sedation should be minimized to avoid respiratory depression. Supplemental oxygen at the same FiO_2 used at home is given en route to the OR, with an ideal SpO_2 goal between 90% and 95%.

Donor lung preservation requires precise fluid administration to prevent pulmonary edema. Central venous pressures ideally should be maintained at less than 10 mm Hg, with a wedge pressure less than 12 mm Hg.

The total lung capacity depends on the size differential between the donor lung and the recipient. If the donor lung is large compared to the space in the patient's chest, it may interfere with venous return by compressing the heart. Height is the single most important indicator of total lung capacity, followed by inframammary chest circumference ratio.

Lung function will vary depending on the ischemic time—that is, the length of time between clamping and removal of the lung from the donor to the time of vascular anastomosis in the recipient. Once the lung vessels are connected in the recipient, "wash-out" of ischemic by-products will occur, and preservative fluid will flow into the circulation. This shock to the system can cause sudden hypotension and increased peak inspiratory pressure. This side effect is generally short-lived but may require boluses of ephedrine (sympathomimetic) to maintain the patient's systolic blood pressure.

Lung transplant patients often exhibit a large ventilation/perfusion mismatch owing to the degree of hypoxic pulmonary vasoconstriction (HPV) after the new lung(s) is transplanted. These patients can be extremely difficult to ventilate; thus good communication between the anesthesia provider and the surgeon regarding oxygen saturations and carbon dioxide levels is required. Both $PaCO_2$ and $ETCO_2$ should be carefully monitored.

Temperature loss is common with an open-chest procedure. Upper- and lower-body warming blankets are needed as well as fluid warmers. The ambient temperature in the room may also need to be warmed.

Monitors and IV Access

- Radial arterial line, preferably on the side opposite from operative lung.
- Central line with central venous pressure monitoring.
- Pulmonary artery catheter. For single-lung transplant patients, the tip of the pulmonary artery catheter should be positioned in the contralateral lung.
- Transesophageal echocardiography (TEE).

- Fiberoptic bronchoscope.
- One or two large-bore peripheral IVs.

IV Vasoactive Agents
- IV pump: phenylephrine, nitroglycerin
- Syringe for bolus: phenylephrine, ephedrine, esmolol (Brevibloc), labetalol, hydralazine

Volume Requirements
Limit fluids. These patients may need diuretics postoperatively.

Induction
A slow, controlled induction is achieved utilizing etomidate 0.2–0.3 mg/kg if the patient's ejection fraction (EF) is less than 30%, thiopental 2–4 mg/kg in 50 mg increments, or ketamine 1–2 mg/kg.

Succinylcholine (Anectine) may be given with a defasiculating dose of rocuronium on induction.

Fentanyl 50–100 mcg/kg should be give for the duration of the case. Place an epidural for postoperative pain control.

Maintenance
Maintenance is accomplished with the judicious use of opioids with a volatile agent. Nitrous oxide is avoided. Transesophageal echocardiography is used to monitor right ventricular function and intracardiac air.

Mechanical ventilation should support tidal volumes of 7–10 mL/kg at a respiratory rate of 10–20 breaths per minute. A slower respiratory rate may be necessary to allow adequate expiratory time so as to prevent gas trapping.

The FiO_2 should be titrated to maintain SpO_2 at more than 96%. Hypercarbia and hypoxia are common problems during removal of the native lung. If oxygen saturation is difficult to maintain, the CRNA, in collaboration with the surgeon, may add CPAP to the nonventilated lung or PEEP to the ventilated lung. Pressure-control ventilation is ideal to minimize trauma to the nontransplanted lung and to decrease pressure on the suture lines of the transplanted lung.

Use intermediate- to long-acting muscle relaxants. Their effects are not reversed at the end of the case.

Emergence
Muscle relaxants may be helpful during transport to the ICU to prevent patient movement.

Postoperative Measures
The patient will remain intubated postoperatively.

CARDIAC SURGERY PEARLS

Have heparin and protamine available for all vascular surgeries. An activated clotting time (ACT) device should be available anytime these drugs are given, to monitor heparin and protamine effect.

KEY CARDIAC SURGERY ANATOMY

- Cardiac baroreceptors: specialized neurons in the aortic arch and carotid sinuses that regulate blood pressure through a negative feedback system (called the baroreflex) mediated by the autonomic nervous system. These mechanoreceptors detect pressure in blood vessels, sending messages to the central nervous system to increase or decrease peripheral resistance and cardiac output.
- Cardiac chemoreceptors: sensory receptors in the aortic arch and carotid artery that can detect chemical stimuli in the arterial blood and create changes in respiratory rate, heart rate, cardiac output and blood pressure.
- Right ventricle (RV): perfused during systole.
- Left ventricle (LV): perfused during diastole.
- Coronary arteries: perfused during diastole and systole; peak perfusion during diastole.

HEART PRESSURES

RAP: right atrial pressure (also known as CVP); range 8–10 mm Hg

RVP: right ventricular pressure; range 15–25/0–8 mm Hg

PAP: pulmonary artery pressures; range 15–25/8–15 mm Hg

PAS: pulmonary artery systolic; range 15–25 mm Hg

PAD: pulmonary artery diastolic; range 8–15 mm Hg

- PAD can be used as an index of left ventricular end diastolic pressure.
- PAD is equal to wedge when the PVR is normal.
- PAD is greater than wedge if the PVR is elevated.

MPAP: mean pulmonary artery pressure; range 10–20 mm Hg

PCWP: pulmonary capillary wedge pressure; range 8–12 mm Hg

LAP: left atrial pressure; range 8–10 mm Hg

FORMULAS

- CO: cardiac output = SV × HR/1000; normal range 4–8 L/min.
- CI: cardiac index = CO/BSA; × normal range 2.0–4.0 L/min/m^2.
- SV: stroke volume; CO/HR × 1000; normal range 60–90 mL/contraction.

  Cause of high SV: bradycardia, decreased afterload, increased venous return, inotropes

  Cause of low SV: acidosis, tamponade, decreased CO/preload, vasodilation, increased afterload

- EF: ejection fraction = SV/EDV; range 0.6–0.7 (60–70%).

  EF < 30%: affects activities of daily living

  EF < 20%: severe effect on activities

- Mean arterial blood pressure:

$$MAP = \frac{SBP + 2(DBP)}{3};$$

normal range 70–105 mm Hg

- Systemic vascular resistance:

$$SVR = \frac{MAP - CVP}{CO} \times 80;$$

normal 900–1500 dynes/sec/cm^5

Cause of high SVR: cardiogenic shock, hypovolemic shock, left ventricular failure, inotropes

Cause of low SVR: anemia, hypoxemia, septic/neurogenic shock, vasodilation

- Pulmonary vascular resistance:

$$PVR = \frac{MPAP - PCWP}{CO} \times 80;$$

normal 50–200 dynes/sec/cm^5

Cause of high PVR: adult respiratory distress syndrome, alveolar hypoxia, mitral stenosis, pulmonary emboli

Cause of low PVR: vasodilation; medications such as Inocor, aminophylline, nitroglycerin, phosphodiesterase

- CPP: Coronary perfusion pressure = DBP − PAD; normal 50–70 mm Hg; PCWP can be substituted for PAD.
- SVO$_2$: venous oxygen content: (MVO$_2$: mixed venous oxygen saturation); an index of cardiac output and overall tissue perfusion. This measure allows minute-to-minute assessment of total tissue oxygen balance (delivery versus consumption) at the tissue level.

MVO$_2$ varies directly with cardiac output, hemoglobin levels, and oxygen saturation.

MVO$_2$ varies inversely with tissue oxygen requirements and oxygen consumption (VO$_2$).

Normal is 65–75%: 25% is extracted and utilized in body tissues. Under normal conditions, if there is 1000 mL of oxygen, 350 mL of oxygen is used by the body's tissues and 650 mL is returned to the lungs; thus normal SVO$_2$ is 65%.

Cause of increased MVO$_2$: check for wedged pulmonary artery catheter (common cause), increased FiO$_2$, methemoglobinemia, sepsis, hypothermia, elevated cardiac output with left-to-right shunts, neuromuscular paralysis (muscles less active), or inotropic drugs.

Cause of decreased MVO$_2$: decreased hemoglobin level, low oxygen saturation (arterial hypoxia), or low cardiac output with myocardial damage, congestive heart failure, hypovolemia, hypoxia, or inadequate pulmonary gas exchange; or increased tissue demand owing to malignant hyperthermia, thyroid storm, shivering, fever, exercise, or agitation.

If the MVO$_2$ falls below 30%, the oxygen balance is compromised and anaerobic metabolism ensues.

- Oxygen consumption of the heart: For every 10°C drop in temperature, metabolic demand requirement decreases by half.

  Normal heart at 37°C: 8–10 mL/100 g of heart muscle/min

  Fibrillating heart at 27°C: 4–5 mL/100 g of heart muscle/min

  Heart in systole at 17°C: 2–2.5 mL/100 g of heart muscle/min

  Heart in ventricular fibrillation: extreme increase in oxygen consumption with decreased supply; must defibrillate quickly

- Myocardial oxygen balance: Myocardial ischemia occurs when demand is greater than supply. The primary anesthetic management goal in patients with coronary artery disease is to maintain the balance between myocardial oxygen supply and demand.

  Improving myocardial oxygen balance by decreasing oxygen demand:
  - Decrease contractility. Negative inotropes: beta-blockers, calcium-channel blockers, sympatholytics. Clonidine is an alpha$_2$ agonist.
  - Decrease the wall tension by decreasing the chamber size (use a vasodilator, diuretic).
  - Slow the heart rate: An increased heart rate causes the greatest increase in myocardial oxygen consumption. Two-thirds of the heart cycle is diastole: When the coronary arteries are filling, by slowing the heart rate, the coronary arteries have more time to fill, so they get more oxygen (use beta-blockers).

Improving myocardial oxygen balance by increasing oxygen supply:
  - Increase FiO$_2$.
  - Keep hematocrit within acceptable levels.
  - Slow the heart rate.

ANESTHETICS AND THE HEART

Assessment of LV function (ejection fraction) determines the patient's cardiac reserve and suggests the best anesthetic to use. It also predicts the type of support needed for separation from cardiopulmonary bypass.

The primary effect of all volatile anesthetics is myocardial depression, through depression of SA node automaticity. In terms of their ability to produce myocardial depression, anesthetic agents have the following strengths: enflurane > halothane = desflurane > isoflurane = sevoflurane. Some studies suggest that all volatile anesthetics depress cardiac contractility by decreasing the entry of calcium into cells during depolarization.

Coronary vasodilators have the following strengths: isoflurane > halothane = enflurane > sevoflurane. Minimal vasodilation occurs with desflurane and nitrous oxide.

Opioids, especially fentanyl and sufentanil, can depress cardiac conduction. Ketamine has the least effect on cardiac contractility, but is still a negative inotrope.

CONDUCTION DISTURBANCES

Preoperatively, the patient's current medications should be continued and electrolyte levels

MYOCARDIAL OXYGEN SUPPLY	MYOCARDIAL OXYGEN DEMAND (CAUSE OF CONSUMPTION)
Heart rate	Contractile state
Hemoglobin levels	Increased heart rate (increased work, decreased coronary artery filling time)
Coronary artery oxygen	Myocardial wall tension
	Increased preload or afterload
	Increased contractility

(especially potassium levels) should be reviewed to look for any potential effects that may impair pacemaker capture or enhance arrhythmias.

General Pacemaker Information

Pacing electrodes are attached to an electrical pulse generator that is preset to deliver an impulse at a specific rate and amplitude. Some pacemaker generators are set up so that they can also sense the heart's intrinsic electrical activity and suppress its next impulse. A generator's sensing threshold can be altered so that it can function in a fixed mode (asynchronous—provides electrical impulses without regard to intrinsic electrical activity) or demand mode (synchronous—senses the intrinsic electrical activity and provides impulses or inhibition).

Pacemaker Terms

Output: pulse amplitude.

Rate: frequency.

Pulse width: duration.

mA (milliamps): the threshold to pace. To test the threshold, increase the pacemaker heart rate higher than the native rhythm with the mA at maximum setting, then decrease the mA level at which loss of capture occurs. Give the lowest mA possible to achieve the desired result.

Automatic Interval (AI): time in milliseconds between successive pacemaker impulses. Divide AI into 60,000 to determine the heart rate.

Hysteresis: difference between the escape and automatic interval that allows the patient's HR to decrease below the automatic interval before the pacemaker is activated. For example, a 10-beat hysteresis allows the patient's rate to fall to 65 before activating pacing at 75.

R-wave sensitivity: number of R-wave millivolts required to activate the sensing circuit and, in turn, inhibit the pacing circuit. The amplitude of the R wave sensed must be greater than the programmed R-wave sensitivity.

Slew rate: rate of voltage change of the R wave of the ventricular electrocardiogram. It allows T waves and myopotentials, such as those associated with shivering, *not* to be recognized as R waves.

Triggered pacemaker: a pacemaker that detects R waves (spontaneous depolarization) and instantaneously triggers an impulse that delivers an electrical pulse to the heart exactly at the peak of every R wave on the ECG.

Inhibited pacemaker: a pacemaker that detects R waves, compares them to the programmed standard, and inactivates the pacing circuit (withholds the stimulus) upon sensing a spontaneous depolarization.

Pacemaker Lead Types

- Unipolar lead system: a negative electrode in the heart; positive electrode in the generator.
- Bipolar lead system: both electrodes are located 1–2 cm apart in the heart.

Types of Pacemakers

- *Asynchronous:* stimulates ventricular contraction when a specified rate of pacing is required.
- *Demand:* initiates ventricular contraction only when the heart rate falls below a preset rate.
- *Physiologic:* synchronizes atrial and ventricular activity to improve cardiodynamics.
- *Rate adaptive pacing:* ensures that the heart rate increases when the patient exercises or experiences stress.

When the transvenous leads attach to the endocardium, the generator is usually placed over the pectoral muscle. If the leads are epicardial, the generator is usually placed in the abdominal wall.

Rate Adaptive Pacing	
TECHNOLOGY	**SENSED PARAMETER**
Piezoelectric crystal	Vibration acceleration
Impedance	Respiratory rate Minute ventilation RV pre-ejection period
Thermistor	RV temperature
Pressure	RV pressure
Optical reflectance	Oxygen saturation

Pacemaker Naming Function

- The first letter indicates which chamber is paced.
- The second letter indicates which chambers are sensed.
- The third letter identifies the response to the sensed signal: 0 = no sensing, I = inhibit (i.e., the pulse is suppressed and the internal clock reset); T = trigger (i.e., a pulse is administered); D = both triggering and inhibiting functions exist.
- The fourth letter indicates the unit's programmable functions.
- The fifth letter designates the device's antitachycardia features.

The simplest pacemaker provides asynchronous ventricular pacing (no sensing, no inhibition) and is designated VOO.

> AOO: fixed-rate atrial pacer
>
> VOO: fixed-rate ventricular pacer

DOO: fixed-rate atrial/ventricular pacer

AAI: demand atrial pacer, inhibited by the patient's intrinsic atrial depolarization

VVI: demand ventricular pacer, inhibited by the patient's intrinsic atrial depolarization

DDD: paces and senses in atria and ventricle

Operating Room Issues
Pacemakers

When a patient with a pacemaker is scheduled to come to the operating room, find out as much as possible about the device before the patient arrives in the OR (i.e., make and model).

What happens when a magnet is placed over a pacemaker device can vary among manufacturers as well as within the models themselves. *Contact the pacemaker representative to obtain specific information regarding the patient with a pacemaker who is coming to the operating room for surgery.* In most cases, placement of a magnet over a unit will convert a demand pacemaker to an asynchronous pacemaker (DOO, VOO, or AOO) and, therefore, prevent asystole. Having the pacemaker in asynchronous mode will create a rhythm that will compete with the heart's intrinsic rhythm (as it cannot detect intrinsic ventricular depolarization), so the use of a magnet will likely be necessary only in pacemaker-dependent patients who exhibit bradycardia or asystole during electrocautery use. Ventricular tachycardia can be initiated if pacing occurs on a T wave that is conducted.

CHAMBER PACED	CHAMBER SENSED	RESPONSE TO SENSING	PROGRAMMABLE FUNCTIONS	ANTITACHYCARDIA FEATURES
V: ventricle	V: ventricle	T: triggered	P: simple programmable	P: pace
A: atrium	A: atrium	I: inhibited	M: multiprogrammable	S: shock
D: dual (A + V)	D: dual (A + V)	D: dual (T + I)	C: communicating	D: dual (P + S)
O: none	O: no sensing	O: none	R: rate modulating	O: none
S: single (A or V)	S: single (A or V)		O: none	

Automatic Implantable Cardioverter-Defibrillators

When a patient with an AICD comes to the operating room, find out as much as possible about the device before the patient arrives in the OR (i.e., make and model).

Contact the AICD representative to obtain specific information regarding the patient with an AICD who is coming to the operating room for surgery. Have the ICD turned completely off prior to surgery and turned back on as soon after the surgery as possible, as ICD units are extremely sensitive to electrocautery. The device should be enabled before transport to the recovery area or an external defibrillator should accompany the patient during transport.

For patients receiving general anesthesia, the ICD may need to remain activated until induction is complete. Prior to deactivation of the ICD, rescue defibrillation pads must be placed on the patient. Depending on the location of the planned surgical incision sites, the selected locations of the defibrillation pads can vary. If a mediastinal incision is anticipated, then a left and right lateral chest placement is appropriate. For potential incision sites involving the left or right subclavicular areas, the anterior–posterior placement is best. The defibrillation pads function best with the least amount of distance the electric current must travel. The current must transverse the heart musculature, which is best achieved with one "defib" pad placed on the patient's back in the left subscapular area, the other pad on the left anterior chest adjacent to the patient's sternal midline, and the top of the pad 1 cm below the left nipple line.

Of significant concern is whether the patient is undergoing surgical removal of pacing or ICD leads that provide pacing for dependent patients. As a precaution, these patients must have an additional set of EKG leads placed, which, in conjunction with the defibrillation pads, can provide an additional means of monitoring the patient.

Thresholds on the pacemaker monitor are established prior to prepping the patient's skin and sharing the space with the OR staff in the event the patient should need to be urgently paced as well as defibrillated.

In our practice (please check with your AICD representative for information specific to your own practice), we have found that if a magnet is used over an ICD to disable tachyarrhythmia detection, and the patient has V-fib in the OR, just taking the magnet off could quickly result in the ICD defibrillating the patient. For Medtronic ICDs, a magnet will suffice for deactivating the device; however, most anesthetists and surgeons are uncomfortable with this practice and opt for the traditional method of deactivation.

Anesthetic Implications for the Patient with an Implantable Device Coming to the Operating Room

While protective mechanisms in pacemakers help to defend these devices against external electrical energy, high-strength signals from electrosurgical equipment (electrocautery) can exceed these safe limits. Therefore, anytime an electrical current is applied to the body, there is a potential for harm both to the unit itself and to the patient. In addition, electrical surges can decrease the long-term battery power of such a device.

Electromagnetic interference (EMI)—that is, Bovie electrocautery—generates an electrical current that may be identified as noise or misidentified as intrinsic heart activity by an AICD or pacemaker; this can reprogram a device, or damage the device or circuitry so that it is unable to deliver pacing capability or AICD shocks. With a pacemaker, electrocautery could inhibit pacing: The pacemaker incorrectly interprets these electric signals as intrinsic activity of the heart and does not generate a signal. That possibility explains why a change to asynchronous pacing (VOO or DOO) is necessary. Unfortunately, asynchronous pacing can induce ventricular arrhythmias and/or fibrillation.

For the AICD, the device may sense the induced voltage as a cardiac signal and may defibrillate the patient.

To minimize cautery interference with a pacemaker's or AICD's function, follow these guidelines:

- The grounding pad should be placed between the site of electrocautery and the device, if possible, as this arrangement provides an energy pathway to the pad and away from the device. Cautery should never touch the pacemaker or wires; electrosurgery should remain 6 inches or farther away from the device and lead system.
- Prepare the pulse generator appropriately for the use of electrocautery using a programmer or magnet. Placing a magnet over the device causes it to go into asynchronous pacing mode (no sensing— just paces).
- Deactivate the AICD just before surgery starts (reactivating it as soon as possible after surgery). Have emergency temporary pacing, defibrillation equipment, and emergency drugs available. If external defibrillation is necessary on these patients, position the paddles as far from device as possible—at least 6 inches away.
- Always monitor the patient during electrosurgery. If the EKG is not clear due to interference, a means of audible pulse detection (i.e., pulse oximetry, Doppler, or an arterial line) that is not affected by electrocautery is *mandatory* to help monitor the heart rhythm.
- Use a bipolar electrocautery system when possible. Use short, intermittent, and irregular bursts at the lowest feasible energy levels.
- If unipolar electrocautery is necessary, the current path should be as far from the device and leads as possible.

- If programming changes were made, the pulse generator should be reprogrammed back to the desired settings immediately following the procedure.

In regard to *radiofrequency ablation* (i.e., ESWL for kidney stones), for the patient with a pacemaker, contact the pacemaker representative to determine whether the pacer should be shut off. For the patient with an AICD, deactivate the device before the procedure begins; reactivate it as soon as possible after the end of the case.

Acute hypokalemia or respiratory alkalosis can increase the threshold for ventricular capture, which could result in a loss of pacing. Hypokalemia can also markedly increase the risk of ventricular fibrillation. (normal potassium level 3.7–5.0 mEq/L; "less than 4, give more.")

Acute hyperkalemia and acidosis decrease the fibrillation threshold, which can make the patient vulnerable to ventricular fibrillation. Calcium administration decreases potassium levels by shifting potassium into the cells, which can restore normal pacemaker function. Calcium chloride can be administered faster than calcium gluconate and provides greater bioavailability of calcium.

Contact Information for Implantable Cardiac Device Manufacturers

Biotronik, Inc.
1-800-547-9001
www.biotronik.com

Guidant-Boston Scientific
1-800-227-3422
www.guidant.com

Medtronic
1-800-328-2518
www.medtronic.com

St. Jude Medical
1-800-777-2237
www.sjm.com

Safe Procedures with Pacemakers and AICDs

- Electrocautery—but note that the AICD must be deactivated before any procedure if electrocautery is used within 6 to 8 inches of the device. See safety guidelines above.
- Diagnostic radiation: X-rays, fluoroscopy, mammogram.
- CT scan.
- Ultrasound.
- Laser surgery: an AICD should be deactivated.
- Radiofrequency ablation: pacemakers have been reset with radiofrequency ablation; an AICD should be deactivated.
- Lithotripsy: an AICD should be deactivated.

Contraindicated Procedures with Pacemakers and AICDs

MRI is contraindicated in any patient with a pacemaker or AICD.

Cardiac Conduction Pathway

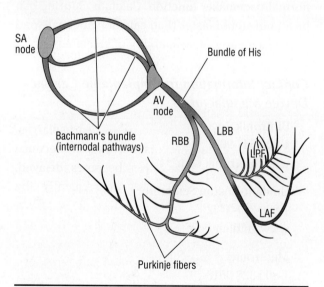

Figure 15-1 *The Cardiac Conduction Pathway*
Source: From Arrhythmia Recognition: The Art of Interpretation, *by Tomas B. Garcia, MD.*

HEART BLOCKS

First-degree AV block: PRI > 0.20.

Second-degree AV block (also known as Wenchebach or Mobitz I): PRI progressively lengthens until a QRS is dropped. ("Longer, longer, longer, drop—Wenchebach.")

Second-degree AV block (also known as Mobitz II): P waves are regular; ventricles (R to R) are irregular; PRI remains constant. One or more (but not all) of the atrial impulses fail to conduct to the ventricles; will see several P waves between QRS complexes. May progress quickly to complete heart block.

Third-degree AV block (complete heart block): The P-P interval and R-R intervals are consistent but P waves have no relationship to QRS; PRI is never constant. ("No electrical relationship between atria and ventricles.")

BUNDLE BRANCH BLOCKS
Right Bundle Branch Block (RBBB)

EKG: VI: RSR' (triphasic)

L1: wide S wave; QRS > 0.12

V6: wide S wave; QRS > 0.12

Left Bundle Branch Block (LBBB)

EKG: V1: monophasic, downward deflection

Lead I: RSR

V6: no Q wave, wide S wave

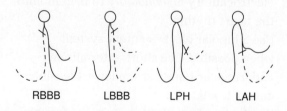

Figure 15-2 *Bundle Branch Blocks*

HEMIBLOCKS

Left Anterior Hemiblock

Supplied by LAD

EKG: left axis deviation

Leads II, III, AVF: small R wave, deep S wave

Leads I, AVL: small Q wave, tall R wave

QRS not significantly widened

V5–6: deep S wave

Left Posterior Hemiblock

EKG: right axis deviation

Leads I, AVL: small R wave, deep S wave

Leads II, III, AVF: small Q wave, tall R wave

Bifasicular Block

EKG: RBBB, left axis deviation

Leads II, III, AVF: small R wave, deep S wave

Trifasicular Block

EKG: Bifasicular block with first-degree or second-degree AV block

CARDIAC SURGERY: PERMANENT PACING AND AICD

Biventricular Pacing (Cardiac Resynchronization)

This form of cardiac pacing involves placement of transvenous (both right atrial and ventricular) and/or epicardial (through a thoracotomy) left ventricular pacemaker leads to synchronize discoordinated ventricular contractions. Both ventricles are stimulated to "beat" at the same time, decreasing septal wall displacement and decreasing mitral regurgitation. The goal is for the patient to have increased contractility, cardiac output, and stroke volumes with improved exercise tolerance, decreased shortness of breath, improved regional perfusion defects, shorter QRS intervals, lower mortality from sudden death, and a better quality of life with fewer hospital admissions.

Biventricular pacing is used to treat heart failure. This progressive disorder results from any process that damages myocardial cells, such as ischemia, infarction, and viral and bacterial infections. It leads to dilatation and enlargement of the ventricles (ventricle remodeling), resulting in decreased contractility, mitral regurgitation, ventricular dyssynchrony during depolarization, and prolonged QRS interval (longer than 120 milliseconds). As the heart continues to fail, further adverse remodeling occurs, causing more regional ischemia and further dyssynchrony of the ventricles.

Biventricular pacing is done if the ejection fraction is less than 35%, patients have moderate to severe symptoms of heart failure (New York Heart Association [NYHA] Classes III and IV heart failure), the QRS interval is longer than 120 milliseconds, and ventricular dyssynchrony (measured by echocardiography) persists despite optimal drug treatment. This type of pacing is not appropriate for bradycardia.

Normally, systole in the left ventricle occurs either simultaneously or just before systole in the right ventricle. In heart failure, as the heart enlarges, the ventricles become discoordinated because interventricular depolarization becomes delayed, resulting in a prolonged QRS. Consequently, the interventricular septum moves into the noncontracting ventricle, decreasing cardiac output and increasing pulmonary capillary wedge pressures.

Biventricular pacing differs from standard pacing for bradycardia in relation to the placement of the left ventricular lead(s), timing of ventricular stimulation, and atrioventricular settings (shorter than in intrinsic timing).

Operative Procedure

Transvenous

Going through an infraclavicular subclavian vein incision, leads are threaded into the right atrial appendage and the right ventricular apex (anterior wall). A second ventricular lead is placed, if possible, into the left ventricular posterolateral wall via a lateral vein of the coronary sinus.

Thoracotomy

A small thoracotomy incision is made at the transaxillary or mid-clavicular line; a small portion of rib is usually removed, and the left ventricular epicardial lead is sewn onto the epicardium. The proximal end of the lead is threaded up through the chest wall to the generator. Only one left ventricular lead is needed when placed epicardially. This approach is used if the transvenous approach for the left ventricular pacing lead is not possible; the atrial lead (and right ventricular lead) can still be placed transvenously.

Subcutaneous Generator

Usually placed below the left clavicle, a subcutaneous generator can be programmed to deliver simultaneous left and right ventricular pacing. The atrioventricular delay (between the atrial and ventricular leads) is programmed to override the patient's intrinsic conduction by setting the paced PRI shorter than the intrinsic PRI.

Anesthetic

For the transvenous approach, monitored anesthesia care (MAC) is commonly used with local anesthesia. For thoracotomy, general endotracheal anesthesia (GETA) is used. A double-lumen endobronchial tube may be needed, but is not always essential.

For patients requiring a thoracotomy, an epidural may be placed preoperatively so that it can be bolused for pain control postoperatively.

Positioning

The patient is placed supine for the transvenous approach; he or she is placed in a slight bump-up position on the thoracotomy side when that technique is used. The arm may be placed at the side or brought over the head. The surgeon may prefer to be present during positioning and draping.

Anesthetic Implications

Patients presenting for biventricular pacing are usually on beta-blockers, angiotensin-converting enzyme (ACE) inhibitors, and/or aldosterone antagonists.

The ventricular lead at the left posterolateral wall can come near the course of the left phrenic nerve, causing hiccoughs or painful stimulation of the diaphragm. The lead can be repositioned if this reaction occurs during surgery; postoperatively, the generator can be reprogrammed.

The surgeon may request anesthesia personnel to hold ventilations when screwing in the epicardial lead.

A sling should be placed around the arm on the side where the generator is implanted before the patient leaves the operating room, to prevent the patient from moving the arm. The patient's arm should not be lifted above the shoulder level to prevent lead dislodgement.

Postoperatively, the patient should remain in an ICU for 24 hours. These patients all have a history of a decreased ejection fraction, and congestive heart failure is a concern. Fluids should be carefully monitored; diuretics are usually given on the first postoperative day.

Insertion of a Permanent Pacemaker

The implantation of a permanent pacemaker—a small electronic device—is intended to help stabilize and regulate electrical problems with the heart. An electrode lead is passed through a large vein (usually the subclavian or cephalic vein), through the superior vena cava, and into the right atrium and right ventricle. It is secured so that it is in contact with and attached to the endocardium; the electrode is then connected to a pulse generator. The pacemaker ensures that the heartbeat will not go lower than a preset level.

An electrode lead can also be threaded through a pacing pulmonary artery catheter with a pacing wire to the heart as a temporary measure.

A permanent pacemaker is used to treat bradycardia; sick sinus syndrome; second-degree type 2 or third-degree heart blocks; and bifasicular or trifasicular heart block.

Operative Procedure

The pacemaker leads are threaded percutaneously into the heart, usually via the subclavian vein. A single lead is placed into the right ventricle; alternatively, dual chamber leads are placed in the right atrium and in the right ventricle, with their positioning guided under fluoroscopy. The electrode is then attached to an external pacemaker for testing. A pulse generator unit is inserted into a subcutaneous pocket formed by the surgeon, usually in the upper left chest. A tunneling instrument is used to make a path for the electrode, which is then attached to the pulse generator. The generator is programmed and tested intraoperatively.

Anesthetic

Anesthesia usually consists of sedation with a local anesthetic. Depending on the surgeon's preference and the patient's status, a general anesthetic with an oral endotracheal tube (OETT) may be needed.

Positioning

The patient is placed in a supine position, with at least one arm tucked at the side. The head is turned away from the operative side.

Anesthetic Implications

Continue antiarrhythmic therapy perioperatively. Reliable IV access is necessary, and transcutaneous pacing pads should be placed on the patient's chest with an external defibrillator monitor on and ready for use. Chronotropic drugs should also be available—specifically, atropine, epinephrine, and isoproterenol.

Minimize sedation, which may depress spontaneous respirations. Avoid the use of negative inotropes.

Carefully monitor the EKG in leads 2 and 5, and notify the surgeon if any sustained cardiac dysrhythmias occur.

There may be a need to deepen sedation during tunneling, as this part of the procedure is very stimulating.

Document the pacemaker manufacturer and settings on the operative record for future anesthetic information.

Insertion of an Implantable Cardioverter-Defibrillator (AICD)

A cardiac defibrillator is implanted to provide a defibrillatory impulse to people with documented ventricular arrhythmias or with a strong potential for malignant cardiac rhythms. Two defibrillator electrodes are placed in contact with the myocardium; they are then connected to a small battery and computerized device placed in a subcutaneous pocket of the chest (usually the left chest, though it can also be placed in the abdomen). Separate electrodes are used for pacing and sensing.

ICDs deliver an electrical discharge to the myocardium when they sense either ventricular fibrillation or ventricular tachycardia. They are used for *primary prevention* of sudden cardiac death caused by asymptomatic coronary artery disease and nonsustained ventricular arrhythmias, following coronary artery bypass graft (CABG) in patients with severe left ventricular dysfunction (ejection fraction < 30%), and for patients waiting for heart transplantation. ICDs may also be used for *secondary prevention* in cases of coronary artery disease, in patients with a family history of sudden death, and for inducible sustained ventricular arrhythmias. Single- or dual-chamber therapy is possible; that is, one can have just defibrillator therapy or have both defibrillator and pacemaker.

Operative Procedure

Multiple detection zones for antitachycardia pacing, cardioversion shocks, and defibrillation capability with tiered shocks are tested during surgery. During the intraoperative testing phase, ventricular tachycardia or fibrillation is induced by the surgeon and the ICD is tested for sensing, charging, and successful defibrillation. The surgeon may need to do several tests. If the ICD defibrillation is unsuccessful, rescue with external defibrillation starting at 200 J, then increasing joule strength to 300 J and to 360 J (monophasic) or up to 200 J (biphasic) if needed.

Anesthetic
Anesthesia consists of MAC or a GA with an OETT. Muscle relaxants may be given during general anesthesia. Jet ventilation may be used to help decrease the heart shifting in the chest from intrathoracic pressure changes during ventilations.

Monitors
An arterial line is required even if sedation anesthesia is used; personnel need to verify blood pressure with aberrant rhythms. A central line may also be needed.

Positioning
The patient is placed supine with bilateral arms tucked at the sides.

Anesthetic Implications
These patients usually have very little cardiac reserve and may have coronary artery disease, ventricular dysfunction, cardiomyopathy, and valvular heart disease.

Always have emergency equipment and drugs available and ready to use. External defibrillator pads should be placed on the patient and connected to a monitor. Drugs should be drawn up and available: lidocaine 100 mg, atropine 1 mg, calcium chloride 2 g, epinephrine 10 mcg/mL, amiodarone, magnesium. Use oral airways and endotracheal tubes as necessary. Deepen the anesthetic level for the testing phase of ICD firing.

See: detection of 8 to 10 fast beats.

Think: delay of 2.5 to 10 seconds before charging (Will this rhythm stop on its own?).

Charge: charge for 6 to 15 seconds to 0.1 to 31 J and then discharge.

Intraoperative defibrillator testing is intended to establish the defibrillation threshold—that is, the minimal energy required to defibrillate the heart to a stable rhythm. Internal paddles should be readily available. External patches should be placed preoperatively.

The newer AICDs are also combined with a pacemaker.

CARDIAC SURGERY: TEMPORARY PACING
Temporary pacing can be established by transcutaneous, transesophageal, transvenous, or epicardial electrodes. Temporary pacing may serve as a bridge until permanent pacing can be established or as a temporary measure until cardiac condition stabilizes.

Transcutaneous Pacing

In transcutaneous pacing, pacing pads are placed on the chest, both anterior and posterior, to stimulate myocardial ventricular contraction. This technique is used to pace patients without an underlying heart rate; as part of minimally invasive direct coronary artery bypass (MIDCAB); and placed for a redo CABG or initial CABG.

Operative Procedure
Place the pads over the left chest anteriorly and the left back (between the scapula and spine, while avoiding the scapula bone) per the package directions.

Anesthetic
Sedation is used if general anesthetic has not been given.

Positioning
Turn the patient from side to side or have him or her sit up for pad placement, then place the patient supine.

Anesthetic Implications

It is very uncomfortable to have electricity surge through the chest if awake. These patients must be sedated.

Transesophageal Pacing

In transesophageal pacing, a flexible electrode is placed into the esophagus to pace the atrium only. This type of pacing is useful only for symptomatic sinus bradycardia and for terminating some supraventricular tachyarrhythmias.

Insertion of a Transvenous Pacing Electrode

In transvenous pacing, an electrode lead is placed through a large vein (usually the subclavian or cephalic vein), through the superior vena cava, and into the right atrium and right ventricle. It is secured so that it is in contact with and attached to the endocardium; the electrode is then connected to a pulse generator.

An electrode lead can also be threaded through a pacing pulmonary artery catheter with a pacing wire to the heart. Both techniques are used to treat a heart block that either persists or occurs intermittently.

Operative Procedure

An incision is made over the chosen vein—usually the jugular, subclavian, or cephalic vein. A pacing electrode is inserted and advanced under fluoroscopy guidance into the right ventricle. This electrode is attached to an external pacemaker for testing. An incision is made into the chest wall with a pocket formed down into the fascia, creating a place for the pulse generator. A tunneling instrument is used to make a path for the electrode, which is then attached to the pulse generator.

Anesthetic

Usually sedation and MAC are used. Some cases may need general anesthesia and an OETT.

Positioning

The patient is positioned supine, with the head turned away from the operative side.

Anesthetic Implications

Continue antiarrhythmic therapy preoperatively. Reliable IV access is needed, and transcutaneous pacing pads should be placed on the patient's chest with an external defibrillator monitor turned on and ready to use. Chronotropic drugs should be available—specifically, atropine, epinephrine, and isoproterenol. Watch the EKG monitor closely during advancement of the pacing electrode and alert the surgeon to ectopy.

Sedation may need to be deepened during the tunneling part of the procedure, as it is very stimulating.

Insertion of an Epicardial Pacing Electrode

An atrial or ventricular pacing electrode lead is placed on the myocardium when the thorax has been opened. This procedure is performed in preparation for a cardiopulmonary bypass, or when the patient has a heart block, asystole, or bradycardia. It is possible to increase cardiac output by increasing the heart rate (without catecholamines) in patients with perioperative bradyarrhythmias.

Operative Procedure

The epicardial pacing lead is placed on the myocardium during open heart surgery; the wires are externalized.

Anesthetic

GETA is used during this procedure.

Positioning

The patient is placed in the supine position with bilateral arms tucked at the sides.

Anesthetic Implications

Check pacemaker box before leaving the operating room. Make sure that both the atrial and ventricular leads work correctly.

Cardiac Mapping and Ablation

Cardiac mapping and ablation is performed to isolate and ablate areas of the heart that give rise to supraventricular arrhythmias—such as atrial fibrillation, atrial flutter, AV nodal reentry tachycardia, AV reentrant tachycardia (Wolf-Parkinson-White syndrome), or atrial tachycardia.

Operative Procedure

In the *percutaneous/transvenous* approach, femoral vessels are accessed and guide wires are passed through them. Arrhythmia mapping can be completed in 1 hour but can also last 4 or more hours. Involves using direct current radiofrequency to ablate (via high-energy current) diseased atrial or ventricular electrical pathways that have led to arrhythmias.

An *open chest* procedure with sternotomy is still sometimes required.

Mapping of the target foci and accessory pathways requires inducing a reentry tachycardia using a stimulator to initiate dysrhythmias. Have a defibrillator available during this process, including external chest pads or paddles (internal for surgical ablation).

Anesthetic

This procedure is often done under conscious sedation. If GETA is used, jet ventilation is useful. Lidocaine should not be given during induction.

Positioning

The patient is placed in the supine position. Careful positioning and padding of all body prominences is important because of the length of the case.

Anesthetic Implications

During or after ablation, the patient may have pain, arrhythmias (bradycardia, asystole, and ventricular arrhythmias), bleeding, pneumothorax, MI, or CVA. He or she should be transferred to a monitored inpatient bed at the end of the case.

Antiarrhythmic medications are usually discontinued prior to surgery to make the dysrhythmias more inducible.

Cardiac mapping and ablation is usually a very long procedure—3 to 5 hours in duration.

CARDIAC SURGERY: CORONARY ARTERY DISEASE

Percutaneous Transluminal Angioplasty

In percutaneous transluminal coronary angioplasty (PTCA), the plaque is not removed (increased risk with attempted removal if a piece of plaque breaks off and becomes embolus); the plaque is compressed like "foot prints in the snow." PTCA is done for coronary artery blockage amenable to balloon compression.

Operative Procedure

PTCA is a mainstay of interventional cardiology. A balloon catheter is positioned across the area of stenosis and inflated to compress the coronary artery blockage.

Anesthetic

All patients receive aspirin preoperatively and heparin during the case; an activated clotting time (ACT) device is used to monitor anticoagulation.

Monitors

Femoral venous and arterial lines are needed for all patients.

Positioning

The patient is placed in the supine position, with the arms tucked at the sides.

Anesthetic Implications

Clarify whether the patient has an allergy to IV dye, contrast, shrimp, or other relevant allergens: As part of this procedure, radiopaque dye is injected into the coronary arteries to locate and quantify occlusions.

An *atherectomy* can also be accomplished by the same route. The catheter used for this procedure has a rotary cutting device to shave away and suction away the obstruction.

Postoperative anticoagulation is needed (e.g., Plavix, aspirin).

Coronary Artery Bypass Graft Conduits

Grafts used to bypass occluded coronary arteries include the left internal mammary artery (LIMA), saphenous vein graft (SVG) from the leg, right internal mammary artery (RIMA), radial artery, and/or epigastric artery (gastroepiplocic).

A "pedicle graft" refers to a graft where the proximal end is not cut, thereby maintaining natural blood flow, while the distal end is cut and sutured onto a new area (i.e., the LIMA maintains its proximal blood flow at the left subclavian, while the distal end is severed and sutured to the left anterior descending artery, past the coronary artery blockage). The pedicle graft may have some tissue surrounding the distal end so that it can be sewn onto the heart to prevent it from twisting or flipping. A "free graft" means that both the proximal and distal ends of the graft have been severed.

Coronary Artery Bypass Graft

CABG involves the grafting of the internal mammary artery (right or left) and/or segments of autologous saphenous vein (SVG), or other vessels as needed, to bypass coronary artery obstruction. This described procedure is done on cardiopulmonary bypass. Also, see "off-pump" procedures this chapter.

CABG is performed when a significant coronary artery blockage is creating symptoms owing to ischemia of the heart muscle. The left and right coronary arteries originate through the coronary ostia (two openings in the aortic sinus) at the root of the aorta.

Operative Procedure

Approach is through a median sternotomy. The SVG portion, taken from the leg, is sewn onto the distal coronary artery (past the blockage) and then proximally sewn onto the aorta. The internal mammary usually maintains its blood supply proximally and the distal end is sewn onto the coronary artery, bypassing the blockage.

Anesthetic

General anesthesia is used with a single-lumen ETT; muscle relaxants are given. Neuromuscular blockade is not reversed at the end of the case as the patient is taken, still intubated, to the ICU.

Positioning

The patient is placed in a supine position, with a shoulder roll used to slightly extend the head. Arms are placed on padding and tucked at the patient's sides. After the arms are tucked at the sides, check the function of both the arterial line (Can you draw blood back? Is there a good waveform?) and IVs (Is the IV running without difficulty?).

Changing the patient from a Trendelenburg to reverse Trendelenburg position can help to increase or decrease preload and maintain blood pressure within specific parameters. Positioning changes during the surgery are common.

Anesthetic Implications
Anesthetic Goals
- The patient is moved to the operating room table.
- Arterial and central lines and monitors are usually placed while the patient is sedated, but before general anesthesia is initiated. Oxygen is given by nasal cannula (looped up to the top of the head so that it will not be in the way during internal jugular CVP and PAC placement).
- Any IVs placed preoperatively may be of a small gauge. Do not remove them, but rather

cap them and start larger lines. Bleeding can occur or a hematoma may form after heparinization. Any attempted IV should be managed with a pressure dressing.

- The preference for an arterial line is for right radial placement if a left internal mammary artery (LIMA) is to be dissected because the sternal retractor can compress the left subclavian artery. If the LIMA won't be used, the arterial line should be placed in the radial artery of the arm that has a BP that is more than 15 mm Hg higher than the other. Notify the surgeon if the BP difference between the arms is greater than 15–20 mm Hg.
- Central venous line and pulmonary artery catheter are usually inserted through the right internal jugular vein.

Induction

The agent choice is based on left ventricular function. The following technique is recommended, although others are used:

- Oxygen at 100% FiO_2.
- Etomidate 0.2–0.3 mg/kg if CO is less than 35%.
- Sodium thiopental 2–4 mg/kg if CO is more than 35%.
- Midazolam 2–3 mg (or more) before sternotomy.
- Fentanyl 5–10 mcg/kg initially (can slow heart rate).
- Narcotics decrease the stress hormone response but can produce chest rigidity. If this occurs, give muscle relaxants and intubate the patient.
- Rocuronium 5 mg/kg defasiculating dose, if succinylcholine (Anectine) is given.
- Succinylcholine (Anectine) 1–2 mg/kg.

A patient with poor LV function may not tolerate a high concentration of an inhalation agent (although a small concentration is appropriate), whereas a patient with good LV function (more than 50%) can tolerate a narcotic and inhalation agent for anesthesia.

Maintenance

- Oxygen at 100% FiO_2 or air/oxygen. Avoid nitrous oxide (increases air bubble size in arterial system).
- Fentanyl 50–100 mcg/kg for entire case if LV function is good; use a dose of less than 50 mcg/kg if the EF is low.
- Vecuronium 10 mg IV; titrate to peripheral nerve stimulator 0/4.
- Pancuronium is used if the heart rate is low.
- Isoflurane, sevoflurane, or desflurane, titrated to 0.5 MAC.

Pre-bypass Period

Maintain systolic blood pressure at 100–115 mm Hg throughout the pre-bypass time. Maintain hemodynamics to avoid exacerbations of myocardial ischemia.

Draw a baseline ACT.

Minimize IV fluids in the pre-bypass period (500 mL is a good goal). The patient will receive 1.5 L fluid with cardiopulmonary bypass.

It is a period of low stimulation during prep and draping. If the patient becomes hypotensive, check for the cause and treat or put the patient in Trendelenburg position. Consider lowering the anesthetic depth. If the cardiac index is more than 2.0, you can give phenylephrine or ephedrine. Dobutamine or dopamine may be needed, as the venous capacitance system is sequestering volume in these cases and the heart rate may be low due to use of beta-blockers and/or narcotic administration.

Antifibrinolytics

Antifibrinolytics may not be used in all CABG cases with cardiopulmonary bypass. Check with the surgeon before giving these agents or refer to your institutional guidelines.

Fibrinolysis is the normal path to dissolve clots: plasminogen → plasmin → fibrin → fibrin split products (FSP). Antifibrinolytic therapy is given because millions of tiny clots form when the patient's blood supply is exposed to body trauma—in this case, a chest incision or cardiopulmonary bypass. The by-products of clot breakdown should not circulate in the blood.

If an antifibrinolytic is to be given, it is started before the clotting cascade begins (with the chest incision). Antifibrinolytics prevent the breakdown of fibrin by preventing attachment of plasmin to fibrin. It inhibits plasmin from stimulating fibrin breakdown. Amicar (aminocaproic acid) is one example of an antifibrinolytic; its loading dose is 5–10 g over 30–60 minutes; the infusion dose is 1–2 g/hr in surgery.

Skin Incision

Have adequate depth of anesthesia before the skin incision is made. Prevent tachycardia-induced ischemia. The use of high-dose opioids (e.g., Fentanyl) in cardiac anesthesia helps to decrease the stress response; there is a lack of myocardial depression with high-dose opioids. High-dose opioids are acceptable if you do not plan to extubate the patient in the OR or in the first few hours in the ICU. Precedex (Dexmedetomidine) may be helpful in modulating narcotic administration and decreasing response to surgical stimulation.

Sternotomy

A sternotomy provokes extreme stimulation. This procedure requires deep anesthesia plus vasodilators to decrease blood pressure. With first-time sternotomy (using a reciprocating saw), the patient's lungs must be deflated and the patient must be off the ventilator (disconnect the bag). Chart whether the lungs are up or down during sternotomy. The patient must be 100% muscle relaxed for sternotomy.

Conduit Harvesting

The left internal mammary artery (LIMA), saphenous venous graft (SVG), and radial artery may be harvested. During the internal mammary dissection, decrease the tidal volume (to decrease the lung inflation, as it may affect the surgeon's view of the mammary bed) and increase the respiratory rate to maintain the end-tidal CO_2 within normal levels.

If the graft is an artery, it is prone to spasm with manipulation. Papaverine, Cardizem, and nitroglycerin can be used to dilate and relax the smooth muscle of the artery. If the radial artery is to be used as a graft for bypass, place no IV, arterial line, or BP cuff on the chosen arm. A pulse oximetry probe *must* be placed on the arm that the radial artery is harvested from; in the initial portion of the harvest, ulnar blood flow can then be confirmed by the continuous readout indicating that the saturation has not dropped on that arm. After harvesting, the arm is closed and tucked at the patient's side.

Diltiazem drips 1–2 mg/hr are routinely used in free arterial graft patients. The drip needs to be started prior to harvest and continued perioperatively and postoperatively.

Anticoagulation

Heparin 300–400 units/kg body weight is given through the central line with known blood return; it is administered before cannulation. Check the ACT 3–4 minutes after giving heparin, ACT needs to be more than 480 seconds for the patient to go on bypass. If this goal is not met, additional heparin may be given. Anticoagulants may prevent acute clot formation or disseminated intravascular coagulation (DIC) while the patient is on the bypass machine.

Aortic Cannulation

Decrease the patient's systolic blood pressure to 85–100 mm Hg for aortic cannulation (to help prevent aortic dissection if the cannula separates the intimal wall from the media and adventitia). The aortic cannula is usually placed in the ascending aorta proximal to the innominate artery, but can also be placed in the femoral artery.

Venous Cannulation

The venous cannula is placed in the right atrium after aortic cannulation. Typically a multistage venous cannula is placed through an opening in the right atrium and passed into the inferior vena cava. If the patient becomes hypotensive or has atrial/ventricular arrhythmias, treat him or her with drugs or place the patient on bypass. Malposition of venous cannulas can interfere with venous return and impede venous drainage from the head and neck, which causes distention of head and neck blood vessels.

Aortic Clamp

The surgeon will call for "aortic flow down" just before the cross-clamp is applied.

The arterial waveform will become nonpulsatile when the aortic clamp is on. This step is considered the initiation of "ischemia time" for all tissues.

Stop Ventilation

Stop ventilation when the PA and arterial waveforms are flattened and the patient is on full-flow cardiopulmonary bypass. Check with the perfusionist regarding their use of inhalational agents.

Cardioplegia

Diastolic arrest ensures myocardial preservation; cardioplegia stops the heart with a hyperkalemic solution at 8°C. This solution is given intermittently by the perfusionist through a direct line from a plegia administration system on the bypass pump via the antegrade and retrograde lines. It is used to perfuse and cool areas of the myocardium so as to maintain heart arrest and reduce the oxygen requirements of the heart. If the heart fibrillates, cardioplegia is given to still the heart.

- *Antegrade cardioplegia perfusion:* via coronary aortic root or coronary ostia. An ostial catheter (aortic vent) increases pressure to shut the aortic valve and push cardioplegia down the coronary arteries in a normal direction at a pressure of 75–100 Torr.
- *Retrograde cardioplegia perfusion:* via coronary sinus, perfuses "backward" into the coronary veins. Retrograde flow is needed if high-grade lesions prevent normal flow from carrying the

cardioplegia solution to the tips of the coronary arteries (past blockages). The catheter is placed through the right atrium and directly into the coronary sinus (venous system). Pressure of 30–50 Torr pushes the solution backward into the venous side, then to the capillaries, and then to the distal ends of the coronary arteries *up* to the blockage.

Perfusionist

Full-flow cardiopulmonary bypass runs at 2–2.5 L/min/m^2.

While the patient is on full bypass, all IV and volatile agents are given by the perfusionist. If volume is needed in the pump, the perfusionist will check the HCT levels. If the HCT falls below 20, washed cells or PRBC will be added. If the HCT is in the low to middle 20s (ideal levels are 22–25 during CPB), crystalloids or colloids (hetastarch, albumin) can be added. The perfusionist gives 0.5% isoflurane through the bypass machine. The patient's body temperature is cooled as hypothermia itself is an anesthetic and an excellent myocardial protectant.

Once On Bypass

IVF is slowed to a minimal rate to "keep vein open," as most intravascular fluid is given through the bypass pump. Vasoactive agents are turned off; inotropes, antiarrhythmics, and insulin are continued.

Withdraw the pulmonary artery catheter to 2–3 cm to prevent wedging of the catheter on bypass. Check the patient's neck for thrill (from a malpositioned arterial cannula) and the pupils. Arterial cannula malposition can cause the bypass outflow to be directed *into* carotid artery, which can cause ipsilateral pupil dilation; bilateral fixed and dilated pupils indicate hypoxia. In such a case, inform the surgeon to reassess the bypass circuitry.

- Organ perfusion is the goal while on bypass; it is best when MAP is in the range of 30–60 mm Hg. A higher pressure may be needed if patient has carotid stenosis. Patients who are perfused with a MAP greater than

70 mm Hg have better neurologic outcomes. The surgeon will tell the perfusionist where the MAP should be maintained.

- Ventricular fibrillation often occurs as the heart is rapidly cooling; fibrillation rapidly consumes the myocardial oxygen supply and protection. More cardioplegia will be given to still the heart from fibrillating.
- The surgeon sews the distal grafts first, and then sews the proximal ends of the grafts to the aorta.
- The surgeon will ask the perfusionist to "fill the heart" to test the conduit size.
- Recalibrate all lines before taking the patient off bypass.
- Measure the urinary output every 30 minutes—this is an especially important consideration while the patient is on bypass. Urinary output should be greater than 1 mL/kg/hr.

Gradual Rewarming

Rewarming starts when the distal anastomosis is complete. Give IV amnestic and narcotic agents when starting to rewarm the patient; the patient's maximum temperature on bypass should have been at 34°C or less to help prevent intraoperative awareness. Additional dosing may be needed during rewarming to cover the period of separation from bypass when no inhalational agent is used.

- Lung ventilation must start before bypass separation. The surgeon will request ventilation for de-airing and then again prior to separation from bypass. When lung ventilation is resumed; several breaths are given to recruit and inflate pulmonary alveoli while watching lung tissue enlarge through the sternal opening. Use care to not overinflate and put a strain on the internal mammary grafts. Provide FiO_2 at 100%. (There is some question as to the value of 100% FiO_2 coming off cardiopulmonary bypass. Check with your institutional guidelines. Recent research has suggested that the FiO_2 should be decreased to 80% if the patient is on amiodarone.)

Bypass Termination Requirements

- Rectal body temperature should show that the patient is rewarmed to at least 35°C for at least 5 minutes, and for 7–10 minutes in elderly patients. A body temperature that is less than 34°C can cause fibrillation and death.
- For a stable EKG rhythm, normal sinus rhythm is preferred. Internal defibrillation at 10–20 J may be necessary to achieve this rhythm. If asystole occurs or if the heart rate is inadequate, the pacemaker can be started at a rate of 80–100. Initiate both atrial and ventricular mA at 20, decrease the mA until capture is lost, and then turn the rate back up as necessary. May give lidocaine 1 mg/kg; or magnesium 2 g after the cross-clamp is off.
- Assess the heart contractility to determine if inotropic support is necessary. A calcium chloride 250–1000 mg bolus through the central line may be needed. Pump volume can be given to supplement body fluid volume and maintain filling pressure; it is given via the arterial cannula in the aorta by the perfusionist. The patient becomes volume dependent with separation, and volume is needed to maintain a constant SVR, blood pressure, and cardiac output.
- Normal potassium value should be less than 5.0; hematocrit should be in the range of 22–25% or greater.
- Air is evacuated from the heart and grafts. Trendelenburg to reverse Trendelenburg position changes are often requested by the surgeon to facilitate air evacuation.
- The aortic clamp is removed marking the *end of ischemia time.* Note the aortic clamp time and bypass time on and off; chart both on the patient's record.

Bypass Separation

Watch the patient's blood pressure as bypass flow decreases. If the blood pressure is too low when the patient is off bypass, maintain a partial bypass, start appropriate infusions, adjust the ventricular volume, and then try to wean the patient off bypass again.

A SBP of 90–110 mm Hg is necessary to minimize bleeding yet still perfuse organs adequately. The surgeon may lift the heart to check the posterior wall for bleeding which will temporarily drop the blood pressure. The perfusionist will return bypass reservoir blood, with an HCT goal of 22–30%. The atrial cannula (venous) is removed first; the arterial cannula is the last to be removed.

Coming Off Bypass Support

In case of post-bypass low cardiac output:

- Low pulmonary artery pressure (low filling pressures): give volume, increase preload.
- Low ejection fraction: increase contractility with inotropes.
- High afterload (SVR > 1200): decrease afterload, can use sodium nitroprusside (SNP).
- Low heart rate: increase heart rate; program pacemaker.

- Arrhythmias (loss of atrial kick): atrial/ventricular pacing; intra-aortic balloon pump set at 1:1.

In case of post-bypass hypotension, assess LV volume/function. Check CVP, PAD, CO/CI, and TEE for wall movement abnormalities. Treat the patient with volume, calcium, vasopressors, or inotropes as necessary.

Alpha agonists may be needed. A ventricular assist device may be needed for the right or left ventricle, or both ventricles.

In case of post-bypass hypertension, assess whether the level of anesthesia is deep enough. Treat the patient with narcotics and volatile (inhaled) agents as necessary; some patients may need vasodilators.

Post-bypass Period

Protamine 1.3–1.5 mg (per 100 units of heparin that was given) can be administered once hemostasis is controlled, the aortic and vena cava cannulae have been removed, and hemodynamic stability is achieved. Protamine binds and inactivates heparin. Check the patient's ACT 3 minutes after giving this agent; it should be the same or less than the baseline ACT. Give Protamine slowly

Preload		Contractility		Afterload	
CVP	PCWP	SVI	LVSWI	PVR	SVR
LOW	**HIGH**	**LOW**	**HIGH**	**LOW**	**HIGH**
Volume	Dilators	+ Inotrope	Beta-blocker	Vasopressor	Dilator
Colloids	NTG	Dobutrex	Labetalol	Epinephrine	Nipride
Blood	Nipride	Dopamine	Lopressor	Norepinephrine	Amrinone
Crystalloids	Diuretic	Epinephrine		Dopamine	IABP 1:1
		Inocor		Vasopressin	Isuprel
		Levophed		Phenylephrine	
		Neosynephrine		IABP 1:1	
		Primacor			

to prevent hypotension or pulmonary hypertension; it can provoke severe hemodynamic reactions. The risk of anaphylaxis is increased for patients with diabetes who have received NPH (Neutral *Protamine* Hagedorn) insulin and/or vasectomized males. Have epinephrine 10 mcg/mL ready to treat reactions that result in pulmonary hypertension with systemic hypotension.

Uncontrolled bleeding may be caused by inadequate surgical control of bleeding, inadequate heparin reversal, thrombocytopenia, platelet dysfunction, hypothermia if the patient's body temperature is less than 35°C, or newly acquired coagulopathy. In such cases, it may be necessary to give more Protamine, fresh frozen plasma, platelets, DDAVP, or Factor VII.

Finish giving Protamine before starting to give cell-saver (BRAT) blood; then give blood products.

Do not hyperventilate the patient, as this process causes alkalosis. Oxyhemoglobin dissociation shifts to the left, causing less oxygen release to the tissues. If the patient is alkalotic, first decrease the intravascular volume, then decrease the respiratory rate to decrease minute ventilation: 8 mL/kg + 150 mL (dead space) should be an adequate tidal volume.

Shoot a cardiac output both before closing the chest and after the chest is closed with sternal wires. Intrathoracic pressure can increase significantly (decreasing preload and cardiac output) once the chest is closed. Inform the surgeon of the closed-chest CO and document it.

Redo CABG and Sternotomy Issues

Blood must be in room to start the case.

The patient must be ventilated and maintained during sternotomy. This practice keeps the chest wall farther away from the heart, thereby decreasing the risk of the saw hitting the pericardium; the heart may be adhered to the sternum. An oscillating saw is used in a redo sternotomy.

If the heart is cut during sternotomy and catastrophic bleeding occurs, the patient must be placed on "sucker bypass" (draining venous blood by pump "suckers" and returning flow by a femoral cannula). Administer heparin 400 U/kg to prepare for CPB and start cardiopulmonary bypass as soon as possible.

These patients have scar tissue from their last surgery, making the surgery more difficult, with a higher blood loss potential. These patients are also usually sicker, requiring longer bypass times and longer aortic cross-clamp time with associated difficulties.

Off-Pump Coronary Artery Bypass Graft

Coronary artery bypass grafting may be done without cardiopulmonary bypass. Although cardiopulmonary bypass is not planned with an off-pump coronary artery bypass (OPCAB) procedure, the patient should be fully prepped and draped in preparation to go on bypass at any time in case of emergency.

The ideal candidate for off-pump CABG is a hemodynamically stable patient with coronary arteries that can be stabilized on the anterior wall of the heart. OPCAB is promoted in patients at increased risk for stroke, severe lung disease, severe vascular disease, and renal dysfunction.

OPCAB can be used to perform multi-vessel bypass, to carry out redo CABG, and in patients with aortic disease in whom cannulation of the aorta poses significant embolic risk. However, the surgeon may have more difficulty accessing the circumflex vessel in an OPCAB procedure, due to the cardiac tilting needed to access the lateral wall. Major difficulties related to this surgery include hemodynamic alterations with cardiac manipulation/tilting and intraoperative myocardial ischemia.

Indications for OPCAB include single- to multiple-vessel CABG on patients where the side effects of cardiopulmonary bypass are especially undesirable.

Contraindications to this procedure include cardiomegaly, small or deep coronary arteries, left main artery disease, severe LV dysfunction (less than 30% ejection fraction), and hemodynamic instability.

Operative Procedure

The heart vascular system is accessed through a standard median sternotomy. OPCAB is closer to the surgeon's usual coronary artery bypass surgical routine and allows for the standard technique used for mammary artery harvesting. The LIMA's proximal blood flow originates from the left subclavian artery, and the distal attachment is anastomosed to the coronary artery past the coronary blockage.

Opposite from the CABG procedure on bypass, the proximal anastomosis is done first—that is, the conduit is sewed to the aorta and *then* the coronary artery is clamped to sew the distal anastomosis—to decrease ischemic time. SBP maintained at 90–100 mm Hg, and MAP is kept greater than 60 mm Hg during the *proximal* anastomosis. Avoid tachycardia to maximize coronary perfusion.

For the distal anastomosis, the coronary artery to be grafted has a tourniquet or snare placed around the artery to occlude it so as to ensure bloodless anastomotic conditions, resulting in brief periods of ischemia. During this time, the MAP should be maintained greater than 70 mm Hg and monitoring of myocardial ischemia is crucial. Document the time the coronary vessel is occluded and the time it is reopened again: this period is the "ischemic" time for that vessel. If a tourniquet or snare is not placed (based on the surgeon's preference), to minimize myocardial ischemia, an intracoronary shunt can be inserted by the surgeon to redirect blood flow to the distal myocardium.

No matter what method is used, protecting the myocardium from ischemia during coronary artery flow interruption (while the surgeon performs the anastomosis) is imperative. The goal is to provide a bloodless surgical field and maintain myocardial oxygen balance by decreasing oxygen demand—decrease heart rate, contractility, and myocardial wall tension—and increasing supply—increase arterial oxygen concentration, keep MAP greater than 70 mm Hg, and maintain coronary perfusion pressure (CPP) = DBP − LVEDP.

Calcium antagonists, magnesium, and beta-blockers can be given to improve myocardial oxygen balance. Begin by decreasing heart rate and contractility while increasing the myocardial oxygen supply.

Stabilizing Devices

Heart wall motion can be decreased by the placement of a stabilizing device onto the heart muscle. Because the heart is still beating during the grafting, stabilizing devices have been created to reduce the motion of the heart muscle (and thus the coronary vessel) during the cardiac and respiratory cycles. Stabilizing devices include *compression devices,* which compress the myocardium, restricting the motion of that area but also causing a decrease in stroke volume; these devices can decrease cardiac output minimally to moderately. Also, *suction stabilizers* may be used; they attach to and lift the epicardium, pulling the area taut. These devices do not decrease stroke volume, giving greater hemodynamic stability and allowing greater flexibility in accessing vessels on the inferior and posterior surface of the heart.

When the heart is tilted in a vertical position (for the surgeon to access the posterior or lateral wall), blood flow must travel *upward* to the ventricle, which creates a marked decrease in cardiac output. It is important to increase the preload before lifting the heart out of the pericardial cradle. Leg elevation appears to be the best way to increase preload. Another method of cardiac manipulation includes placing multiple stitches in the pericardium, which act as levers to manipulate the heart. This reduces the hemodynamic instability of cardiac manipulation by hand.

Prepare for improved hemodynamics when blood flow is restored to the coronary artery. Prepare to decrease or discontinue vasoactive agents.

Positioning

The patient is placed in a supine position, with a shoulder roll used to slightly extend the head.

Arms are placed on padding and tucked at the patient's sides. Bed position is changed frequently. The use of a 20-degree tilt Trendelenburg position is useful in reducing some of the hemodynamic instability during the procedure, but steep head-down positions should be avoided due to the severe decrease in functional residual capacity (FRC). This reduction may not be tolerated in a patient who is not supported on bypass.

After arms are tucked at sides, check the function of both the arterial line (Can you draw blood back? Is there a good waveform?) and IVs (Is the IV running without difficulty?).

Surgical prep done is like the prep for CABG, plus both groins are prepared for emergent cannulation if bypass becomes necessary.

Moving the patient from the Trendelenburg position to a reverse Trendelenburg position can help to increase or decrease preload and maintain blood pressure within specific parameters.

Anesthetic

GETA is given with insertion of a single-lumen OETT; muscle relaxants are given. Isoflurane, Sevoflurane, or Desflurane may be used. Fentanyl 15–20 mcg/kg is given. No antifibrinolytics are usually given.

Anesthetic Goals

- Control blood pressure and heart rate. Expect wide swings in hemodynamics while the surgeon lifts and moves the heart to sew grafts.
- Avoid tachycardia. Increase the diastolic time by slowing the heart rate to maximize coronary perfusion and make suturing easier for the surgeon. Keep the heart rate in the low normal range (approximately 60 beats per minute).
- The goal is for the patient to be extubated shortly after surgery. Using lower-dose narcotics and short- to medium-acting muscle relaxants is beneficial.
- Antifibrinolytics are not typically ordered for off-pump CABG, although this is surgeon specific.

- When blood flow is restored to the coronary artery, the blood pressure will increase and the patient's hemodynamics will improve. Be ready to titrate/turn off inotropes at this point.

Monitors
- TEE is invaluable
- Arterial line (usually left radial)
- Pulmonary artery catheter
- Central venous line
- Two large-bore peripheral IVs
- Have pacing/defibrillation pads on

Temperature
Normothermia should be maintained. All measures are taken to avoid hypothermia. Room temperature, fluid warmers, a sterile warming blanket over the legs (sterile if the saphenous conduit is to be excised; the blanket can be applied after graft removed), humidifier, cover head, and low gas flows can all be utilized. When cardiopulmonary bypass is not done, blood cannot be warmed through the pump; thus it is harder to keep and get patient warm.

IV Fluids and Volume Requirements
Keep the patient in a state of euvolemia. It is very important to maintain an adequate intravascular volume for these patients as a first-line defense to maintain blood pressure and cardiac output.

IV Bolus and Drips
IV drips to have ready include phenylephrine (Neo-Synephrine), nitroglycerine, sodium nitroprusside (SNP), and Levophed.

IV bolus drugs to have ready include heparin, protamine, calcium chloride, and ephedrine.

Call for heparin—usually 300–400 units/kg body weight, delivered IV through the central line. The goal is for ACT to be 480 seconds or longer. Perform an ACT check every 30 minutes to ensure that this level is maintained. If additional heparin is required, recheck the ACT in 3 minutes. Reversal of heparin with protamine is optional. If protamine is needed, give 1.3–1.5 mg per 100 units of heparin (dose is calculated based on both the total heparin dose and the ACT values).

Maintain the potassium (K$^+$) level within normal limits (WNL). If K$^+$ is WNL and arrhythmias occur, administer magnesium sulfate. During CPB, the perfusionist will usually give mannitol to help the patient diurese all the fluid given during heart surgery. If CPB is not done, the patient will not be given mannitol and will not diurese as much; therefore, there is no need to replace potassium with as large a dose as when CPB is performed.

Anesthetic Implications

The surgical team must be prepared to place the patient onto cardiopulmonary bypass at any time.

The atrial pacing wire is connected to a pacemaker. A ventricular pacing wire is placed if the RCA vessel is to be interrupted.

The anesthetic goal is to protect the myocardium from ischemia during coronary artery flow interruption while the surgeon performs the anastomosis. Maintain a MAP of 70 mm Hg. ST-segment elevation indicates ischemia; its significance depends on the degree of stenosis of the target vessel and the degree of collateral vessels. Severe ischemia to the RCA can result in dangerous arrhythmias due to interruption of blood flow to the AV node; complete heart block can be seen. Severe ischemia to the LAD can result in a severe decrease in left ventricular pumping ability and be manifested by hypotension, ST-segment elevation, elevated pulmonary artery pressures, and decreased CO and SVO$_2$; the TEE can assess regional wall abnormalities. Therefore, it is important to know the heart catheterization report results preoperatively and to determine which vessels are occluded and by what percentage they are occluded.

Minimally Invasive Direct Coronary Artery Bypass Graft

Minimally invasive direct (without sternotomy approach) coronary artery bypass (MIDCAB) grafting is done without cardiopulmonary bypass. Usually only the left anterior descending coronary artery is operated on with a MIDCAB; however, the surgeon is able to work on *all* the coronary vessels if necessary (even those on the inferior and posterior surfaces of the heart). These procedures are typically short cases, with the goal being to extubate the patient at the end of the case or shortly after the patient arrives in the CTSU. Cardiopulmonary bypass is not used with a MIDCAB, but *the surgical team must be prepared to place the patient on cardiopulmonary bypass at any time.* The patient should be fully prepped and draped in preparation to go on cardiopulmonary bypass in case of emergency.

MIDCAB is used to perform single- to multiple-vessel CABG on a patient where the side effects of cardiopulmonary bypass are especially undesirable. This technique allows for decreased use of blood products and faster recovery from surgery, and it enables patients to avoid the complications associated with CPB.

Operative Procedure

An incision is made at the left thorax at the fourth intercostal space, from approximately 2 cm to the left of the sternum along the inframammary line, usually 6 cm long. Thus, this procedure is sometime called a "mini-thoracotomy." The fourth intercostal space muscles are divided, a 5-cm segment of costal cartilage is removed, and the pleural space is entered. The pericardium is incised and retracted out of the way. The LIMA is dissected free; proximal blood flow originates from the subclavian artery and the distal attachment is anastomosed to the coronary artery past the coronary blockage.

Because the heart is still beating during the grafting, stabilizing devices have been created to reduce the motion of the heart muscle and thus the coronary vessel during the cardiac and respiratory cycles. Stabilizing devices include *compression devices* (which compress the myocardium, restricting the motion of that area but also causing a decrease in stroke volume; can decrease cardiac output minimally to moderately) and *suction stabilizers* (which attach to and lift the epicardium, pulling the area taut, but do not decrease stoke volume giving greater hemodynamic stability; this allows greater flexibility in accessing vessels on the inferior and posterior surfaces of the heart). To minimize myocardial ischemia, shunts inserted by the surgeon can be placed to provide blood flow to the distal myocardium.

After the anastomosis is complete, the flow through the mammary artery is allowed to return prior to removing the tourniquet from the vessel. The integrity of the anastomosis is inspected, and its patency and flow are assessed. The pedicle is then secured to the epicardium.

Call for heparin—usually 300–400 units/kg body weight delivered through a central line. The goal is for the ACT to be 480 seconds or greater.

Check the ACT every 30 minutes to maintain this level. If additional heparin is required, recheck the ACT 3 minutes after each dose is given.

Reversal of heparin with Protamine is optional. If Protamine is needed, give 1.3–1.5 mg per 100 units of heparin (the dose is calculated based on both the heparin dose and ACT values).

Lidocaine 1 mg/kg IV is given before occluding the coronary artery.

If grafts other than the LIMA to the LAD are needed, the proximal anastomosis is done first—the conduit is sewed to the aorta (before the coronary artery is clamped to sew the distal anastomosis)—to decrease the ischemic time. Heart motion can be decreased by the placement of a stabilizing device onto the heart muscle. The MAP should be maintained greater than 60 mm Hg during proximal anastomosis.

The coronary artery to be grafted has a tourniquet or snare placed around the artery to occlude it to ensure bloodless anastomotic conditions, resulting in brief periods of ischemia. During this time, the MAP should be greater than 70 mm Hg and monitoring of myocardial ischemia is crucial. Assess ischemia via EKG, TEE, and new large "V"

waves on the pulmonary artery wedge. Document the time the coronary vessel is occluded and the time it is reopened; this period is the "ischemic" time for that vessel.

Protecting the myocardium from ischemia during coronary artery flow interruption (while the surgeon performs the anastomosis) is imperative. The goal is to maintain myocardial oxygen balance by decreasing oxygen demand (decreasing heart rate, contractility, and myocardial wall tension) and increasing supply (increasing arterial oxygen concentration, keeping MAP greater than 70 mm Hg, maintaining coronary perfusion pressure: DBP–LVEDP, normal 50–70 mm Hg).

After completing the anastomosis, the blood flow through the mammary is allowed to return prior to removal of the occluding device. Anastomotic integrity is checked for patency (by Doppler) and bleeding.

Anesthetic
General anesthesia with a single-lumen endotracheal tube is usual, but the surgeon may require placement of a DLEBT; muscle relaxants are given. The goal is to extubate the patient in the OR at the end of the procedure or early in the ICU stay.

Monitors
- Radial arterial line, preferably right side
- CVP and PAC in RIJ
- TEE
- External defibrillator pads must be on; cannot use internal pads in an emergency

IV Vasoactive Agents
- IV pump: phenylephrine, nitroglycerin
- Diltiazem 125 mg in 100 mL NSS = 1 mg/mL
- Syringe for bolus: vasopressor, vasodilator

IV Fluids and Volume Requirements
- One or two large-bore IVs
- No fluid limits; patients may need diuretics postoperatively

Induction

Here is one suggested technique:

- Etomidate 0.3 mg/kg with EF < 30%, or
- Thiopental 2–4 mg/kg if EF > 30%, or
- Propofol 1–1.5 mg/kg if EF > 30%

Fentanyl 25 mcg/kg or less for the entire case. Use smaller amounts of short-acting opioids for earlier potential extubation at the end of the case.

Succinylcholine (Anectine) is given with a defasiculating dose of Rocuronium on induction.

Maintenance

- Desflurane, sevoflurane, or isoflurane
- Avoid pancuronium due to vagolytic effect
- Short- to intermediate-acting muscle relaxants for reversal at the end of the case

Emergence

- Reverse the muscle relaxant.
- 100% FiO$_2$.

Positioning

The patient is placed in a supine position, with a shoulder roll to slightly extend the head. Arms are placed on padding and tucked at the patient's sides. The bed position is changed frequently. The use of a 20-degree tilt Trendelenburg position is useful in reducing some of the hemodynamic instability during the procedure, but steep head-down positions should be avoided due to the severe decrease in FRC. This reduction may not be tolerated in a patient who is not supported on bypass.

After the patient's arms are tucked at the sides, check the function of both the arterial line (Can you draw blood back? Is there a good waveform?) and IVs (Is the IV running without difficulty?).

Surgical prep done is as for CABG, plus both groins are prepared for emergent cannulation if the patient must go on bypass.

Moving the patient from Trendelenburg position to reverse Trendelenburg position can help to increase or decrease preload and maintain blood pressure within specific parameters.

Anesthetic Implications

No antifibrinolytics (e.g., Amicar) are given.

All measures should be taken to avoid hypothermia. Room temperature, fluid warmers, a sterile warming blanket over the legs (sterile if the saphenous conduit is to be excised—the blanket can be applied after graft removed), humidifier, cover head, and low gas flows can all be utilized. When cardiopulmonary bypass is not done, blood cannot be warmed through the pump; in such a cases, it is more difficult to keep and get the patient warm.

Laser Transmyocardial Revascularization

Laser transmyocardial revascularization (TMR) involves the creation of transmural channels that improve myocardial perfusion through collateral vessels. This procedure must be done on a beating heart. TMR can be performed in conjunction with a CABG on CPB.

TMR is used to treat severe coronary artery disease that is not amenable to standard CABG and angioplasty and that is refractory to medical treatment. Patients may be sicker after this surgery until collateral circulation is formed.

Operative Procedure

An incision is made either by sternotomy or left anterior thoracotomy at the fifth through sixth intercostal spaces. The pericardium is entered anteriorly, and the heart is suspended in the pericardial cradle. The carbon dioxide laser is aimed and placed against the epicardium and fired. The transmural channels, 1 mm in diameter and 1 cm apart, that are created act as conduits for the flow of oxygenated blood from the LV into the ischemic myocardium. The number of channels varies, depending on the size of the heart. The average number is 25.

The laser is triggered to fire on the R wave of the EKG when the ventricle is maximally dilated. This minimizes the risk of collateral damage to heart structures and decreases the risk of induction of arrhythmias.

Success is measured by the TEE. The new flow of oxygenated blood appears as a stream of air bubbles in the ventricle.

The channels become endothelialized (a clot is formed on the epicardium) and remain open with improved perfusion through collateral formation, especially in the subendocardial areas. After TMR, perfusion scans will show the creation of new blood vessels or modeling of existing blood vessels that indicates improved collateral flow to the ischemic myocardium.

Anesthetic

For the thoracotomy approach, GA is given with insertion of a double-lumen endobronchial tube. The tube is changed to a single-lumen ETT at the end of the case.

For the sternotomy approach, GA is given with insertion of a single-lumen endobronchial tube.

Positioning

The patient is placed in a partial right lateral position, with a sheet roll running the length of the back so that the upper body is turned partially but the hips are supine (groin vessels can be accessed for CPB or IABP).

Moving the patient from Trendelenburg to reverse Trendelenburg position can help to increase or decrease preload and maintain blood pressure within specific parameters.

Anesthetic Implications

Decrease FiO_2 from 100% to 40% when the laser is being used. Use eye pads soaked with saline. Keep a basin of water with a bulb syringe at the head of the OR table in case of fire. Eye protection is required for both the patient and all staff in the room.

Temperature

Maintain normothermia for the patient. All measures should be taken to avoid hypothermia. Room temperature increased, fluid warmers, a warming blanket over the patient's legs, a warmed humidifier, head cover, and low gas flows can all be utilized. When cardiopulmonary bypass is not done, blood cannot be warmed through pump; in such cases, it is more difficult to keep and get the patient warm.

Monitors and IV Access
- One or two large-bore peripheral lines
- CVP and usually a PAC in RIJ
- Radial arterial line, right preferred

Induction
The induction regimen includes etomidate, fentanyl, midazolam, succinylcholine, rocuronium, and 100% FiO_2.

Maintenance
- Recommended regimen: oxygen/air, isoflurane, fentanyl, muscle relaxant of choice.
- Have magnesium and lidocaine available.
- The goal is early extubation in the CTSU.
- The patient may need some inotropic support because the channels created need some time to develop and increase myocardial perfusion.

Complications

Potential complications of TMR include ventricular fibrillation, bleeding leading to pericardial tamponade, accidental perforation of great vessels or epicardial coronary arteries, damaged chordae tendinae or cusp of the mitral or aortic valve if laser power is insufficient to create a hole through the pool of blood in the LV, and damage to the Purkinje network.

Minimally Invasive Cardiac Surgery

"Minimally invasive cardiac surgery" can refer to OPCAB, MIDCAB, and even robotic-assisted CABG. In such a procedure, a full sternotomy is not done and there is limited or slow access to the heart in an emergency.

External defibrillator pads should be placed on the anterior and posterior chest. The patient can be defibrillated, cardioverted, or externally paced through these pads.

HEART VALVES

Left Ventricular Vent Use in Aortic or Mitral Valve Surgery or Closure of a Ventricular Septal Defect

During cardiopulmonary bypass, if the left heart valves are closed, there is a danger of over-distention of the myocardium due to blood build-up. This blood comes from the coronary venous and coronary sinus (i.e., bronchial, thesbian, and azygous veins) system, which drains into the heart and does not go through the vena cava to the bypass machine. This blood needs to be drained to prevent myocardial stretch. Distention can lead to myocardial warming and subsequent ischemia from an increase in MVO_2; surgical exposure can be compromised. The LV vent is placed to drain this blood, remove air to prevent embolism, and decompress the left side of the heart. This vent is also used for antegrade perfusion of cardioplegia.

Valve Disease: Treatment Goals

- The only time a decrease in preload is desirable is with *acute* MR.

- In a patient with stenotic valves, the goal is to increase the SVR to feed the coronary arteries.
- With regurgitation, the goal is to decrease SVR so as to unload blood more easily; and to increase the heart rate to push blood through with less time for back flow.

Hypertrophic Cardiomyopathy

Patients with hypertrophic cardiomyopathy (HOCM) have an increased myocardial oxygen need. They are prone to left bundle branch block and left anterior hemiblock.

These patients complain of dyspnea, angina, pre-syncope, and syncope on exertion but most patients are asymptomatic before their sudden death.

Factors that exacerbate the outflow obstruction include conditions that decrease ventricular cavity size, such as enhanced contractility, decreased ventricular volume (decreased preload), and decreased afterload.

Treat HOCM with beta-blockers and calcium-channel blockers, both of which decrease contractility. Maintain a slower heart rate, a decreased

	AS	AR	MS	MR	Tamponade	HOCM
Preload	Full	Full	Full	Full	Full	Full
Heart rate	Slower normal sinus rhythm	Faster normal sinus rhythm	Slower normal sinus, avoid tachycardia	Faster normal sinus rhythm	Increase	Slow
Afterload	Constrict	Dilate	Maintain normal, don't overdilate	Dilate	Constrict	Maintain
Contractility					Increase	Decrease
Treatment	Neosynephrine	Ephedrine	Volume	Nipride	Epinephrine	Volume
		Increase heart rate	Beta-blocker		Volume	Beta-blocker
	Avoid NTG	Atropine and SNP OK to give			Pericardial tap or window	Avoid inotropes and NTG

contractility, and a reduced left ventricular ejection—all of these measures increase left ventricular size by widening the left ventricular outflow tract diameter. Volatile agents cause a dose-dependent myocardial depression, reducing the degree of left ventricular outflow obstruction.

Atrial fibrillation or a junctional rhythm are poorly tolerated in HOCM patients due to the loss of atrial kick. Amiodarone is effective for both supraventricular and ventricular arrhythmias. Digoxin is unsuitable because of its positive inotropic effects.

Hypotension is managed best with alpha agonists (phenylephrine, Levophed), intravascular volume, and Trendelenburg position.

Avoid the use of inotropes (which increase outflow obstruction), ketamine, and Pancuronium (which causes tachycardia).

Regional anesthesia is contraindicated with HOCM.

Heart Rate
Avoid tachycardia.

Preload
Maintain adequate preload. Give fluids to maintain volume. Avoid the use of nitroglycerin.

Afterload
Maintain adequate afterload by using phenylephrine.

CARDIAC SURGERY: AORTIC VALVE

Aortic valve disease may present as stenosis, regurgitation, or both.

Aortic Stenosis

Aortic stenosis (AS) may occur as a valvular, sub-valvular, or supravalvular condition. When the valve is stenotic, it causes a pressure gradient between the left ventricle and the aorta. The more stenotic the valve, the higher the gradient (pressure overloads in left ventricle). This imbalance causes the ventricle to hypertrophy, with

decreased compliance occurring in response to the increased pressures. Chronic obstruction to left ventricular ejection results in left concentric ventricular hypertrophy with a myocardium that is very susceptible to ischemia. The LV is vulnerable to ischemia due to increased oxygen need and consumption along with decreased subendocardial perfusion, not as a result of coronary artery disease.

- Normal: valve area is 3–4 cm^2; gradient 10–25 mm Hg
- Moderate stenosis: valve area is 1.5–1.8 cm^2; gradient is 25–40 mm Hg
- Critical stenosis: valve area is less than 0.7 cm^2; gradient is more than 50 mm Hg

Patients with aortic stenosis may have angina, syncope, or heart failure related to an increase in left ventricular systolic pressure. They may also experience dyspnea, decreased exercise tolerance, sudden death, decrease in LV compliance, and LV hypertrophy. The oxygen demands of a hypertrophied myocardium may be more than the heart can supply.

The primary goals in treatment of aortic stenosis are to maintain normal sinus rhythm, avoid tachycardia, and maintain normovolemia and SVR. A decreased SVR can mean a decreased blood pressure and decreased coronary perfusion pressures. Avoid hypovolemia. Diastolic blood pressure must be maintained to preserve coronary artery blood flow. Systemic pressure must be maintained to perfuse the myocardium.

Spinal and epidural anesthesia are contraindicated with aortic stenosis.

Heart Rate
Maintain a slow to normal heart rate. A longer systole is needed to get the blood out. However, too slow a heart rate lengthens diastole and decreases the blood volume moved to the ventricle.

Preload
Maintain high preload; do not use nitroglycerin.

Afterload

An increased SVR is needed to maintain coronary perfusion (which explains why spinal and epidural anesthesia are contraindicated in patients with AS). Use volume and phenylephrine to achieve this goal.

Aortic Regurgitation

In aortic regurgitation (AR), blood flow backs into the left ventricle due to a floppy aortic valve, increasing the heart's workload and gradually increasing compliance.

Maintain NSR at a slightly increased heart rate; this lessens diastolic time and decreases regurgitation time. A decreased SVR will help the heart empty with each contraction. Maintain myocardial contractility; a slight increase in cardiac preload is acceptable. Aortic regurgitation results in chronic volume overload of the left ventricle with eccentric hypertrophy.

Patients with aortic regurgitation may have dyspnea, angina, LV failure, and widened pulse pressure. The diastolic blood pressure is usually low *because the valve does not clamp shut.*

Heart Rate

The heart rate should be normal to slightly increased.

Preload

Maintain a normal to slightly increased preload.

Afterload

Lower the afterload by vasodilation; can use sodium nitroprusside (SNP). Avoid any increase in SVR.

Aortic Valve Repair

Stenotic aortic valve (AV) repair is usually performed in a cardiac catheterization lab where a balloon valvotomy procedure can be performed. Open chest aortic valve repair is almost exclusively limited to patients with aortic regurgitation (AR) without aortic stenosis.

Operative Procedure

Aortic valvotomy is not curative but should relieve many of the symptoms associated with damage to this valve. A guide wire is introduced into the femoral artery and advanced into the aorta and into the left side of the heart. A sheath is passed over the guide wire; through the sheath, a balloon catheter is introduced and positioned across the narrowed aortic valve. The balloon is inflated and deflated several times (visualized using a dilute contrast dye) to widen the opening. If there is difficulty maintaining the balloon in the aortic valve during inflation, temporary ventricular pacing at a high heart rate can reduce the cardiac output, giving stability to the balloon. There is a small but significant risk of pulmonary edema due to severe aortic regurgitation with this procedure. When the cardiologist/surgeon believes the valve is wide enough, the catheter is removed.

In the open chest aortic valve repair a median sternotomy is done, and cardiopulmonary bypass is initiated. A transverse aortotomy is done above the sinotubular junction. A reduction annuloplasty is done.

Anesthetic

General anesthesia is given with insertion of an OETT; muscle relaxants are given.

Monitors

An arterial line, a central line, and a PA catheter are needed. A TEE monitor is very helpful.

IV Vasoactive Agents
- IV pump: phenylephrine, nitroglycerin
- Syringe for bolus: vasopressor, vasodilator; phenylephrine or ephedrine should be available.

Positioning

The patient should be placed in a supine position, with a shoulder roll placed to extend the head.

Moving the patient from Trendelenburg position to reverse Trendelenburg position can help to increase or decrease preload and maintain blood pressure within specific parameters.

Anesthetic Implications

Prophylactic antibiotics should be administered before skin incision.

Aortic Valve Replacement

Aortic valve replacement (AVR) involves the excision and replacement of the diseased aortic valve with a mechanical or pig valve. It is done with the patient on cardiopulmonary bypass (CPB); see the section on CABG for a discussion of CPB-related issues.

AVR may be performed in case of a stenotic or regurgitive valve. The patient may have had rheumatic heart disease, a congenital bicuspid valve, endocarditis, or calcified degeneration of the valve.

Operative Procedure

The heart is approached through a median sternotomy. Vents are placed in the heart to remove the venous drainage still emptying into the heart (even though the patient is on CBP—that is, blood return from bronchial, thesbian veins, pulmonary retrograde flow, and aortic insufficiency).

The aorta is cross-clamped distal to the valve. The aortic root is opened, and the valve is excised. The annulus is measured and the appropriate-size prosthesis is inserted and sutured into place. Rewarming starts after the valve is sutured into place. Air is vented from the left ventricle and the aorta before the aorta is unclamped. Pacing wires are placed. The heart is closed and purged of air.

Anesthetic

General anesthesia is given with insertion of an OETT; muscle relaxants are given.

Monitors

An arterial line, a central line, and a PA catheter are needed. A TEE monitor is very helpful.

Drugs

Phenylephrine, ephedrine and beta-blockers should be drawn up and ready.

Vasoactives

IV drips to have ready include phenylephrine (Neo-Synephrine), nitroglycerine, and sodium nitroprusside (SNP)

Positioning

The patient is placed in a supine position, with a shoulder roll placed to extend the head.

Moving the patient from Trendelenburg position to reverse Trendelenburg position can help to increase or decrease preload and maintain blood pressure within specific parameters.

Anesthetic Implications

Prophylactic antibiotics should be administered before skin incision.

Systemic arterial vasodilation with hypotension must be avoided and treated quickly and aggressively if it does occur. However, postoperative hypertension places stress on the new valve.

These patients require a higher than normal filling pressure after coming off CPB.

CARDIAC SURGERY: MITRAL VALVE

The mitral valve is a bi-leaflet valve, with a normal surface area of 4–6 cm^2.

Mitral Stenosis

In mild mitral stenosis (MS), the mitral valve surface area is greater than 1.5 cm^2, with a gradient pressure of less than 5 mm Hg. Symptoms usually start when valve closes to less than 2.5 cm^2. In severe stenosis, the mitral valve surface area is less than 1.0 cm^2, with a gradient pressure of more than 25 mm Hg.

MS prevents the left ventricle from becoming fully filled. The left atrium hypertrophies, resulting in increased pulmonary pressures.

In treating MS, it is important to maintain NSR, avoid tachycardia (the LV does not have time to fill), and maintain normovolemia and preload. A beta-blocker or calcium-channel blocker may be needed to keep the heart rate at 60–80 beats/min. Digitalis may be used to control the ventricular rate response if the patient is in atrial fibrillation.

Patients with mitral stenosis may have shortness of breath with exertion, pulmonary edema, pulmonary hypertension, increased left atrial pressures, and right ventricular hypertrophy and/or failure.

Heart Rate
Maintain a normal heart rate, and avoid tachycardia (which causes a decreased CO). Bradycardia increases CO.

Preload
Maintain adequate intravascular volume but avoid pulmonary vascular congestion.

Pulmonary Vascular Resistance
Avoid increases in pulmonary vascular resistance (PVR). PVR increase may be due to use of nitrous oxide, acidosis, or hypoxia. Treat this condition with nitroglycerin (to decrease preload), diuretic, and reverse Trendelenburg position. Consider giving nitric oxide.

SVR/Afterload
Avoid increases in SVR but do not overdilate.

Mitral Regurgitation

Mitral regurgitation (MR) causes dilation of the left ventricle and cardiomyopathy. Acute mitral valve regurgitation can cause a severe increase in left atrial pressures and possibly pulmonary edema. Reflex sympathetic stimulation leads to tachycardia. Chronic development of MR leads to left atrial hypertrophy, along with left ventricular overload and eccentric hypertrophy.

In patients with MR, maintain NSR to a slightly more rapid rhythm. A decreased SVR helps the left ventricle pump blood out, and normovolemia

is necessary. Volatile agents can be especially deleterious in patients with CHF; determine whether their use is appropriate based on each patient's hemodynamics.

Patients with MR may have dyspnea, palpitations, fatigue, left ventricular hypertrophy and/or failure, increased left atrial pressures, atrial fibrillation, and/or pulmonary edema.

Heart Rate
Maintain a slightly more rapid normal sinus rhythm.

Preload
Maintain normovolemia to slightly full volume.

Afterload
Decrease afterload.

Acute MR
Stabilize the patient by decreasing the amount of regurgitation, increasing forward cardiac output, and reducing pulmonary veno-congestion.

Give vasodilating drugs:

- Nitroprusside: In a normotensive patient, it may accomplish all three of the previously mentioned goals. It should not be administered alone in a hypotensive patient, as it may decrease diastolic blood pressure and coronary perfusion pressure.
- Dobutamine: Inotropic agent.
- Milrinone: Inodilator agent (both an inotropic and vasodilator).
- IABP increases forward flow while decreasing regurgitant volume.
- Prepare the patient for surgery.

Chronic MR
Treatment of patients with asymptomatic chronic MR is controversial. They may need to be managed surgically before deterioration of left ventricular function occurs. Manage the ventricular response rate if the patient is in atrial fibrillation with digoxin, calcium-channel blockers, beta-blockers, or

Amiodarone. The risk of embolism is less in chronic MR than in MS, but still present; thus the patient's INR should be maintained between 2 and 3.

Severe mitral regurgitation in the presence of congestive heart failure (even with normal LV function and an ejection fraction greater than 60%) requires surgical repair.

Mitral Valve Repair

Mitral valve (MV) repair is necessary to treat a moderately to severely stenotic or regurgitive valve.

Operative Procedure

Mitral balloon valvotomy doubles the valve area, decreases the pressure gradient, and improves overall function of the heart. It will decrease the left atrial pressure to less than 18 mm Hg if successful. This procedure is performed in a cardiac catheterization lab. Valvotomy is not curative but should relieve many of the symptoms associated with MS or MR.

A catheter is inserted (usually) through the femoral vein and advanced into the right atrium (RA). A tiny hole is created in the septum between the RA and the left atrium (LA); the catheter is positioned into the narrowed mitral valve. The balloon is inflated and deflated several times to widen the opening. The catheter is then removed. Valve repair may also be performed as an open procedure. It is done to separate fused valve leaflets, sew torn leaflets, or reshape parts of the valve. The surgeon will place a bi-caval cannula through the right atrium into the inferior vena cava and a right-angle cannula directly into the superior vena cava, allowing unobstructed access to the dome of the left atrium for the valve work.

Anesthetic

General anesthesia is given with insertion of an OETT for an open procedure; muscle relaxants are given.

Monitors

An arterial line, a central line, and a PA catheter are needed. A TEE monitor is very helpful.

Drugs

Phenylephrine or ephedrine should be drawn up and ready to treat hypotension. Beta-blockers should be available to decrease the patient's heart rate.

Vasoactives

IV drips to have ready include phenylephrine (Neosynephrine), nitroglycerine, and sodium nitroprusside (SNP).

Positioning

The patient is placed in a supine position; for an open procedure a shoulder roll is placed to extend the head. Bilateral arms are placed on pads and tucked at the patient's sides.

Moving the patient from Trendelenburg position to reverse Trendelenburg position can help to increase or decrease preload and maintain blood pressure within specific parameters.

Anesthetic Implications

Prophylactic antibiotics should be given before skin incision.

Continue preoperative digoxin and beta-blockers to maintain a slower heart rate. Avoid ketamine, as it will increase the heart rate.

Mitral Valve Replacement

Mitral valve replacement (MVR) consists of the excision and replacement of a diseased mitral valve. It is done while the patient is on cardiopulmonary bypass.

MVR is used to treat a moderately to severely stenotic or floppy regurgitive valve. Valve replacement with a mechanical or biological valve is reserved for valves that are damaged beyond repair.

Operative Procedure

An open mitral valve commissurotomy is approached through a median sternotomy. Moderate hypothermic cardiopulmonary bypass is initiated, the ascending aorta is cross-clamped, and cardioplegia is infused. An atriotomy is performed to expose the mitral valve. The valve is excised, the annulus is measured, and the appropriate prosthesis is inserted and sutured into place. Rewarming then starts. Pacing wires are placed. The replacement valve can be a preserved biological valve (porcine) or an artificial prosthesis of various sizes, shapes, and mechanics.

Anesthetic
General anesthesia is given with insertion of a single-lumen OETT; muscle relaxants are given.

Positioning
The patient is placed in a supine position, with a shoulder roll placed to extend the head.

Moving the patient from Trendelenburg position to reverse Trendelenburg position can help to increase or decrease preload and maintain blood pressure within specific parameters.

Anesthetic Implications
Prophylactic antibiotics should be given before skin incision.

PERICARDIAL SURGERY
Pericardiectomy/Pericardial Window

Pericardiectomy is the subtotal or total removal of the pericardium. The pericardial window is the piece of the pericardium being removed.

Pericardial disease can be divided into constrictive pericarditis and effusive pericarditis. Constrictive pericarditis involves inflammation affecting both the parietal and visceral pericardium, whereas effusive pericarditis is the accumulation of fluid within the pericardial sac. Both conditions produce cardiac compression to some degree.

Acute *tamponade* is a situation in which effusion recurs or cannot be drained satisfactorily with effusion pericarditis. It may also occur with constrictive pericarditis, when the pericardium becomes fibrous and impairs contractility, thereby restricting preload.

Pericardial pressure is normally subatmospheric, but becomes more negative during inspiration. A rapid increase in intrapericardial fluid will increase systemic venous pressure, reduce chamber volumes, narrow the difference between systolic and diastolic pressure, and cause an overall reduction in the heart's ability to pump blood out. A decrease in arterial pressure of more than 10 mm Hg may be seen during inspiration (pulsus paradoxus).

Operative Procedure
A left anterolateral thoracotomy or a median sternotomy is used to access the pericardium. The pericardium is opened vertically and flaps dissected; the pericardial flaps are excised approximately 1 cm anterior to the phrenic nerves. The outer pericardial layer may then be separated from the pleura, which contains the phrenic nerves.

Cardiopulmonary bypass may be used and accessed through the femoral vessels.

Anesthetic
General anesthesia is used with a double-lumen endobronchial tube (DLEBT); muscle relaxants are given. If a flexible bronchoscopy will be performed, initially insert a single-lumen endotracheal tube; place at least an 8.0-size tube. The single-lumen ETT may be changed to a double-lumen tube to facilitate one-lung ventilation. Confirm placement of the double-lumen tube with fiberoptic bronchoscopy. At the end of the case, if the patient does not meet the extubation criteria, change out the DLEBT to a single-lumen tube. (See Chapter 3 on DLEBT for more information.)

Positioning
The patient is placed in a supine position, with bilateral arms tucked at the sides.

Moving the patient from Trendelenburg position to reverse Trendelenburg position can help to increase or decrease preload and maintain blood pressure within specific parameters.

Anesthetic Implications

Induction of anesthesia can really decrease blood pressure because of the pressure already present on the heart. Have ephedrine ready for hypotension; do not use phenylephrine (Neosynephrine) as it is undesirable to increase the SVR.

Once the pericardium open, the effusion is suctioned away and the blood pressure can increase.

The EKG will show nonspecific ST-T changes in the majority of patients; some will have a low QRS voltage or atrial arrhythmia.

CARDIAC SURGERY: THORACIC AORTA

ATA: ascending thoracic aneurysm; proximal to innominate artery; affects cerebral perfusion.

Arch: between origins of innominate and left subclavian artery.

DTA: descending thoracic aneurysm; affects spinal cord perfusion; distal from origin of left subclavian artery.

Aortic Dissection

An aortic dissection is a tear or rupture of the intimal layer of the aorta. Such intramural separation may occur due to the force of blood. The aneurysm progresses distally, with dilation involving all three layers of the vessel wall. Any artery take-off from the aorta may also become involved (e.g., iliac, common carotid, innominate, left subclavian, renal).

Classifications of Aortic Dissection

Stanford Classification of Thoracic Aortic Dissection

Type A: involves the ascending aorta and aortic arch regardless of its extent.

Type B: descending aorta distal to the left subclavian.

Proximal lesions are considered surgical emergencies.

DeBakey Classification of Thoracic Aortic Dissection

Type I: dissects all of aorta (ascending, arch, descending); only type I deals with arch.

Type II: ascending aorta only, stops proximally to the innominate artery.

Type IIIa: distal subclavian to above diaphragm.

Type IIIb: distal subclavian to past diaphragm.

Crawford Classification of Thoracic Aortic Dissection

I: proximal to above renal arteries.

II: proximal to aortic bifurcation.

III: above the renal arteries to beyond the aortic bifurcation.

IV: at the renal arteries to below the aortic bifurcation; "abdominal."

Clinical Presentation

Aortic dissection can be asymptomatic if very small. If there are symptoms, they may include the following:

- Interscapular (between shoulder blades) back pain or left-sided pleuritic pain; sudden-onset severe chest or neck pain; abdominal pain.
- Chest pain: anterior chest pain for ascending dissection; posterior chest pain for descending dissection.
- Hoarseness, stridor, dysphagia, dyspnea. The recurrent laryngeal nerve [RLN] loops around the aorta on the left; when the aorta increases in size it can stretch the RLN with tracheal/esophageal compression.
- Tearing sensation.
- Acute HTN.
- Feeling of impending doom.
- Signs of MI, CNS dysfunction, renal failure, visceral ischemia (blood in stool), paraplegia, lower extremity claudication or absent lower extremity pulses.

TEE can be used to diagnose aortic dissection.

It is crucially important to assess and document the neurologic, cardiovascular, and pulmonary systems prior to surgery.

Medical Management
- Beta-blockers may be given to decrease the heart rate to the goal of 60–80 beats/min: labetalol, esmolol (Brevibloc), Inderal, Lopressor (metoprolol).
- Vasodilators may be given to decrease the systolic pressure to the goal of 100–115 mm Hg: sodium nitroprusside (SNP), nitroglycerin, fenoldopam, hydralazine.

Preoperative Measures
Give a nonparticulate antacid or Reglan if possible.

Surgical and Anesthetic Goals
- Address the airway first.
- Place an arterial line and two large-bore IVs. If time permits, place a PA catheter and CVP.
- Lower the systolic BP to 105–115 mm Hg.
- Control acute hemorrhage; decrease ejection velocity. The heart rate goal is 60–80 beats/min.
  - Propranolol: Administered as IV bolus of 1 mg; additional doses up to 4–8 mg may be required until results are seen.
  - Labetalol: combined alpha and beta-blocker. Give a 20 mg loading bolus and allow several minutes until effects are seen. If no effect occurs, double the dose and wait. If no effect is observed, repeat 40–80 mg every 10 minutes until a total of 300 mg has been given. An infusion of 1 mg/min or a small bolus may be used every 10–30 minutes for control.
  - Esmolol (Brevibloc): short-acting, short-half-life beta-blocker. Give a bolus of 500 mcg/kg over 1 minute; an infusion of 50 mcg/kg/min may also be given up to 300 mcg/kg/min. This agent is a good choice in patients with obstructive lung disease, as it is beta1 selective.

- Monitor for organ ischemia (CNS, heart, lungs, kidney, liver, and gut).
- Repair the diseased aorta and restore the relationships among the major arterial branches.
- Control postoperative bleeding and coagulopathy.
- Give barbiturates to ensure non-awareness and flat EEG activity.
- Have 8 or more units of typed and cross-matched blood available in the operating room.

Vasodilators
- Sodium nitroprusside (SNP): agent of choice. Starting dosage is 0.5–1 mcg/kg/min and titrate.
- Nitroglycerin: direct vasodilator, but less potent than SNP. Use in cases of myocardial ischemia with ascending aortic pathology. Dosage is 1–4 mcg/kg/min.
- Fenoldopam: rapid-acting vasodilator D_1-receptor agonist. Causes vasodilation with increased renal blood flow (RBF). Starting dosage is 0.05–0.1 mcg/kg/min. Maximum dose is 0.8 mcg/kg/min.

Induction
Use a rapid-sequence induction.

Repair of Ascending Thoracic Aortic Aneurysm or Dissection

Surgery is needed to repair the ascending portion of an aortic dissection. The aortic valve may also need to be repaired if it is involved. The coronary arteries can also be affected, usually due to the compression from the dissection, and their repair will require bypass grafts to be done. The patient is placed on full cardiopulmonary bypass for this procedure. The aortic arch vessels, which provide the blood supply to the brain, need to be temporarily isolated to repair the ascending aortic dissection. Techniques that allow for brain protection and cerebral perfusion are required because of the increased potential for cerebral ischemia. Deep hypothermic cardiac arrest (DHCA) and both antegrade and retrograde cerebral perfusion are utilized for cerebral protection. (See Chapter 3 for more information on cerebral protection.)

Atherosclerosis, advanced syphilis, and Marfan syndrome are all diseases associated with aortic dissection or aneurysm. Signs and symptoms of an ascending aortic aneurysm reflect extension of the aneurysm to the trachea, esophagus, laryngeal nerves, vessels of the aortic arch, coronary arteries, and pericardium. See "clinical presentation in aortic dissection" above for more possible signs and symptoms.

Operative Procedure

A median sternotomy is used, and the patient is typically placed on cardiopulmonary bypass and performed with deep hypothermic cardiac arrest (DHCA). It is not possible to place an aortic cannula due to the area associated with the dissection, but cardiopulmonary bypass can be done through an atriofemoral or femoral–femoral approach. Proximal and distal aortic clamps are placed. During DHCA, the ascending aorta is opened, debris is removed, the proximal aortic root is reconstructed, and suturing of the graft begins. The aortic valve is either resuspended (85%) or replaced. Working distally into the arch, the aortic layers are reapproximated with a Teflon strip supporting the medial and adventitial layers. Once the distal graft is completed, the graft is clamped and cardiopulmonary bypass is started. The heart is then de-aired, the cross-clamp is removed, and the coronary arteries are allowed to perfuse. Reimplantation of coronary arteries into the aortic graft is necessary with ascending aortic dissections.

Anesthetic

General anesthesia is given with insertion of a double-lumen endobronchial tube (DLEBT); muscle relaxants are given.

Positioning

The patient is placed in a supine position, with a shoulder roll to extend the head. Bilateral arms are tucked at the sides.

Moving the patient from Trendelenburg position to reverse Trendelenburg position can help to increase or decrease preload and maintain blood pressure within specific parameters.

Anesthetic Implications

Monitors and Lines

Blood pressure control is paramount. Two or more large-bore IVs are placed due to the hemorrhage risk.

Arterial lines are placed in the left radial (due to clamping of the innominate artery) *and* femoral arteries (above and below the aneurysm, which allows the surgical team to assess perfusion pressures to both the brain and kidneys during cross-clamping). These lines should be placed in an artery whose flow does not depend on the segment of the aorta to be clamped.

Place a pulse oximetry clip on the patient's right hand. The waveform will be lost if the innominate artery is compressed or if there is inadequate blood supply from the false lumen of a dissected aorta or obstruction by an intimal flap.

Venous cannulation consists of a single cannula to right atria.

TEE is invaluable to visualize the dissection (i.e., to identify site of intimal tears and extent of dissection) and monitor ventricular function, valvular function, and wall motion changes that might reflect ischemia.

A pulmonary artery catheter helps to precisely control systemic and intracardiac pressures in patients with a significant aortic lesion and underlying HTN. This information is used to guide fluid management and blood product replacement during complex aortic resection complicated by hypothermia and coagulation disturbances.

SSEP is monitored during cross-clamping to identify important intercostal arteries that will need to be anastomosed to the aortic graft.

Barbiturates and corticosteroids may offer further spinal cord and cerebral protection with prolonged cross-clamp time. (See Chapter 3 for more information on cerebral protection.)

EEG and BIS are used to monitor the depth of hypothermia and ensure electrical silence during DHCA.

Monitor the urinary output every thirty minutes, and watch for hematuria.

Monitor the nasal temperature to verify brain cooling.

Key Points

It is of paramount importance to control hyperdynamic responses to intubation and surgical stimulation that may increase aortic shear forces and worsen dissection, precipitate aneurysm rupture, or cause myocardial ischemia. Moderate doses of short-acting opioids (fentanyl or sufentanil IV boluses, or a remifentanil infusion) provide satisfactory analgesia while allowing for an early neurologic assessment and patient wake-up in the ICU. Barbiturates and volatile anesthetics used for cerebral protection will provide further hypnosis in the OR.

Repair of an Aortic Arch Aneurysm or Dissection

Surgical repair of an aortic arch aneurysm or dissection is performed with the patient on cardiopulmonary bypass with deep hypothermic cardiac arrest (DHCA). DHCA is necessary because arch surgery must interrupt cerebral blood flow; see Chapter 3 for more information on DHCA.

Atherosclerosis, advanced syphilis, and Marfan syndrome are all diseases associated with aortic dissection or aneurysm.

Operative Procedure

A median sternotomy is performed, with the patient placed in deep hypothermic circulatory arrest (DHCA). An atriofemoral or femoral–femoral bypass may be used. The aneurysm and possible dissection can extend from the origin of the

innominate artery to the distal origin of the left subclavian artery; preserving brain blood flow is crucial when the arch is affected in this way.

Anesthetic

GETA is given with insertion of a single-lumen OETT or a DLEBT; muscle relaxants are given.

Positioning

The patient is placed in a supine position, with a shoulder roll.

Moving the patient from Trendelenburg position to reverse Trendelenburg position can help to increase or decrease preload and maintain blood pressure within specific parameters.

Anesthetic Implications

The anesthetic goals with this procedure are to control the patient's blood pressure, preserve the myocardium and reduce myocardial stress, preserve CNS integrity by maintaining cerebral blood flow, and reduce the risk of hemorrhage. Rewarm the patient slowly.

Monitors and IV Access

- Arterial line: left radial (due to clamping of the innominate) or femoral catheter (a femoral arterial line may be the only option)
- Pulmonary artery catheter, CVP, TEE, cell-saver technology
- Multiple peripheral IV sites
- SSEP
- EEG and BIS; transcranial Doppler
- Nasal temperature to verify brain cooling

Induction

Agents are given to control the patient's hemodynamics—narcotics, beta-blockers, and volatile agents.

Repair of a Descending Thoracic Aortic (Thoracoabdominal) Aneurysm or Dissection

Surgical repair is needed to treat a descending thoracic or thoracoabdominal aortic aneurysm or possible dissection. Atherosclerosis, advanced syphilis, and Marfan syndrome are all diseases associated with aortic dissection or aneurysm. Patients with descending thoracic aortic disease are usually hypertensive.

Operative Procedure

A left lateral thoracotomy incision is made at the fourth through fifth or seventh through eighth intercostal space. This procedure is usually done without placing the patient on cardiopulmonary bypass. Commonly, a cross-clamp is applied above and below the aneurysm, the aorta is opened, and the diseased segment is replaced with a graft. A synthetic graft may be placed inside the opened aorta and sewn into place; the old aorta wall is then closed over the graft. The clamps are removed, bleeding is controlled, and the chest is closed.

Three surgical methods are used:

- *Simple cross-clamp.* The proximal aorta is clamped, with the surgeon sewing as quickly as possible. This technique requires excellent surgical skills and speed to reduce the ischemia time.
- *Shunt.* Blood is shunted distally in an attempt to maintain spinal cord, renal, and lower extremity perfusion. It is usually shunted from the proximal aorta to the femoral artery, which decompresses the proximal segment and perfuses the distal segment. Systemic heparinization is not required with a shunt.
- *Cardiopulmonary bypass.* The aorta is clamped, and blood is circulated to the lower body via femoral–femoral bypass or left atrial–femoral bypass.

Anesthetic

One-lung ventilation with a left double-lumen endobronchial tube is used to deflate the left lung, thereby decreasing pulmonary contusion and improving surgical access. CPAP is used for the upper lung (patient in lateral decubitus position);

PEEP is used for the lower lung. Change to a single-lumen endotracheal tube at the end of the case for postoperative ventilation. Note that facial and airway edema can be severe at the end of the case, so have a tube changer, fiberoptic scope, Glidescope, jet ventilator, and other equipment readily available to manage the tube change.

Induction

Many of these patients will be considered to have full stomachs and should have a rapid-sequence induction (RSI). Agents to control hemodynamics should be available—narcotics, beta-blockers, and volatile agents.

Maintenance

Isoflurane does not inhibit hypoxic pulmonary vasoconstriction (HPV) with one-lung ventilation, so PaO_2 does not drop. Fentanyl and muscle relaxation are given.

Pre-clamp Period

Approximately 30 minutes before the cross-clamp is applied, give mannitol 0.5–1.0 g/kg to protect the spinal cord and the kidneys. See Chapter 3 for more information regarding aortic cross-clamping and spinal cord issues.

Aortic Cross-clamp On

Maintain MAP at more than 70 mm Hg after the aortic cross-clamp is applied. The mean arterial pressure distal to the aortic clamp will decrease and the distal spinal cord will be at risk of ischemia. Several techniques can be used to increase the distal arterial perfusion pressure, such as the placement of a simple shunt (a shunt is placed above and below the cross-clamp) and a partial (femoral vein to femoral artery) or full (left atrium to femoral artery) cardiopulmonary bypass. Heparin is usually not given during these cases because of the patient's coagulopathy, unless partial or full cardiopulmonary bypass is used.

The use of nitroprusside can be detrimental to spinal cord perfusion, as this agent decreases systemic vascular resistance, thereby shunting blood away from the spinal cord vessels and collateral branches.

Positioning

The patient is placed in a right lateral decubitus position.

Moving the patient from Trendelenburg position to reverse Trendelenburg position can help to increase or decrease preload and maintain blood pressure within specific parameters.

Anesthetic Implications

Massive blood loss with ensuing coagulopathy may occur during this procedure. Blood products and clotting factors should be available and ready in the operating room.

CXR should be available in the operating room. Evidence of an aneurysm compression of the left main stem bronchus may necessitate a different intubation technique.

Monitors and IV Access

- Two arterial lines to read proximal and distal pressures. These lines should include right radial (right side due to clamping of the subclavian artery and radial to read the upper body pressures, above the aneurysm) and femoral arterial catheters (femoral arterial line required in descending aneurysm surgery to monitor distal pressures).
- Two large-bore peripheral IVs and right internal jugular or femoral cordis introducer. Several large-bore central access sites should be available with fluid warmers; they must be ready to massively transfuse and give fluids. A pulmonary artery catheter may be inserted through the already placed cordis postoperatively.
- TEE.

Key Points

The patient's blood pressure must be controlled to prevent rupture. Have bolus doses of beta-blockers and vasodilators at the ready. IV drips of phenylephrine (Neo-Synephrine) and nitroglycerin are also important.

Maintain adequate brain hypothermia using surface and core cooling.

Hemodilution is important: The HCT should be decreased to 18–20% to prevent blood viscosity with colder temperatures.

Maintain pH and PCO_2.

Use muscle relaxants to reduce total-body oxygen consumption.

Hyperglycemia is more common due to adrenal stress with cooling. Avoid IV solutions with glucose before and after DHCA. Hyperglycemia can exacerbate cerebral ischemia and edema.

TRANSPLANTATION

Heart Transplant

In a heart transplant, the surgeon removes the patient's damaged native heart and transplants a donor heart. This procedure may be performed with any form of end-stage cardiac disease where survival cannot be assured with conventional forms of therapy, such as idiopathic dilated cardiomyopathy, ischemic heart disease, valvular heart disease, congenital heart disease, or a redo transplantation. To be candidates for heart transplant, patients must also demonstrate an absence of concomitant disease that might limit survival, such as pulmonary hypertension, malignancy, or advanced liver or kidney disease.

Operative Procedure

In the *donor* heart, the SVC, IVC, aorta, and pulmonary veins are transected. The recipient's chest is opened with a median sternotomy, and the pericardium is opened. The aorta (arterial) and bi-caval (venous) cannulation is done; bypass is established.

Removal of the native heart is done, leaving the posterior right atrium attached to the superior and inferior vena cava, and the posterior interatrial septum with the posterior left atrium. (A modification of this technique allows the anatomic integrity of the right atrium to be maintained to better preserve the SA node and tricuspid valve function.) The initial anastomosis of the donor heart is made to the recipient's left atrial free wall, followed by the right atrium to the free right atrial wall and septum. Finally, the aortic and pulmonary artery anastomosis is done. Epicardial pacing wires are always placed by the surgeon to ensure pacing capability post-operatively.

During transplantation, sympathetic postganglionic, parasympathetic preganglionic, and afferent nerves to the heart are transected. The loss of sympathetic innervation prevents the heart from rapidly changing its rate and contractility in response to exercise, hypovolemia, or vasodilation. The renin–angiotensin, vaso-regulatory systems are then impaired, along with the elimination of the signals that allow the native heart to perceive angina.

Anesthetic

General anesthesia is given with insertion of an OETT; muscle relaxants are given.

Positioning

The patient is placed in a supine position, with arms padded and tucked at the sides. A rolled towel along the upper spine or shoulder roll are used to widen the chest and extend the patient's head.

Anesthetic Implications

Strict aseptic precautions are needed with IV insertion, invasive monitoring, drug administration, airway management, and blood sampling.

Preoperative

Antibiotics and immunosuppressive drugs are given according to the center's protocol.

Patients will usually be considered to be "full-stomach" cases and a rapid sequence induction is needed. Ranitidine is given to decrease pH. Metoclopramide is given to increase gastric emptying.

Midazolam 1–2 mg and fentanyl 50 mcg IV can be given to sedate the patient for line placement if the hemodynamic condition is stable. Oxygen may be given by nasal cannula during this time.

Monitors and IV Access
- Two large-bore peripheral IVs.
- Arterial line.
- CVP placed in the *left* internal jugular (the right jugular is used for postoperative ventricular biopsies).
- Pulmonary artery catheter: inserted until the tip is in the superior vena cava. Once the transplantation is complete, the PAC can be advanced into the pulmonary circulation.
- TEE probe: placed after induction; used to assess ventricular volume and contractility. With discontinuation of CPB, the TEE is used to evaluate adequate de-airing of the heart.

Although invasive lines can be placed, induction must wait until the go-ahead is given by the harvesting surgeon. Be cautious of overmedicating these patients, even when they are very nervous, as these patients have no cardiac reserve.

Induction
The choice of anesthetics is based on the patient's physical status. One suggested technique is the following (although others are also used):

- Midazolam 2–3 mg, total 5 mg before sternotomy; additional 5 mg on rewarming.
- Etomidate 0.2–0.3 mg/kg if cardiac output is less than 35%.
- Sodium thiopental 2–4 mg/kg: given if cardiac output is more than 35%.
- Rocuronium 5 mg/kg defasiculating dose, if succinylcholine (Anectine) is given.
- Succinylcholine (Anectine) 1–2 mg/kg. If succinylcholine is not given, a longer-acting nondepolarizing neuromuscular blocking agent can be used.
- Fentanyl 5–10 mcg/kg initially.
- Oxygen at 100% FiO_2.

A patient with poor LV function may not tolerate a high concentration of an inhalation agent (although a small concentration is appropriate). Patients with chronically low cardiac output have longer circulation times and a potential smaller volume of distribution, so decrease all anesthetic drug doses and allow for longer circulation times for the drugs to take effect in these individuals.

Maintenance

- Oxygen at 100% FiO_2 or air/oxygen
- Fentanyl 50–100 mcg/kg for the entire case if LV function is good; give less than 50 mcg/kg if EF is low
- Vecuronium 10 mg IV; titrate to maintain peripheral nerve stimulator TOF 0/4
- Pancuronium: used if heart rate is low
- Isoflurane, sevoflurane, or desflurane: titrate to 0.5 MAC

Skin Incision

Have an adequate depth of anesthesia before the skin incision is made. Prevent tachycardia-induced ischemia.

Pre-bypass Period

A careful balance between organ perfusion and sufficient inotropic support is required to maintain the native heart until CPB is started. However, sufficient systemic perfusion outweighs any negative effects on the native heart.

Sternotomy

A sternotomy provides extreme stimulation. To counteract this effect, deep anesthesia is needed; vasodilators may be used to decrease blood pressure. With a first-time sternotomy, the patient's lungs are usually deflated and off ventilator (disconnect the bag), though this choice depends on the surgeon's preference. For redo sternotomy, the patient's lungs are left inflated—again, the choice depends on the surgeon's preference. The patient must be 100% muscle relaxed for sternotomy.

Anticoagulation

Heparin 300–400 units/kg is given IV through the central line. Check the ACT 3–4 minutes after giving heparin; it needs to be more than 480 seconds for the patient to go on bypass.

Aortic Cannulation

Decrease the patient's systolic blood pressure to 85–100 mm Hg to help prevent bleeding from aorta during cannulation. A cannula is usually placed in the ascending aorta proximal to the innominate artery, although it can also be placed in the femoral artery.

Bicaval Venous Cannulation

Placed after aortic cannulation.

If the patient becomes hypotensive or has atrial/ventricular arrhythmias, treat the condition with drugs or place the patient on CPB.

IV Fluids and Volume Requirements

Maintain the patient in a state of euvolemia to hypovolemia. Cardiac output is sensitive to the filling pressures in the right atrium. The ideal IV fluid volume infused prior to bypass should be approximately 500 mL total.

Full-Flow Cardiopulmonary Bypass

During CPB, IVF slowed to a minimal KVO rate; most IVF is given through the bypass pump. If volume is needed in the pump, the perfusionist will check the HCT levels. If the HCT falls into the teens, washed cells or PRBCs are usually added (based on surgeon preference). If the HCT is in the low to middle 20s (the ideal level is in the range of 22–25% during CPB), crystalloids or colloids (hetastarch, albumin) can be added.

Take the patient off the ventilator. The perfusionist gives 0.5% isoflurane and oxygen through the bypass machine; hypothermia itself is anesthetic. *Once the patient is on full bypass, all IV fluids and volatile agents are given by the perfusionist.*

The CRNA should check the patient's neck for thrill for a malpositioned arterial cannula. He or she should also monitor the pupils: arterial cannula malposition can cause the bypass outflow to be directed *into* the carotid artery, which can cause ipsilateral pupil dilation; bilateral fixed and dilated pupils indicate hypoxia. In either case, inform the surgeon to reassess the bypass circuitry.

Ongoing adequate organ perfusion is the goal. *MAP greater than 70 mm Hg is the best pressure for maintaining adequate perfusion.* Again, while on CPB, this is the done by the perfusionist.

Ventricular fibrillation occurs as the heart is rapidly cooling; it consumes myocardial oxygen reserves and protection.

Recalibrate all lines before the patient comes off bypass.

Reperfusion

After the pulmonary anastomosis is done, the heart is reperfused and allowed to warm, usually for at least 10 minutes, to ensure that the cardioplegia has been washed out and that myocardial contractility is becoming normal.

Termination of CPB Requirements

- Core body temperature rewarmed to at least 36°C (or surgeon preference).
- Stable EKG rhythm—preferably normal sinus rhythm. The patient may need internal defibrillation at 10–20 J. If asystole occurs or if the heart rate is inadequate, the pacemaker can be started at a rate of 80–100. Initiate both atrial and ventricular mA at 20, decrease the mA until capture is lost, and then turn the mA back up.
- Heart contractility assessment: determine if inotropic support is necessary. A calcium chloride 250–1000 mg bolus through the central line may be needed. Pump volume can also be given to supplement the existing volume and to maintain filling pressure; it is

given via the arterial cannula in the aorta by the perfusionist.

- Normal potassium value of less than 5.5.
- Air evacuated from heart and grafts.
- Lung ventilation resumed. Recruit several breaths to inflate the alveoli, while watching the lung tissue enlarge through sternal opening. Use care to not overinflate and rip pericardial sutures. FiO_2 at 100% is appropriate.

Coming Off Bypass Support

- A junctional rhythm is common in a transplanted heart and may require isoproterenol 2–6 mcg/min to increase the heart rate to 100–120 beats/min. The cardiac output of the denervated heart is solely heart rate dependent, and the heart rate is unresponsive to physiologic compensation (i.e., carotid massage). The denervated heart loses all vagal tone effects on both the SA node and the AV node, resulting in an increased resting heart rate of 90–100 beats/min.
- Sympathetic stimulation leads to a delayed heart rate increase in response to hypoxemia, hypercarbia, hypotension, or pain.
- Hypertension can cause a reflex bradycardia.
- Parasympathetic stimulation does not produce any heart rate change.

Only drugs that act directly on the heart will be effective after a heart transplant. Drugs acting through the autonomic nervous system do not work. Alpha- and beta-adrenergic receptors are intact.

- Propranolol works by blocking the effect of isoproterenol and norepinephrine at the SA node.

Alpha agonists that may be used include phenylephrine and norepinephrine (Levophed):

- Phenylephrine: minimal increase in heart rate; some vasoconstriction.

- Norepinephrine: maximum attempt to increase SVR.

Inotropes that may be used include dobutamine, epinephrine, milrinone, and dopamine. The goal of hemodynamic support is to maintain systemic perfusion with an adequate cardiac output while preventing right heart failure. To do this, we must maintain the balance of end-organ perfusion, systemic arterial BP, and pulmonary vascular resistance (PVR).

- Dopamine increases contractility.
- Dobutamine increases contractility.
- Epinephrine increases contractility and heart rate.
- All will increase heart rate: epinephrine > dopamine > dobutamine.
- Ephedrine: direct cardiac stimulator. Dilators may also be used:
- Nitroglycerin: 1–4 mcg/kg/min; titrate to dilate coronary arteries in ischemia and decrease PVR.
- Nitroprusside: 0.5–1 mcg/kg/min; titrate to decrease afterload (SVR) and decrease BP, which decreases stress on the suture line and decreases bleeding.
- Fenoldopam: 0.05–0.1 mcg/kg/min; rapid-acting vasodilator; dopamine-receptor agonist that increases renal blood flow.

The following agents *do not work* after heart transplant: atropine, neostigmine, digoxin (does not work with acute use); pancuronium (does not exert its vagolytic effect in a transplanted heart).

An intra-aortic balloon pump may be needed to assist ventricular ejection of blood.

The CVP should be maintained at 5–10 mm Hg with volume transfusion while the patient is coming off bypass.

Because portions of both the native and recipient right atria are present, the EKG may show two P waves, although the SA node from the donor determines the heart rate. While electronically there is a P wave, there is no synchronization between the recipient and the donor's atria which leads to the loss of normal contribution to stroke volume (approximately 30%). Epicardial pacemaker wires are placed during surgery, although pacing does not produce the same improvement in CO as does isoproterenol.

Post-bypass Period

When hemostasis is controlled and the cannulas are removed, protamine 1.3–1.5 mg to 100 units heparin may be given IV; this agent binds to and inactivates heparin. Give protamine *slowly* to prevent hypotension or pulmonary HTN. Note that this agent carries an anaphylaxis risk; there is also risk for severe hypotension if the patient has received protamine in the past year.

Check ACT 3 minutes after giving protamine. It should be the same or less than the baseline ACT.

If the patient develops hypotension, assess LV volume/function. Check the CVP, PAD, CO/CI, TEE for wall movement abnormalities; give volume, vasopressors, or inotropes as necessary.

If the patient develops hypertension, confirm that the anesthesia is deep enough. Give narcotics or volatile agents, if necessary. Alternatively, vasodilators—nitroglycerin, sodium nitroprusside (SNP), fenoldopam, nicardipine may be given.

If bleeding occurs, the patient may need more protamine, or fresh frozen plasma, platelets, or DDAVP. Infuse cell-saver blood. Finish giving all of the protamine before starting infusion of cell-saver or blood products.

Arrhythmias are more common in transplanted hearts, especially in the early postoperative period. Sinus bradycardia, which occurs in 50% of patients in the first few weeks postoperatively, can significantly reduce cardiac output. Atrial pacing will be needed in this event. Atrial fibrillation or flutter, premature atrial contractions (PACs) and premature ventricular contractions (PVCs) are also common, albeit not necessarily related to organ rejection.

Arrhythmias associated with rejection consist of sustained or complex ventricular arrhythmias or a sudden death episode. Standard antidysrhythmic drugs and cardioversion are used to treat these dysrhythmias.

Hyperacute rejection occurs within minutes or hours of the transplant. This condition is caused by an exaggerated immune response thought to be due to donor-specific antibodies in the recipient. Despite this risk, 80% of heart transplant patients survive the first year.

Abdominal and Gastrointestinal Surgery

16

ABDOMINAL AND GASTROINTESTINAL SURGERY PEARLS

- Avoid nitrous oxide with bowel surgery. Nitrous oxide is 30 times more soluble than nitrogen, and diffuses into closed gas spaces faster than nitrogen diffuses out. Because this build-up of gases increases the volume or pressure of any closed spaces, it is contraindicated in the presence of closed spaces such as small bowel obstruction.
- Bowel preps (to cleanse the entire bowel) are usually given only for colon resections involving the transverse, descending (left), sigmoid colon, or rectum. Bowel preps are not given for a small bowel surgeries or ascending (right) colon resection because the bacterial load is so low in the small intestine and the ascending colon that postoperative infection is not a concern.
- Check coagulation studies and platelet levels if the patient is taking anticoagulants (e.g., Plavix) before planning a spinal for neuraxial anesthesia.

Abdominal Laparotomy

In abdominal laparotomy, an opening is made through the abdominal wall into the peritoneal cavity by an incision, usually 5–7 inches long. The incision cuts through the skin, subcutaneous tissue, fascia, and muscles into the peritoneum. This technique is used to explore, diagnose, and treat abdominal and GI conditions. GETA and muscle relaxation are needed for this procedure.

Surgical movement of the peritoneum and internal organs may cause a vagal response with a decrease in heart rate.

Abdominal Laparoscopy

Chapter 3 discusses laparoscopy in depth. If the patient's oxygen saturation decreases after insufflation of the abdomen, check for bilateral breath sounds. The tracheal tube can go into the right main stem bronchus, with the pressure of insufflation pushing the diaphragm upward. If breath sounds are decreased on the left, pull the endotracheal tube back until breath sounds are audible bilaterally and retape the tube.

Postoperative Nausea and Vomiting

The following characteristics are associated with increased risk of PONV following abdominal or GI surgery:

- Female
- Motion sickness history
- Pediatrics (6–10 years of age): 34% PONV occurrence
- Pediatrics (11–14 years of age): 35–50% PONV occurrence
- Nonsmoker
- Anxiety
- Surgery length greater than 45–60 minutes

ESOPHAGUS SURGERY

Esophageal Dilation

Esophageal dilation with a dilator is done to remedy abnormal narrowing or tightening of the esophagus. The majority of esophageal strictures are caused by gastroesophageal reflux disease (GERD), but strictures can also be due to cancer, surgery, and aging. The patient may present with difficult or painful swallowing and/or weight loss.

Operative Procedure

Several methods are used to dilate the esophagus. A soft rubber bite block is inserted between the upper and lower teeth before proceeding.

Dilator: Bougie

A series of rigid, but flexible, cone-shaped rubber tubes are lubricated with a water-based jelly and passed through the mouth and into the esophagus, one at a time. Sequentially larger tube sizes are used to dilate the obstructed area; the entire length of the esophagus is dilated with this method. Each tube is left in place for approximately 15 seconds before removing and inserting the next larger size.

Bougie dilation is especially useful for long esophageal strictures. This tube is inserted through the esophagus without direct visualization unless fluoroscopy is done.

Wire

A flexible wire is passed through the mouth, into the esophagus, and across the stricture through an endoscope. The endoscope is removed slowly while maintaining the wire in the same position. A bougie dilator (e.g., Savary dilator, which has a hole passing from end to end) is lubricated with a water-based jelly and then guided over the wire and across the stricture. Fluoroscopy is used with this technique.

Balloon

A deflated balloon is passed through an endoscope and out the end. The balloon is inflated at the stricture, enlarging the narrowing. These balloons can be inflated from 6 to 30 mm in size.

After dilation is finished, an esophageal stent may be placed with the help of an endoscope.

Anesthetic

A local anesthetic gel can be used with IV sedation. GETA with insertion of an OETT may be needed.

Positioning

The patient is placed in a supine position, with bilateral arms tucked at the sides. A slight left lateral position may be helpful.

Anesthetic Implications

If the patient is intubated, hold the OETT to secure it with bougie dilator insertion and removal to prevent dislodging the tube. If the surgeon asks the CRNA to insert the bougie, lubricate with a water-based jelly; do *not* push the bougie in if it meets with resistance.

These patients require special eye care if intubated. Paper tape is used to close the eyes to prevent corneal drying or abrasions; eye pads are then placed over both eyes to protect them.

Eye ointment can be instilled before taping for patients who will remain intubated postoperatively.

Complications

Potential complications include esophageal injury or rupture: There is a high risk of death if rupture occurs. Have IV fluid and blood tubing available and ready in case of bleeding, along with at least one peripheral IV.

Transhiatal (Approach) Esophagectomy

Transhiatal esophagectomy is the surgical removal of at least two-thirds to the entire thoracic and abdominal esophagus. This procedure is performed to treat benign or malignant esophageal lesions; including Barrett's esophagus (esophageal dysplasia, a pre-cancerous state); trauma; chronic inflammation; or motility disorders. Surgery may be done for curative or palliative reasons.

Operative Procedure

In the transhiatal approach, a left neck (above the clavicle) incision and an upper abdominal incision are usually made. Blunt dissection of the esophagus is made between these two incisions.

With any approach, the proximal stomach and entire esophagus are dissected free of the surrounding tissues; the diseased esophagus is resected and removed. The stomach, stapled at the greater curvature to create a tubular shape, is pulled up through the chest to reach the remaining portion of the esophagus to create a cervical esophagogastric anastomosis. If the remaining esophagus after resection is too short to attach to the stomach, a small segment of the colon may be used as a conduit between these two structures. Accessible lymph nodes are removed for staging.

A vagal-sparing esophagectomy may be done to preserve the vagus nerve branches so that acid production and digestive functions are maintained.

Transhiatal esophagectomy may also be done by a VATS procedure or abdominal laparoscopy; these techniques are not detailed here.

Anesthetic

GETA is given with insertion of a single-lumen OETT; a double-lumen endobronchial tube may be needed if a thoracotomy is done; muscle relaxants are given. Avoid the use of nitrous oxide. A rapid-sequence induction is prudent if the patient has any symptoms of gastric reflux. An epidural may be placed for postoperative pain control. If an epidural is placed, pain issues should be addressed by anesthesia postoperatively.

Monitors and IV Access
- An arterial line is needed.
- Central venous lines are usually needed for volume resuscitation and fluid monitoring.
- Multiple large-bore peripheral IVs are needed if no CVP is placed or present.
- A pulmonary artery catheter may also be required.

IV Fluids and Volume Requirements
These patients are usually somewhat dehydrated and require crystalloid fluid replacement at a rate as high as 8–10 mL/kg/hr. Crystalloid, hextend, and blood products may be used. The goal is to maintain the patient in a euvolemic to slightly dry state.

Positioning

The patient is placed in a supine position, with arms tucked at the sides. The left neck will also be in the operative field, turn the head away from the surgical side.

Anesthetic Implications

Two of the major risk factors for esophageal disease are heavy alcohol consumption and tobacco use, both of which can affect the anesthetic course. These patients are often quite sick and malnourished.

These patients require special eye care. Paper tape is used to close the eyes to prevent corneal drying or abrasions; eye pads are then placed over both eyes to protect them. Eye ointment can be instilled before taping for patients who will remain intubated postoperatively.

A feeding tube may be placed during this surgery to allow the patient to be fed postoperatively while the esophagus rests. These patients may be very malnourished from dysphagia.

This is a long-duration surgery. It is key to keep patients warm during the procedure.

Because the operative field is in the vicinity of the endotracheal tube and oxygen, care must be taken to avoid airway/OR fires. See Chapter 1 on safety concerns for more information.

Complications

There is a risk of pneumothorax occurring during this procedure. Also, there is a risk of great vessel or airway injury during blunt dissection.

Esophagectomy: Transthoracic or Abdominothoracic Approach

Transthoracic/abdominothoracic esophagectomy is the surgical removal of the middle to distal thoracic or abdominal esophagus. This procedure is performed to treat a benign or malignant esophageal lesion, at the middle to lower third of the esophagus; Barrett's esophagus (esophageal dysplasia, a precancerous state); trauma; chronic inflammation; or motility disorders. Surgery may be done for curative or palliative reasons.

Operative Procedure

- Low-esophageal lesions: accessed through the left chest or a single thoracoabdominal incision
- Mid-esophageal lesions: accessed through the abdomen and right chest
- Upper-esophageal lesions: accessed through the right chest, abdomen, and neck

With any approach, the proximal stomach and entire esophagus are dissected free and the remaining portion of the esophagus is connected to the remaining portion of the stomach. The whole stomach, colon, and jejunum (vascularized grafts) may be used as grafting substitutes for the resected esophagus.

This approach allows for complete lymph node dissection.

A vagal-sparing esophagectomy may be done to preserve the vagus nerve branches so that acid production and digestive functions are maintained.

Part or all of this procedure may be done laparoscopically.

Anesthetic

GETA is given with insertion of a double-lumen endobronchial tube for one-lung ventilation if the right or left chest is accessed (see Chapter 3 for more information on DLEBT); muscle relaxants are given. Avoid the use of nitrous oxide. A rapid-sequence induction is prudent if the patient has any symptoms of gastric reflux. An epidural may be placed for postoperative pain control. If an epidural is placed, pain issues should be addressed by anesthesia postoperatively.

Monitors
- Arterial line
- Central line
- Multiple large-bore peripheral IVs are needed if a CVP is not placed.
- PA catheter—may be indicated but is rarely placed

IV Fluids and Volume Requirements
Fluid shifts can be quite dramatic during this procedure, and patients may require crystalloid fluid replacement at a rate up to 10 mL/kg/hr. The goal is to maintain the patient in a euvolemic to slightly dry state.

Positioning

The patient is placed supine for the abdominal portion of the procedure, and then repositioned in semi-lateral position for thoracotomy approaches.

Anesthetic Implications

Type and cross-match the patient's blood. Blood may need to be available in the operating room depending on the patient's condition.

These patients require special eye care. Paper tape is used to close the eyes to prevent corneal drying or abrasions; eye pads are then placed over both eyes to protect them. Eye ointment can be instilled before taping for patients who will remain intubated postoperatively.

This is a long-duration surgery, so it is key to keep patients warm during the procedure. Upper- and lower-body warming blankets are needed as well as fluid warmers. The ambient temperature in the room may also need to be increased.

These patients are usually sick and may present as malnourished. Their albumin/protein levels may be low, and the bio-distribution of the anesthetic agents may be affected by their condition. Two of the major risk factors for esophageal disease are heavy alcohol consumption and tobacco use, both of which affect the anesthetic course.

These patients may be very malnourished from dysphagia. A feeding tube may be placed during this surgery to allow the patient to be fed postoperatively while the esophagus rests.

These patients are usually left intubated at the end of the case and transported to the ICU.

Complications

There is a risk of pneumothorax occurring during this procedure.

Excision of Esophageal Diverticulum

This procedure comprises the surgical closure of one or multiple diverticula of the esophagus. A diverticulum is a localized outpouching of the upper, middle, or most distal portion of the esophageal wall. To propel food into the stomach, the esophagus generates internal pressure. That pressure can herniate the esophageal lining through a weakness in the wall, creating a pouch. Food and saliva can collect in all of these pouches. Most diverticula are the result of a functional obstruction to the peristaltic wave, usually due to an abnormal *lower* esophageal sphincter. Esophageal diverticula occur primarily in older adults.

A *Zenker's diverticulum* is caused by a tonically contracted *upper* esophageal sphincter that impedes the forward movement of swallowed food. An increased intraluminal pressure forces the esophageal mucosa to herniate through the posterior midline of the inferior pharyngeal muscle, which causes pockets to form that collect small amounts of food.

Operative Procedure for Zenker's Diverticulum

In the *closed/endoscopic approach,* after placing a bite block, an endoscope is inserted into the esophagus. A stapler is then introduced and used to connect one wall of the diverticulum to the esophageal wall.

In the *open approach,* with the patient's head turned to the right side for a left neck approach, an incision is made along the anterior border of the left sternocleidomastoid muscle (SCM) down to approximately 2 cm above the substernal notch. The SCM is divided and the larynx retracted medially; the carotid sheath is retracted laterally. The posterior esophagus is dissected away from the prevertebral fascia at or below the level of the cricoid cartilage. A bougie dilator is first lubricated with a water-based jelly and then inserted to dilate and stent the esophagus. The diverticulum is grasped and either stapled or sutured shut across the neck of the sac. The bougie dilator is then removed.

Anesthetic

GETA is used with a single-lumen OETT. Muscle relaxants are used. An epidural may be placed for postoperative pain control. If the epidural is put in, pain issues should be addressed by anesthesia specialists postoperatively.

Positioning

The patient is placed in a supine position, with the head turned away from the operative site, with a shoulder roll to extend the head. Bilateral arms are placed on padded armboards, with the shoulders at a less than 90 degree angle. The head of the bed will be 90–180 degrees away from the anesthetist.

Anesthetic Implications

These patients usually have had difficulty in eating and will have had poor nutrition prior to surgery. Lowered albumin and protein levels will affect the anesthetic action. Also, these patients are at increased risk for infection. A feeding tube may be placed into the patient's stomach to deliver postoperative nutrition, especially if the patient is weak and malnourished.

Aspiration can result from esophageal diverticula. A thorough preoperative lung auscultation should be done to rule out wheezing, rales, or rhonchi.

These patients require special eye care. Paper tape is used to close the eyes to prevent corneal drying or abrasions; eye pads are then placed over both eyes to protect them. Eye ointment can be instilled before taping for patients who will remain intubated postoperatively.

Hold the OETT to secure it during bougie insertion and removal to prevent dislodging the tube. If the surgeon asks the CRNA to insert the bougie, first lubricate with a water-based jelly; do *not* push bougie in if it meets with resistance.

Do not place an esophageal or orogastric/nasogastric tube.

Diverticula of the mid- or lower esophagus are usually addressed through the right or left chest.

Complications

Potential complications include damage to the recurrent laryngeal nerve. The thyroid gland and the carotid artery are both retracted during this case with a possibility of injury and blood loss.

Nissen Procedure: Laparoscopic Fundoplication

The Nissen procedure involves the laparoscopic wrapping of the gastric fundus around the lower esophagus to tighten the lower esophageal sphincter. The fundoplication procedure is performed to correct gastroesophageal reflux, a paraesophageal hernia, or a hiatal hernia (also known as a diaphragmatic hernia). It seeks to reestablish the gastroesophageal angle and to establish a barrier to intrathoracic gastric displacement; it also reinforces the lower esophageal sphincter (LES), which stops acid from backing up into the esophagus.

Operative Procedure

Laparoscopic pneumoperitoneum is established; traction is applied to the esophagus by a laparoscopic grasper, and the vagus nerve branches are preserved. A 50–60 Fr. esophageal dilator (bougie) is lubricated with a water-based jelly then passed transorally to provide a stent that the surgeon can use to tighten the gastric fundus (upper curve of the stomach) around the lower esophagus. (A lighted endoscope is an alternative to the bougie.) The gastric fundus is manipulated circumferentially around the esophagus and then sutured or stapled to itself. This maneuver causes the lower portion of the esophagus to pass through a small tunnel of stomach muscle. The circumferential fundus creates the fundoplication or "wrap."

Another surgical approach to gastroesophageal reflux is an "anti-reflux valve"—a doughnut-shaped prosthetic implant that is placed around the esophagus under the diaphragm and is sutured in place. It allows food to pass down the esophagus and into the stomach, but prevents the stomach from sliding up into the chest.

Anesthetic

GETA is given with insertion of an OETT; muscle relaxants are needed. Avoid using nitrous oxide to minimize gastric/bowel distention. These patients are considered as having a full stomach; thus they should receive aspiration prophylaxis and undergo rapid-sequence induction. Use caution when removing the esophageal dilator from the mouth so as to not extubate the patient's endotracheal tube at the same time.

Positioning

The patient is placed in a supine position, with arms tucked bilaterally. A lateral position may be needed if the LES cannot be accessed by an abdominal approach.

Monitors and IV Access
- An arterial line may or may not be used.
- A single peripheral IV is usually all that is needed.

Anesthetic Implications

An orogastric tube can be placed immediately after induction to suction the stomach but must be removed for esophageal dilator placement. A nasogastric tube is placed after the dilator is removed and before the patient's emergence from anesthesia.

These patients require special eye care. Paper tape is used to close the eyes to prevent corneal drying or abrasions; eye pads are then placed over both eyes to protect them.

Surgical pneumothorax is possible. If it occurs, a chest tube is inserted into the pleural space at the end of the case to allow for lung reexpansion.

Pressure-controlled ventilations are helpful. In such a case, use lower tidal volumes and provide for higher respiratory rates to control end-tidal CO_2 within normal ranges.

Hold the OETT to secure it with bougie dilator insertion and removal so as to prevent dislodging the tube. If the surgeon asks the CRNA to insert the bougie, lubricate with a water-based jelly; do *not* push the bougie in if it meets with resistance.

STOMACH SURGERY

Subtotal Gastrectomy: Billroth I and Billroth II

Subtotal gastrectomy entails removal of the lower two-thirds of the stomach and reestablishment of the continuity of the gastrointestinal tract. Gastrointestinal continuity is reestablished by anastomosing the gastric remnant to the proximal duodenum (Billroth I; also known as gastroduodenostomy); alternatively, the duodenum may be left in place and the stomach anastomosed end-to-end with the proximal jejunum (Billroth II; also known as gastrojejunostomy). This procedure is performed to treat peptic ulcer disease or gastric cancer of the distal stomach.

Operative Procedure

A large midline incision is made, and the peritoneal cavity is examined. The stomach is freed from its attachments, and the surgeon removes the lower two-thirds portion of the stomach. The surgeon then sutures the remaining portion of the stomach to either the proximal duodenum or the proximal jejunum. The abdominal wound is closed in layers.

Anesthetic

General anesthesia is used with a single-lumen OETT; muscle relaxants are given. Patients should be treated as if they have a full stomach and undergo rapid-sequence induction. Avoid using nitrous oxide to minimize gastric/bowel distention.

Monitors and IV Access
- An arterial line is needed.
- A central venous line is preferred.
- A pulmonary artery catheter is rarely placed but may be needed based on the patient's cardiovascular history.
- If no central line is placed, have at least two large-bore peripheral IVs.

Positioning

The patient is placed in a supine position, with bilateral arms tucked at the sides.

Anesthetic Implications

These patients may be malnourished due to their disease, so check their preoperative electrolyte, H&H, albumin, BUN, creatinine, and glucose levels. If they also have any liver disease, check coagulation study results.

Type and cross-match the patient's blood, as there is a potential for blood loss with this procedure.

These patients require special eye care. Paper tape is used to close the eyes to prevent corneal drying or abrasions; eye pads are then placed over both eyes to protect them. Eye ointment can be instilled before taping for patients who will remain intubated postoperatively.

A nasogastric tube is placed intraoperatively; the surgeon can help to guide distal end placement internally. Secure the tube well and document "tube not to be allowed to move"; relay this information in your report to the receiving RN postoperatively as well.

Large third-space fluid shifts are common during subtotal gastrectomy procedures. Consider using albumin or hetastarch fluid boluses to manage volume issues.

Temperature loss is also common with open abdomen procedures. Upper- and lower-body warming blankets are needed as well as fluid warmers; the ambient temperature in the room may also need to be increased.

Total Gastrectomy

Total gastrectomy entails the surgical removal of the stomach and reestablishment of the continuity of the gastrointestinal tract between the esophagus and the jejunum. This procedure is performed to treat malignancy of the stomach (along with adjacent lymph node metastasis) or uncontrolled bleeding. If gastrectomy is done for malignancy, then lymph nodes, adjacent organs (including the spleen), and the greater omentum are removed.

Operative Procedure

A thoracoabdominal approach incision may be necessary; bilateral subcostal incisions can also be done. After the abdomen is opened, the surgeon thoroughly explores the cavity for masses or lesions. Blood vessels connecting the spleen to the stomach are divided, with the blood supply to the spleen being maintained. The stomach is loosened from the surrounding structures. Proximally, the esophagus is clamped; distally, clamping is done past the pylorus. Gastric fluid spillage is avoided. The stomach is removed and the tissues behind where the stomach was positioned are examined for evidence of metastasis.

A portion of the duodenum (that was removed) is sutured closed at one end, with the other end being anastomosed (end-to-side) to the jejunum. Anastomosis of the distal esophagus to the proximal jejunum is then done; the bile duct is inserted into the duodenum so that bile juices can be brought into the digestive process.

Total gastrectomy can also be done laparoscopically.

Anesthetic

GETA is given with insertion of a single-lumen OETT; muscle relaxants are given. Avoid using nitrous oxide to minimize gastric/bowel distention.

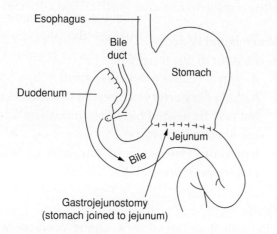

Figure 16-1 *Billroth II*

Positioning

The patient is placed in a supine position, with bilateral arms tucked.

Anesthetic Implications

These patients may be malnourished due to their disease, so check their preoperative electrolyte, H&H, albumin, BUN, creatinine, and glucose levels. If they also have any liver disease, check coagulation study results.

Has the patient already had chemotherapy or radiotherapy? If so, that treatment may affect intubation, as tissues may be more friable. Anticipate larger blood loss in such cases.

Type and cross-match the patient's blood, as there is a potential for blood loss with this procedure.

These patients require special eye care. Paper tape is used to close the eyes to prevent corneal drying or abrasions; eye pads are then placed over both eyes to protect them. Eye ointment can be instilled before taping for patients who will remain intubated postoperatively.

A nasogastric tube is placed intraoperatively; the surgeon can help to guide distal end placement internally. Secure the tube well and document "tube not to be allowed to move"; relay this information in your report to the receiving RN postoperatively as well.

Large third-space fluid shifts are common with gastrectomy. Consider using albumin or hetastarch fluid boluses to manage volume issues.

Temperature loss is also common with open abdomen procedures. Upper- and lower-body warming blankets are needed as well as fluid warmers. The ambient temperature in the room may also need to be increased.

Monitors and IV Access

- An arterial line is usually placed.
- CVP and/or a pulmonary artery catheter may be needed based on the patient's history.
- If no central line is placed, have at least two large-bore peripheral IVs.

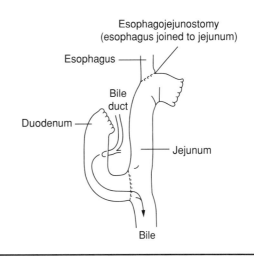

Figure 16-2 *Total Gastrectomy*

Gastrostomy or Jejunostomy Tube Insertion

This surgery involves establishment of a temporary or permanent artificial opening and tube placement into the stomach (gastrostomy) or jejunum (jejunostomy) exiting onto the skin of the abdominal wall. When done at the time of an open operation, it is called "open tube placement". If a gastrostomy and tube insertion is performed with an endoscope, it is referred to as a percutaneous endoscopic gastrostomy tube placement (PEG) procedure (detailed below).

Such a tube is used to either drain the stomach or provide liquid nutrition and medications to a person who is unable to eat, drink, or swallow normally. In addition, some patients require a feeding method that bypasses the pharynx and esophagus. Typically, patients who require this procedure will have experienced a stroke or head injury, will have dementia, or will have another comorbid condition.

Operative Procedure

After injecting local anesthesia into the skin, a small ½-inch incision is made into the skin of the upper left or midline abdomen and then into the wall of the stomach. The gastrostomy tube is placed into the stomach and secured with a balloon to the inside. Traction is placed on the tube to elevate the stomach against the abdominal wall, where it is secured with sutures. A small tube may be threaded through the gastrostomy tube, inserted until the distal end is in the jejunum, and secured there; such a tube reduces the risk of reflux of the stomach contents. The stomach (around the gastrostomy tube) and abdominal wall incision are then sutured closed.

The procedure is performed in a similar manner with the use of *laparoscopy*.

A *permanent* gastrostomy tube (G-tube) is created with a stomach flap formed around the catheter to decrease wound healing difficulties.

Anesthetic

Local anesthesia is used with IV sedation. GETA and muscle relaxants may be needed. Avoid using nitrous oxide to minimize gastric/bowel distention.

Positioning

The patient is placed in a supine position, with arms extended on armboards or tucked at the sides.

Anesthetic Implications

Tape the patient's eyes closed to prevent corneal abrasion or drying.

The anesthetic issues with this procedure are similar to those that arise with any laparotomy. In addition, anesthetic considerations related to these patients' typically poor nutritional state should be included in planning.

These patients are often in poor condition owing to chronic diseases and arrive to the operating room already intubated.

Make sure tube feedings have been stopped at least 8 hours prior to surgery.

One peripheral IV is usually all that is needed. If TPN is infusing, keep it infusing through a dedicated IV and start another IV to deliver anesthetic drugs and IV fluids.

Gastrostomy: Percutaneous Endoscopic Tube Placement

Gastrostomy establishes a permanent or temporary artificial opening into the stomach that exits onto the skin of the abdominal wall. The Percutaneous Endoscopic Tube (PEG) procedure is performed with a flexible fiberoptic gastroscope.

A gastrostomy is done either to drain the stomach or to allow for liquid feedings for patients who are unable to take nutrition by mouth. A rubber catheter, which exits out of the abdominal wall, maintains the patency of the gastrostomy tract.

Operative Procedure

After a bite block is placed into the patient's mouth, a gastroscope is passed into the stomach, which is then distended with air. The lighted tip of the scope touches the gastric wall so that the light can be seen externally; a percutaneous stab wound is then created by a large needle aimed at the gastroscope tip. This cut is viewed through the endoscope to ensure proper placement. A wire is passed through the needle and grasped by the endoscope; the gastroscope and the wire is then withdrawn from the stomach (up through the esophagus) and removed from the patient. The PEG tube is "threaded" over the wire. Traction is applied to the wire that exits the patient's belly wall, and the PEG tube is pulled through the patient's mouth and esophagus into the stomach. The distal end of the gastrostomy tube has a mushroom-shaped end that prevents it from being pulled out through the belly wall. The catheter is secured to the skin.

Anesthetic

This procedure is performed with IV sedation and local anesthesia to the back of the throat. General anesthesia may be needed.

Positioning

The patient is placed in a supine position, with bilateral arms at the sides.

Anesthetic Implications

Both insufflation of the stomach and the sedation required for the procedure can increase risk of aspiration.

These patients are often in poor condition owing to chronic diseases and may arrive to the operating room already intubated.

These patients require special eye care if general anesthesia is given. Paper tape is used to close the eyes to prevent corneal drying or abrasions; eye pads are then placed over both eyes to protect them. Eye ointment can be instilled before taping for patients who will remain intubated postoperatively.

Make sure tube feedings have been stopped at least 8 hours prior to surgery.

One peripheral IV is usually all that is needed. If TPN is infusing, keep it infusing through a dedicated IV and start another IV to deliver anesthetic drugs and IV fluids.

Hold the endotracheal tube in a secure position when the surgeon inserts and withdraws the gastroscope to avoid accidental extubation.

Peptic Ulcer Closure

Surgical closure may be necessary to treat a perforated gastric or duodenal ulcer. Presentation of a perforated gastric ulcer can span the range between perforation with spontaneous closure needing medical treatment to perforation with extensive gastric acid spillage into the abdominal contents and life-threatening peritonitis.

Operative Procedure

The abdominal cavity is entered via *laparotomy* (midline abdominal incision) or *laparoscopy*. The site of perforation is found. The perforation is closed with sutures or staples, or is simply patched with omentum, called a "Graham patch."

Anesthetic

GETA is given with insertion of an OETT; muscle relaxants are given. Avoid using nitrous oxide to minimize gastric/bowel distention.

Positioning

The patient is placed in a supine position, with arms possibly tucked bilaterally.

Anesthetic Implications

These patients often have a history of alcohol abuse and cigarette smoking with the associated comorbid conditions.

Limitations to the laparoscopic approach include the risk of peritonitis and dense adhesions. Diffuse peritonitis can cause massive fluid shifts. ICU care is often needed in such cases. The patient may not be safe to extubate if large-volume fluid resuscitation is anticipated in the postoperative period.

An arterial line and a central venous line would likely be needed to deliver such fluids. At least two peripheral IVs are needed if a central line is not placed.

Type and cross-match the patient's blood, in preparation for possible blood loss.

Tape the patient's eyes closed to prevent corneal abrasion or drying.

These patients are often in poor condition owing to chronic diseases and may arrive to the operating room already intubated.

Vagotomy: With or Without Pyloroplasty

Vagotomy is a transection of the vagus nerves that is used to treat peptic ulcer disease. This procedure is done to interrupt the parasympathetic innervation so as to reduce gastric acid secretion and allow ulcer healing.

The vagus nerve can be transected at the main vagal trunks (*truncal*), which interrupts all the branches to the stomach and other abdominal viscera (liver, gallbladder, bile duct, pancreas, all of small intestine, and part of large intestine). Pyloroplasty is done in conjunction with a truncal vagotomy to decrease pressure across the pyloric sphincter and enhance gastric emptying, which is otherwise delayed after a vagotomy.

The transection may also be *selective,* in that only gastric vagal nerves are interrupted. Selective vagotomy permits gastric emptying without the need for pyloroplasty unless underlying pylorus stricture or disease is present. With this technique, transection of the vagus nerves is done at the level of the distal esophagus, or at the gastric cardia.

Operative Procedure

A small midline incision is made and the esophagus retracted. The vagus trunk and nerves are identified, ligated, and resected. Hemoclips can also be applied to the severed nerve trunks (instead of ligating them). Small sections of nerve tissue are sent to pathology to confirm that the nerve was actually divided. The pyloroplasty is then done if the truncal branches are truly severed.

Vagotomy can also be done using a *laparoscopic* approach.

Anesthetic

GETA and muscle relaxants are given. Avoid using nitrous oxide to minimize gastric/bowel distention.

Positioning

The patient is placed in a supine position. The arms may be extended on armboards but are usually tucked at sides.

Anesthetic Implications

In a laparoscopic vagotomy, pneumoperitoneum is established. Esophageal dilators are passed orally to facilitate traction on the stomach. Hold the endotracheal tube in a secure position when the surgeon inserts and withdraws the esophageal dilators to avoid accidental extubation.

These patients require special eye care. Paper tape is used to close the eyes to prevent corneal drying or abrasions; eye pads are then placed over both eyes to protect them.

Another procedure that can be done laparoscopically is the *vagotomy with anterior seromyotomy.* The organization of the branches of the anterior vagus nerve, which are often embedded within the seromuscular layer of the stomach, may prevent division of the individual branches in some patients. In these cases, a seromyotomy is made (with care taken to avoid penetration of the mucosa) to transect these vagal branches. Methylene blue may be instilled into the stomach via an orogastric tube to verify gastric repair integrity.

Testing for gastric acidity may be done intraoperatively. Pentagasitrin 6 mcg/kg is given subcutaneously; this agent stimulates gastric acid production. The surgeon lavages sodium bicarbonate to remove residual acid through the laparoscope port. Red dye is instilled into the stomach to coat the gastric mucosa. If vagotomy is complete, the red dye will remain unchanged. If even partial innervation remains, however, the affected area will turn black (seen via the scope) and additional nerve transection may be done.

A nasogastric tube is placed after induction.

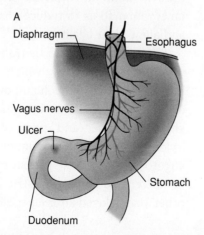
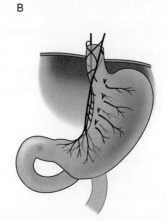

A
Diaphragm — — Esophagus

Vagus nerves —

Ulcer —

— Stomach

Duodenum

B

Figure 16-3 *Vagotomy*

Patients who present for this surgery have peptic ulcer disease and may be actively bleeding. Type and cross-match their blood; blood products may need to be available in the operating room depending on the patient's preoperative hematocrit level.

Have one or two peripheral IVs.

BARIATRIC SURGERY

Bariatric surgery is performed to help obese patients lose weight.

Ideal body weight formula: centimeters − 100 = kilograms

Body mass index (BMI) = kilograms ÷ meters^2

Obesity Pearls

- Morbidity and mortality increase sharply with increasing BMI and age.
- Preoperative testing: along with standard preoperative laboratory values, a chest x-ray and a 12-lead EKG should be obtained. If the patient has a cardiac history, the patient should also have had a cardiac stress test along with an arterial blood gas analysis.
- Potential complications of bariatric surgery include hemorrhage, injury to the gastrointestinal tract, deep venous thrombosis, pulmonary embolism, anastomotic leaks, infection, and small bowel obstruction.
- Check the operating room table weight limits and know your patient's kilogram weight before bringing the patient into the OR.

BMI (kg/m^2)	Classification
< 18.5	Underweight
20–25	Normal weight
26–30	Overweight
> 30–34.9	Obese
> 35	Morbidly obese

Figure 16-4 *Body Mass Index (BMI)*

- Anesthetic challenges in obese patients include a potentially difficult airway, a large tongue and thicker neck, and limited cervical neck range of motion. To facilitate intubation, place the patient in the "sniffing position": Place blankets or pillows under the upper shoulders and head to elevate the patient's head by approximately 10 cm, which extends the head at the atlanto-occipital joint to align the oral, pharyngeal, and laryngeal axis. When aligned, the visualization from the lips to the glottis and vocal cords is almost straight. A difficult airway cart may need to be in the room while intubation is performed.
- Obese patients often have poor gastric emptying from increased abdominal weight and intra-abdominal pressures. Rapid-sequence induction may need to be done because the risk of aspiration is higher in such cases.
- Obese patients tend to have decreased functional residual capacity (FRC), vital capacity (VC), and tidal volumes with increased carbon dioxide production and levels. Chronic hypoxia and hypercarbia, possible right ventricular hypertrophy and failure, and pulmonary hypertension are other factors complicating anesthesia management in these patients.
- Obese patients can desaturate quickly and easily. Before induction, with the patient in the sniffing position, have the patient take deep breaths for a few minutes longer than normal to oxygenate the individual as well as possible. Use preoperative sedation very cautiously, if at all.
- During emergence, place the patient in reverse Trendelenburg position. If he or she is spontaneously breathing, set the pop-off valve to airway pressures of 5–10 cm H_2O to keep the airway open. Insert a lubricated soft-rubber trumpet into one side of the nose. If possible, transfer the (still intubated) patient to the bed or stretcher. After giving full neuromuscular reversal and once the

patient is fully awake and following commands, pull the OETT and immediately place the ventilator mask over the patient's mouth and nose. If the respiratory effort is effective and oxygen saturations are greater than 96%, insert a nasal cannula or place a face mask and position the head of the bed up by 30–45 degrees to help gravity pull the abdomen away from the lungs.

- Pharmacokinetics are affected by obesity: There is an increased volume of distribution and increased elimination half-life for lipophilic drugs in obese patients, but normal volume of distribution and elimination half-life for hydrophilic drugs. Increase the succinylcholine (Anectine) dose in such cases because of increased pseudocholinesterase activity.

- Most bariatric surgery is performed laparoscopically. Most patients who are scheduled for a laparoscopic bariatric procedure will have had a bowel prep and will be dehydrated. IV fluids should be given preoperatively to prevent hypotension during anesthesia induction.

- Associated medical comorbidities with the morbidly obese patient include these and others:

Pulmonary: obstructive sleep apnea (OSA), obesity hypoventilation syndrome (Pickwickian syndrome), restrictive lung disease, asthma, and/or pulmonary hypertension

Cardiovascular: hypertension, LV hypertrophy and cardiomegaly, coronary artery disease, peripheral vascular disease, congestive heart failure

Gastrointestinal: gastroesophageal reflux, hiatal hernia, poor gastric emptying, increased abdominal pressure and increase in gall bladder and biliary tree diseases, increased risk of aspiration

Endocrine: type 2 diabetes, Cushing's disease, cholecystitis, hypothyroidism, and resistance to insulin

Musculoskeletal: osteoarthritis

Adjustable Gastric Banding

Gastric banding is a restrictive surgery carried out for the purposes of weight loss in the morbidly obese patient unable to lose weight by diet and exercise. This procedure effectively narrows the distal esophagus. The band can be adjusted or temporarily placed if necessary. The goal is for the patient to eat only ½ to 1 cup of food before feeling full.

Operative Procedure

Gastric banding may be done as an open abdomen procedure or a laparoscopic procedure.

In an *open procedure,* the liver is retracted; an adjustable gastric band (several products are on the market) is placed and sutured around the upper part of the stomach, creating a smaller stomach pouch. The band can be adjusted in size by inflating or deflating the band through a port placed just below the skin and fat surface of the abdomen. Depending on the size of the band placed, some fluid may be inserted into the band intraoperatively; alternatively, this adjustment may be made after the patient is discharged. Fluid in the band is inserted or withdrawn based on how hungry the patient feels.

If this procedure is done *laparoscopically,* once the trocars have been inserted and pneumoperitoneum established, the surgeon may come to the head of the bed to place an EGD scope down the patient's esophagus. The surgeon uses this scope to visually inspect for stomach perforations from the trocar insertion. The band is placed around the proximal portion of the stomach and secured in place. The filling port is implanted in the same way as in the open procedure.

Anesthetic

GETA and muscle relaxants are given. Anesthetic dosages should be calculated on the patient's ideal body weight and not the actual weight. The "sniffing position" is used for intubation. Rapid-sequence induction is commonly employed in the obese patient. Avoid using nitrous oxide to minimize gastric/bowel distention.

Positioning

The patient is placed supine, in reverse Trendelenburg position. Bilateral arms are placed on padded armboards, with the shoulders at an angle less than 90 degrees. Secure the arms so they do not fall off the armboards when the head of the bed is tilted. The legs may also need to be padded and taped (at the thighs and at the ankles) to prevent falling off the table. Special attention must be paid to positioning to avoid stress or pressure to joints and areas of the body that press against parts of the bed and other equipment.

Anesthetic Implications

An orogastric tube can be inserted immediately after induction and intubation to empty the stomach; then it should be withdrawn. This practice ensures that the stomach is empty and flat to help avoid puncture during trocar insertion in a laparoscopic approach.

These patients require special eye care. Paper tape is used to close the eyes to prevent corneal drying or abrasions; eye pads are then placed over both eyes to protect them.

Hold the endotracheal tube in a secure position when the surgeon inserts and withdraws the EGD scope to avoid accidental extubation.

The obese patient has associated issues with difficult intubation and intravenous placement.

Keeping these patients warm can be especially difficult due to their body mass index.

If the patient uses CPAP at home, check whether the patient brought their machine and what the usual settings are.

Make sure that the patient is in a head-up position and wide awake before attempting extubation. Before extubating the individual, place a lubricated red-rubber nasal trumpet to prevent airway obstruction. Use a non-rebreather face mask (which delivers close to 100% oxygen) or Ventimask (which delivers approximately 55% oxygen) when patient is first extubated to maximize oxygen delivery.

Complications

Potential complications include stomach perforation and liver injury.

Gastric Bypass (Roux-en-Y)

Gastric bypass is the surgical formation of a stomach pouch to limit the amount of food taken in and bypass sites of food absorption. This pouch is permanently separated and divided from the rest of the stomach. The lower part of the stomach is bypassed, and food enters the small intestine within 10 minutes after food is ingested. Also known as Roux-en-Y surgery, this procedure is used to treat the morbidly obese patient who is unable to lose weight by diet and exercise. After undergoing Roux-en-Y surgery, the patient will feel full after eating only ¼ to ½ cup of food.

Operative Procedure

In *open bariatric surgery,* an incision is made below the sternum, ending just above the navel. In *laparoscopic bariatric surgery,* multiple small incisions are made, trocars are inserted into the peritoneal cavity, and a pneumoperitoneum is created.

With either technique, the stomach is separated into two parts. The stomach is sutured or stapled just below the esophagus, forming a 20- to 30-mL pouch above the staples. The small bowel is divided about 1 foot below the stomach. The intestines form a "Y" as one end of the small intestine is attached to the stomach pouch (a 1.5-cm stoma is created in the stomach pouch) and the other end is attached farther down, bypassing five feet of intestines so calories are not absorbed until moving beyond that area. The lower portion of the stomach is not removed and remains functioning. When this procedure is complete, food and fluids will pass from the new stomach pouch into the small bowel.

Anesthetic

General anesthesia is given with insertion of an OETT; muscle relaxants are given. Anesthetic dosages should be calculated on the patient's ideal body weight and not the actual weight. Place the patient in the "sniffing position" for intubation. Rapid-sequence induction is commonly performed in the obese patient. Avoid using nitrous oxide to minimize gastric/bowel distention.

Positioning

The patient is placed supine, in a reverse Trendelenburg position. Bilateral arms are placed on padded armboards, with the shoulders at an angle less than 90 degrees. Secure the arms so they do not fall off the armboards when the head of the bed is tilted. The legs may also need to be padded and taped (at the thighs and at the ankles) to prevent falling off the table. Special attention must be paid to positioning to avoid stress or pressure to joints and areas of the body that press against parts of the bed and other equipment.

Anesthetic Implications

Obesity is present if the body mass index is greater than 25 kg/m^2.

The obese patient can make both intubation and intravenous line placement difficult.

Keeping these patients warm can be especially difficult owing to their body mass index.

If the patient uses CPAP at home, check whether the patient brought their machine and what the usual settings are.

Tape both of the patient's eyes closed to prevent corneal abrasion or drying.

No esophageal tubes should be placed.

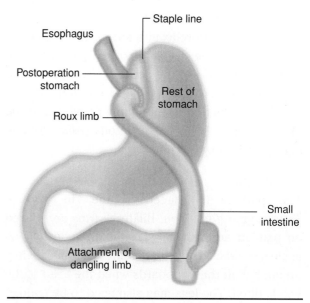

Figure 16-5 *Roux-en-Y Gastric Bypass*

Make sure that the patient is in a head-up position and wide awake before attempting extubation. Before extubating the individual, place a lubricated red-rubber nasal trumpet to prevent airway obstruction. Use a non-rebreather face mask (which delivers close to 100% oxygen) or Ventimask (which delivers approximately 55% oxygen) when the patient is first extubated to maximize oxygen delivery.

Vertical Banded Gastroplasty (Stomach Stapling)

Vertical banded gastroplasty (VBG) makes the stomach smaller by stapling off an upper section of the stomach; swallowed food then enters this pouch. The outlet of the pouch is restricted by a band of synthetic mesh, which slows emptying and gives a "full" sensation to the patient after he or she takes only a few bites. Stomach stapling may be used to treat the morbidly obese patient who is unable to lose weight by diet and exercise. When the procedure is complete, the patient can eat only ½ to 1 cup of food before feeling full.

Operative Procedure

An incision is made in the abdomen. Surgical staples and a plastic band are used to create a small pouch at the top of the stomach. This pouch is not completely closed off from the rest of the stomach; instead, a small opening allows the partially digested food to move into the rest of the stomach and then into the intestines.

Anesthetic

GETA and muscle relaxants are given. Anesthetic dosages should be calculated on the patient's ideal body weight and not the actual weight. Place the patient in the "sniffing position" for intubation. Rapid-sequence induction is commonly performed in the obese patient. Avoid using nitrous oxide to minimize gastric/bowel distention.

Positioning

The patient is placed supine, in a reverse Trendelenburg position. Bilateral arms are placed on padded armboards, with the shoulders at an angle less than 90 degrees. Secure the arms so they do not fall off the armboards when the head of the bed is tilted. The legs may also need to be padded and taped (at the thighs and at the ankles) to prevent falling off the table. Special attention must be paid to positioning to avoid stress or pressure to joints and areas of the body that press against parts of the bed and other equipment.

Anesthetic Implications

The obese patient can make intubation and intravenous line placement difficult.

No esophageal tubes should be placed.

Keeping these patients warm can be especially difficult due to their body mass index.

If the patient uses CPAP at home, check whether the patient brought their machine and what the usual settings are.

Make sure that the patient is in a head-up position and wide awake before attempting extubation. Before extubating the individual, place a lubricated red-rubber nasal trumpet to prevent airway obstruction. Use a non-rebreather face mask (which delivers close to 100% oxygen) or Ventimask (which delivers approximately 55% oxygen) when the patient is first extubated to maximize oxygen delivery.

SMALL INTESTINE SURGERY

Open Appendectomy

An open appendectomy is the surgical excision of the appendix—a finger-like projection from the cecum located in the right lower abdominal quadrant. It may be carried out to remove an acutely inflamed or ruptured appendix; alternatively, this procedure may be performed as an incidental removal during an open abdominal procedure.

Operative Procedure

The appendix projects from the terminal ileum of the small intestine. An incision is made just above the right groin, down through the peritoneum. The appendix is carefully ligated from the ileocecal valve and its mesentery, and removed from the body. The stump is sutured and closed.

This procedure is often done laparoscopically (discussed in the next subsection).

Anesthetic

General anesthesia is given with insertion of an OETT; muscle relaxants are given. Avoid using nitrous oxide to minimize gastric/bowel distention. Perform a rapid-sequence induction if the abdomen is distended or an ileus is present. An open appendectomy is usually done as an emergency case, so patients should be considered to have a full stomach and requires a rapid-sequence induction. If a spinal/epidural is placed, it needs be at the T6–T8 analgesia level.

Positioning

The patient is placed in a supine position. Although the arms may be tucked bilaterally, usually just the left arm is tucked.

Anesthetic Implications

These patients have usually been feeling nauseous for some time and may be quite dehydrated. Supplement volume with crystalloid infusion.

If the appendix is severely inflamed, is infected, or has burst, peritonitis can occur and cause volume shifts. Patients in such cases are often quite ill and the appendectomy is done in an open approach.

Insert an orogastric tube to suction out the stomach (patient may already have a nasogastric tube). For a perforated appendix and possible peritonitis, the surgeon may want a nasogastric tube to stay in the patient for 24 hours.

Laparoscopic Appendectomy

Laparoscopic excision of the appendix may be performed in cases of uncomplicated appendicitis. This technique is appropriate in the setting of an acutely inflamed appendix without the presence of acute peritonitis.

Operative Procedure

A small incision is made at the umbilicus, and other entry ports (usually two more) can be made anywhere in the belly to allow access for instruments. Pneumoperitoneum is achieved. The appendix is located at the terminal ileum of the small intestine. The appendix is carefully ligated from the ileocecal valve and its mesentery, and removed from the body. The stump is sutured and closed. The abdomen is irrigated and suctioned out; bleeding is cauterized. The trocars are removed and the abdomen desufflated. The trocar incision sites are sutured or closed with surgical glue. Small gauze dressings are placed over larger incision sites.

Anesthetic

General anesthesia is given with insertion of an OETT; muscle relaxants are given. Avoid using nitrous oxide to minimize gastric/bowel distention.

Perform a rapid-sequence induction if the abdomen is distended or an ileus is present.

Positioning

The patient is placed in a supine position. The left arm will often be tucked.

Anesthetic Implications

If an abscess or significant adhesions are encountered, conversion to an open procedure would be necessary.

Peritonitis can cause volume shifts.

Once pneumoperitoneum is achieved, the anesthesist may switch to pressure ventilation to achieve appropriate tidal volumes. Adjust the respiratory rates to maintain $ETCO_2$ levels between 33 and 36 mm Hg. When the insufflation is released, the pressure against the lungs is decreased; quickly decrease the set pressure volumes so as not to give too high a tidal volume.

Diverticulectomy (Meckel's Diverticulum)

Diverticulectomy is the surgical excision of a diverticulum of the small intestine.

Operative Procedure

In the *open* approach, an incision is made on the abdomen (usually right side or midline), the diverticulum is identified and removed, and the wall of the small bowel is sutured closed. If it is large, a piece of small bowel may need to be resected, with the ends anastomosed back together.

In the *laparoscopic* approach, a pneumoperitoneum is created after several small incisions are made over the abdomen. A 2- to 3-inch long incision may also be made so the surgeon can place a hand into the operative field to aid in dissection and retraction.

Anesthetic

GETA and muscle relaxants are given. Avoid using nitrous oxide to minimize gastric/bowel distention.

Positioning

The patient is placed in a supine position.

Anesthetic Implications

Patients may have had black, tarry stools preoperatively. A preoperative hematocrit may be done to ascertain hematocrit levels.

Peritonitis can cause volume shifts.

Some patients may have received a bowel prep and be dehydrated; this practice is surgeon specific.

At least two large-bore peripheral IVs are needed.

Enterostomy: Ileostomy or Jejunostomy

Enterostomy is the creation of a passage between the small intestine and the abdominal wall—that is, the creation of a stoma. It is done to bypass an obstruction, to prevent intestinal contents from crossing a more distal anastomosis (to provide "bowel rest"), or because the colon and rectum have been removed. The procedure is named according to the section of the small intestine that is used to form the stoma (jejunum = jejunostomy; ileum = ileostomy). The stoma may be temporary or permanent.

Operative Procedure

A midline abdominal incision is made to expose the entire small bowel and peritoneum for examination. The portion of small intestine is cleared of its mesentery, and the proximal end (of either the ileum or jejunum) is passed through a stoma (a disc of skin and subcutaneous fat) onto the abdominal wall. The bowel wall is everted on itself and sutured circumferentially. The distal end of the intestine may be sutured or stapled closed; alternatively, it may be left open to create a "loop." An ostomy bag is placed over the stoma.

Part of this procedure can be done laparoscopically.

For a *continent ileostomy,* a resected section of small intestine is fashioned into a pouch. This pouch (called a K-pouch) allows for the collection of stool so that it does not drain continuously through the stoma. The distal end of the intestine, just past the pouch, is brought to the abdominal surface and a stoma is formed. A valve is fashioned by suturing the intestine in a certain way so that stool does not leak out. An indwelling catheter is placed through the stoma into the pouch at the end of the surgery. This catheter will remain for approximately 3 weeks to allow the stool to drain continuously while the pouch matures.

After the pouch matures, the patient must insert a catheter when it is time to empty the pouch. How often the pouch is drained is patient specific but the interval usually becomes longer over time. If the pouch is not emptied when it becomes full, pressure can build up and pull at the suture line; the pouch can perforate or tear, or the valve could leak.

Anesthetic

GETA is given with insertion of an OETT; muscle relaxants are given. Avoid using nitrous oxide to minimize gastric/bowel distention. Perform a rapid-sequence induction if the abdomen is distended or an ileus is present.

Positioning

The patient is placed in a supine position, with arms tucked at the sides bilaterally.

Anesthetic Implications

These patients are often chronically sick. Consequently, they may have a high medication need and/or be quite ill.

Nasogastric tube placement should be done with surgeon assistance. The tube is placed, the surgeon checks its placement internally, and then the tube is taped securely.

Monitors and IV Access

- An arterial line may be needed.
- A central venous catheter may be needed.
- At least two large-bore peripheral IVs are needed if a central line is not placed.

Resection of Small Intestine (Small Bowel Resection)

This procedure involves excision of a specific segment of the small intestine. The proximal edge of small bowel is then anastomosed to a distal piece of small bowel or colon. Resection of the small intestine is performed in cases of small bowel obstruction (SBO), gangrene, herniation, perforation, trauma, hemorrhage, diverticulum, Crohn's disease, adhesions interfering with normal bowel function, inflammatory bowel disease, rare primary tumors, and mesenteric infarctions.

Operative Procedure

A midline abdominal incision is made to expose the entire small bowel and peritoneum for examination. The mesentery is divided, and the entire small bowel is examined along its length. The affected segment is excised and continuity of the bowel is restored.

Anesthetic

GETA is given with insertion of an OETT; muscle relaxants are given. Avoid nitrous oxide. These patients are considered to be "full stomach" cases, and a rapid-sequence induction is needed. An epidural may be placed for postoperative pain control. If an epidural has been placed, then pain issues should be addressed by anesthesia specialists postoperatively.

Positioning

The patient is placed in a supine position, with arms tucked at the sides bilaterally or extended onto padded armboards.

Anesthetic Implications

The patient may have been vomiting and be very dehydrated. If small bowel surgery is done on an emergency/urgent basis, the patient may be quite sick.

Nasogastric tube placement should be done with surgeon assistance. The tube is placed, the surgeon checks its placement internally, and then the tube is taped securely; the tube will remain in postoperatively.

Type and cross-match the patient's blood prior to surgery.

Preoperatively, check the patient's electrolyte levels, especially the potassium level, and give replacement electrolytes if needed.

Antiemetics should be given.

Large third-space fluid shifts are common in the setting of infection, obstruction, and trauma. Consider giving albumin or hetastarch fluid boluses before and during surgery.

Temperature loss is common with an open abdomen procedure. Upper- and lower-body warming blankets are needed as well as fluid warmers. The ambient temperature in the room may also need to be increased.

Monitors and IV Access

- An arterial line may or may not be needed.
- A central venous catheter may or may not be needed.
- At least two large-bore peripheral IVs are needed if a central line is not placed.

LARGE BOWEL SURGERY

Abdominoperineal Resection

Abdominoperineal resection (APR) involves excision of a portion of the distal sigmoid colon and the entire rectum. Organs and structures to avoid include the ureters, bladder, prostate, and vagina. The abdominal and perineal approaches can be performed by two separate teams simultaneously. If one team is performing both procedures, the abdomen is closed before prepping and draping for the perineal approach.

Indications for APR include inflammatory bowel disease (ulcerative colitis or Crohn's disease) of the lower sigmoid colon, rectum, and/or anus; irreversible rectal/sphincter injuries; and malignancy.

Operative Procedure

APR may be done through a midline abdominal approach as well as through a perineal approach. The abdominal incision is a vertical or transverse approach. The distal portion of the colon is transected; the proximal portion is brought through the rectus muscle and sewed circumferentially as a stoma to the abdominal wall to create a permanent colostomy. The perineal tissue is entered, the rectum is dissected from the perineal muscle, the levator muscle is incised, and the previously dissected distal colon and rectum are excised.

Intraoperative placement of ureteral stents may be needed.

Anesthetic

GETA is given with insertion of an OETT; muscle relaxants are given. Perform a rapid-sequence induction if the abdomen is distended. Avoid nitrous oxide.

Positioning

Surgery is begun with the patient in a supine position; this is then changed to a lithotomy position for perineal access.

Anesthetic Implications

The patient may have been vomiting and will have received a bowel prep and be dehydrated. If this procedure is done on an emergency/urgent basis, the patient may be quite sick.

Nasogastric tube placement should be done with surgeon assistance. The tube is placed, the surgeon checks its placement internally, and then the tube is taped securely.

This surgery can last for many hours. Large third-space fluid shifts are common; consider giving albumin or hetastarch fluid boluses along with a crystalloid infusion.

Temperature loss is common with an open abdomen procedure. Upper- and lower-body warming blankets are needed as well as fluid warmers.

The ambient temperature in the room may also need to be increased.

The anesthestist may need to assist the ureteral identification with methylene blue injection.

Type and cross-match the patient's blood prior to surgery. Bleeding can be moderate to large with this procedure.

Monitors and IV Access

- An arterial line is normally placed.
- A central venous catheter may or may not be needed.
- At least two large-bore peripheral IVs are needed if a central line is not placed or present.

Anterior Resection of Sigmoid Colon (Low) and Rectosigmoidostomy

In this procedure, the sigmoid colon and proximal rectum are excised and removed either through the abdomen or transanally via the distal rectal remnant. The proximal rectal remnant and the distal descending colon are anastomosed to provide for bowel continuity.

Indications for anterior resection of the sigmoid colon and rectosigmoidostomy include benign (polyps or diverticulitis) or malignant disease of the sigmoid/left colon/upper rectum. Organs and structures to avoid include the urethra, bladder, prostate, and vagina.

Operative Procedure

Anterior resection of the sigmoid colon is similar to abdominoperineal resection with the exception that the mid- and distal rectum and anal sphincters are left in place. Sigmoidoscopy may be added to check the integrity of the anastomosis. Intraoperative placement of ureteral stents may be needed.

This procedure may also be done using a laparoscopic-assisted approach.

Anesthetic

General anesthesia is given with insertion of an OETT; muscle relaxants are given. Perform a rapid-sequence induction if the abdomen is distended. Avoid nitrous oxide.

Positioning

The patient is placed in a lithotomy position, with bilateral arms tucked at the sides.

Anesthetic Implications

The patient will have received a bowel prep and be dehydrated.

Nasogastric tube placement should be done with surgeon assistance. The tube is placed, the surgeon checks its placement internally, and then the tube is taped securely.

Large third-space fluid shifts are common with this procedure; consider giving albumin or het-astarch fluid boluses along with a crystalloid infusion.

Type and cross-match the patient's blood prior to surgery. Moderate to large blood loss is possible with this procedure.

Temperature loss is common with an open abdomen procedure. Upper- and lower-body warming blankets are needed as well as fluid warmers. The ambient temperature in the room may also need to be increased.

The anesthesist may need to assist the ureteral identification with methylene blue injection.

These patients may be quite ill due to a major underlying condition.

Monitors and IV Access

- An arterial line is normally placed.
- A central venous catheter may be placed to monitor fluid status.
- At least two large-bore peripheral IVs are needed if a central line is not placed.

Colostomy

Colostomy is the formation of a temporary or permanent connection from the colon to the abdominal wall as a stoma; the goal is to divert stool from the distal colon. A colostomy can be created in the transverse or descending sigmoid colon. The portion of the proximal colon is pulled up into a stoma (a disc of skin and subcutaneous fat) and onto the abdominal wall, and then the bowel wall is everted on itself and sutured circumferentially.

Colostomy may be performed in cases involving inflammation, tumor/malignancy, rectal stricture, or unrepairable anal incontinence—in essence, any condition that requires the colon to "rest."

Operative Procedure

Loop Colostomy

A loop colostomy is a temporary colostomy where the proximal and distal portions of the colon remain connected. The bowel is loosened from its surrounding mesentery and omentum. A piece of a soft rubber hose or the surgeon's finger is looped under the colon to tent and elevate the colon up to the left of the midline onto the abdomen. A loop ostomy bridge is placed underneath the loop of colon to maintain its position on the abdomen. This bridge is made of a plastic or glass rod with a rubber hose attached to both ends of the rod to prevent it from slipping or retraction. The loop is covered with petroleum gauze. Approximately 48 hours after the loop is formed, the surgeon will "ventilate" (open) the externalized apex of the colon loop with electrocautery. The omentum acts as a seal around the colon to reduce spillage into the peritoneal cavity when the colon lumen is opened. An ostomy bag is applied.

Double-Barrel Colostomy

In double-barrel colostomy, the portions of the colon are separated to form two side-by-side ostomies. The feces from the proximal loop does not spill into the distal loop.

Terminal Colostomy

In terminal colostomy, the distal portion of the colon is removed completely; the proximal end is brought up on the abdominal wall and a stoma is formed. This is a permanent colostomy with complete diversion of fecal matter. The abdominal wall is closed.

Anesthetic
General anesthesia is given with insertion of an OETT; muscle relaxants are given. Avoid nitrous oxide to prevent distention of the bowel. Perform a rapid-sequence induction if the abdomen is distended.

Positioning
The patient is placed in a supine position.

Anesthetic Implications
The patient will have received a bowel prep and be dehydrated.

The surgeon will mark the proposed placement for the stoma preoperatively.

If not already placed preoperatively, a nasogastric tube should be placed with surgeon assistance. The tube is placed, the surgeon checks its placement internally, and then the tube is taped securely.

The patient presenting for a colostomy may be quite ill and possibly have chronic pain issues. If this patient has already received chemotherapy and/or radiation, there is an increased risk of friable tissues with blood loss.

Monitors and IV Access
- An arterial line may need to be placed to monitor blood pressure and for serial arterial blood gases.
- A central venous catheter may be placed to monitor fluid status.
- At least two large-bore peripheral IVs are needed if a central line is not placed.

Colostomy Closure
Colostomy closure is performed when there is no further need for fecal diversion; it reestablishes colon continuity and repairs the abdominal wall. The viscera is closed, but the skin and subcutaneous tissue can be left open and packed to prevent wound infection.

Operative Procedure
A circumferential incision is made around the stoma to free the skin margin, and the proximal and distal ends of the colon are anastomosed together.

Anesthetic
GETA is given with insertion of an OETT; muscle relaxants are given.

Positioning
The patient is placed in a supine position; the arms may be tucked bilaterally.

Anesthetic Implications
The patient will have received a bowel prep and be dehydrated.

Nasogastric tube placement should be done with surgeon assistance. The tube is placed, the surgeon checks its placement internally, and then the tube is taped securely as it exits the nares.

Large fluid shifts and loss are possible with this procedure. For this reason, a minimum of two peripheral IVs are needed.

Colectomy
Colectomy is the excision of a segment of the large intestine. This surgery is usually performed for adenocarcinomas, obstruction, ulcerative colitis, trauma, or diverticulitis. The laparoscopic approach is used only if tumors are benign.

Operative Procedure
Using either a laparoscopic or open approach, the surgeon mobilizes the colon and ligates the corresponding blood vessels. The diseased or damaged bowel is resected and removed; the remaining ends of the distal and proximal colon may be anastomosed together or a (permanent or temporary) colostomy or ileostomy may be formed.

A lymphadenectomy may also be performed if the colectomy is done as a treatment for colon cancer.

The abdominal cavity is irrigated and suctioned, and the incision lines are closed.

Anesthetic

General anesthesia is used with an OETT; muscle relaxants are given. Perform a rapid-sequence induction if the abdomen is distended. Avoid nitrous oxide to prevent bowel distention.

Positioning

The patient is placed supine; a steep Trendelenburg position is used for the laparoscopic approach.

Anesthetic Implications

The patient will have received a bowel prep and be dehydrated.

Nasogastric tube placement should be done with surgeon assistance. The tube is placed, the surgeon checks its placement internally, and then the tube is taped securely as it exits the nares.

Large fluid shifts and loss are possible with this procedure. For this reason, a minimum of two peripheral IVs are needed.

Hartmann Procedure

Use of the Hartmann procedure is usually limited to emergency situations in which immediate anastomosis of the left colon is not possible or not safe to complete due to infection. This surgery is performed when colon cancer or diverticulitis has perforated the bowel wall or when the bowel is too injured for safe anastomosis.

Operative Procedure

Using either an open or laparoscopic approach, the diseased portion of the colon is resected. A sigmoid colostomy is formed, and the distal end of the colon is either brought out to the abdominal wall as a mucous fistula or closed and

returned intraperitoneally. The colostomy is usually performed as a temporary procedure.

Anesthetic

General anesthesia is given with insertion of an OETT; muscle relaxants are given. Avoid nitrous oxide. Rapid-sequence induction is appropriate when done as an emergency procedure.

Positioning

The patient is placed in a supine position, with arms tucked at both sides.

Anesthetic Implications

The patient may have received a bowel prep and be dehydrated.

Nasogastric tube placement should be done with surgeon assistance. The tube is placed, the surgeon checks its placement internally, and then the tube is taped securely as it exits the nares.

Monitors and IV Access

- An arterial line may need to be placed to monitor blood pressure and for serial arterial blood gases. An arterial line is usually necessary, as these patients may be septic or well on their way to getting there.
- A central venous catheter may be placed to monitor fluid status.
- Large fluid shifts and loss are possible with this procedure. For this reason, a minimum of two peripheral IVs are needed if a central line is not placed.

Right Hemicolectomy and Ileocolostomy

Right hemicolectomy and ileocolostomy involve resection of the terminal ileum (end of the small intestine), the appendix, their mesenteries, and the right half of the colon (all of the ascending and part of the transverse colon). This surgery is performed to treat tumors, bleeding, inflammation, and trauma. Obstruction is less often encountered in the right half of the colon.

Operative Procedure

The ileum and the remaining portion of the transverse colon are anastomosed together. Other organs and structures at risk with this operation include the right ureter, duodenum, and inferior vena cava.

This procedure can be done through a laparoscopic-assisted approach.

Anesthetic

GETA is used with an OETT; muscle relaxants are given. Perform a rapid-sequence induction if the abdomen is distended. Avoid nitrous oxide to prevent bowel distention. An epidural catheter is often placed for postoperative pain control.

Positioning

The patient is placed in a supine position, with both arms padded and tucked bilaterally.

Anesthetic Implications

Most patients will not have received a bowel prep, as this surgery focuses on the ascending colon.

Nasogastric tube placement should be done with surgeon assistance. The tube is placed, the surgeon checks its placement internally, and then the tube is taped securely.

Transverse Colectomy

Transverse colectomy consists of resection of a segment of the transverse colon with anastomosis of both the proximal and distal ends to establish continuity. Surrounding structures at risk during this procedure include the stomach, pancreas, spleen, and superior mesenteric vessels. This surgery is performed to treat inflammatory bowel disease, strictures, and malignant tumors.

Operative Procedure

The ascending colon is anastomosed to the descending colon after the transverse colon has been excised. The mesentery and the peritoneum are sutured closed, and the abdominal incision is then closed.

Transverse colectomy may also be done through a laparoscopic-assisted approach.

Anesthetic

General anesthesia is used with an OETT; muscle relaxants are given. Perform a rapid-sequence induction if the abdomen is distended. Avoid nitrous oxide to prevent distention of the bowel.

Positioning

The patient is placed in a supine position, with both arms padded and tucked bilaterally.

Anesthetic Implications

The patient will have received a bowel prep and be dehydrated.

Nasogastric tube placement should be done with surgeon assistance. The tube is placed, the surgeon checks its placement internally, and then the tube is taped securely as it exits the nares.

RECTUM SURGERY

Lateral Internal Sphincterotomy

Lateral internal sphincterotomy is intended to help heal a chronic, longitudinal anal tear (fissure). Such difficulties are caused by stretching of the anus beyond normal capability, such as is seen in women following childbirth, after difficult bowel movements or constipation, or following anal intercourse. Surgery is usually done only after medical interventions have failed.

An internal sphincterotomy (division of the internal anal sphincter) may be indicated to lower the resting pressure of the internal sphincter, which can help with healing. The internal sphincter is one of two muscles that control the sphincter; it is the involuntary muscle that controls that passage of stool. Fecal and flatulence incontinence are common side effects after this operation.

Operative Procedure

A speculum is inserted into the anal canal. A 2- to 3-cm incision is made over the internal anal sphincter. Forceps are used to secure the sphincter, and a small portion is cauterized, opening the internal sphincter. The edges of the fissure are removed and the incision line is closed.

Anesthetic

General anesthesia is used with an OETT. Neuraxial (spinal or epidural), local, or combination anesthesia may be employed; a hypobaric spinal is appropriate if the jack-knife position is used.

IV Fluids and Volume Requirements

Crystalloid infusions are given to supplement the patient who is in a dehydrated state.

Positioning

The patient is placed in a jack-knife, lithotomy, or lateral decubitus position, with the upper leg bent forward to access the perineum.

Anesthetic Implications

The patient will have received a bowel prep and be dehydrated.

Fistulotomy

A fistula-in-ano (commonly caused by infection or perirectal abscess) is an abnormal connection from the rectum to the skin that bypasses the anus. In a fistulotomy, the surgeon opens and drains this tract, clearing away any infected tissue.

Recurrent perirectal abscess in the same location may indicate a communication with the rectum; fistulotomy is performed in such cases.

Operative Procedure

Both openings of the fistula are identified. Tissue overlying the tract is divided to allow the tract to heal. If the tract is deep and division of tissue will impair fecal continence, a cutting seton (a rubber vessel loop) maybe placed through the fistula and tied to itself; this will slowly divide the tissues over time and allow the fistula to heal.

Anesthetic

General anesthesia is used with an OETT. Neuraxial (spinal or epidural), local, or combination anesthesia may be employed; a hypobaric spinal is appropriate if the jack-knife position is used.

IV Fluids and Volume Requirements

Crystalloid infusion may be used to supplement the patient who is in a dehydrated state.

Positioning

The patient may be placed in a jack-knife, lithotomy, or lateral decubitus position, with the upper leg bent forward to access the perineum.

Anesthetic Implications

The patient will have received a bowel prep and be dehydrated.

Hemorrhoidectomy

Hemorrhoidectomy consists of the excision of enlarged veins of the anus along with any overlying skin and mucous membrane. It is performed in cases involving pain or bleeding from enlarged veins of the anus that have not responded to medical treatment.

Operative Procedure

This procedure may be done with a sigmoidoscope. Tissue for resection is identified and excised, using a circular stapler, cryotherapy, radiofrequency ligation, heater-probe coagulation, or laser.

Anesthetic

GETA is used with an OETT. Neuraxial (spinal or epidural), local, or combination anesthesia may be employed; a hypobaric spinal is appropriate if the jack-knife position is used. The patient may need muscle relaxants with GA to relax the anal sphincter.

Positioning

The patient is placed in a jack-knife, lithotomy, or lateral decubitus position, with the upper leg bent forward to access the perineum.

Anesthetic Implications

The patient will have received a bowel prep and be dehydrated.

Check preoperative H&H levels.

Check coagulation studies and platelet levels if the patient is taking anticoagulants (e.g., Plavix) before planning a spinal for neuraxial anesthesia.

When a laser procedure is done, care must be taken to avoid OR fires. See Chapter 1 on safety concerns for more information.

Pilonidal Cyst and Sinus Excision

This procedure removes a pilonidal cyst and its accompanying sinus—that is, the channel that originates from the cyst and opens to the skin to drain the infection. It is performed to treat a pilonidal cyst and sinus, or infection in the hair follicle of the sinus tract. Such cysts may be found in the sacrococcygeal region just above the gluteal cleft (crack between the buttocks) on the lower sacrum and can be quite deep. They can contain hair, skin, necrotic tissue, and other tissue debris and can range in severity from a draining pilonidal sinus to an acute abscess. This condition can be a recurrent problem if the cyst and sinus are not totally removed. Total surgical excision of both the cyst and the sinus is done when an acute process is not present.

Operative Procedure

In the presence of acute infection, the wound will be drained and can be left open and packed.

For surgical excision, the buttock cheeks are pulled apart and taped to secure them for surgical exposure. A probe is inserted into the sinus to identify the sinus direction. An elliptical incision is made over the sinus tract and cyst, but usually off the midline (to remove the focus of shearing stress when sitting postoperatively); cautery is used for hemostasis. If the wound is left open, it is packed. If the wound is closed, sutures are used. A dressing is placed over the incision.

Anesthetic

GETA is used with an OETT. Regional, local, or combination anesthesia (spinal or epidural) may be employed; a hypobaric spinal is appropriate if the jack-knife position is used.

Positioning

The patient is placed in a jack-knife, prone, lithotomy, or lateral decubitus position, with the upper leg bent forward to access the perineum.

Anesthetic Implications

One peripheral IV is usually all that is needed.

Methylene blue or indigo carmine should be available. The surgeon injects this dye into the sinus; it stains the cyst but not the surrounding tissues. This information helps to guide the complete excision of the cyst and sinus tract.

Rectal Prolapse (Presacral Rectopexy)

Presacral rectopexy is performed to correct complete rectal prolapse.

Operative Procedure

An abdominal approach is used to mobilize the rectum within the abdomen and pelvis, by fixing it to the presacral fascia and periosteum with a mesh material.

Positioning

The patient is placed in a lithotomy or supine position, with arms tucked at the sides bilaterally.

Anesthetic

GETA is used with an OETT; muscle relaxants are given.

Anesthetic Implications

The patient will have received a bowel prep and be dehydrated.

One peripheral IV is usually sufficient.

ENDOSCOPY SURGERY PEARLS

- The patient may need to hold products containing aspirin or NSAIDs (e.g., Motrin) for at least seven days before the procedure. Notify the gastroenterologist if the patient is taking any blood thinners, such as Coumadin, Plavix, Lovenox, or heparin.
- The physician can "tattoo" a questionable area in the gastrointestinal tract with indigo carmine (India ink) to help relocate the spot in a future scope procedure or during a laparoscopic or laparotomy procedure.
- Endoscopy can be done through a stoma.

Anesthesia for All Endoscopic Procedures

The vast majority of endoscopic procedures are performed in an outpatient setting with anesthesia consisting of a narcotic (Demerol or fentanyl) and a benzodiazepine. Currently, there is a trend toward using more sedation with hypnotic agents. The primary anesthetics used are Versed (midazolam) and propofol for anxiety and sedation. In our practice, we have found that using just propofol as the sole anesthetic is sufficient and safe, with good amnesia effects in most endoscopic procedures.

Benadryl may be used as an adjunct to increase sedation. This agent has a synergistic effect with Versed and propofol and may help to decrease the amounts of other anesthetics needed. Because it depresses the central nervous system, patients who are given Benadryl should be closely monitored during and after the procedure.

There is an increased risk of respiratory depression with opioid administration if sedatives have been given. Nevertheless, it may be beneficial to administer opioids, such as fentanyl at 0.25–0.5 mcg/kg to blunt sympathetic response and aid in MAC anesthesia. Reversal agents, such as flumazenil (for benzodiazepine reversal) and Narcan (for opioid reversal), should be available and administered if needed.

Some local anesthetics (e.g., prilocaine, benzocaine, cetacaine) can cause a fatal methemoglobinemia reaction if used in excess of the maximum dosages.

Methemoglobinemia renders the hemoglobin incapable of carrying oxygen or carbon dioxide. In addition, the oxy-hemoglobin dissociation curve shifts to the left, impairing the delivery of oxygen at the tissue level. Methylene blue 2 mg/kg can be used in the treatment of methemoglobinemia, along with high-flow oxygen.

Robinul 0.1–0.2 mg IV can be given to decrease mouth and oropharynx secretions. Lidocaine 1 mg/kg IV can be given to help decrease airway reactivity, oropharynx sensitivity, and gagging.

Anesthesia for Pediatric Endoscopic Patients

Lidocaine lollipops, if available, can be used to prepare a child for an upper gastrointestinal procedure. Oral, nasal, or rectal benzodiazepines are utilized before IV sedation is given. Potentially serious airway complications are even more of a risk with this patient population because their tongues are much larger and their airways are much smaller; even small amounts of mucous or edema can increase this resistance even further. The surgical procedure often takes longer in children, with greater sedation needs, because it is difficult to get a good bowel cleansing on these patients. As a consequence, the risk of aspiration and often the need for general anesthesia are greater.

Depending on the patient's acuity and reason for the procedure, pediatric endoscopy may be done in either an outpatient surgical center or in the hospital. A thorough preoperative evaluation and history and physical are important in either case.

The local anesthetic, prilocaine, is not recommended for use in infants.

COLONOSCOPY

Colonoscopy is an endoscopic procedure that uses a lighted, flexible endoscopic tube to transmit images of an examination of the entire large colon (approximately 5 feet in length from the rectum to the ileocecal valve) and the distal part of the small bowel to a video screen. It may be performed for either diagnostic or therapeutic purposes.

- *Diagnostic:* detect and biopsy ulcers and bleeding, polyps, diverticuli, tumors, and inflammation; detect the early signs of colon or rectal cancer; follow up after abnormal barium X-rays; for complaints of diarrhea, constipation, a change in bowel patterns, rectal bleeding, or anemia.
- *Therapeutic:* cauterization or laser treatments of polyps, tumors, or bleeding; dilation.

Operative Procedure

The colonoscope is inserted into the rectum and advanced rather quickly to the cecum and the appendiceal opening or until the ileocecal valve (where the large and small intestine meet at the lower right quadrant) is visualized. The physician then slowly withdraws the scope, carefully examining all sides of the colon. (In some centers, the anesthetist is required to document the time the scope is at the ileocecal valve to confirm that the gastroenterologist has allowed enough time to properly examine the bowel on withdrawal of the scope.) A snare or forceps "bite" of tissue is taken to biopsy any unusual polyps, growths, or mass. A grounding pad may need to be placed for cautery excision, if needed. Either at the beginning of the procedure or at the end, the scope is folded into a U-shape to visualize the distal rectum and anal canal, which cannot be examined completely with the antegrade view. Usually a sigmoidoscopy is done in conjunction with a colonoscopy.

If a mass or an unresectable lesion is found, an ink tattoo can be placed with an injection catheter to mark the exact location of the lesion for relocation at a future endoscopy or to help the surgeon locate the lesion at the time of a laparotomy or laparoscopy.

Anesthetic

Conscious sedation is typically used to provide amnesia and to decrease patient movement. A propofol drip, Versed (midazolam), ketamine, and a narcotic can all be used.

Positioning

The patient is placed in a left lateral position, with knees pulled up and legs bent as though in the sitting position. This position may need to be changed during the procedure.

Anesthetic Implications

Minimal monitoring includes pulse oximetry, EKG, and blood pressure, readings should be measured and recorded at least every 5 minutes during the procedure. Oxygen is given via nasal cannula or simple face mask. CO_2 monitoring is a helpful adjunct, accomplished by placing the CO_2 sample line within the face mask or in the proximity of the nasal cannula.

These patients are NPO for 12 hours (except for the bowel prep itself) prior to the procedure. As a consequence, they are likely to present with dehydration and may manifest hypovolemia.

A colonoscopy is becoming a routine screening test for people ages 50 years and older. Rescreenings, after one normal colonoscopy, are done every 5 to 10 years.

ENDOSCOPIC RETROGRADE CHOLANGIOPANCREATOGRAPHY

Endoscopic retrograde cholangiopancreatography (ERCP) is a diagnostic endoscopic procedure that uses a specially designed side-viewing endoscope that permits visualization and cannulation of the ampulla, and thereby the pancreatic duct and common bile duct. As with other endoscopy techniques, images of the stomach, duodenum, pancreatic, and biliary ductal systems are transmitted to a video screen. ERCP combines endoscopy with fluoroscopy; thus the patient will lie on an X-ray table. "Retrograde" refers to the direction in which the contrast dye is injected to visualize the bile duct system and the pancreas.

ERCP is performed to diagnose problems in the liver, gallbladder, bile ducts, and pancreas. The drainage ducts from these organs are called the biliary tree. Thus, ERCP may be used to discover the reason for jaundice, pancreatitis, upper abdominal pain, and unexplained weight loss. A stone may be obstructing the common bile duct, for example.

Operative Procedure

Local anesthetics are given to numb the back of the throat. A mouthpiece is inserted between the upper and lower teeth to prevent the patient from biting down on the scope. Lowering the chin down toward the sternum can aid the physician in passing the scope through the oropharynx. If passage is still difficult, thrusting the jaw forward can help.

The lighted flexible endoscope is passed through the esophagus, stomach, and duodenum, until it reaches the very small opening into the biliary tree where the gallbladder, liver, and pancreas drain into the duodenum (common bile duct entrance); these images are transmitted to a video screen. A small tube is passed through the endoscope so that dye can be injected into the biliary tree and X-rays can be taken. If the exam shows a stricture of the ducts or gallstones, instruments can be threaded through the scope to remove a stone or dilate a stricture; biopsies can also be taken. A papillotomy is an incision in the common bile duct distal muscle that enlarges the duct opening, thereby facilitating stone removal. A catheter may be left in the duct for temporary drainage.

Anesthetic

Conscious sedation is typically used to provide amnesia and to decrease patient movement. A propofol drip, Versed (midazolam), ketamine, and a narcotic can all be used.

Positioning

The patient is placed in a left lateral, partially prone, position. The left arm is extended above the head, and the right arm is tucked at the side of the body. If at all possible, have the patient put themselves in this position, ask if they are comfortable and if they have any numbness and tingling of the arms before sedating. This position may need to be changed during the procedure.

Anesthetic Implications

Minimal monitoring includes pulse oximetry, EKG, and blood pressure, readings should be measured and recorded at least every 5 minutes during the procedure. Oxygen is given via nasal cannula. CO_2 monitoring is a helpful adjunct, accomplished by placing the CO_2 sample line within the proximity of the nasal cannula.

Patients must be NPO for 8 hours before this procedure. A bowel prep is not needed.

Prior to the procedure, clarify that the patient is not allergic to iodine or shrimp, as contrast dye is used during this procedure.

An anticholinergic agent (Robinul, atropine) can be given to decrease oral or gastric secretions.

ERCP can take anywhere from 30 minutes to several hours. Placing the intravenous needle in the hand/arm closest to the anesthetist (e.g., with the anesthetist standing at the patient's head with the left arm extended above the head) can make it easier to assess and access the IV site.

The most stimulating parts of the case are when the physician inserts the endoscope over the tongue and through the oropharynx, when the physician blows air into the duodenum, and when balloon dilation of the duct is performed.

Biliary flow from the common bile duct into the duodenum in controlled by the sphincter of Oddi. Some physicians use glucagon to inhibit intestinal motility and to reduce tone in the sphincter of Oddi, thereby decreasing biliary pressure. Glucagon may also be given to reduce gastroduodenal motility and produces a significant reduction in sphincter contraction: 1 unit = 1 mg glucagon, 0.25–2 mg given IV or 1–2 mg given IM.

All opioids can cause spasm of the sphincter of Oddi; thus their use should be avoided until the end of the exam. If an opioid is needed, give Demerol, as it produces the least spasm of the sphincter of Oddi.

Of all the endoscopic procedures, adequate sedation is most important in ERCP. This procedure involves the delicate placement of a catheter into a specific duct (pancreatic or common bile duct) for dye injection; the associated ampullary sphincterotomy involves the cautery destruction of the ampullary sphincter to allow common bile duct stone extraction.

Complications

Potential complications of ERCP include cardiopulmonary complications (due to deep sedation, long duration of ERCP, partial prone position, along with frequent comorbid conditions) along with bleeding and perforation of the duodenum.

ESOPHAGOGASTRODUODENOSCOPY

Esophagogastroduodenoscopy (EGD) is a diagnostic endoscopic procedure that uses a lighted, flexible endoscopic tube to transmit images of the upper part of the gastrointestinal tract (esophagus, stomach, proximal duodenum) to a video screen. It may be performed for either diagnostic or therapeutic purposes.

- *Diagnostic:* anemia, upper GI bleeding, nausea and vomiting, abdominal or chest pain, dyspepsia, chronic reflux that can lead to Barrett's esophagus (precancerous lesions), difficult or painful swallowing, confirmation of celiac disease by biopsy
- *Therapeutic:* esophageal varices, sclerotherapy, injection of epinephrine into bleeding lesions, biopsy of polyps or any other abnormal tissue, laser therapy, removal of foreign bodies, cauterization of bleeding tissue, tamponade of bleeding esophageal varices, photodynamic therapy to esophageal malignancies, drainage of pancreatic pseudocyst, dilation or stenting of a stricture, placement of a percutaneous gastrostomy feeding tube

Operative Procedure

Local anesthetics are given to numb the back of the throat. A mouth piece is inserted between the upper and lower teeth to prevent the patient from biting down on the scope. Lowering the chin down toward the sternum can aid the physician in passing the scope through the oropharynx. If passage is still difficult, thrusting the jaw forward can help. The lighted flexible endoscope is passed through the esophagus; biopsies can be done.

If a gastrostomy feeding tube (PEG tube) is to be placed, see Chapter 16, Abdominal and Gastrointestinal Procedures, for more information.

Anesthetic

Conscious sedation is typically performed to provide amnesia and to decrease patient movement. A propofol drip, Versed (midazolam), ketamine, and a narcotic IV can all be used.

If general anesthetic is given and the patient requires intubation, a reinforced ETT may be used to prevent endotracheal compression as the endoscope is passed into the esophagus.

Positioning

The patient is placed in a left lateral position, with the head of the bed elevated 30–45 degrees. This position may need to be changed during the procedure. Position the patient so that his or her shoulders are at the break of the table so that the head can be flexed or extended for surgical access.

Anesthetic Implications

Minimal monitoring includes pulse oximetry, EKG, and blood pressure, readings should be measured and recorded at least every 5 minutes during the procedure. Oxygen is given via nasal cannula. CO_2 monitoring is a helpful adjunct, accomplished by placing the CO_2 sample line within the proximity of the nasal cannula.

Patients must be NPO for 8 hours for solids and 4 hours for liquids before the procedure. A bowel prep is not needed.

ESOPHAGOSCOPY: UPPER GASTROINTESTINAL ENDOSCOPY

Esophagogastroduodenoscopy is really the same procedure as esophagoscopy or gastroscopy and includes evaluation of the entire upper gastrointestinal (UGI) tract. It is unusual to look just at the esophagus (as described here for esophagoscopy), because complete evaluation of the esophagus needs to include the retroflexed view of the gastric fundus/gastroesophageal junction (GEJ) performed within the stomach.

Esophagoscopy is a diagnostic endoscopic procedure that uses a lighted, flexible endoscopic tube to transmit images of the fiberoptic examination of the esophagus and the stomach onto a video screen.

This procedure is used to assess upper GI bleeding and dyspepsia; monitor or diagnose gastroesophageal reflux disease (GERD) and Barrett's esophagus; investigate the cause of difficult or painful swallowing; perform esophageal varices sclerotherapy; inject epinephrine in bleeding lesions; biopsy polyps or any other abnormal tissue; remove foreign bodies, cauterize bleeding tissue, tamponade bleeding esophageal varices; deliver photodynamic therapy for esophageal malignancies; dilate or stent a stricture; and assist in the placement of a percutaneous gastrostomy feeding tube.

An EGD or upper GI endoscopy can also be used to perform procedures that tighten the lower esophageal sphincter (LES) by placing sutures around the lower esophagus or by injecting substances around the LES to limit reflux.

Operative Procedure

After spraying local anesthesia into the throat, a bite guard is inserted between the upper and lower teeth to prevent the patient from biting down on the scope. The fiberoptic scope is advanced down the patient's throat to examine the esophagus and upper stomach. Injections, tissue cauterization, and biopsies can be done at this time.

Anesthetic

Sedation is used to provide amnesia and to decrease movement. Midazolam and propofol are commonly given together. Fentanyl can be added, although it may cause more respiratory depression.

If general anesthesia is given and the patient requires intubation, a reinforced ETT may be used to prevent endotracheal compression as the endoscope is passed into the esophagus.

Positioning

The patient is placed in a left lateral position, with the head of the bed elevated 30 degrees. This position may need to be changed during the procedure. Position the patient so that his or her shoulders are at the break of the table so that the head can be flexed or extended for surgical access.

Anesthetic Implications

A jaw-thrust maneuver may be needed to assist passage of the scope into the esophagus.

Lidocaine 1 mg/kg IV may be given to decrease airway reactivity. The anesthetist can also give Robinul 0.1–0.2 mg IV to decrease airway secretions.

Minimal monitoring includes pulse oximetry, EKG, and blood pressure, readings should be measured and recorded at least every 5 minutes during the procedure. Oxygen is given via nasal cannula. CO_2 monitoring is a helpful adjunct, accomplished by placing the CO_2 sample line within the proximity of the nasal cannula.

Patients must be NPO for 8 hours for solids and 4 hours for liquids before the procedure. A bowel prep is not needed.

Complications

Potential complications from this procedure include esophageal or stomach perforation, which can lead to pneumothorax and/or hemorrhage.

GASTROSCOPY

Gastroscopy is a diagnostic endoscopic procedure that uses a lighted, flexible endoscopic tube to transmit images of the stomach to a video screen. It is performed to assess upper GI bleeding and dyspepsia, inject epinephrine in bleeding lesions, biopsy polyps or any other abnormal tissue, remove foreign bodies, cauterize bleeding tissue, and assist in the placement of a percutaneous gastrostomy feeding tube.

Operative Procedure

A mouth piece is inserted between the upper and lower teeth to prevent the patient from biting down on the scope. The fiberoptic scope is advanced down the patient's throat to examine the stomach. Injections, tissue cauterization, and biopsies can be done at this time.

Anesthetic

Sedation is used to provide amnesia and to decrease movement. Midazolam and propofol are commonly given together. Fentanyl can be added, although it may cause more respiratory depression.

Positioning

The patient is placed in a left lateral or supine position. This position may need to be changed during the procedure. Position the patient so that his or her shoulders are at the break of the table so that the head can be flexed or extended for surgical access.

Anesthetic Implications

Minimal monitoring includes pulse oximetry, EKG, and blood pressure, readings should be measured and recorded at least every 5 minutes during the procedure. Oxygen is given via nasal cannula. CO_2 monitoring is a helpful adjunct, accomplished by placing the CO_2 sample line within the proximity of the nasal cannula.

Patients must be NPO for 8 hours for solids and 4 hours for liquids before the procedure. A bowel prep is not needed.

Complications

Potential complications of gastroscopy include puncture of the esophagus and stomach, as well as bleeding, especially if this procedure is done with a rigid scope.

SIGMOIDOSCOPY

Sigmoidoscopy is a diagnostic endoscopic procedure that uses a lighted, flexible fiberoptic endoscopic tube to transmit images of the sigmoid colon (the rectum through the most distal part of the descending colon) to a video screen. It allows for examination of the sigmoid colon only.

This procedure is used to evaluate patients with colitis, diarrhea, constipation, abdominal pain, or early signs of cancer. Polyps can be removed during the examination.

Operative Procedure

Sigmoidoscopy can be done using either a flexible or rigid sigmoidoscope, although the flexible scope procedure is often preferred. The scope is inserted and the sigmoid colon is inspected; biopsies may also be taken.

Anesthetic

Sedation is used to provide amnesia and to decrease movement. Midazolam and propofol are commonly given together.

Positioning

The patient is placed in a left lateral position; the same position is generally used for both flexible and rigid scope procedures. This position may need to be changed during the procedure.

Anesthetic Implications

Minimal monitoring includes pulse oximetry, EKG, and blood pressure, readings should be measured and recorded at least every 5 minutes during the procedure. Oxygen is given via nasal cannula. CO_2 monitoring is a helpful adjunct, accomplished by placing the CO_2 sample line within the proximity of the nasal cannula.

These patients are NPO for 12 hours and have taken a bowel prep. Thus they are likely to present with dehydration and may manifest hypovolemia.

Complications

Potential complications of sigmoidoscopy include puncture of the colon and bleeding.

SMALL BOWEL ENTEROSCOPY

Small bowel enteroscopy is a diagnostic endoscopic procedure that uses a lighted, flexible endoscopic tube to transmit images of the small intestine onto a video screen. It is used to check for bleeding ulcers, inflammation, infection or disease, and anemia along with normal colonoscopy and gastroscopy. Also, this procedure may be performed to check for amyloidosis, celiac disease, Crohn's disease, vitamin B_{12} deficiency, infectious gastroenteritis, lymphoma, tropical sprue, lactose intolerance, and unexplained diarrhea and/or gastrointestinal bleeding.

Operative Procedure

A mouth piece is inserted between the upper and lower teeth to prevent the patient from biting down on the scope. The endoscope is then advanced.

A pediatric or adult colonoscope or a "push" enteroscope can be used to access the small intestine through the anus. Most often, the small bowel abnormalities can be reached with a standard endoscope, however, a longer instrument, called an enteroscope, can reach farther into the small intestine. The enteroscope—a flexible tube with *one* balloon—is advanced through the large intestine to the small intestine. As with a colonoscopy, the scope is advanced as far as it can go initially, then slowly withdrawn to allow for complete examination of the walls of the small intestine. An enteroscope/endoscope allows the physician to treat any cause of bleeding and biopsies can be done.

In a double-balloon enteroscopy, *two* balloons attached to the endoscope can be alternately inflated and deflated. This process creates a temporary anchor to pull the endoscope forward (caterpillar-type action) to allow the physician to view the entire small bowel.

Several major difficulties can be encountered when attempting an enteroscopic procedure of the small intestine. This organ is in constant movement (peristalsis), the small intestine is much more mobile than the colon. Adding to the difficulty is the fact that the small intestine is 17 feet long, making it more difficult to reach and posing more difficulty in pinpointing the exact locations of abnormalities for further study or surgical resection. Tattoos can be placed if abnormal anatomy is located; finding the tattoo is easier than trying to find the lesion itself.

Capsule endoscopy is an outpatient procedure that requires no sedation. It is a diagnostic procedure only—no therapeutic actions can be taken during this type of endoscopy. This procedure involves a 1–1/8-inch long × 3/8-inch wide capsule (vitamin-sized) with a 6-hour battery lifespan that contains a light source, a tiny wireless endoscopic camera, and a small transmitter. After the patient swallows this "large pill," the capsule takes thousands of pictures as it moves through the digestive tract. These images are transmitted to a receiver worn by the patient. The capsule passes through the colon and is eventually eliminated. At that point, the patient returns the receiver to the gastroenterologist, who can review the images in detail, looking for abnormalities or areas of bleeding. Research has found this capsule to be better than routine endoscopy or small bowel X-rays for locating abnormalities or the source of bleeding.

Whether diagnosed by routine endoscopy, enteroscopy, or capsule endoscopy, once the cause of small bowel bleeding is determined, the treatment is planned. In cases of arteriovenous malformations (AVM), a small amount of electric current can be delivered through an endoscope to destroy the abnormality. If the AVM is discovered during endoscopy, the treatment can be applied immediately without requiring further diagnostic testing. If found with the capsule, the options include a repeat endoscopy or an enteroscopy if the AVMs are within reach, or surgical assistance as described earlier to help reach the site. Polyps can be removed with an endoscope. Cancers require

surgical removal. Other causes of small bowel bleeding (e.g., Crohn's disease) can be treated medically or surgically.

Anesthetic
Conscious sedation is usually done (no sedation required for "capsule" endoscopy). A propofol drip, Versed (midazolam), ketamine, and a narcotic can all be used. Small bowel enteroscopy may also be done under general anesthesia.

Positioning
The patient is placed in a left lateral position, with the head of the bed elevated 30–45 degrees. This position may need to be changed during the procedure.

Anesthetic Implications
Minimal monitoring includes pulse oximetry, EKG, and blood pressure, readings should be measured and recorded at least every 5 minutes during the procedure. Oxygen is given via nasal cannula. CO_2 monitoring is a helpful adjunct, accomplished by placing the CO_2 sample line within the proximity of the nasal cannula.

This procedure can be quite long in duration. As a consequence, keeping the patient warm is a concern.

Patients should not eat any solid foods or milk products after midnight prior to the procedure, but may have clear liquids until 4 hours before the exam. Some physicians still require NPO after midnight. Thus, they are likely to be dehydrated.

If push enteroscopy is done through the anus, the physician may request metoclopramide IV to increase peristalsis in the intestine as the enteroscope is withdrawn.

Complications
Potential complications from a small bowel enteroscopy include excessive bleeding from the biopsy site, bowel perforation, infection, and aspiration pneumonia.

Liver, Biliary Tract, Gallbladder, Pancreas, and Spleen Surgery

LIVER SURGERY PEARLS

- The liver has four lobes, which make up eight surgical zones.
- Normal portal vein pressure is 5–10 mm Hg. A pressure greater than 10 mm Hg is considered portal hypertension.
- Temperature loss is common with an open abdominal or thoracic procedures. Upper- and lower-body warming blankets are needed as well as fluid warmers. The ambient temperature in the room may also need to be increased.

FUNCTIONS OF THE LIVER

- Blood reservoir
- Formation of lymph
- Filtration of bacteria, old RBCs, hormones, and toxins
- Synthesis of amino acids, alpha and beta globulins, and all plasma proteins
  - Albumin: 10–15 g produced per day; normal level is 3.5–5.5 g/dL; half-life is 14–21 days; makes up 70% of oncotic pressure.
- Synthesis of blood-clotting Factors I, II, V, VII, IX, and X, prothrombin, fibrinogen; not F8 and gamma globulin.
  - Prothrombin time (PT) does not become abnormal until more than 80% of liver synthetic capacity is lost
  - Vitamin K needed to make Factors II, VII, IX, and X (and protein C and S)
- Secretion of bilirubin, cholesterol, electrolytes, lipoproteins, and phospholipids
- Production of bile salts (emulsification and absorption of fats)
  - Released by parenchymal cells of liver → hepatic ducts → cystic duct → gallbladder for storage.
  - Upon stimulation, the gallbladder secretes bile into the duodenum.
  - Bile salts must be present in the small bowel for fat-soluble vitamins to be absorbed.
- Vitamin storage: fat-soluble vitamins (A, D, E, K) and water-soluble vitamins (B_{12} and folate)

- Drug metabolism (CYP 450 system)
- Metabolism of products of carbohydrates, fat, and protein
- Production of pseudocholinesterase (plasma cholinesterase)
    - Half-life: 8–16 hours
    - Function is to hydrolyze exogenous esters (for example, metabolizes local anesthetics and succinylcholine). May be decreased in chronic liver disease and cause longer half-life of succinylcholine; normally, succinylcholine is rapidly metabolized by plasma cholinesterase into succinylmonocholine
- Conversion of ammonium (NH_4) into urea (picked up in large intestine); NH_4 is transported to the liver to be detoxified
- Detoxification of drugs, hormones, and toxic substances
- Conversion of glucose into glycogen (glycogenesis); storage and breakdown of glycogen as needed
    - Enhanced by insulin. The liver can store 75 g glycogen; stores are depleted with starvation within 24–48 hours.

- Glycogenolysis: breakdown of glycogen (enhanced by epinephrine and glucagon)
- Glycolysis: breakdown of glucose into carbon dioxide and water
- Gluconeogenesis: conversion of non-glucose molecules (i.e., amino acids) into glucose

    Inhibited by insulin

    Enhanced by glucocorticoids, catecholamines, and glucagon

- Deamination of amino acids for glucose availability (see gluconeogenesis)
- Formation of ketone bodies and acetate from fatty acids
- Hormone synthesis: T_3 and T_4

SPHINCTER OF ODDI

Spasm of the sphincter of Oddi may be caused by the following agents (listed in order of causing most to least spasm): fentanyl > morphine > Demerol. To treat sphincter of Oddi spasm, give glucagon, Narcan, nitroglycerin, nifedipine, or atropine.

LIVER BLOOD FLOW

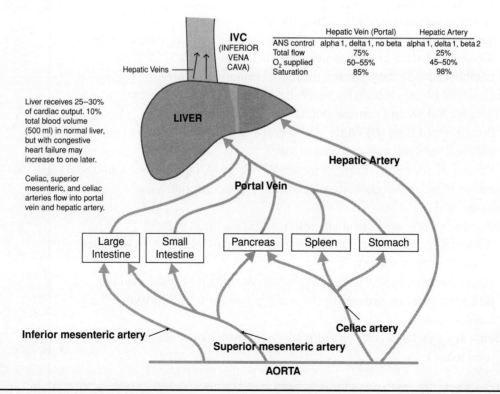

Figure 18-1   *Blood Flow to the Liver*

LIVER DISEASE

Patients with liver disease are often *hyperdynamic,* with increased cardiac outputs and decreased systemic vascular resistance; they have increased blood volumes and anemia. They may experience decreased albumin concentrations (increasing free drug levels in plasma) and increased volume of distribution. In addition, these patients can be very sensitive to sedation. Hypotension and low cardiac output states should be avoided in all individuals with liver disease.

Patients with liver disease can have *affected pulmonary function.* Consequently, they may present with respiratory alkalosis occurring secondary to hyperventilation, chronic hypoxia as a result of shunting and ventilation–perfusion ratio (V/Q) mismatch, a decreased functional residual capacity (FRC), and pleural effusions.

Patients with cirrhosis also have a decreased responsiveness to exogenous cardiovascular stimulants.

Portal hypertension is defined as increased blood pressure in the veins of the abdominal organs. The primary vein of the liver is the portal vein. If this vein develops clots or scar tissue, the blood pressure in the vein increases and portal hypertension develops. Consequently, the blood that normally drains into the liver from the abdominal organs begins to back up. This build-up of blood causes the typical symptoms of portal hypertension, including ascites, hypersplenism, gastrointestinal bleeding, hemorrhoids, and esophageal varices.

Considerations in patients with liver disease include altered metabolism of drugs, vasodilatation, potential for encephalopathy with dehydration, bleeding tendency, and large fluid shifts during surgery. Such patients are also prone to hypoglycemia. In all such cases, healthcare providers must look for concurrent disease states.

ANESTHETICS IN PATIENTS WITH LIVER DISEASE OR DURING HEPATIC SURGERY

All anesthetics potentially decrease hepatocellular function by decreasing portal flow and inhibiting hepatic arterial buffer response.

- Volatile agents: careful titration is needed to keep cardiac output up.
- Isoflurane, sevoflurane, desflurane, and nitrous oxide: either increase hepatic blood flow or do not affect it.
- Halothane and enflurane: decrease hepatic blood flow. Halothane can cause hepatotoxicity and necrosis of the liver.
- Induction agents: Propofol, thiopental and etomidate can decrease hepatic blood flow somewhat. Ketamine is metabolized by the liver's CYP 450 system.
- Vecuronium and rocuronium: metabolized by the liver and have prolonged excretion in patients with cirrhosis.
- Pancuronium, pipecurium, and doxacurium: excreted through the biliary system.
- Atracurium and cisatricurium: undergo Hoffman elimination and can be used in patients with liver disease.
- Succinylcholine: metabolized by plasma cholinesterase, whose levels may be decreased in liver disease. This agent should be used only in very-long-duration surgery.
- Fentanyl: undergoes microsomal hepatic metabolism and can be used in liver surgery cases.
- Remifentanil: metabolized by pseudocholinesterase and can be used in liver surgery cases.
- Anticholinesterase drugs: are only partially metabolized by the liver.

ANESTHETIC CONSIDERATIONS IN PATIENTS WITH LIVER DISEASE OR DURING HEPATIC SURGERY

Rapid-sequence induction is needed, with cricoid pressure applied, when patients have increased abdominal pressure. Use maximum preoperative precautions (i.e., Reglan, sodium citrate).

Maintain blood pressure and cardiac output, and avoid hypotension. Avoid the use of alpha agonists and any vasoconstrictors. Keep the patient's FiO_2 up to maintain the oxygen supply to the hepatocytes and keep the HCT greater than 30%.

Avoid hypovolemia. To do so, perfusion pressure should be adequate.

Preoperative lab results and studies are especially important in patients with liver disease and in patients undergoing hepatic surgery. Check CBC with platelets, electrolytes, liver function tests (ALT, AST, total and indirect bilirubin, LDH), ammonia, albumin, serum protein, lactate, BUN and creatinine, blood glucose, and coagulation studies including PT/INR/PTT. A 12-lead EKG, chest X-ray, pulmonary function tests, and ABGs may also be needed.

VIRAL HEPATITIS

Hepatitis A

Hepatitis A spreads very easily in crowded, unsanitary conditions. It is most contagious 10–14 days before signs and symptoms appear and during the first week after signs and symptoms become manifest. Symptoms include fever, malaise, anorexia, dark urine, and jaundice.

The incubation period for hepatitis A is 15 to 45 days. If antibodies develop, cannot get this infection again.

Transmission
- Fecal–oral route
- Milk, water, or shellfish in infected water
- Sexual activity, oral–anal contact

Hepatitis B

Hepatitis B has an incubation period of 6 to 26 weeks. Groups at increased risk of developing this infection include healthcare workers and sexually active persons (heterosexual, homosexual, or bisexual). Transmission occurs through blood and other bodily fluids (e.g., saliva, semen). If a pregnant woman becomes infected in her third trimester, the infection may be passed to her baby.

Hepatitis C

Most cases of hepatitis C occur following transfusion of blood products. Manifestations of this disease include nausea/vomiting, headache, cough, low-grade fever, right upper quadrant pain, and a weight loss of 2–4 kg. These signs and symptoms occur in three stages:

- *Prodromal:* begins 2 weeks after exposure and ends when signs and symptoms start to show. The person feels terrible, but does not know why.
- *Icteric:* start of jaundice. In the acute phase, the infected individual has abdominal pain and fatigue. The liver is enlarged and tender, and hepatocellular damage occurs.
- *Recovery:* fewer signs and symptoms. The liver is still enlarged, but the person begins to have resolution of the jaundice.

HEPATIC SURGERY

Hepatic Resection

Surgical resection of a portion of the liver may range from a small wedge biopsy to lobe resection. Hepatic resection is indicated for trauma; cysts; tumors—either benign (hemangioma) or primary or malignant tumors; chronic, active hepatitis B or C; or cirrhosis. Note that the majority of liver metastases come from the colon.

Operative Procedure

The incision site is determined by the section of liver to be resected. Often, a right subcostal incision is made, though it may be extended to a left subcostal incision. Most hepatic resections can be performed by a trans-abdominal approach, but some need to be done by a thoraco-abdominal approach. An argon beam laser coagulator may be used, especially during a thoraco-abdominal approach.

Anesthetic

General anesthesia is given with insertion of an oral endotracheal tube (OETT); muscle relaxants are required. A rapid-sequence induction is usually done as these patients often have increased abdominal pressure. An epidural may be placed for postoperative pain control.

These patients may need to remain intubated for 24 hours.

Positioning

The patient is placed in a supine position for a trans-abdominal approach. For major resection, the approach is thoraco-abdominal and the patient is placed in a modified lateral position, right side up.

Preoperative Measures

Check the patient's hematocrit, electrolytes, platelets, BUN and creatinine, blood glucose, and PT/INR/PTT. A chest X-ray may also be needed.

The patient's blood should be typed and cross-matched prior to the procedure, blood units may need to be available in the operating room at the start of the case.

Monitors and IV Access

- Multiple, large peripheral IV lines
- Arterial line
- Central venous catheter usually needed
- Pulmonary artery catheter may be needed, depending on the patient condition and history

IV Fluids and Volume Requirements

The isotonic IV fluid 0.9% normal saline is preferred rather than lactated Ringer's solution: Patients with liver disease are not able to metabolize the lactate ion.

Anesthetic Implications

This surgery has the potential for a large amount of blood loss. Cell-saver technology may be used. A rapid infusion system (RIS) should be available in case of large blood loss and the need for massive blood product transfusions.

Coagulopathy is common in such cases. Replace the blood loss and/or treat coagulopathy with blood products early on.

A nasogastric tube should be placed after induction of anesthesia.

Pulmonary insufficiency is a common comorbidity with liver disease.

Transjugular Intrahepatic Porto-systemic Shunt

In a transjugular intrahepatic porto-systemic shunt (TIPS), a tunnel is made through the liver to connect the portal vein to one of the hepatic veins; a stent is placed in this tunnel to maintain patency.

The portal vein is a large vein that carries blood from the digestive organs to the liver. The three hepatic veins carry blood away from the liver back to the heart. The TIPS procedure decreases portal venous pressure and decreases the formation of ascites; it is intended to produce the same physiologic result as open porto-systemic shunt abdominal surgery.

The TIPS procedure is indicated for patients who have liver disease with portal hypertension and porto-systemic varices (multiple sites are possible, but are most often gastroesophageal) and ascites. These conditions emerge as pressure from the liver radiates up through the inferior vena cava, increasing filling pressures and cardiac output. Gastroesophageal varices rupture can cause massive hemorrhage.

Operative Procedure

The TIPS procedure is done by percutaneous approach through the jugular vein. It involves the surgical creation of a new connection between the hepatic and portal veins along with the placement of one or more expandable metal stents in the intrahepatic tract to maintain patency of this vessel (or vessels).

This procedure can be done by interventional radiology.

Anesthetic

General anesthesia may be given with insertion of an OETT; rapid-sequence induction may be needed. Use of a local anesthetic at the jugular insertion site, along with IV sedation, may be appropriate for very-short-duration cases in some patients.

Positioning
The patient is placed in a supine position.

Anesthetic Implications
Type and cross-match the patients for 4 units of packed cells; keep 2 units ahead.

The TIPS procedure is a radiologic-assisted procedure.

Complications
Potential complications of the TIPS procedure include portal vein rupture, perforation of the liver capsule, complete heart block, and congestive heart failure.

LIVER TRANSPLANTATION

Liver Transplant Recipient: Cadaveric and Live Donor (Orthotopic)

A diseased liver may be replaced with a healthy liver from either a cadaveric donor or a living donor. In case of an adult donor to a very small adult patient or child, the recipient gets the left lobe of the liver (i.e., the smaller lobe); in the case of an adult donor to an adult patient, the recipient gets the right lobe of the liver.

Liver transplant is performed in case of end-stage liver disease, acute liver failure, or any irreversible liver dysfunction. These patients may have portal hypertension, esophageal varices, splenomegaly, ascites, hepatic encephalopathy, jaundice, chronic hepatitis B and/or C, severe coagulopathy, sclerosing cholangitis, biliary atresia, biliary cirrhosis, and hepatorenal syndrome (hepatic dysfunction causes decreased blood flow to the kidneys causing renal failure). HIV status is no longer an absolute contraindication to hepatic transplantation.

Operative Procedure
A large bilateral subcostal is one type of incision made in the upper abdomen. There are three stages to liver transplantation.

Preanhepatic Stage
This stage involves mobilization of the native liver to prepare for its removal. The diseased liver is divided away from the supporting ligaments, as well as the common bile duct, the hepatic artery and vein, and the portal vein. This can be a long, tedious process, and significant blood loss can occur during this stage. Issues to be considered by the surgical team include bleeding due to decreased clotting factors, decreased and sequestered platelets in the spleen; metabolic acidosis; and fibrinolysis. Issues for anesthesia include keeping the patient warm; volume status; lines placed; and the potential need for placement of bypass cannulas. Colloids and fresh frozen plasma may be given as indicated to minimize the decrease in preload when the liver vessels and the inferior vena cava (IVC) are cross-clamped.

The complete cross-clamping of the IVC is usually not tolerated due to the sudden decrease in venous return and cardiac output and venous engorgement proximal to the clamp. Thus, before the vena cava is clamped, extracorporeal venovenous bypass (VVB) cannulas may be placed. This bypass of blood from the lower to the upper part of the body is used to improve hemodynamic stability and reduce bleeding from the engorged portal system. VVB can improve hemodynamics, delay the onset of metabolic acidosis, decrease blood loss, and preserve renal function. However, it can also cause air embolism or thromboembolism—complications that can be fatal.

VVB cannulas are placed in the common iliac vein and the portal vein. The common iliac vein cannula drains blood coming from the lower extremities, whereas the transected portal vein cannula drains blood coming from the viscera. These cannulas are joined at a Y-junction, and blood is drained to centrifugal pump. The blood is returned to the body through a central venous cannula to the axillary vein or jugular vein (Figure 18-2). No additional heparin is added, other than what is already in bypass system.

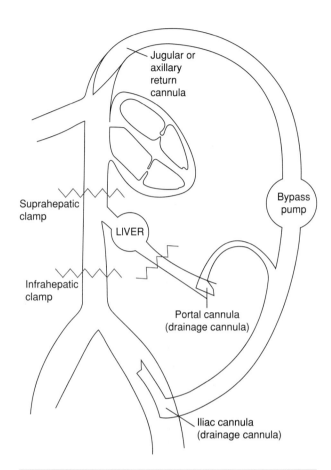

Figure 18-2   *Veno-Venous Bypass*

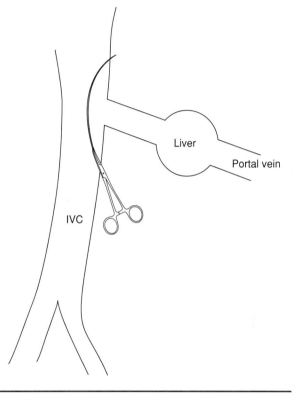

Figure 18-3   *Piggyback Modification*

In a "piggyback" modification (Figure 18-3), the donor's vena cava is left in situ. This approach has the advantage that the venous return is not compromised during the anhepatic phase and, therefore, bypass is not needed.

With or without veno-venous bypass, the suprahepatic and infrahepatic portions of the IVC are both clamped and transected. This action decreases the venous return to the heart from the portal vein and inferior vena cava.

Anhepatic Stage
Occlusion of the portal vein marks the onset of the anhepatic phase, in which the native liver is removed. Implantation of the donor graft proceeds with anastomosis of the suprahepatic and the infrahepatic vena cava before anastomosing the hepatic artery.

To prepare the patient for reperfusion, give steroids (methylprednisolone), calcium chloride, and sodium bicarbonate IV, and ventilate the patient with 100% FiO_2. Have atropine, epinephrine, defibrillator, and a rapid infusion system available before reperfusion begins. The patient should have adequate intravascular filling volumes before flushing the portal vein.

Revascularization/Reperfusion (Postanhepatic) Stage
The postanhepatic stage begins when the portal vein and hepatic artery are unclamped and ends when the surgery is completed. The liver is flushed with blood and the vena cava clamps are removed. After stabilizing the patient, reconstruction of the hepatic artery ensues: All blood vessels are anastomosed, restoring blood flow; hemostasis is achieved. Maintain a mean blood pressure of

70 mm Hg to prevent hepatic artery thrombosis. *The blood pressure should not be too high, as hypertension can cause bleeding.*

The donor and recipient's common bile duct (CBD) is anastomosed in an end-to-end fashion or the CBD is anastomosed to the jejunal portion of the small intestine during biliary reconstruction. The gallbladder is also removed.

Bypass is discontinued and the abdomen is closed.

Reperfusion Syndrome

Reperfusion of the donor liver, during which the portal vein is flushed, can be the most critical stage of the transplant process. During this phase, the ischemic metabolic by-products of a non-perfused liver and preservative fluid (including cytokines, cold-temperature products, and products of ischemic metabolism) are flushed out into the recipient's bloodstream. The result may be volume overload, hemodynamic instability, severe systemic hypotension, bradycardia, increased peak inspiratory pressures, supraventricular and ventricular arrhythmias, decreased cardiac output and systemic vascular resistance, pulmonary emboli (of either clot or air), profuse bleeding, pulmonary edema, coagulopathy, and pulmonary hypertension with right ventricular failure. Occasionally, complete cardiac arrest can occur. There is often extreme cardiac demand during this time, so it is important to monitor the patient for ST-segment changes and arrhythmias. Give the patient a bolus of ephedrine (a sympathomimetic) or epinephrine, if needed, to maintain MAP and stabilize hemodynamics.

Hyperkalemia occurs on reperfusion, so the anesthetist should keep the patient's potassium level below 4.0 mEq/L before beginning reperfusion. Elevated potassium levels after reperfusion usually return to normal levels within 10–20 minutes. Calcium chloride and sodium bicarbonate are the drugs of choice for the acute treatment of hyperkalemia.

Hypocalcemia can lead to profound myocardial depression. Even so, *hypercalcemia* should be avoided, as intracellular calcium overload can cause harm to the transplanted liver.

Fibrinolysis usually reaches its most severe level after reperfusion, driven by abrupt increases in tissue plasminogen activator levels as this product is released from the graft endothelial cells. Antifibrinolytic (Amicar) and cryoprecipitate (contains fibrinogen, von Willebrand factor, Factor VIII, fibrin, and Factor XIII) may be required to counteract this fibrinolysis. Reperfusion coagulopathy can also occur from diffuse activation of the clotting cascade; platelets may also need to be given.

Anesthetic

General anesthesia is given with insertion of an OETT; muscle relaxants required. These patients are usually considered emergency cases, except with living-related donors. As such, rapid-sequence induction is appropriate.

Give 100% FiO_2 before induction. Note that these patients are often hypoxic, with a decreased FRC.

Positioning

The patient is placed in a supine position, with bilateral arms tucked at the sides.

Anesthetic Implications

Type and cross-match the patient's blood; 2–4 units of cross-matched blood and FFP should be available in the operating room. These patients are very coagulopathic (with decreased levels of clotting factors and vitamin K deficiency), and they typically lose large amounts of blood during this operation. A prolonged prothrombin time (PT) correlates with the severity of the disease. Accurate determination of blood loss is next to impossible. Instead, intravascular volume is assessed by an increase in heart rate with a decrease in blood pressure, central venous pressure, and urinary output.

Liver transplantation is usually a very long surgery (6–12 hours). During this procedure, patients lose heat through massive fluid replacement and transfusion of blood products, delivered through the extracorporeal circuit, and the placement of a cold donor liver into the abdominal cavity. Keep these patients warm by decreasing fresh gas flow on the ventilator, increasing the room temperature, and using warming blankets (over the upper chest/head and the lower extremities) and fluid warmers.

Post-transplant liver function will vary depending on the ischemic time—that is, the length of time between clamping and removal of the liver from the donor to the time of vascular anastomosis in the recipient).

Immunosuppressants are an essential part of preventing rejection of the donor kidney.

A nasogastric tube should be placed after induction of anesthesia.

Anesthesia Goals for the Liver Transplant Recipient

Maintaining an adequate perfusion pressure is important during these cases. Keep the intravascular volume up and the urine output high.

Strict aseptic precautions are needed with IV insertion, invasive monitoring, drug administration, airway management, and blood sampling.

Preoperative Labs and Tests

Check preoperative lab results carefully.

Comorbidities

Patients with end-stage liver disease have dysfunction to virtually every other organ system. In particular, they may have ascites, peripheral edema, and portal hypertension with splenomegaly. The following comorbidities are also possible:

- *Heart:* Patients may be in a hyperdynamic state characterized by increased cardiac output and low systemic vascular resistance (SVR); they may also have cardiomyopathy. Monitor these patients carefully for arrhythmias.

- *Neurologic:* As many as 80% of acute liver failure patients have cerebral edema and an increased intracranial pressure with cerebral encephalopathy.
- *Renal:* Patients may have "hepatorenal syndrome," which leads to hypoperfusion of the kidney with increased BUN and creatinine levels. This syndrome is caused by renal vasoconstriction.
- *Pulmonary:* The pulmonary status of these patients is usually affected by their liver disease; for example, they may exhibit pulmonary hypertension, ventilation–perfusion mismatching, atelectasis, and pleural effusions. Patients may have received a prostaglandin infusion to treat the pulmonary hypertension when coming to the OR. Another condition associated with liver disease is hepato-pulmonary syndrome, a type of oxygen-resistance hypoxemia. These patients will often need to remain intubated postoperatively to ensure that their oxygen levels increase.

Intraoperative Labs

Keep potassium levels less than 4.0 mEq/L in anticipation of high potassium influx with reperfusion. A glucose/regular insulin infusion may be necessary to help push potassium back into the cells.

Check labs at least every 30 minutes if the patient is unstable, and every hour if the patient is stable. Check serum levels of potassium, sodium (keep within 10 mEq/L of the normal sodium level), calcium (citrate toxicity is possible with multiple blood transfusions, binding the citrate to the calcium), glucose, lactate, and hematocrit.

In the preanhepatic and anhepatic phases, progressive thrombocytopenia may result from a dilutional process, platelet consumption, or splenic sequestration. In the post-reperfusion phase, fibrinolysis occurs. Alterations in coagulation can be dramatic during liver transplant. For this reason, coagulation studies should be evaluated frequently during this surgery.

Monitors and IV Access

Place an arterial line. Check with the surgeon regarding the plan for veno-venous bypass and the possibility of using the axillary vein; if the axillary vein is to be used for VVB, use the radial artery in the other arm. Usually, patients will have an arterial line in one radial artery and the other in the right femoral artery.

A central line is required.

A pulmonary artery catheter is required. Have a cardiac output pulmonary artery catheter that has REF/EDV/SVO$_2$ continuous monitoring capability, if possible.

Perform TEE monitoring.

Thromboelastogram (TEG) results should be used to guide blood product transfusion.

A rapid infusion system can deliver 500–1500 mL/min of warmed fluid, blood, or blood products through a central line.

Have multiple peripheral and central IV access lines available. Have two dedicated volume lines. Ensure that blood tubing and normal saline lines are hung and connected to the patient before the surgery starts.

IV Vasoactive Agents

- IV pump: phenylephrine; epinephrine; norepinephrine; nitroglycerin; dopamine; dobutamine; amiodarone; lidocaine; and/or isoproterenol (decreases pulmonary vascular resistance)
- Syringe for bolus: ephedrine; esmolol (Brevibloc); calcium chloride; atropine; sodium bicarbonate; heparin; Amicar; tromethamine (THAM: a parenteral systemic alkalizer and fluid replenisher; acts as an osmotic diuretic; to treat acidosis—along with sodium bicarbonate—but does not contain any additional sodium, unlike sodium bicarbonate); vasopressin 0.5–1 mcg (specifically constricts the splanchnic bed, which includes the mesenteric, splenic, and hepatic bed—the first two comprising the

major part of the inflow to the third); does not cause tachycardia
- Other drugs to have available: methylene blue (free-radical scavenger); SoluMedrol 1 g

IV Fluids and Volume Requirements

Colloids and FFP should be given as indicated to minimize the decrease in preload when the liver vessels are clamped.

Do not give lactated Ringer's solution to any patient with liver disease. Instead, give 0.9% normal saline, and watch for the emergence of hyperchloremic metabolic acidosis.

Induction

A "high-low" OETT (made by Mallinckrodt) may need to be placed for postoperative use. This tube contains an added suction port that helps decrease the risk of aspiration.

Consider giving etomidate for induction if the patient is unstable or if the ejection fraction is less than 30%. Thiopental, propofol, and fentanyl can be given as well.

Succinylcholine (Anectine) is avoided in patients with severe liver disease. In such cases, patients' pseudocholinesterase levels are decreased, leading to an increased half-life for this drug.

Narcotics are all metabolized by the liver except remifentanil (which is metabolized by pseudocholinesterase).

Rapid-sequence induction should be used with all liver transplant recipients due to their increased abdominal pressures and delayed gastric emptying.

Intraoperative/Maintenance Measures

Muscle relaxants that do not require liver metabolism should be used: cisatricurium or atricurium. (Rocuronium, vecuronium, pancuronium, pipecuronium, and doxacurium are eliminated through either biliary or hepatic excretion.) Because the abdominal muscles are cut during this surgery, muscle relaxants are given to keep the patient still during this part of the procedure. More muscle relaxation is needed at the end of the case to help with closing the abdominal musculature.

Isoflurane, sevoflurane, or desflurane may be used in liver transplant recipients.

Avoid the use of nitrous oxide to prevent bowel distention. Avoid the use of halothane: 20–45% of this agent is metabolized by the liver and halothane can cause hepatotoxicity. Enflurane decreases hepatic blood flow.

Benzodiazepines and high-dose fentanyl (25–75 mcg/kg) may be used in liver transplant recipients. When muscle relaxants and high-dose narcotics are given, inhaled anesthetics can be run at half-MAC.

Avoid direct-acting vasopressors (i.e., phenylephrine) in organ transplants.

Patients with liver disease will have an altered response to drugs due to their increased volume of distribution combined with their decreased ability to metabolize drugs.

Monitor blood glucose levels intraoperatively, keeping tight control over them. An insulin drip may be needed to keep the blood glucose between 80 and 110 mg/dL.

Emergence

The patient will remain intubated and should be transferred to the ICU on full monitors and 100% FiO_2.

Postoperative Measures

Postoperative issues may include bleeding, biliary leaks, vascular thrombosis (hepatic artery or portal vein), and infection. Graft function and rejection are also essential concerns:

- *Immediate rejection* is termed "hyper-acute." In this type of rejection, preformed antibodies are present and microvascular clots and thrombosis develop.
- *Acute rejection* occurs after 5 days post transplant.

Signs of graft function include increased serum ionized calcium (citrate metabolism), correction of acidosis, correction of serum glucose (glycogen release), bile formation, reduced need for hemodynamic support, and metabolism of muscle relaxant.

After either living-related or cadaveric liver transplantation, the patient continues to receive immunosuppressive drugs, which are first administered in the operating room. The initial 48 hours following the transplantation are critical—even if the liver looks healthy immediately following the surgery. Within 24 to 48 hours, the transplant team will know whether the organ is functioning properly.

Hint: Keep IV bags and blood product bags in stacks on a blanket folded on the floor. This practice helps to keep track of fluids and blood products. You can even separate piles according to the IV site where they are infused.

Liver Transplant Donor: Live Donor Liver Transplantation (LDLT)

Live donor liver transplantation (LDLT) is a procedure in which a living person donates a portion of his or her liver to another. In the case of an adult donor to a child (or small adult patient), the recipient gets the left lobe of the liver (the smaller portion). In the case of an adult donor to an adult patient, the recipient gets the (larger) right lobe of the liver.

The donor's surgery takes about 4 hours.

Strict aseptic precautions are needed with IV insertion, invasive monitoring, drug administration, airway management, and blood sampling.

After living-related liver transplantation, the patient continues to receive immunosuppressive drugs, which are first administered in the operating room. The initial 48 hours following the transplantation are critical—even if the liver looks healthy during surgery. Within 24 to 48 hours, the transplant team will know whether the organ is functioning properly.

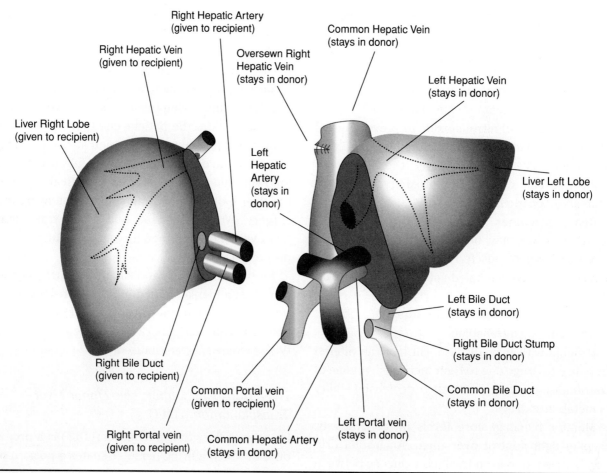

Figure 18-4   *Liver Anatomy Involved in Living Liver Donor*

BILIARY TRACT AND GALLBLADDER SURGERY

Intraoperative Cholangiogram

An intraoperative cholangiogram is performed prior to ligation of a cystic duct. A radiopaque dye is injected through a catheter into the common bile duct (CBD), and the CBD is evaluated for patency and location/size of any stones. X-rays of the gallbladder are done to check for stones and strictures of the biliary tree.

Anesthetic Implications

Preoperatively, check the patient for any allergy to contrast dye.

Open Cholecystectomy

Open cholecystectomy involves the surgical removal of the gallbladder through an abdominal incision. This procedure may be performed to treat chronic or acute cholecystitis, to treat cholelithiasis, or to remove malignancy or polyps. Open cholecystectomy is done (instead of a laparoscopic approach) if the patient has intra-abdominal adhesions, an infection, or complicated medical problems.

Operative Procedure

The gallbladder lies behind the liver. A right subdiaphragmatic incision is made to expose the gallbladder. The liver is carefully retracted upward and the duodenum is retracted downward to expose the biliary structures. The cystic artery and cystic duct are divided and ligated, and the gallbladder is removed.

This procedure is often done laparoscopically (discussed later in this chapter).

Anesthetic

GETA; muscle relaxants are given. A rapid-sequence induction may be needed if the abdomen is distended.

Positioning

The patient is placed in a supine position, with the arms tucked or placed at a shoulder angle less than 90 degrees on padded armboards.

Anesthetic Implications

An orogastric tube should be passed to decompress the stomach.

An intraoperative cholangiogram may be performed to visualize the CBD and to assess its patency—a process that requires fluoroscopy. Clarify whether the patient is allergic to contrast dye preoperatively.

Postoperative narcotics are needed. Check with the surgeon regarding his or her intraoperative narcotic preference given the potential for biliary spasm with the use of narcotics. The open procedure is quite painful, as the incision goes through multiple muscle layers that are strained by respiration; these patients are at high risk for postoperative atelectasis and pneumonia.

Patients requiring cholecystectomy are often dehydrated from vomiting. Intravenous fluids and antiemetics should be given.

Glucagon may be requested by the surgeon; it has a spasmolytic effect in the gastrointestinal system and can relax the sphincter of Oddi. In higher doses, this agent is a positive inotrope and chronotrope, increasing myocardial contractility and heart rate. Glucagon may cause nausea and vomiting, especially when it is given in doses greater than 2 mg.

Laparoscopic Cholecystectomy

Laparoscopic cholecystectomy is the endoscopic excision of the gallbladder. It is performed to treat gallstones and diseases of the gallbladder.

Operative Procedure

An incision is made at the umbilicus, an introducer scope with a camera is inserted, and carbon dioxide is used to insufflate the abdomen. Several other stab incisions are made to create additional ports used for retractors and cautery. The cystic artery and duct are divided and clipped. The fundus and the neck of the gallbladder are freed from the liver bed, placed in a removable bag, and pulled out through one of the larger laparoscopic ports. If the gallbladder is too large to remove through a laparoscopic port, it is removed through a small incision made in the abdomen.

Anesthetic

GETA; muscle relaxants are given. A rapid-sequence induction may be needed if the abdomen is distended.

Positioning

The patient is placed in a supine position, with the arms tucked or placed at a shoulder angle of less than 90 degrees on padded armboards. The patient will be moved from a Trendelenburg position to reverse Trendelenburg position to change internal organ placement to facilitate organ exposure for the surgeon.

Anesthetic Implications

See Chapter 3 for more information on laparoscopy.

An orogastric tube should be passed to decompress the stomach. Antiemetics should be given.

An intraoperative cholangiogram may be performed to visualize the CBD and to assess its patency—a process that requires fluoroscopy. Clarify whether the patient is allergic to contrast dye preoperatively.

Check with the surgeon regarding his or her intraoperative narcotic preference because of the potential for biliary spasm.

Glucagon may be requested by the surgeon; it has a spasmolytic effect in the gastrointestinal system and can relax the sphincter of Oddi. In higher doses, this agent is a positive inotrope and chronotrope, increasing myocardial contractility and heart rate. Glucagon may cause nausea and vomiting, especially when it is given in doses greater than 2 mg.

PANCREAS SURGERY

Pancreatectomy: Partial or Complete

Partial pancreatectomy usually refers to the removal of the distal portion, or tail, of the pancreas. A subtotal pancreatectomy involves resection of the pancreas from the mesenteric vessels distally, leaving the head and uncinate process (the portion of the head of the pancreas that hooks behind the superior mesenteric vessels) intact. If a tumor or mass is restricted to the very distal portion of the pancreas, a very small portion of the head may remain and be attached to the duodenum along with the common bile duct.

Pancreatectomy is performed in cases involving ductal obstruction, pancreatic stones or cysts, trauma, benign or malignant tumors, chronic pancreatitis, and endocrine tumors. In a large majority of pancreatic cancer cases, the cancer consists of a ductal adenocarcinoma, which occurs in the head of the pancreas. Complete surgical resection is the only definitive treatment of ductal pancreatic cancer.

Operative Procedure

The pancreas is dissected away from the mesenteric and portal vessels and removed. These procedures can be quite long—4 to 6 hours in duration.

In a partial pancreatectomy, part of the pancreas, the duodenum, the gallbladder, and part of the bile duct are removed. The tail of the pancreas is joined to a portion of small bowel.

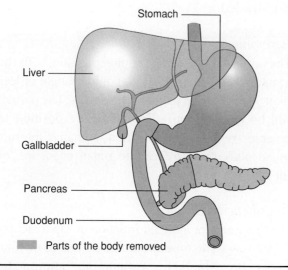

Figure 18-5   *Partial Pancreatectomy: What is Removed*

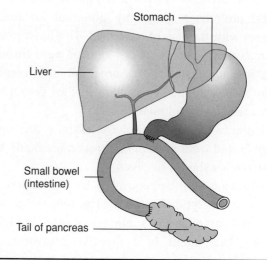

Figure 18-6   *Partial Pancreatectomy: What is Left Behind*

In a total pancreatectomy, the entire pancreas and duodenum, the distal portion of the stomach, the gallbladder, part of the bile duct, the spleen, and the surrounding lymph nodes are removed. The remaining distal portion of the stomach is anastomosed to a portion of the small intestine.

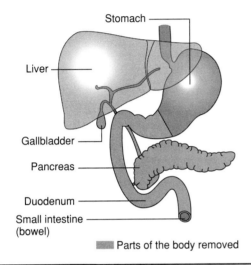

Figure 18-7 *Total Pancreatectomy: What is Removed*

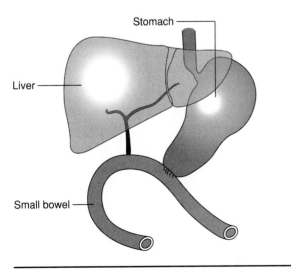

Figure 18-8 *Total Pancreatectomy: What is Left Behind*

Anesthetic

GETA; muscle relaxants are given. A rapid-sequence induction should be used with these patients due to their increased abdominal pressures; such patients may be considered emergency cases. Avoid the use of nitrous oxide to prevent bowel distention. An epidural may be placed for postoperative pain control.

Positioning

The patient is placed in a supine position. Bilateral arms tucked at the sides.

Preoperative Measures

Check the preoperative lab results carefully. Check hematocrit, electrolytes, liver function tests (ALT, AST, total and indirect bilirubin, LDH), albumin, platelets, BUN and creatinine, blood glucose, and PT/INR/PTT. A chest X-ray may also be needed. Severe electrolyte disturbances may be present with pancreatitis.

Anesthetic Implications

Type and cross-match the patient's blood. These patients can lose large amounts of blood during this operation.

Monitor and maintain tight controls on blood glucose levels, using a regular insulin drip or $D_{50}W$.

A nasogastric tube should be placed after induction of anesthesia.

Patients with acute pancreatitis are usually hypotensive and hypovolemic. As such, they require aggressive intravascular volume resuscitation with crystalloid and/or blood products perioperatively. These patients usually experience large third-space fluid shifts.

Keep these patients warm by using warming blankets and fluid warmers.

The pulmonary status of these patients is affected by their pancreatic disease. Pleural effusions, ventilation–perfusion mismatching, and atelectasis may be seen, all of which can progress to respiratory failure.

Pancreaticoduodenectomy (Whipple Procedure)

These procedures involve removal of the head of the pancreas, the entire duodenum, the proximal portion of the jejunum, the distal third of the stomach, the gallbladder and the distal half of the common bile duct. The biliary, pancreatic, and gastrointestinal tracts are reestablished for continuity. Such surgeries are performed to treat either regional malignancy (head of the pancreas), malignant tumors of the common bile duct, traumatic injury to the pancreas, or benign, obstructive, chronic pancreatitis.

Operative Procedure

Through a large midline, abdominal incision, the surgeon dissects down to the retroperitoneum. The pancreas is assessed for resectability. If the mesenteric vessels or the liver is infiltrated with cancer, the Whipple procedure is not done; instead, the patient's incision is simply closed. If the tumor is resectable, the head of the pancreas is mobilized, the common bile duct is transected, and the gall bladder is removed. Once the superior mesenteric vein is freed from the pancreas, it is transected. The jejunum is first transected, and then anastomosed to the distal pancreas, the bile duct, and the stomach. A stent may be placed to maintain congruity of the anastomosis. Drains are placed and the incision is closed.

Anesthetic

GETA; muscle relaxants are given. A rapid-sequence induction should be used with these patients due to their increased abdominal pressures; such patients may be considered emergency cases. Avoid the use of nitrous oxide to prevent bowel distention. An epidural may be placed for postoperative pain control.

Positioning

The patient is placed in a supine position. Bilateral arms are tucked at the sides.

Preoperative Measures

Check the preoperative lab results carefully. Check hematocrit, electrolytes, liver function tests (ALT, AST, total and indirect bilirubin, LDH), albumin, platelets, BUN and creatinine, blood glucose, and PT/INR/PTT. A chest X-ray may also be needed. Severe electrolyte disturbances may be present with pancreatitis. Monitor and maintain tight controls on blood glucose levels, using a regular insulin drip or $D_{50}W$.

Patients with acute pancreatitis are usually hypotensive and hypovolemic (and may have received a bowel prep). As such, they require aggressive intravascular volume resuscitation with crystalloid and/or blood products perioperatively. These patients usually experience large third-space fluid shifts.

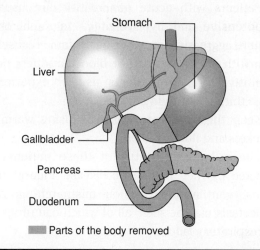

Figure 18-9   *Whipple: What is Removed*

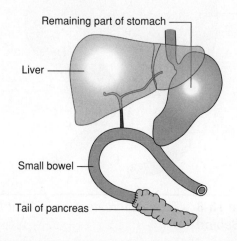

Figure 18-10   *Whipple: What is Left Behind*

Monitors and IV Access

• An arterial line is needed.
• A CVP may also be needed.

Anesthetic Implications

Type and cross-match the patient's blood. These patients can lose large amounts of blood during this operation.

The pulmonary status of these patients is affected by their pancreatic disease. Pleural effusions, ventilation–perfusion mismatching, and atelectasis may be seen, all of which can progress to respiratory failure.

Once the peritoneum is opened, the operability of the findings is assessed.

Keep these patients warm by using upper and lower body warming blankets and fluid warmers.

A nasogastric tube should be placed after induction of anesthesia.

Pancreas Transplantation

In pancreatic transplant, a cadaveric transplantation of a pancreas or a partial pancreas from a living donor is transplanted into a recipient whose pancreas makes no insulin. Recipients of such transplants have end-stage type 1 diabetes with severe end-stage renal disease. Often, both a pancreas and a kidney (from the same donor) are transplanted during the same surgery.

Operative Procedure

A low abdominal incision is made. Because the pancreas is a vital organ, performing functions necessary in the digestion process, the recipient's native pancreas is left in place, and the donated pancreas is attached in a different location. A donor pancreas is grafted to the recipient's iliac vessels, while the pancreatic duct is connected to the bladder.

Anesthetic

General anesthesia is given with insertion of an OETT; muscle relaxants are needed. Avoid the use of phenylephrine with any organ transplant, which is a direct vasoconstrictor.

Monitors and IV Access

• An arterial line is necessary.
• A central line is necessary.
• A pulmonary artery catheter may be warranted as well.

Positioning

The patient is placed in a supine position, with arms tucked at sides.

Anesthetic Implications

Strict aseptic precautions are needed with IV insertion, invasive monitoring, drug administration, airway management, and blood sampling.

Type and cross-match the patient's blood preoperatively.

A nasogastric tube should be placed after induction of anesthesia.

Maintaining an adequate perfusion pressure is important during these cases. Keep the intravascular volume up and the urine output high.

Monitor the patient's blood glucose levels intraoperatively, keeping tight control. An insulin drip may be needed to keep the blood glucose between 80 and 110 mg/dL.

Pancreas function will vary depending on the ischemic time—that is, the length of time between clamping and removal of the pancreas from the donor to the time of vascular anastomosis in the recipient. Once the pancreas vessels are connected in the recipient, a "wash-out" of ischemic by-products and preservative fluid will sweep these elements into the circulation. This shock to the system can cause a sudden hypotension and increased peak inspiratory pressure. Although this side effect is generally short-lived, a bolus of ephedrine (a sympathomimetic) may be needed to maintain the patient's systolic blood pressure.

Immunosuppressants are an essential part of preventing rejection of the donor pancreas.

SPLEEN SURGERY

Open Splenectomy

Splenectomy is the surgical removal of the spleen. The need for removal usually arises due to trauma with uncontrolled bleeding. Other indications for this procedure include hematologic disorders, tumors, cysts, idiopathic thrombocytopenic purpura (ITP), hemolytic anemia, thrombosis of the splenic blood vessels, presence of an accessory spleen, splenomegaly (spleen greater than 20 centimeters longitudinally), and staging of Hodgkin's and non-Hodgkin's disease.

The spleen helps the body fight infection and filters foreign substances from the blood; it also regulates blood flow to the liver and can sequester (store) platelets. *Splenectomy should be avoided due to the body's need for indefinite protection from pneumococcal pneumonia.*

Operative Procedure

A midline or left subcostal incision is made. A thoraco-abdominal approach may be necessary. The splenic artery is ligated and the splenic vein is tied; the ligaments supporting the spleen are detached and the spleen removed. The spleen can be removed in pieces or as a whole.

Laparoscopic removal is possible if the spleen is only slightly larger than normal or of normal size.

Anesthetic

GETA; muscle relaxants are needed. Avoid the use of nitrous oxide to prevent bowel distention. A rapid-sequence induction is usually needed. An epidural catheter may be placed for postoperative pain control.

Positioning

The patient is placed in a supine position. The left side may be bumped up with a blanket or roll under the patient's flank. Surgeon preference may dictate use of the lateral decubitus position.

Anesthetic Implications

A nasogastric tube is usually inserted. The surgeon may help to confirm NGT placement internally; once confirmed, tape the tube securely to the patient's nose.

Large volume blood loss is possible with splenectomy, so the patient's blood should be typed and cross-matched. Cell-saver technology may also be used.

A surgically created pneumothorax is possible if the surgeon punctures through the diaphragm. In such a case, a chest tube may need to be inserted.

Patients with ITP may present with a very low platelet count or platelet dysfunction. Regional anesthesia may be contraindicated in these patients.

Assess and rehydrate these patients before and during surgery with crystalloid solutions and blood products as indicated.

These patients may have received chemotherapy and have multiple systemic difficulties. A thorough preoperative history, laboratory tests, CXR, and EKG may all be needed. Lab tests should include a CBC, electrolytes, PT/PTT/INR, platelet count, BUN and creatinine, and blood glucose.

Monitors and IV Access

- An arterial line may or may not be placed.
- Central line placement is possible.
- Two large-bore peripheral IVs are needed if a central line not placed.

Genitourinary and Renal Surgery

19

GENITOURINARY AND RENAL SURGERY PEARLS

The injectable dyes used in genitourinary (GU) and renal surgery are considered interchangeable. They are mainly used to look for ureteral or bladder injury (iatrogenic).

- *Indigo carmine:* causes a temporary increase in blood pressure and a drop in the pulse oximetry saturation; in rare cases, may provoke an allergic reaction.
- *Methylene blue:* can cause hypotension.

FUNCTIONS OF THE KIDNEY

- Performs acid–base regulation:

  Fluid balance (Approximately 60% of the total weight of an adult is water.)

  pH

  Volume

  Concentration

- Maintains electrolytes. Electrolytes refer to substances such as sodium, potassium, and chloride ions, all of which are found in the blood. Levels of these electrolytes must be maintained within certain limits.

  Aldosterone is secreted by the adrenal gland and is released when the renin reaction is started or there is a change in electrolytes and fluid.

  Parathyroid hormone (PTH) is secreted by the parathyroid gland in response to the body's calcium level. Calcium reabsorption is related to a form of vitamin D made by the kidney. As the kidney function decreases, more calcium is excreted, causing levels of this ion to drop. PTH is then secreted, making the kidneys reabsorb more calcium.

- Regulates blood pressure. By correctly regulating the amount of fluid retained by the body and through the production of certain hormones, the kidneys help to regulate the blood pressure. The kidneys produce a hormone called renin that raises blood pressure. Renin is released when the volume of blood decreases to a dangerous level. The production of renin is also stimulated by a decrease in the sodium content of the blood.

- Carries out erythropoietin production. The kidneys produce another hormone called erythropoietin, which stimulates the bone marrow to produce red blood cells (RBCs; also called erythrocytes). Erythropoietin production is also stimulated by hypoxia (creating more RBCs to carry hemoglobin).
- Regulates vitamin D production.
- Excretes waste products. The kidneys regulate three main toxic end-metabolites:

Urea formed from ammonia and protein metabolism

Creatinine from muscle metabolism

Uric acid from protein metabolism

BASIC ANATOMY OF THE KIDNEYS

Each kidney has two layers: an outer cortical layer (85% of the total organ) and a medullary inner portion (15%). The kidneys are seated between T12 and L3.

Fluid flows through the kidneys at a rate of 1–2 L/min. These organs receive 20–25% of the total cardiac output. In addition, 1.2 million nephrons are located in each kidney.

Commonly Encountered GU/Renal Abbreviations

- CRF: chronic renal failure
- ARF: acute renal failure
- GFR: glomerular filtration rate
- RBF: renal blood flow

DIURETIC AGENTS

DIURETIC	SITE OF ACTION	MECHANISM	EFFECT
Osmotic: mannitol	Proximal tubule, descending loop, collecting duct	Increases osmosis into proximal tubule	Volume expansion and increased GFR
Loop agents: furosemide and Edecrin	Ascending loop of Henle	Decreases reabsorption of sodium chloride	Increased water loss
Thiazides: hydrochlorothiazide	Early segments of thedistal tubule	Decreases reabsorption of sodium chloride	Increased water loss
Potassium-sparing agents: spironolactone	Distal tubule	Inhibits aldosterone	Increased sodium loss and subsequently water; retention of potassium

RENAL DISEASE

- *Pre-renal oliguria:* inefficient perfusion to the kidneys resulting from dehydration or cardiac output problems
- *Renal oliguria:* may occur from pre-renal problems and ultimately results from parenchymal diseases such as acute tubular necrosis
- *Post-renal oliguria:* obstructive problems to urine outflow

Complications of Renal Disease

Metabolic considerations in renal patients:

- Metabolic acidosis: hyperkalemia and acidosis secondary to the inability to excrete acid metabolite
- Diabetes

Hematological considerations in renal patients:

- Anemia: caused by decreased erythropoietin production

- Bleeding: decreased RBC lifespan, increased bleeding times from dysfunctional platelet aggregation (not thrombocytopenia), coagulopathies, decreased Factor III production, and decreased vitamin K dependent factors

GI considerations in renal patients:

- Increased gastric acid and volume production
- Increased nausea and vomiting
- Gastric paresis
- Delayed emptying
- Friable mucous membranes
- GI bleeding

Cardiovascular considerations in renal patients:

- Hypertension: may cause or be the result from increased renin excretion
- Increased cardiac output due to anemia
- Fluid overload
- Advanced coronary artery disease
- Left ventricular hypertrophy
- Ischemic heart disease
- Congestive heart failure (CHF)

Immunological considerations in renal patients:

- Leukocyte dysfunction leading to higher infection risks

Major electrolyte imbalances associated with renal failure:

- K^+: hyperkalemia. (To treat hyperkalemia, give IV calcium, IV regular insulin/glucose, and hyperventilation.)
- Ca^+: hypocalcemia.
- Po_4: hyperphosphatemia.
- Mg^{++}: hypermagnesemia. (All muscle relaxants are potentiated with increased Mg^+ levels.)

Acute Risk Factors for Renal Failure

- Volume depletion.
- Nephrotoxic agents (especially with dehydrated patients):

    Antibiotics: tetracycline, aminoglycosides, gentamycin, amphotericin B

    Chemotherapeutic agents: cisplatin and cyclosporine; cardioglycosides

- IV contrast dye. Radiocontrast dye causes microvascular obstruction through creation of crenated RBCs in a direct insult to the tubules.
- Septic shock
- NSAIDs (e.g., Toradol). By inhibiting prostaglandin synthesis, these agents ablate the vasodilatory effects, thereby aggravating renal underperfusion.
- Rhabdomyolysis and myoglobinemia

Rhabdomyolysis is the rapid breakdown and necrosis of skeletal muscle tissue due to injury from physical, chemical, or biologic causes. This muscle destruction causes myoglobin to be released into the plasma (myoglobinemia). Myoglobin is renal toxic: it clogs the renal tubules. Rhabdomyolysis accounts for as much as 25% of all acute renal failure.

Rhabdomyolysis is related to the following conditions:

- Direct, acute trauma
- Ischemia
- Compartment syndrome
- Increased metabolism
- Prolonged fever
- Status epilepticus
- Intravascular hemolysis from mismatched blood transfusion

To treat rhabdomyolysis, maintain increased renal blood flow and urine flow through the use of IV fluids and diuretics. Alkalinization of urine with sodium bicarbonate should keep the pH of urine greater than 5.6 (but only if the acid–base balance is appropriate). Give calcium to decrease elevated potassium levels.

Chronic Risk Factors for Renal Failure

- Preexisting renal disease
- Advanced age
- Hypertension
- Cirrhosis

- CHF
- Diabetes

Medical Management of Patients with Renal Failure

- Restriction of protein intake
- Correction of acidosis
- Management of hypertension
- Fluid restriction
- Restriction of intake of nonexcretable elements
- Minimization of calcium and phosphorus imbalances
- Treatment to improve anemia

GU/RENAL SURGERY FOR PATIENTS WITHOUT RENAL DISEASE

Anesthetic methods for GU surgery include general anesthesia (GA), spinal anesthetic with IV sedation, or local sedation (LA) with IV sedation. Anesthetics alter renal function by altering renal blood flow, glomerular filtration rate, and renal vascular resistance.

The goals of anesthetic management in regard to renal function in the surgical patient include the following:

- Evaluation of renal function and detection of renal insufficiency
- Preservation of renal integrity
- Prevention of acute renal failure

To accomplish these goals, the following measures are important:

- Adequate hydration is the key to preserving renal function.
- Give diuretics after rehydration.
- Avoid hypotension and use of nephrotoxic agents.
- Give dopaminergic agonists.
- Maintain systemic blood pressure within a range of 80–180 mm Hg to prevent changes in GFR, thereby augmenting renal blood flow and perfusion pressure.

Anesthetics directly alter renal function:

- They cause renal vascular resistance, decreasing renal blood flow.
- They affect GFR and renal tubular function.

Anesthetics also indirectly alter renal function:

- They decrease cardiac output.
- They activate the sympathetic nervous system, which increases renal vascular resistance and increases endogenous secretion of antidiuretic hormone (ADH).

ANESTHESIA IN PATIENTS WITH RENAL DISEASE

Preoperative evaluation and labs should focus on the following considerations:

- Fluid balance
- Current CBC
- Electrolytes (especially potassium and BUN/creatinine level)
- Coagulation (include a PT/INR/PTT)
- Acid–base status
- Potential for infection

These patients often have comorbid conditions, including poor nutritional status and decreased albumin levels. It is not unusual for these patients to have other coexisting conditions as well, such as hypertension, anemia, coagulopathies, GI disturbances, neuropathies and paresthesias, hyperkalemia, acidosis, edema, poor digestion, and diabetes.

Questions to Ask Preoperatively for the Patient with Renal Disease on Dialysis

- What kind of dialysis is the patient on?
- When was the patient's last dialysis treatment? (To ascertain how urgently dialysis is needed and possibility of fluid overload.)
- How often does the patient get dialysis?
- What is the location and quality of dialysis access? Assess and document bruit and

thrill preoperatively and postoperatively. The arm with an arteriovenous fistula or shunt should not be tucked tightly or at all during surgery; rather, secure it on an armboard. Do not take a blood pressure, perform a venipuncture, or place any IV in the extremity used for dialysis access. (For the patient undergoing nephrectomy, this surgery may render the patient hemodialysis dependent postoperatively. Check with the surgeon as to the side on which hemodialysis access is planned, if not already in place.)

- Has the patient experienced hemodynamic instability during dialysis? If so, you can anticipate that the individual will also become unstable on induction of anesthesia.
- Does the patient make urine?
- What is the patient's dry weight? (The weight *before* dialysis.)

How Renal Failure Alters Drug Actions

- Water-soluble drugs are cleared to a lesser extent.
- Acidosis increases the amount of free drug present in the body by altering protein binding and ionization. (Renal patients should not be allowed to hypoventilate, as this condition will worsen acidosis.)
- Hypoalbuminemia (loss through nephrons) increases the amount of free drug present even more.
- Peripheral edema from intravascular volume overload can occur from a decreased oncotic pressure caused by proteinuria and hypoalbuminemia.

Major Considerations for Renal Patients' Anesthesia

IV fluids to give include 0.9% or 0.45% normal saline. Hang only 500-mL bags to avoid accidental overhydration; use microdrip tubing. Try to run the fluid at a rate less than 30 mL/hr; keep fluid amounts to a minimum. Do not overload the patient's fluid levels: don't rehydrate and replace losses. Replace volume loss with a component transfusion if the hematocrit is low. Treat hypotension more with vasopressors and not IV fluids. Mannitol and loop diuretics work only if the patient is already hydrated and makes urine.

Do not give IV fluid that contains electrolytes. For example, do not use lactated Ringer's solution (which contains potassium and lactate) or Plasmalyte (which contains magnesium), as both of these fluids can worsen renal failure.

Maintain an appropriate *electrolyte balance.* Maintain cardiac output because it is what is driving electrolyte production; alter dosages of depressant drugs as necessary.

Other key considerations include the potential for *infection* and *coagulopathies.*

General Anesthesia and the Patient with Renal Disease

- Avoid elective surgery unless patients' serum potassium is less than 5.5 mEq/L.
- The elimination pathway is the key to selecting anesthesia agents.
- Drugs will have altered protein binding in patients with renal disease due to decreased protein levels and acidosis.
- These patients have electrolyte disorders with altered volume of distribution.
- If general anesthetic is used, consider patients with renal disease to be "full stomach" cases. A rapid-sequence induction with cricoid pressure should be done.
- Use anesthetics judiciously; start at low doses and change the doses slowly.
- Narcotics, sedatives, and barbiturates will have a prolonged effect in patients with renal failure.
- Patients with CRF are cardiac output (CO) "driven," so it is essential to maintain CO. Volatile agents decrease cardiac output; use them judiciously.

- Succinylcholine (Anectine) can be given to patients with renal disease if the serum potassium is not elevated.
- Dialysis can lower serum cholinesterase levels, thereby producing a prolonged response to succinylcholine.
- Critically ill patients in acute renal failure can present for surgery with sepsis, severely acidotic, and/or in shock.
- Document fistula placement and function preoperatively and postoperatively.
- Document paresthesias and neuropathies preoperatively.
- Leave the arm used for dialysis access untucked to prevent compression.

Which muscle relaxants are safe to give in renal patients?

- Atracurium: metabolized by Hoffman elimination
- Cisatracurium: metabolized by Hoffman elimination
- Rocuronium: metabolized by the liver
- Vecuronium: decrease the dose by 30%; metabolized by the liver

Pancuronium, doxacurium, and pipecuronium have a significantly prolonged effect in patients with renal failure. Reversal agents have a (beneficial) prolonged elimination pattern. If patients have hypermagnesemia levels, muscle relaxation may be prolonged.

Special considerations are necessary when general anesthesia is used in patients with anemia. Most likely, a compensatory tachycardia will occur due to the anemia with the use of inhalation agents; the FiO_2 level may need to be increased to compensate for the blood's decreased oxygen-carrying capacity.

Regional Anesthesia and the Patient with Renal Disease

If regional anesthesia is used, give intravenous colloids (instead of crystalloids) due to the likelihood of hypotension. Use of such anesthesia may be contraindicated by coagulopathy and neuropathy (chart any such deficits preoperatively).

Regional anesthesia has the least effect on renal function (versus general endotracheal anesthesia [GETA]). However, neuraxial anesthesia can cause a significant decrease in blood pressure, which *can* affect renal blood flow and glomerular infiltration rate, which *does* affect renal function.

Spinal/Epidural Levels for GU surgeries

T6–T7: bladder stretch, peritoneal, radical cystectomy

T8: ureters

T8–T9: TURP/TURB

T9–T10: cystoscopy; (less invasive) procedure involving the bladder

GU Irrigating Solutions

Isotonic and non-electrolyte irrigating solutions may be used in patients undergoing GU/renal surgery. Such fluids may have side effects, however.

- Sorbitol or dextrose can cause hyperglycemia.
- Glycine can cause circulatory depression and transient postoperative visual impairment due to neurotransmitter inhibition in the CNS. Hyperammonemia can occur from glycine degradation.
- Mannitol causes intravascular volume expansion and fluid overload.
- Distilled water can cause hemolysis and hyponatremia. It provides good visibility and is hypotonic. The risk of significant absorption is possible.

Irrigating fluids should never be electrolyte solutions, as such fluids will disperse the electrocautery current. Do not use water as an irrigating fluid. While it provides great visibility, it is hypotonic; thus, red blood cells become hemolyzed if a large amount of water is absorbed.

Irrigating fluids should be warmed to prevent hypothermia.

Careful monitoring of the amount of irrigating fluid instilled and returned is important.

GU/RENAL SCOPE PROCEDURES

Cystoscopy

Cystoscopy is the endoscopic examination of the interior of the lower urinary tract: Through a cystoscope, the bladder (cystoscopy), urethra (urethroscopy), and ureteral orifices (ureteroscopy) can be visualized. A small catheter can be passed through a cystoscope and advanced farther up through the ureters into the kidneys' collection system.

A *resectoscope* is a wide-angle telescope with an electrically activated wire loop that can be inserted into the bladder to biopsy lesions from the bladder, prostate, or urethra. It is capable of transmitting both cutting and coagulating currents to resect tissue.

Cystoscopy is performed to visualize the urethra or bladder when the patient has experienced urinary tract symptoms (e.g., pain, burning, hematuria, difficult urination). It may be used for diagnostic purposes, to treat lesions, for stent placement access, to dilate strictures or the urethra, to collect a sterile urine sample, for biopsy, or for stone removal with a laser, basket, or forceps. In addition, it allows for instillation of chemicals (i.e., hyaluronic acid) to treat interstitial and hemorrhagic cystitis.

Operative Procedure

Either a flexible or a rigid cystoscope or resectoscope, or both types, may be used. The scope is connected to an irrigating system to dilate the bladder for visualization. For visualization of the kidneys' collecting system (transurethral ureteropyeloscopy), a radiopaque dye is injected through small catheters, which are passed through the cystoscope and placed into the distal ureters.

For examination up to the kidneys, a guide wire is inserted through the bladder and up into the proximal ureter and kidney under fluoroscopic guidance. A ureteroscope is then passed over the guide wire.

In cases involving large stones in the bladder, the stones must be fragmented before they are removed—a procedure called litholapaxy.

Anesthetic

A topical anesthetic agent (lidocaine jelly), regional anesthesia (analgesia to T9), or GETA can be given with insertion of a laryngeal airway mask (LMA); GA is used with an OETT in pediatric patients. These patients are usually not very uncomfortable after the surgery. If pain-relief is needed, use small amounts of short-acting opioids.

Positioning

The patient is placed in a lithotomy position.

Anesthetic Implications

Obtain a preoperative CBC and electrolyte panel for all patients undergoing cystoscopy.

Bladder perforation can be caused by manipulation of the cystoscope or resectoscope during this procedure; ureteral perforation can occur with transurethral ureteroscopy/nephroscopy. Suspect perforation if irrigation fluid fails to return or a patient under general anesthesia starts to exhibit hypertension and tachycardia, followed by hypotension and bradycardia. An awake patient will experience suprapubic fullness and pain in the upper abdomen or referred from the diaphragm to the precordial region or shoulders, along with nausea and diaphoresis. Large perforations can lead to unexplained hemodynamic changes, such as sudden hypotension or hypertension, vagal response (bradycardia), or cardiovascular collapse. Perforation is an emergency: patients need GETA and an exploratory laparotomy for bladder repair in most instances.

Diagnostic dyes may be used to colorize urine so as to indicate perforation of bladder or ureters. Cystograffin (a sterile radiopaque contrast agent) is often used to determine the extent of perforation. X-rays and fluoroscopy are done during this procedure.

Retrograde Pyelogram

In a retrograde pyelogram, contrast is injected into the ureter so that the ureter and kidney can be fluoroscopically visualized. This procedure is performed to identify bladder-filling defects or to delineate renal anatomy and abnormality.

PENIS AND URETHRA SURGERY

Excision of Condylomata Acuminata

Laser ablation or a plain "Bovie" may be used to fulgurate condylomas of the penis. This procedure involves laser removal of "genital warts" due to human papillomavirus (HPV), a sexually transmitted disease.

Operative Procedure

After application of local anesthetic, laser ablation is used to remove condyloma lesions. Antibiotic ointment is placed over the lasered sites; a dressing is usually not needed.

Anesthetic

Local anesthetic is used, along with IV sedation.

Positioning

The patient is placed in a supine position, and may need to be frog-legged.

Penectomy: Partial or Total

Penectomy is the surgical removal of part of the penis or the entire penis. It is considered a partial penectomy if 2 cm or more of the proximal shaft is left intact. This length allows for directable and upright urination. If this margin cannot be achieved, total penectomy with perineal urethrostomy is required.

Penectomy is performed to treat advanced penile cancer or necrosis. It may also be done for sexual reassignment purposes.

Operative Procedure

Penectomy may be done as a two-part surgery. The ideal procedure removes the disease with adequate margins while preserving sexual and urinary function. Advanced-stage tumors may require a scrotectomy (surgical removal of part of the scrotum) or orchiectomy (surgical removal of one or both testes) along with a penectomy.

For total penectomy, a circumferential incision is made at the base of the penis and carried down to the base of the corpora (corpora cavernosa [singular = cavernosum])—a pair of sponge-like regions of erectile tissue in the penis containing most of the blood during erection. The surgeon then creates a new opening for the urethra between the scrotum and the anus. The urethra is mobilized, grasped, and brought down through the perineal urethrostomy. The urethral mucosa is then sutured to the perineal skin; an indwelling catheter will be inserted into the urethrostomy site at the end of the case. Groin lymph nodes may also be removed depending on the stage of the cancer.

Following penectomy, urination is still controlled by the natural valve at the base of the bladder, as it is above the level of the penis.

Anesthetic

General anesthesia is given with insertion of an OETT; muscle relaxation is not required. Neuraxial anesthesia may be used, consisting of epidural anesthesia to T8–T9.

Positioning

The patient is placed in a supine position, and may need to be frog-legged.

Anesthetic Implications

A type and screen of the patient's blood is usually all that is needed, unless the patient has coagulopathies or is severely anemic.

If the patient is alert and oriented, he may require more anxiolytic/sedation preoperatively.

Penile Implant

Penile implant entails insertion of a prosthesis into the penis. This procedure is performed as a treatment for erectile dysfunction.

Operative Procedure

Many types of prostheses are available. The selection of a device depends on both the cause of impotence and patient choice.

A urethral catheter is inserted into the penis after induction of anesthesia.

If a *malleable penile prosthesis* is used, based on the man's penile dimensions, the largest and longest prosthesis is inserted into a small incision at the base of the penis at the penis–scrotal junction. The prosthesis can be bent in the desired direction for either intercourse or concealment.

An *inflatable penile prosthesis* involves two paired cylinders inserted into both sides of the penis (into the corpora). It is inserted through an incision, approximately 3 cm long, made at the base of the penis into the scrotum. A fluid reservoir is inserted and secured into the suprapubic region next to the bladder. Fluid movement between the reservoir and the cylinders is controlled by a pump placed in the scrotum (usually on the dominant hand side) next to the testis.

Blunt dissection is done to insert the cylinders into the penis, while small incisions are made into the scrotum and suprapubic area.

Anesthetic

GETA; OETT or an LMA are used. Neuraxial anesthesia consists of a spinal anesthetic.

Positioning

The patient is placed in a supine position. He may need to be frog-legged for scrotal access. Lithotomy may be done.

Anesthetic Implications

Manipulation of the genitals can cause a sudden and profound vagal bradycardia. Have glycopyrrolate and atropine drawn up for these cases. Notify the surgeon if bradycardia occurs.

Infection is a serious concern with penile implants. To guard against this possibility, the anus should be isolated completely from the surgical area. The prosthesis parts should not touch any part of the skin when they are inserted into the body.

Blood glucose levels should be obtained preoperatively, as these patients are often diabetic.

Urethral Meatotomy

In urethral meatotomy, the urethral meatus is incised. This procedure may be performed to relieve congenital or acquired stenosis of the external urethral meatus or to enlarge the urethral opening.

Operative Procedure

An incision is made to enlarge the meatus; the mucosal layer is then sutured to the skin. Petroleum gauze is placed over the incision.

Anesthetic

A local anesthetic is used along with IV sedation for adults. Pediatric patients require general anesthesia. Can be done with volatile agents by mask or with insertion of an LMA or an OETT.

Positioning

A male patient is placed in a supine position. A female patient is placed in a lithotomy position.

Anesthetic Implications

Urethral meatotomy is usually a very short case.

Urethroplasty

Urethroplasty involves reconstruction of the urethra for narrowing or strictures of the lumen. This surgery is performed to repair an injury or a defect in the walls of the urethra.

Operative Procedure

In the male, a U-shaped incision is made in the perineum between the scrotum and the anus to access the urethra. Placing a sound into the urethra (a sound has a curved tip that is designed to be passed through the urethra) up to the stricture helps to identify where the stricture ends. An incision is made into the dorsal side of the penis, the bulbocavernosus muscle is dissected, and the tissue surrounding the strictured urethra is excised around the placed sound. Anastomosis of the severed urethral ends can be done.

The procedure for women involves the development of an inverted U-shaped vaginal flap with its apex at the urethral meatus. A Foley catheter is inserted into the urethra; the stricture is incised until the entire structure is open. The vaginal flap is then sutured to the proximal urethrotomy to augment the urethra. A 16 Fr. Foley catheter is placed and left in place for 7 to 10 days.

In more complex cases, free skin grafts or mobilized vascular grafts are necessary to bridge larger urethral defects. A buccal mucosal graft may be harvested from the mouth in these situations.

A urinary diversion may need to be created to allow for urethral "rest" after this surgery.

Anesthetic

GETA is given with insertion of an OETT; muscle relaxants are given.

Positioning

The patient is placed in an exaggerated lithotomy position. The anus must be isolated away from the surgical site.

Anesthetic Implications

Urethroplasty is usually a long case, so it is important to keep the patient warm.

There are obvious airway implications if a buccal free skin graft is needed.

SCROTUM AND TESTICLES SURGERY
Epididymectomy

Excision of the epididymis from a testis is known as epididymectomy. This procedure is performed when chronic scrotal pain localized to the epididymis is still present after all nonsurgical treatments have been attempted. It is an operation of last resort, as nearly half of all patients who have this surgery continue to have "phantom pain."

The epididymis is a structure within the scrotum attached to the backside of the testis. This coiled segment of the spermatic ducts serves to store, mature, and transport spermatozoa between the testis and the vas deferens. Chronic epididymitis can occur from bacterial infection, after a severe case of epididymitis, or from cysts on the epididymis.

Epididymectomy does not make a man sterile if done on only one side. If it is done bilaterally, however, sperm can no longer travel to the ejaculatory duct.

Operative Procedure

In this procedure, the entire epididymis is removed through a transverse scrotal incision. The testicle is first removed through the scrotal incision and the epididymis meticulously dissected free from the testicle. The testicle is then returned to the scrotum. The incision lines are sutured closed in layers.

Anesthetic

GETA, spinal, or a local anesthetic with IV sedation may all be used. These patients are usually treated on an outpatient basis. If narcotics are given, use small amounts of short-acting opioids.

Positioning

The patient is placed in a supine, frog-legged position.

Anesthetic Implications

CBC and chemistry 7 lab results should be obtain preoperatively, especially if the patient has an infection.

Manipulation of the genitals can cause a sudden and profound vagal bradycardia. Have glycopyrrolate and atropine drawn up for these cases. Notify the surgeon if bradycardia occurs.

A scrotal support strap is applied at the end of the case.

Hydrocelectomy

Hydrocelectomy is the excision of a hydrocele through the tunica vaginalis of testis (serous covering of testis). A hydrocele is a painless enlargement in the scrotum, caused by an accumulation of serous fluid around the testis in the tunica vaginalis. It can occur spontaneously or be the result of trauma or infection.

Operative Procedure

An inguinal or scrotal incision is made, and the accumulated fluid is evacuated. The tunica edges are sutured together to prevent reaccumulation of fluid. A hydrocele may be accompanied by an inguinal hernia that can be repaired during the same procedure.

Anesthetic

GETA is given with insertion of an OETT. These patients are usually treated on an outpatient basis. If narcotics are given, use small amounts of short-acting opioids.

Positioning

The patient is placed in a supine, frog-legged position.

Anesthetic Implications

Manipulation of the genitals can cause a sudden and profound vagal bradycardia. Have glycopyrrolate and atropine drawn up for these cases. Notify the surgeon if bradycardia occurs.

A hydrocele can be associated with an inguinal hernia; if both are repaired in the same surgery, the case can go longer than anticipated. Keep the patient warm.

A scrotal support strap is applied at the end of the case.

Orchiectomy

Orchiectomy is the removal of one (testis) or both (testes) testicles. It may be necessary in cases involving trauma, irreversible vascular compromise after testicular torsion, the need for endocrine control of prostate cancer, or primary tumors of the testes.

Operative Procedure

An incision is made on the scrotum and dissected through the tunica vaginalis for benign conditions. If a tumor is suspected, an inguinal approach is used. The spermatic cord is ligated, and the testis is removed unilaterally or bilaterally for benign disease or endocrine control. For malignant disease, high ligation of the spermatic cord is done. A testicular prosthesis may be placed at the time of the original surgery, at a later date, or not at all.

Anesthetic

GETA may be given with insertion of an OETT. Spinal anesthesia may also be used with IV sedation.

Positioning

The patient is placed in a supine position, with legs apart or frog-legged. The arms may be extended on armboards bilaterally.

Anesthetic Implications

If the patient is elderly, perform an EKG or other indicated cardiac studies preoperatively.

Manipulation of the genitals can cause a sudden and profound vagal bradycardia. Have glycopyrrolate and atropine drawn up for these cases. Notify the surgeon if bradycardia occurs.

A sterilization consent form should be signed by the patient if both testes are to be removed.

A scrotal support strap is applied at the end of the case.

Testicular implants can be surgically inserted, but implantation is usually not done until several months after an orchiectomy is done. The patient's testes should be measured preoperatively so that the appropriate size of prosthesis is ordered.

Spermatocelectomy

Spermatocelectomy is the excision of a cyst of the epididymis. Such a benign cystic swelling of the sperm-conveying ductal system typically originates from the superior head of the epididymis.

Operative Procedure

A scrotal incision is made, and the cystic mass is dissected free and excised. If the spermatic duct is interrupted and fertility is a consideration, anastomosis is performed. Methylene blue dye may be used to test the patency of the anastomosis.

Anesthetic

Sedation is used with local anesthetic; GETA may be needed, insertion of an LMA or OETT.

Positioning

The patient is placed in a supine position, with either the legs apart or up in stirrups.

Anesthetic Implications

Manipulation of the genitals can cause a sudden and profound vagal bradycardia. Have glycopyrrolate and atropine drawn up for these cases. Notify the surgeon if bradycardia occurs.

Methylene blue should be available.

A scrotal support strap is applied at the end of the case.

Testicular Biopsy

In this procedure, a small piece of a testicle is excised and biopsied to discern whether testis function is normal—that is, whether sperm production is normal. The biopsy can be unilateral or bilateral depending on the reason for the biopsy.

Operative Procedure

A small incision is made over the anterior wall of the scrotum, and a small piece of testicle tissue is excised. The small opening in the testicle is sutured, and then the scrotal skin is sutured closed.

Anesthetic

Sedation is given with a local anesthetic; GA may be needed, with insertion of an LMA. Spinal anesthesia may also be used.

These patients are usually treated on an outpatient basis. If narcotics are given, use small amounts of short-acting opioids.

Positioning

The patient may be placed in either a lithotomy position or supine with legs in frog-legged position.

Anesthetic Implications

Testicular biopsy is a very quick procedure.

Manipulation of the genitals can cause a sudden and profound vagal bradycardia. Have glycopyrrolate and atropine drawn up for these cases. Notify the surgeon if bradycardia occurs.

A scrotal support strap is applied at the end of the case.

Testicular Torsion

Testicular torsion is an emergency procedure to untwist and secure a torsed testicle. This condition results in ischemia of the testicle secondary to the interruption in blood flow.

Torsion of a testicle and spermatic cord is an anatomic abnormality that allows the spermatic cord to twist more easily, resulting in compromise of the blood supply to the testicle. In a "bell-clapper deformity," the tunica vaginalis covers not only the testicle and the epididymis, but also the spermatic cord, allowing the testis to rotate freely within the tunica. The degree of ischemia depends on how long the testicle is torsed and what the degree of rotation of the spermatic cord is (the testicular artery is contained in the spermatic cord).

Operative Procedure

If the testicle is detorsed successfully, it will be sutured within the scrotum to prevent further twisting (orchiopexy). Given that approximately 40% of men who have this abnormality have it bilaterally, the surgeon will affix the other testicle in the same manner during the same operation.

Anesthetic

A rapid-sequence induction should be done as this is an emergency procedure; GETA is given with insertion of an OETT.

Positioning

The patient is placed in a supine position.

Anesthetic Implications

Before surgery, the patient is in acute pain. Testicular torsion is considered a surgical emergency.

Manual detorsion is possible, but restoration of blood flow must be confirmed following the maneuver.

The testicle must be detorsed within 6–8 hours or else it is rarely salvageable. In the latter case, it must be surgically removed (orchiectomy).

Torsion is characterized by severe unilateral testicular pain and sudden swelling. Patients may also have abdominal pain and nausea and vomiting. Epididymitis is a common misdiagnosis.

Manipulation of the genitals can cause a sudden and profound vagal bradycardia. Have glycopyrrolate and atropine drawn up for these cases. Notify the surgeon if bradycardia occurs.

A scrotal support strap is applied at the end of the case.

Varicocelectomy

Varicocelectomy could also be termed "internal spermatic vein ligation," as the dilated gonadal veins of the testis are actually ligated during this surgery. Such a procedure is performed to reduce venous backflow of blood, which raises the same issues as varicose veins of the leg.

A varicocele is an abnormal dilation of the veins of the spermatic cord that can result in a progressive decline in sperm quality and infertility. Clinical diagnosis can be made when a varicocele is present with Valsalva maneuver; this abnormality can be seen through the scrotal skin and referred to as a "bag of worms."

Operative Procedure

The affected spermatic veins are tied off above the varicocele; blood is rerouted through unaffected veins.

An *open inguinal, subinguinal, or retroperitoneal approach* allows the surgeon to easily identify the spermatic cord and access the testis. Often a microscope or surgical loupes are used to perform the identification.

Laparoscopic approach can be done through the abdominal cavity.

In *percutaneous venous embolization,* an angiographic catheter is inserted through the femoral vein and advanced into the spermatic vein. The dilated veins can be occluded with balloons, coils, or glue.

Anesthetic

GETA is given with insertion of an LMA; spinal anesthesia may also be used.

Positioning

The patient is placed in a supine, frog-legged position.

Anesthetic Implications

Manipulation of the genitals can cause a sudden and profound vagal bradycardia. Have glycopyrrolate and atropine drawn up for these cases. Notify the surgeon if bradycardia occurs.

A scrotal support strap is applied at the end of the case.

Vasectomy

Vasectomy involves the ligation of a segment of the vas deferens in the bilateral scrotum. A vasectomy is performed for voluntary sterilization. The vas deferens carries the sperm from the testes, inside the spermatic cord, to the ejaculatory ducts in the urethra. Ligating the vas deferens will prevent sperm from entering the seminal stream.

Operative Procedure

A small incision is made into the scrotum on both sides. The vas deferens is isolated and ligated. Following this surgery, the testicles will continue to produce sperm, but the sperm will be reabsorbed by the body.

Anesthetic

Anesthesia options include spinal anesthesia or IV sedation and local anesthesia.

These patients are usually treated on an outpatient basis. If narcotics are given, use small amounts of short-acting opioids.

Positioning

The patient is placed in a supine position, with either legs apart or legs in stirrups.

Anesthetic Implications

A sterilization consent form should be signed by the patient, along with the consent for surgery.

Manipulation of the genitals can cause a sudden and profound vagal bradycardia. Have glycopyrrolate and atropine drawn up for these cases. Notify the surgeon if bradycardia occurs.

A scrotal support strap is applied at the end of the case.

Vasovasostomy

Vasovasostomy involves the anastomosis of the ligated ends of the vas deferens. The procedure is performed when a patient seeks to reestablish continuity of the vas deferens to restore fertility or to alleviate chronic testicular pain after vasectomy.

Operative Procedure

After a small incision is made into the scrotum, the testicle, epididymis, and vas deferens are brought out of the scrotal sac. A microscope is used; scar tissue at the separated ends of the vas deferens is excised. The mucosal lining of the lumen is approximated with sutures.

Anesthetic

Either regional anesthesia or sedation plus local anesthesia may be used.

These patients are usually treated on an outpatient basis. If narcotics are given, use small amounts of short-acting opioids.

Positioning

The patient is placed in a supine position, with either legs apart or legs in stirrups.

Anesthetic Implications

Manipulation of the genitals can cause a sudden and profound vagal bradycardia. Have glycopyrrolate and atropine drawn up for these cases. Notify the surgeon if bradycardia occurs.

A scrotal support strap is applied at the end of the case.

PROSTATE GLAND SURGERY

Transrectal Cryosurgical Ablation of the Prostate Gland

In transrectal cryosurgical ablation of the prostate gland, probes (cryoneedles) are inserted through the perineum into the prostate gland; needle insertion is assisted by transrectal ultrasound. Gas-driven probes allow highly pressurized gas (argon to freeze tissue; helium to thaw it) to destroy prostate tissue by sequentially freezing and thawing the gland, causing cell destruction and cell membrane rupture.

This procedure is performed to relieve urinary obstruction caused by benign or malignant prostate disease. These patients may have post-radiotherapy localized prostate cancer.

Operative Procedure

To begin, the surgeon will insert a cystoscope into the bladder and may insert a suprapubic catheter (which is clamped to keep the bladder full). The cystoscope is removed, and a silicone catheter is inserted into the urethra. Next, the entire catheter length is filled with aerated jelly and sterile water, allowing the urethra to be clearly visualized by ultrasound. The scrotum is fixed away from the anus using two stay sutures.

A probe (covered and lubricated) inserted into the rectum provides the surgeon with longitudinal and transverse views of the prostate. Measurements are taken, and the cryoneedles are inserted through the peritoneum into the prostate. Cryosurgery utilizes high-pressure argon and helium gases whose supply sources are linked by a computer-controlled delivery system to the cryoneedles. Between the freezing cycles, which use argon, the prostate gland is allowed to thaw first passively, then actively by application of helium. Each cycle of freezing lasts for approximately 10 minutes. Once the entire prostate gland has been treated, the needles are removed.

A warmer is kept in position for 20 minutes until the gland has thawed entirely. During this time, pressure is applied to the perineum to reduce the amount of bruising postoperatively. If a suprapubic catheter was introduced earlier, it is removed. Finally, a urethral catheter is inserted; it will remain in place for as long as 2 weeks postoperatively. A gauze dressing is applied over the perineum.

Anesthetic
GETA is given with insertion of an LMA or an OETT.

Positioning
The patient is placed in either an exaggerated lithotomy position or a lateral decubitus position.

Anesthetic Implications
Care is taken not to damage the rectal wall, bladder neck, and tissues below the pelvic floor.

A scrotal support strap is applied at the end of the case.

Transurethral Resection of the Prostate Gland or Lesions of the Bladder

Transurethral resection of the prostate gland (TURP) entails removal of prostatic tissue through a cystoscope. Transurethral resection of lesions of the bladder (TURB) involves removal of such lesions in the same manner. These procedures are performed for prostate or bladder biopsy or excision of a benign, symptomatic prostate gland. The goal is to relieve urinary obstruction caused by benign or malignant disease of an enlarged prostate gland.

Operative Procedure
A resectoscope is inserted, and electrodissection is done to remove pieces of prostatic tissue or a bladder lesion (usually the lesion is taken along with underlying muscle) until all desired material is evacuated. The prostate capsule is left intact. A coagulating current then seals the vessels. A three-way urethral catheter is inserted after the cystoscope is removed. A lesion that has deeply invaded into the bladder wall must be treated with an open bladder procedure and cannot be removed transurethrally.

In *laser resection,* no irrigation fluid is needed. This technique is also less painful than the standard resection. A laser fiber is passed through a cystoscope and is used to heat prostate tissue or a bladder lesion (and coagulate the tumor bed) until it is vaporized. Laser resection is also a quicker procedure than standard resection, usually taking only 15–30 minutes.

A urethral catheter is placed at the end of the surgery.

Anesthetic
A spinal or epidural to T10 is the preferred anesthetic because these types of anesthesia make it easier to identify transurethral resection (TUR) syndrome and there tends to be less blood loss with these options; they are also associated with a decreased incidence of postoperative venous thrombus or embolus. Neuraxial anesthesia needs

to be at the T10 level, because the stretch receptors in the distended bladder cause pain higher than the coverage needed for bladder surgery. If regional anesthesia is used, make sure the patient stays very still: movement can cause injury or perforation.

GETA with an OETT or LMA may also be used.

Positioning
The patient is placed in a lithotomy position.

Anesthetic Implications
These patients are usually elderly males with multiple comorbidities. A thorough preoperative history and physical assessment should be done. An EKG and a chest X-ray should also be performed preoperatively. These patients are at increased risk for perioperative myocardial infarction, pulmonary edema, and acute renal failure.

Lab tests—CBC, chemistry, platelets, coagulation panel, BUN and creatinine, glucose levels—should be completed preoperatively. If the patient is anemic, getting a type and screen of his blood is useful (given the risk of blood loss with these procedures) and makes it easier to get blood products if the need arises.

Give minimal amounts of IV fluids through a peripheral IV to minimize fluid overload due to possible irrigation absorption.

Complications: TUR Syndrome
TUR syndrome is a term applied to a constellation of signs and symptoms caused primarily by excessive absorption of the irrigating fluid; it is also called irrigation fluid solute toxicity. Symptoms can become manifest either intraoperatively or postoperatively.

During a TURP procedure, the bladder is continuously irrigated with a solution to maintain visibility through the cystoscope and to distend the urethra. The prostate gland has an extensive plexus of venous sinuses (the dorsal venous plexus), which can absorb the irrigating fluid. Normally, 20 mL/min is absorbed during a TURP, and the procedure usually lasts 45–60 minutes.

Factors Affecting Absorption of Irrigating Fluids
- Type of irrigating fluid
- Duration of resection (should not exceed 2 hours)
- Height of irrigation fluids
- Blood loss

Signs and Symptoms of TUR Syndrome
Absorption of a large volume of fluid can result in signs of "water intoxication": hypervolemia and dilutional hyponatremia leading to hemolysis of red blood cells, cerebral edema, congestive heart failure, and pulmonary edema, plus hypertension, tachycardia, and ventricular fibrillation (if the sodium level is less than 120 mEq/L).

Symptoms of TUR syndrome in an awake patient include restlessness, headache, dyspnea, agitation, nausea and vomiting, visual disturbances, mental confusion, and coma. Note that the first sign of hyponatremia is confusion.

Symptoms of TUR syndrome in an anesthetized patient include seizures, cyanosis, arrhythmias, bradycardia (vagal response), and unexplained hypotension or hypertension. These symptoms can become rapidly fatal.

Prevention of TUR Syndrome
Irrigating solutions should not be hung higher than 30 cm above the operating table at the beginning of the procedure and higher than 15 cm above the table during the final stages. Hanging fluid bags at a higher level could result in increased fluid absorption.

Treatment of TUR Syndrome
Early recognition is key to successful treatment of TUR syndrome.

Maintain oxygenation and perfusion at adequate levels. If the patient's level of consciousness changes, intubate and ventilate the individual.

If dilutional hyponatremia occurs, stop or rapidly complete the procedure.

Eliminate absorbed water, give the patient diuretic agents and hypertonic saline.

If the sodium level is less than 120 mEq/L, give IV 3% sodium chloride. Increase the sodium level by no more than 12 mEq/L in a 24-hr period. A severely low sodium level can cause ventricular fibrillation and unconsciousness.

Other Complications with Cystoscopy and TURP

Bladder perforation can be caused by a cystoscope or resectoscope during a TURP procedure. Suspect this problem if irrigation fluid fails to return. Symptoms include hypertension and tachycardia, followed by hypotension and bradycardia. An awake patient will experience suprapubic fullness and pain in the upper abdomen or referred from the diaphragm to the precordial region or shoulders, along with nausea and diaphoresis. Large perforations can lead to unexplained hemodynamic changes such as sudden hypotension or hypertension, vagal response (bradycardia), or cardiovascular collapse. Perforation is an emergency: Patients need GETA and an exploratory laparotomy for bladder repair.

Warm irrigating fluids should be used to prevent *hypothermia*. Warming blankets, warmed IV fluids, and a warm room temperature are also measures that can prevent this complication.

Blood loss can be very difficult to monitor because the irrigating fluid dilutes and washes the blood away. Preoperative typing and cross-matching of the patient's blood is suggested.

Patients who have undergone TURP can develop *coagulopathy* and *disseminated intravascular coagulation* (DIC) postoperatively. Though rare, these complications are caused by the release of thromboplastin from the prostate and dilutional thrombocytopenia.

Septicemia is possible because the prostate can harbor colonized bacteria that are let loose during the TURP procedure.

Simple Perineal Prostatectomy

Simple perineal prostatectomy is the removal of a prostate gland through an open approach so that surrounding tissues and lymph nodes can be tested for metastasis; radical perineal prostatectomy

(discussed in the next section) may follow a positive pathology report. The simple perineal approach is completed when the pathology reports come back as negative for metastasis.

This procedure is intended to relieve urinary obstruction caused by benign disease. It is most often performed if the cancer is confined to the capsule.

Operative Procedure

A curved "retractor" is placed through the urethra to lift the prostate upward. From the base of the scrotum, a midline incision is made down the perineum, connecting to a curvilinear incision made above the rectum; the rectourethral muscle is retracted downward, helping to expose the prostate gland. A biopsy is taken from the prostate gland for frozen section. If the pathology results are negative, the benign prostate is removed. If the pathology results are positive, a radical perineal (total) prostatectomy is done.

A drain is placed and the prostate capsule incision is repaired; the tissue is closed in layers. A three-way urethral catheter is inserted through the urethra into the bladder for continuous irrigation of the bladder postoperatively.

Anesthetic

GETA and muscle relaxation are given. An epidural catheter may be placed preoperatively and not bolused until the end of the case for postoperative pain management.

Positioning

The patient is placed in an exaggerated lithotomy position, with a pad under the buttocks. A slight Trendelenburg position facilitates surgeon access.

Anesthetic Implications

Nerve injury may occur while the patient is in the lithotomy position, especially with extreme hip flexion. There is also an increased risk of deep venous thrombosis (DVT) with the lithotomy position.

Prostatectomy can result in impotency. The risk of rectal injury is also increased.

It is not possible to perform iliac node dissection with this approach.

The volume of packed cells to have typed and cross-matched depends on the size of the prostate to be removed: The larger the gland/mass, the more blood loss expected.

A scrotal support strap is applied at the end of the case.

Radical (Total) Perineal Prostatectomy

Total perineal prostatectomy is the radical excision of the prostate and linked tissues, including the prostate, prostate capsule, seminal vesicles, and portions of the vas deferens through an incision in the perineum; the pelvic lymph nodes are also removed. This approach, which is used to remove a cancerous prostate gland, allows the surgeon better visualization and access to the prostate and seminal vesicles than simple perineal prostatectomy (discussed in the previous section). In benign disease, the prostate is enucleated from its capsule during this surgery.

Operative Procedure

A curvilinear incision (an upside-down "U") is made in the perineum. The prostate gland is then carefully dissected away from the bladder, urethra (bladder is separated from the urethra), rectum, and vas deferens. Local lymph nodes can be biopsied for frozen section; only if these lymph nodes are negative for metastasis will the surgery continue.

After the prostate and the other structures are removed, the bladder neck is anastomosed to the urethra over an indwelling urethral catheter. The catheter will stay in place for as long as two weeks postoperatively.

The radical approach is accompanied by a laparoscopic or low abdominal node dissection. The laparoscopic approach may precede the perineal prostatectomy.

Anesthetic

GETA is given with insertion of an OETT. Muscle relaxation is necessary if laparoscopic or open node dissection is done.

Positioning

The patient is placed in a lithotomy position, with knees touching the chest, or an exaggerated lithotomy position, with a pad under the buttocks. A slight to steep Trendelenburg position facilitates surgeon access. The patient is placed supine for laparoscopic node dissection.

Anesthetic Implications

Prostatectomy can result in impotency. The risk of rectal injury is also increased with this procedure.

It is not possible to perform iliac node dissection with this approach.

The volume of packed cells to have typed and cross-matched depends on the size of the prostate to be removed: The larger the gland/mass, the more blood loss expected.

Limit IV crystalloids in patients who experience blood loss; use colloids as blood replacement products instead. Have at least two large-bore peripheral IVs available. A central line and an arterial line may also be needed.

A scrotal support strap is applied at the end of the case.

Nerve-Sparing, Radical Retropubic Prostatectomy with Pelvic/Retroperitoneal Lymphadenectomy

Radical retropubic prostatectomy is the surgical removal of the prostate gland, the prostate capsule, seminal vesicles, and ampulla of the vas deferens through an incision in midline lower abdominal area. This approach avoids incising and entering the bladder. Also removed are all of the bilateral pelvic lymph nodes (external iliac, obturator, and hypogastric nodes en bloc).

Radical lymphadenectomy is a bilateral resection of the pelvic and retroperitoneal lymph nodes.

In this procedure, the lymphatic structures are dissected away from the aorta, vena cava, and the kidneys and sent to the pathology lab for evaluation.

This procedure is performed to remove an organ-confined cancerous prostate gland. "Nerve-sparing" refers to sparing the posterolateral neurovascular bundles that supplies the corpus cavernosa nerve involved with erectile potency.

Operative Procedure

A urethral catheter is inserted at the beginning of the case. The lymphadenectomy is done first so that the nodes can be sent off for frozen section. While the surgical team is waiting for the pathology report, the veins traveling over the prostate are ligated; the prostate is exposed in the prevesical space and enucleated by digital dissection. The urethra is cut both above and below the prostate.

The posterolateral nerve bundles (which are responsible for erections) are examined for disease. If no disease is apparent, the surgeon may not remove them (nerve-sparing radical prostatectomy). If the nerves must be removed, they are severed near the urethra.

After the prostate and the other structures are removed, the bladder neck is trimmed and anastomosed to the urethra over an indwelling urethral catheter.

Anesthetic

GETA is given, possibly along with muscle relaxation. Check with the surgeon before giving muscle relaxants, especially in cases involving nerve-sparing surgery. An arterial line is needed, and possibly a CVP catheter. If the patient has a cardiac/pulmonary history, a pulmonary artery catheter may also be required.

Positioning

The patient is placed in a supine position. Kidney rest may be elevated to hyperextend the patient's body slightly.

Anesthetic Implications

Temperature loss is common with a retropubic prostatectomy procedure, especially if lymph node dissection is performed during the same surgery. Upper- and lower-body warming blankets are needed as well as fluid warmers. The ambient temperature in the room may also need to be increased.

The volume of packed cells to have typed and cross-matched depends on the size of the prostate to be removed: The larger the gland/mass, the more blood loss expected.

The pelvic wall contains many blood vessels and nerves. Caution must be used during the lymph node dissection to prevent injury to these structures.

Complications

This procedure can cause several undesirable and serious side effects and complications, including damage to urinary sphincters, causing incontinence, and damage to penile nerves, leading to impotence.

Robotic-Assisted Laparoscopic Prostatectomy

The prostate gland may be removed in a prostatectomy using a robot-assisted laparoscopic approach. The bladder neck, seminal vesicles, and ampullae of the vas deferens are also removed through an incision during such a procedure. Laparoscopic prostatectomy is performed to relieve urinary obstruction caused by benign or malignant disease and to remove a localized, cancerous prostate gland.

Advantages of using the robot include availability of improved nerve-sparing techniques with less blood loss and a shorter hospital length of stay. These advantages, in turn, lead to improved continence and impotency rates.

Operative Procedure

The laparoscopic approach to robot-assisted radical prostatectomy provides the surgeon with a three-dimensional image of the prostate and a

10-fold magnification that allows for better control, finer movement, and greater precision.

After the prostate and the other structures are removed, the bladder neck is anastomosed to the urethra over an indwelling urethral catheter. At this point, the robotic-assisted portion is complete. The patient is flattened out of the steep Trendelenburg position, the laparoscopic trocars are removed, and the small incisions closed.

Anesthetic

GETA is given with insertion of an OETT; muscle relaxants are given. The anesthetist can use pressure-controlled ventilation, smaller tidal volume settings, and an increased respiratory rate to maintain ETCO$_2$ within normal limits. Pressure-controlled ventilation is an especially good choice in patients who are obese, have COPD, or are more difficult to ventilate while in a steep Trendelenburg position.

Monitors and IV Access

An arterial line is often preferred due to the length of these cases. A central venous line may also be needed.

IV Fluids and Volume Requirements

Keep IV fluids to a minimum until the end of the case, so as to minimize the risk of urine spilling out into the abdominal cavity until the urethra is anastomosed. Excess urine output can affect the surgeon's view as well. A urethral catheter to drain urine is not inserted until the end of the case. Once the anastomosis is complete, IV fluids can be given freely.

If patients have received a bowel prep, they will be dehydrated prior to surgery. Maintain blood pressure at an adequate level with vasopressors—not IV fluid—until the end of the case (when the urethra is reestablished with the bladder).

Positioning

The patient is placed in a supine position, with legs in stirrups or boots for lithotomy position. A steep Trendelenburg position is needed for optimal internal organ visualization by the surgeon. Bilateral arms should be carefully padded and tucked at the sides.

Patients are kept in steep Trendelenburg position for the duration of the surgery, which is usually 3–6 hours long. They are placed directly on a warmed gel pad (when moved from the stretcher to the OR table) and key portions are taped to the bed frame (after induction) to prevent the body from moving cephalad while the bed is in steep Trendelenburg position. It is of paramount importance to meticulously position and pad all pressure points to prevent nerve injury. The bed should be tested in all extreme positions (before draping) to make sure the patient's body does not move.

Both the steep Trendelenburg position and laparoscopic pneumoperitoneum have effects on body systems:

- *Respiratory* effort is hampered by the limitations on normal lung and diaphragmatic movement, decreased functional residual capacity, decreased pulmonary compliance, and reduced lung volume. These changes can lead to hypoxia, hypercapnia, and atelectasis. Setting the ventilator on pressure-controlled ventilations can help to maximize tidal volume while minimizing peak inspiratory pressures.

- The *cardiovascular* system is strained by the decreased cardiac output (by 10–30%), decreased mean arterial pressures, and increased pulmonary wedge pressures and central venous pressures. In patients with preexisting heart disease, these changes can lead to myocardial ischemia and dysrhythmias. Pneumoperitoneum can also lead to profound bradycardia or asystole. If either problem occurs, notify the surgeon at once, decrease the insufflation pressure, and treat the patient with Robinul and/or atropine.

- *Renal* blood flow and glomerular filtration rates are decreased, while antidiuretic and aldosterone hormones are released, leading to decreased urinary output.

- Facial, eyelid, and conjunctival *swelling* may occur with increased intracranial pressures.

Anesthetic Implications

Use a warming blanket and fluid warmers to help maintain normothermia.

Preoperative lab values should be checked, such as CBC, PT/INR/PTT, and electrolytes with glucose.

Type and cross-match the patient's blood pre-operatively.

Simple Retropubic Prostatectomy

The simple retropubic prostatectomy surgically removes a prostate tumor that is too large to be resected transurethrally. The hypertrophic prostate tissue is brought out through the incision made into the anterior prostate gland. The bladder is not entered (extravesical approach).

This procedure is done to relieve a urinary obstruction caused by benign or malignant disease. It is most often performed if the cancer is confined to the capsule.

Operative Procedure

A cystoscopy is done prior to an open prostatectomy. After the cystoscope is removed, a three-way urethral catheter is inserted into the bladder and the balloon inflated; the catheter is clamped off.

The retropubic approach is through a low midline abdominal incision. The dorsal vein complex, the main arterial supply to the prostate gland, and the bladder neck are visualized. Once the blood supply has been controlled, the anterior prostate capsule is opened and the central bulk of the prostate mass is excised, leaving the outer capsule and associated structures intact. A urethral catheter is inserted at the end of the case. Hemostasis is achieved, a drain is placed, and the wound is closed. A suprapubic catheter—in addition to urethral catheter—is usually inserted.

Anesthetic

GETA and muscle relaxation are given.

Positioning

The patient is placed in a supine position.

Anesthetic Implications

The volume of packed cells to have typed and cross-matched depends on the size of the prostate to be removed: The larger the gland/mass, the more blood loss expected.

Patients will have received a bowel prep and be dehydrated; for this reason, consider giving albumin/hetastarch fluid boluses along with a crystalloid infusion. These patients will have an exaggerated drop in their blood pressure on induction of anesthesia.

Suprapubic Prostatectomy (Transvesical Prostatectomy)

Suprapubic prostatectomy is the surgical removal of the prostate gland, the bladder neck, seminal vesicles, and ampullae of the vas deferens through an incision into the bladder. This procedure is not used to treat malignancy, but rather to relieve urinary obstruction caused by benign disease. The primary advantage (relative to the retropubic approach) is that the suprapubic route allows for direct visualization of the bladder neck and mucosa. The main disadvantage is the challenge in controlling bleeding beneath the symphysis pubis.

Operative Procedure

A cystoscopy is done prior to an open prostatectomy. After the cystoscope is removed, a three-way urethral catheter is inserted into the bladder and the balloon inflated; the catheter is clamped off. A low midline abdominal incision is made from the navel to the pubic area or transverse abdominal incision. An incision is made into the dome of the anterior bladder wall, and the bladder is inspected. The prostate tumor is enucleated by finger dissection and removed through the cavity of the bladder. Only the prostate tissue itself is cored and removed—the prostate capsule is not excised. The surgeon may need to place a finger in the rectum to push the prostate gland forward for easier dissection. A drain is placed; the bladder and abdominal incisions are closed.

After the procedure, a suprapubic catheter exits the bladder (on the bladder dome) and abdominal wall. The three-way urethral catheter also remains in the bladder.

Anesthetic

GETA can be given, and the patient may need muscle relaxation. Spinal or epidural anesthesia to T10 is the preferred anesthetic option.

Positioning

The patient is placed in a supine position.

Anesthetic Implications

IV fluids do not have to be kept at a minimum with this type of prostatectomy (as in the robotic-assisted prostatectomy) and can be given freely. A urethral catheter is not inserted until the end of the case; urine output is part of the fluids suctioned from the abdominal cavity during the surgery. These patients will have received a bowel prep and will be dehydrated.

Type and cross-match the patient's blood preoperatively, as moderate to large blood loss is possible.

The insertion of a central venous line may be important so that the filling pressure and fluid volumes can be monitored; urine cannot be measured with this approach.

Transrectal Seed Implantation (Interstitial Radiotherapy with Brachytherapy)

Brachytherapy refers to a form of radiotherapy where a radioactive source is placed inside or next to the area requiring treatment. In this case, it is used to treat prostate cancer.

Transrectal seed implantation is the ultrasound-guided permanent placement of radioactive seeds into the prostate gland. These seeds can deliver a much higher radiation dose to the prostate but with limited radius of penetration; thus this therapeutic approach produces only limited tissue injury surrounding the rectum and the bladder (as with external beam radiation).

Operative Procedure

Transrectal seed implantation is considered a radiation oncology treatment; it is an optional treatment for prostate cancer.

A urethral catheter is inserted into the bladder, the bladder is filled with sterile saline, and the drainage tubing is clamped to keep the bladder full. Contrast medium may also be instilled to allow the surgeon to visualize the bladder more clearly.

A probe (covered and lubricated) inserted into the rectum provides the surgeon with longitudinal and transverse views of the prostate. Measurements are taken, and the lead-lined needles are then inserted through the perineum into the midportion of the prostate. Seeds may be encased in lead-lined tubes that are attached to lead-lined placement needles. The seeds are permanently implanted directly into the prostate gland. Cystoscopy is done at the end of the case to remove any seeds placed inadvertently into the urethra or bladder. A urethral catheter is left in at the end of the case.

Fluoroscopy or ultrasound imaging may be used intraoperatively to assist the surgeon in needle positioning.

Anesthetic

Spinal block to T8 is used for single seed placement; an epidural is used for repeated procedures. This procedure can last two hours, so GETA may also be necessary.

Positioning

The patient is placed in a lithotomy position.

Anesthetic Implications

Patients will have received an enema (not a bowel prep).

One large-bore peripheral IV is usually all that is needed.

Some seeds may pass in the urine for the first few days. Urine must be strained for this reason, and any seeds retrieved should be returned to the oncologist.

Some seed types may already be embedded in a type of suture that allows them to remain positioned where placed by the surgeon. This practice minimizes seed movement and the risk of passing seeds in the urine.

A scrotal support strap is applied at the end of the case.

Special protection must be worn by operating room staff during transrectal seed implantation due to the risk of radiation exposure.

BLADDER AND URETHRA SURGERY

Bladder Augmentation (Augmentation Cystoplasty)

Bladder augmentation is a reconstructive surgery that seeks to increase the bladder reservoir capacity and lower the pressure within the bladder. It involves tissue grafts that are anastomosed to the bladder (ileum—ileocystoplasty; stomach—gastrocystoplasty; ureter—ureterocystoplasty), or other substitutes that are sewn to the urinary bladder.

This procedure is done in children and adults who have inadequate or abnormal bladder capacity or detrusor muscle compliance (the detrusor muscle pushes down during urination, helping to expel urine from the bladder). These problems may be due to neuropathic causes (e.g., multiple sclerosis, spina bifida/myelodysplasia, or spinal cord injury) or non-neuropathic causes (e.g., interstitial or radiation cystitis, bladder exstrophy, bladder obstruction, or detrusor instability).

Operative Procedure

A midline abdominal laparotomy incision is made for lower abdominal grafts (e.g., ileum, colon); the incision will extend to the xyphoid process for upper abdominal grafts (e.g., stomach). An incision is then made over the top and around the upper dome of the bladder. The graft is prepared (the portion of stomach, ileum, or other tissue is removed and repair is done to the graft site) and anastomosed to the dome. A drain is placed and the incisions closed in layers. A suprapubic catheter is placed and brought out through a small abdominal incision; a three-way urethral catheter is also placed into the bladder through the urethra for irrigation fluids.

Anesthetic

GETA and muscle relaxation are given. Children may have a caudal block placed at the end of the case for postoperative pain control. Adults may have an epidural catheter inserted preoperatively but not bolused until the end of the case.

Positioning

The patient is placed in a supine position.

Anesthetic Implications

These patients may have been on anticholinergic medications to help increase detrusor stability and decrease symptoms of urinary urgency. Urethral sphincter support may also have been employed (e.g., Botox or a piece of fascia placed around the urethra). Other procedures may be done in conjunction with bladder augmentation, including sling procedures, urethral lengthening, and ureteral reimplantation.

If any portion of the small or large intestine is used for augmentation, a nasogastric tube should be placed after induction of anesthesia.

This surgery can last from 4 to 8 hours, during which temperature loss is common. Upper- and lower-body warming blankets are needed as well as fluid warmers. The ambient temperature in the room may also need to be increased.

Simple Cystectomy

Simple cystectomy is the surgical removal of the bladder. It is done for benign conditions such as hemorrhagic or radiation cystitis.

Operative Procedure

A transverse or midline vertical incision is made in the lower abdomen. The bladder is separated from its surrounding tissues; nerves, arteries, and veins are identified and ligated, and the bladder is removed. An ileal conduit (urinary diversion) is then performed.

A partial cystectomy can be done if a lesion is localized at the dome of the bladder. *This does not require urinary diversion surgery.* The cancerous portion of the dome is excised and, if a small area is left open, the remaining walls of the bladder are anastomosed. A mucosal/tissue graft may be sewn to replace a larger piece of removed bladder wall.

Anesthetic
GETA and muscle relaxation are given. An epidural catheter can be placed preoperatively for postoperative pain control.

Positioning
The patient is placed in a supine position.

Anesthetic Implications
Type and cross-match the patient's blood and have two units of packed red cells available; this surgery carries a risk of moderate blood loss. Establish at least two large-bore peripheral IVs. A CVP may be needed to monitor fluid status, as a urethral catheter is not placed during simple cystectomy.

An arterial line may be needed based on patient history and due to the length of the surgery. These can be very long cases.

Keep these patients warm with fluid warmers and warming blankets. Increase the room temperature if necessary.

If a piece of colon is to be used as a graft, the patient will have received a bowel prep. These patients are also NPO for at least 8 hours (except for the bowel prep itself) and present with dehydration. They may also manifest hypovolemia, especially on anesthetic induction. Check CBC and electrolyte levels preoperatively, as these individuals may have electrolyte disturbances.

Radical Cystectomy: With or Without Pelvic Lymphadenectomy
Radical cystectomy is the removal of the urinary bladder, distal ureters, urethra, local lymph nodes, and other tissues that may contain cancer cells.

With a radical cystectomy in women, in addition to the anatomy listed previously, the uterus, cervix, fallopian tubes, ovaries, and a portion of the vagina are removed. The vagina may be packed at the end of the case to help prevent bleeding.

With a radical cystectomy in men, in addition to the anatomy listed previously, the ampulla of the vas deferens, prostate, and seminal vesicles may be removed.

Radical cystectomy is done to treat neurologic disorders, radiation injury (radiation cystitis), congenital defects, intractable infection, severe trauma, severe hemorrhage, and cancer in which the lesion has infiltrated the bladder wall with evidence of metastases. The depth of infiltration and overall condition of the patient will dictate the extent of the procedure (i.e., whether a pelvic lymphadenectomy is done).

Operative Procedure
Prior to a cystectomy, if it has not been done before, a permanent urinary diversion procedure is performed. The lymphadenectomy is carried out first so that the nodes can be sent off for frozen section. The bladder is loosened from the surrounding tissues; arteries, veins, and ligaments are transected and tied off; and the bladder and urethra are removed.

Anesthetic
GETA is given with insertion of an OETT; muscle relaxants are given. An epidural may be placed for postoperative pain control (to the T4 level). A combination of anesthetic techniques may be used.

Positioning
Male patients are placed in a supine position. Female patients are placed in a lithotomy position

while the urethra and bladder are mobilized; they are then moved into a supine position for a midline abdominal incision for the cystectomy.

Anesthetic Implications

Type and cross-match the patient's blood, and have at least two units of packed red cells available; the surgery carries a risk of moderate to severe blood loss.

These patients are NPO for at least 8 hours (except for the bowel prep itself) and present with dehydration. They may also manifest hypovolemia, especially on anesthetic induction. Check CBC and electrolyte levels preoperatively, as these individuals may have electrolyte disturbances.

Monitors and IV Access
- Two large-bore peripheral IVs
- Arterial line—usually necessary
- Central venous line—usually necessary to monitor fluid status

IV Fluids and Volume Requirements

Crystalloid and colloid IV infusions at a rate of 5–10 mL/kg/hr are used for maintenance and deficit fluid requirements. Monitor urinary output through a urostomy pouch.

Suprapubic Cystolithotomy

Suprapubic cystolithotomy is an open bladder procedure to remove bladder calculi (stones). It is performed when the patient has bladder calculi that cannot pass due to their size or owing to an obstruction.

Operative Procedure

A urethral catheter is inserted at the beginning of the procedure. Water or normal saline is instilled to distend the bladder and the catheter is clamped.

A transverse low abdominal suprapubic incision is made, and tissue is incised down to the urinary bladder. Two stay sutures are applied onto the anterior bladder wall; they are used to pull up and tent the bladder. A stab incision is made into the tented bladder wall, with the opening being enlarged as needed (based on the size of the stone). Forceps are used to grab the stone and remove it. The bladder is inspected for other pathology and then closed. A suprapubic catheter/drain is inserted to drain urine in combination with the urethral catheter.

Anesthetic

Anesthetic options consist of neuraxial (spinal) anesthesia or GETA with an OETT or LMA.

Positioning

The patient is placed in a supine position.

Anesthetic Implications

Suprapubic cystolithotomy is usually a very quick case.

Suprapubic Cystostomy

In suprapubic cystostomy, an opening is made into the bladder through a low abdominal incision. This procedure allows for urinary diversion to relieve obstruction or to allow a site more distal to the bladder to "rest" after, for example, vesicourethral anastomosis.

Operative Procedure

A low suprapubic incision is made. The bladder may be distended by clamping off a urinary catheter. The dome of the bladder is incised; a catheter is inserted and secured with absorbable sutures to obtain a watertight closure. The catheter exits the skin and is secured with a stitch.

Anesthetic

Anesthetic options include spinal anesthesia, topical anesthesia with sedation, and GETA with LMA.

Positioning

The patient is placed in a supine position.

Anesthetic Implications

Suprapubic cystostomy may be done either percutaneously or during a laparotomy.

Implantation of Sacral Nerve Stimulator

A neurostimulator may be implanted to help control an overactive bladder. Such a sacral nerve stimulator is used in people with urge incontinence caused by an overactive bladder, whose condition has not responded to medications or behavioral modification. The implanted neurostimulator sends mild electrical pulses to the sacral nerve, which influences the bladder control muscles. The effectiveness of the therapy is tested with an external device before the stimulator is actually implanted.

Operative Procedure

The neurostimulator is implanted under the skin in the upper buttock or under the skin in the abdomen. A lead is placed near the sacral nerve and then tunneled under the skin to the stimulator. Adjustments to the programming device can be made as needed at the physician's office.

Anesthetic

GETA; no muscle relaxants are given. Local anesthesia may also be used with IV sedation.

Positioning

The patient is placed in a prone or lateral decubitus position.

Anesthetic Implications

Sedation should be deepened when the surgeon is tunneling the lead to the neurostimulator, as this process is very stimulating.

Fluoroscopy is done with lead placement.

As after any implanted device, this patient should not have an MRI study after this surgery. In addition, the neurostimulator should be turned off before the patient undergoes any surgery where electrocautery is used.

Complications

Potential complications include infection, change in bowel function, and an unpleasant sensation during stimulation.

URINARY DIVERSIONS

Ileal Conduit Diversion (Noncontinent Diversion; Cutaneous Diversion)

To create a urinary diversion, an isolated intestinal conduit may be used to create a channel that connects both ureters to a surgically created stoma that exits the abdominal wall; an ostomy bag is attached to collect the urine. The most common conduit diversion is an ileal conduit (distal section of the small intestine; described here) but the conduit can also be made from a piece of the large intestine. Urinary diversion is appropriate in cases involving disease of the bladder or distal ureters necessitating their removal.

Operative Procedure

Ileal conduit diversion is performed in conjunction with a cystectomy. After an incision is made in the lower abdomen, the ureters are loosened from surrounding tissue and dissected from the bladder. A retroperitoneal tunnel is created so that the farthest ureter (usually the left ureter) can be brought over to the conduit.

A small urine reservoir is surgically created from a small segment (approximately 15 cm long) of ileum of the small intestine. The proximal end of the ileal conduit is sutured closed and secured to the posterior peritoneum to prevent movement; the distal end is brought up to the abdominal wall to form a stoma (right lower quadrant of the abdomen) and sutured to the skin. The ureters are implanted into the ileal segment. Stents are placed in both ureters to prevent them from closing. A drain is placed and the incision is closed. A urostomy pouch is applied.

Anesthetic

General anesthesia is given with insertion of an OETT; muscle relaxants are given.

Positioning

The patient is placed in a supine position, with arms extended on armboards.

Anesthetic Implications

Type and cross-match the patient's blood, as this surgery carries a risk of moderate blood loss.

A CVP and/or arterial line may be necessary based on the patient's history. Establish at least two large-bore peripheral IVs.

Ileal conduit diversion can be a very long surgery, and the potential for heat loss is very high. Keep this patient warm with upper- and lower-body warming blankets, fluid warmers, and other measures.

Contrast studies are done to look for anastomotic leakage or obstruction at the end of the case.

If the stoma can be catheterized by the patient to empty the reservoir, it is called a continent cutaneous reservoir.

Bladder Substitution Surgery (Continent Diversion)

Two types of internal continent reservoirs may be created, using a segment of the intestine or the stomach to create a storage pouch.

- *Abdominal diversion reservoir:* A pouch inside the abdomen connects directly to the stoma with a small opening. Both ureters are implanted into the pouch. No pouch is worn; the patient must catheterize the stoma several times every day and night.
- *Bladder substitution diversion:* A pseudo-bladder is constructed from a rectal reservoir. A piece of large intestine, with its blood supply intact, is sewn to resemble a pouch-shaped reservoir. Both ureters are implanted into the top of the pouch, whereas the urethra is implanted in the lowest part of the pouch. Stents are placed in the ureters. This type of bladder substitution allows for the collection of urine and helps the patient avoid having an

external appliance. It lets the patient urinate through the urethra normally; alternatively, the patient may have to empty the reservoir with a catheter through the native meatus. This is a longer, more difficult surgery than the abdominal diversion reservoir procedure, and there are more complications and longer hospitalizations with this type of diversion.

These patients are NPO for at least eight hours (except for the bowel prep itself) and present with dehydration. They may also manifest hypovolemia, especially on anesthetic induction. Check CBC and electrolyte levels preoperatively, as these individuals may have electrolyte disturbances.

Estimated blood loss (EBL) and urinary output is difficult to ascertain during bladder substitution surgery, as blood mixes with urine in such cases and is suctioned out from the abdominal cavity during the surgery. A CVP may be needed to monitor fluid status; an arterial line is usually inserted to monitor blood pressure and provide access for serial arterial blood gases and labs. At least two large-bore peripheral IVs should be established if a CVP is not placed.

SURGERY FOR URINARY INCONTINENCE
Slings

Creation of a sling is the surgical restoration of the genitourinary tissue/organ positioning in a woman. This procedure may be performed to treat female stress incontinence, urethral hypermobility, or intrinsic sphincter deficiency (ISD). The goal of this treatment is to create sufficient urethral compression to achieve bladder control and to provide support for a sagging urethra and/or bladder. Slings can be from the patient's own fascia, cadaveric fascia, or polypropylene mesh.

Operative Procedure

A cystoscopy is usually done throughout these procedures, with a suprapubic catheter being placed at the end of the case. If a vaginal incision is made, the vagina may be packed at the end of the case to help prevent bleeding.

Needle Suspension

The approach can be percutaneous or vaginally. Sutures are placed through the pubic skin or a vaginal incision into the anchoring tissues on each side of the bladder neck and tied to the fibrous tissue or pubic bone.

Percutaneous Approach

A pubovaginal sling is made of a strip of strong connective tissue taken from the patient's abdominal fascia. After infiltrating local anesthesia into the abdominal wall incision sites, an incision is made above the pubic bone and a strip of rectus fascia is harvested to make a sling. Another incision is made in the vaginal wall, through which the sling is grasped and adjusted around the bladder neck and the urethra. The sling is secured by two sutures loosely tied to each other above the pubic bone incision, thereby providing a hammock to support the bladder neck. The sling is positioned at the mid-urethra and allows the urethra to compress itself shut to hold back urine during coughing or laughing.

While synthetic mesh material can be used for the sling, it often causes urethral erosion.

Tension-Free Vaginal Tape

Tension-free vaginal tape is a synthetic mesh-like tape that is placed under the mid-urethra like a sling (called a pubourethral sling) to keep it in its normal position. This approach is performed under local anesthesia with IV sedation, spinal anesthesia, or GETA; it takes less than an hour to perform. Vaginal tape prevents urine leakage by reinforcing the ligaments and tissues that support the urethra. It provides support only when needed, creating a "tension-free" solution that reduces the risk of over-correction.

Transvaginal Anchor

A transvaginal anchor is a device that returns the urinary anatomy to its proper position and restores urinary function. A small incision is made in the vaginal wall. Two small tacks are placed in the pubic bone, and a sling is inserted into the vagina and attached to the tacks with sutures. This arrangement allows the bladder neck to be suspended to the pubic bone instead of utilizing abdominal fascia fixation. The sling supports the bladder, bladder neck, urethra, and urethral sphincter so urine can flow and be consciously controlled by the patient. This approach prevents Valsalva-induced tension on the suspension sutures.

Anesthetic

Spinal or epidural anesthesia may be used; GETA is another option. Local anesthetic and IV sedation may be preferred, as the surgeon may need for the patient to be able to cough on command during this surgery.

Positioning

The patient is placed in either a lithotomy or supine position.

Complications

Complications are rare during sling surgery, but may include bladder or pelvic visceral perforation, hematoma, bleeding, urinary retention, and infection.

Vesicourethral Suspension (Marshall-Marchetti-Krantz Procedure)

Vesicourethral suspension, also known as the Marshall-Marchetti-Krantz (MMK) procedure, involves the elevation and suspension into the pelvic space of the bladder neck and the proximal urethra by suturing paraurethral, vaginal tissue, and the pubococcygeal muscle to the back of the symphysis pubis. It differs from the sling procedure in that it can require an abdominal incision and retropubic dissection

Vesicourethral suspension is performed to treat urinary stress incontinence. In such cases, poor muscle tone of the perineal muscles causes the bladder to sag, creating an abnormal urethrovesical angle;

this phenomenon can cause urinary incontinence during coughing, sneezing, or physical activity.

Operative Procedure

Vaginal Approach

An incision is made into the anterior vaginal wall and extended to the urethra and the bladder. The anterior vaginal wall is fixed to the Cooper's ligament. If a vaginal incision is made, the vagina may be packed at the end of the case to help prevent bleeding.

Abdominal Approach

A low transverse suprapubic abdominal incision is made, and the bladder and urethra are dissected away from surrounding structures. Sutures are placed around the paraurethral tissue; these tissues are then pulled back into the pelvis. The free ends of the sutures are anchored to surrounding cartilage and the back of the symphysis pubic bone.

Vaginal Wall Sling

A part of the anterior vaginal wall is mobilized and used to support the vesicourethral segment.

When suturing the prevaginal connective tissue, the surgeon will place his or her hand in the vagina to make sure the suture needle does not enter the vagina and is not stitched closed.

Suspension alone may be inadequate; in many cases, sling procedures are also required.

Burch Retropubic Colposuspension

In the Burch retropubic colposuspension, the vagina and bladder neck are suspended to the lateral ligaments to treat urinary stress incontinence. This procedure is usually done when the abdomen is opened for another surgery, though it can also be done laparoscopically. The bladder neck and urethra are separated from their surrounding tissues. The bladder neck is then elevated by lateral sutures that pass through the vagina and Cooper's ligaments from each side.

Anesthetic

GETA is given with insertion of an OETT; muscle relaxants are given.

Positioning

The patient is placed in a lithotomy position, with arms extended on armboards bilaterally.

Anesthetic Implications

A urethral catheter will be placed.

Urinary Sphincters

Artificial urinary sphincters may be needed in cases involving urinary incontinence or birth defects affecting the urinary tract.

Operative Procedure

Artificial Prosthetic Urethral Sphincter

This urinary prosthetic device has three components: a pump, a balloon reservoir that is placed in the pelvis, and a single or double cuff that fits around the proximal urethra close to the bladder. All three components are filled with sterile saline.

Through a low transverse abdominal incision, the balloon reservoir is placed and secured under the abdominal rectus muscle. The pump is surgically implanted in the scrotum (in men) or in the lower belly, labia, or leg (in women). The urethra must be mobilized for cuff placement.

The cuff is deflated by squeezing or pressing a button connected to the pump. The fluid in the cuff empties into the reservoir, the urethra opens, and the bladder empties. Fluid from the reservoir returns to the cuff every 90 seconds automatically, which again closes the urethra.

Urethral Bulking Agents

An artificial urinary sphincter may also be created through simple periurethral injection of bulking material such as Teflon or collagen around the opening of the bladder.

Anesthetic

Anesthesia options include neuraxial (spinal) anesthesia and GETA.

Positioning

The patient is placed in a lithotomy position.

Anesthetic Implications

An artificial urinary sphincter is used only if a sling procedure cannot be done.

Complications

Potential complications include infection, tissue breakdown, and mechanical failure.

KIDNEY AND URETER SURGERY

Extracorporeal Shock Wave Lithotripsy

Lithotripsy is used to disintegrate kidney and urinary tract calculi. Extracorporeal shock wave lithotripsy (ESWL) is used for large, multiple stones, It breaks apart upper urinary tract calculi by means of precisely directed shock waves delivered to a patient (outside the body) immersed in a water bath. Disintegrated stones pass out of the patient's body in the urine. ESWL, which is considered to be first-generation lithotripsy, is a noninvasive procedure.

Human tissue has similar acoustical density and properties as water. These properties ensure that shock waves go through tissue with little change in impedance and little to no damage.

Operative Procedure

Multiple shock (sound) waves pass through the water into the body, pulverizing the calculus into sand-like particles that are eliminated via the urine. A calculi piece must be 2 mm or less in diameter to pass through urinary system. The actuation of the triggering mechanism by the EKG and respiratory motion may decrease the number of shock waves required and decreased radiation exposure.

Water-proofed EKG leads are imperative in ESWL, as the release of the shock waves must appropriately coincide with the cardiac cycle. The shock wave is set to be triggered 20 milliseconds after the R wave of the EKG—the absolute refractory period of the ventricle—to avoid ventricular or supraventricular arrhythmias. The timing of the shock is triggered 1:1 by the heart rate, or 1:2 if the heart rate is greater than 120 beats/min. The EKG leads should be placed so they are not in the shock wave's path.

If the stone is located in the proximal ureter, the bony structures may prevent visualization and impede the shock wave. In such a case, the surgeon may reposition the stone back into the kidney.

While there are more potential complications related to the bath-immersion method, some physicians believe that this lithotripsy technique ensures better stone fragmentation. These shock waves are more painful than the second-generation lithotripsy method, however, and may require general anesthesia. The pain felt is from the shock wave hitting the skin.

Anesthetic

Several anesthesia options are available. Intercostal blocks may be used with IV sedation. Alternatively, spinal/epidural anesthesia to the T6 level with IV sedation may be used; tape the epidural on the side of the patient's back away from shock path, and ensure that there are no air bubbles under tape. Finally, GETA may be given with insertion of an OETT. Intubation can be performed while the patient is on the stretcher before placing on the gantry stretcher.

Positioning

For the water-immersion technique, the patient is safety-strapped onto a gantry stretcher, which is then lowered into the immersion tub. The patient is positioned in the water so that the kidney stone lies exactly in the path of the machine's focal point of shock wave discharge. The shock generated passes fairly easily into the body tissues, and the energy is released when the stone is encountered, fragmenting it. The body can then expulse the fragments through the urinary tract.

The head of the gantry stretcher is elevated so that the patient's head never goes in the water.

Anesthetic Implications

An epidural catheter must be protected from the water. Keep it safe with a sterile 2 × 2 piece of gauze covered with a watertight plastic occlusive adhesive seal.

Taping the EKG leads on can help prevent them from becoming loose during water immersion. Keep EKG leads out of the sound wave path. The blood pressure cuff and oximeter connects should also stay out of water. A pulse oximeter should be placed on the patient's ear lobe, where it can remain out of the water. Use water wings to float the patient's arms.

Placing the patient in the water-immersion bath for lithotripsy increases SVR (decreasing cardiac output), venous return, and PA pressures. The CVP may increase by as much as 10–14 cm H_2O. Hypotension and a vagal response can occur due to vasodilation from the warm water, so have vasoactive bolus drugs and Robinul and/or atropine available and ready for use. The water pressure may affect the pulmonary system as well, decreasing FRC and vital capacity and causing a ventilation–perfusion (V/Q) mismatch.

Spontaneous respirations or full ventilatory breaths can lead to changes in the intrathoracic pressures causing the stone to move out of the shock wave's path; this would be counterproductive to successful treatment. Increasing the respiratory rate and lowering the tidal volume to maintain $ETCO_2$, or the use of high-frequency jet ventilation may be helpful in reducing stone movement and minimizing the number of shock waves needed to pulverize the stone.

X-ray or fluoroscopy is done in conjunction with ESWL.

The total number of shock waves required depends on the size, location, and composition of the stone as well as the patient's physique. While injury to renal structures is minimal with this technique, there is a limit to the number of shocks (maximum 2000/day for each kidney) that can be given in a 24-hour period. Be aware that hematuria and perirenal hematoma can occur with this technique.

Monitor the bath temperature carefully. If it is too cold, the patient may become hypothermic and vasoconstricted. Shivering can confound the EKG monitoring and render the wave generator ineffective; it also increases oxygen consumption. If the bath temperature is too warm, peripheral vasodilation can occur and the patient may become hypotensive.

Oral anticoagulants should be discontinued in enough time to allow normalization of clotting parameters. Antiplatelet therapy should be discontinued at least 7 days before the patient undergoes ESWL.

To shorten the procedure time, atropine or Robinul can be given (if there are no contraindications). These medications increase the heart rate, causing the shock waves to be fired faster.

ESWL is not performed in the operating room. Anesthesia providers should ensure that a ventilator and fully stocked anesthesia cart are available at the site to handle any situation or emergency that might arise.

The circuitry of a pacemaker or AICD can be damaged with ESWL. An AICD should be turned off before undergoing ESWL.

Hypothermia can occur if the bath water is too cold and when the patient is brought out of the immersion bath. Quickly dry and cover the patient with warm blankets.

Absolute contraindications to shock wave therapy include pregnancy, abnormal coagulation disorders, an active urinary tract infection or urosepsis, staghorn calculi, ureteral obstruction distal to the stone, body weight more than 275 pounds, and abdominal aortic aneurysm greater than 6 cm in size. *Relative contraindications* to shock wave therapy include small aortic aneurysm, spinal tumors, hemangioma in vertebral canal, uncontrolled arrhythmias, and metal instrumentation in lumbar area.

Extracorporeal Shock Wave Lithotripsy without Water Bath

Second-generation lithotripsy provides for the disintegration of upper urinary tract calculi (ureteral and renal) by means of precisely directed shock waves generated by an electromagnet through self-contained water-filled cushions; this method does not involve patient immersion into a water bath. The shock waves used with this variation of lithotripsy are lower in wattage and less painful than those used with first-generation (water-immersion) lithotripsy. Having the patient *not* lowered into a water bath also alleviates the physiologic changes associated with that process.

Operative Procedure
In this non-immersion technique, two X-rays (anterior and posterior views) are taken. These X-rays, along with fluoroscopic imaging capabilities, allow for precise low-pressure shock waves to break up urinary calculi without being painful to the patient.

Anesthetic
Sedation and MAC are used for the non-immersion lithotripsy technique.

Positioning
The patient is placed in a supine or prone position based on the stone location and the patient's body habitus.

Anesthetic Implications
Alert patients to the start of the shocks so they don't jump.

A ureteral stent may be placed to allow the fragments to pass easily and with less pain.

Electrohydraulic Lithotripsy
In this lithotripsy variant, fragmentation of urinary tract calculi found in the bladder is accomplished by means of electrohydraulic shock waves delivered via a probe inserted transcystoscopically. Electrohydraulic lithotripsy is considered a minimally invasive procedure.

Operative Procedure
Cystoscopy is performed. An electrohydraulic lithotripter is passed through the cystoscope and can produce a series of sharp, high-amplitude shock waves that fragment the bladder calculi.

These fragments may be eliminated in the urine or, if too large, retrieved with a grasper. These shock waves have no effect on the bladder wall because of its high tissue flexibility.

Anesthetic
IV sedation or GETA with insertion of an OETT.

Positioning
The patient is placed in a lithotomy position.

Anesthetic Implications
Saline solution irrigation is necessary.

Do not use an electrohydraulic lithotripter on any patient with a pacemaker or AICD.

Laser Lithotripsy
In this variant of lithotripsy, fragmentation of urinary tract calculi found in the ureter or bladder is accomplished by means of light from a holmium laser. Laser lithotripsy is considered a minimally invasive procedure.

Operative Procedure
A cystoscope, ureteroscope, or nephroscope is inserted. A thin fiberoptic catheter is inserted through the endoscope and advanced until it reaches the stone. Laser light then fragments or disintegrates the stone. Small fragments may be retrieved with a basket or, if very small, may be eliminated in the urine.

Anesthetic
Anesthesia options include neuraxial (spinal) anesthesia and IV sedation and local anesthetic. GETA may be required in some cases.

Positioning
The patient is placed in a lithotomy position.

Anesthetic Implications
All personnel in the room and the patient must use proper eye covering.

A ureteral stent may be placed to allow the fragments to pass easily and with less pain.

Ultrasonic Lithotripsy

In this variant of lithotripsy, fragmentation of urinary tract calculi found in the ureter or bladder is accomplished by means of ultrasonic waves. Ultrasonic lithotripsy is considered a minimally invasive procedure.

Operative Procedure

A cystoscope, ureteroscope, or nephroscope is inserted. A thin catheter is inserted through the endoscope and advanced until it reaches the stone. An ultrasound catheter is then advanced through the endoscope until it reaches the stone. The mechanical vibrations of the ultrasound fragment and pulverize the stone. Small fragments may be retrieved with a basket or, if very small, may be eliminated in the urine.

Anesthetic

Anesthesia options include neuraxial (spinal) anesthesia and IV sedation and local anesthetic. GETA may be required in some cases.

Positioning

The patient is placed in a lithotomy position.

Anesthetic Implications

A ureteral stent may be placed to allow the fragments to pass easily and with less pain.

Laparoscopic Nephrectomy

Laparoscopic nephrectomy involves the surgical removal of the kidney and the ureter. It may be performed either to remove a kidney for organ donation or to treat kidney cancer.

Operative Procedure

Three or four small incisions are made along the abdomen (start in midline abdomen and rotate out and down towards iliac crest) for laparoscopic trocar insertion. A pneumoperitoneum is created. Through these ports, the kidney to be removed is separated from its anatomic moorings. Once the kidney dissection is complete, a 3- to 4-inch midline incision is made to remove the kidney from the body.

Anesthetic

GETA and muscle relaxation are used. While the donor has healthy kidneys, their renal function is about to be decreased by half; thus it is important to avoid giving vasoconstrictors (e.g., phenylephrine).

Positioning

The patient is placed in a lateral decubitus position, with his or her waist over the middle break in the OR table. An axillary roll is placed.

Anesthetic Implications

Kidney donor patients should have donated several units of autologous blood several weeks before the surgery. The night before the surgery, the donor is hydrated with IV crystalloids to promote active diuresis. During the surgery, maintain donor urinary output at a rate of 1 mL/min or more. Mannitol and/or furosemide may need to be given. Heparin will be given IV before removal of the donor kidney to limit intrarenal clotting.

Strict aseptic precautions are needed with IV insertion, invasive monitoring, drug administration, airway management, and blood sampling.

Monitors and IV Access

An arterial line is standard, and a central line may be needed.

Open Nephrectomy

Open nephrectomy is the surgical removal of the kidney, along with the ureter. It is indicated in cases involving trauma, hydronephrosis, pyelonephritis, renal artery stenosis, renal atrophy, or kidney donation.

Operative Procedure

When a flank approach (i.e., incision from the 12th rib to the iliac crest) is used with the nephrectomy, a lower flank or inguinal incision is used to expose the distal ureter extraperitoneally. The kidney and ureter are mobilized; the ureter is divided and the distal end ligated. The distal ureter is dissected free of surrounding tissues, and a small cuff of the bladder is excised with the intramural portion of the ureter. The kidney is brought out; the bladder incision is repaired. A suprapubic catheter may be placed. A drain is placed and the incision is closed.

Anesthetic

GETA is given with insertion of an OETT; muscle relaxants are given. A rapid-sequence induction is needed if the patient is in renal failure or has delayed gastric emptying.

Positioning

The patient is placed in a supine position for an abdominal approach; he or she is placed in a lateral decubitus position, with an axillary roll, for a flank approach. The patient's waist should be placed over the middle break in the OR table.

Anesthetic Implications

Preoperative Measures

Check the patient's H&H, potassium, blood glucose, PT/INR/PTT, BUN and creatinine, and platelet levels. If the patient is on dialysis, clarify when the patient had the last dialysis treatment; it should have been done with 24 hours of surgery to maximize fluid withdrawal and electrolyte stability.

Monitors and IV Access
- An arterial line is usually needed.
- A central venous line may be needed.
- At least two large-bore peripheral IVs are needed to deliver crystalloids/colloids and/or blood products if a CVL is not placed.

IV Vasoactive Agents
- IV pump: renal-dose (2–3 mcg/kg/min) dopamine infusion

- Syringe for bolus: mannitol, furosemide for maintaining urinary output

IV Fluids and Volume Requirements

Use of colloids helps to keep the crystalloid amounts required to a minimum, as evaporative losses are minimal with colloids. Avoid use of lactated Ringer's solution, as it may increase potassium levels. If the patient is in renal failure, hang the crystalloid IVF bag on microdrip tubing.

Induction

Do not use succinylcholine if the patient is in renal failure and has an elevated potassium. Give atricurium or cisatricurium for muscle paralysis. Propofol and etomidate are metabolized by the liver and excreted in the urine.

Radical Nephrectomy

Radical nephrectomy is the removal of a kidney, adrenal gland, ureter, fascia, and surrounding fat and lymph node tissue. It is performed in cases involving malignant disease of the kidney.

Operative Procedure

An abdominal or flank approach (transperitoneal or anterior retroperitoneal) is used. A transthoracic approach with rib resection may be necessary for large upper-pole lesions. The surgeon will tie off all renal arteries and veins before manipulating the organ to prevent blood loss and malignant cell cascade to the rest of the body. A lymphadenectomy is usually done on lymph nodes surrounding the affected kidney.

Anesthetic

GETA is given with insertion of an OETT; muscle relaxants are given.

Positioning

The patient is placed in a supine position for the abdominal approach; he or she is placed in a lateral decubitus position, with an axillary roll, for the flank approach. The patient's waist should placed over the middle break in the OR table.

Anesthetic Implications

This surgery may render the patient dependent on hemodialysis postoperatively. Check with the surgeon as to which arm will be used for hemodialysis access, if it is not already in place.

Moderate blood loss is possible with this surgery. Type and cross-match the patient's blood, and have two units of packed red blood cells available. Note that tumor can be present in vessels that may experience bleeding/blood loss issues.

Preoperative Measures

Check the patient's H&H, potassium, blood glucose, PT/INR/PTT, BUN and creatinine, and platelet levels. If the patient is on dialysis, clarify when the patient had the last dialysis treatment; it should have been done within 24 hours of surgery to maximize fluid withdrawal and electrolyte stability.

Monitors and IV Access

- An arterial line is usually needed.
- A central venous line may be needed.
- At least two large-bore peripheral IVs should be established for crystalloids/colloids and/or blood products.

IV Vasoactive Agents

- IV pump: renal-dose (2–3 mcg/kg/min) dopamine infusion
- Syringe for bolus: mannitol, furosemide for maintaining urinary output

IV Fluids and Volume Requirements

Use of colloids helps to keep the crystalloid amounts needed to a minimum, as evaporative losses are minimal with colloids. Avoid use of lactated Ringer's solution, as it may increase potassium levels. If the patient is in renal failure, hang the crystalloid IVF bag on microdrip tubing.

Induction

Do not use succinylcholine (Anectine) if the patient is in renal failure or has an elevated serum potassium. Give atricurium or cisatricurium for muscle paralysis. Propofol and etomidate are metabolized by the liver and excreted in the urine.

Kidney Nephrostomy: Ureteral or Percutaneous

Kidney nephrostomy is the aspiration or drainage of pus in the renal pelvis. It is also done to remove kidney or proximal ureteral stones.

Operative Procedure

A stent or drainage tube can be placed percutaneously or cystoscopically into the ureter.

For the *cystoscopic approach,* a guide wire is inserted into the ureteral orifice. The stent is advanced over the wire up to the renal pelvis, where the stent is positioned.

For the *percutaneous approach,* a stab wound is made at the costovertebral angle. A drainage tube is then introduced into the kidney under fluoroscopic guidance.

Anesthetic

Spinal or epidural anesthesia with sedation is usually used. Some patients may require general anesthesia with insertion of an OETT or LMA.

Positioning

The patient is placed in a lithotomy position for ureter placement; he or she is placed in a prone or lateral decubitus position for percutaneous placement.

Anesthetic Implications

X-ray or fluoroscopy is used during this procedure.

Patients presenting for a kidney nephrostomy procedure may be very sick from the kidney infection. They may have been through multiple procedures that were not successful in remedying the underlying illness.

Complications

Bladder or ureteral perforation is possible during this procedure.

Pyelolithotomy, Nephrolithotomy, and Ureterolithotomy

These procedures involve removal of calculi from the ureter, renal pelvis, and kidney:

- Pyelolithotomy: renal pelvis stones
- Nephrolithotomy: renal parenchyma stones
- Ureterolithotomy: proximal ureter stones

These lithotomy variants may be used if lithotripsy (extracorporeal shock wave, laser, or ultrasonic) treatments have been unsuccessful.

Operative Procedure
Proximal Calculi

A flank incision is made, with rib resection also being possible. Blood flow to the kidney may need to be temporarily interrupted (by occluding the main vessels atraumatically) if stones are present in the renal parenchyma. Stones in the renal pelvis or in the proximal ureter are extracted through incisions overlying the stones. A clamp is placed over the distal ureter to occlude it, thereby preventing migration of stone fragments. The collecting system is irrigated and sutured closed.

Distal Calculi

These calculi are approached retroperitoneally by inguinal, lower midline abdominal, or transverse oblique incision. Control of the ureter distal and proximal to the stone is done with clamps. An incision is made in the ureter and the stone retrieved.

If the surgeon can palpate the calculus, he or she may inject a mixture of calcium chloride, thrombin, and cryoprecipitate to form a clot around the calculus and prevent its migration. The incision is made over the affected anatomy; the stone is then manipulated so that it can be removed.

Percutaneous Nephrolithotomy

A fiberoptic nephroscope is inserted into the kidney through a small flank incision.

Anesthetic
GETA is given. Some patients may need muscle relaxants.

Positioning
The patient is placed in a lateral decubitus position for removal of proximal calculi. He or she is placed in a supine position for removal of distal calculi.

Anesthetic Implications
Euvolemia may occur owing to the additional IV fluid given to flush the kidney.

Ureterectomy

Ureterectomy is the excision of all or part of a ureter. It is performed to treat ureteral and/or renal pelvic cancer.

Operative Procedure
A *partial* ureterectomy preserves existing urinary function. It can be done if the cancer has not spread to the surrounding tissues. In a segmental ureterectomy, the diseased portion of the ureter is removed, with the opened ends then being reanastomosed. If the cancer is confined to the distal ureter, it is resected and the remaining ureter anastomosed to the bladder.

In a *radical* ureterectomy, the entire ureter is removed, usually in conjunction with the removal of other tissues and organs.

Ureterectomy can be done as a laparoscopic or laparoscopic-assisted robotic procedure.

Anesthetic
GETA and muscle relaxation are given.

Positioning
The patient is placed in a supine position, with bilateral arms either extended or tucked.

Anesthetic Implications
A ureterectomy is usually done in conjunction with the removal of other uro-renal structures, such the kidney and upper bladder.

Cutaneous Ureterostomy

Cutaneous ureterostomy establishes a ureteral stoma on the abdominal wall for urinary diversion.

It is performed in cases of distal ureteral obstruction caused by tumor, radiation injury, fibrosis, or intractable infection. The ureterostomy is usually temporary, as the stoma may later be incorporated into an ileal-loop conduit or the affected ureter anastomosed to the opposite ureter (ureter-oureterostomy).

Operative Procedure

The affected ureter is exposed and dissected free as distally as possible. It is then brought out to the stoma site and sutured to the abdominal skin. A urostomy pouch is placed.

Anesthetic

GETA is given with insertion of an OETT.

Positioning

The patient is placed in a supine position, with the arms extended on armboards.

Anesthetic Implications

One large-bore peripheral IV is usually all that is needed.

DIALYSIS ACCESS

See the discussions of arteriovenous (AV) fistulas and shunts and venous access to dialysis catheters in Chapter 22.

Peritoneal Dialysis Catheter Placement

This procedure involves the surgical placement of a dialysis catheter (known as a Tenckhoff catheter) for peritoneal dialysis (PD). Peritoneal dialysis seeks to establish a balance of electrolytes and remove metabolites from the body in patients who are experiencing chronic renal failure or insufficiency. This technique uses the peritoneal membrane as the dialyzing membrane.

Operative Procedure

Placement of a PD catheter is usually done by laparoscopic approach. Laparoscopic trocars are inserted into the abdomen. A dialysis catheter is then inserted into the peritoneal cavity of the abdomen, typically near the naval. This process can be complicated by adhesions or prior infections in the abdomen, which may cause the patient to experience increased pain and bleeding.

Anesthetic

PD catheter placement can be done under local anesthetic and sedation if not done laparoscopically. General anesthesia with insertion of an OETT is needed for laparoscopy. Rapid-sequence induction should be done to avoid problems with renal failure–associated gastroparesis.

Positioning

The patient is placed in a supine position.

Anesthetic Implications

The most stimulating portion of PD catheter placement is when the peritoneum is entered and during tunneling of the catheter. Deepen sedation before this part of the surgery is performed.

PD uses hyperosmolar glucose solutions (ranging from 4% to 25%). This solution pulls large amounts of fluid from the cells; it is essential to check patients' glucose levels frequently. Observe patients for an insulin reaction or hyperglycemia after dialysis.

It is essential to maintain the sterility of the catheter, as the risk of catheter infection and peritonitis is very high with PD.

Monitor patients' vital signs, abdominal girth, and mental status during PD.

Phases of Peritoneal Dialysis

- Inflow time: dialysis fluid enters the peritoneal cavity.
- Dwell time: diffusion phase; extra fluid and waste diffuse across the membrane from the underlying blood vessels into the dialysis fluid. The longest phase of PD, dwell time lasts several hours.
- Outflow time: fresh fluid is replaced back into the peritoneal cavity. Two liters is kept in the

abdomen at all times. During this phase, which lasts approximately 20 minutes, healthcare providers must monitor and measure outflow.

Types of Peritoneal Dialysis

- Continuous ambulatory peritoneal dialysis (CAPD): outlined above. PD is usually completed 4–6 times per day.
- Continuous cycling peritoneal dialysis (CCPD), also known as automated peritoneal dialysis (APD): a machine fills and drains the dialysate automatically while the patient is sleeping. Cycles occur so that there are 3–10 dwells per night. This process takes approximately 10 hours.

Complications

Potential complications include less predictable fluid removal, access complications such as peritonitis and catheter infection, reduced diaphragmatic compliance, decreased functional residual capacity, and fluid retention. PD is less efficient at removing wastes from the body than hemodialysis but does allow for greater mobility and fewer symptoms.

TRANSPLANTATION

Kidney Transplant Donor

In this procedure, a healthy kidney is removed for donation purposes.

Operative Procedure

This procedure can be done laparoscopically. See the discussion of laparoscopic nephrectomy earlier in the chapter for more information.

In an *open* procedure, a lateral flank incision is made; the kidney, artery, vein, and ureter are identified and ligated. The organ is removed and immediately taken to a waiting recipient, who is in a nearby operating room.

Anesthetic

General anesthesia is given with insertion of an OETT. While the donor has healthy kidneys, their renal function will be decreased by half; thus it is important to avoid the use of vasoconstrictors (e.g., phenylephrine).

Positioning

The patient is placed in a lateral decubitus position. The table is flexed upward, with kidney rest up. An axillary roll is placed.

Anesthetic Implications

Donors are usually young and healthy.

The donor should have donated several units of autologous blood several weeks before the surgery.

The night before the surgery, the donor is hydrated with IV crystalloids to promote active diuresis. During the surgery, maintain donor urinary output at a rate of 1 mL/min or more. Mannitol and/or furosemide may need to be given.

Heparin will be given IV before removal of the donor kidney to limit intrarenal clotting.

Strict aseptic precautions are needed with IV insertion, invasive monitoring, drug administration, airway management, and blood sampling.

Monitors and IV Access

An arterial line is standard, and a central line may be needed.

Kidney Transplant Recipient

A kidney transplant patient may receive either a cadaveric or live-donor kidney, in either a laparoscopic or open procedure. Kidney transplants are performed in patients with various forms of end-stage renal disease, including chronic pyelonephritis, polycystic kidney disease, renal trauma, and glomerulonephropathy. They are intended to replace renal dialysis after chronic renal failure. These patients are usually uremic and acidotic; they have electrolyte abnormalities and fluid overload.

Operative Procedure

Immunosuppression is started in the preoperative area.

The donor kidney is placed outside the peritoneal cavity in the right or left iliac fossa.

Regarding the new kidney, the surgeon first performs venous anastomosis to the recipient's external iliac vein, followed by arterial anastomosis to the external iliac artery. Next, the donor ureter is implanted directly into the recipient's bladder. The surgeon also needs to sew on three other veins: renal, gonadal, and inferior phrenic.

After the new kidney is completely connected, the surgeon usually orders Lasix (furosemide) 1 mg/kg, mannitol 1 g/kg, and methylprednisolone 1 g to be given and the systolic blood pressure maintained at 140 mm Hg. It may take a while for the new kidney to start making urine, however.

Anesthetic

General anesthesia is given with insertion of an OETT. Muscle relaxants are given, maintain twitches to ½ twitch out of four (moving is disastrous). A rapid-sequence induction should be done, as these patients have delayed gastric emptying and increased abdominal pressures.

The time of vessel anastomosis is not very stimulating, so the patient's blood pressure may decrease during this part of the surgery. Decrease anesthetic agents to prevent hypotension.

An epidural catheter is placed for postoperative pain control.

Positioning

The patient is placed in a jack-knife position, with either the left or right side up (according to the operative side).

Anesthetic Implications

Clarify when the patient had the last hemodialysis treatment; it should have been done within 24 hours of surgery to maximize fluid withdrawal and electrolyte stability. Reconfirm the preoperative laboratory data, especially the patient's potassium and hematocrit levels.

Preoperative Measures

Assess and document the active arteriovenous fistulas.

Monitors and IV Access

An arterial line is required.

A central line is usually needed. The goal is to have CVP at approximately 10 mm Hg upon unclamping of the vessels; this rate allows for good perfusion.

Peripheral IV access is usually limited due to the patient's chronic dialysis. Do not establish an IV, take blood samples, or measure a blood pressure on an extremity with a fistula, as it may be necessary to do hemodialysis postoperatively. Do not use a dialysis catheter without a direct order from the surgeon/dialysis physician.

IV Fluids and Volume Requirements

Use of colloids helps to keep the crystalloid amounts needed to a minimum. If the donated kidney does not work, the body will have no way to get rid of any excess surgical IV fluid.

When infusing maintenance crystalloids, use hypotonic crystalloid solutions: D_5W or $D_{5½}$ NS. Replacement fluids may consist of 0.9% NS—but this fluid can increase sodium levels. Avoid use of lactated Ringer's solution, as it may increase the patient's potassium levels. Any crystalloid should be delivered via microdrip tubing. In general, limit the volume of fluids given.

The anesthesia goal is to maintain a high perfusion pressure throughout the surgery by maintaining a slightly higher than normal mean arterial pressure. Urinary output should be maintained at a rate of 1 mL/min or more. Give mannitol or furosemide as necessary.

Treat hypotension with vasopressors early, these patients cannot handle hydration measures. Do *not* used alpha agents to treat blood pressure abnormalities. The goal is to maintain a stable blood pressure in the normal to slightly elevated range for better perfusion—for example, SBP in the range of 130–140 mm Hg.

The new kidney's function will vary depending on the ischemic time—that is, the length of time between clamping and removal from the donor to the time of vascular anastomosis in the recipient.

When this process lasts less than 30 minutes, rapid diuresis may occur; in contrast, with ischemic times greater than 2 hours, oliguria or anuria can occur.

Once the kidney vessels are connected in the recipient, a flood of ischemic by-products and preservative fluid will be washed out into the circulation. This shock to the system can cause sudden hypotension and increased peak inspiratory pressure. This side effect is generally short-lived but you may need to give a bolus of ephedrine (sympathomimetic) to maintain systolic blood pressure.

Keep the patient warm by using warming blankets and fluid warmers.

Preoperatively, the patient's potassium level should be less than 5.5 mEq/L. Preoperative dialysis should be performed, with packed red blood cells given to minimize anemia. Also, coagulation studies, including platelets, PTT, PT, and INR, should be within normal limits prior to surgery. Mannitol is often used in transplant protocols and should be considered with volume assessment.

Immunosuppressants are an essential part of preventing rejection of the donor kidney.

Type and cross-match the patient's blood preoperatively, and have two units of blood available in the operating room. Note that uremic patients' hematocrit levels are usually in the range of 18–24 g/dL.

Strict aseptic precautions are needed with IV insertion, invasive monitoring, drug administration, airway management, and blood sampling.

GYNECOLOGICAL SURGERY PEARLS

- Preoperative H&H, potassium, and glucose lab values are blood tests commonly performed before gynecological surgery.
- Patients will most likely have a straight catheter placed to drain urine at the beginning of gynecological surgery.
- Have gynecological patients void before surgery if a urethral catheter will not be inserted intraoperatively.
- Perform a human chorionic gonadotropin (HCG) test—a pregnancy test—on all women of childbearing age prior to surgical procedures, but especially when surgery is done on the uterus or surrounding structures.
- A common position in gynecological surgery is the lithotomy position, which requires special considerations (see Chapter 2). Special vigilance is needed regarding hand and finger placement when lowering or raising the foot of the bed. The legs should be carefully placed in sling or boot stirrups to prevent nerve damage or vascular changes; this precaution is necessary in either low or high lithotomy.
- A spinal or epidural neuraxial block for gynecological procedures is done to level T10—usually the only level needed for gynecological surgery.
- A vasovagal reaction can occur in response to traction on the uterus or with cervical dilation. Atropine and Robinul should be available.
- A sterilization consent form may need to be signed by the patient if sterilization is planned or if there is any risk of surgical sterilization with the surgery.

POSTOPERATIVE NAUSEA AND VOMITING

The following characteristics are associated with increased risk of PONV following gynecological surgery:

- Female
- Motion sickness history
- Nonsmoker

- Anxiety
- Surgery length greater than 45–60 minutes

PREEMPTIVE ANALGESIA

- Gabapentin (Neurontin) 1200 mg PO × 1
- Celecoxib (Celebrex) 400 mg PO × 1
- Acetaminophen (Tylenol) 1000 mg PO × 1 (Do not exceed 4000 mg of acetaminophen in 24 hours, from all sources. In patients with liver impairment or chronic liver disease, acetaminophen intake should not exceed 2000 mg in 24 hours.)

DRUGS TO HAVE AVAILABLE FOR GYNECOLOGICAL SURGERY

Oxytocics

Oxytocic agents improve uterine contractility and decrease bleeding by stimulation of smooth muscle.

- Pitocin (oxytocin): 10–40 units/1L bag; 10 units/mL in vial. A recommended ratio is 20 units per 1 L crystalloid solution. If severe bleeding continues or the uterus is not contracting sufficiently, give 40 units/L.
- Methylergonovine maleate (Methergine): 0.2 mg IM given to contract uterus and decrease bleeding. Can cause hypertension and myocardial ischemia.
- Prostaglandin 200–500 mcg IM or intramyometrially.

Tocolytics

Tocolytic agents decrease uterine contractility, thereby preventing preterm labor.

- Ritodrine (Yutopar): 0.05–0.1 mg/min IV
- Terbutaline (Brethine): 2.5–10 mcg/min IV
- Magnesium sulfate: loading dose, 4–6 g in 100 mL IV bag over 20 min; maintenance dose, 2–4 g/hr

IV Dyes

- Methylene blue: 0.1–0.2% mL/kg IV slow push. An indicator IV dye used to test the patency of the ureters or in hysterosalpingogram. While it is a treatment for methemoglobinemia, methylene blue can cause anemia or make methemoglobinemia worse.
- Indigo carmine: 40 mg indigotindisulfonate in water for injection; 5 mL ampule given IV to detect patent ureters. Used with a cystoscope in place. Indigo carmine is the preferred medication due to its small risk of side effects; usually only a mild pressor effect is observed.

Elimination of either dye begins soon after injection, with the dye appearing in the urine within 10 minutes in average cases. The half-life is 4 to 5 minutes following IV injection. Larger quantities are necessary when IM injection is employed. Appearance time and elimination are delayed following intramuscular injection.

VULVA SURGERY

Excision of Condylomata Acuminata

Condylomata acuminata, also known as genital warts, are caused by infection with human papillomavirus (HPV); HPV is transmitted by direct genital contact during sexual activity. The most common types of HPV to infect the anogenital tract are HPV-6, HPV-11, HPV-16, and HPV-18; more than 90% of condylomas are caused by HPV-6 and HPV-11, the "low-risk" HPV types. A vaccine has been developed against these four most common types of HPV.

Condylomas may be associated with dysplasia and/or cervical, vaginal, and anal cancer. Small, pinkish, raised growths, they sometimes have a cauliflower-like appearance and appear externally on the genitalia, in the anal area, internally in the vaginal vault, or cervix.

Operative Procedure

Condylomas can be removed using cold (cryotherapy or liquid nitrogen), heat, or excision by a scalpel or carbon dioxide laser vaporization. The type of excision is based on the type and extent of the lesions; wide local excision of the vulva is frequently done. After local anesthetic is infiltrated at the base of the lesions, the condylomas are removed. Antibiotic ointment is placed over the excised sites.

Anesthetic

A local anesthetic is used along with IV sedation. For excision of large numbers of condyloma or if lesions are larger than 2 cm, GETA is usually necessary.

Positioning

The patient is placed in a lithotomy position.

Anesthetic Implications

If laser ablation of genital warts is done, all personnel should wear special facemasks to protect against inhalation of aerosolized HPV.

There is also risk of fire with a laser procedure. See Chapter 1 on safety concerns for more information.

NSAIDs may be given intravenously to supplement other pain management measures.

Simple Vulvectomy

Simple vulvectomy is the surgical resection of both the labia majora and the labia minora of the vulva. The protective hood of the clitoris (glans clitoris) and perianal tissue may also be removed.

This procedure is performed in cases involving cancerous lesions of the vulva. Such lesions are often linked to condylomata acuminata (HPV infection), which can lead to cancer of the vulva and vagina.

Operative Procedure

Usually an area 2 cm outside the tumor margin is excised. A frozen section may be sent to the pathology lab during surgery to confirm the HPV infection diagnosis. A simple vulvectomy may be a bilateral procedure.

Anesthetic

Usually GETA is given, although spinal anesthesia with IV sedation is another option.

Positioning

The patient is placed in a lithotomy position.

Anesthetic Implications

NSAIDs can be given intravenously to help with postoperative pain control.

There is potential for significant blood loss with this procedure, so at least a type and screen of the patient's blood should be performed preoperatively.

Radical Vulvectomy with Groin Lymphadenectomy

Radical vulvectomy is the surgical resection of the bilateral labia minora and majora from the perineum to an upper margin of the mons pubis (circumferential incision), outward to the iliac crests, including the bilateral inguinal/femoral regions. The clitoris, mons pubis, distal portions of the urethra, and vagina may also need to be excised. This procedure may be done using one encompassing incision, or vulva and groin incisions may be done separately. It can be unilateral or bilateral.

Indications for radical vulvectomy include invasive vulvar carcinoma that has not metastasized. This condition is often linked to condylomata acuminata (HPV infection), which can lead to cancer of the vagina.

Operative Procedure

A low transverse abdominal incision is made over the symphysis pubis bone. The sentinel nodes are examined first. A frozen section is sent to the pathology lab to confirm and ensure clear margins (usually an area of tissue 2 cm beyond the tumor margin is taken) if metastasis is not found. If metastasis is identified, a full, deep pelvic lymph node dissection is done.

The vulvar and perineal resection is done and the tissue is sent to the pathology lab for analysis.

Reconstruction of the vaginal walls and pelvic floor is done. Different types of tissue flaps can be used, including gracilis myocutaneous flap, inferiorly based transverse rectus abdominis (TRAM) flap, and omentum and delayed skin grafting.

Meticulous hemostasis is achieved; drains are placed and the incision line(s) closed. One or more skin or myocutaneous grafts may be necessary.

A urethral catheter is inserted at the end of the case.

Anesthetic
GETA is used. An epidural may be placed for postoperative pain control.

Positioning
The patient is placed in a lithotomy position.

Anesthetic Implications
Type and cross-match the patient's blood preoperatively. There is a moderate risk of blood loss with this procedure, as the genitalia and perineum are very vascular. There is also a risk for femoral vessels to be compromised if the inguinal/femoral regions are resected.

Because these tissues are quite vascular, maintaining a slight decrease in the mean arterial blood pressure (MAP of approximately 60–70 mm Hg) can help to minimize bleeding.

An arterial line and/or central venous line may be needed, depending on the patient's condition.

Patients will have received a bowel prep and be dehydrated. Consider giving albumin/hetastarch fluid boluses along with a crystalloid infusion.

VAGINAL APPROACH
Conization and Biopsy of Cervix
Conization is the excision of a cone-shaped wedge of tissue at the cervix—specifically, at the cervical os. *Cold* conization refers to scalpel and scissor excision (also known as a "cold-knife" procedure), plus cryosurgery. *Hot* conization refers to the use of electrocautery or laser. (Also, see the discussion of loop electrosurgical excision procedures [LEEP] later in this chapter.)

Conization removes abnormal cells of the cervix, which are then analyzed (biopsy). This procedure is performed to diagnose or treat cervical dysplasia or cancer of the cervix (carcinoma in situ [CIS]).

Operative Procedure
A dilation and curettage (D&C) procedure may be performed before the conization.

- *Cryosurgery:* freezing technique with liquid nitrogen or carbon dioxide to ablate (destroy, rather than cut away) abnormal cervical tissue.
- *Excision:* scalpel or scissor dissection; LEEP procedure.
- *Laser:* high-energy light to ablate the tissue. General anesthesia is typically used with this technique to make sure the patient holds absolutely still during the laser portion of the procedure.

Cryosurgery and laser dissection are both considered ablation techniques. Thus, a biopsy cannot be taken with these methods, as the tissue is destroyed during the ablation. Excision procedures allow the taking of a tissue sample for pathology examination.

Anesthetic
Anesthesia options include sedation with local anesthesia or neuraxial block to T10. Usually local anesthesia with sedation is all that is needed in conjunction with a paracervical or intracervical block. Alternatively, general anesthesia may be used with an endotracheal tube or LMA if the patient is not pregnant. If the patient is pregnant, she is considered to have a full stomach and requires rapid-sequence induction if general anesthesia is used.

Positioning
The patient is placed in a lithotomy position. A slight Trendelenburg position may also be helpful. The patient's arms are extended on armboards bilaterally.

Anesthetic Implications

There is a fire risk if a laser is used. See Chapter 1 on safety concerns for more information.

If the patient is pregnant, a more superficial wedge of the cervical os is removed, as there is an increased risk of bleeding due to the increased vascularity of the pregnant uterus and cervix.

A local anesthetic and epinephrine solution may be injected around the cervix before an incision is made to decrease swelling and to prevent bleeding. Watch for an increase in heart rate or blood pressure or EKG changes during infiltration.

Colporrhaphy: Anterior and/or Posterior

Colporrhaphy is the surgical repair of a defect in the vaginal wall. It provides for reinforcement of musculofascial support anteriorly in case of bladder prolapse (cystocele), posteriorly in case of rectal prolapse (rectocele), and the upper wall of the vagina in case of small intestine prolapse (enterocele). These defects can push against the wall of the vagina or can come out and through the opening of the vagina.

This surgery is done to prevent protrusion of the bladder, intestine, and/or rectum into the vaginal space. Such prolapse typically occurs in women who have had multiple vaginal births, have decreased estrogen levels, are obese, have chronic constipation, had undergone an inadequate episiotomy, or do strenuous work. Colporrhaphy can be performed in conjunction with other procedures, including vaginal hysterectomy.

A *cystocele* (protrusion of the bladder into the anterior vagina due to a defect in the pubocervical fascia that separates the bladder and vagina) may present with urinary retention and stress incontinence. In this case, colporrhaphy seeks to restore the urethrovesical angle and give the bladder adequate support.

A *rectocele* (protrusion of the rectum into the posterior vagina) can present with difficulties in defecation. The rectum may have torn from the fascial and muscular attachment of the pelvic wall; the levator ani muscles can become stretched or torn. Several layers of sutures are placed to plicate the pararectal fascia to allow reduction of the rectocele.

An *enterocele* (herniation of small intestine through the vagina, due to tearing of the fascia and muscles of female pelvic floor) can result in uterine prolapse. This is a defect in the myofascial layer of the posterior vaginal wall.

Operative Procedure

A speculum is inserted into the vagina. An incision is made into the vagina over the prolapse. The vaginal mucosa is separated from the fascia, and the defect is folded over (plicated) and sutured; mesh may be placed to help reinforce the fascia and muscle layer. A urethral or suprapubic catheter is placed, and vaginal packing is placed at the end of the case to reduce bleeding.

Anesthetic

A spinal to the T10 sensory level with sedation. Alternatively, GETA and an OETT may be used.

Positioning

The patient is placed in a dorsal lithotomy position, with the arms extended on armboards bilaterally.

Anesthetic Implications

Give patients prophylactic antiemetics in an effort to avoid PONV (see Chapter 4).

NSAIDs may be given intravenously to supplement other pain management measures (see Chapter 4).

Colpotomy (Culdotomy; Vaginotomy)

In colpotomy, an incision is made into the vagina to visualize pelvic structures, remove or biopsy pelvic cysts or masses, or perform surgery on the fallopian tubes or ovaries. This procedure is performed to check for intraperitoneal bleeding, obtain access to the ovaries (e.g., for aspiration of ovarian cysts), perform tubal sterilization, remove an intrauterine device (IUD) that has migrated to an extrauterine location, perform myomectomy, or as part of a vaginal hysterectomy.

Operative Procedure

An incision is made into the posterior wall of the vagina and advanced into the peritoneum behind the cervix. The cul-de-sac is explored; the *cul-de-sac* refers to the rectouterine pouch (pouch of Douglas), which lies between the back wall of the uterus and the rectum. After the procedure, the peritoneum and the vagina are sutured closed. A urethral catheter and vaginal packing may be inserted.

Culdoscopy is the endoscopic visualization of the peritoneal space, so as to provide visualization of pelvic structures through an incision into the vagina.

Culdocentesis is the aspiration of fluid from the cul-de-sac.

Anesthetic

Anesthesia options include a spinal or epidural to the T10 sensory level, GETA, or local anesthesia with IV sedation.

Positioning

The patient is placed in a lithotomy position.

Anesthetic Implications

One peripheral IV is usually sufficient.

Anticipate a vasovagal response with traction on the uterus. If it occurs, it may be necessary to give the patient Robinul and/or atropine.

NSAIDs may be given intravenously to supplement other pain management measures.

Dilation and Curettage

In a D&C procedure, the surgeon opens the cervix and scrapes to remove endocervical/endometrial tissue. This surgery may be performed to control abnormal uterine bleeding, relieve dysmenorrhea, evaluate infertility, or take a biopsy to diagnose cervical or uterine cellular abnormality or malignancy.

Operative Procedure

A speculum is inserted into the vagina; local anesthetic is injected into the cervix. The cervix is grasped with a clamp to secure it, and the cervix is dilated. A progressively larger dilating curette is then moved in and out of uterus to loosen and scrape away the endometrial lining.

Anesthetic

Sedation with a local anesthetic is often used. A spinal anesthetic to the T10 level may also be used. As always, GETA may be needed. If the patient is more than 16 weeks (4 months) pregnant, consider the patient to be a "full stomach" case. (See the discussion of the dilation and evacuation procedure in the next section for more information.)

Positioning

The patient is placed in a lithotomy position, with the arms extended on armboards bilaterally. If GETA is used, after intubation and induction, the patient will need to be moved so that the buttocks are at the lower leg break of table. If the patient is pregnant, a rapid-sequence induction should be done.

Anesthetic Implications

A local anesthetic and epinephrine solution may be infiltrated at the cervix to decrease swelling, with the ultimate goal of preventing bleeding. Watch for an increase in heart rate or blood pressure or EKG changes.

An HCG lab test (urine test for pregnancy) should be done preoperatively.

The patient's bladder will be drained by an in-and-out catheter. Document the amount of urine collected by this means.

The most stimulating portion of a D&C occurs during cervical dilatation and curettage, and during suctioning. Deepen the sedation before these two parts of the procedure are started to avoid patient movement.

Have Pitocin or ergonovine maleate available. Pitocin (oxytocin) 10–20 units/1 L bag or ergonovine maleate 0.2 mg IM may be given to contract the uterus and decrease bleeding.

Anticipate a vasovagal response with traction on the uterus and during cervical dilation. If it occurs, it may be necessary to give Robinul and/or atropine.

Complications

Uterine perforation is a possible complication of D&C.

Dilation and Evacuation (Therapeutic Abortion)

Dilation and evacuation (D&E) involves dilation of the cervix, plus scraping and vacuum suction of uterine contents. It is performed to remove the artifacts of an incomplete or missed abortion, to remove benign gestational trophoblastic disease (GTD; hydatidiform mole), or to remove fetal contents for pregnancy termination.

Operative Procedure

A speculum is inserted into vagina; local anesthetic is injected into the cervix. The cervix is grasped with a clamp and dilated. Suction curettage with pregnancy more than 12 weeks (representing the majority of cases) or a sharp curette (rarely) may be used. Vacuum aspiration is used to remove the uterine contents.

Anesthetic

Sedation is used in conjunction with a local anesthetic. A rapid-sequence induction is needed if the patient is greater than 16 weeks pregnant.

General anesthesia and an OETT may be used if the patient is more than 10–12 weeks pregnant, due to the gastroparesis and potential for aspiration associated with this gestation period. If the patient is more than 16 weeks (4 months) pregnant, consider her to be a "full stomach" case.

Positioning

The patient is placed in a lithotomy position, with the arms extended on armboards bilaterally. If GETA is used, after intubation and induction, the patient will need to be moved so that the buttocks are at the lower leg break of table.

Anesthetic Implications

A local anesthetic and epinephrine solution may be infiltrated at the cervix to decrease swelling, thereby preventing bleeding. Watch for an increase in heart rate or blood pressure or EKG changes.

The most stimulating portion of a D&E occurs during cervical dilatation and curettage, and during suctioning. Deepen the sedation before these two parts of the procedure are started to avoid patient movement.

An HCG lab test (urine test for pregnancy) should be done preoperatively. In cases involving unexpected fetal demise, the mother may require more anxiolytics (midazolam).

The patient's bladder will be drained by an in-and-out catheter. Document the amount of urine collected by this means.

Have Pitocin and ergonovine maleate available. Pitocin (oxytocin) 10–20 units/1 L bag or ergonovine maleate 0.2 mg IM may be given to contract the uterus and decrease bleeding.

The further along the pregnancy, the greater the amount of blood loss possible.

Anticipate a vasovagal response with traction on the uterus and cervical dilation. If it occurs, it may be necessary to give the patient Robinul and/or atropine.

Complications

Uterine perforation is a possible complication of D&E.

Endometrial Ablation

Endometrial ablation is performed to create endometrial fibrosis or stenosis of the uterine cavity so as to stop dysfunctional uterine bleeding. It is indicated for dysfunctional uterine bleeding in patients who do not desire further pregnancy (there is no guarantee of sterilization). Ablation destroys the endometrium, resulting in scarring of the uterine lining. It will also reduce or stop all further menstrual periods.

Operative Procedure

The cervix is grasped and dilated. Next, the uterus is "sounded"; a sound is a probe with measuring indicia, inserted to accurately determine the depth of the uterus. Wetness or mucus level is noted after withdrawing the sound.

Novasure System

The surgeon measures the length of the cervix and the uterus, and then inserts a hysteroscope into the uterus. The Novasure wand is placed through the hysteroscope and the distal gold-plated mesh is expanded. The radiofrequency current is then delivered to the endometrium.

Radiofrequency

Through a hysteroscope, a probe, covered with an insulated sleeve to protect the bladder, is passed into the uterine cavity; it may be rotated during the procedure to ensure uniform tissue destruction. The endometrial tissues are heated to 62–65°C for several minutes. Uterine blood flow, thermal non-conductivity of the myometrium, and the geometrically proportional fall-off of the heating effect combine to protect the surrounding organs.

Hydrothermal Ablation

The surgeon inserts a hysteroscope into the vagina, allowing heated saline solution to flow freely over the inside surface of the uterus. Hydrothermal ablation (HTA) takes approximately 30 minutes and can be done under local or general anesthesia. A concern when this method is used is the possibility of hot water leaking out into the fallopian tubes and/or burning the intestines.

Cryoablation

A cryoprobe is inserted into the uterus, and the endometrial tissue is scraped and removed.

Wire-Loop Resection

A resectoscope is inserted into the uterus, for visualization purposes. It has a built-in wire loop that uses high-frequency electrical energy to cut or coagulate endometrial tissue. The resectoscope has the advantage of also being able to remove polyps and small internal fibroids.

Hot Water Balloon

A Thermachoice balloon is placed through the cervix into the uterus. Hot water is circulated inside the balloon to destroy the endometrium. Some experts have expressed concerns that the balloon might not be able to reach the corneal (top corners) of the uterus.

Anesthetic

MAC is used with deep sedation, with the anesthesia being deepened before increased stimulation associated with ablation. Neuraxial anesthesia with a spinal to the T10 level and IV sedation may also be used. Some cases may require GETA.

Positioning

The patient is placed in a lithotomy position.

Anesthetic Implications

The most stimulating part of the surgery occurs when the cervix is grasped and dilated and when the uterine tissues are heated.

A local anesthetic and epinephrine solution may be infiltrated at the cervix to decrease swelling, thereby preventing bleeding. Watch for an increase in heart rate or blood pressure or EKG changes.

Anticipate a vasovagal response with traction on the uterus and cervical dilation. If it occurs, it may be necessary to give the patient Robinul and/or atropine.

The patient's bladder may be drained by an in-and-out catheter. Document the amount of urine collected by this means.

NSAIDs may be given intravenously to supplement other pain management measures.

Complications

Potential complications include uterine perforation, bowel or bladder injury, and cervical lacerations.

Vaginal Hysterectomy

Vaginal hysterectomy is the removal of the uterus through an incision made into the vaginal wall; no abdominal incision is made. This surgery is performed to remove a uterus that is not greatly enlarged or for benign uterine conditions, including tumors, pelvic relaxation, endometriosis, and dysfunctional uterine bleeding. It is done vaginally if the patient has poor pelvic muscular support and an anterior and posterior colporrhaphy also needs to be done.

Operative Procedure

Two types of vaginal hysterectomy are possible:

- *Total:* removal of the uterine body, fundus, and cervix
- *Partial (supracervical):* removal of the uterine body only; leaves the cervical stump (supracervical)

This type of hysterectomy is done completely through the vagina. The labia may be retracted with sutures to keep it out of operative field. A suture may also be placed in the cervix to allow for traction.

The surgeon loosens the uterus and dissects it away from the cervix. The uterosacral and cardinal ligaments and uterine arteries are ligated to allow for removal of the uterus. The surgeon then loosens the uterus through the vaginal vault and removes it through an incision in the vagina. Laparoscopic ports may be used at the end of the case to enter the abdomen to check for bleeding. See "Laparoscopic-Assisted Hysterectomy with Transvaginal Manipulation" later in this chapter for more information.

A urethral or suprapubic catheter is placed. Vaginal packing is inserted, and a perineal pad is placed.

Anesthetic

Neuraxial anesthesia consists of a spinal or epidural to the T10 level, with IV sedation. Some cases may require general anesthesia with an OETT and muscle relaxation.

Positioning

The patient is placed in a lithotomy position, with the arms extended on armboards bilaterally.

Anesthetic Implications

Increases in heart rate may be due to a vasoconstrictor injected into the vaginal incision sites. Monitor the EKG and blood pressure for changes.

Notify the surgeon of any bleeding in the urine.

A sterilization consent form should be signed by the patient, along with the consent form for surgery.

Anticipate a vasovagal response with traction on the uterus and cervical dilation. If it occurs, it may be necessary to give the patient Robinul and/or atropine.

Type and screen the patient's blood preoperatively.

Smooth emergence from anesthesia is important with this surgery. The goal is to avoid coughing, bucking, or nausea/vomiting or retching so as to prevent increased risk of bleeding, hematoma formation, or suture line disruption from the increased abdominal pressures. Antiemetics should be given (see Chapter 4).

Hysteroscopy

Hysteroscopy involves the use of a hysteroscope to examine the uterine cavity. A rigid, lighted, fiberoptic endoscope is commonly used in this procedure. Flexible scopes are becoming more popular for diagnostic procedures.

Hysteroscopy is used to diagnose the cause of intrauterine bleeding, perform a biopsy, perform an infertility evaluation, and remove an intrauterine device. A fluid (saline or glycine) is used to distend the uterus for visualization. Carbon dioxide is rarely used for this purpose in the United States.

Operative Procedure

A vaginal speculum is inserted. A paracervical block with local anesthetic without epinephrine is the usual anesthetic option injected for postoperative pain control and to decrease bleeding. The cervix is grasped with a clamp, and the hysteroscope is inserted into the uterine cavity. The intrauterine cavity is visualized; biopsies may also be taken.

Anesthetic

Anesthetic options include GETA with an OETT; local anesthesia with IV sedation (usually done); and neuraxial anesthesia (spinal to the T10 level).

Positioning

The patient is placed in a lithotomy position, with the bilateral arms on padded armboards and the shoulders at an angle less than 90 degrees.

Anesthetic Implications

Anticipate a vasovagal response with traction on the uterus and cervical dilation. If it occurs, it may be necessary to give the patient Robinul and/or atropine.

Bags of instilled glycine or saline for intrauterine distention are hung on an IV pole and delivered by gravity; this fluid can be absorbed by the open vessels. Surgical staff will measure the fluid going in and out; monitor the patient for signs of fluid overload. Sodium and potassium levels should be assessed preoperatively, before the hysteroscopy begins. Signs and symptoms of hyponatremia include agitation, confusion, lethargy, nausea and vomiting, and hypertension followed by hypotension.

It is important to minimize the amount of peripheral IV fluids given to patients because so much fluid can potentially be absorbed through the uterus. If a fluid deficit of more than 500 mL occurs with uterine instillation, the procedure should be stopped.

NSAIDs may be given intravenously to supplement other pain management measures.

Complications

Potential complications of hysteroscopy include uterine or bowel perforation, infection, bleeding, cerebral edema, and death. Gas embolism is possible if carbon dioxide is used to insufflate the bladder (see Chapter 3).

Loop Electrosurgical Excision Procedure

Loop electrosurgical excision procedure (LEEP) is an electrosurgical procedure to remove a cone-shaped wedge at the cervical os. (Also see the discussion of conization and biopsy of the cervix earlier in this chapter.) This approach helps to decrease risk of bleeding.

LEEP is performed to remove abnormal cells of the cervix. It may be undertaken to either diagnose or treat cervical dysplasia or cancer of the cervix (carcinoma in situ [CIS]).

Operative Procedure

A thin wire loop is inserted into the vagina. An electric current is then used to remove a wedge of the cervix.

Anesthetic

Anesthesia options include neuraxial block to the T10 level; although usually local anesthesia with sedation is all that is needed in conjunction with a paracervical or intracervical block. Alternatively, general anesthesia may be used with an OETT. If the patient is pregnant, she is considered to be a "full stomach" case and requires rapid-sequence induction if a general anesthetic is given.

Positioning

The patient is placed in a lithotomy position. A slight Trendelenburg position may also be helpful. The arms are extended on armboards bilaterally.

Anesthetic Implications

The patient's bladder will be drained by an in-and-out catheter. Document the amount of urine collected by this means.

If the patient is pregnant, a more superficial wedge of the cervical os is removed, as there is an increased risk of bleeding due to the increased vascularity of the pregnant uterus and cervix.

A local anesthetic and epinephrine solution may be injected around the cervix before an incision is made to decrease swelling and to prevent bleeding. Watch for an increase in heart rate or blood pressure or EKG changes.

NSAIDs may be given intravenously to supplement other pain management measures.

Complications

Perforation of the uterus is a possible complication of this procedure.

Marsupialization of Bartholin Duct Cyst or Abscess

Marsupialization of a Bartholin duct cyst or abscess entails the incision and drainage of a recurrent vulva/vaginal cyst. The Bartholin glands, which are normally present on each side of the vaginal opening at the 4 o'clock and 8 o'clock positions, are normally neither visible nor palpable. If the duct draining a gland becomes blocked, however, normal secretions cannot drain, and swelling and possible infection can ensue. A simple cyst or abscess of the Bartholin duct of the vulva or vagina can be simply drained in the physician's office.

A patient with a recurrent Bartholin cyst may need to have marsupialization of the cyst to prevent a recurrence.

Operative Procedure

In this procedure, the labia are retracted and the cyst is exposed. An incision is made over the cyst and the contents evacuated. The wall of the abscess is then sutured to the skin of the vaginal mucosa (medially) and the outer edge of the vaginal canal (laterally). This allows the cut skin cell fibroblasts to spread down into the cyst, permitting secretions to escape and the wound to granulate and reepithelialize outward for healing.

Anesthetic

Anesthesia may consist of sedation with local anesthesia or a pudental block.

Positioning

The patient is placed in a lithotomy position, with the arms extended on armboards bilaterally.

Anesthetic Implications

The patient's bladder may be drained by an in-and-out catheter. Document the amount of urine collected by this means.

NSAIDs may be given intravenously to supplement other pain management measures.

Radical Trachelectomy

Radical trachelectomy is a procedure used in cases of early-stage cervical cancer to save the uterus. The surgeon removes the cervix, parametrium, vaginal cuff, and surrounding lymph nodes. The uterus is then attached to the vagina. A cervical cerclage is done to allow the patient to carry a pregnancy. This surgery may be performed either transabdominally or transvaginally.

If a woman who has had a radial trachelectomy becomes pregnant, she must give birth via cesarean section. Such women have a slightly higher risk of miscarriage than women in the general population.

Trachelorrhaphy

Trachelorrhaphy is the removal of torn surfaces or suture repair of the cervical neck and the reconstruction of the cervical canal. It is performed in cases involving cervical lacerations from trauma.

Operative Procedure

A speculum is inserted into the vagina; local anesthetic is injected into the cervix. The cervix is grasped with a tenaculum and dilated. The affected surface tissue is removed, and cervical flaps are undermined to loosen them. A small cone is removed from the cervical canal and then covered with mucosal flaps. Bleeding is cauterized or ligated. A urethral catheter is inserted into the bladder; packing is placed in the vagina.

Anesthetic

Anesthesia options include local anesthesia with IV sedation; GETA; and a spinal to the T10 sensory level.

Positioning

The patient is placed in a lithotomy position, with the arms extended on armboards bilaterally.

Anesthetic Implications

The most stimulating part of this surgery is when the cervix is grasped and local anesthetic is injected into the cervical tissue.

Typing and cross-matching of the patient's blood may be needed. These patients can potentially lose a significant amount of blood depending on the degree of the tear.

The patient's bladder may be drained by an in-and-out catheter. Document the amount of urine collected by this means.

A local anesthetic and epinephrine solution may be injected around the cervix before an incision is made to decrease swelling and to prevent bleeding. Watch for an increase in heart rate or blood pressure or EKG changes.

NSAIDs may be given intravenously to supplement other pain management measures.

Transvaginal Oocyte Retrieval

Transvaginal oocyte retrieval (TVOR) collects oocytes after a woman has undergone ovarian stimulation. This procedure is done on women 35 to 36 hours after they are injected with human chorionic gonadotropin (HCG), an ovulation-inducing agent. Surgery must be performed in this time frame. If TVOR is done after ovulation, oocyte retrieval would not be possible.

Operative Procedure

A sterile speculum is inserted into the vagina and is prepped. The speculum is withdrawn, and an ultrasound probe with a 16-gauge needle is inserted through the vaginal fornix to the ovary. Once the needle is in the ovary, the ovarian follicles are aspirated. The procedure is then repeated on the other ovary. After removal of the ultrasound probe, a speculum is inserted in the vagina to check for hemostasis of the vaginal wall and cervix.

Anesthetic

IV sedation is typically used. In rare cases, local, regional, or general anesthesia may be given.

Positioning

The patient is placed in a dorsal lithotomy position, with bilateral arms on padded armboards.

Anesthetic Implications

Patients receive anxiolytics preoperatively. This procedure is associated with minimal blood loss and minimal postoperative pain. Given the risk of PONV, it is wise to treat patients prophylactically with antiemetics.

NSAIDs may be given intravenously to supplement other pain management measures.

Complications

Potential complications include nerve injury from hyperflexion of the hip or pressure on the nerve over the fibula.

Urinary Stress Incontinence Operation

Suspension of the bladder is one option for treating urinary stress incontinence. Such surgery may be performed to restore continence in older or multiparous women, or to treat a disorder of the musculofascial support to the bladder neck and pelvic floor. See Chapter 19 for more information on female stress incontinence and surgical restoration.

Operative Procedure

Vaginal Approach

The vaginal approach involves urethral plication. The bladder is emptied and a weighted speculum is placed in the vagina. The extent of the cystourethrocele is determined, after which the mucosa is injected with a vasoconstrictive solution to decrease bleeding. The mucosa is dissected, and vertical mattress sutures are placed to elevate the posterior urethra to a high retropubic position. Extra mucosa is excised.

Abdominal Approach

Abdominal approaches are performed with a urinary catheter in place. A low transverse abdominal incision is made to allow the surgeon to reach the area between the parietal peritoneum and the rectus fascia (space of Retzius). Blunt dissection is used to open and extend this area, with the surgeon raising the anterior vagina and bladder neck and suturing tissue lateral to the urethra to Cooper's ligament.

Urethral Sling

Construction of a urethral sling is reserved for women with low urethral pressure and/or a history of failed incontinence operations. During this procedure, a urethral catheter is placed. The vaginal mucosa is incised and dissected away from the paravesicle and paraurethral fascia. A low transverse abdominal incision is made, and a strip of rectus fascia is brought through the vagina, around the urethra, and back to the abdomen, where it is attached to the rectus fascia. This process creates a sling for the bladder neck. The incisions are closed, and a suprapubic catheter is inserted.

Anesthetic

GETA is given; muscle relaxation is needed.

Positioning

For a vaginal approach, the patient is placed in a dorsal lithotomy position. For an abdominal approach, she is placed in a frog-legged position.

Anesthetic Implications

Type and cross-match the patient's blood preoperatively. There is a risk of significant bleeding with both the vaginal and abdominal approaches, albeit more so with the abdominal approach.

A local anesthetic and epinephrine solution may be infiltrated to decrease bleeding. Watch for an increase in heart rate or blood pressure or EKG changes.

Vesicovaginal Fistula Repair

Vesicovaginal fistula repair encompasses the surgical repair and closure of the fistula between the bladder and the vagina. This surgery is performed when communication between the bladder and the vagina allows urine to be involuntarily discharged into the vaginal vault. A vesicovaginal fistula can be caused by prolonged labor in childbirth or can occur following pelvic surgery, radiation therapy, or rape.

Operative Procedure
Vaginal Approach

After inserting a percutaneous suprapubic tube and urethral catheter, a vaginal speculum is placed. The bladder must be mobilized away from the vagina to reduce the risk of suture placement into the bladder wall. The fistula is identified. A small urethral catheter is then inserted through the fistula and into the bladder to allow the fistula to be moved and the bladder to be filled to identify anatomical planes while suturing.

A small incision is made into the vaginal wall, and blunt dissection is used to separate the anterior vaginal wall away from the bladder. An incision is made to circumscribe the fistula, and the anterior vaginal wall is dissected off the underlying fascia. The fistula tract is closed in a watertight fashion, followed by suturing the fascia closed. At this point, redundant vaginal mucosa can be excised and the incision closed. Pelvic drains and a suprapubic and/or urethral catheter are placed. The vagina is packed to prevent bleeding.

Open Approach

With the patient in a modified lithotomy position, a urethral catheter is inserted. A small incision is made under the umbilicus and carried down into the peritoneal cavity. The bladder must be completely mobilized to excise the fistula and separate the bladder from the vagina. After separating the two, the surgeon places omental tissue (taken from the abdomen) between the vagina and the bladder to reinforce the tissue. The bladder is closed in layers and the vagina is closed, both using absorbable sutures. Pelvic drains and a suprapubic catheter are placed.

Ureteral reimplantation may need to be done in conjunction with a vesicovaginal fistula repair.

Anesthetic
Either a spinal block to T10 with IV sedation or GETA may be used.

Positioning
The patient is placed in a lithotomy position.

Anesthetic Implications
Pelvic drains and a suprapubic and/or urethral catheter are placed. The choice of catheters is surgeon dependent: Some surgeons will place both, but usually only one is inserted.

Complications
Injury to the bladder is possible with this surgery.

ABDOMINAL APPROACH

Laparoscopic-Assisted Hysterectomy with Transvaginal Manipulation

This form of hysterectomy entails the laparoscopic-assisted removal of the uterus with transvaginal manipulation. The laparoscopic approach is used in patients in whom an abdominal incision would increase morbidity and a vaginal hysterectomy would be technically difficult.

Operative Procedure
For the laparoscopic portion of the surgery, a pneumoperitoneum is created by using carbon dioxide to insufflate the abdomen. Moist packing or a urethral catheter with an inflated balloon is placed in the vaginal cuff to maintain the pneumoperitoneum. The uterus is separated from all the surrounding tissues.

If the cervix is left (called a "supracervical hysterectomy"), the uterus can be removed through one of the laparoscopic ports or through the vaginal colpotomy. The vaginal cuff is sutured closed after the uterus is removed.

The uterus is removed through the vagina, during which the pneumoperitoneum may be decreased or lost. If the ventilator is set on pressure ventilation and pneumoperitoneum is lost, lung volumes will increase dramatically.

This procedure may be done either laparoscopically or with robotic-assisted laparoscopy.

Anesthetic
GETA is given with insertion of an OETT; muscle relaxants are required.

Positioning
The patient is placed in a low lithotomy position, with the arms tucked at the sides bilaterally. A slight Trendelenburg position is useful.

Anesthetic Implications
A sterilization permit must be signed by the patient, along with the surgical consent form.

A type and screen of the patient's blood may be all that is needed.

An orogastric tube is inserted after induction and intubation to drain the patient's stomach contents.

Smooth emergence from anesthesia is important with this surgery. The goal is to avoid coughing, bucking, or nausea/vomiting or retching so as to prevent increased risk of bleeding, hematoma formation, or suture line disruption from the increased abdominal pressures. Antiemetics should be given (see Chapter 4).

At the end of the case, a cystoscope is inserted to examine the bladder to assess for bladder perforation (after laparoscope trocars have been introduced transabdominally).

Radical Hysterectomy

Radical hysterectomy is the removal of the uterus, cervix, fallopian tubes, ovaries, upper vagina, and supporting vaginal and uterine ligaments, along with all pelvic lymph nodes. It is indicated for gynecologic malignancy.

Operative Procedure
After placing a urethral catheter, a midline abdominal incision is made. The anatomy listed previously is dissected away from surrounding structures that are to remain and removed. All removed tissue is sent for pathology analysis. The remaining upper

third of the vagina is sutured closed. The abdominal wound is closed in layers; a drain is placed. A suprapubic catheter may be inserted (based on surgeon preference).

Anesthetic

GETA and muscle relaxation are used.

Positioning

The patient is placed in a supine position.

Anesthetic Implications

A sterilization permit must be signed by the patient, along with the surgical consent form.

Type and cross-match the patient's blood preoperatively, and have 2 units of packed red blood cells available.

An orogastric tube is inserted after induction and intubation to drain the patient's stomach contents. A nasogastric tube may need to be inserted instead, check with the surgeon.

Smooth emergence from anesthesia is important with this surgery. The goal is to avoid coughing, bucking, or nausea/vomiting or retching so as to prevent increased risk of bleeding, hematoma formation, or suture line disruption from the increased abdominal pressures. Antiemetics should be given (see Chapter 4). Have a team member hold gentle pressure over the suture lines if the patient does cough or vomit.

Total Abdominal Hysterectomy: With or Without Bilateral Salpingo-oophorectomy

Total abdominal hysterectomy (TAH) is the removal of the uterus and the cervix. It is performed to treat a benign or malignant condition of the uterus including tumors, endometriosis, and dysfunctional uterine bleeding. It may also be used to diagnose, stage, or treat cervical or enodometrial cancer that has not metastasized outside the uterus. Another common preoperative diagnosis is pelvic relaxation, including any of the following conditions: uterine prolapse, enterocele (intrusion of the intestine into the pouch of Douglas), cystocele (intrusion of the bladder into the anterior wall of the vagina), urethrocele (intrusion of the urethra into the anterior wall of the vagina), or rectocele (intrusion of the rectum into the posterior wall of the vagina).

Operative Procedure

Once an incision is made into the abdomen, but before any tissue is excised, the lymph nodes are meticulously examined; any suspicious nodes are excised and sent for frozen section or pathology analysis. If signs of malignancy are found, the case may be stopped and incisions closed to prevent cancerous cells from being released by tissue manipulation and forced into the peritoneum and bloodstream. If malignancy is not found, the uterus is freed from the surrounding tissues (i.e., ureters, bladder, uterine ligaments) and removed. The upper third of the vagina and all parametrial tissues (to the pelvic side wall) are excised. Multiple drains are placed and all incisions are closed.

An open hysterectomy *without* a bilateral salpingo-oophorectomy (BSO) may be done to preserve ovarian hormone function. BSO may be performed in conjunction with a hysterectomy, in which case the procedure is called a *complete hysterectomy*.

TAH may be done laparoscopically or with robotic-assisted laparoscopy. Lymph node inspection and biopsies can also be carried out using this approach. In addition to the trocar insertion site incisions, a small, 2- to 3-inch incision may be made to facilitate removal of an abnormally large uterus. A cystoscopy may be performed at the end of the case to assess for bladder perforation.

Anesthetic

GETA is given with insertion of an OETT; muscle relaxants are given. An epidural block may be inserted preoperatively for postoperative pain control.

Positioning

For the laparoscopic or robotic approach, the patient is placed in a lithotomy position, with the arms tucked at the sides bilaterally. A steep

Trendelenburg position is useful. For the abdominal approach, the patient is placed supine.

Anesthetic Implications

A sterilization permit must be signed by the patient, along with the surgical consent form.

These patients may have anemia preoperatively owing to chronic bleeding. Even if the patient's hematocrit is within normal levels, type and cross-match her blood preoperatively. Have 2–4 units available, as there is a potential for a large blood loss if the great vessels are injured.

A bowel prep is usually given. Thus, these patients will be quite dehydrated, with subsequent hypotension occurring on induction of anesthesia. Maintain vascular hydration; colloids may be needed for this purpose.

Orogastric tube placement should be done for a laparoscopic procedure. Nasogastric tube placement may be warranted due to slow or stopped peristalsis accompanying the laparotomy procedure.

Monitor the patient's urinary output during the surgery for the presence of hematuria with possible ureteral/bladder injury.

Hypothermia is a major issue with an open abdominal procedure. Use fluid warmers, upper-body and leg warming blankets, and other measures to prevent heat loss.

Indigo carmine is given intravenously (wear gloves when drawing up, as this dye stains) to check ureteral patency. It will make the patient's urine turn blue.

Smooth emergence from anesthesia is important with this surgery. The goal is to avoid coughing, bucking, or nausea/vomiting or retching so as to prevent increased risk of bleeding, hematoma formation, or suture line disruption from the increased abdominal pressures. Antiemetics should be given (see Chapter 4).

Myomectomy

Myomectomy is a procedure to remove uterine fibroids that cause bleeding and pain. The open approach allows the surgeon to palpate the uterus to find deeper fibroids.

Operative Procedure

Open Approach

A lower abdominal transverse or vertical midline incision is made for an open procedure. The fibroid tumor is separated from the uterine wall by dissection or laser. The uterus is closed in multiple layers; the incision is closed.

Laparoscopic Approach

The laparoscopic approach may be used to remove fibroids that are attached by a stalk (subserous myomas) to the outside of the uterus.

Robotic Laparoscopic Approach

A robotic-assisted procedure is now used to remove intramural and subserosal fibroids with minimal blood loss.

Vaginal Approach: Colpotomy

A hysteroscope is inserted into the uterus to remove fibroids on the submucous layer (inside) of the uterus. This procedure is rarely done.

Anesthetic

General anesthesia with an OETT is used with the open and laparoscopic myomectomy approaches. For the colpotomy approach, neuraxial anesthesia consisting of a spinal or epidural to the T10 level, local anesthesia, and IV sedation are used.

Positioning

The patient is placed in a supine position.

Anesthetic Implications

Because the tissues of the uterus are quite vascular, maintaining a slightly decreased mean arterial blood pressure (60–70 mm Hg) can help to minimize bleeding.

Type and cross-match the patient's blood before surgery starts; there is a risk of blood loss with a myomectomy.

If a laser is used to remove the fibroid, fires and burns are a potential problem. See Chapter 1 on safety concerns for more information.

Smooth emergence from anesthesia is important with this surgery. The goal is to avoid coughing, bucking, or nausea/vomiting or retching so as to prevent increased risk of bleeding, hematoma formation, or suture line disruption from the increased abdominal pressures. Have a team member hold gentle pressure over any suture lines if the patient does cough or vomit. Antiemetics should be given (see Chapter 4).

Pelvic Exenteration

Pelvic exenteration is the total excision and removal of the internal genitalia, cervix, uterus and upper vagina, a portion of the levator muscles, the bladder and distal ureters, rectum, distal sigmoid colon, pelvic lymph nodes, and para-aortic lymph node; it includes pelvic peritoneum dissection. Excision of the fallopian tube(s) and ovaries may also be done (salpingo-oophorectomy). A fecal and urinary diversion must also be created; see Chapter 19 for more information on the cutaneous ureterostomy, ileal conduit, and colostomy procedures. Pelvic exenteration may also include a partial omenectomy and appendectomy. The surgical area stretches from the infrarenal to anterior to lumbar vessels.

While this surgery is extreme, it is considered curative if all cancerous tissue is removed. It may be performed to explore the abdominal cavity, provide for cancer staging, debulk any tumor, remove residual tumor, and obtain cytologic washings from multiple areas in the peritoneal cavity. The goal is the meticulous examination of all abdominopelvic cavities.

Pelvic exenteration is performed in patients with cervical, fallopian tube, peritoneum, and/or ovarian carcinoma, either radio resistant or recurrent, and in patients with rectal malignancy. *Ovarian cancer can spread directly to other organs in the pelvis and lymphatics or can seed cancer cells into the peritoneum.*

Patients undergoing this procedure are usually quite ill, with significant morbidity and mortality.

Operative Procedure

A large midline incision is made. All organs and tissues listed previously are removed through the abdominal portion of this surgery, except for the distal rectum and the anus, which are removed through the perineum. The pelvic floor is then closed. The bladder and rectum may be able to be preserved if no tumor is present in these areas. The vagina may need to be reconstructed. An omental pelvic carpet/sling and gracilis myocutaneous flap are created as part of vaginal and perineal reconstruction.

The lymph nodes throughout the peritoneum and organs surrounding the uterus are meticulously inspected and palpated. Any suspicious nodes are removed and sent for frozen section analysis. Ureters are cut as distal (close to the bladder) as possible, and the bladder is removed.

Pelvic exenteration may be done laparoscopically. Lymph node inspection and biopsies can also be done with this approach as well. A 2- to 3-inch abdominal incision may be needed to remove an abnormally large uterus.

A continent urinary diversion is created using an ileocolonic segment, ileal loop, or transverse colon conduit, with the colon being transected at the appropriate level. Vaginal reconstruction is done; the pelvic floor is covered with a muscle flap. A suprapubic catheter is placed. Multiple drains are placed and all incisions are closed.

A *second-look laparotomy* may be performed in patients who have undergone chemotherapy after a radical hysterectomy was done. The only true and reliable method to evaluate the status of tumor growth or presence, this procedure involves a hands-on visual inspection of the remaining peritoneal contents. It can be done laparoscopically.

Anesthetic

GETA is given with insertion of an OETT; muscle relaxants are given. An epidural catheter may be placed for postoperative pain control.

Positioning

The patient is placed in a supine position for the abdominal portion of the surgery, and in the lithotomy position for the perineal portion.

Anesthetic Implications

These patients may be anemic preoperatively owing to chronic bleeding. Even if the patient's hematocrit is within normal levels, type and cross-match the blood prior to surgery. Have 2–4 units available in the operating room, as there is a potential for a large blood loss if the great vessels are injured. Anticipate a large blood loss and fluid shifts by establishing multiple IV access sites.

A nasogastric tube, if not already present, should be inserted.

Temperature loss is a major concern with this procedure. Upper- and lower-body warming blankets are needed as well as fluid warmers. The ambient temperature in the room may also need to be increased.

Maintain urinary output at a rate of 1 mL/kg/hr or more.

Obtain at least the following preoperative labs: CBC, chemistry with BUN and creatinine, and PT/INR/PTT. Obtain an EKG.

Postoperative ventilation may be required. These patients usually require care in an ICU for several days.

If the patient is to be extubated, smooth emergence from anesthesia is important with this surgery. The goal is to avoid coughing, bucking, or nausea/vomiting or retching so as to prevent increased risk of bleeding, hematoma formation, or suture line disruption from the increased abdominal pressures. Have a team member hold gentle pressure over the suture lines if the patient does cough or vomit. Antiemetics should be given (see Chapter 4).

Once the surgery is completed, cover the patient with warmed blankets to prevent shivering.

Monitors and IV Access

- Arterial line placement is required to monitor continuous blood pressure. It readily permits arterial sampling for blood gases and labs.
- Place two large-bore peripheral IV lines.
- CVP may be needed if urgent fluid resuscitation is anticipated because of extensive blood loss.
- A PA catheter may be needed if the patient has cardiac history or is hemodynamically unstable.

Salpingo-oophorectomy

Salpingo-oophorectomy is the removal of a fallopian tube and ovary; it can be bilateral. This procedure is indicated for a benign or malignant condition of the fallopian tube or ovary, including benign or malignant tumor, acute or chronic infections, tubal pregnancy, and hemorrhage.

Operative Procedure

In an open procedure, a laparotomy incision is made. The infundibulopelvic ligaments that extend out from the ovary to the wall of the pelvis and support the ovaries are ligated. The connection between the uterus and the fallopian tubes (uterine cornu) is excised. The fallopian tube(s) and ovary(ies) are removed. The abdominal incision is closed in layers.

This procedure can be done using a laparoscopic approach.

Anesthetic

GETA, muscle relaxation are used.

Positioning

The patient is placed in a supine position.

Anesthetic Implications

A sterilization permit must be signed by the patient, along with the surgical consent form.

Tubal Ligation (Sterilization)

Tubal ligation is the surgical interruption of the fallopian tubes, resulting in sterilization.

Operative Procedure

The fallopian tubes can be clipped shut or ligated and separated. The goal in either case is the complete closure of both fallopian tubes.

This surgery can be done by *posterior colpotomy* by retracting the cervix anteriorly, with a transverse incision then being made into the posterior vaginal mucosa. Forceps enter the peritoneum and grasp both fallopian tubes. The patient may have a straight catheter procedure to drain urine during this surgery.

With a *laparoscopic approach,* coagulation of 3 cm of the fallopian tube can be done, or two spring clips (placed closed together) can be placed across the entire tube.

Closure of the tubes is done at least 3 cm away from the uterine–fallopian tube juncture.

Tubal ligation may be done in conjunction with a cesarean section. After a vaginal delivery, tubal ligation is usually done on the first or second postpartum day.

Anesthetic

GETA is given with insertion of an OETT; muscle relaxants may be given. A skilled surgeon can be very quick with the laparoscopic approach; muscle relaxation may not be needed.

Positioning

The patient is placed in either a supine or lithotomy position.

Anesthetic Implications

The patient, along with the surgical consent form, must sign a sterilization permit.

This surgery usually lasts 20–45 minutes. If a muscle relaxant is given, keep 1/4 twitch train of four (TOF) so that a second twitch can return in a timely manner for reversal.

NSAIDs may be given intravenously to supplement other pain management measures.

Ectopic Tubal Pregnancy

In an ectopic pregnancy, the product of conception becomes lodged and grows outside of the endometrial cavity. The fallopian tube is the most common site for ectopic pregnancies, although they can occur in the ovary or peritoneal cavity as well. Ectopic pregnancy is diagnosed based on the presence of elevated HCG serum levels and the absence of a gestational sac on ultrasound.

Operative Procedure

Treatment of an ectopic pregnancy can usually be done *laparoscopically* if the bleeding is controlled, with the product of conception/ectopic pregnancy being removed through salpingostomy (opening into the fallopian tube). A salpingectomy to remove the affected fallopian tube may also need to be done.

A *ruptured ectopic pregnancy* is considered a surgical emergency. In such a case, the patient may be actively bleeding into the peritoneal cavity.

Anesthetic

GETA and muscle relaxation are used. Rapid sequence induction should be done.

Positioning

The patient is placed in a lithotomy, Trendelenburg position.

Anesthetic Implications

A D&C procedure may be done in conjunction with ectopic pregnancy.

Methotrexate 15–30 mg IM, may be used with ectopic pregnancy in the perioperative setting. This agent is given to interrupt cell division and prevent the growth of any embryonic or fetal cells left behind after surgery to end an ectopic pregnancy.

Smooth emergence from anesthesia is important with an open approach to this surgery. The goal is to avoid coughing, bucking, or nausea/vomiting or retching so as to prevent increased risk of bleeding, hematoma formation, or suture line disruption from the increased abdominal pressures. Have a team member hold gentle pressure over the suture lines if the patient does cough or vomit.

Antiemetics should be given (see Chapter 4).

Tuboplasty: Fallopian Tubes

Tuboplasty reestablishes the patency of the fallopian tubes. This procedure is performed when the patient seeks to establish continuity of the tubes in hopes of conceiving. Obstruction of the fallopian tubes can be caused by infection, tubal ligation, and scarring. Tubal anastomosis is primarily undertaken to reverse previous tubal ligation and is usually performed with an operating microscope.

Operative Procedure

Using a small urinary catheter inserted into the uterine cavity, a dilute solution of methylene blue or indigo carmine may be injected into the fallopian tubes to determine the patency (chromotubation) of the tubes and the placement of tube closure. Through either a laparotomy incision or a laparoscopy portal, the closed portions of the tube are isolated and freed from the fold of the peritoneum surrounding the tubes. While maintaining as much length of the open fallopian tube as possible, the closed portion is excised away. Luminal patency is checked by injecting dye toward and into the uterus and outward through the distal tube. Once the fallopian tube's patency is ascertained, the excised ends are anastomosed (end-to-end tuboplasty anastomosis) through the muscularis wall only (no suture material passing through the mucosa).

This surgery can be carried out as a laparoscopy, robotic-assisted, or laparotomy procedure; it may include lysis of adhesions. Techniques to open an obstructed fallopian tube include microsurgery, laser, dissection, excision and anastomosis, and electrocautery. The chances of success depend on the amount of tube scarring and destruction.

Anesthetic

GETA is given with insertion of an OETT; muscle relaxants are given.

Positioning

The patient is placed in a supine position, with the arms extended on armboards bilaterally. Trendelenburg position is done to facilitate injection of dye into the cervix.

Anesthetic Implications

Smooth emergence from anesthesia is important with an open approach. The goal is to avoid coughing, bucking, or nausea/vomiting or retching so as to prevent increased risk of bleeding, hematoma formation, or suture line disruption from the increased abdominal pressures. Have a team member hold gentle pressure over the suture lines if the patient does cough or vomit. Antiemetics should be given (see Chapter 4).

Uterine Fibroid Embolization (Uterine Artery Embolization)

In uterine fibroid embolization (UFE), the blood vessels supplying a fibroid tumor (myoma) are occluded. Blocking the blood flow to the fibroid causes the fibroid cells to die and shrink, thereby causing the fibroid to shrink.

Operative Procedure

A sheath is inserted into the femoral artery. A tiny catheter is advanced through the femoral sheath, directed by arteriography of the pelvic vasculature, to the uterine artery. An embolic agent—polyvinyl alcohol (PVA) particles, a gelatin sponge, or microspheres—is injected through this catheter to embolize the arteries that send blood to the fibroid. Arteriography will indicate whether the vessels feeding the fibroid have been occluded.

Collateral circulation maintains blood supply to the myometrium.

Anesthetic
Two types of anesthesia may be used: local anesthesia with IV sedation or a spinal block.

Positioning
The patient is placed in a supine position.

Anesthetic Implications
The patient should be informed of the possible warm flushed feeling with injection of radiologic contrast, even if she is to be sedated.

The affected leg should be kept straight (at the groin) for six hours following removal of the femoral artery sheath.

OBSTETRIC SURGERY

Cervical Cerclage (Cervical Ligature)

Cervical cerclage is the placement of an encircling suture ligature at the level of the internal cervical os in an effort to maintain the integrity of an incompetent cervix from mid- to late pregnancy. The goal is to prevent cervical dilatation that might result in spontaneous abortion. Thus, cervical ligature is intended to reinforce and secure an incompetent cervix, and to prevent premature dilation.

Operative Procedure
Cervical cerclage is usually done through a vaginal approach. An incision is made in the vaginal mucosa at the anterior and posterior aspects of the cervix. A non-absorbable suture is stitched around the cervix and tightened. The suture is usually removed around the 38th week of gestation.

In rare cases, an abdominal approach may be used.

Anesthetic
Anesthesia options include neuraxial anesthesia (spinal or epidural); GETA; or sedation/MAC with local anesthetic. Avoid the use of midazolam and nitrous oxide. Give minimal amounts of all IV drugs,

as most of these agents will cross the placental barrier. See Chapter 3 for more information on anesthesia and the pregnant patient.

Positioning
The patient is placed in a lithotomy position, with the arms extended on armboards bilaterally. While she is in the supine position, a wedge should be placed under the mother's right hip for left uterine displacement (LUD) after the 20th week of gestation, so as to keep the fetus's weight off the mother's aorta. Venous return and cardiac output to the mother decrease and ureteroplacental insufficiency in the baby (from aortocaval compression) occurs if the mother lies in the supine position.

Anesthetic Implications
It is best to perform a cervical cerclage procedure before actual dilation of the cervix occurs.

Cesarean Section Birth

Cesarean section is the delivery of a fetus through an incision in the mother's abdomen and uterus. Indications for this procedure include planned delivery by the mother's choice, previous uterine surgery precluding the possibility of vaginal birth, cephalopelvic disproportion, failure to progress, fetal breech presentation, malrotated fetus, placenta previa/abruption, and emergency conditions in which the safety of the fetus or the mother (or both) is in jeopardy. A cesarean may also be done if the mother has an active case of genital herpes or another vaginal infection that may jeopardize the baby's health in the event of vaginal delivery.

Operative Procedure
After the insertion of a urinary catheter, a low transverse abdominal incision (planned cesarean) or vertical incision from umbilicus to mons pubis is made on the abdomen. The abdominal wall is opened in layers; the peritoneum is opened. A transverse incision is made over the uterus and enlarged with the surgeon's hands applied laterally. External fundal pressure may be applied to the upper abdominal

area (above the uterus) as the fetal head is gently elevated and brought out of the uterus. After the head is delivered, the nares and mouth of the fetus are suctioned before bringing out the rest of the fetus. The cord is clamped and cut; the fetus is handed off to the neonatal nurse and brought to the warmer for assessment and/or resuscitation.

In the event of a breech or transverse presentation, the fetus's foot and leg are brought out of the incision first. As with a "head-first" presentation, as soon as the head is delivered, the neonate's nose and mouth are suctioned out.

The uterus is brought out of the wound to be sutured. This step often causes the mother a lot of pressure and pain in the abdomen, chest and shoulder (especially the right shoulder). Letting the mother know that these feelings are normal is comforting to many women. If the patient becomes anxious or complains of pain, it is acceptable to give her benzodiazepines or narcotics (given only after the baby has been delivered). The uterus is replaced into the abdominal cavity, and the wound is closed in layers. After a dressing is placed, the surgical nurse will massage the patient's fundus to help push out any blood or clots from the vagina before moving the mother off the operating room table to the bed.

Anesthetic

A spinal/epidural block is given. GETA and an OETT are appropriate if the neuraxial block is refused, contraindicated, ineffective or in an emergency (see Emergency Cesarean Section below). The anesthesia team must always be prepared to implement general anesthesia in an obstetric operating room.

Positioning

The patient is placed in a supine position, with the arms extended on armboards bilaterally. The arms should be secured on armboards if neuraxial anesthesia is given and the patient is awake. While she is in the supine position, a wedge should be placed under the mother's right hip for

left uterine displacement (LUD) after the 20th week of gestation, so as to keep the fetus's weight off the mother's aorta. Venous return and cardiac output to the mother decrease and ureteroplacental insufficiency in the baby (from aortocaval compression) occurs if the mother lies in the supine position. LUD can be discontinued after the baby is delivered.

Anesthetic Implications

All pregnant patients are considered "full stomach" cases and require a nonparticulate antacid by mouth before neuraxial anesthesia.

Fetal heart tones (FHT) are usually checked before and after neuraxial anesthesia is implemented. The findings are documented on the anesthesia record.

Before implementing a neuraxial block, unless contraindicated, 500–1000 mL of fluid should be infused intravenously to prevent the hypotensive response to the sympathectomy.

Check the level of paresthesia from the neuraxial block before draping the patient; it should be at the T4 level bilaterally. The surgeon should check that the mother is insensate (usually via a pinch test) at the incision line before making the initial incision. The mother should be instructed that although she should not feel "sharp pain," she will feel some movement and pressure. The pressure sensation will be most acute when the surgeon is applying manual pressure to deliver the fetal head (pressure felt across the abdomen) and when the uterus is external to the abdominal cavity so that the surgeon can sew the uterus closed (pressure felt across the abdomen, the chest, and up to the shoulders—especially in the right shoulder from phrenic nerve irritation).

If the patient complains of shortness of breath or difficulty breathing, have the mother blow air into your hand or squeeze your fingers as hard as possible. If either response is weak, the neuraxial anesthesia may be too high. Such a patient may need to receive a general anesthetic with oral intubation to maintain adequate oxygenation.

If the patient complains of nausea or "not feeling good," the blood pressure may have dropped due to the spinal or epidural. Immediately treat the patient for hypotension and give an antiemetic. Ephedrine and phenylephrine (Neosynephrine) are vasopressors commonly given in these circumstances.

Document the time of case start, uterine incision, and time of birth(s) on the anesthetic record.

Pitocin (oxytocin), 20–40 units added to a 1-L bag of IV fluid, given to the mother after the baby is separate from the mother and the placenta has been delivered; this medication will facilitate uterine contraction. A second 1-L bag with Pitocin is usually given after the first is infused. Check with the surgeon or hospital protocol to determine the preferred approach.

Any drug given to the pregnant mother may potentially affect the fetus. Drugs to avoid in pregnant women include nitrous oxide, benzodiazepines, and opioids. In some cases, ketamine may be given to awake, anxious mothers to help calm them before the fetus is delivered by cesarean section.

Antiemetics should be given to all patients undergoing cesarean section.

Tubal ligation may be performed at the time of a cesarean section if that procedure is planned in advance.

Emergency Cesarean Section

With an emergency cesarean section, the goal is to get the baby out of the uterus as quickly as possible through a surgical incision. This surgery is necessary in case of fetal distress/bradycardia, non-reassuring fetal heart tones (FHT), hemorrhage, uterine rupture, or a prolapsed umbilical cord.

Operative Procedure

A vertical incision from umbilicus to mons pubis is made. The abdominal wall is opened in layers; the peritoneum is opened. A transverse incision is made over the uterus and enlarged with the surgeon's hands applied laterally. External pressure is applied to the uterine fundus as the fetal head is elevated and quickly brought out of the uterus. After the head is delivered, the nares and mouth of the fetus are suctioned before bringing out the rest of the fetus. The cord is clamped and cut; the fetus is handed off to the neonatal nurse and brought to the warmer for assessment and/or resuscitation. After being stabilized in the operating room, the baby is taken to the intensive care nursery for evaluation.

Anesthetic

Anesthesia consists of GETA with rapid-sequence induction.

Have the patient take 4–5 deep breaths with 100% FiO_2 prior to induction.

Thiopental is the drug of choice for induction purposes in obstetric emergencies.

Give the succinylcholine (Anectine) dose for intubation.

Place a smaller than calculated OETT, as the patient's mucous membranes will be swollen.

These cases are usually so quick that a nondepolarizing muscle relaxation is not needed; if such an agent is given, use only a small amount. Run inhaled anesthesia at ½ MAC with 100% FiO_2 until the baby is delivered.

Positioning

The patient is placed supine in the "sniff position." While she is in the supine position, a wedge should be placed under the mother's right hip for left uterine displacement (LUD), so as to keep the fetus's weight off the mother's aorta. Venous return and cardiac output to the mother decrease and ureteroplacental insufficiency in the baby (from aortocaval compression) occurs if the mother lies in the supine position. LUD can be discontinued after the baby is delivered.

Anesthetic Implications

If possible, the mother should receive a clear antacid by mouth preoperatively to decrease the level of acid in the stomach in the event of regurgitation.

Type and cross-match the patient's blood. A trauma pack of un-cross-matched blood may be needed if the mother is hemorrhaging. Anticipate and prepare for moderate to massive blood loss.

Check fetal heart tones (FHT) as soon as the mother is supine on the operating room table. It may be necessary to monitor for FHT throughout the entire emergency cesarean section.

Once the baby is delivered and the umbilical cord is clamped, you can give the mother narcotics and midazolam as necessary.

Monitor the mother's urinary output for blood. Extubate this patient when all criteria are met.

Monitors

• An arterial line is recommended.
• A central venous line may be needed.
• Two large-bore PIVs should be placed if a CVP is not inserted.

Vasoactive Agents

• IV vasoactive agents: ephedrine, phenylephrine (Neo-Synephrine)
• Other drugs to have available: Pitocin (oxytocin); methylergonovine maleate (Methergine), 0.2 mg IM; prostaglandins

Complications
Potential complications of an emergency cesarean section include bladder injury.

Postpartum Tubal Ligation

Postpartum tubal ligation (PPTL) is a surgical procedure in which a woman's fallopian tubes are blocked, tied, or cut. It is usually performed 24–36 hours postpartum in women who desire permanent sterilization.

Operative Procedure
The fallopian tubes are typically located higher in the abdomen immediately after pregnancy. An incision is made just below the belly button (navel). The fallopian tubes are brought out of the incision and ligated and severed bilaterally.

See the discussion of tubal ligation earlier in this chapter for more information.

PPTL can be done during a cesarean section with the abdominal incision still open.

Anesthetic
Anesthesia options include GETA or neuraxial anesthesia (spinal or epidural to the T4 level).

Positioning
The patient is placed in a lithotomy position, with the arms secured at an angle less than 90 degrees on armboards. She may be placed in Trendelenburg during surgery so that gravity displaces the abdominal contents cephalad, per surgeon request.

Anesthetic Implications
A consent form for sterilization must be signed, along with the consent form for the cesarean section.

If PPTL is performed under general anesthesia, use a smaller ETT, as the patient's airway will be engorged and friable.

Anesthetic requirements in postpartum patients are reduced.

If PPTL is performed under spinal block, give lactated Ringer's solution, 500–1000 mL bolus, prior to placing the spinal. Have phenylephrine (Neosynephrine) and ephedrine ready to treat hypotension.

Check the patient while she is in the Trendelenburg position to make sure her arms don't fall off the armboards.

Retained Placenta Removal

After delivery of the fetus, manual or surgical removal of a retained placenta in the uterus is sometimes necessary. A retained placenta may be one that has actually separated from the uterus but is engulfed by the cervix, or the placenta may still be adhered to the uterine wall. Severe bleeding often occurs in both of these instances, so blood transfusions are common in patients with a retained placenta. For significant bleeding with placenta accreta, an emergency hysterectomy (discussed later in this chapter) is required.

Operative Procedure
If the placenta is adhered to the uterine wall, it may need to be removed manually in total or removed in fragments by a curette. In some cases, the placenta may have grown into the uterine wall (placenta accreta), so that the uterus (with the placenta) must be surgically removed.

Anesthetic
For manual or curette removal of the placenta in whole or in fragments, spinal or epidural neuraxial anesthesia, or GETA, is needed. For a TAH, GETA with muscle relaxation is needed.

Positioning
The patient is placed in a lithotomy position for manual extraction of the placenta. She is placed in a supine position for TAH.

Anesthetic Implications
The uterus may be massaged to help it contract.

A retained placenta can cause significant blood loss.

Vasoactive Agents
- IV vasoactive agents: ephedrine, phenylephrine (Neosynephrine); nitroglycerin infusion to relax the smooth muscle of uterus
- Other drugs to have available: Pitocin (oxytocin); methylergonovine maleate (Methergine), 0.2 mg IM; prostaglandins to help prevent or decrease bleeding from the uterus

Uterine Inversion Management

Uterine inversion management seeks to return a partially or completely inverted uterus to its natural position. Uterine inversion occurs when the uterine fundus collapses into the endometrial cavity and possibly out through the cervix. It is a potentially life-threatening complication of vaginal

and (rarely) cesarean delivery. Treatment should begin as soon as the inversion is recognized to replace the uterus and prevent significant blood loss and maternal instability. Inversion can occur anywhere from within hours of delivery to more than a month postpartum. An inversion can also occur when attempts to deliver the placenta cause the uterus to turn inside out.

In case of uterine inversion, you will see the fundus of the uterus (a large, dark red mass) coming out of the cervix. The mother will be in extreme pain and often hemodynamically unstable. This scenario can range from an inverted fundus that has not come through the cervix (*incomplete inversion*) to a *total inversion* in which both the vagina and the uterus are inverted and outside the body.

Operative Procedure
Manual Uterine Inversion
The physician will attempt to push the fundus back through the dilated cervix slowly and steadily. General anesthesia may be required. If the uterus cannot be manually replaced, an open abdominal procedure must be done.

Open Uterine Inversion
A midline laparotomy incision is made, and the uterus is repositioned. The wound is then closed in layers.

Anesthetic
GETA is used with rapid-sequence induction; ketamine may be the induction agent of choice for a hemodynamically unstable mother. Succinylcholine (Anectine) can be used as well.

Positioning
The patient is placed in the lithotomy position for manual uterine inversion. She is placed in a supine position for an open procedure.

Anesthetic Implications
For manual attempts to manage inversion, administer tocolytics: IV nitroglycerin (0.25–0.5 mg IV

over 2 minutes), terbutaline (0.1–0.25 mg IV over 2 minutes; has a rapid onset of action), or magnesium drip (4–6 mg loading dose IV over 20 minutes to relax the uterus and uterine vessels). Note that magnesium cannot be given if the mother's blood pressure is low.

Oxytocin and methylergonovine are usually needed to help the uterus contract, but should not be given until after the uterus has been successfully replaced in the pelvis. The uterus may also be massaged from inside the vagina and on the abdomen to help it contract.

If the placenta has not been delivered when the uterus inverts, do not attempt to remove the placenta until the uterus is positioned normally.

Antibiotics should be given.

Significant blood loss is common with uterine inversion, and administration of blood products is usually necessary. Multiple large-bore peripheral IVs should be established.

Complications

Potential complications of uterine inversion management include endometritis and damage to the uterus or intestines.

Emergency Obstetrical Hysterectomy

Emergency obstetrical hysterectomy is an emergency procedure to remove the uterus during labor and delivery. It may be performed in cases involving antepartum hemorrhage, usually from uterine atony and placenta accreta, or uterine rupture. It represents a last resort to save the mother's life.

Operative Procedure

See the discussions of total abdominal hysterectomy and emergency cesarean section earlier in this chapter for more information.

Anesthetic

Have the patient take 4–5 deep breaths with 100% FiO_2. Anesthesia options include GETA and cricoid pressure with rapid-sequence induction. If GETA is used, ketamine may be the induction agent of choice for a hemodynamically unstable mother. Succinylcholine (Anectine) can be used as well.

The patient may already have neuraxial anesthesia but endotracheal intubation is required to control the airway and for skeletal muscle relaxation.

Positioning

The patient is placed in a supine position with left uterine displacement until the fetus is delivered.

Anesthetic Implications

Significant blood loss is common in these cases, and administration of blood products is usually necessary. Un-cross-matched blood may be needed if typed and cross-matched blood is not available.

Multiple large-bore peripheral IVs should be established.

Complications

Potential complications include sepsis and DIC.

Orthopedic Surgery

21

ORTHOPEDIC SURGERY PEARLS

- If open reduction and internal fixation are performed with rigid fixation, in general the likelihood of union is high. In a few types of fractures, the blood supply to the bone is poor and closed reduction techniques are advantageous for bone healing, but these are the exception.
- Patients who present to the operating room with orthopedic injuries may have sustained high-force trauma; it is of critical importance to fully evaluate these patients for coexisting neurologic, thoracic, or abdominal trauma before giving anesthesia. Any patient coming for surgery under these circumstances should be considered a "full stomach" case and should be intubated with an oral endotracheal tube (not a laryngeal mask airway [LMA] tube) with general anesthesia, using rapid-sequence induction. NPO time is counted from when the patient last ate until the time of trauma, as GI motility stops (with decreased gastric emptying) at trauma time.
- Alcohol (ETOH) is involved in 50% of cases requiring emergency orthopedic procedures. Factors related to alcohol use that should be taken into account by the anesthetist include decreased anesthetic requirements, dieresis, hypothermia, and vasodilation.
- Ketamine can be used for orthopedic patients who have received a spinal or epidural when sedation or anxiolysis is given. This agent helps to keep the patient still and breathing.
- The patient must be kept asleep until the splint or external fixator is applied.
- Patients with rheumatoid arthritis may have cervical nerve root compression or atlanto-occipital instability. Assess the patient's ability to extend the neck and ask about any numbness or tingling with neck movement. Check the neck X-ray for subluxation of the cervical spine. These patients may require awake fiberoptic intubation. They may be on chronic steroid therapy, so that an intraoperative "stress dose" of steroids may need to be given.

- Deep venous thrombosis (DVT) is a *major* concern during orthopedic surgery; regional anesthesia decreases the risk of DVT. DVT prophylaxis must be used in these patients.
- When the patient is in a sitting position, the danger of brachial plexus and forearm neuropathies is decreased compared to when the patient is in the lateral decubitus position. Also, when the patient is in the sitting position, the arm's weight helps to distract the shoulder joint and avoids distortion of the intra-articular anatomy.
- Trauma patients should be maintained in a C-collar with spinal precautions until cleared.
- Neurovascular compromise is possible with an orthopedic injury. Assess the area distal to the separation for circulation, sensation, and motor function preoperatively and postoperatively, and document the findings.

FAT EMBOLISM SYNDROME

Fat embolism syndrome is most often seen with long bone fracture, total joint replacement, or multiple fractures with pelvic injury. Immobilizing fractures as soon as possible is important to decrease secondary injuries, decrease pain, and minimize chance of fat emboli occurring.

RHABDOMYOLYSIS

Rhabdomyolysis (muscle necrosis) is a rapid breakdown of skeletal muscle tissue due to injury (from physical, chemical, or biologic causes), acute ischemia, dramatically increased metabolism (status epilepticus), or compartment syndrome. This muscle destruction causes a release of myoglobin into the plasma, which is toxic to the kidneys (renal system). It is worsened by hypovolemia. Rhabdomyolysis accounts for as much as 25% of all cases of acute renal failure. It is diagnosed based on increased serum levels of muscle enzymes (CPK, SGOT, SGPT, and LDH levels) as well as the presence of hyperkalemia, hyperphosphatemia, brown urine, and (sometimes) urine myoglobin.

Rhabdomyolysis may lead to compartment syndrome—that is, muscle injury may lead to swelling and increased pressure in a confined space (a compartment). The resulting compromised circulation can endanger the affected tissue. Compartment syndrome is most common after injury in the lower leg or the muscles of the abdominal wall and can require emergency fasciotomy.

Kidney failure is another possible complication of rhabdomyolysis. In such cases, myoglobin is excreted by the glomeruli but precipitates in the proximal convoluted tubules of the nephrons.

Treatment for rhabdomyolysis includes hydration, mannitol, diuretics, and bicarbonate (given to increase urine pH) to help the body excrete myoglobin more effectively. Hemodialysis may be necessary to clear myoglobin from the bloodstream. Keep urinary output at a rate of 100–150 mL/hr.

The overall prognosis when rhabdomyolysis occurs is favorable as long as this condition is recognized and treated promptly.

Fasciotomy

A fasciotomy is done to treat compartment syndrome. It becomes necessary when intracompartmental (IC) pressure (measured by tonometry; normal intracompartmental pressure < 30 mm Hg) within the confined space of the fascial compartment increases to the point that it exceeds capillary perfusion pressure and impairs blood supply to the limb. If the diastolic blood pressure is less than 30 mm Hg from the intracompartmental pressure, this is also considered a sign of increased IC pressure and a fasciotomy is indicated.

Other signs to assess for in an awake, alert, and oriented patient include pain with passive stretch of the muscle (most sensitive clinical exam): "pain out of proportion."

Without prompt surgical release of the pressure within 6–8 hours, nerve damage and muscle necrosis occurs. Compartment syndrome is considered a true emergency.

Compartment syndrome is most commonly seen in the anterior lower leg and in the deep volar forearm. Nevertheless, it can occur anywhere in the body with a confined compartment (e.g., the abdomen).

Compartment syndrome is caused by any process which increases pressure within a closed space:

- Internal causes: fractures, hemorrhage, vascular puncture
- External causes: prolonged limb compression, crush injuries, burns

It is believed that ischemia is possible at compartment pressures greater than 30 mm Hg. This condition is considered an emergency warranting immediate surgical intervention for preservation of the limb and can be fatal if not treated.

Treatment of Compartment Syndrome

Operative Procedure
An incision is made in the skin, and a small area of fascia is removed where it will best relieve pressure. The incision is usually left open for 24–48 hours and then closed. If the wound cannot be closed, it is often covered with a vacuum dressing for closure later.

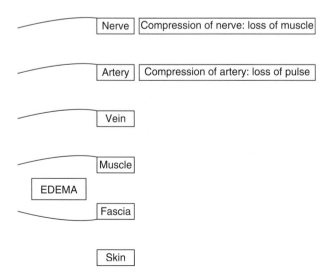

Anesthetic
General anesthesia is most common. If the patient has no underlying issues such as trauma, necrotizing fasciitis, or sepsis, spinal anesthesia is appropriate because the procedure is short.

Positioning
The patient is placed in a supine or lateral decubitus position, depending on the location of the pressure.

DEFINITIONS

Arthrodesis: surgical resection of the articular surfaces of a joint with bony stabilization resulting in bony fusion. Done to relieve pain or restore alignment in a diseased, unstable, or injured joint.

Arthroscopy: extensive visualization of the intra-articular aspect of a joint is possible. Can be used to diagnose a condition or to perform specific surgeries.

Arthrotomy: incision into a joint.

Closed reduction: a surgical procedure in which the physician realigns the fracture without needing to cut the skin. X-ray or fluoroscopy is used to verify placement. Sedation is usually all that is required, but note that trauma patients are considered to be full-stomach cases. If general anesthesia is used, rapid-sequence induction and an endotracheal tube are warranted.

Dislocation: separation of two bones around a joint with loss of articular contact. Often results in ligament and capsule damage.

External fixation: a surgical treatment used to stabilize fractures when a cast will not allow for proper alignment of the fracture. In this kind of fixation, holes are drilled into uninjured areas of bones around the fracture and threaded pins are screwed into the bone. Outside the body, a rod or a curved piece of metal with special ball-and-socket joints joins the pins to provide stability to the fractured bone or unstable joint. External fixation is commonly limited to patients with open fractures who also suffer from bone loss and vascular and soft-tissue injuries. Risks with external fixation include pin tract infections to soft tissue and/or bone, and injury to neurovascular structures.

Fracture: structural break in bone continuity.

Intramedullary nailing (intramedullary rods): devices that are used to align and stabilize fractures of the long bones of the extremities (i.e., femur, tibia). Intramedullary (IM) nails are inserted into the bone marrow canal in the center of the bone and share the load with the bone (rather than just support the bone), allowing the patient to be able to use the extremity more quickly. They cannot be used for all fractures. The IM nail can stay inside the bone forever, but if it causes pain, it may need to be surgically removed.

The IM nail does not involve placement of multiple screws for plate fixation, which may disrupt the periosteal blood supply. While it does not significantly damage the viability of the bone, IM nailing is believed to destroy the intramedullary blood supply.

Osteotomy: a surgical procedure in which the bones around a joint are cut, reoriented, and fixed in a new position.

Subluxation: partial loss of articular contact between two bones in a joint.

Synovectomy: excision of all or a portion of the synovial membrane of the knee.

LEVELS OF ORTHOPEDIC SURGERY

- **True emergency:** threatens a neurovascular structure and can produce loss of "life or limb." Immobilization of a fractured extremity is _key_ to decrease the chance of secondary injury, to decrease pain, and minimize chance of fat emboli. If more than 6 hours pass from injury to surgical intervention, infection risk may preclude closure of open, traumatic wounds. True emergency examples include:
  - Joint dislocations
  - Digit replantation
  - Compartment syndrome
  - Fracture with vascular injury
  - Unstable pelvic ring disruption
  - Spine injury with progressive neurologic deficit
  - Open fractures
- **Urgent:** open fractures; long bone fractures of the femur or tibia; multiple trauma.
- **Elective:** knee scope procedures; anterior cruciate ligament (ACL) tear.

ANESTHETICS FOR ORTHOPEDIC PROCEDURES

Anesthetics for orthopedic procedures include general anesthesia, neuraxial (spinal or epidural), and peripheral nerve blocks (PNB; continuous or single dose), used either singly or in combination.

Peripheral Nerve Blocks

- Shoulder: interscalene
- Above the elbow: supraclavicular, infraclavicular, interscalene, intercostobrachial
- At or below the elbow: supraclavicular, infraclavicular, axillary, Bier block
- Thigh, leg, ankle, or foot: femoral, sciatic
- Posterior knee, leg, or lower leg (if a thigh tourniquet is not used): sciatic

Interscalene Block

An interscalene block is done to anesthetize the shoulder and proximal arm. It can occasionally cross the elbow and anesthetize part of the forearm (and rarely the fingers).

This block generally misses the ulnar branch (the most inferior portion of the brachial plexus), which feeds cutaneous sensation of the fourth and fifth fingers of the hands. The ulnar branch is also involved with fine motor movement of the fingers, as it innervates the lumbrical muscles.

Hemidiaphragmatic paralysis is a consequence of an interscalene block; do not use this anesthesia option if the patient has preexisting respiratory compromise. An interscalene block is placed near the spinal cord and can get a high spinal effect; it can affect the phrenic nerve.

Supraclavicular Block

A supraclavicular block provides anesthesia to the entire upper extremity. It is most likely to block all nerves for the entire arm, especially from the mid-humerus to the fingers. It can also be used to anesthetize the shoulder if the local anesthesia spreads in a cephalad manner.

A supraclavicular block is supplemented with a superficial cervical plexus block to anesthetize the skin overlying the shoulder.

Infraclavicular Block

An infraclavicular block provides anesthesia from the hand up to the mid-humerus (just like the supraclavicular block, although coverage of the axillary nerve supplying the shoulder is less common). Called a "high axillary block," it provides anesthesia to the elbow, forearm, or hand.

Coverage of the axillary nerve supplying the shoulder is less common.

To block the medial aspect of the arm, perform an intercostobrachial block.

Intercostobrachial Block

An intercostobrachial block is not part of the brachial plexus. Rather, this type of anesthetic is used to perform a ring block in the axilla or a T2 paravertebral block. It provides anesthesia to the medial and posterior portions of the upper part of the upper arm.

Axillary Block

An axillary block provides anesthesia below the elbow to numb the hand and forearm. It typically misses the musculocutaneous branch.

Bier Block

Bier block is done for surgery of the hand and lower forearm.

Femoral Block

A femoral block provides anesthesia for surgery to the femur or knee.

Femoral and Sciatic Block

Anesthesia for surgery to the femur, lower leg, ankle, or foot may consist of a femoral and sciatic block.

Popliteal Block

A popliteal block affects the tibial and peroneal nerves. It is used for surgeries of the foot and ankle.

Sciatic Nerve Block

Few surgical procedures can be performed with a sciatic block alone.

ORTHOPEDIC SURGERY: SHOULDER GIRDLE

Anatomy that can be injured during surgery in the shoulder girdle includes the brachial plexus, great vessels (subclavian), axillary nerve, and musculocutaneous nerve. Pneumothorax is a possible complication.

Correction of Acromioclavicular Joint Separation

This surgery involves open reduction and internal fixation of the acromioclavicular (AC) joint. The AC joint is located at the distal end of the clavicle and attaches to the acromion of the scapula. With AC joint separation, the ligamentous support of the distal clavicle is disrupted due to athletic injuries or trauma. Most AC joint separations can be treated nonoperatively but Grades IV–VI AC separations are usually treated surgically.

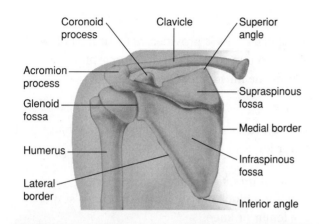

Figure 21-1 *Anatomy of the Acromioclavicular Joint and Shoulder*
Source: AAOS, 2004.

Operative Procedure

A curved incision made over the AC joint and distal end of the clavicle. The surgeon typically cuts off the end of the clavicular portion, partially sacrifices the coracoacromial ligament, and then sutures the acromial end to the lateral aspect of the clavicle for increased stability.

Keep the patient asleep until the sling is on.

Anesthetic

General anesthesia is used with an oral endotracheal tube (OETT); muscle relaxation is given. A peripheral block (placed with IV sedation) or a combination of peripheral and general anesthesia may be used. The endotracheal tube is taped on the opposite side of the mouth from the side of surgery to keep out of the surgeon's working area.

An interscalene block is the most commonly performed block for shoulder surgery. A supraclavicular brachial plexus block can also be performed, as local anesthesia will spread in a cephalad direction (and anesthetize the axillary nerve).

Positioning

The patient is usually placed in a beach-chair position, but can be lateral decubitus or supine with the arm flexed over the chest. A sandbag or folded sheet is tucked under the affected shoulder. The head is turned away from the surgical side. If the beach-chair position is used, see Chapter 3 for more information on the risks of venous air embolism with this position.

Anesthetic Implications

If the beach-chair position is used, careful attention to stabilization of the patient's head is necessary. It may be difficult to see the patient's face after the drapes are up and the lights are turned down. Tape the ETT securely, as access to the patient's head will be limited after surgery begins.

These patients require special eye care. Paper tape is used to close the eyes to prevent corneal drying or abrasions; eye pads are then placed over both eyes. Consider using protective goggles.

The IV and blood pressure cuff should be placed on the nonoperative arm.

The surgeon may request a SBP of less than 100 mm Hg to prevent bleeding and improve visualization during arthroscopic surgery.

Neurovascular compromise is rare with this injury. The axillary, musculocutaneous, brachial plexus, and subclavian vessels are at risk, however.

Repair of Dislocated Anterior Shoulder

Surgery may be necessary to strengthen the anterior joint capsule and musculotendonous support of the shoulder when recurrent anterior shoulder dislocation occurs. The glenohumeral joint can dislocate anteriorly, posteriorly, or inferiorly relative to the glenoid. (See also the "Correction of Recurrent Anterior Shoulder Dislocation" section later in this chapter.)

Operative Procedure

The anterior joint capsule cushions and supports the humeral head. Surgery to repair dislocations in this area can be done either arthroscopically or as an open procedure.

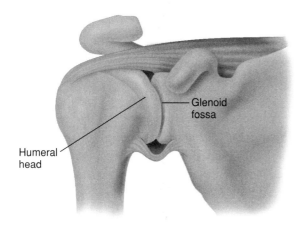

Normal

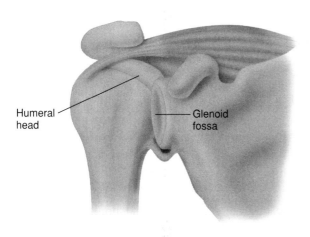

Posterior dislocation

Figure 21-2   *Posterior Dislocation of the Shoulder, Showing Anatomy of the Glenoid Fossa*
Source: AAOS, 2004.

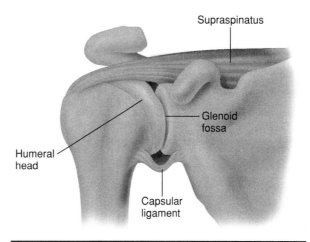

Figure 21-3   *The Shoulder Capsule*
Source: AAOS, 2004.

In an open procedure, an anterior incision is made over the pectoral groove. There are several modifications of this procedure.

- *Bankart:* The glenoid labrum and the anterior capsule are reattached to the rim of the glenoid cavity.
- *Putti-Platt:* The subscapularis tendon and the capsule are detached from the humerus and sutured laterally on the humeral neck to support the anterior supporting structures and to prevent excessive external rotation of the shoulder.
- *Bristow:* The coracoid process and attached muscles are detached, inserted into the neck of the scapula, and fixed. The transferred muscular origins serve as a buttress across the anterior and inferior aspect of the joint and also anchor the lower half of the subscapularis. An anterior incision is made over the pectoral groove. The joint capsule is exposed and the coracoid process is osteotomized from the scapula.

The patient is kept asleep until a sling is placed.

Anesthetic

If general anesthesia is given with insertion of an ETT; muscle relaxants can be given.

Alternatively, IV sedation with an interscalene block is the most commonly performed block for shoulder surgery. A supraclavicular brachial plexus block can also be performed, as local anesthesia will spread in a cephalad direction (and anesthetize the axillary nerve).

A combination of general and peripheral block anesthesia may be used for postoperative pain control.

Positioning

The patient is placed in a supine position, with the affected shoulder elevated on a folded sheet or blanket. The elbow is flexed over the chest; the head is turned away from the surgical side. A beach-chair position or lateral decubitus may also be used. If the beach-chair position is used, see Chapter 3 for more information on venous air embolism.

Anesthetic Implications

Injury to the axillary nerve or artery may occur with this procedure. Check the patient's sensation over the lateral deltoid region to assess the axillary nerve.

The IV and blood pressure cuff should be placed on the nonoperative arm.

Rotator cuff injuries are a common associated injury after shoulder dislocation in adults.

If the beach-chair position is used, careful attention to stabilization of the patient's head is necessary. It may be difficult to see the patient's face after the drapes are up and the lights are turned down. Tape the ETT securely, as access to the patient's head will be limited after surgery begins.

These patients require special eye care. Paper tape is used to close the eyes to prevent corneal drying or abrasions; eye pads are then placed over both eyes. Consider using protective goggles.

The surgeon may request an SBP of less than 100 mm Hg to prevent bleeding and improve visualization during arthroscopic surgery.

Brachial Plexus Surgery

Anatomy of the Brachial Plexus

The brachial plexus is an arrangement of nerve fibers that come from the spine; it is formed by the ventral rami of the C5–C8 nerves and T1 nerve (and may contain C4 and T2 as well). The brachial plexus travels through the neck and the axilla and into the arm as three distinct nerve trunks, located between the anterior and middle scalene muscles (the subclavian artery also runs between these muscles).

These three distinct nerve trunks are named the superior, middle, and inferior trunk. The superior is primarily derived from C5–C6; the middle trunk is derived from C7; and the inferior trunk is derived from C8–T1.

As the plexus passes over the lateral edge of the first rib and under the clavicle, the fibers form three cords that are named according to their relationship to the axillary artery: lateral, medial, and posterior. At the lateral border of the pectoralis minor muscle, each cord terminates in a major nerve.

Surgery and Indications

Procedures performed on the brachial plexus include neurolysis, nerve grafting, nerve transfer, and neurotization (implantation of a nerve into a paralyzed muscle) with intraoperative nerve testing. Denervated muscle can lead to deformities of the muscles and skeletal system. Although the brachial plexus can be damaged in high-impact conditions such as motor vehicle accidents, it is commonly injured when a baby's shoulder becomes stuck during the birth process and excessive force is applied to the baby's head and neck, resulting in the brachial plexus being stretched or torn.

Operative Procedure

Surgical incision is made above the clavicle similar to anterior neck dissection or below the clavicle. For axillary nerve dissection, a posterior approach is done.

The patient should be kept asleep until the sling is on.

Anesthetic

General anesthesia is given with insertion of an ETT. Rapid-sequence induction should be used if the case involves a trauma patient. No muscle relaxation is given. These patients may require

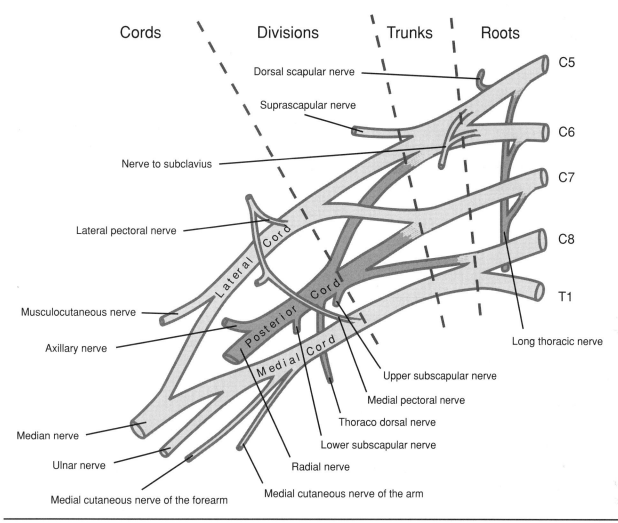

Figure 21-4 *Brachial Plexus*

fiberoptic intubation, especially if the patient is wearing a hard cervical collar brace.

Supraclavicular, infraclavicular, axillary, or interscalene brachial plexus blocks can be placed with this type or surgery (with the choice depending on the specific site of surgery). As always with any block, but particularly for this surgery, check with the surgical team as to whether neurological testing is needed immediately postoperatively.

Positioning
Patient positioning varies depending on the exact procedure performed. The patient is usually placed

supine with the head of the bed elevated, but can be lateral decubitus. If the beach-chair position is used, see Chapter 3 for more information on venous air embolism.

Anesthetic Implications
Intraoperative nerve testing will be performed, so no muscle relaxants are given.

The IV and blood pressure cuff should be placed on the nonoperative arm if the patient has a unilateral injury.

There is a potential for significant blood loss with this surgery. Place two or more large-bore peripheral IVs in case fluid/blood resuscitation is required.

Traumatic brain injury, occult pulmonary, cardiac, and mediastinal injuries may be present in any trauma patient. A hard C-collar should be placed on any trauma patient until the cervical spine is cleared.

Secure the ETT well, as access to the patient's head will be limited after surgery begins. Consider protective goggles or eye pads for patient.

The surgeon may request a SBP of less than 100 mm Hg to prevent bleeding and improve visualization during arthroscopic surgery.

Complications

Potential complications include brachial plexus injury, hemo-pneumothorax, and pneumothorax.

Neurovascular compromise is possible with an injury to the brachial plexus, especially if a fracture has occurred. Assess the upper extremity for circulation, sensation, and motor function preoperatively and postoperatively, and document the findings.

Clavicular Fracture Repair

A clavicle fracture rarely requires surgical intervention; instead, the affected shoulder is immobilized in a splint. Internal fixation of a clavicular fracture usually involves the middle or distal third of the clavicle. Surgery is required for non-union of the bones, associated scapular fracture, open fracture, severe displacement, and neurovascular compromise with vessels and nerves of brachial plexus.

Operative Procedure

The clavicle is an S-shaped bone that acts as a support between the sternum and the glenohumeral joint. A plate, screw, or intramedullary pin fixation can be used for surgical reduction of a clavicular fracture. Keep the patient asleep until the sling is placed.

Anesthetic

General anesthesia is given with insertion of a LMA or OETT, with rapid-sequence induction and an OETT being used if the patient is a trauma case. If the patient is intubated, tape the tube on the side of the mouth opposite from the surgical side.

An interscalene block can be done for clavicle surgery, but is usually not helpful for proximal clavicular surgery. General anesthesia may be combined with a peripheral block for postoperative pain control.

Positioning

The patient is placed in either a supine or beach-chair position; a sandbag or folded sheet is tucked under the affected shoulder. The patient's head is turned away from the surgical field. If the beach-chair position is used, see Chapter 3 for more information on venous air embolism.

Anesthetic Implications

The clavicle lies in close proximity to the pleura and major blood vessels, so monitor this area for injury.

Place the IV and blood pressure cuff on the non-operative arm.

Neurovascular compromise is possible with a clavicle fracture. Assess the area distal to the fracture for circulation, sensation, and motor function preoperatively and postoperatively, and document the findings. If the beach-chair position is used, careful attention to stabilization of the patient's head is necessary. It may be difficult to see the patient's face after the drapes are up and the lights are turned down. Tape the ETT securely, as access to patient's head will be limited after surgery begins.

These patients require special eye care. Paper tape is used to close the eyes to prevent corneal drying or abrasions; eye pads are then placed over both eyes. Consider using protective goggles.

The surgeon may request SBP of less than 100 mm Hg to prevent bleeding and improve visualization during arthroscopic surgery.

Complications

Brachial plexus or subclavian artery injury may occur during surgery.

Open Reduction of Humeral Head Fracture

Most humeral head fractures are treated nonsurgically. In some cases, however, realignment and fixation of the humeral head are performed through a surgical incision. If the fracture is severely comminuted, a total shoulder joint replacement may be necessary.

Operative Procedure

A deltopectoral approach—between the deltoid (laterally) and the pectoralis (medially)—is used. Fixation may be achieved with wire, screws, and/or special plates. The fracture fragment is repaired with wire, and the soft-tissue injuries are repaired. If the humeral head is also fractured, wire and a plate may be needed. A drain may be placed.

Keep the patient asleep until the sling is placed.

Anesthetic

General anesthesia is given with insertion of an OETT; rapid-sequence induction is appropriate for a trauma patient. Muscle relaxants are given. Interscalene block would be the peripheral block of choice for this location. Supraclavicular block could also be considered, but it sometimes will miss the proximal upper arm.

General anesthesia may be combined with a peripheral block for postoperative pain control.

Positioning

The patient is placed in a supine or slightly lateral position, with a bump-up by folded blanket or sheet; the beach-chair position may also be used. If the beach-chair position is used, see Chapter 3 for more information on venous air embolism.

Anesthetic Implications

Place the IV and blood pressure cuff on the nonoperative arm.

Injury to the subclavian/radial artery or ulnar nerve injury is possible with humeral head fracture. This fracture can also be associated with rib fractures and pneumothorax.

If the beach-chair position is used, careful attention to stabilization of the patient's head is necessary. It may be difficult to see the patient's face after the drapes are up and the lights are turned down. Tape the ETT securely, as access to patient's head will be limited after surgery begins.

These patients require special eye care. Paper tape is used to close the eyes to prevent corneal drying or abrasions; eye pads are then placed over both eyes. Consider using protective goggles.

The surgeon may request a SBP of less than 100 mm Hg to prevent bleeding and improve visualization during arthroscopic surgery.

Correction of Rotator Cuff Tear

Various methods are used to reconnect the supraspinatus tendon—that is, to reattach it to the proximal humeral head from which it was torn. Such surgery is usually done arthroscopically, but can be done as an open procedure.

The rotator cuff comprises a group of muscles and four tendons that surround the head of the humerus—namely, the supraspinatus, infraspinatus, teres minor, and subcapularis tendons. These muscles and tendons stabilize the shoulder joint (a ball-and-socket joint made up of the humerus, clavicle, and scapula) by keeping the humerus seated in the scapula, and allow the arm to be raised and rotated.

Surgery is indicated for tears that do not respond to nonsurgical management and that are associated with paresis, diminished function, and limited movement. Partial tears are usually due to degenerative processes, whereas complete tears occur with trauma.

Operative Procedure

- *Arthroscopy:* The surgeon percutaneously anchors the rotator cuff to the greater tuberosity of the proximal humerus.
- *Open procedure:* A small incision is made into the deltoid muscle to view the shoulder while repairing it. The rotator cuff is sutured back to

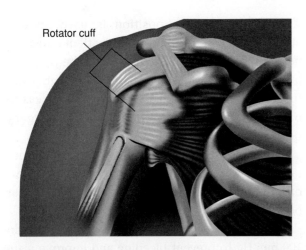

Figure 21-5 *Rotator Cuff*

the greater tuberosity. A tendon flap can be used to bridge a defect.

- *Mini-open procedure:* A lateral incision is made, and the deltoid muscle is retracted. The rotator cuff is sutured.

A sling is placed immediately after the dressing is secured. Keep the patient asleep until the sling is on.

Anesthetic
General anesthesia, an ETT, and rapid-sequence induction are used with trauma patients; ETT intubation is appropriate if muscle relaxation is needed.

Interscalene block is the most commonly performed peripheral block for shoulder surgery. Supraclavicular block can also be performed, as local anesthesia often will spread in a cephalad direction (and anesthetize the axillary nerve).

A combination of general anesthesia with a peripheral block is used for postoperative pain control.

Positioning
The patient is placed in a beach-chair or lateral decubitus position, with the head turned away from the operative side. A sandbag or folded towel is placed under the affected shoulder. If the beach-chair position is used, see Chapter 3 for more information on venous air embolism.

Anesthetic Implications
If the beach-chair position is used, careful attention to stabilization of the patient's head is necessary. It may be difficult to see the patient's face after the drapes are up and the lights are turned down (for arthroscopy). Tape the ETT securely, as access to patient's head will be limited after surgery begins.

These patients require special eye care. Paper tape is used to close the eyes to prevent corneal drying or abrasions; eye pads are then placed over both eyes. Consider using protective goggles.

Place the IV and blood pressure cuff on the nonoperative arm.

The surgeon may request a SBP of less than 100 mm Hg to prevent bleeding and improve visualization during arthroscopic surgery.

Correction of Recurrent Anterior Shoulder Dislocation
The gross anatomy of the shoulder consists of three main components: muscle, ligaments, and bone. The glenohumeral ligaments, function is to limit the lateral rotation of the shoulder. The rotator cuff muscles (supraspinatus, infraspinatus, teres minor, and subscapularis) supply additional stability. Finally, the humeral head articulates in a shallow socket provided by the glenoid fossa. It is composed of the bony glenoid and the glenoid labrum.

The shoulder is the most commonly dislocated joint in the body, with dislocations being caused by either trauma or muscle laxity. A piece of the shoulder cartilage, called the labrum, can be injured with shoulder trauma, causing dislocation. The labrum circles the glenoid bone, making the socket deeper and the joint much more stable.

Surgery is performed to correct shoulder laxity, which can lead to recurrent subluxation or dislocation. The rate of recurrence is 70% in patients younger than age 30, but the rate of recurrence decreases with increasing age. Anterior dislocations account for approximately 95% of shoulder dislocations.

Operative Procedure

Correction of recurrent anterior shoulder dislocation is usually performed as an open procedure but can be done arthroscopically.

Keep the patient asleep until the sling is placed.

Anesthetic

General anesthesia, an ETT, and rapid-sequence induction is appropriate for a trauma patient.

Regional blockade may or may not be given. Interscalene block is the most commonly performed peripheral block for shoulder surgery. Supraclavicular brachial plexus block can also be performed, as local anesthesia often will spread in a cephalad direction (and anesthetize the axillary nerve).

A combination of general anesthesia with regional anesthesia may be used for postoperative pain control.

Positioning

The patient may be placed in a beach-chair, lateral decubitus, or supine position with the operative arm over the chest. If the beach-chair position is used, see Chapter 3 for more information on venous air embolism.

Anesthetic Implications

If the beach-chair position is used, careful attention to stabilization of the patient's head is necessary. It may be difficult to see the patient's face after the drapes are up and the lights are turned down (for arthroscopy). Tape the ETT securely, as access to patient's head will be limited after surgery begins.

These patients require special eye care. Paper tape is used to close the eyes to prevent corneal drying or abrasions; eye pads are then placed over both eyes. Consider using protective goggles.

Place the IV and blood pressure cuff on the non-operative arm.

The surgeon may request a SBP of less than 100 mm Hg to prevent bleeding and improve visualization during arthroscopic surgery.

Correction of Sternoclavicular Dislocation

Sternoclavicular dislocation is usually treated nonoperatively with manual traction. If surgery is required, ligament repair with reconstruction is the most widely accepted type of surgery. Surgical fixation with wires is not recommended because of case reports of lethal hardware migration.

Sternoclavicular dislocations are infrequent and are typically due to trauma. Prompt diagnosis and treatment are necessary to prevent complications of vessel rupture or thoracic outlet syndrome (compression of major vessels, trachea, and esophagus within the superior mediastinum).

Anesthetic

General endotracheal anesthesia (GETA) with rapid-sequence induction is appropriate for a trauma patient. No brachial plexus block is effective in anesthetizing the medial aspect of the clavicle; instead, consider giving general anesthesia alone.

Positioning

The patient is placed in a supine position. The head of the bed may be slightly raised.

Anesthetic Implications

Place the IV and blood pressure cuff on the nonoperative arm.

Keep the patient asleep until the sling is on.

Secure the ETT well, as access to patient's head will be limited after surgery begins. Consider protective goggles or eye pads for patient.

The surgeon may request a SBP of less than 100 mm Hg to prevent bleeding and improve visualization during arthroscopic surgery.

Complications

Damage to mediastinal structures can occur during this surgery. Pneumothorax is the most frequently observed complication.

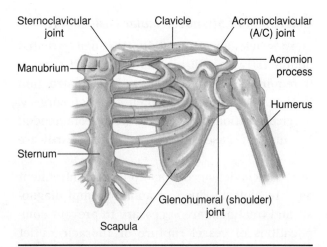

Figure 21-6 *Sternoclavicular Joint*
Source: AAOS, 2004.

ORTHOPEDIC SURGERY: HUMERUS, RADIUS, AND ULNA

Closed Reduction of Humerus, Radius, or Ulna Fracture

Realignment and fixation are used to repair nondisplaced fractures of the upper extremity. Such fractures are usually distal, and closed reduction and immobilization minimize the risk of non-union and infection with these injuries.

Operative Procedure
The surgeon applies traction to realign the bones, and a cast is applied. A sling will be needed if the arm is set in a cast.

Anesthetic
GETA, an OETT, and rapid-sequence induction are appropriate for a trauma patient.

Supraclavicular, infraclavicular, or axillary brachial plexus blocks can also be performed. Proximal humerus surgery requires an interscalene block.

A combination of general anesthesia with a peripheral block may be used for postoperative pain control.

Positioning
The patient is placed in a supine position.

Anesthetic Implications
Keep the patient asleep until the repair cannot be disrupted by movement. A sling will be needed.

Place the IV and blood pressure cuff on the non-operative arm.

Neurovascular compromise is possible with this injury. Assess the area distal to the fracture for circulation, sensation, and motor function preoperatively and postoperatively, and document the findings.

Open Reduction of Humerus Fracture

This surgery involves realignment and fixation of a fracture of the humerus through an incision. A variety of fractures of the humerus can occur.

Operative Procedure
Incision placement will be made based on the place and type of fracture. Intramedullary nailing is rarely done. Open reduction and internal fixation using compression plates and screws is more commonly employed. External fixation may also be done.

In open reduction and internal fixation, screws are placed, both distal and proximal to the fracture, that maintains the plate. A bone graft may be done if a non-union is persistent and the fracture needs to be stabilized. Care is taken to avoid nerves and neurovascular structures. If a mal-union has occurred, osteotomy is performed to restore alignment. For condylar fractures, threaded wires or screws may be placed. A drain may be inserted, and the wound is closed.

Keep the patient asleep until the repair cannot be disrupted by movement. A sling will be needed.

Anesthetic
General anesthesia, an ETT, and rapid-sequence induction are appropriate for a trauma patient.

Proximal humerus surgery requires an interscalene block. Anesthesia for surgery to the distal humerus can consist of supraclavicular, infraclavicular, or axillary nerve blocks.

A combination of general anesthesia with a peripheral block may be used for postoperative pain control.

Positioning
The patient is placed in a lateral decubitus or supine position, with the shoulder near the edge of the table. The head of the bed may be raised.

Anesthetic Implications
Place the IV and blood pressure cuff on the nonoperative arm.

Splints and braces are rarely applied after open reduction and internal fixation. The plates and screws are strong enough to allow immediate range of motion.

Methylmethacrylate may be needed in rare cases.

Neurovascular compromise is possible with this injury. Assess the area distal to the fracture for circulation, sensation, and motor function preoperatively and postoperatively, and document the findings. Humeral shaft fractures can cause radial nerve injury.

Repair of Distal Humeral Fractures: Supracondylar, Epicondylar, Intercondylar

This surgery involves realignment and fixation of a displaced fracture of the distal third of the humerus through an incision. A variety of distal humeral fractures or combination of fractures are possible.

Operative Procedure
An incision is made in the posterior or lateral part of the upper arm; fixation is done with plates and screws. It is a surgical emergency if the displacement compresses the neurovascular bundle.

Intercondylar fractures can be very difficult to repair. Surgery time in such cases can be extended.

A comminuted distal humerus fracture is repaired with plates and screws. A plate is often used to bridge fracture fragments without rigid fixation.

If a cast is applied, then allow it to set and a sling to be put around the patient prior to waking the patient up.

Anesthetic
GETA, an OETT, and rapid-sequence induction are appropriate for a trauma patient.

Alternatively, peripheral block anesthesia with IV sedation may be used. Distal humerus surgery can be completed under supraclavicular, infraclavicular, or axillary nerve blocks.

A combination of general anesthesia with a peripheral block may be used for postoperative pain control.

Positioning
The patient is placed in a supine position, with the operative arm draped across the patient's chest; provide a bump-up with a folded blanket. If the patient is placed in a prone position, the elbow is then flexed over a small table. The lateral decubitus position may also be used.

Anesthetic Implications
Place the IV and blood pressure cuff on the nonoperative arm.

Keep patient warm, as this surgery can have a long duration.

If a compression tourniquet is used, it is usually set at 50–100 mm Hg above the patient's systolic blood pressure; the maximum setting is less than 300 mm Hg in the upper extremity. Chart both the tourniquet time and setting. The tourniquet should be released after 2 hours to prevent injury.

Neurovascular compromise is possible with this injury, especially radial or ulnar nerve injury. Assess the area distal to the fracture for circulation, sensation, and motor function preoperatively and postoperatively, and document the findings. A supracondylar humerus (distal) fracture poses a specific risk of injury to the brachial artery.

Repair of Olecranon (Elbow) Fracture

Realignment and fixation of fractures of the elbow (the proximal piece of the ulna) are performed through a surgical incision.

Operative Procedure

When a fracture produces bone fragments of the elbow or separate larger pieces of bone, open reduction is indicated. Small fragments may be excised and the triceps tendon reattached to the proximal ulnar shaft. Larger fragments are aligned and fixed with a figure-of-eight wire loop, plates, screws, and/or intramedullary pins.

Keep the patient asleep until the cast is set and a sling is placed to support the arm.

Anesthetic

General anesthesia, an OETT, and rapid-sequence induction are appropriate for a trauma patient.

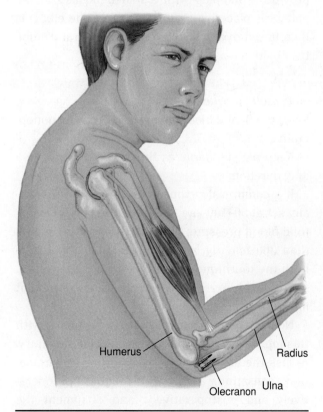

Figure 21-7 *Olecranon Repair*
Source: AAOS, 2004.

Peripheral block anesthesia with IV sedation may also be used. A supraclavicular or infraclavicular brachial plexus block can be done.

A combination of general anesthesia with a peripheral block may be used for postoperative pain control.

Positioning

The patient is placed in a prone (with elbow flexed over a small table), supine, or lateral decubitus position.

Anesthetic Implications

Place the IV and blood pressure cuff on the nonoperative arm.

If a compression tourniquet is used, it is usually set at 50–100 mm Hg above the patient's systolic blood pressure; the maximum setting is less than 300 mm Hg in the upper extremity. Chart both the tourniquet time and setting. The tourniquet should be released after 2 hours to prevent injury.

Keep the patient asleep until the cast is applied and hardened or a splint is applied.

Neurovascular compromise is possible with this injury. Assess the area distal to the fracture for circulation, sensation, and motor function preoperatively and postoperatively, and document the findings. Monitor the patient for compartment syndrome of the forearm.

Open Reduction of Radius or Ulnar Fracture

Realignment and fixation of fractures of the forearm are performed through a surgical incision. Closed reduction of non-comminuted fractures of the radius and ulna is usually only done in children; adults usually require open reduction with internal fixation (ORIF).

A functioning radial head is needed for rotation (pronate and supinate) of the forearm at the elbow. Fractures involving the radial head often result in loose bony fragments or mal-alignment that can limit pronation and supination. Removal of the fragments with repair of the radial head restores motion. Removal of the radial head is also an acceptable treatment in older patients and usually results in complete return of motion.

When the radial head is excised in a younger patient, the patient may permanently lose the ability to supinate or pronate the forearm. If the radial head is excised, it is done proximal to the radial tuberosity.

Open reduction with internal fixation is required with distal radial fractures if there is severe shortening, angulation, or unstable comminution of a distal radius fracture.

Operative Procedure

The surgeon starts the incision 5 cm distal to the radial head and cuts down to lateral humeral condyle. Anatomic reduction and stabilization of the fragments may be done with pins, wires, plates, and/or screws. A bone graft also may be performed if non-union exists.

X-ray guided percutaneous pinning may be done for bone stabilization.

Radial head excision must be done for severely comminuted radial head fractures in adults. Excision of the radial head is usually not performed in the pediatric population.

A cast is applied, and the arm is maintained in a 90-degree flexion at the elbow. Keep the patient asleep until the cast is set and a sling is placed to support the arm.

Anesthetic

General anesthesia, an ETT, and rapid-sequence induction are appropriate for a trauma patient. Alternatively, peripheral block anesthesia with IV sedation may be used. Supraclavicular, infraclavicular, or axillary brachial plexus blocks can be done.

A combination of general anesthesia with a peripheral block may be used for postoperative pain control.

Positioning

The patient is placed in a supine position, with the operative arm extended on a hand table. The nonoperative arm is either tucked at the patient's side or secured on a padded armboard, with the angle at the shoulder being less than 90 degrees.

Anesthetic Implications

If a compression tourniquet is used, it is usually set at 50–100 mm Hg above the patient's systolic blood pressure; the maximum setting is less than 300 mm Hg in the upper extremity. Chart both the tourniquet time and setting. The tourniquet should be released after 2 hours to prevent injury.

Place the IV and blood pressure cuff on the nonoperative arm.

Keep the patient asleep until the cast is applied and hardened or a splint is applied.

A distal radius fracture can cause a median nerve injury or a compartment syndrome. Assess the area distal to the fracture for circulation, sensation, and motor function preoperatively and postoperatively, and document the findings.

Repair of Proximal Third Fractures of the Ulna

The procedure involves realignment and fixation of fractures of the bones of the proximal ulna. Proximal third fractures of the ulna typically occur when the person falls with the arm hyperextended. If the proximal head of the ulna is fractured, the radial head is also dislocated.

Operative Procedure

Operative treatment with internal fixation is required in nearly all cases. The incision is made over the fractured bone. A plate is centered over the fracture so that six screws can be placed—three distally and three proximally to the fracture—to stabilize the bone. Closed reduction may be attempted (with sufficient sedation and analgesia, with or without muscle relaxants) if acute neurovascular compromise is present. A cast is applied, with the arm flexed in a 90-degree angle. Keep the patient asleep until the cast is applied and hardened or a splint is applied and a sling placed to support the affected arm.

Anesthetic

GETA with rapid-sequence induction is appropriate for a trauma patient; alternatively, peripheral block anesthesia with a supraclavicular or infraclavicular brachial plexus block can be done. If an axillary block is used, all nerves need to be anesthetized around the axillary artery to ensure a surgical block.

A combination of general anesthesia and a peripheral block may be used for postoperative pain control.

Positioning

The patient is placed in a supine position. The operative arm is extended on a side-table.

Anesthetic Implications

Place the IV and the blood pressure cuff on the nonoperative arm.

If a compression tourniquet is used, it is usually set at 50–100 mm Hg above the patient's systolic blood pressure; the maximum setting is less than 300 mm Hg in the upper extremity. Chart both the tourniquet time and setting. The tourniquet should be released after 2 hours to prevent injury.

Keep the patient asleep until the cast is applied and hardened or a splint is applied.

Neurovascular compromise is possible with this injury. Assess the area distal to the fracture for circulation, sensation, and motor function preoperatively and postoperatively, and document the findings.

Transposition of the Ulnar Nerve

Transposition of the ulnar nerve (subcutaneous or submuscular) allows for more slack in the nerve course. Subcutaneous placement can result in painful paresthesias with simple local trauma. Submuscular transposition involves placing the nerve in a well-vascularized bed and may help prevent recurrent symptoms.

Transposition of the ulnar nerve is performed to alleviate pain in the forearm that radiates in the distribution of the ulnar nerve. In such cases,

numbness and tingling occur in half of the ring finger and the whole of the little finger. There is also weakness of intrinsic hand muscles.

Traumatic ulnar neuritis can lead to claw-hand formation. Damage to the ulnar nerve can occur with trauma to the elbow.

Operative Procedure

The ulnar nerve supplies the dorsal and palmar aspects of the medial half of the ring finger and the whole of the little finger. In nerve transposition surgery, the incision is made over the medial elbow, from the medial epicondyle down to the proximal forearm. Surgical methods focus on releasing the nerve along its course at sites of compression, preventing subluxation over the medial epicondyle, and preventing traction or tension on the nerve with elbow motion.

Keep the patient asleep until the cast is applied and hardened or a splint is applied and the sling is placed to support the operative arm.

Anesthetic

General anesthesia with an OETT or LMA, peripheral block anesthesia, or a combination is commonly used. Supraclavicular, infraclavicular, or axillary brachial plexus blocks can be performed effectively.

A combination of general anesthesia with a peripheral block may be used for postoperative pain control.

Positioning

The patient is placed in a supine position, with the operative arm extended on a hand surgery table.

Anesthetic Implications

Place the IV and the blood pressure cuff on the nonoperative arm.

Nerve repairs must be protected with splints prior to the patient's emergence from anesthesia.

If a compression tourniquet is used, it is usually set at 50–100 mm Hg above the patient's systolic blood pressure; the maximum setting is less than 300 mm Hg in the upper extremity. Chart both the tourniquet time and setting. The tourniquet should be released after 2 hours to prevent injury.

Neurovascular compromise is possible with this condition. Assess the area distal to the ulnar nerve for circulation, sensation, and motor function preoperatively and postoperatively, and document the findings. Ulnar nerve injury presents with "claw-hand," evidenced by hyperextended metocarpophalangeal joints and flexed interphalangeal joints. These changes are more obvious at the ring and little fingers, because the first and second lumbrical muscles are not paralyzed.

ORTHOPEDIC SURGERY: HAND AND WRIST

Open Reduction of Carpal Bone Fracture

Most fractures of the wrist are treated by closed reduction and immobilization. Open reduction may occasionally be used for realignment and fixation of fractures of the bones of the wrist.

The wrist is made up of eight separate carpal bones; they connect the radius and ulna to the metacarpal bones. The scaphoid is the most frequently fractured carpal bone.

Operative Procedure

Open-reduction surgery is required when the fracture is displaced or dislocated, or when non-union of the bones occurs. The incision site depends on the fracture site, but is usually over the palmar surface of the wrist when repairing a scaphoid fracture. Fixation may be done with pins, wires, plates, and/or compression screws. A bone graft (from the elbow or radius bone) may be performed if non-union is persistent. More severe injuries may require excision of carpal bones and the radial or ulnar styloid process to prevent arthritis. Small bone fragments are excised, and larger fragments are aligned and fixed.

Keep the patient asleep until the cast is applied and hardened, a splint is applied, or an external fixator is applied and the sling is placed to support the operative arm.

Anesthetic

GETA and rapid-sequence induction are appropriate for a trauma patient. A combination of general anesthesia with peripheral block anesthesia (for postoperative pain control) is commonly used.

Brachial plexus block via the supraclavicular, infraclavicular, or axillary sites can be done. For short-duration procedures involving the wrist and hand, brachial plexus blocks are preferred.

Complex fractures may take longer periods of time for repair. In such cases, general anesthesia may be more appropriate.

Positioning

The patient is placed in a supine position. The affected arm is extended on a hand table, with the patient's torso near the edge of the table.

Anesthetic Implications

Place the IV and blood pressure cuff on the nonoperative arm.

If a compression tourniquet is used, it is usually set at 50–100 mm Hg above the patient's systolic blood pressure; the maximum setting is less than 300 mm Hg in the upper extremity. Chart both the tourniquet time and setting. The tourniquet should be released after 2 hours to prevent injury.

Surgery may occur around the radial artery (near the scaphoid bone) or the ulnar artery (if the fracture is on the little-finger side of the hand). Inadvertent injury to these vessels may produce extensive blood loss.

Keep the patient sedated or asleep until the cast is applied and hardened or a splint is applied. The thumb is incorporated into a cast, or a thumb spica is used.

Neurovascular compromise is possible with this injury. Assess the area distal to the fracture for circulation, sensation, and motor function preoperatively and postoperatively, and document the findings.

Carpal Tunnel Release

Carpal tunnel release involves decompression of the median nerve on the volar (palm side) surface of the wrist. It is performed to treat carpal tunnel syndrome, which presents with symptoms such as pain, numbness, and tingling of the fingers (especially the thumb, index, and middle fingers) and weakness of the thumb muscles due to medial nerve entrapment. Carpal tunnel syndrome is caused by trauma, repetitive injuries, or occupational injuries involving thickened muscles. Carpal tunnel release may also be done to treat rheumatoid synovitis or with a distal radius fracture.

Operative Procedure

In an *open* procedure, a curved incision is made parallel to the thenar crease and angled toward the ulnar side of the wrist. After the skin and subcutaneous tissue are excised and reflected, the transverse carpal ligament is divided. Care is taken to avoid injury to nerve branches. Surgical excision of part or all of the synovial membrane of the flexor tendons may be done at the same time.

In an *endoscopic* procedure, a skin incision is made at the wrist and a trocar is inserted. The release is performed with probes and endoscopic knives. The incision is closed. There is an increased risk of nerve laceration during endoscopic carpal tunnel release.

A splint is applied at the end of surgery.

Anesthetic

MAC sedation and a local anesthetic may be used. For regional anesthesia, Bier blocks are commonly performed with 50 mL of 0.5% lidocaine *without* epinephrine for soft-tissue procedures of short duration (45–60 minutes). It is usually necessary to keep the patient sedated until the compression tourniquet is released and the splint is applied.

Bier Block

A 20- to 22-gauge IV catheter is placed in the surgical arm on the dorsum of the hand; a second catheter is placed in the nonsurgical arm for sedation and resuscitation purposes. Cotton batting is placed around the operative arm; a pneumatic tourniquet is placed on the upper arm but not inflated. Elevate the arm to promote venous drainage while an Esmarch bandage is applied tightly for further exsanguination. After exsanguination, while still holding the arm up into the air, the double pneumatic tourniquet is inflated (50–150 mm Hg greater than the SBP, 2 × SBP, or a maximum of 300 torr).

1. Inflate the distal cuff.
2. Inflate the proximal cuff.
3. Deflate the distal cuff.

Test the radial artery for occlusion, making sure no pulse is present. If surgery is longer than 1 hour, the surgical arm IV catheter can be left in and reinjected after 90 minutes; it can be retained for a maximum of 2 hours.

Never use Bupivacaine with a Bier block (it is too cardiotoxic).

Local Anesthetic

A local anesthetic is delivered into the operative arm (with the tourniquet inflated). Inject 50 cc of either 0.5% lidocaine PF solution plain (no epinephrine) or prilocaine plain solution.

Some local anesthetic may slip under the cuff; tourniquet pain is the limiting factor in how long it may remain in place (surgery time is limited to 45 minutes). The patient will experience a pins-and-needle sensation; discoloration will occur. Local anesthetic can be released into systemic circulation if the tourniquet is released before 20 minutes.

Patients with rheumatoid arthritis can have cervical nerve root compression and/or atlanto-occipital instability. If general anesthesia is required, assess the patient's ability to extend the neck and ask about any numbness or tingling with neck movement. Check the neck X-ray for subluxation of the cervical spine. These patients may require awake fiberoptic intubation.

Positioning

The patient is placed in a supine position, with the affected arm extended on a hand table.

Anesthetic Implications

Place the blood pressure cuff on the nonoperative arm.

If a compression tourniquet is used, it is usually set at 50–100 mm Hg above the patient's systolic blood pressure; the maximum setting is less than 300 mm Hg in the upper extremity. Chart both the tourniquet time and setting. The tourniquet should be released after 2 hours to prevent injury.

A splint is applied at the end of the case.

Neurovascular compromise of the hand nerve is possible with the endoscopic approach to carpal tunnel release. Assess preoperative and postoperative sensation of the hand and fingers, and document the findings.

Flexor Tendon Laceration Repair

Repair of a flexor tendon laceration involves approximation of the severed ends of the flexor tendon on the palm side of the hand. This surgery is performed in case of either new injury to a tendon or a failed previous tendon repair.

The common flexor tendon is shared by a number of flexor muscles in the forearm; its origin is attached to the medial epicondyle of the humerus. It serves as the origin for several muscles of the anterior forearm.

Flexor tendons allow the fingers to bend. If the flexor tendon is cut completely in half, the end connected to the muscle may pull back into the palm and must be corrected surgically.

Operative Procedure

An incision is made according to the injury site. If a large gap exists between the severed ends, a graft is needed; often the palmaris longus tendon or extensor tendons of the toe are used for this purpose. The tendon ends are retrieved and sewn together. Nerve repair is done at the same time if needed.

A splint is applied at the end of the case; the fingers are splinted in the flexed position to minimize mechanical stress on the repaired tendon. Keep the patient asleep (an especially important consideration whenever nerves and tendons are repaired) until the splint is on; a sling may be placed to support the operative arm.

Anesthetic

General anesthesia, an OETT, and rapid-sequence induction are appropriate for an emergency procedure.

Peripheral block anesthesia is commonly used if surgery is not an emergency procedure. Brachial plexus block via the supraclavicular, infraclavicular, or axillary sites can be done.

A combination of a general anesthetic and a peripheral nerve block may be used to help control postoperative pain.

Positioning

The patient is placed in a supine position, with the unaffected arm on an armboard and the affected arm on a side table.

Anesthetic Implications

Place the IV and blood pressure cuff on the nonoperative arm.

If a compression tourniquet is used, it is usually set at 50–100 mm Hg above the patient's systolic blood pressure; the maximum setting is less than 300 mm Hg in the upper extremity. Chart both the tourniquet time and setting. The tourniquet should be released after 2 hours to prevent injury.

Ganglion Excisions

Ganglion excision is the surgical removal of a ganglion cyst. Aspiration is a simpler procedure, but the cyst recurs in approximately half of all such cases.

A ganglion is a cystic dilation of a joint capsule or tendon sheath that contains synovial fluid. Ganglions are usually attached by a stalk of tissue to a joint capsule, tendon, or tendon sheath. The sites in which ganglions are most frequently found include the dorsum of the wrist and the palm of hand, although these cysts can occur in almost any joint.

Operative Procedure
An incision is made over the ganglion. The joint is entered, and the ganglion is secured and removed, including excising the stalk of the cyst from its origin. Care is taken to avoid injury to nerve branches. Complete excision makes recurrence rare.

Excision can be done arthroscopically.

A volar wrist ganglion (palm side of the wrist, just below the thumb) can grow around the radial artery. Care must be taken to avoid damaging this artery during excision.

A compression dressing is applied; it is covered with an elastic bandage at the end of the case.

Anesthetic
MAC sedation and local anesthesia are used. Keep the patient sedated until a pressure dressing is applied. Brachial plexus blocks are rarely performed, as the postoperative pain is limited. If a peripheral block is needed, a Bier block can be done.

A splint may be applied if the ganglion was at a joint, to keep the patient from moving or bending the joint.

Positioning
Patient positioning depends on the location of the ganglion. Most patients are placed supine, with the affected arm on a hand table.

Anesthetic Implications
Place the IV and blood pressure cuff on the nonoperative arm.

If a compression tourniquet is used, it is usually set at 50–100 mm Hg above the patient's systolic blood pressure; the maximum setting is less than 300 mm Hg in the upper extremity and less than 400 mm Hg in the lower extremity. Chart both the tourniquet time and setting. The tourniquet should be released after 2 hours to prevent injury.

Elevation of the forearm postoperatively helps to minimize swelling.

Wrist Arthrodesis
Wrist arthrodesis is the surgical fixation of the wrist bones, sometimes using a bone graft. This procedure is generally done when other treatments have been unsuccessful and wrist movement cannot be preserved. Usual indications include post-traumatic degenerative arthritis following fractures and dislocations, osteoarthritis and rheumatoid arthritis, carpal bone instability due to ligament tears, and aseptic necrosis of the lunate carpal bone of the wrist.

Operative Procedure
Intramedullary fixation is achieved using pins, plates, and/or screws. The distal radius may be used for fixation of the wrist.

Anesthetic
General anesthesia is used with an OETT or LMA, along with a peripheral block for postoperative pain control. A brachial plexus block via the supraclavicular, infraclavicular, or axillary approach can be performed.

Patients with rheumatoid arthritis can have cervical nerve root compression and/or atlanto-occipital instability. Assess the patient's ability to extend the neck and ask about any numbness or tingling with neck movement. Check the neck X-ray for subluxation of the cervical spine. These patients may require awake fiberoptic intubation.

Positioning
The patient is placed in a supine position, with the operative arm extended on a side table. The nonoperative arm is secured on a padded

armboard, with the shoulder at an angle of less than 90 degrees.

Anesthetic Implications

These patients may be on chronic steroid therapy, so that an intraoperative "stress dose" of steroids may need to be given.

Place the IV and blood pressure cuff on the nonoperative arm.

If a compression tourniquet is used, it is usually set at 50–100 mm Hg above the patient's systolic blood pressure; the maximum setting is less than 300 mm Hg in the upper extremity. Chart both the tourniquet time and setting. The tourniquet should be released after 2 hours to prevent injury.

ORTHOPEDIC TRANSPLANTATION

Digit and Hand Replantation

Surgical replantation in the adult is carried out for amputations involving the thumb, multiple digits, and the palm. In children, nearly all amputations are replanted.

Operative Procedure

Microsurgical replantation is an emergency procedure. Incisions will extend both proximal and distal to the traumatic amputation, allowing for neurovascular exploration. Lower extremities may be prepped in preparation for both vein and skin grafts.

Once arterial blood flow is reestablished, normothermia must be maintained to prevent vasospasm. Other ways to prevent vasospasm include administration of antithrombotics, smooth muscle relaxants (e.g., Papaverine), or vasodilators.

Anesthetic

Anesthesia consists of rapid-sequence induction and general anesthesia with an OETT. A concurrent brachial plexus block (supraclavicular, infraclavicular, or axillary) can be used for postoperative pain control. This can be a very long procedure and "single-shot" blocks may incur more risk than benefit.

IV catheter placement should be done prior to induction of general anesthesia in a pediatric patient.

Positioning

The patient is placed in a supine position, with the operative arm extended on a hand table. The nonoperative arm is either secured to a padded armboard or tucked at the patient's side.

Anesthetic Implications

Place the IVs and the blood pressure cuff on the nonoperative arm.

Euvolemia to hemodilution is needed to achieve a hematocrit level in the range of 30–35%.

Heparin and dextran can be administered to prevent thrombosis.

Keep the patient's blood pressure within 10–20% of normal to maintain adequate perfusion pressure.

If a compression tourniquet is used, it is usually set at 50–100 mm Hg above the patient's systolic blood pressure; the maximum setting is less than 300 mm Hg in the upper extremity. Chart both the tourniquet time and setting. The tourniquet should be released after 2 hours to prevent injury.

A routine volar hand splint is applied at the end of the case. Keep the patient asleep until a splint is applied.

The patient requires ICU monitoring postoperatively.

ORTHOPEDIC SURGERY: PELVIS

The pelvis is also referred to as the pelvic ring or girdle. It is composed of three bones: the sacrum and two innominate bones. The sacrum is joined to the innominate bones by the strongest ligaments in the body—the iliosacral ligaments. The innominate bones are joined anteriorly by the cartilage of the pubic symphysis. As this description suggests, multiple bones, joints, and ligaments can be injured in the pelvic girdle, including the symphysis pubis, pubic rami, sacroiliac joint, iliac wing, and sacrum. There is also enormous risk to internal organs with pelvic injuries—to the bladder and urethra, iliac and femoral arteries, aorta, and so on. The goal of surgery is to restore anatomic alignment.

Pelvic fracture treatment is based on the type of fracture. Treatment ranges from closed reduction with external fixation to internal, open reduction and stability of injuries.

Closed Reduction and External Fixation of the Pelvis

Multiple fractures can occur in the pelvic ring; these injuries range from stable to life threatening. Application of an anterior external fixator is intended to restore the anatomical position and provide stability for the pelvis in open-book injuries. In general, severe open-book pelvic injuries are life threatening. Expect the patient with this type of injury to be hemodynamically unstable, with average 24-hour blood requirements in excess of 20 units. Lower-extremity IV access is typically ineffective because the pelvic venous system is commonly completely disrupted.

Operative Procedure

In an "open-book" pelvic injury, the pubic symphysis is disrupted and the innominate bones are externally rotated. This results in a significant increase in pelvic volume and precludes the tamponade of pelvic bleeding. The volume of the pelvis is reduced by closing down the open anterior injury, thereby creating an environment for tamponade of bleeding surfaces (i.e., reduced pelvic volume). External fixator pins are inserted into the iliac crest bones percutaneously or through multiple small incisions to stabilize the anterior pelvis. Transiliac rods are used to reduce sacral disruptions in the posterior pelvis. An external crossbar is attached to 5-mm pins that are then placed into the stable section of the pelvis to maintain alignment and reduction.

Anesthetic

GETA is used with rapid-sequence induction on the patient's bed. Move the patient to the OR table after induction to minimize pain during transfer and positioning. Muscle relaxation is required for fracture reduction procedures.

Positioning

The patient is placed in the supine position.

Anesthetic Implications

Neurovascular compromise is possible with this injury. Assess the bilateral legs and feet for circulation, sensation, and motor function preoperatively and postoperatively, and document the findings.

Monitor for—and expect—occult blood loss in the pelvis and legs. Monitor serial hematocrit levels frequently.

Pelvic Fracture and Disruption

This surgery involves realignment and fixation of fractures of the pelvis. It is indicated in case of nonunion or mal-union of the pelvis.

Operative Procedure

Open reduction of displaced bony fragments is performed through incisions, utilizing X-ray images as a guide to align and fix the pelvis in an anatomic position, using plates and screws.

- *Anterior* approaches to the pelvis are used for reductions and fixations of fractures and dislocations of the symphysis pubis, pubic rami, iliac wing, acetabulum, and anterior aspect of the sacroiliac joint.
- *Posterior* approaches to the pelvis are used for reductions and fixation of fractures and dislocations of the sacrum and acetabulum.

Anesthetic

General anesthesia is used with an OETT, with rapid-sequence induction taking place on the patient's bed. Move the patient to the OR table after induction to minimize pain during transfer and positioning. Muscle relaxation is required for fracture reduction procedures.

Neuraxial anesthesia is rarely employed in such cases, as it is inappropriate for pelvic fracture surgery. The patient positioning necessary for spinal anesthesia may compromise bony stability and disrupt any pelvic hematoma; also, aggressive coagulation for thrombosis prevention is often initiated on the day of surgery.

If a neuraxial block is absolutely needed, place a spinal or epidural with IV sedation. IV ketamine and propofol can be used to help sedate the patient for the block as well as positioning on OR table.

Positioning

The patient is placed supine for the anterior approach and prone for the posterior approach.

Anesthetic Implications

Expect large blood losses; indeed, life-threatening blood losses are associated with pelvic fractures. Cell-saving techniques are useful. Deliberate hypotension or hemodilution may be necessary to control blood loss. Blood loss may sometimes be hidden, with a large amount of blood settling into the pelvis and/or legs.

Prevent nerve injury with meticulous padding to the patient's chest, pelvis, and extremities.

Neurovascular compromise is possible with these injuries. Assess and document the bilateral legs and feet for circulation, sensation, and motor function preoperatively and postoperatively.

Patients with pelvic injuries will have sustained high-force trauma; thus, it is of critical importance to fully evaluate each patient for other injuries. Injuries from the trauma as well as complications from a pelvic fracture may affect major vessels, nerves, and visceral organs contained within the pelvic girdle.

ORTHOPEDIC SURGERY: HIP

Open Reduction of Acetabulum Fractures

The acetabulum is contained within the bony pelvis; it is the rounded cavity at the base of the ilium into which the ball-shaped head of the femur fits. Surgical treatment of acetabulum fractures focuses on hip joint preservation by accurately reconstructing the supporting bony anatomy. Surgery may also be performed to repair non-union or mal-union of the acetabulum.

Fractures of the acetabulum may be the result of either low- or high-energy injuries. Typically, younger patients with dense bone require high-energy trauma to disrupt the acetabulum. By comparison, elderly patients with osteopenia are susceptible to acetabular fractures as a consequence of a fall from a standing height. In either type of injury, traumatic force is transmitted through the femoral head from the greater trochanter. Associated injuries to the surrounding pelvic bone are not unusual.

Operative Procedure

The patient must be fully evaluated and stabilized before internal fixation is performed. Typically, skeletal traction (femoral traction pin) has been placed to immobilize the fracture until internal fixation can be done.

The incision site is based on surgeon preference and the site and type of fracture. Three approaches are commonly used: ilioinguinal (anterior approach), extended iliofemoral (lateral approach), and Kocher-Lagenbeck (posterior approach). Internal fixation utilizes plates, screws, wires, and pins. Once the fracture is stabilized, external traction is no longer required.

If an acetabular fracture cannot be repaired or reduced, a total hip arthroplasty with bone grafting must be done.

Anesthetic

GETA is used with an OETT; rapid-sequence induction is necessary for trauma patients. Muscle relaxation is needed to reduce the fracture. Induction can be done on the OR table if the patient is able to tolerate the move; however, in many cases it may need to be done on the stretcher or patient's bed so that the move to the OR table is tolerated.

Spinal neuraxial anesthesia should not be used for acute treatment of fractures, owing to the need to perform an accurate neurovascular exam immediately postoperatively.

Positioning

The patient may be placed in a supine (anterior approach), lateral decubitus, or prone (posterior approach) position.

Anesthetic Implications

Expect large blood losses with this surgery. Cell-saving techniques are useful. Deliberate hypotension or hemodilution may be necessary to control blood loss.

Prevent nerve injury with meticulous padding to the patient's chest, pelvis, and extremities.

Keep the patient asleep until the hip is immobilized.

Neurovascular compromise is possible with this injury. Assess the area distal to the fracture for circulation, sensation, and motor function preoperatively and postoperatively, and document the findings. A posterior hip dislocation can cause a sciatic nerve injury.

Arthrodesis of Hip

Arthrodesis of the hip is surgery that fuses the femur to the acetabulum. It is indicated for severe osteoarthritis of the hip in a person with contraindications to total hip arthroplasty, neuromuscular disease, or recurrent dislocation of the hip. Osteoarthritis is common in young adults who experience hip trauma and local infection; it typically presents with back and/or ipsilateral hip pain.

Operative Procedure

The incision can be made anterior, posterior, and lateral when an internal fixation is performed. Internal fixation is done using a plate secured by screws. The hip is usually fused in a 30-degree flexion; a spica cast may be placed at the end of the case.

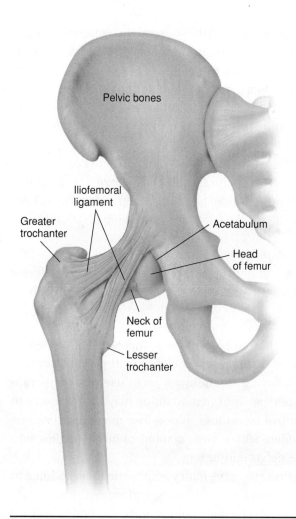

Figure 21-8   *Anatomy of the Hip Joint*
Source: AAOS, 2004.

Anesthetic

Neuraxial block may consist of a spinal or epidural with IV sedation. IV ketamine and propofol can be used to help sedate the patient for the block as well as for positioning on the OR table. Internal fixation of a fractured hip is associated with less blood loss when a spinal or epidural anesthesia has been given.

Alternatively, general anesthesia is given with insertion of an OETT; induction can be done on the OR table if the patient is able to tolerate the move. General anesthesia may also be combined with an epidural placed for postoperative pain control.

Positioning

The patient is placed in a supine or lateral decubitus position. Meticulous padding is important, as this procedure can last 3–4 hours.

Anesthetic Implications

Major blood loss is possible with this procedure. Cell-saver technology can be used. Controlled hypotension (do not allow the mean arterial pressure to fall below 60 mm Hg) can be used to help decrease blood loss.

Keep the patient warm.

An arterial line is usually needed.

A central venous pressure line may or may not be inserted.

When deciding whether to do a hemiarthroplasty (reconstruction of one side of the joint) versus total hip reconstruction, the patient's age, medical condition, and level of activity must be considered.

Complications

This procedure carries a high risk for postoperative complications such as non-union or malposition of the joint.

ORTHOPEDIC SURGERY: FEMUR

Subtrochanteric femur fractures occur distal to the level of the lesser trochanter, within 5 cm of the lesser trochanter. Below this level, the fracture is considered a femoral shaft fracture.

Prosthetic Replacement of Femoral Head (Hemiarthroplasty of Hip)

Hemiarthroplasty of the hip entails placement of a prosthesis to substitute for the femoral head. It is used for the treatment of displaced femoral neck fractures in the elderly or medically compromised patient. One advantage of this procedure over other treatments is that immediate weight bearing is allowed; however, the surgery itself is more extensive.

Operative Procedure

Either a posterior or anterolateral exposure may be used. Both approaches are performed with the patient in the lateral decubitus position. Methylmethacrylate may be used to seat the prosthesis into the femoral shaft.

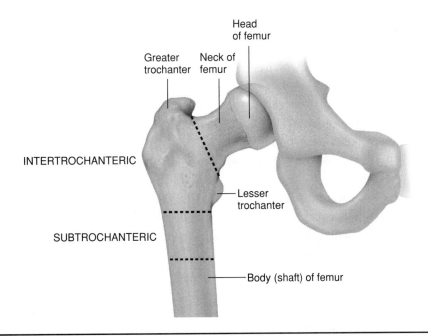

Figure 21-9 *Anatomy of the Proximal Femur*
Source: AAOS, 2004.

Anesthetic

The neuraxial block consists of a spinal or epidural with IV sedation. IV ketamine and propofol can be used to help sedate the patient for the block as well as for positioning on the OR table.

General anesthesia is used with an OETT.

Positioning

The patient is placed in a lateral decubitus position.

Anesthetic Implications

See the discussion of methylmethacrylate bone cement in Chapter 3.

Open Reduction and Internal Fixation of Femoral Fracture: Intertrochanteric (Proximal Femur) Fracture

Open reduction and internal fixation (ORIF) of a proximal femur fracture is performed to realign broken bones. Surgical hardware is used to hold the bones in place.

Proximal femur fractures are commonly referred to as hip fractures. These fractures involve the uppermost portion of the femur just adjacent to the hip joint. Proximal hip fractures include femoral neck, intertrochanteric, and sub-trochanteric fractures. Nondisplaced femoral neck and any intertrochanteric fractures usually require ORIF, as do all subtrochanteric fractures.

Buck's traction may be used to stabilize the leg until surgery can be done and to minimize muscle spasms in elderly patients. Skeletal traction is used in younger patients with high-energy injuries. Anatomic reduction is necessary before surgical repair to reduce the risk to surrounding structures.

Falls are the most common cause of hip fractures in older adults. Motor vehicle collisions and high-force trauma are the usual causes of these injuries in the younger population.

Operative Procedure

The incision is made over the fracture site, usually proximal to the lateral thigh. It must be large enough to accommodate a plate if it is used. Screws,

pins, and plates or intermedullary nails (or IM devices) are used for fixation of the bone fractures. Once a compression plate and a screw are used to achieve interfragmental compression (lag screw), the traction can be released. For comminuted fractures of the femoral head or displaced femoral neck fractures, total hip arthroplasty may be required.

Percutaneous pinning can be used with nondis-placed femoral neck fractures.

One or more drains are occasionally placed. The incision line is then closed.

Anesthetic

A neuraxial block consists of a spinal or epidural with IV sedation. IV ketamine and propofol can be used to help sedate the patient for the block as well as for positioning on the OR table. Internal fixation of a fractured hip is associated with less blood loss when a spinal or epidural anesthesia has been given.

General anesthesia, an OETT, and rapid-sequence induction are appropriate in a trauma patient. Induction can be done on the OR table if the patient is able to tolerate the move; however, induction may need to be done on the stretcher or patient's bed so that the move to the OR table is tolerated.

Positioning

The patient is placed in a supine or lateral decubi-tus position. These surgeries can be long-duration procedures, so meticulous care in positioning and padding of all body prominences is required. The surgery is performed on a fracture table.

Anesthetic Implications

Preoperative lab tests should include CBC and PT/INR/PTT measurements. A 12-lead EKG should be obtained with older patients.

Type and cross-match the patient's blood pre-operatively. Moderate blood loss is possible with this procedure.

An arterial line may be indicated.

Minimal to moderate IV fluids should be given. Maintain urinary output at a rate of 0.5 mL/kg/hr. Keep the patient warm.

Open Reduction and Internal Fixation of Femoral Fracture: Femur Shaft Fracture

Open or closed realignment and fixation are used to treat a fracture of the femur shaft. This procedure is indicated for fracture or non-union of the femoral shaft. Such injuries are common in young males due to trauma; pathologic fractures can also occur. An external fixator or skeletal traction may be placed temporarily until an open reduction can be done.

IM fixation devices are increasingly becoming the preferred method of treatment for femoral fractures because they increase the weight-bearing capacity, decrease the risk of implant failure, and reduce complications compared to an ORIF with plates and screws. A nail can be placed either proximal-to-distal or distal-to-proximal from the lesser trochanter to the distal femur (within 7 cm of the articular surface).

Operative Procedure

Depending on the fracture type and associated injuries, either an external fixator or an open procedure is needed.

An *intertrochanteric intramedullary nail* is the most common method of fixation. With an IM nail is used, the procedure is typically performed percutaneously, with small incisions being made at the proximal and distal ends of the femur. The fracture is manually reduced by the surgeon, and femur continuity is confirmed by X-ray. A small incision is made, and a guide pin is placed in the proximal or distal femur under X-ray guidance. The intramedullary canal is reamed over a guide wire. A rod is then seated over the guide pin, introduced into the distal segment, and secured into the condylar region. The IM nail connects the two ends of the femur; screws are placed above and below the fracture point to secure the rod in place.

Anesthetic

Spinal neuraxial anesthesia should not be used for acute treatment of fractures, owing to the need to perform an accurate neurovascular exam immediately postoperatively.

General anesthesia, an OETT, and rapid-sequence induction are appropriate in trauma patients. Induction can be done on the OR table if the patient is able to tolerate the move; however, induction may need to be done on the stretcher or patient's bed so that the move to the OR table is tolerated.

Positioning

The patient is placed in a supine position.

Anesthetic Implications

Temporary traction devices are removed prior to skin preparation.

Fluoroscopy is done during the procedure.

Neurovascular compromise is possible with a femoral shaft fracture. Assess the area distal to the femur for circulation, sensation, and motor function preoperatively and postoperatively, and document the findings. Open femur fractures are associated with a 1–2% incidence of limb-threatening femoral artery or sciatic or femoral nerve injuries.

Open Reduction and Internal Fixation of Femoral Fracture: Supracondylar (Distal Femur) Fracture

ORIF is used to achieve anatomical reduction, alignment, and stabilization of the articular surface and alignment of the distal femur to provide joint stability following supracondylar fractures (also known as condyle and epicondyle fractures). This procedure performed for various types of fractures of the distal femur: displaced fractures, open fractures, and those associated with a vascular injury.

Distal femur fractures are often involved with the knee joint and cartilage and with proximal tibial plateau surfaces. Condylar fractures often result in multiple bone fragments. Even with perfect surgical alignment of the bone and cartilage surfaces, there is an increased risk of developing arthritis due to damage of the articular surface.

Supracondylar femur fractures are more common in patients with severe osteoporosis and in patients who have previously undergone total knee replacement surgery. In these persons, the bone just above the knee joint may be weaker than in normal individuals and, therefore, more prone to fracture. However, patients may also sustain supracondylar femur fractures after high-energy injuries.

Distal femur fractures occur at approximately one-tenth the rate of proximal femur fractures.

A bone graft is needed in the setting of non-union and bone loss, but is rarely performed in the acute setting.

Operative Procedure

Treatment is highly variable. Possible procedures include closed reduction with a cast or brace, an external fixator, or an intramedullary nail. Alternatively, an open procedure with pins, screws, nails, and plates may be done to repair the fracture. An incision is made along the femur for the open procedure.

Anesthetic

Spinal neuraxial anesthesia should not be used for acute treatment of fractures, owing to the need to perform an accurate neurovascular exam immediately postoperatively.

General anesthesia, an OETT, and rapid-sequence induction are appropriate for trauma patients. Induction can be done on the OR table if the patient is able to tolerate the move; however, induction may need to be done on the stretcher or patient's bed so that the move to the OR table is tolerated.

Positioning

The patient is placed in a supine position.

Anesthetic Implications

Cruciate ligaments may also require repair with distal femur fracture.

If a compression tourniquet is used, it is usually set at 50–100 mm Hg above the patient's systolic blood pressure; the maximum setting is less than 400 mm Hg in the lower extremity. Chart both the

tourniquet time and setting. The tourniquet should be released after 2 hours to prevent injury.

Neurovascular compromise is possible with this injury. Assess the area distal to the fracture for circulation, sensation, and motor function preoperatively and postoperatively, and document the findings.

Trauma patients may have more than one fracture and require more than one type of orthopedic surgery.

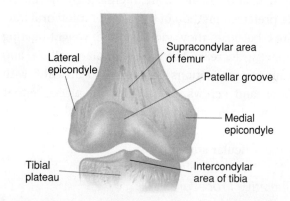

Figure 21-10 *Bones of the Knee Joint (Patella Removed)*
Source: AAOS, 2004.

ORTHOPEDIC SURGERY: KNEE

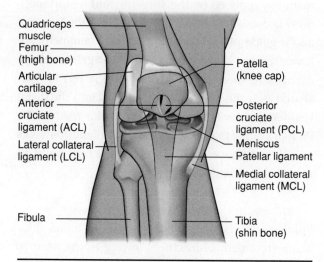

Figure 21-11 *Anatomy of the Knee Joint*

Arthrodesis of Knee

Arthrodesis of the knee is surgical bone fusion resulting in fixation of the knee joint. It is performed to relieve pain and to provide support to a diseased or injured joint.

Operative Procedure

An anterior midline knee incision is made; anterior arthrotomy, cartilage, and a small amount of bone are excised. Bones are stabilized with plates, screws, and an intramedullary rod, or an external fixator. A cast or splint is placed at the end of the case; keep the patient asleep until the cast is applied and hardened or a splint is applied.

Anesthetic

The neuraxial block consists of a spinal or epidural with IV sedation. IV ketamine and propofol can be used to help sedate the patient for the block as well as for positioning on the OR table.

Alternatively, general anesthesia is used with an OETT. A femoral and/or sciatic nerve block may be placed for postoperative pain control.

Positioning

The patient is placed in a supine position, with the arms extended on padded armboards.

Anesthetic Implications

If a compression tourniquet is used, it is usually set at 50–100 mm Hg above the patient's systolic blood pressure; the maximum setting is less than 400 mm Hg in the lower extremity. Chart both the tourniquet time and setting. The tourniquet should be released after 2 hours to prevent injury.

Repair of Cruciate or Collateral Ligament Tears

ACL repair provides for reconstruction of torn ligaments of the knee that are causing instability and pain. Trauma is the major common cause of knee ligament tears, though osteoarthritis and rheumatoid arthritis can also cause such tears.

The cruciate and collateral ligaments are crucial to maintenance of a stable knee joint. The collateral ligaments support the knee medially and laterally, while the cruciate ligaments support the knee anteriorly and posteriorly. Autografts (portion of the patellar tendon or hamstrings) or allografts, bovine xenografts, and artificial substitutes may all be used to augment or reconstruct these ligaments when they are damaged.

Operative Procedure

In an *open* procedure, a longitudinal incision is made either medially or laterally, contingent on the involved ligament.

- *Cruciate ligaments.* Tears of the anterior cruciate ligament (ACL) and posterior cruciate ligament (PCL) are generally repaired only if bone is avulsed at one end of the ligament with direct suture, staples, or screws. Repair of avulsions is most common in children.
- *Collateral ligaments.* The medial collateral ligament (MCL) is rarely repaired because it often heals with nonoperative treatment. Lateral collateral ligament (LCL) rupture occasionally requires reconstruction. If a reconstruction is performed, an incision is made over the ligament either medially or laterally. The torn ligament is repaired by direct suture or by stapling the torn ligaments to bone.

ACL repair can be done *arthroscopically* unless multiple tears and fractures are present. With this approach, standard knee arthroscopic portals are made and a diagnostic knee arthroscopy is performed. The torn ACL is identified and removed. Examination of the menisci, chondral surfaces, and PCL is also undertaken. Tunnels for reconstruction are drilled in the tibia and femur.

Autografts (patellar tendon or hamstring), homografts, or allografts are then passed through a small incision in the proximal tibia. The graft is secured with large screws.

Anesthetic

The neuraxial block consists of a spinal or epidural with IV sedation. IV ketamine and propofol can be used to help sedate the patient for the block as well as for positioning on the OR table.

Alternatively, general anesthesia is used with an OETT. A femoral nerve block with or without a sciatic nerve block can be employed for postoperative pain control.

Positioning

The patient is placed in a supine position, with knees extending over the lower break in the table. The operative knee may be positioned differently. The foot of the bed is lowered when the surgeon is ready. The patient's arms are extended on padded armboards.

Anesthetic Implications

If a compression tourniquet is used, it is usually set at 50–100 mm Hg above the patient's systolic blood pressure; the maximum setting is less than 400 mm Hg in the lower extremity. Chart both the tourniquet time and setting. The tourniquet should be released after 2 hours to prevent injury.

Keep the patient asleep until a knee immobilizer has been applied to maintain knee immobilization. There is possibility of injury to the repair if the patient moves the leg or bends it before a splint is applied.

Knee Manipulation Under Anesthesia

Knee manipulation may be employed to release abnormal scar formation within the joint. This treatment is used for arthrofibrosis—abnormal scar formation within the joint after knee surgery or knee fracture.

Operative Procedure

The knee is straightened and flexed to release the scar tissue until a fuller range of motion is appreciated.

Anesthetic

IV sedation is usually all that is required.

Positioning

The patient is placed in a supine position, with arms extended on padded armboards.

Anesthetic Implications

This is usually a very quick procedure.

Lateral or Medial Menisectomy

Menisectomy is the excision of a torn meniscus, which frequently results from trauma.

Operative Procedure

Standard knee arthroscopy portals are created. A diagnostic knee arthroscopy is performed, and the medial and lateral menisci are visualized. Probes are used to identify tears. The meniscal tears are usually treated with removal of the torn tissue (menisectomy). Small biters and shavers are used to trim the torn cartilage.

Anesthetic

The neuraxial block consists of a spinal or epidural with IV sedation. IV ketamine and propofol can be used to help sedate the patient for the block as well as for positioning on the OR table.

Alternatively, general anesthesia is used with an OETT or LMA. A femoral or sciatic nerve block can be done for postoperative pain control.

Keep the patient asleep until a cast is applied and hardened or a leg immobilizer is placed.

Positioning

The patient is placed in a supine position, with knees extending over the lower break in the table. The operative knee may be positioned differently. The foot of the bed is lowered when the surgeon is ready. The patient's arms are extended on padded armboards.

Anesthetic Implications

If a compression tourniquet is used, it is usually set at 50–100 mm Hg above the patient's systolic blood pressure; the maximum setting is less than 400 mm Hg in the lower extremity. Chart both the tourniquet time and setting. The tourniquet should be released after 2 hours to prevent injury.

Patella Dislocation Correction (Patellar Realignment)

An open surgical procedure is used to realign the extensor mechanism of the knee, realign the patella in its normal position, and prevent chronic dislocation of the patella. Traumatic dislocations of the patella can occur, although dislocations (subluxation) more commonly result from underlying anatomical abnormalities. The patella tracks more lateral than normal in such cases, so the medial soft tissues can be tightened or the tibial tubercle moved.

Operative Procedure

Multiple surgical procedures have been designed to shift the insertion of the patellar tendon back to its original position at the tibia; all involve incising the lateral quadriceps tendon.

In severe mal-alignment of the extensor mechanism, the insertion of the patellar tendon may be moved to a more medial location.

Anesthetic

The neuraxial block consists of a spinal or epidural with IV sedation. IV ketamine and propofol can be used to help sedate the patient for the block as well as for positioning on the OR table.

Alternatively, general anesthesia is used with an OETT or an LMA. A femoral or sciatic nerve block can be performed for postoperative pain control.

Positioning

The patient is placed in a supine position, with arms extended on padded armboards.

Anesthetic Implications

If a compression tourniquet is used, it is usually set at 50–100 mm Hg above the patient's systolic blood pressure; the maximum setting is less than 400 mm Hg in the lower extremity. Chart both the tourniquet time and setting. The tourniquet

should be released after 2 hours to prevent injury.

Patella Tendon Rupture Repair

The patellar tendon connects the tibia and the patella. This tendon affects movement to the extensor mechanism of the knee, so complications from its rupture can be very disabling. Rupture usually occurs due to trauma.

Operative Procedure

The incision is made over the tendon; the tendon sheath is opened. The tendon ends are reapproximated with an interlocking stitch technique, usually done through bone tunnels within the patella or tibial tubercle. Fascia can be used to augment the suture line. The sheath is sutured and the skin closed.

Anesthetic

The neuraxial block consists of a spinal or epidural with IV sedation. A femoral nerve block can be performed for postoperative pain control.

General anesthesia, an OETT, and rapid-sequence induction may be used in trauma cases.

Keep the patient asleep until a cast is applied and hardened or a splint is applied.

Positioning

The patient is placed in a supine position.

Anesthetic Implications

If a compression tourniquet is used, it is usually set at 50–100 mm Hg above the patient's systolic blood pressure; the maximum setting is less than 400 mm Hg in the lower extremity. Chart both the tourniquet time and setting. The tourniquet should be released after 2 hours to prevent injury.

Patellectomy

Patellectomy is the removal of the patella ("knee cap"—a triangular bone that articulates with the femur and covers and protects the knee joint). This bone may be removed due to a comminuted fracture of the patella or painful degenerative arthritis. Removing the patella can significantly reduce the knee's ability to extend fully and can cause atrophy and decreased strength of the quadriceps muscle.

Patellar Fracture Reduction

Open reduction and internal surgical repair of patellar fragments are performed in cases involving displaced fractures of the patella. The goal is to restore the extensor mechanism and reconstruct the articular surface of the patella. The extensor mechanism can fail in one of three places—quad tendon, patella, or patellar tendon.

Operative Procedure

A longitudinal pre-patellar incision is made, with exploration of the joint and patellar tendon following. The fracture site is exposed, and debris and small fragments are irrigated. Major fracture fragments are approximated and repaired with a tension band, bone screws, and/or wires (circumferential loop technique). All of these devices are designed to produce compression forces across the fracture site(s).

If the whole patella is broken in smaller fragments, they can be excised, albeit with shortening of the patellar tendon (patellar tendon repair). The wound is closed.

A quadriceps tendon repair may also be done.

Anesthetic

Spinal neuraxial anesthesia should not be used for acute treatment of fractures, owing to the need to perform an accurate neurovascular exam immediately postoperatively.

General anesthesia, an OETT, and rapid-sequence induction are appropriate in trauma patients. Muscle relaxation is needed to reduce the fracture. Induction may need to be done on the stretcher or patient's bed so that the move to the OR table is tolerated.

Positioning

The patient is placed in a supine position, with arms extended on padded armboards.

Anesthetic Implications

Keep the patient asleep until a cast or splint is applied to stabilize the knee.

If a compression tourniquet is used, it is usually set at 50–100 mm Hg above the patient's systolic blood pressure; the maximum setting is less than 400 mm Hg in the lower extremity. Chart both the tourniquet time and setting. The tourniquet should be released after 2 hours to prevent injury.

Popliteal Cyst Excision (Baker's Cyst)

Excision of a popliteal cyst in the posterior knee joint may become necessary in the aftermath of a meniscal tear. A popliteal cyst is formed by the herniation of the synovial membrane or the accumulation of synovial fluid of the knee joint into one of several bursae in the popliteal space.

Operative Procedure

After an oblique incision of the popliteal space is made, the deep fascia is separated, exposing the cyst. The cyst is then dissected free. The cyst and its pedicle are traced back to the posterior knee joint, the pedicle is ligated, and the cyst excised. The wound is closed, and a splint is applied.

Anesthetic

GETA may be required; MAC anesthesia is typically utilized for this procedure, as postoperative pain control is well managed with IV/PO medications.

Spinal anesthesia with a short-acting local anesthetic can be efficacious, however, if a neuraxial block is done.

Positioning

The patient is placed in a prone position, with a roll underneath the ankles.

Anesthetic Implications

These cysts can be quite painful.

If a compression tourniquet is used, it is usually set at 50–100 mm Hg above the patient's systolic blood pressure; the maximum setting is less than 400 mm Hg in the lower extremity. Chart both the tourniquet time and setting. The tourniquet should be released after 2 hours to prevent injury.

Tibial Plateau Fracture

Tibial plateau fracture occurs at the top of the shin bone, and involves the cartilage surface of the knee joint.

ORTHOPEDIC SURGERY: LOWER LEG

Achilles Tendon Repair

The Achilles tendon is part of the posterior leg, attaching the calf muscle (gastrocnemius and soleus muscles) to the posterior aspect of the calcaneus. The Achilles tendon facilitates walking, and the Achilles muscle reflex tests the integrity of the S1 spinal nerve root. A rupture of this tendon may be either partial or complete, and requires either immobilization or surgery as treatment. Rupture may be caused by a sudden forced plantar flexion of the foot, unexpected dorsiflexion of the foot, or violent dorsiflexion of a plantar flexed foot.

Operative Procedure

Two surgical methods are commonly used: open (one large incision is made in the back of the leg) and percutaneous (several small incisions are made). In both procedures, the surgeon sutures the Achilles tendon back together. The differences between the two methods relate to their wound complications and re-rupture rates. Open surgery is more likely to result in wound complications, whereas percutaneous surgery has higher tendon re-rupture rates.

In recent years, less invasive treatments for Achilles tendon repair have emerged that provide for speedier recovery times. Tissue graft products often consist of a part of another tendon; used as a bridge to link the severed tendon lengths, they provide a scaffold on which new tissue grows, increasing the overall strength of the repair. Bone anchors are screws that are drilled into the heel bone to secure the tendon and tissues. New arthroscopic procedures have been introduced as well.

Anesthetic

A neuraxial block consists of a spinal or epidural with IV sedation. Alternatively, general anesthesia may be used with an OETT, or MAC anesthesia with a popliteal fossa block for intraoperative and postoperative pain control. A femoral block with sciatic block may also be used.

Keep the patient asleep until a cast is applied and hardened or a splint is applied.

Positioning

The patient is placed in a prone position.

Anesthetic Implications

If a compression tourniquet is used, it is usually set at 50–100 mm Hg above the patient's systolic blood pressure; the maximum setting is less than 400 mm Hg in the lower extremity. Chart both the tourniquet time and setting. The tourniquet should be released after 2 hours to prevent injury.

Open Reduction of Tibial Fracture

Realignment and fixation of the tibia are accomplished through a surgical incision. This procedure is used for open tibial fractures accompanied by severe soft-tissue injury.

Three types of tibial fractures are distinguished:

- Tibial plateau fractures (proximal)
- Tibial shaft fractures (repaired by IM nailing)
- Distal tibia fractures (ankle and articular fractures that also include fibula fractures)

Open fractures of the tibia are more common, as one-third of this bone's surface is subcutaneous. Blood supply to the tibia is more precarious than that of other long bones, because it is not enclosed by heavy muscle. Rotational deformities often occur in conjunction with trauma. Delayed union, non-union, and infection are common complications of an open tibial fracture.

Operative Procedure

The type of fixation device is determined by the type of fracture. An *open* surgical approach is needed if multiple fractures are present, especially to the knee and ankle joints. A longitudinal incision is made over the fractured bone. Transverse bone screws or plates are applied to reduce fracture fragments; bone grafting may be done to repair a non-union.

If an intramedullary nail is employed, an incision about the tibial tuberosity is made. A drill reamer penetrates the medullary canal. The nail is inserted and aligned to avoid malrotation. It is then driven past the fracture site into the distal bone. The wound is closed.

In *closed* reduction and external fixation, two or three pins are percutaneously placed, both proximally and distally to the fracture, after aligning the bones under fluoroscopy guidance.

Anesthetic
Spinal neuraxial anesthesia should not be used for acute treatment of fractures of the tibia, owing to the need to perform an accurate neurovascular exam immediately postoperatively.

General anesthesia, an OETT, and rapid-sequence induction are appropriate in trauma cases. Induction can be done on the OR table if the patient is able to tolerate the move; however, induction may need to be done on the stretcher or patient's bed so that the move to the table is tolerated. IV ketamine and propofol can be used to help sedate the patient for positioning on the OR table.

Positioning
The patient is placed in a supine position, with arms extended on padded armboards.

Anesthetic Implications
Keep the patient asleep until the cast is applied and hardened or a splint is applied.

Generally, surgery is undertaken to fix a fractured fibula bone only when the tibial fracture involves the distal articular surface.

If a compression tourniquet is used, it is usually set at 50–100 mm Hg above the patient's systolic blood pressure; the maximum setting is less than

400 mm Hg in the lower extremity. Chart both the tourniquet time and setting. The tourniquet should be released after 2 hours to prevent injury.

Trauma to the lower leg bones can cause compartment syndrome.

Neurovascular compromise is possible with this injury. Assess the area distal to the tibial fracture for circulation, sensation, and motor function preoperatively and postoperatively, and document the findings. Monitor the patient for any signs and symptoms of compartment syndrome.

ORTHOPEDIC SURGERY: ANKLE AND FOOT
Open Reduction of Ankle Fracture
This surgery includes realignment and fixation of the medial malleolus (tibia), lateral malleolus (fibula), and/or posterior malleolus (posterior aspect of distal tibia). It is performed as acute fracture repair.

Operative Procedure
Open reduction and internal fixation of an ankle fracture rely on pins, plates, and/or screws to hold the bones in proper alignment until the bones heal.

For open repair of any or all of these bone fractures, an incision is made over the involved fracture site. Typically, two incisions are made—one medial and one lateral. The fracture is aligned and fixed with screws that stabilize the fractured fragments to the tibia and fibula. After the wound is closed, a short leg splint is applied.

Anesthetic
The neuraxial block consists of a spinal or epidural with IV sedation. Alternatively, a sciatic nerve block (at either the gluteal or popliteal fossa area) may be used, along with a saphenous nerve block to cover the medial portion of the ankle. IV ketamine and propofol can be used to help sedate the patient for the block(s) as well as for positioning on the OR table.

General anesthesia, an OETT, and rapid-sequence induction are appropriate for trauma cases. Induction can be done on the OR table if the patient is able to tolerate the move; however, induction may need to be done on the stretcher or patient's bed so that the move to the OR table is tolerated.

Keep the patient asleep until the cast is applied and hardened.

Positioning

The patient is placed in a supine position, with arms extended on padded armboards. A folded sheet is placed under the surgical-side hip, rotating the ankle inward, if the lateral ankle is involved.

Anesthetic Implications

If a compression tourniquet is used, it is usually set at 50–100 mm Hg above the patient's systolic blood pressure; the maximum setting is less than 400 mm Hg in the lower extremity. Chart both the tourniquet time and setting. The tourniquet should be released after 2 hours to prevent injury.

Complications

The superficial peroneal nerve is at risk from the lateral/fibular incision. Because it is totally exposed, it must be protected during the surgery.

Arthrodesis of Ankle

Arthrodesis of the ankle comprises fusion of the ankle. Multiple joints may be fused—tibiotalar, talocalcaneal, talonavicular, and calcaneocuboid. This procedure is performed to relieve pain, provide stability, and stop a joint-destroying disease process, such as is seen with poliomyelitis, rheumatoid or traumatic arthritis, clubfoot, and post-traumatic deformity. This surgery will limit the patient's ability to dorsi-flex or plantar-flex the ankle.

Operative Procedure

Multiple incisions about the ankle may be employed. The joints to be fused are exposed, cartilage surfaces resected, and bones apposed and internally fixed in a stable fashion with screws and/or plates. A drain is usually placed, and the skin closed.

Anesthetic

The neuraxial block consists of a spinal or epidural with IV sedation. Alternatively, a sciatic nerve block (at either the gluteal or popliteal fossa area) may be used, along with a saphenous nerve block to cover the medial portion of the ankle.

Alternatively, general anesthesia is used with an OETT.

Positioning

The patient is placed in a supine position, with arms extended on padded armboards.

Anesthetic Implications

Keep the patient asleep until the short leg cast or splint is applied.

If a compression tourniquet is used, it is usually set at 50–100 mm Hg above the patient's systolic blood pressure; the maximum setting is less than 400 mm Hg in the lower extremity. Chart both the tourniquet time and setting. The tourniquet should be released after 2 hours to prevent injury.

Bunionectomy (Exostectomy), with or without Fusion (Hallux Abductus Valgus Repair)

Bunionectomy is the removal of a soft-tissue or bony mass at the medial site of the first metatarsal head (on the big toe). Such a mass is associated with a deformity of the big toe.

Bunionectomy is performed as a treatment for pain and swelling of the big toe, in which a painful plantar callus (build-up of skin on the ball of the foot) radiates pain to the leg and/or knee. A bunion is caused by a structural defect of the foot, but is accentuated by wearing high-heels with pointed toes.

Operative Procedure

A 2- to 3-inch incision is made on the top or side of the great toe joint. The surgeon will excise soft tissue and/or a bony mass, providing for realignment of the ligaments around the great toe joint. If the joint is deformed, tiny wires, screws, plates, or Kirschner wire may be needed to stabilize the area.

The incision is closed with sutures. Multiple variations of this procedure exist.

Bunionectomy may or may not be done with a fusion. The decision to fuse the toe joint depends on the patient's activity level.

Keep the patient asleep until a cast or walking boot is placed to maintain stability.

Anesthetic

General anesthesia is the most common plan. If the patient has extensive comorbidities, spinal anesthesia should be considered. Postoperative pain is usually controlled by the surgeon infiltrating the surgical site with local anesthetic agents and through IV/PO medications.

Positioning

The patient is placed in a supine position, with arms extended on padded armboards.

Anesthetic Implications

If a compression tourniquet is used, it is usually set at 50–100 mm Hg above the patient's systolic blood pressure; the maximum setting is less than 400 mm Hg in the lower extremity. Chart both the tourniquet time and setting. The tourniquet should be released after 2 hours to prevent injury.

Correction of Hammer Toe Deformity, with or without Fusion

The term "hammer toe" is used to describe an abnormal flexion of the proximal interphalangeal (middle) joint of the second, third, or fourth toes. Initially, hammer toes are flexible and can be corrected with simple interventions. If left untreated, however, they can become fixed and require surgery to repair. These deformities are caused by a muscle imbalance.

Operative Procedure

Correction of a hammer toe may or may not be done with a fusion of the joint. An incision is made across the deformed proximal interphalangeal joint. The surgeon will incise the long extensor tendon to the toe, and excise the bony deformity. Depending on the severity of the deformity, a

Kirschner wire may be inserted to fuse the joint and stabilize the toe during the postoperative period.

Anesthetic

General anesthesia with OETT or LMA is the most common plan. If the patient has extensive comorbidities, spinal anesthesia should be considered. Postoperative pain is usually controlled by the surgeon infiltrating the surgical site with local anesthetic agents and through IV/PO medications.

Positioning

The patient is placed in a supine position, with arms extended on padded armboards.

Anesthetic Implications

If a compression tourniquet is used, it is usually set at 50–100 mm Hg above the patient's systolic blood pressure; the maximum setting is less than 400 mm Hg in the lower extremity. Chart both the tourniquet time and setting. The tourniquet should be released after 2 hours to prevent injury.

Repair of Metatarsal Fracture

This surgery provides for internal fixation of fractures of the long bones of the foot (metatarsals). Such injuries are usually the result of direct trauma.

There are five metatarsals in each foot that attach to the phalanges (toe bones). The fifth metatarsal is especially vulnerable to avulsion injuries in which the peroneus brevis muscle pulls off the bone; this condition is treated nonoperatively. An ORIF is often necessary if a fracture to the proximal fifth metatarsal goes through the proximal metaphysic, due to the high rates of non-union in such cases.

Operative Procedure

Incision placement is based on the site of the fracture. Kirschner wires are driven into the canal of the fractured bone.

Anesthetic

The foot is primarily innervated by the sciatic nerve. The exception relates to the saphenous nerve (a branch of the femoral nerve), which innervates the medial superficial structures of the lower calf, ankle, and foot. With metatarsal fractures, both the sciatic and saphenous nerves need to be anesthetized. Depending on the density of the block, general or spinal anesthesia may be necessary, instead of MAC anesthesia.

GETA with an OETT is used with rapid-sequence induction in trauma cases.

Keep the patient asleep until a cast is applied and hardened or a foot boot is applied.

Positioning

The patient is placed in a supine position, with arms extended on padded armboards.

Anesthetic Implications

If a compression tourniquet is used, it is usually set at 50–100 mm Hg above the patient's systolic blood pressure; the maximum setting is less than 400 mm Hg in the lower extremity. Chart both the tourniquet time and setting. The tourniquet should be released after 2 hours to prevent injury.

Metatarsal Head Resection

Excision of the metatarsal heads is performed to relieve pain related to prominence of the metatarsal heads. These patients usually have rheumatoid

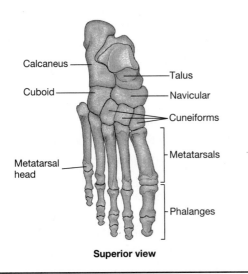

Superior view

Figure 21-12 *Bones of the Foot*
Source: Clark, 2005.

arthritis and an enlarged metatarsal head of the great toe, as is seen with bunions (see the earlier discussion of bunionectomy).

Operative Procedure

A longitudinal incision is made in the interspace adjacent to the particular metatarsal head to be excised. Contracted soft tissue is released. The end of the metatarsal is smoothed with a bone rasp. A Kirschner wire is inserted through the medullary canal of the metatarsal stump, aligning it in proper relation to the appropriate toe. The wire is capped and the wound is closed. A bulky dressing is applied.

Anesthetic

The foot is primarily innervated by the sciatic nerve. The exception involves the saphenous nerve (a branch of the femoral nerve), which innervates the medial superficial structures of the lower calf, ankle, and foot. With metatarsal fractures, both the sciatic and saphenous nerves need to be anesthetized. Depending on the density of the block, general or spinal anesthesia may be necessary.

Patients with rheumatoid arthritis can have cervical nerve root compression and/or atlanto-occipital instability. Assess the patient's ability to extend the neck and ask about any numbness or tingling with neck movement. Check the neck X-ray for subluxation of the cervical spine. These patients may require awake fiberoptic intubation.

Positioning

The patient is placed in a supine position, with arms extended on padded armboards. The operative ankle is supported off the OR table on a pillow.

Anesthetic Implications

If a compression tourniquet is used, it is usually set at 50–100 mm Hg above the patient's systolic blood pressure; the maximum setting is less than 400 mm Hg in the lower extremity. Chart both the tourniquet time and setting. The tourniquet should be released after 2 hours to prevent injury.

Tendon Lengthening

This procedure involves surgical lengthening or moving of the tendon to a new insertion site to help to restore balance or normalize joint motion. The contraction of the muscle may be due to either neuromuscular disease or trauma.

Operative Procedure
Lengthening

An incision is made over the tendon, and the tendon sheath is opened. A Z-type incision is made over the tendon, allowing it to be elongated while keeping the proximal and distal insertion sites to be maintained in a normal place. The tendon is reapproximated by suturing it together.

Tendon Transfer

An incision is made over the tendon, cutting close to the insertion site. A new incision is made at the intended bony insertion site, and the tendon is then transferred. The tendon is secured at the new site with sutures or staples to the bone.

Anesthetic

The neuraxial block consists of a spinal or epidural with IV sedation. IV ketamine and propofol can be used to help sedate the patient for the block as well as for positioning on the OR table.

Alternatively, general anesthesia is used with an OETT or an LMA.

The patient should be kept asleep until the cast is applied and hardened or a splint is applied.

Positioning

Patient positioning depends on the tendon placement.

Anesthetic Implications

If a compression tourniquet is used, it is usually set at 50–100 mm Hg above the patient's systolic blood pressure; the maximum setting is less than 400 mm Hg in the lower extremity. Chart both the tourniquet time and setting. The tourniquet should be released after 2 hours to prevent injury.

AMPUTATION OF THE LOWER EXTREMITY

Amputation: Disarticulation of the Hip

This amputation of an entire lower extremity is done through the hip joint. It may be performed in cases involving a malignant tumor of the femur, hip, or pelvis; traumatic amputation to the femur, hip, or pelvis; or uncontrollable infection to leg, hip, or pelvis.

Operative Procedure

An anterior oblique-shaped incision is made, detaching all the muscles surrounding the hip joint. Vessels, muscles, and nerves are located and ligated. A gluteal flap is sewn anteriorly. A compression dressing is applied.

Anesthetic

General anesthesia with an OETT is necessary due to the duration and extent of the surgery. A rapid-sequence induction is needed if the patient has been involved in a trauma. Place an epidural catheter to T6 for postoperative pain control, with boluses of medications being given postoperatively. Aggressive anticoagulation for thrombosis prevention is often initiated the day of surgery, which can complicate catheter removal. Regional anesthesia is rarely employed for these procedures.

Positioning

The patient is placed in a supine or lateral decubitus position.

Anesthetic Implications

Expect large blood losses. Type and cross-match the patient's blood; it may be necessary to have 2–4 units available in the operating room at the start of the case. Establish multiple large-bore peripheral IVs or a central venous line. An arterial line is needed to monitor blood pressure and blood draws for serial hematocrit levels and arterial blood gases. A pulmonary artery catheter may be needed if the patient's condition warrants it.

Cell-saving techniques are useful (except when amputation is done due to tumor).

Deliberate hypotension or hemodilution may be necessary to control blood loss. Lower the systolic blood pressure to approximately 30% of the patient's baseline, but do not decrease the mean arterial pressure to less than 60 mm Hg.

Temperature control may be difficult when the lower extremity from the waist down is uncovered. Warming blankets (one over the upper body and one over the nonoperative leg) and fluid warmers should be used; the room temperature should be increased if these measures prove ineffective.

Above-the-Knee Amputation

Severance of the distal femur and the lower leg may be necessary in cases involving gangrene, vascular insufficiency, trauma, and malignancy.

Operative Procedure

A musculocutaneous flap (muscle, overlying skin, and subcutaneous tissue) is created for femoral stump coverage. The saphenous nerve, superficial femoral artery and vein, and sciatic nerve are ligated and divided; leg muscles are transected circumferentially. The femur is transected with a saw. Bone edges are smoothed with a rasp. Hemostasis is achieved and the wound is closed. A closed suction device may be inserted. A plaster cast or temporary prosthesis is used to minimize postoperative edema and to help shape the stump for a permanent prosthesis (created later).

A guillotine amputation can also be done. With this approach, a stump is not created and the wound is not closed until a later date. The femur is transected with a saw, the leg is left open, and a compression dressing is applied.

Anesthetic

GETA with an OETT is commonly employed, as postoperative pain is usually well controlled with IV/PO medications. Induction can be done on the OR table if the patient is able to tolerate the move.

Neuraxial anesthesia, including a spinal or epidural block, can be done; epidural placement can help with phantom pain postoperatively.

Positioning

The patient is placed in a supine position, with arms extended on padded armboards.

Anesthetic Implications

Maintain anesthesia until a cast can be placed and is set.

Patients are usually elderly diabetics with failed bypass grafts or patients with post-traumatic complications. These patients have atherosclerotic changes to all vessels, especially the coronary arteries and the carotid arteries. They are at very high risk for perioperative myocardial ischemia.

If a compression tourniquet is used, it is usually set at 50–100 mm Hg above the patient's systolic blood pressure; the maximum setting is less than 400 mm Hg in the lower extremity. Chart both the tourniquet time and setting. The tourniquet should be released after 2 hours to prevent injury.

Below-the-Knee Amputation

Severance of the lower leg below the knee may be necessary in cases involving gangrene, vascular insufficiency, trauma, and malignancy.

Operative Procedure

The soft tissue is cut; large vessels, nerves, and muscles are ligated; and small vessels are cauterized. A saw is used to cut the tibia and fibula. The muscles are folded up; a longer posterior flap is brought forward to cover the stump. The skin is sutured closed. Gauze is wrapped around the stump, and a stocking is placed over it. A compression stocking or a cast is then applied.

A guillotine amputation can also be done. With this approach, a stump is not created and the wound is not closed until a later date. The tibia and fibula are transected with a saw, the leg is left open, and a compression dressing is applied.

Anesthetic

GETA with an OETT is commonly employed, as postoperative pain is usually well controlled with IV/PO medications. Induction can be done on the OR table if the patient is able to tolerate the move.

Neuraxial anesthesia, including a spinal or epidural block, can be done; epidural placement can help with phantom pain postoperatively.

Positioning

The patient is placed in a supine position.

Anesthetic Implications

Tourniquets may not always be used, but should be placed in case of bleeding.

If a compression tourniquet is used, it is usually set at 50–100 mm Hg above the patient's systolic blood pressure; the maximum setting is less than 400 mm Hg in the lower extremity. Chart both the tourniquet time and setting. The tourniquet should be released after 2 hours to prevent injury.

Toe or Foot Amputation

A toe or foot amputation may be necessary in cases involving vascular disease, diabetes complications, and trauma.

Operative Procedure
Foot

Amputation of the foot can be more complicated and last longer than an above- or below-the-knee amputation, as the foot anatomy is more complex. Amputation of the foot is usually done through the ankle. The heel pad, with its blood supply left intact, is sutured directly to the distal tibial edge to cover the bone and prevent migration. A posterior flap of skin is fashioned so that it is longer and can be brought over the stump and sutured to the anterior skin of the leg.

Toe

Amputation of the toe can be much faster than a foot amputation. If done at the midmetatarsal level, the patient will be able to walk without a prosthesis. A dorsal incision is made over the toe(s) at the transmetatarsal level. A skin flap is created and brought over the ends of the bones and sutured to the dorsal flap.

A bulky compression dressing is applied at the end of the case.

Anesthetic

An ankle block with sedation is recommended for a toe amputation, if possible, on this patient population (often neuropathy contributes to the primary process, which itself reduces the need for a dense block). If a dense block is required, a neuraxial technique (spinal or epidural) or a popliteal fossa block would be effective. With the ankle and foot, the medial portion is innervated by the saphenous nerve, which would also need to be anesthetized.

If the upper part of the foot, closer to the ankle, is also amputated, sciatic and saphenous nerve blocks would be required for complete analgesia of the ankle.

Positioning

The patient is placed in a supine position.

Anesthetic Implications

These patients usually have COPD, so avoid intubating them if possible.

Although blood loss is usually minimal with these surgeries, a thigh tourniquet may be placed so that it is already in place in the event of increased blood loss. If a thigh compression tourniquet is inflated, it is usually set at 50–100 mm Hg above the patient's systolic blood pressure; the maximum setting is less than 400 mm Hg in the lower extremity. Chart both the tourniquet time and setting. The tourniquet should be released after 2 hours to prevent injury.

ORTHOPEDIC SURGERY: TOTAL JOINT REPLACEMENT

See the discussion of methylmethacrylate bone cement in Chapter 3.

Many patients who require a joint replacement have been on chronic pain medications and/or steroids. As a consequence, they may have a higher opioid requirement and may require a stress dose of a steroid during surgery.

Total Ankle Arthroplasty

In total ankle arthroplasty, a dysfunctional ankle joint surface is surgically replaced with a prosthesis. The distal tibial and talus articular surfaces are replaced with high-density prosthesis components and fixed with methylmethacrylate.

This surgery is indicated for degenerative and rheumatoid arthritis. Rarely done, it is performed on older patients or those who are sedentary.

Operative Procedure

An anterolateral incision is made. Osteotomy incisions for the tibia and talus are made with an oscillating saw. A section of tibia is cut, with trial insertion of the prosthesis being attempted. Holes are made in the talus to provide fixation points for the bone cement. The tibial prosthesis and the talar prosthesis are then seated permanently with methylmethacrylate (see the discussion of methylmethacrylate in Chapter 3). A splint is applied over a bulky dressing.

Anesthetic

The neuraxial anesthesia consists of a spinal or epidural with IV sedation; sciatic and saphenous nerve blocks would be required for complete analgesia of the ankle.

Alternatively, general anesthesia is used with an OETT.

A combination of general and regional anesthesia may also be employed.

Patients with rheumatoid arthritis can have cervical nerve root compression and/or atlanto-occipital instability. Assess the patient's ability to extend the neck and ask about any numbness or tingling with neck movement. Check a neck X-ray for subluxation of the cervical spine. These patients may require awake fiberoptic intubation.

Positioning

The patient is placed in a supine position.

Anesthetic Implications

Laminar air flow in the room should be used.

Maintain anesthesia until the splint is applied.

If a compression tourniquet is used, it is usually set at 50–100 mm Hg above the patient's systolic blood pressure; the maximum setting is less than 400 mm Hg in the lower extremity. Chart both the tourniquet time and setting. The tourniquet should be released after 2 hours to prevent injury.

Total Elbow Arthroplasty

In total elbow arthroplasty, a dysfunctional elbow joint surface is surgically replaced with a prosthesis. This procedure restores movement and relieves pain from rheumatoid arthritis, osteoarthritis, or degenerative disease of the synovium or cartilage of the elbow. It is indicated only for elderly patients, with low-demand activity.

Operative Procedure

Methylmethacrylate may or may not be used, depending on the quality of the diseased bone and implant design. A sling should be placed before fully waking the patient.

Anesthetic

Supraclavicular or infraclavicular approaches would be the peripheral blocks of choice. The intercostobrachial nerve needs to be anesthetized as well (because surgical stimulation is often present on the proximal posterior surface of the upper arm for this procedure). Interscalene or axillary blocks could be considered; however, the density of these blocks in the elbow can often be less than the two more proximal blocks.

General anesthesia with an OETT or a combination of general anesthesia and a peripheral block may also be used.

Patients with rheumatoid arthritis can have cervical nerve root compression and/or atlanto-occipital instability. Assess the patient's ability to extend the neck and ask about any numbness or tingling with neck movement. Check a neck X-ray for subluxation of the cervical spine. These patients may require an awake fiberoptic intubation.

Positioning

The patient is placed in either a prone, lateral decubitus, or supine position.

Anesthetic Implications

Place IVs and the blood pressure cuff on the non-operative arm.

If a compression tourniquet is used, it is usually set at 50–100 mm Hg above the patient's systolic blood pressure; the maximum setting is less than 300 mm Hg in the upper extremity. Chart both the tourniquet time and setting. The tourniquet should be released after 2 hours to prevent injury.

Hemi-arthroplasty of the elbow is also known as radial head replacement.

Total Hip Arthroplasty or Total Hip Replacement

Total hip arthroplasty (THA) or total hip replacement (THR) entails placement of a prosthesis to replace the femoral head and neck and reconstruction of the acetabulum with an acetabular cup. This surgery restores movement and relieves pain. Indications for these procedures include rheumatoid arthritis, osteoarthritis, degenerative disease of the synovium or cartilage, avascular necrosis, damage caused by infection, severe femoral head fractures, hip arthrosis, benign and malignant tumors of the hip joint, congenital deformity/dislocation of the hip, and failed reconstruction.

Two types of fixation can be done:

- Young, active patients are ideal candidates for noncemented THR. Fixation with a noncemented prosthesis depends on a tight fit of implants within strong bone. Roughened surfaces and biologically active coatings promote in-growth of bone into the prosthesis as the fixation method.

- Elderly patients with poor-quality bone usually receive cemented components. Polymethylmethacrylate (PMMA) is used for the cement.

The position and incision are the same for both cemented and noncemented hip replacements.

Operative Procedure

A long incision is made across the iliac crest to the thigh; the fascia is incised and the muscle fibers separated. The femoral head is dislocated from the acetabulum by adduction and internal rotation. The femoral neck is osteotomized, and the femoral head and a portion of the femur neck are excised and extracted. The proximal femur is trimmed and the medullary canal reamed to accept the prosthesis. The acetabulum is then exposed, and the capsule is detached from the anterior and inferior margins. Acetabular reamers are employed to prepare the acetabulum to accept the cup prosthesis, and then anchoring holes are drilled.

For the cemented procedure, polymethylmethacrylate is used to seat the femoral prosthesis, with the excess being trimmed. (See the discussion of methylmethacrylate in Chapter 3.) When the cement is set, the hip is relocated.

For the noncemented version, the acetabular cup and the femoral component can be cementless. The acetabular cup is fixed to the acetabulum with screws or by "interference fit" (also known as "press fit"—a fastening between two parts that is achieved by friction after the parts are pushed together).

The soft tissues and tendons are reattached, and the wound is closed. A closed drainage system may be employed.

An abduction pillow is secured between the patient's thighs to prevent dislocation of the femur in the acetabulum.

Anesthetic

The neuraxial block consists of a spinal or epidural with IV sedation. IV ketamine and propofol can be used to help sedate the patient for the block as well as for positioning on the OR table. The rate of deep venous thrombosis is less with a THR when epidural anesthesia is used. Neuraxial blocks can also help reduce the incidence of deep vein thrombosis and blood volume losses (via sympathectomy).

Alternatively, general anesthesia is used with an OETT. Induction can be done on the OR table if the patient is able to tolerate the move; however, induction may need to be done on the stretcher or patient's bed so that the move to the table is tolerated.

A combination of general anesthesia and an epidural may be used for postoperative pain control.

Patients with rheumatoid arthritis can have cervical nerve root compression and/or atlanto-occipital instability. Assess the patient's ability to extend the neck and ask about any numbness or tingling with neck movement. Check a neck X-ray for subluxation of the cervical spine.

These patients may require awake fiberoptic intubation.

Positioning

The patient is placed in a lateral decubitus position for the lateral/posterior approach, and in a supine position for the anterior approach.

Anesthetic Implications

Type and cross-match the patient's blood preoperatively. Blood may need to be available in the operating room.

Two large-bore peripheral IVs are preferred.

During reaming of both the femur and the acetabulum, venous sinuses are opened. Large blood losses can occur, and venous air embolism and fat embolism are risks.

Vasoactive drugs—both vasopressors and dilators—should be available. A hypotensive technique can be useful in keeping MAP around 60 mm Hg to help prevent blood losses. Vasoconstrictor drugs may be needed to keep the patient at the same MAP level. These patients are often on daily antihypertensive therapy; when sedated, their pressures may dip lower than acceptable levels.

Complications

Potential complications of THR include fat embolism, air embolism, thromboembolism, pulmonary embolism, bone marrow embolism, hip dislocation, and/or infection.

Deep vein thrombosis is a very common complication after hip arthroplasty. Intraoperative and postoperative prophylaxis for this condition should be initiated and carried out.

Minimally Invasive Total Hip Arthroplasty

Minimally invasive total hip arthroplasty (MITHA) is associated with less damage to the muscles and tendons around the hip joint than traditional THA. It also results in less surgical trauma, less intraoperative blood loss, less pain, minimal scarring, and decreased hospital lengths of stay and rehabilitation times.

Operative Procedure

The *single-incision MITHA* requires the patient to be in the lateral decubitus or supine position. It involves an anterior or posterior approach, employing a shorter incision and tighter surgical field, and remains centered on the greater trochanter. The limited surgical area requires the use of specialized instruments.

For the *double-incision MITHA*, the patient is placed supine. One 2-inch anterolateral incision creates access for osteotomy of the femoral head and placement of the acetabular prosthesis. A second posterior incision accommodates introduction of the prosthetic femoral head.

Anesthetic

The neuraxial block consists of a spinal or epidural with IV sedation.

Total Knee Arthroplasty or Total Knee Replacement

Total knee arthroplasty (TKA) or total knee replacement (TKR) entails replacement of the knee joint by prosthesis; that is, a dysfunctional knee joint surface is surgically replaced with a prosthesis to restore movement and relieve pain. A TKR resurfaces the distal femur with a metal prosthesis that articulates with a polyethylene surface that is attached to the tibia.

These surgeries are done for pain, deformity, and instability of the knee secondary to rheumatoid arthritis, osteoarthritis, and post-traumatic conditions.

Operative Procedure

Few surgeons are doing noncemented knees today. Instead, all patients—young and old—get cemented knee replacements. Polymethylmethacrylate (PMMA; see Chapter 3) is used for the cement.

The distal femur, patella, and tibia are exposed through an anterior or anteromedial incision. The articular surfaces of the femoral condyles, tibial plateau, anterior trochlear surface of the femur, and articular surface of the patella are trimmed to accept the prosthesis. The prosthesis is bonded to the femoral and tibial bones with methylmethacrylate. Next, the surgeon seats the prosthesis using a mallet. The high-density polyethylene patellar component is cemented and seated with a vise-like clamp. The medial and lateral menisci are replaced with a wedge of high-density polyethylene.

Occasionally, only a single component of the knee articular surface needs to be replaced. More commonly, the entire surface requires replacement.

A closed drainage system is inserted. An ice wrap is curved around the knee and filled with ice water. A dressing is applied and covered with an Ace wrap. A knee binder (which prevents inadvertent knee bending) is then wrapped around the leg and Velcro-strapped shut.

Anesthetic

The neuraxial block consists of a spinal or epidural with IV sedation.

A femoral nerve block with or without a sciatic nerve block can be employed for postoperative pain control. Many orthopedic surgeons prefer the sciatic nerve block not to be performed, as a foot drop is present for the duration of the block. The current trend is to ambulate the patient early after surgery, which is obviously made more difficult when a foot drop is present.

General anesthesia is used with an OETT; muscle relaxants are needed.

A combination of general anesthesia and an epidural may also be used.

Patients with rheumatoid arthritis can have cervical nerve root compression and/or atlanto-occipital instability. Assess the patient's ability to extend the neck and ask about any numbness or tingling with neck movement. Check a neck X-ray for subluxation of the cervical spine. These patients may require awake fiberoptic intubation.

Positioning

The patient is placed in a supine position, with arms extended on padded armboards.

Anesthetic Implications

Laminar air flow in the room should be used.

Type and cross-match the patient's blood preoperatively. A large blood loss is possible even with compression tourniquet use.

Establish two large-bore peripheral IVs.

If a compression tourniquet is used, it is usually set at 50–100 mm Hg above the patient's systolic blood pressure; the maximum setting is less than 400 mm Hg in the lower extremity. Chart both the tourniquet time and setting. The tourniquet should be released after 2 hours to prevent injury.

Keep the patient asleep (with general anesthesia) or sedated (with neuraxial anesthesia) until the knee immobilizer is on.

A procedure called a "uni" knee involves replacement of a single compartment.

Complications

Deep vein thrombosis is a very common complication after knee arthroplasty.

Total Shoulder Arthroplasty

In total shoulder arthroplasty, a dysfunctional shoulder joint surface is surgically replaced with a prosthesis. This surgery is performed to restore movement and relieve pain from end-stage rheumatoid arthritis or osteoarthritis (glenohumeral arthritis), degenerative disease of the synovium or cartilage of the shoulder joint, avascular necrosis of humeral head, or non-union of the proximal humerus following trauma.

Operative Procedure

A deltopectoral incision is made, the shoulder capsule incised, and the muscles of the shoulder are reflected medially. Attachment of major tendons is preserved with adequate bone fragments, while loose fragments are excised. Shoulder arthroplasty

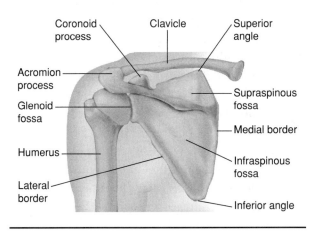

Figure 21-13 *Total Shoulder Arthroplasty*
Source: AAOS, 2004.

involves excision of the head of the humerus. The prosthesis is driven into the humeral shaft and the fragments are wired to the prosthesis. Methylmethacrylate (see Chapter 3) may be used to secure the prosthesis. The rotator cuff and soft tissue are closed over the wire sutures. The long head of the biceps tendon may be sutured to the repaired rotator cuff or implanted into the bicipital groove. The deltoid muscle is reattached. A drain is placed and the incision is closed.

Shoulder *hemiarthroplasty* involves reconstruction of the humeral head only and not the glenoid (seen with proximal humeral fractures or avascular necrosis of humeral head). *Total arthroplasty* entails humeral head replacement with a stemmed prosthesis and resurfacing of glenoid, sometimes with methylmethacrylate.

Anesthetic

An interscalene approach is the block of choice for this procedure. This issue can be addressed with the surgeon; otherwise, general anesthesia can be included in the plan. A continuous scalene catheter may be placed for an infusion of local anesthetic.

General anesthesia with an OETT may be used either alone or with a peripheral block for postoperative pain control. Muscle relaxants may be required by the surgeon, and endotracheal intubation is required.

Patients with rheumatoid arthritis can have cervical nerve root compression and/or atlanto-occipital instability. Assess the patient's ability to extend the neck and ask about any numbness or tingling with neck movement. Check a neck X-ray for subluxation of the cervical spine.

These patients may require awake fiberoptic intubation.

Positioning

The patient is placed in a beach-chair position, with the head of the bed raised 30–40 degrees; alternatively, a lateral decubitus position may be used.

The head of the bed will be positioned 90 degrees away from the anesthetist. If the beach-chair position is used, see Chapter 3 for more information on venous air embolism.

Anesthetic Implications

Laminar air flow in the room should be used.

Keep the patient asleep until a sling is placed.

Place IVs and the blood pressure cuff on the nonoperative arm.

Type and cross-match the patient's blood preoperatively. Blood loss can be significant with this procedure.

If an arterial line is placed, make sure to level the transducer at the external ear meatus.

If the beach-chair position is used, careful attention to stabilization of the patient's head is necessary. It may be difficult to see the patient's face after the drapes are up and the lights are turned down. Tape the ETT securely, as access to patient's head will be limited after surgery begins.

These patients require special eye care. Paper tape is used to close the eyes to prevent corneal drying or abrasions; eye pads are then placed over both eyes. Consider using protective goggles.

ORTHOPEDIC ARTHROSCOPY

Arthroscopy of the Ankle

In this minimally invasive surgery, a small camera and instruments are placed through small incisions to examine or treat an injured or diseased ankle joint. This procedure may be performed for either for diagnostic or therapeutic indications; patients may have osteoarthritis or rheumatoid arthritis.

Operative Procedure

Three anterior ports and three posterior ports may be inserted, although the usual number are two anterior ports and one posterior port. A clear solution is infused to maintain distention and to clear the area of blood for visualization purposes. The soft tissue can be debrided, a osteochondral lesion shaved, synovectomy performed, or pins inserted. A local anesthetic with epinephrine solution can be injected at the port entry sites or into the joint distention fluid to help decrease bleeding and minimize postoperative discomfort.

A compression wrap may be wrapped around the ankle.

Anesthetic

The most common anesthetic plan for this procedure is general anesthesia with an OETT; muscle relaxation may be required.

Neuraxial anesthesia (spinal or epidural) or popliteal fossa sciatic nerve block anesthetizes all but the medial portion of the ankle.

Assess for rheumatoid arthritis and possible cervical subluxation. Such patients may require fiberoptic intubation.

Positioning

The patient is placed in a supine position, with arms extended on padded armboards; the foot of the bed is lowered. The operative ankle is positioned per surgeon preference. The unaffected extremity may be flexed at the knee. Support stockings and/or wraps are used for intermittent insufflation in an effort to prevent thrombus.

Anesthetic Implications

If a compression tourniquet is used, it is usually set at 50–100 mm Hg above the patient's systolic blood pressure; the maximum setting is less than 400 mm Hg in the lower extremity. Chart both the tourniquet time and setting. The tourniquet should be released after 2 hours to prevent injury.

Remanipulation of the ankle/foot may be necessary 2 weeks postoperatively.

Local anesthetic with or without epinephrine may be instilled into the joint being examined. Local anesthesia may also be injected at the arthroscopy port incision sites.

Arthroscopy of the Elbow

In this minimally invasive surgery, a small camera and instruments are placed through small incisions to examine or treat an injured or diseased elbow joint. This procedure may be performed for either diagnostic or therapeutic indications; patients may have osteoarthritis or rheumatoid arthritis. The surgery may also include removal of loose bodies from a previous fracture or injury that are causing pain or stiffness, contractures, treatment of arthritis or lysis of adhesions, and synovectomy.

Operative procedure

Placement of the scope portals depends on the result of the findings on MRI, X-ray, or other diagnostic tests. A clear solution is infused to maintain distention and to clear the area of blood for visualization purposes. The soft tissue can be debrided, an osteochondral lesion shaved, synovectomy performed, or pins inserted. A local anesthetic with epinephrine solution can be injected at the port entry sites or into the joint distention fluid to help decrease bleeding and minimize postoperative discomfort.

A compression wrap may be wrapped around the elbow.

Anesthetic

An interscalene, supraclavicular, infraclavicular, or axillary block may be placed. An interscalene block can occasionally be set up higher in the brachial plexus, which results in sparing of the radial nerve (and consequently poor posterior anesthesia). Supraclavicular and infraclavicular blocks have the best chance of achieving surgical anesthesia for the elbow.

Alternatively, general anesthesia is used with either a LMA or OETT.

Assess for rheumatoid arthritis and possible cervical subluxation. Such patients may require fiberoptic intubation.

Positioning

The patient is placed in a supine position, with the affected arm across the body, usually suspended. Alternatively, the patient may be placed in a prone position with the affected upper arm supported, but the elbow flexed at a 90-degree angle. A lateral decubitus position is also possible.

Anesthetic Implications

Although elbow arthroscopy is not a new procedure, it is used less frequently than other arthroscopic procedures.

Place IVs and the blood pressure cuff on the nonoperative arm.

Because of the tight area where the nerves pass through the elbow, there is potential for nerve damage. This area should be assessed preoperatively and postoperatively.

If a compression tourniquet is used, it is usually set at 50–100 mm Hg above the patient's systolic blood pressure; the maximum setting is less than 300 mm Hg in the upper extremity. Chart both the tourniquet time and setting. The tourniquet should be released after 2 hours to prevent injury.

Local anesthetic with or without epinephrine may be instilled into the joint being examined. Local anesthesia may also be injected at the arthroscopy port incision sites.

Arthroscopy of the Hip

In this minimally invasive surgery, a small camera and instruments are placed through small incisions to examine or repair tissues of the hip joint. This procedure may be performed for either diagnostic or therapeutic indications; patients may have osteoarthritis or rheumatoid arthritis.

Operative Procedure

A clear solution is infused to maintain distention and to clear the area of blood for visualization purposes. The soft tissue can be debrided, an osteochondral lesion shaved, synovectomy performed, or pins inserted. A local anesthetic with epinephrine solution can be injected at the port entry sites or into the joint distention fluid to help decrease bleeding and minimize postoperative discomfort.

Anesthetic

The neuraxial block consists of a spinal or epidural with IV sedation. IV ketamine and propofol can be used to help sedate the patient for the block as well as for positioning on the OR table.

Alternatively, general anesthesia is used with an OETT.

Assess for rheumatoid arthritis and possible cervical subluxation. Such patients may require fiberoptic intubation.

Positioning
The patient is placed in a supine or lateral decubitus position.

Anesthetic Implications
Local anesthetic with or without epinephrine may be instilled into the joint being examined. Local anesthesia may also be injected at the arthroscopy port incision sites.

Arthroscopy of the Knee

In this minimally invasive surgery, a small camera and instruments are placed through small incisions to examine or repair tissues of the knee joint. This procedure may be performed for either diagnostic or therapeutic indications; patients may have osteoarthritis or rheumatoid arthritis. It is indicated for repair or removal of the meniscus, synovectomy, patellar shaving, repair of ligaments, ACL reconstruction, biopsies, and removal of loose bodies.

Operative Procedure
An inflow port is inserted laterally into the suprapatellar pouch adjacent to the superior pole of the patella. The knee joint is then infused with a clear solution to distend the structures and to keep the area clear of blood, allowing the surgeon to visualize the anatomy. An incision is made over the anterolateral aspect of the joint, with a trocar and sheath being inserted. An obturator replaces the trocar in the sheath and is advanced into the joint. Once the obturator is in position, it is withdrawn and an arthroscope with a camera is inserted. Additional ports can be placed as necessary to accommodate other instruments.

As part of this procedure, soft tissue can be debrided, a osteochondral lesion shaved,

synovectomy performed, or pins inserted. A local anesthetic with epinephrine solution can be injected at the port entry sites or into the joint distention fluid to help decrease bleeding and minimize postoperative discomfort.

A compression wrap may be wrapped around the knee. A knee immobilizer is placed.

Anesthetic
Usually, the anesthetic plan involves general anesthesia. Spinal or epidural anesthesia should be considered in patients with certain comorbidities.

General anesthesia can be used with insertion of an OETT.

Assess for rheumatoid arthritis and possible cervical subluxation. Such patients may require fiberoptic intubation.

Positioning
The patient is placed in a supine position, with the knees extending over the lower break in the table; the arms are secured on armboards. Both legs will be flexed at the knees to 90 degrees, with the foot of the bed lowered. The nonoperative leg should have support stockings and/or wraps for intermittent insufflation in an effort to prevent thrombus.

Anesthetic Implications
If a compression tourniquet is used, it is usually set at 50–100 mm Hg above the patient's systolic blood pressure; the maximum setting is less than 400 mm Hg in the lower extremity. Chart both the tourniquet time and setting. The tourniquet should be released after 2 hours to prevent injury.

Local anesthetic with or without epinephrine may be instilled into the joint being examined or injected at the arthroscopy port incision sites.

Arthroscopy of the Shoulder

In this shoulder surgery, a small camera is placed through small incisions to examine or repair tissue around the shoulder joint. This procedure may be performed for either diagnostic or therapeutic indications; patients may have osteoarthritis or rheumatoid arthritis. Indications include removal of loose bodies, lysis of adhesions, synovectomy, bursectomy, biopsy of the synovium, stabilization of dislocation, correction of rotator cuff tears, and decompression of the subacromial area; all of these conditions may result from either arthritis or trauma.

Operative Procedure

Three ports are usually utilized. The posterior port is placed 2 cm inferior and 1 cm medial to the posterolateral corner of the acromium process. The anterior port is placed (under direct visualization) inferior to the biceps tendon. The lateral port is inserted 2 cm distal to the lateral border of the acromium. A clear solution is infused to maintain distention and to clear the area of blood for visualization purposes. The soft tissue can be debrided, an osteochondral lesion shaved, synovectomy performed, or pins inserted.

A compression wrap may be wrapped around the shoulder. Keep the patient asleep until the sling is placed.

Anesthetic

General anesthesia is used with an OETT or LMA if patient positioning allows for this option. A combination of GETA with an interscalene brachial plexus block may be used to reduce postoperative pain.

Assess for rheumatoid arthritis and possible cervical subluxation. Such patients may require fiberoptic intubation.

An intra-articular catheter may be threaded for a local anesthetic infusion for postoperative pain control. A local anesthetic with epinephrine solution can be injected at the port entry sites or into the joint distention fluid to help decrease bleeding and minimize postoperative discomfort.

Positioning

The patient may be placed in a supine position, with the head of the bed elevated. Alternatively, a beach-chair or lateral decubitus position may be used. If the beach-chair position is used,

see Chapter 3 for more information on venous air embolism.

Anesthetic Implications

Place IVs and the blood pressure cuff on the non-operative arm.

If the beach-chair position is used, careful attention to stabilization of the patient's head is necessary. It may be difficult to see the patient's face after the drapes are up and the lights are turned down. Tape the ETT securely, as access to patient's head will be limited after surgery begins.

These patients require special eye care. Paper tape is used to close the eyes to prevent corneal drying or abrasions; eye pads are then placed over both eyes. Consider using protective goggles.

ORTHOPEDIC SURGERY: SPINAL COLUMN

Pedicle Fixation of the Spine

Pedicle screw fixation is used to internally immobilize targeted spinal segments and enhance fusion. This surgery is performed to fuse and stabilize the spine when patients have degenerative spinal disorders such as spondylolisthesis, neoplastic instability, infection, degenerative disc disease, and recurrent disc herniation.

Operative Procedure

A midline incision is made; the spinal column and the disc space are exposed by removing the facet joints (joints of spine) while protecting the nerve roots. The disc space is entered and the disc material is removed. A spacer is placed in the disc space to maintain the disc height. Pedicle screws are attached to rods or plates. A bone graft is usually taken from the iliac crest. A suction drain is placed, and the wound is closed with sutures.

Anesthetic

General anesthesia is given with insertion of an ETT. Induction may take place on the patient's bed or stretcher, with the patient being turned prone after induction.

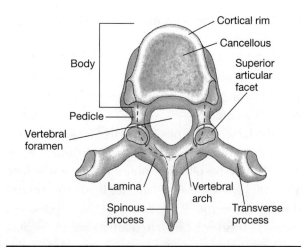

Figure 21-14   *Anatomy of Thoracic Vertebrae*
Source: Clark, 2005.

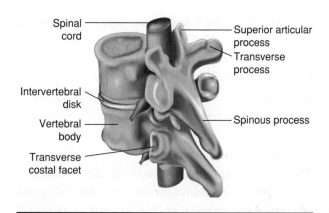

Figure 21-16   *Posterior Spinal Segment*

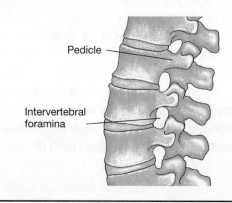

Figure 21-17   *Lateral View of Normal Spine*
Source: Clark, 2005.

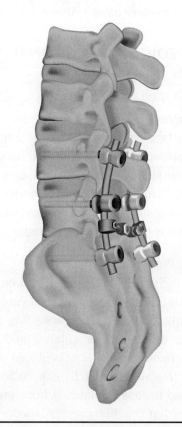

Figure 21-15   *Pedicle Fixation of the Spine*

Positioning

The patient is placed in a prone position, with arms either in the swimmer's position or tucked at the sides. Protect the patient's eyes and face.

Anesthetic Implications

Assess pain and/or weakness preoperatively, and document the findings.

Somatosensory evoked potentials (SSEPs) may be monitored during the procedure.

Have adequate IV access in case crystalloids, colloids, or blood replacement is needed.

A type and cross-match of the patient's blood is needed.

The surgeon may request that a hypotensive technique be employed to control blood loss. Use of a beta blocker (labetalol) or nipride may be necessary.

Be conscious of patient positioning and check it often during the case. Keep the spine neutral during the turn to the prone position. Keep the shoulders less than 90 degrees in the swimmer's position (elbows flexed). Protect the patient's face (eyes, nose, chin) from pressure. Protect the eyes from corneal abrasion by using paper tape to close the eyelids; eye pads may then be placed over the taped eyes.

Surgical Treatment of Scoliosis

Surgical repair of scoliosis consists of the insertion of internal splints—by way of compression and distraction rods, frames, wires, and other fixation devices—to a curved spine. It is done to straighten the spine (which is characterized by both bending and twisting) as much as possible in a safe manner and prevent further curvature.

This surgery may be performed for cosmetic reasons and/or compromised physiologic processes such as musculoskeletal and respiratory functions (restrictive disease). Scoliosis is a three-dimensional deformity; with lateral and rotational deformity of the thoracolumbar spine accompanied by a deformity of the rib cage. The bigger the angle of curvature of the spine, the more serious the systemic manifestations. Scoliosis can be congenital, idiopathic, neuromuscular, or myopathic. Cor pulmonale is the principal cause of mortality in patients with uncorrected scoliosis.

Operative Procedure

A long, vertical midline incision is made over the curved region of the spine, exposing the lamina on both sides. This approach requires cutting through the muscles of the back. Spinal fusion may also be done; an iliac crest bone graft may be taken for fusion.

A new procedure involves a *thoracoscopic* minimally invasive correction. The patient is positioned laterally. Several small incisions are made along the lateral edge of the thorax; intervertebral discs are removed along the curvature of the spine. Pieces of removed rib are ground up and used for bone graft to fuse along the curvature. Screws are inserted into the vertebrae, and a rod is attached to correct the curvature. Recovery time, blood loss, and pain levels are about the same with this procedure as with the posterior fusion. The major advantage is the smaller incisions and the ability to preserve spinal levels.

The *spinal stapling technique* is considered largely experimental but is used in younger children. Small incisions are made along the spinal cord; smaller metal brackets are attached to the vertebrae that can be adjusted every 6 months. The staple binds the growth center on the convex side so that the concavity may catch up in terms of growth and length. This procedure can be done thoracoscopically, which allows for smaller adjustments with less damage potential to the spinal cord; the incision is smaller and less invasive.

The *Harrington rod* procedure is not often used but is described here. The segmental instrumentation involves placing anchor points at the top, bottom, and selected mid-portion of the spine. Rods are used to connect the anchor points. The anchor points are distracted on the concave side to correct the curve. The rods are then derotated to correct the rotation abnormality of the spine.

An anterior approach by *anterolateral thoracotomy* is used for a thoracolumbar deformity.

Anesthetic

General anesthesia is used with an OETT. Muscle relaxants are given if neurologic monitoring is not to be done; check with the surgeon before giving these agents. Avoid succinylcholine (Anectine) if the patient has muscle disease. Avoid heavy premedication or sedation.

ANGLE CURVATURE (DEGREES)	CLINICAL SIGNIFICANCE
< 10	Normal
> 40	Surgical intervention
> 65	Restrictive lung disease (see the discussion of pulmonary function tests later in this chapter)
> 120	Alveolar hypoventilation (ventilation/perfusion mismatch); pulmonary hypertension is also common

Keep the patient's blood pressure from becoming too high to prevent increased bleeding, but maintain MAP at more than 60 mm Hg to avoid compromising spinal cord blood flow.

Positioning

The patient is placed in a prone position, with arms in the swimmer's position. Extra care should be taken owing to the padding of the chest wall deformity and abnormal extension of limbs. Protect the patient's eyes.

Anesthetic Implications

The need for a thorax/body cast postoperatively varies with the surgery performed.

These patients require special eye care. Paper tape is used to close the eyes to prevent corneal drying or abrasions; eye pads are then placed over both eyes to protect them. Eye ointment can be instilled before taping for patients who will remain intubated postoperatively. Be aware that patients who have ointment in their eyes will sometimes rub their eyes (to clear their vision postoperatively) and accidentally scratch their eyes or face.

The surgeon may prefer use of a hypotensive technique to keep blood loss at a minimum. In such cases, you can use a labetalol IV bolus or a nitroglycerin or sodium nitroprusside (SNP) drip to maintain a MAP at approximately 60 mm Hg.

Take aggressive temperature conservation steps. Warming blankets, fluid warmers, and warm room temperature should all be used.

Type and cross-match the patient's blood preoperatively. Two to four units of blood may need to be in the operating room, as there is increased blood loss with vertebral surgery. Cell-saver collection is usually done.

Assess the patient's neurologic status, and document any deficits and symptoms preoperatively. Because the curve of the spine can reach 65 degrees, the stretching of the spinal cord can result in an alteration in the arterial supply, nerves, and muscles owing to spinal cord compression.

This can cause neurologic deficits which must be ascertained preoperatively. In addition, surgical straightening or correcting of spinal abnormalities can cause ischemia to the spinal cord from blood supply compression.

Careful preoperative assessment of the cardiovascular and pulmonary systems is also important, as these systems can be affected by the rib cage deformity with lung compression and decreased chest wall compliance. Cardiovascular disease may include congestive heart failure, right ventricular hypertrophy, and cor pulmonale.

Pulmonary disease states associated with scoliosis include restrictive lung disease, increased pulmonary vascular resistance and pulmonary hypertension, and airway abnormalities.

Pulmonary Function Tests

Patients with restrictive disease have the following PFT findings:

- Decreased FRC
- Decreased VC
- Decreased TLC
- Normal FEV_1/FVC

These patients may also have a decreased PaO_2 and an increase in physiologic dead space. They are usually hypoxemic (with secondary polycythemia) and hypercapnic.

Monitors and IV Access

- An arterial line may be needed.
- A central venous pressure line *may or may not be needed.*
- Multiple large-bore peripheral IVs should be established.

SSEPs may be monitored during the procedure to assess the posterior spinal cord. Limited use of volatile anesthetics and muscle relaxants may be necessary. Motor evoked potentials (MEPs) may be monitored to assess the anterior cord. A "wake-up" test may also be required. See the discussion of neurophysiologic monitoring in Chapter 3 for more information.

IV Vasoactive Agents
- IV pump: nitroglycerin, sodium nitroprusside (SNP)
- Syringe for bolus: phenylephrine (Neosynephrine)

IV Fluids and Volume Requirements
Have blood tubing with normal saline and multiple IV access sites available for giving blood products.

Anticipate a large blood loss, and plan on aggressive fluid and blood replacement. These patients have large third-space fluid shifts.

VASCULAR SURGERY PEARLS

Heparin and Protamine

Have heparin and protamine available for all vascular surgeries. An activated clotting time (ACT) machine should be available anytime these drugs are given, to monitor their effects. See the discussion of coagulation and anticoagulation in Chapter 4 for more information.

Protamine use may result in an unwanted allergic-type reaction. The incidence is small with responses as follows:

- *Anaphylaxis:* mediated by immunoglobulin E (IgE) antibodies, which bind to the surface of mast cells and basophils. Prior sensitization to protamine is needed to provoke this reaction. With re-exposure, these cells release histamine, prostaglandins, and chemotactic factors, resulting in vascular collapse.

Anaphylactic reactions are more common in patients who are sensitized to protamine, including members of the following groups:

  - Patients with a fish allergy: 24.5-fold risk increase for allergic reaction
  - Diabetics maintained on NPH (neutral protamine Hagedorn) insulin: 8.2 fold risk increase for allergic reaction
  - Allergy to any drug: 3-fold risk increase for allergic reaction
  - Patients with previous exposure to protamine: for example, through previous cardiac catheterization or hemodialysis

- *Anaphylactoid reaction:* non-immunologic; does not require prior exposure to protamine. The complement system is activated with generation of anaphylatoxins and thromboxane. Patient reactions may range from mild hypotension to acute cardiovascular collapse, decreased SVR, marked pulmonary hypertension, and increased CVP.

Peripheral Vascular Disease

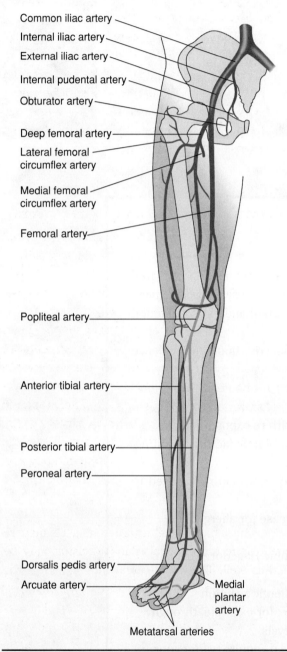

Figure 22-1 *Vascular Anatomy Lower Extremity*
Source: Clark, 2005.

Acute Blockage of Distal Vessels

Acute blockage can be caused by embolism, aneurysm, thrombosis, trauma, or intra-arterial injection of noxious substances. Irreversible damage can occur with acute occlusion within 4–6 hours.

The "five P's" of acute peripheral vascular disease (PVD) symptoms are pain, paralysis, paresthesia, pulselessness, and pallor.

- Calf pain (claudication) is caused by superficial femoral artery occlusion.
- Thigh and calf pain is caused by ileo-femoral occlusion.
- Hip and buttock pain is caused by aorto-iliac occlusion.

These patients will most likely already have had angiography, anticoagulants, and thrombolytics before coming for an embolectomy or bypass.

Atherosclerotic Arterial Insufficiency

Atherosclerotic arterial insufficiency, a chronic blockage of distal vessels, ranges from intermittent claudication (insufficient flow to meet exercise demands) to limb-threatening ischemia (blood flow is insufficient to meet the resting metabolic demands of an extremity). It is most commonly caused by *atherosclerosis,* a disease of the intima (innermost wall) of an artery. This condition can progress to tissue gangrene when spontaneous necrosis occurs due to inadequate perfusion.

Non-atherosclerotic causes of arterial insufficiency include the following conditions:

- *Immune arteritis:* multiple diseases that cause a transmural inflammatory response. Immune complexes are released into the arterial endothelium, the complement cascade is activated, white blood cells release lysosomal enzymes, and the arterial wall becomes damaged and thromboses the artery. This leads to eventual necrosis beyond the vascular bed.
- *Buerger's disease (thromboangiitis obliterans):* chronic arterial insufficiency to the hands and feet; directly linked with tobacco use, particularly affecting Jewish or Asian males aged 20–40 years. This painful disease can lead to gangrene of the fingers and toes. It does not seem to affect other organs of the body.

- *Giant cell arteritis (temporal arteritis):* specifically affects the vessels supplying the head, eyes, and optic nerves. This disease occurs most frequently in persons older than the age of 70. Although persons of Scandinavian descent are more commonly affected, giant cell arteritis may be found in all racial groups.
- *Takayasu's arteritis:* a rare, chronic inflammatory condition of the aorta and its major branches. Vascular changes cause dilatation of the aorta and narrowing of other vessels, which in turn leads to stenosis, thrombosis, and aneurysms. Takayasu's arteritis is sometimes called "pulseless disease" because of an inability to feel pulses in the upper extremities. It most commonly affects Asian women younger than the age of 40.
- *Popliteal entrapment syndrome:* an uncommon, congenital abnormality typically affecting young athletic males, who present with symptoms of calf claudication. It is caused by abnormal positioning of the popliteal artery in relation to its surrounding muscles, resulting in extrinsic arterial compression and vascular damage.
- *Homocysteinemia:* an inborn error of metabolism resulting in a variant of premature atherosclerosis. Excess homocysteine alters the arterial wall and prostaglandin metabolism, which interferes with platelet function. Patients may present with serious vascular events (stroke or heart attack) despite the absence of common risk factors such as hypertension, smoking, or diabetes.

Surgical Interventions for Arterial Occlusive Disease

Surgical interventions for arterial occlusive disease include early restoration of blood flow and the management of reperfusion consequences. These methods include thrombolysis, endovascular procedures, surgical thromboembolectomy, and arterial bypass procedures. For bypass grafts, the patency of a saphenous vein graft exceeds that of all synthetic grafts, such as those made of Dacron or Teflon (polytetrafluoroethylene [PTFE]). The vein can be excised from its bed and reversed so that the native proximal vein is anastomosed to the distal arterial site and the native distal vein is anastomosed to the proximal arterial site. The vein can also be left in situ (in its native bed) and the valves lysed. Cryopreserved human saphenous vein has also been used successfully. Heparin is given during vessel bypass surgery.

VASCULAR SURGERY

Abdominal Aortic Aneurysm Resection: Open

With the open approach, repair of an abdominal aortic aneurysm (AAA) takes place through an abdominal or flank incision (retroperitoneal). AAA is caused by medial layer degeneration and circumferential bulging of the abdominal aorta.

The abdominal aorta begins in the diaphragm at T12 and ends at L4 (at the aortic bifurcation). Vessel defects most commonly occur below the renal arteries and may extend to involve the bifurcation and common iliac arteries. Surgical repair is done when the diameter of the AAA exceeds 5 cm. The hallmark presentation for ruptured AAA is severe back/abdominal pain, accompanied by systolic blood pressure of less than 90 mm Hg.

Operative Procedure

An incision is made midline abdominal; a transperitoneal or retroperitoneal (flank) incision may be used as well. The intestines are mobilized to the side and packed out of the field. The posterior parietal peritoneum is incised and the aorta is exposed. Cross-clamping and resection are usually an infrarenal procedure; the proximal and distal control of the aneurysm is done with vascular clamps. The aneurysm is opened, and atheromatous and thrombotic material is removed.

Occasionally, the aneurysm may not contain any atheromatous material, but is instead just filled with blood. Bleeding from the lumbar arteries, which feed into the posterior wall of the aneurysm, is controlled with sutures.

Reconstruction requires placement of a prosthetic graft, the aneurysm is usually not removed. The aorta can be anastomosed or the graft sewn to the intact posterior wall of the aorta. The inferior mesenteric artery (distally) and/or the renal artery(ies) (proximally) may need reimplantation. After the proximal graft is in place, the suture line is tested for leakage. The aortic clamp may be repositioned onto the graft, particularly if the initial cross-clamping occurred above the renal arteries—this restores blood flow to the kidneys as soon as possible. The distal graft is then sutured in place. The graft used may be straight (tubular) or bifurcated, depending on iliac involvement.

When the surgeon is satisfied with hemostasis, cross-clamps are released. At this time, the surgeon may elect to manually control the rate at which blood flow is restored to the extremities to avoid a sudden drop in blood pressure. The walls of the aneurysm may be closed over the graft to protect it from contact with the intestines and avoid development of a fistula.

Spinal cord perfusion in the thoracolumbar area is derived from the artery of Adamkiewicz, which joins the anterior spinal artery in sending flow to the lower thoracic and lumbar segments, as well as the celiac artery, the superior mesenteric artery, and the inferior mesenteric arteries. This anatomy can be important, especially in thoracoabdominal aneurysm repair, where the cross-clamp is applied above these structures. Risk of paraplegia, mesenteric/bowel ischemia/infarction, renal ischemia/failure, and hepatic ischemia with coagulopathy is increased if thoracolumbar blood flow is decreased when systemic pressures are low. See the discussion of aortic cross-clamping in Chapter 3 for more information.

Anesthetic

A spinal or epidural can be done; most commonly, general anesthesia (GETA) is used with insertion of an oral endotracheal tube (OETT). Use drugs that do not require renal clearance.

Positioning

The patient is placed in either a supine (midline abdominal incision), with arms extended on armboards; or lateral decubitus (retroperitoneal exposure) position.

Anesthetic Implications

The preoperative administration of cyclooxygenase inhibitors (aspirin or ibuprofen) may help to maintain a stable cardiac output after cross-clamping.

Coexisting diseases with AAA often include hypertension, angina, myocardial ischemia, history of myocardial infarction, congestive heart failure, diabetes, COPD, and chronic renal insufficiency. Death with elective AAA usually occurs from myocardial infarction.

Acute renal failure can follow suprarenal or infrarenal aortic cross-clamping. Hydration with 0.9% normal saline and prompt blood product replacement may help to maintain intravascular volume and renal function.

Type and cross-match the patient's blood preoperatively; have two units available. The surgeon may also require the use of cell-saver technology.

Monitor renal function; document urinary output every 30 minutes.

Anesthetic Goals for AAA Resection

The anesthetic should minimize any organ dysfunction, but especially problems within the myocardial, renal, and pulmonary systems.

The overall choice for the anesthetic is geared toward ensuring a smooth induction and cardiovascular stability. Keep the patient's blood pressure within 20% of the baseline. Medications used for this purpose may include atenolol 50–100 mg PO preoperatively, atenolol 5 mg IV, or esmolol (Brevibloc) infusion; high-dose narcotics (fentanyl, sufentanil); clonidine 400–600 PO preoperatively; and/or epidural local anesthetics with narcotics. Hypotension may follow induction, in which case you should elevate the patient's legs (or place the patient in Trendelenburg position) and administer blood and fluids. The patient may need to receive phenylephrine or dopamine until the aorta can be cross-clamped.

Bradycardia is considered better than tachycardia. It is best to keep pulmonary artery pressures at a low-normal level. It is also essential to keep the patient warm. EKG monitored for signs of ischemia. Do not let any aspect of the patient's condition change dramatically during induction or emergence; keep the patient hemodynamically stable.

Monitors and IV Access

- An arterial line is routinely inserted.
- A central venous pressure (CVP) line is routinely inserted.
- A pulmonary artery (PA) catheter is indicated in some patients.
- Peripheral IVs should be established in the upper extremities or neck.
- ST-segment analysis is performed, using EKG leads 2 and 5 or 4 and 5.

IV Vasoactive Agents

The following vasoactive agents are frequently used in AAA repair: phenylephrine (Neosynephrine), nitroglycerine, sodium nitroprusside (SNP), and/or fenoldopam.

IV Fluids and Volume Requirements

Keep the patient in a state ranging from euvolemia to hypovolemia until cross-clamp is about to come off the aorta.

Induction

Decrease stress on induction, and keep SPB within 20% of the baseline pressure.

Intraoperative Measures/Maintenance

Isoflurane may actually protect the patient from spinal cord ischemia; Sevoflurane and Desflurane are also acceptable.

Keep IV drugs ready: heparin, protamine.

Prostacyclin and thromboxane release occurs when the surgeon begins abdominal exploration and traction of the small intestine; this effect can also be evoked with aortic cross-clamping. Mesenteric mast cells release histamine. Signs and symptoms of these imbalances include facial flushing, decreased systemic vascular resistance (SVR), hypotension, tachycardia, and increased cardiac index.

Preoperative, preventative treatment consists of cyclooxygenase inhibitors—aspirin (ASA) or ibuprofen; intraoperatively, vasoconstrictors to increase SVR; and beta blockers to treat tachycardia. Histamine blockers may be given preoperatively to help avoid histamine release if this syndrome occurs.

Aortic Cross-Clamp Issues

See Chapter 3 for more information on aortic cross-clamping.

Before the cross-clamp is applied, the surgeon will call for heparin—usually 100 units/kg IV through central line. Heparin is given and allowed to circulate for 3 minutes before the cross-clamp is placed. Notify the surgeon when 3 minutes has passed.

Keep the patient in a hypovolemic state and use the hypotension technique to decrease MAP right before cross-clamp application. SPB should be in the vicinity of 90 mm Hg prior to clamp placement.

Once the cross-clamp is on, if the normal preoperative SBP is in the range of 160–180 mm Hg, maintain SBP at 140–160 mm Hg to perfuse organs.

The distal aorta is clamped first (so plaque pieces don't break off and flow to the legs). This step produces an immediate increase in blood pressure, SVR (afterload), and coronary blood flow above the clamp; a decreased venous return (preload) to the heart, with passive recoil occurring distal to the clamp. While coronary blood flow will be increased, so will the myocardial oxygen demand; thus ischemia and myocardial dysfunction can occur. Assess myocardial function immediately prior to and after clamp application—watch for left ventricular failure and myocardial ischemia.

Myocardial stress is related to the level of the clamp: A clamp placed higher than the renal arteries (suprarenal) will increase the mean blood pressure by 50%. If so, it may be necessary to deepen the anesthetic and use vasodilators: nipride (sodium nitroprusside), nitroglycerine, and/or fenoldopam to decrease the blood pressure. Watch for left ventricle failure and myocardial ischemia. Assess renal function and urinary output, check cortical function with an EEG, and check the patient's pupils. If there is evidence of organ ischemia, the surgeon may need to remove clamp either fully or partially.

The hemodynamic response to *infrarenal* aortic cross-clamping is influenced by fluid volume and the preoperative cardiac status; the hemodynamic response is usually not as severe as *suprarenal* clamping.

Document the cross-clamp time; this is start of ischemic time.

Before the cross-clamp removed, implement volume loading. Have vasopressors ready. Prepare for hypotension (MAP drops 40–60 mm Hg), hypovolemia, and metabolic washout from ischemic extremities → acidosis → ETCO$_2$ increases. Prepare for this situation by turning off vasodilators (i.e., nipride), lightening the anesthetic, and implementing volume loading (but do so judiciously and do not overload the patient). Aortic release after occlusion can lead to sympathetic nervous system (SNS) activation with release of prostaglandins, platelet sequestration, complement activation, and cytokine release that produces oxygen-derived free radicals. Mannitol may be given before aortic unclamping to decrease the production of thromboxane.

Once the cross-clamp is off, if hypotension continues for more than 4 minutes, the surgeon may need to reclamp the aorta and recheck for bleeding or myocardial dysfunction.

Chart the cross-clamp removal time; this is the end of "ischemic time."

Emergence
The goal is smooth emergence and a hemodynamically stable patient. Coughing and bucking will cause the patient's blood pressure to spike.

Distal circulation should be evaluated for embolization. Contrast may be needed for angiography.

Abdominal Aortic Aneurysm Resection: Endovascular Repair

For an endovascular repair, the patient should have an infrarenal abdominal aneurysm with an aortic neck length (from renal arteries to aneurysm) more than 1.5 cm (depending on the endograft used), that has limited tortuosity, and is 5 cm in diameter and 1.5 to 10 cm long.

Operative Procedure
A minimally invasive technique, an endoscopic approach may be used to repair an infrarenal AAA by positioning a collapsible Dacron graft with metal support (similar to a stent) above and below the aneurismal area to exclude the aneurysm from the circulation. The graft self-expands as it is deployed by the surgeon. Some grafts have little hooks that grab onto the vessel wall. The graft may be in sections that combine to form a bifurcated graft; alternatively, a one-piece bifurcated graft may be used. The surgeon will use balloons to ensure that the graft is fully expanded. Additional sections or extensions of graft may be placed as needed; these will also be ballooned. The procedure is done with fluoroscopy throughout. No aortic cross-clamp is used with this type of endovascular repair.

Anesthetic
IV sedation with a spinal or epidural with sedation may be used. Alternatively, general anesthesia is given with insertion of an OETT.

Positioning
The patient is placed in a supine position, with arms either extended on armboards or padded and tucked (according to surgeon preference).

Anesthetic Implications
Type and cross-match the patient's blood preoperatively. It may be necessary to have blood in the operating room.

Have heparin and protamine available.

Be prepared to convert to an emergency open AAA repair if an adverse situation develops.

The goal is for the anesthetic to minimize any organ dysfunction, but especially damage to the myocardial, renal, and pulmonary systems.

IV contrast is used, so check for allergy to IV dye, shellfish, preoperatively. It may be necessary to give Benadryl, steroids, and IV fluids to preserve renal function and prevent histamine release.

Anesthesia Goals for Endovascular Repair of an AAA

The overall choice for the anesthetic is based on the need for a smooth induction and cardiovascular stability. Keep stress low, with the goal of keeping blood pressure within 20% of the baseline measurement. Have nitroglycerin, sodium nitroprusside, and phenylephrine drips ready. Bradycardia is considered better than tachycardia. Do not let any aspect of the patient's condition change dramatically during induction or emergence; keep the patient hemodynamically stable.

The hypotension technique is typically used with deployment of a graft.

Also, it is important to keep the patient warm.

Monitors and IV Access

- An arterial line is needed. A central line with cordis needed as well.
- ST-segment analysis is necessary, using EKG leads 2 and 5 or 4 and 5.
- Place peripheral IVs in the upper extremities or neck.

IV Fluids and Volume Requirements

Keep the patient in a state of euvolemia to hypovolemia.

Abdominal Aortic Aneurysm Rupture: Emergency Surgery

When an AAA ruptures, patients can present as either stable with a slow leak or in extremis with a very high mortality rate. Ruptures most commonly occur in the retroperitoneum, which can permit tamponade of the hemorrhage. Such patients are more likely to present in a more stable condition, allowing for a controlled induction. However, even though these patients have a hemorrhage that is at least partially contained, rapid exsanguination can occur at any time. A smaller percentage of aneurysms rupture into the peritoneal cavity, which is associated with a larger degree of exsanguination. The overall mortality rate for AAA rupture is 50%.

The hallmark presentation of AAA rupture is severe back pain, abdominal pain, syncope or frank collapse; and/or vomiting.

Operative Procedure

The time it takes to get proximal aortic clamp on to control bleeding is crucial to patient survival. See the discussion of open AAA resection earlier in this chapter for more information.

Anesthetic

GETA with a rapid-sequence induction and insertion of an OETT, scopolamine (amnestic) is used. Induction must take place quickly, with the incision being made immediately after the patient is asleep. If the patient's condition allows for a controlled induction, GETA with rapid-sequence induction is also used but in a slower and more controlled manner. For either, use etomidate and paralytics.

Positioning

The patient is placed in a supine position. Bilateral arms are usually tucked at the patient's side.

Anesthetic Implications

The goals with this surgery are to control blood loss, have and maintain a BP, and preserve organ function. Volume resuscitation consists of IV fluids, colloids, and blood products. There is rarely enough time to type and cross-match the patient's blood, so blood replacement will likely consist of noncrossed blood or O-negative blood. Vasoactive drugs to be given may include phenylephrine (Neosynephrine) and epinephrine.

No heparin is given with emergency rupture.

Peripheral IVs should be placed in the upper extremities or neck. An arterial line and central venous catheter must be inserted.

Arteriovenous Fistula or Shunt

An arteriovenous (AV) fistula or shunt is created surgically to allow for permanent vascular access for hemodialysis. This procedure is performed to provide large-bore IV, usually frequent, access to a patient's vascular system for venipuncture during renal dialysis or infusion chemotherapy.

Operative Procedure

A *fistula* consists of an anastomosis and direct communication between an artery and a vein. The increased blood flow causes the vein to grow larger and more thick-walled, permitting easy access during hemodialysis. *The fistula is considered the best long-term access method, as it has a lower complication rate and lasts longer than any other type of access.*

To create a fistula, a selected artery is anastomosed to the vein. Typically, the radial artery to cephalic vein in a side-by-side approach at the wrist is used, but other options include anastomosis of the basilic vein to radial artery, the brachial artery to cephalic vein, or the axillary vein to brachial artery. Vascular clamps or elastic loops around the vessels (vessel loops) control blood flow while an incision is made into the lumen of the artery.

Historically, four types of anastomosis between the artery and vein have been employed: side to side, end to end, end of vein to side of artery, and end of artery to side of vein. Most commonly, the side-to-side and end of vein-to-side of artery approaches are used. These procedures are done months before hemodialysis can be started, to allow the fistula or shunt to "mature"; it can take up to a year to mature. This access should allow continuous high volumes of blood flow. An intraoperative arteriogram or Doppler may be done to confirm blood flow.

A *shunt* (also known as a *graft*) is created using a graft; prosthetic loop communication is part of this technique. All synthetic grafts, such as Dacron or Teflon (PTFE) grafts, and heterografts (grafts from another species such as bovine) are anastomosed to the artery and the vein in an end-to-side manner; the loop of the graft connects the artery and the vein. This surgical method requires tunneling of the graft for placement. *A shunt does not need to mature as long as a fistula and can be used soon after placement.*

Anesthetic

Anesthesia options include MAC with local anesthesia or GETA with insertion of an OETT. An axillary block helps with sympatholysis on the artery being operated on. Use drugs that are *not* metabolized by the kidneys—such as cisatricurium or atracurium—for muscle relaxation.

Positioning

The patient is placed in a supine position. The patient's upper body is placed at the edge of operating room table toward the affected arm; the surgeon will position the arm. Place the nonsurgical arm on the OR table or on an armboard at an angle less than 45 degrees.

Anesthetic Implications

Heparin 1000 units/mL and protamine 10 mg/mL should be available. Heparin is given before clamping the artery; protamine is very seldom needed but should be on hand.

Most of these patients are stable. The unstable patients usually get a subclavian dialysis catheter for dialysis until they are stable.

To protect the dialysis graft, no blood pressure readings or venipuncture should be performed in the extremity with the graft. Even if the graft is nonfunctional, the vessels remain arterialized and IVs may not run in that arm. A fistula or shunt can clot if the patient becomes hypotensive. A warming pad may help prevent vasoconstriction.

Place peripheral IVs in the nonoperative arm.

Important Anatomy of Carotid Arteries

Carotid Sinus

The carotid sinus is located at a slight dilation in the carotid artery at its bifurcation into the external and internal carotids. The sinus contains baroreceptors that are sensitive to arterial pressure; when stimulated, they cause a reflexive decrease in heart rate and blood pressure and subsequent decrease in cerebral blood flow (CBF). (Arterial pressure is also sensed in the aortic arch.)

The carotid sinus is innervated by the afferent CN9 and efferent CN10 nerves. During carotid surgery, manipulation of this area can cause bradycardia and hypotension. The surgeon can inject lidocaine 10–20 mg at the carotid sinus to prevent a fluctuation in the blood pressure.

Carotid Bodies

The carotid bodies sense arterial pO_2 and H^+ concentration (pH). They are located at the bifurcation of the carotids, are innervated by CN9, and are integrated in the medulla (respiratory center).

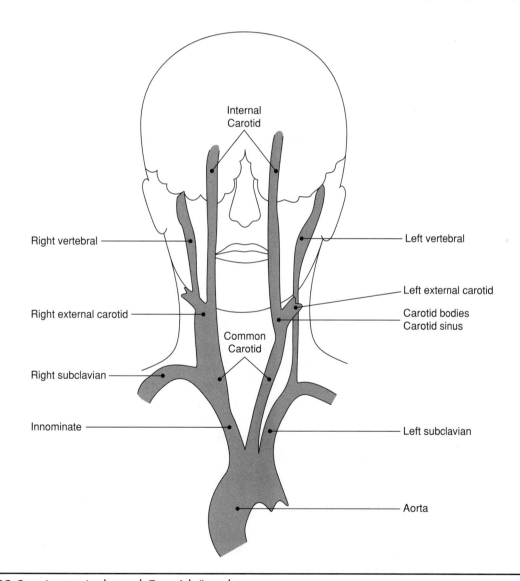

Figure 22-2 *Aorta, Arch, and Carotids/Jugulars*

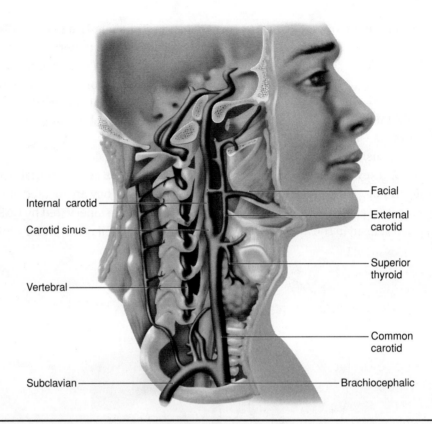

Figure 22-3   *The Arteries of the Head and Neck*
Source: AAOS, 2004.

Common Carotid

The common carotid is the major provider of blood flow to the brain, face, neck, and upper extremities.

External Carotids

The external carotids perfuse the superficial face, ears, scalp, neck and thyroid, mouth and tongue, nasal areas, and dura.

Internal Carotids

The internal carotids perfuse the circle of Willis anterior circulation (80%), eye (ophthalmic artery), side of the forehead, and nose.

Circle of Willis

Circle of Willis vessels include the basilar (flow from subclavians via vertebrals), posterior cerebral, posterior communicating, distal internal carotid, middle cerebral, anterior cerebral, and anterior communicating vessels. Approximately 25% of all patients do not have a complete anastomotic circle of Willis and may need a shunt during carotid endarterectomy (CEA). The circle of Willis is a valve-less system that allows retrograde flow. See Chapter 5 for more information on the circle of Willis.

Carotid Endarterectomy

CEA is done to restore carotid artery blood flow and enhance cerebral circulation due to carotid narrowing or stenosis. The procedure attempts to remove plaque at the carotid bifurcation (most commonly) or at the proximal internal carotid artery.

CEA is indicated for 70% stenosis (narrowing) of the carotid (considered severe), in patients with transient ischemic attacks with ipsilateral carotid stenosis (more than 70%), and for minor stroke with ipsilateral carotid stenosis (more than 70%). It may also be performed in symptomatic patients with less than 70% blockage.

Operative Procedure

The surgeon makes an oblique neck incision at the anterior border of the sternocleidomastoid muscle. The carotid sheath is exposed and incised. The carotid bifurcation (at C4), which includes the common internal carotid artery (ICA) and the external carotid artery (ECA), is exposed. The surgeon will announce the dose of heparin and when to give it.

Opening the diseased artery requires occlusion of all feeding arteries. Proximal and distal control of the carotid artery and its bifurcation is achieved with clamps or vessel loops. Surgeon clamps the arteries in this order: internal → common → external. The arteries are unclamped in reverse order: external → common → internal. Once the artery is occluded, the surgeon will ask for the blood pressure to be maintained at a higher level to improve collateral circulation.

An incision is made to open the artery, and atherosclerotic plaque is removed. Notify the surgeon immediately if bradycardia or ectopy occurs during carotid bulb manipulation; the surgeon can inject local anesthetic (usually 1% lidocaine) at the bulb. The artery incision is sutured closed (primary closure) or a patch graft of vein or synthetic material may be used to close the artery. A drain may be placed for excessive oozing. A dressing is placed over the incision.

Stump Pressure

The systolic or mean arterial pressure is measured by a needle placed in the internal carotid artery. It measures cerebral perfusion pressure (CPP) in the circle of Willis and brain, with the surgical team looking for an intact circle of Willis and/or collateral circulation.

A long piece of pressure tubing is connected to the needle. The other end of the tubing is handed off the sterile field to the anesthetist to be connected to a pressure transducer (a second stopcock on the arterial transducer). The transducer is zeroed. The surgeon will note the current mean arterial pressure (MAP) in the artery, perform a trial occlusion, and note the pressure at that point. The cerebral perfusion pressure (CPP) should be more than 50–60 torr. Readings of less than 25 torr indicate the need for placement of a shunt during endarterectomy. CPP can also be measured during surgery by means of an intraluminal Fogarty balloon catheter, which is used in place of a distal internal carotid clamp.

In an awake patient under cervical block, a shunt would need to be placed if the patient's level of consciousness (LOC) changes.

Carotid Shunt

An intraluminal shunt is placed from the proximal (common carotid artery) to the distal (internal carotid artery) to maintain cerebral blood flow during carotid artery cross-clamping. Note and document the shunt time. Use of a carotid shunt seems to provide maximal neuroprotection, but carries risks associated with dislodgement of emboli and intimal wall dissection.

Anesthetic

General Anesthesia

The goals with general anesthesia for a carotid endarterectomy are as follows:

- To maintain hemodynamic stability to ensure cerebral perfusion
- To minimize cardiac depression

A balanced general anesthesia using multiple agents is a common practice—that is, combining intravenous (propofol, thiopental, or etomidate) and volatile (Isoflurane, Desflurane, or Sevoflurane) agents, along with narcotics (fentanyl, sufentanil, or remifentanil). Nitric oxide is not contraindicated; however, it will increase the size of air emboli and is usually not used.

GETA, an OETT, and muscle relaxants guarantee the surgeon a quiet field with better control of vital signs but make it difficult to assess the patient neurologically. Some patients may also experience large blood pressure swings (especially hypertension) during induction and emergence from anesthesia. These patients have widely varying blood pressures during surgery (owing to carotid sinus stimulation or loss of baroreceptors), so you need to be prepared to bolus or titrate vasoactive drugs rapidly. Set the inhaled agent at 1 MAC and titrate vasoactive agents so as to control blood pressure.

Regional Anesthesia

The goals in regional anesthesia for a carotid endarterectomy are twofold:

- To facilitate continuous neurologic assessment of the awake patient
- To maintain blood pressure stability

The neurological examination may include the ability to follow directions, the ability to count backward, the strength of a hand grip, and alertness; there may also be assessment of the mental status (conversing with the patient) and contralateral motor and sensory responses during carotid cross-clamping. If inadequate collateral perfusion develops, it will be signaled within approximately 30 seconds by a deteriorating neurological assessment; a change in level of consciousness indicates that a shunt needs to be placed.

Anesthesia Goals for CEA

No matter which anesthetic technique is used, the following goals apply in CEA:

- Keep blood pressure within 20% of baseline for maintenance of CPP in the high-normal to slightly elevated range (70 mm Hg or higher; keep blood pressure higher to perfuse collateral areas) and MAP in the range of 80–90 mm Hg. Lopressor (metoprolol), labetalol, or hydralazine IV bolus may be given in case of hypertension. Nitroglycerin and phenylephrine IV drips may also be used for blood pressure control. *Blood vessels in ischemic areas have lost normal autoregulation; their functioning is pressure dependent.*
- In treating intraoperative hypotension, keep the preload at normal levels and do not *just* give vasopressors.
- Maintain normocapnia in the patient.
- Provide aggressive blood sugar control, keeping blood glucose in the range of 80–110 mg /dL. *Hyperglycemia can worsen ischemic injury by increasing lactic acidosis from anaerobic glycolysis.*

- Provide for good surgical exposure and a motionless field.
- Keep the patient warm.
- At the end of the case, the patient's blood pressure and heart rate are often elevated, so a longer-acting agent (e.g., labetalol, hydralazine) may be used.
- Rapid wake-up for neurologic examination in the operating room is necessary. The ultimate goal is a pain-free patient.

Preoperative Measures

Optimize the patient's coexisting conditions.

Document the full neurological assessment—specifically, chart neurologic deficits. Position the patient's head similar to the operative position and assess for changes. Avoid large doses of benzodiazepines, as they may produce longer sedation and hypercapnia with depressed respirations. These patients may have been treated medically with platelet anti-aggregates (e.g., aspirin, dipyridamole [Persantine]), so watch for bleeding.

Coumadin should be discontinued 5–7 days prior to surgery while aspirin continues.

Monitors and IV Vasoactive Agents

- Placement of an arterial line is routine.
- A CVP line may or may not be placed in the contralateral internal jugular vein or either femoral vein, if needed.
- Place peripheral IVs in the nonoperative side.

Cerebral Monitoring

Cerebral monitoring (see Chapter 3) is done to assess cerebral perfusion, thereby identifying patients at risk for neurologic injury during cross-clamping of the carotid arteries. Commonly used technologies include EEG, somatosensory evoked potentials (SSEP), transcranial Doppler, and near infra-red spectroscopy (NIRS).

If intraoperative cerebral ischemia is detected, immediate measures should be taken to rectify it, including informing the surgeon, the clamp should be released if the carotid artery has not been opened, a shunt may need to be placed, increasing MAP by 10–20%, and administrating neuroprotective agents. Any changes or suppression in the EEG is helped by raising the blood pressure so as to improve collateral flow through the circle of Willis.

Cerebral oximetry is a noninvasive means of measuring the adequacy of cerebral blood flow. A 10% change or a measurement of less than 4% is significant and results in neurologic compromise to some degree.

Sodium thiopental is the only agent that may provide cerebral protection for focal ischemia when used properly (initial dose of 10–15 mg/kg and then 5 mg/kg every 10–15 min, or guided by EEG of burst suppression). An inotrope and vasopressors are frequently required to counteract its effect of hemodynamic suppression.

No cerebral monitoring modality is as sensitive or specific as assessing an awake patient.

IV Vasoactive Agents

- IV pump: nitroglycerine, phenylephrine (Neo-Synephrine), sodium nitroprusside (SNP)
- Syringe for bolus: ephedrine, phenylephrine (Neo-Synephrine), esmolol (Brevibloc), labetalol, hydralazine

Low-molecular-weight dextran may be given as a plasma expander and can reverse red blood cell aggregation; this effect improves the rate of blood flow in the microcirculation and can help prevent a thrombus from forming at the suture line. Dextran should be started very slowly, as allergic reactions are possible. Some agents, such as Dextran 40 (Rheomacrodex), are associated with a reduced risk of side effects such as allergic responses or hemorrhage.

IV Fluids and Volume Requirements

Keep the patient in a state from euvolemia to slightly dry. Lactated Ringer's solution or 0.9% normal saline may be administered if necessary; colloids may also be given.

Induction

For general anesthesia, etomidate or thiopental is used for induction. Avoid succinylcholine (Anectine), as the fasciculations it produces are undesirable. Give a nondepolarizing muscle relaxant (NDMR; e.g., rocuronium, vecuronium, cisatricurium) once you are able to ventilate the patient by mask. Isoflurane, sevoflurane, or desflurane are appropriate volatile agents. The anesthetic choice should not interfere with any neurophysiologic monitoring.

Intraoperative Measures/Maintenance

Keep the $PaCO_2$ in the range of 35–36 mm Hg; check ABGs. Low-dose narcotics (fentanyl 1–2 mcg/kg or remifentanil infusion 2 mg in 40 mL normal saline at 0.05 mcg/kg/min) allow for quick wake-up and assessment of neurological status. Pentothal may be used for burst suppression, based on EEG monitoring.

Prior to clamping the carotid artery, the surgeon will ask for bolus of heparin 75–100 units/kg or another specific amount. Flush the heparin in through the IV line (a central line, if available) as rapidly as the blood pressure will allow (heparin can cause hypotension). Announce to the surgeon the 3-minute mark, as the carotid clamp is placed at this point.

Decrease the blood pressure before the clamp applied to help prevent a hypertensive spike.

While the carotid is clamped, a deep anesthetic level is needed. The internal carotid will be cross-clamped first.

In this patient population, the CBF is more likely to be pressure dependent. Maintaining MAP at a level 10–20% higher than baseline is recommended during carotid clamping to augment the collateral cerebral perfusion. At the same time, keeping the SBP at less than 160 mm Hg (the surgeon may specifically direct where he or she want the SBP to be) is extremely important to prevent cerebral hyperemia (hyperperfusion), excessive surgical bleeding, and stress on the heart.

When the carotid is being unclamped, increase preload to at or just above baseline by the time the clamp is removed.

Emergence from Anesthesia

The goal is to have a smooth and rapid emergence, with stable hemodynamics being maintained, to facilitate immediate neurologic assessment. The goal is intact cardiovascular, neurological, and respiratory stability; an awake, neurologically intact patient should be realized as soon as possible after surgery. Avoid coughing and bucking on the ETT, can use lidocaine IV or laryngeal (LITA) to attenuate airway reflexes. Esmolol (Brevibloc) 10–50 mg IV may be given to manage hypertensive spikes in blood pressure.

Postoperative Measures

The brain is not used to increased pressure from increased blood flow and the cerebral vessels cannot constrict as needed under these circumstances; thus *hyper-perfusion syndrome* results from long-term loss of autoregulation. Specifically, increased blood pressures may lead to hemorrhage and cerebral edema, as evidenced by confusion and seizures. The post-stenosis epithelial layer is especially vulnerable to post-CEA high pressure shear force. Patient complaints of ipsilateral headache, blurred vision, and facial or eye pain are suggestive of brain hyperemia and demand urgent management.

CEA is also associated with is a high incidence of postoperative hypertension due to *baroreceptor regulation loss.* It may take days to achieve adequate blood pressure control. Very volatile blood pressures can occur if a bilateral CEA is done, and there can be long-term losses of baroreceptor reflexes.

Hypotension following CEA is often volume related. Treat this imbalance with fluids; some patients may need vasopressors. Postoperative hypotension may also be related to myocardial ischemia, so look for ischemic changes on EKG and treat accordingly.

The leading cause of death after CEA is myocardial infarction. Postoperative stroke is also a concern; it can occur from inadequate blood flow through the circle of Willis during carotid clamping or from debris embolization from clamping the carotid. Hematoma formation and bleeding at the incision site are not rare complications (because heparin and dextran are given), and any swelling must be assessed for and treated immediately. Any swelling or blood collection can cause rapid airway compression or edema. If these complications occur, reintubate the patient early with a smaller than calculated endotracheal tube; the patient will probably need to return to the OR so that the surgeon can remove the hematoma and cauterize any bleeding.

Positioning

The patient is placed in a supine position, with a shoulder roll placed. The head of the bed is elevated slightly; the patient's head is slightly extended and tilted away from the operative side. Bilateral arms are tucked at the patient's sides. Secure the ETT on the opposite side of the mouth from the surgical side.

Anesthetic Implications

A CEA may be done in conjunction with coronary artery bypass graft (CABG).

Have the patient's X-rays and angiogram films available in the operating room.

Type and cross-match the patient's blood preoperatively.

Heparin 1000 units/mL and protamine 10 mg/mL should be available in the OR.

Complications

Potential complications of CEA include vocal cord paralysis with recurrent laryngeal nerve damage; damage to the accessory or hypoglossal nerves if there is swelling postoperatively; tension pneumothorax from air dissection into the pleural space from a neck wound; and hematoma.

In case of postoperative cerebrovascular accident (CVA) or loss of consciousness, suspect problems with the intimal flap inside the operative vessel (which prevents blood flow from getting to the brain). Immediate cerebral angiography is indicated with this complication, which may need surgical correction.

Cervical nerve block can result in phrenic nerve paralysis, hemorrhage, and cranial nerve dysfunction.

Dialysis Catheter Placement: Venous Access

A temporary catheter is often placed to provide large-vein access for short-term dialysis treatment. Two types of catheters are used:

- Udall catheter: Y-shaped catheter, usually placed in the subclavian vein
- Shaldon catheter: bilateral femoral vein catheter

Operative Procedure

An IV stick is done percutaneously into the subclavian vein in the neck or chest, or into the femoral vein in the groin. A catheter is then threaded through this site. A tunnel is made from the subclavian vein to the skin surface. Fluoroscopy may be used to assist with catheter placement. The catheter may be ended by a port, or a "pig-tail" catheter may exit through the skin.

Anesthetic

Sedation with local anesthetic is used.

Positioning

The patient is placed in a supine position.

Anesthetic Implications

There is potential for the surgeon to lacerate a great vessel, the thoracic duct, or the atrium, which can lead to hemorrhage or possibly cardiac tamponade.

These catheters are not meant for permanent access and will typically be used only until a permanent fistula can be put in and matures. In patients whose fistula or shunt surgery is unsuccessful, a catheter may be inserted and then tunneled under the skin to increase patient comfort and help to reduce complications.

Place peripheral IVs in the nonoperative side.

Do not use the dialysis catheter as an IV access except in an emergency. These catheters are flushed with a large concentration of heparin and capped. If access is required, do so under sterile conditions, and remove the heparin by withdrawing approximately 20 mL of blood before injecting anything. See Chapter 3 for more information on hemodialysis catheter access and flush guidelines.

Femoral Thrombectomy/Embolectomy

Femoral thrombectomy or embolectomy is done to relieve a lower-extremity vascular occlusion. These cases may require an urgent or emergency approach depending on the presentation.

Acute arterial occlusion may be either intrinsic (e.g., a clot or embolus) or extrinsic (owing to penetrating injuries or iatrogenic injury, such as from arterial cannulation) in nature. Either type of occlusion must be corrected within 4–6 hours or irreversible changes in the skeletal muscle and peripheral nerves will ensue. Acute arterial ischemia characterized by the "five Ps": pain, pallor, paralysis, paresthesia, and pulselessness. *No pain is an especially bad sign.* Collateral blood flow can mitigate the effects of chronic ischemia but cannot compensate for acute occlusion.

Operative Procedure

The vessel is accessed above the occlusion. A thin-diameter Fogarty embolectomy catheter is passed down the vessel past the clot; the balloon at the end is inflated and the catheter pulled back, pulling the clot out.

Anesthetic

A spinal or epidural is the anesthetic of choice. Vasodilation is desirable, as it decreases hypercoagulability and helps with surgical exposure. Postoperative pain management is important as well. Clarify the patient's anticoagulation status before deciding which anesthesia method is appropriate. GETA can be done with insertion of an OETT.

Monitors and IV Access
- An arterial line is preferred.
- A central line may or may not be needed.

Positioning
The patient is placed in a supine position.

Anesthetic Implications
Risk factors for thrombus/embolus formation include smoking, diabetes, hypertension, renal disease, atherosclerotic vascular disease, increased lipid levels, and obesity. Watch for bleeding (it can hide in the surgical drapes), emboli, acidosis with recirculation of an ischemic limb, and compartment syndrome.

Have the patient's X-rays and angiogram films available in the operating room.

Type and cross-match the patient's blood preoperatively; have 2 units of packed cells available.

Heparin 1000 units/mL and protamine 10 mg/mL should be available in the OR.

If the patient becomes hypotensive, consider giving dopamine or another inotropic agent. Phenylephrine is a direct vasoconstrictor and will decrease blood flow to the legs. Do not use this agent until its administration is discussed with the surgeon.

Low-molecular-weight dextran may be given as a plasma expander and can reverse red blood cell aggregation; this effect improves the rate of blood flow in the microcirculation and can help prevent a thrombus from worsening or forming at the suture line. Dextran should be started very slowly, as allergic reactions to this agent are possible. Versions such as dextran 40 (Rheomacrodex) are associated with a reduced risk of side effects such as allergic responses or hemorrhage.

Complications
Potential embolectomy complications include perforation, pseudoaneurysm, and side effects from the washout of free radicals.

DISTAL REVASCULARIZATION

Types of Grafts for Distal Revascularization
- *Autologous reversed saphenous:* removed from the patient's leg. The branches are ligated, and the vein is reversed so that valves do not interrupt the blood flow. This type of graft may be harvested endoscopically.
- *Saphenous vein in situ:* vein remains in place. The valves are disrupted and the venous tributaries are ligated; the proximal vein is then attached to the proximal end of the artery and the distal end of the vein is attached to the distal end of the artery. This type of graft may offer improved patency because it avoids the potential twisting of the saphenous vessel that can occur with placement of a reversed vein graft. It also avoids the size discrepancy that sometimes exists between the distal vein and the proximal artery.
- *Prosthetic graft:* Dacron, Gortex. Patency rates are not as high as with autologous grafts.
- *Allograft:* cryopreserved human (donor) saphenous vein.

Vascular Bypass Grafts
Vascular bypass grafts are done to relieve impaired lower-extremity circulation and to relieve symptoms of claudication. They bypass an occluded segment of an artery.

Operative Procedure
An occluded section of artery is bypassed using either a synthetic (Dacron or Teflon) graft or a harvested saphenous leg vein or arm vein that has had its valves incised (or been placed upside down to prevent valve action).

Anesthetic
- General anesthesia, an OETT, and muscle relaxants: Offers better cardiovascular stability; the patient is kept immobile.

- Neuraxial to T10 with sedation. Side effects of the spinal or epidural include vasodilation with decreased hypercoagulability, which helps the surgeon. This option also provides good postoperative pain management.
- Combination: An epidural can be placed preoperatively for postoperative pain control, with general anesthesia being given for surgical anesthesia.

Get an ABG and labs as soon as possible after induction to obtain a baseline reading of oxygenation, $PaCO_2$ and $ETCO_2$ comparison, and hemoglobin and hematocrit (H&H), potassium, sodium, and glucose levels.

Monitors
- An arterial line is required for blood pressure monitoring.
- A central line may be needed for access for fluids and vasoactive medications.
- A PA catheter may be needed depending on the patient's condition.

Positioning
The patient is placed in a supine position.

Anesthetic Implications
Preoperative labs and tests should include H&H, potassium, glucose, PT/INR/PTT, BUN, and creatinine; also obtain a 12-lead EKG. These patients may be sick enough to require pulmonary function studies and an ABG as well.

Clarify whether the patient has an allergy to IV dye, seafood, or shrimp, as contrast dye is often used in this type of surgery.

Type and cross-match the patient's blood preoperatively, and have 2 units of packed cells available. Bleeding can be dramatic with this procedure.

Keep patient the warm with blankets and fluid warmers.

Heparin 1000 units/mL and protamine 10 mg/mL should be available in the OR. Heparin is usually given prior to the application of the vessel cross-clamp to decrease the risk of thromboembolic incidence. These patients may also be given heparin immediately after surgery to prevent clotting of the new bypass graft. Protamine is generally not used but should be available "just in case."

These patients have atherosclerotic changes to all vessels, but especially the coronary arteries and the carotid arteries. The principal risk with these patients is ischemic heart disease due to atherosclerosis. If the patient becomes hypotensive, consider giving dopamine or another inotropic agent. Phenylephrine is a direct vasoconstrictor and will decrease blood flow to the legs. If phenylephrine must be used, talk to the surgeon before administering this agent. Ephedrine may be used to increase blood pressure if the heart rate is slow. Avoid tachycardia.

Monitor the patient for ST-segment elevation or depression—or any EKG changes throughout surgery. Leads II and V5 are best at monitoring for myocardial ischemia.

Low-molecular-weight dextran may be given as a plasma expander and can reverse red blood cell aggregation; this effect improves the rate of blood flow in the microcirculation and can help prevent a thrombus from forming at the suture line. Dextran should be started very slowly, as allergic reactions to this agent are possible. Versions such as dextran 40 (Rheomacrodex) are associated with a reduced risk of side effects, such as allergic responses or hemorrhage.

Complications
Revascularization complications can include emboli, free radical circulation and lactic acidosis (increasing $ETCO_2$ after reperfusing the blocked extremity), hypotension, myocardial instability, dysrhythmias, and rhabdomyolysis with possible compartment syndrome.

INFLOW RECONSTRUCTION

In-flow reconstruction focuses on the aorto-iliac and aorto-femoral vessels—that is, the big vessels. This is a more stressful surgery, as aortic clamping must be done during the bypass surgery.

Aortobifemoral Bypass Graft

Aortobifemoral bypass graft is similar to elective AAA repair. The abdomen (midline or lower abdomen) and both groins are exposed; the aorta is cross-clamped. A bifurcated synthetic graft is sewn to the aorta. The limbs of the graft are tunneled down to the groins, and then sewn into both femoral arteries. The clamps are then removed. Reperfusion of the legs and its side effects are a major source of concern. Use of cell-saver technology is optional due to the fact that there is less blood loss with this procedure than with open elective AAA repair. Aorto-bifemoral bypass graft is done to reperfuse both lower extremities. See the discussion of vascular bypass grafts earlier in this chapter for more information.

Axillofemoral or Axillobifemoral Bypass Graft

If the patient has conditions that preclude direct aortic reconstruction—such as aortic sepsis, aortoenteric fistula, a high operative risk, or some abdominal pathology—the surgeon may decide to avoid an abdominal incision. Instead of a lengthy, involved abdominal aortic procedure, this kind of bypass is extra-anatomical.

An incision is made below one of the collar bones (subclavian), and a vertical incision is made in one or both groins. A synthetic Gortex graft (usually ringed PTFE) is tunneled from the subclavian incision subcutaneously to the groin on the same side. (It may pass superficially or below the pectoralis major, depending on surgeon preference). An additional small incision below the costal border may be needed to assist in tunneling the graft.

For an axillofemoral bypass, the graft is then anastomosed proximally to the axillary artery (end-to-side) and distally to the femoral artery in the groin (axillofemoral bypass).

For an axillobifemoral bypass, an additional synthetic graft is tunneled suprapubically to the opposite groin and anastomosed from one femoral artery to the other. The blood supply to one arm then provides the blood flow to one or both legs.

The adequacy of subclavian and axillary inflow must be determined preoperatively. The axillary graft end should be placed on the side where the blood pressure is highest. See the discussion of vascular bypass grafts earlier in this chapter for more information.

Place peripheral IVs, arterial line, and blood pressure cuff on the nonoperative arm.

Iliofemoral Bypass Graft

An iliofemoral bypass graft is done for unilateral iliac artery occlusive disease.

Operative Procedure

An iliofemoral bypass graft may be done through a flank incision (retroperitoneal) and a groin incision. A synthetic graft is anastomosed to the iliac artery and tunneled down to the femoral artery in the groin. This procedure may be performed successfully through laparoscopically assisted or totally laparoscopic approaches. The patient must have enough normal iliac artery in the pelvis to anastomose. See the discussion of vascular bypass grafts earlier in this chapter for more information.

Position

The patient is placed supine, with a bump-up under the hip of the affected side.

Femorofemoral Bypass Graft

In a femorofemoral bypass graft, a synthetic graft made from a material such as Dacron or Teflon is typically used due to the high volume of the femoral artery that must be accommodated. Alternatively, an autologous graft may be anastomosed to the donor femoral artery. With either type of graft, it is passed in a suprapubic subcutaneous tunnel to the opposite side, and attached to the recipient femoral artery, bypassing the blockage.

Femorofemoral bypass graft is performed as a treatment for an iliac or femoral occlusion. These patients must have one open iliac artery for this type of graft to be an option. The procedure can be done using local anesthetic if necessary in the appropriate patient.

See the discussion of vascular bypass grafts earlier in this chapter for more information.

OUTFLOW RECONSTRUCTION

Outflow reconstruction occurs distal to the inguinal ligament. It is performed to remedy a distal obstruction.

Femoropopliteal Bypass Graft

Femoropopliteal bypass graft consists of the interposition of an autologous or synthetic graft from the common femoral artery to the popliteal artery. The graft may be the patient's own saphenous vein or a synthetic prosthesis. This procedure is done to treat long occlusions (greater than 10 cm in length) in the superficial femoral or popliteal arteries.

Operative Procedure
A vertical incision is made over the inguinal ligament; there may be interruptions in the incision line as it is extended down the leg. Proximally, the common femoral artery and its bifurcation are exposed. The distal popliteal artery is also exposed. A tunneling instrument is used to make a passage from the femoral triangle to the popliteal space under the Sartorius muscle. The patient is given heparin, and the femoral artery is controlled with a vascular clamp or vessel loop. The graft is first sutured to the common femoral artery. If the graft being used is the saphenous vein, it will be inverted so that the most distal end of the vein is sewed at the femoral artery; this arrangement ensures that the valves of the vein do not interfere with the blood flow. In other words, blood will flow through the graft as if it were an artery that has no valves. The graft is passed through the tunnel and grafted to the popliteal artery. Intraoperative angiography may be performed to check for bypass patency.

Vascular surgeons tend to prefer the saphenous vein graft for femoral–popliteal bypass surgery because it has proven to stay open and provide better performance for a longer period of time than synthetic grafts. See the discussion of vascular bypass grafts earlier in this chapter for more information.

Positioning
The patient will be supine with the hip rotated and abducted, with the knee flexed.

Femorotibial Bypass Graft

A femorotibial bypass graft is done when the superficial femoral or popliteal artery is occluded and the tibial arterial lumen is open and continuous into the foot.

A synthetic or reversed saphenous vein graft can be used. Vascular surgeons tend to prefer the saphenous vein graft for femorotibial bypass surgery because it has proven to stay open and provide better performance for a longer period of time than synthetic grafts. See the discussion of vascular bypass grafts earlier in this chapter for more information.

Positioning
The patient will be supine with the hip rotated and abducted, with the knee flexed.

Popliteal–Tibial Bypass Graft

A popliteal–tibial bypass graft is done when there is an occlusion in a segment of the popliteal or tibial artery.

A synthetic or reversed saphenous vein graft can be used. Vascular surgeons tend to prefer the saphenous vein graft for popliteal–tibial bypass surgery because it has proven to stay open and provide better performance for a longer period of time than synthetic grafts. See the discussion of vascular bypass grafts earlier in this chapter for more information.

Positioning

The patient will be supine with their hip rotated and abducted, with the knee flexed.

Portosystemic Shunt (Portocaval Shunt)

A portosystemic shunt provides for diversion of portal venous blood to the systemic venous system. Portal hypertension is usually treated with a transjugular intrahepatic portosystemic shunt (TIPS) procedure (see Chapter 18). *This open surgical procedure is reserved for patients with a failed TIPS.*

A portosystemic shunt is placed to relieve elevated portal venous pressure (also known as portal hypertension). Portal hypertension causes venous dilatation, leading to esophageal or gastric varices, which can bleed; ascites; and hepatic failure. The primary cause of portal hypertension is cirrhosis.

Portal vein blood may be shunted into the inferior vena cava by various methods (end-to-end or side-to-side):

- *Splenorenal shunt:* an anastomosis between the proximal splenic and left renal veins (the spleen is removed in this procedure).
  A variation of this procedure, called a *Warren shunt,* preserves the spleen by creating the anastomosis between the distal splenic and left renal vein.
- *Mesocaval interpositional shunt (Drapanas shunt):* an interpositional graft from the superior mesenteric vein to the inferior vena cava.

Operative Procedure

A right subcostal or a thoracoabdominal incision is made. The inferior vena cava is exposed by reflecting the duodenum and the head of the pancreas medially. Great care is taken to avoid injury to the nearby structures, such as the gallbladder, cystic and common bile ducts, and hepatic artery and its branches. Anastomosis is made side-to-side by excising a window in both the vena cava and the portal vein, or end-to-end by transecting the portal vein and anastomosing to the vena cava. A ringed synthetic Dacron or Gortex graft (PTFE) or an autologous graft (harvested saphenous or jugular vein) may be used to bypass the obstructed hepatic blood flow.

A portosystemic shunt is a palliative measure that is intended to prevent further hemorrhage from varices. The procedure does not repair the damaged liver.

Anesthetic

General anesthesia is used with an OETT; muscle relaxants are needed.

Positioning

The patient is placed in a supine position, with the right side "bumped up" by a folded sheet or blanket. The arms are extended on armboards.

Anesthetic Implications

Angiography is usually done during surgery.

Type and cross-match the patient's blood preoperatively; blood is usually made available in the operating room. There is a major risk of bleeding with this procedure, as patients usually have a coagulopathy in conjunction with their liver disease. With this disease process, many distended and tortuous veins are found throughout the abdominal cavity; also, the surgical area is extremely vascular.

Varicose Vein (Saphenous) Excision and Stripping

Varicose vein excision and stripping is usually done for cosmetic reasons, but varicose veins can also be painful and make the legs feel full and heavy. Surgery is intended to prevent skin ulceration, edema, pain, and fatigue in the leg.

Varicose veins occur in the superficial veins. Severely varicosed veins have a slightly increased risk of deep vein thrombosis. Varicose vein valves usually do not function normally, resulting in venous distention with weakening and dilation of the vein walls.

Operative Procedure

Small incisions are made in the groin and ankle area. A vein stripper is inserted through the ankle incision, threaded through the affected vein, and exits the groin incision. The saphenous vein is ligated at its junction with the femoral vein after the stripper is in position, so as to avoid inadvertent ligation of the superficial saphenous vein or femoral artery. A specialized "stripper head" is attached to the device and then the stripper is gently pulled back through the leg, removing the diseased vessel. Multiple small incisions may be made along the course of the affected vein to remove accessory feeding veins and superficial vein clusters in the thigh and lower leg. These veins would have been marked with permanent marker by the surgeon prior to surgery. Pressure is applied, and residual clots are milked out. Incisions are closed and a pressure dressing (Ace wrap or compression stockings) is applied.

Anesthetic

GETA can be given with insertion of an OETT or LMA (this anesthetic is used if multiple incisions over a long vein are required). Alternatives include a spinal block or local anesthesia with sedation.

Positioning

The patient is placed in a supine or prone position; both positions may be needed. A slight Trendelenburg position helps to shrink the vein.

Anesthetic Implications

The surgeon will usually mark the patient's veins while the patient is standing in the preoperative area.

These patients are usually treated on an outpatient basis unless both legs are operated on.

Poor circulation from large varicose veins can lead to skin ulcers. The legs may bleed profusely if a prominent vein is injured.

Other methods to treat varicose veins include the following options:

- *Sclerotherapy:* A chemical is injected into the varicose veins. The chemical irritates and scars the vein from the inside out.

- *Ablation:* A flexible catheter with small electrodes at the tip is used to heat the walls of the vein and destroy it.
- *Laser treatment:* A flexible catheter is inserted into the varicose vein; a very small laser fiber is then threaded through the catheter. Laser energy is sent through this fiber, obliterating the lumen of the vein.
- *Avulsion (phlebectomy):* This procedure can be done with vein stripping or alone. Multiple small incisions are made, which allows the surgeon to remove individual vein clusters using hooks.

Vena Cava Filter Insertion

In this procedure, a filter is inserted into the inferior vena cava (IVC) to trap emboli, thereby preventing pulmonary emboli while maintaining blood flow through the lumen. Insertion of a vena cava filter is indicated for recurrent thromboembolism, chronic pulmonary embolism, deep venous thromboembolism, and large clots in the vena cava or iliac veins.

Operative Procedure

The filter is placed endovascularly. A guide wire is inserted into the right femoral vein, arm vein, or internal jugular vein. This wire is then guided into the IVC, and the compressed filter is pushed up through the catheter and deployed at the desired location, usually just below the renal vein.

Anesthetic

Local anesthesia and sedation are used.

Positioning

The patient is placed in a supine position.

Anesthetic Implications

Clarify whether the patient has iodine, IV dye, or shellfish allergies, as IV contrast may be used with this procedure.

IVC filter insertion is done on an X-ray table with angiography or fluoroscopy. A Doppler ultrasound may also be used.

PLASTIC SURGERY PEARLS

LOCAL ANESTHETIC	MAXIMUM DOSE WITHOUT EPINEPHRINE	MAXIMUM DOSE WITH EPINEPHRINE
Bupivacaine (Marcaine, Sensorcaine)	3 mg/kg; maximum total dose of 175 mg	3 mg/kg; maximum total dose of 225 mg
Chloroprocaine (Nesacaine) of 800 mg	11 mg/kg; maximum total dose of 800 mg	14 mg/kg; maximum total dose of 1000 mg
Etidocaine (Duranest)	6 mg/kg; maximum total dose 300 mg	8 mg/kg maximum total dose 400 mg
Lidocaine	4.5 mg/kg; maximum total dose 300 mg	7 mg/kg; maximum total dose 500 mg; 35 mg/kg during liposuction
Mepivacaine	4.5 mg/kg; maximum total dose 400 mg	7 mg/kg; maximum total dose 400 mg
Prilocaine	8 mg/kg; maximum total dose 500 mg	9 mg/kg; maximum total dose 600 mg
Procaine (Novocaine)	7 mg/kg; maximum total dose 600 mg	10 mg/kg
Ropivacaine (Naropin)	3 mg/kg; not to exceed 200 mg for minor nerve block	770 mg total over 24 hours
Tetracaine (Cetacaine)	3 mg/kg; maximum total dose 20 mg	2.5 mg/kg

- Plastic surgery is performed either as a cosmetic procedure to make a patient look younger, to improve their appearance, or as a reconstructive procedure to restore the forma and function of an area injured or altered by a congenital malformation, cancer, or trauma.
- The anesthetic approach (general versus local anesthesia and sedation) for plastic surgeries depends on the length of surgery, proximity of the surgery to the airway, surgeon preference, and patient condition.
- Wounds are typically closed in multiple layers with sutures (rarely with staples) which adds to the length of time for wound closure.
- Patients who smoke have increased difficulty with wound healing. Most plastic surgeons require smokers to sign a preoperative letter acknowledging that they smoke and that they have been informed of the associated risks. For some procedures—facelift, browlift, necklift—smoking cessation for 3 weeks prior to and 3 weeks after surgery is mandatory. A nicotine patch is also prohibited as it has similar vasoconstrictive effects to smoking. A urine continine test (an alkaloid found in tobacco and a metabolite of nicotine, can be found in the urine 2–4 days after nicotine use) can confirm nicotine use prior to surgery.
- Airway fire is a risk if cauterization (Bovie) or a laser is used. To prevent airway fires, use caution with oxygen during this procedure. Good communication with the surgeon is essential, especially as the airway is to be entered and tissue is to be cauterized. Of great concern is oxygen trapping by the surgical drapes. The creation of an "open field" that allows rapid dissipation of trapped oxygen is key. Fires can still occur when the surgeon and anesthesia provider have communicated and the oxygen is off prior to Bovie use, but trapped oxygen from prior use is still present in pockets of the drapes that can ignite rapidly. See the discussion of safety concerns in Chapter 1 for more information.
- Combined procedures can be done before the other: facelift → brow lift → blepharoplasty → rhinoplasty.
- Facial and throat surgery may require different intubating techniques or airway management. Typically, a rhinoplasty will require an oral RAE (a type of preformed "U-shaped" endotracheal tube) to allow the tube to be brought inferiorly so as to not interfere with the surgical approach. Similarly, nasal intubation is best used during a chin implant, resection of buccal fat, or when other oral reconstructive procedures are performed.
- Local anesthetics with epinephrine are given very frequently during plastic surgery to decrease the risk of bleeding and swelling. Whenever epinephrine is given, anticipate an increase in the patient's blood pressure (BP). *Pretreat patients* to prevent blood pressure increases, especially when surgery is done on very vascular areas such as the face and scalp. Also, pretreat any patient who has a history of cardiovascular problems such as hypertension. The goal is to prevent blood pressure spikes, not just to treat the blood pressure once it has already become elevated.
- Beta-blockers and vasodilators can be used to lower the blood pressure. Clonidine can be used as an adjunctive hypnotic and antihypertensive.
- Local anesthetics, with or without epinephrine, may be infiltrated at the surgical site to provide for intraoperative and postoperative analgesia. Monitor the EKG for ST-segment and heart rate changes.
- Mild, controlled hypotension may be requested to facilitate hemostasis.
- For plastic surgery to the nose, it is best to put in an endotracheal tube so that a cuff can be inflated and blood, debris, and mucus do not drain down into the lungs. The surgeon will usually place a throat pack, infiltrate the nose with a local anesthetic with epinephrine,

and place cocaine or Afrin soaked pledgets in the nasal cavity to minimize drainage of blood into the airway or stomach.

- Check with the surgeon regarding muscle relaxation requirements before giving these agents, as nerve monitoring may be done. Nerve monitoring is usually not done in an office setting, however.
- A propofol infusion with ketamine boluses can significantly reduce the need for IV opioids and decrease post-operative nausea and vomiting (very important in an outpatient cosmetic setting).
- With all plastic surgery cases, check for recent aspirin, NSAID, anticoagulant, and over-the-counter herbal supplement use. These agents affect platelet function.
  - Heparin must be stopped at least 4 hours prior to surgery.
  - Coumadin must be stopped at least 48 hours prior to surgery.
  - Plavix must be stopped 5 days prior to surgery.
  - Aspirin must be stopped at least 6 days prior to surgery.
  - All NSAIDS must be stopped one week before surgery, and
  - All herbal supplements two weeks prior to surgery.
- Hematoma and bleeding are a major risk with plastic surgery. Increased bleeding contributes to bruising, swelling and recovery from liposuction. Bleeding after a facelift may result in a hematoma that can expand and apply pressure to the recently undermined facial skin flap causing it to become ischemic with loss of facial tissue—a devastating complication. Bleeding after a blepharoplasty could produce a retrobulbar hematoma potentially compromising the optic nerve and leading to blindness. During a tummy tuck, a large area of skin is undermined which can accumulate a significant amount of blood prior to being recognized and may result in

hypotension and the need for urgent evacuation of the hematoma and hemostasis.

Herbals that Promote Bleeding and other Side Effects

- Garlic: inhibits platelet aggregation; increases INR
- Ginkgo biloba: can cause coagulopathy; enhances the effects of aspirin, NSAIDs, warfarin, and heparin; increases ICP
- Guarana (caffeine): can cause seizures, dysrhythmias, and brain vasoconstriction; inhibits platelet aggregation
- Ginseng: hypertension/CNS stimulation; decreases warfarin effects
- Echinacea: decreases corticosteroid efficacy

Sedating Herbal Agents

- Kava: CNS depressant/sedative; potentiates barbiturates, benzodiazepines, and muscle relaxation; decreases the effect of L-dopa treatment
- Valerian: CNS depressant; increases GABA levels
- St. John's wort: inhibits serotonin reuptake (SSRI); leads to exaggerated blood pressure responses

Herbals that Alter Functioning of the Autonomic Nervous System (and may Prolong Anesthesia)

- Ephedra
- Ginseng
- Guarana
- Licorice
- St. John's wort
- Yohimbe (alpha$_2$ blocker)

Antiemetics for Plastic Surgery

Plastic surgery can increase the risk of postoperative nausea and vomiting (PONV). Some centers have started to given ondansetron 4 mg by mouth the evening before surgery, the evening after surgery, and the morning of the day after surgery, along with ondansetron 4 mg IV 30–60 minutes before emergence from anesthesia during surgery. IV steroids (Decadron 8 mg) are given at the beginning of surgery as an adjunct to antiemetics and to help decrease swelling; these agents are given unless otherwise contraindicated. A scopolamine patch (1.5 mg) application behind the ear beginning the evening prior to surgery and continuing 48 hours post-operatively is an excellent adjunctive medication especially for those patients with a history of motion sickness.

The following characteristics make a person more vulnerable to PONV:

- Female
- Motion sickness history
- Nonsmoker
- Anxiety
- Surgery length greater than 45–60 minutes

Smooth emergence from anesthesia is important with these surgeries. The goal is to avoid coughing, bucking, or nausea/vomiting or retching so as to prevent increased risk of bleeding, hematoma formation, or suture line disruption from the increased head, neck, chest, and abdominal pressures. See Chapter 4 for more information regarding antiemetics.

FACE AND EARS

Blepharoplasty: Cosmetic Eyelid Surgery (Lid Lift)

Blepharoplasty is the excision of a protrusion of supraorbital fat and resection of excessive skin of the eyelids. This procedure is often done in combination with a brow lift. If the two are done together, the brow lift is done first to establish the baseline position of the brows to reveal the true mount of upper eyelid soft-tissue redundancy.

Removal of excessive, redundant skin and tissue of the upper or lower eyelids may be performed for functional or cosmetic reasons, or to reinforce the surrounding muscles and tendons.

Specific conditions treated in this way include blepharochalasis (inflammation and edema of eyelid leading to stretching), blepharoptosis (drooping of the upper eyelid), and Asian eyelid.

Operative Procedure
Open Blepharoplasty
The orbicularis oculi muscle is incised parallel at the apex of the eye bulge. Incisions in the upper lids are closed with fine sutures. This procedure can involve resection of skin, muscle (orbicularis oculi), and fat.

- *Upper lid:* The caudal margin of the excision is marked and the upper eyelid skin is pinched. An elliptical incision is made in the natural skin fold of the external upper lid. Excess fat is removed; the wound is closed.
- *Lower lid:* The procedure may be repeated for the lower lids; the incision is made below the lashes or from the inside surface (conjunctiva). The traditional approach is flap elevation, consisting of just skin or skin with attached muscle. The skin is draped upward and outward, and the surgeon excises the excess skin.

Place the dressing before arousing the patient.

CO_2 Laser Blepharoplasty
The fat and skin are resected with a laser instead of a scalpel.

Anesthetic
This surgery involves a very vascular area. Surgeons usually inject with epinephrine and local immediately after induction and then wait for 20 minutes prior to making a skin incision for maximum vasoconstriction.

The most common anesthetic method is MAC with local anesthesia with epinephrine. If the surgery consists of just blepharoplasty (i.e., no other procedure is done in conjunction with the blepharoplasty), then the surgeon will want the patient to be able to follow commands (open and close the eyes). An example regimen is midazolam given preoperatively and intraoperatively; fentanyl IV given based on the patient's respiratory rate; and propofol and ketamine given as a continuous infusion. For example, propofol 50 mL (500 mg) may be mixed with ketamine 50 mg infusion. If more propofol is needed (more than 500 mg), it is not mixed with ketamine.

The second most common anesthetic method is general anesthesia with a laryngeal airway mask (LMA) or an oral endotracheal tub (OETT); this option is appropriate if the blepharoplasty is done in conjunction with another procedure. An oral RAE to may be placed to minimize intrusion into the surgical field.

The greatest stimulation during blepharoplasty occurs during injection of local anesthetic by the surgeon, and again during excision of the median fat pad. Increase rate of infusion or bolus propofol/ketamine before both of these times. You can decrease the infusion rate after the stimulation is completed.

Short-acting narcotics should be used, as these patients are almost always treated on an outpatient basis.

Positioning
The patient is placed in a supine position, with bilateral arms tucked at the sides. The bed may be turned 90–180 degrees away from anesthetist. The head of the bed is elevated 10–30 degrees.

Anesthetic Implications
Electrocautery is used during this procedure, and airway fire is possible when the cautery is around the face. See the discussion of safety concerns in Chapter 1 for more information. One method to avoid the risks associated with use of oxygen around the face (with MAC anesthesia and use of nasal cannula) is as follows:

- Preoperatively, give the patient a vasoconstrictor nasal spray (phenylephrine [Neosynephrine]) to shrink the mucous membranes.

- Once the patient is sedated, place a nasal trumpet into one of the nares, which should be lubricated with lidocaine gel. Usually a size #7.0 trumpet is appropriate for women and a size #7.5 trumpet for men.
- The circulating RN will pass you a sterile red rubber catheter connected to tubing (like suction tubing but not attached to suction; it is attached to the oxygen source).
- Insert the red rubber catheter through the trumpet down the back of the hypopharynx.
- The other end of the tubing is attached to an oxygen source. You can "blend" your gases with this setup—giving a low percentage oxygen flow.

Whatever anesthetic method you choose, make sure you have a safe delivery of oxygen/air to the patient in an "oxygen-enriched environment."

Assess and document preoperative and postoperative vision. The surgeon will need the eyes untaped for a blepharoplasty procedure and will place eye lubricant for protection before starting. Some surgeons place eye protectors into the eyes (over the cornea) to protect them.

A local anesthetic and epinephrine solution is usually infiltrated to decrease swelling and to prevent bleeding during eyelid surgery. Monitor the total amounts of local anesthesia and epinephrine given. *See the local anesthetic chart at the beginning of this chapter.*

These patients are often women in their 50s and 60s, who commonly have a history of hypertension and possibly cardiovascular disease. Whenever epinephrine is given, anticipate an increase in the patient's blood pressure and monitor for EKG changes. Anticipate hypertension and *pretreat* (i.e., labetalol) to prevent blood pressure increases, especially in any patient who has a history of cardiovascular problems such as hypertension. The goal is to prevent blood pressure spikes, not just to treat the blood pressure once it has become elevated.

Mild controlled hypotension may be requested to facilitate hemostasis.

Smooth emergence from anesthesia is important with this surgery. The goal is to avoid coughing, bucking, or nausea/vomiting or retching so as to prevent increased risk of bleeding, hematoma formation, or suture line disruption from the increased head and neck pressures. Antiemetics should be given (see Chapter 4 and "Plastic Surgery Pearls" section in this chapter for more information).

Caution: The manipulation of periorbital fat can have very serious consequences.

Retrobulbar hematoma and blindness can occur postoperatively, and the oculocardiac reflex can complicate the intraoperative course with bradycardia and asystole. Have atropine and Robinul available.

Complications
Potential complications of blepharoplasty include hematoma and bleeding.

Brow Lift

A brow lift is the surgical resuspension of the eyebrows (for brow ptosis) and elimination of the forehead and glabellar (between eyebrows) creases and wrinkles. It is intended to restore a youthful appearance to the upper face. This procedure may be done in conjunction with a blepharoplasty (eyelid lift).

Operative Procedure
With an *endoscopic* approach, the surgeon works in the relatively avascular subgaleal/subperiosteal plane. Multiple smaller incisions are made within the scalp for access. Very small biting forceps are used beneath the flap. Sutures and fixation are done in the same way as the open brow lift. The endoscopic technique is used most frequently in women and men who do not require a large suspension. Men with very heavy set brows may have a coronal (incision all across the scalp) incision.

With an *open* approach, a complete bicoronal flap (in the hair line) is made; the scalp is elevated from the cranium from the vertex of the head to the orbital rims. Brows are elevated by scalp resuspension and/or resection using "key" fixation sutures. Maximal tension is placed laterally to elevate the lateral brow to a greater extent than the medial brow. The soft tissues may be fixated directly to the cranium with absorbable screws and to the temporal fascia with sutures to maintain their new positions. Release of the periosteum along the superior orbital rims is generally a prerequisite to adequate resuspension when using a subperiosteal approach. The scalp suture closure helps hold the resuspended position.

Incisions in the *subcutaneous plane* may be bicoronal or interrupted elliptical incisions. The incision is made in the hairline or in the hair-bearing scalp (which hides the incision line within the hair). The glabellar lines are improved by resecting the corrugator muscles (same muscles that are targets for Botox—this is akin to permanent Botox).

Anesthetic
These patients are often women in their 50s and 60s, who commonly have a history of hypertension and possibly cardiovascular disease. Plan for and *pretreat patients* for possible hypertension, especially when local anesthetics with epinephrine are given. This surgery involves a very vascular area. The goal is to prevent blood pressure spikes, not just to treat the blood pressure once it has become elevated.

General anesthesia with an OETT can be used. An oral RAE may be used to minimize intrusion into the surgical field.

Another anesthetic option is MAC with local anesthesia with epinephrine. This procedure can be done under IV sedation, but be aware of the potential length of the case when making this decision. An example regimen is midazolam given preoperatively and intraoperatively, fentanyl IV given based on the respiratory rate, and propofol and ketamine given as a continuous infusion. For example, propofol 50 mL (500 mg) may be mixed with ketamine 50 mg infusion. Start the infusion at a rate of 120–140 mcg/kg/min as soon as monitors are on the patient; maintain that rate through local anesthetic infiltration by the surgeon. Decrease the infusion rate to approximately 100 mcg/kg/min during periods of low stimulation. If more propofol is needed (more than 500 mg), it is not mixed with ketamine.

Positioning

The patient is placed in a supine, reverse Trendelenburg position, with the head of the bed elevated 20–25 degrees, and bilateral arms tucked at the sides. The bed is turned 90–180 degrees away from the anesthetist.

Anesthetic Implications

Short-acting narcotics should be used, as these patients are almost always treated on an outpatient basis.

Tape both eyelids closed; keep any tape or occlusive dressing away from the eyebrows. Place eye pads over both eyes, and cover the pads with occlusive clear dressings (Tegaderm) to protect the eyes from cleansing solutions and any movement or grazing of instruments by the surgeon or scrub team as they are working over the face.

Electrocautery is used during this procedure, and airway fire is possible when the cautery is around the face. See the discussion of safety concerns in Chapter 1 for more information. One method to avoid the risks associated with use of oxygen around the face (with MAC anesthesia and use of nasal cannula) is as follows:

- Preoperatively, give the patient a vasoconstrictor nasal spray (phenylephrine [Neo-Synephrine]) to shrink the mucous membranes.
- Once the patient is sedated, place a nasal trumpet into one of the nares, which should be lubricated with lidocaine gel. Usually a size #7.0 trumpet is appropriate for women and a size #7.5 trumpet for men.

- The circulating RN will pass you a sterile red rubber catheter connected to tubing (like suction tubing but not attached to suction; it is attached to the oxygen source).
- Insert the red rubber catheter through the trumpet down the back of the hypopharynx.
- The other end of the tubing is attached to an oxygen source. You can "blend" your gases with this setup—giving a low percentage oxygen flow.

Whatever anesthetic method you choose, make sure you have a safe delivery of oxygen/air to the patient in an "oxygen-enriched environment."

A local anesthetic and epinephrine solution is usually infiltrated to decrease swelling and to prevent bleeding during brow lift surgery. Monitor the total amounts of local anesthesia and epinephrine given. *See the local anesthetic chart at the beginning of this chapter.*

Whenever epinephrine is given, anticipate an increase in the patient's blood pressure and monitor for EKG changes. Anticipate hypertension and *pretreat* (i.e., labetalol) to prevent blood pressure increases, especially for any patient who has a history of cardiovascular problems such as hypertension. The goal is to prevent blood pressure spikes, not just to treat the blood pressure once it has become elevated. Mild controlled hypotension may be requested to facilitate hemostasis.

These patients are at high risk of having postoperative nausea and vomiting. Smooth emergence from anesthesia is important with these surgeries. The goal is to avoid coughing, bucking, or nausea/vomiting or retching so as to prevent increased risk of bleeding, hematoma formation, or suture line disruption from the increased head, neck, chest, and abdominal pressures. Give antiemetics prophylactically (see Chapter 4 and "Plastic Surgery Pearls" section in this chapter for more information).

These patients wake up with severe headaches, especially when the coronal approach is used.

Complications

Potential complications include injury to the supraorbital or the supratrochlear nerve branches, resulting in permanent, or more frequently, paresthesia, and hematoma.

Facelift (Rhytidectomy)

Rhytidectomy is the excision of excessive facial skin and repositioning of subcutaneous and deep plane tissues to restore a more youthful appearance to the face and neck.

Operative Procedure

The surgeon makes an incision that follows the anterior contour of the ear, extending superiorly into the scalp, inferiorly curving behind the posterior aspect of the ear, and extending posteriorly to the scalp. The skin and subcutaneous tissue of the face are elevated and raised as a flap, and then a second layer, the superficial musculoaponeurotic system (SMAS), is elevated and used to lift the deeper structures of the face. Sutures to the superficial musculoaponeurotic system (SMAS) layer are applied to mobilize and resuspend the tissues at the temple, in front of the ear, and behind the ear. The overlying skin is pulled and trimmed before suturing in place. Bleeding is monitored for before closing. A full neck/face wrap is placed before the patient awakens.

Anesthetic

The preferred anesthesia method is MAC with local anesthesia and epinephrine. An example regimen is midazolam given preoperatively and intraoperatively, fentanyl IV given based on the respiratory rate, and propofol and ketamine given as a continuous infusion. For example, propofol 50 mL (500 mg) may be mixed with ketamine 50 mg and given by infusion. Start the infusion at a rate of 120–140 mcg/kg/min as soon as monitors are on the patient; maintain that rate through local anesthetic infiltration by the surgeon. Decrease the infusion rate to approximately 100 mcg/kg/min during periods of low stimulation. If more propofol is needed (more than 500 mg), it is not mixed with ketamine.

Patients have a tendency to get uncomfortable in the bed during a long case. Propofol boluses can be administered as needed to keep the patient sedated.

Another anesthetic option is GETA. Short-acting narcotics should be used, as these patients are almost always treated on an outpatient basis. An oral RAE may be placed to minimize intrusion into the surgical field. The OETT can be tied with sutures around the tube and secured to the teeth to avoid placing tape around the mouth or face.

Positioning

The patient is placed in a supine, reverse Trendelenburg position, with the head of the bed elevated 20–25 degrees. Bilateral arms are tucked at the patient's sides.

Anesthetic Implications

Patients requesting a facelift procedure are usually older and may have multiple comorbid conditions. Medical clearance should be obtained preoperatively for any and all patients with a questionable history. Plan for and *pretreat patients* for possible hypertension, especially when local anesthetics with epinephrine are given. This surgery involves a very vascular area.

Question these patients about over-the-counter medications they take. Aspirin, NSAIDs, anticoagulants, and over-the-counter herbal supplements must all be stopped before surgery (see "pearls" at beginning of this chapter for more information). Hematoma and bleeding are major risks with the facelift procedure.

The surgeon will mark the face while the patient is in an upright position in the preoperative area.

Lubricate both of the patient's eyes. The surgeon will need the eyes untaped for a facelift procedure. Some surgeons place eye protectors into the eyes (over the cornea) to protect them.

One method to avoid the risks associated with use of oxygen around the face (with MAC anesthesia and use of nasal cannula) is as follows:

- Preoperatively, give the patient a vasoconstrictor nasal spray (phenylephrine [Neosynephrine]) to shrink the mucous membranes.
- Once the patient is sedated, place a nasal trumpet into one of the nares, which should have been lubricated with lidocaine gel. Usually a size #7.0 trumpet is appropriate for women and a size #7.5 trumpet for men.
- The circulating RN will pass you a sterile red rubber catheter connected to tubing (like suction tubing).
- Insert the red rubber catheter through the trumpet down the back of the hypopharynx.
- The other end of the tubing can be attached to an oxygen source. You can "blend" your gases with this setup—giving a low percentage oxygen flow.

Whatever anesthetic method you choose, ensure that there is a safe delivery of oxygen/air to the patient in an "oxygen-enriched environment." Electrocautery is used in this procedure, and airway fire is possible due to the use of cautery around the face. See the discussion of safety concerns in Chapter 1 for more information.

The length of the case for just a facelift can be 4–6 hours. If the facelift is done in conjunction with a brow lift, the case can be 6–7 hours in length; it can be 7–8 hours if a facelift, brow lift, and lid lift are done in same surgery. These patients need a urethral catheter to drain urine during the procedure. Patient body temperature is also a major concern: Place warming blankets over nonsurgical areas, administer warm fluids, and keep the room temperature warm.

A local anesthetic and epinephrine solution is usually infiltrated to decrease swelling and to prevent bleeding during rhytidectomy surgery. Monitor the total amounts of local anesthesia and epinephrine given. *See the local anesthetic chart at the beginning of this chapter.*

Whenever epinephrine is given, anticipate an increase in the patient's blood pressure and monitor for EKG changes. Anticipate hypertension and *pretreat* (i.e., labetalol) to prevent blood pressure increases, especially in any patient who has a history of cardiovascular problems such as hypertension. The goal is to *prevent* blood pressure spikes, not just to treat the blood pressure once it has become elevated. Mild controlled hypotension may be requested to facilitate hemostasis.

Hematoma formation is the most common complication with this procedure; any such hematoma must be surgically removed. Hypertension (either episodic or a history of hypertension) can increase the risk of intraoperative bleeding/hematoma formation. Anticipate and quickly treat this complication. Maintaining the patient's blood pressure within 20% of the baseline will help to prevent excessive bleeding and hematoma formation.

Hypotension should be communicated to the surgeon. Many surgeons do not want vasopressors given or "too much" crystalloid. They may want colloid IV solutions given, however; calcium chloride or ephedrine can be used to increase blood pressure.

At the end of the case, the patient's hair is washed to remove the prep solution and any blood.

These patients are at high risk of having postoperative nausea and vomiting. Smooth emergence from anesthesia is important with these surgeries. The goal is to avoid coughing, bucking, or nausea/vomiting or retching so as to prevent increased risk of bleeding, hematoma formation, or suture line disruption from the increased head, neck, chest, and abdominal pressures. Give antiemetics prophylactically (see Chapter 4 and "Plastic Surgery Pearls" section in this chapter for more information).

Patients have increased risk for deep venous thrombosis (DVT) and pulmonary embolism with a facelift procedure. For this reason, they should have compression stockings as well as inflation sleeves through the perioperative period. It is also very important to get the patient up and ambulating as soon as possible after surgery.

Nerve injury is possible to the facial nerve branches and the greater auricular nerve. Assess and document any preexisting facial movement abnormalities preoperatively.

Facial Laser Resurfacing: Dermabrasion

Dermabrasion involves sanding or lasering the skin to smooth it. This procedure is performed to smooth scars and surface irregularities (wrinkled or sun-damaged skin), remove benign skin growths of the facial skin, and treat enlarged oil glands of the nose for cosmetic rejuvenation.

Operative Procedure

The skin is held taut and the epidermis is abraded by a sanding cylinder and/or a wire brush. The area is irrigated with saline during and following the procedure.

Carbon dioxide lasers can also be used. Either very short pulsed or continuous light energy is delivered in a scanning pattern to remove thin layers of skin, with minimal heat damage to the surrounding tissues.

A moistened gauze dressing is applied; the wound should be kept moist for 10–21 days and not be allowed to scab. A compression bandage may be applied.

Anesthetic

Anesthesia consists of IV sedation with local anesthetic infiltrated wherever abrasion is to be done. If room air can be tolerated, this is ideal.

A full-face treatment may be done under GETA. Securely tape the ETT/LMA to the side of the mouth where the surgeon is not working to minimize intrusion into the surgical area.

Positioning

The patient is placed in a supine, reverse Trendelenburg position, with the head of the bed elevated 20–25 degrees, with bilateral arms tucked at the sides.

Anesthetic Implications

There is a fire risk with laser abrasion. See the discussion of safety concerns in Chapter 1 for more information.

Tape both eyelids closed. Place eye pads over both eyes, and cover them with occlusive clear dressings (Tegaderm) to protect the eyes from cleansing solutions and any movement or grazing of instruments by the surgeon or scrub team as they are working over the face. Eye "spoons" may be placed over eyes to protect them from laser light.

Mild controlled hypotension may be requested to facilitate hemostasis. Hypertension should be avoided and treated immediately. Anticipate hypertension and *pretreat patients* with, for example, labetalol. There is the possibility of hypertension and increased risk of bleeding with surgery to this very vascular area.

The anesthesia plan is designed to avoid coughing, bucking, or nausea/vomiting or retching so as to prevent increased risk of bleeding from the increased face and neck pressures. Give antiemetics prophylactically (see Chapter 4 and "Plastic Surgery Pearls" section in this chapter for more information).

Mentoplasty (Chin Prosthesis)

Mentoplasty is the correction of a small chin (micrognathia) with the insertion of an alloplastic chin prosthesis. This surgery is performed for cosmetic reasons.

Operative Procedure

Augmentation with a prosthesis may be either submental (into the submental region) or intraoral (into the labial sulcus). With either approach, a pocket is created just large enough to accommodate the prosthesis. The implant may be fixed with a deep mattress suture or secured with screws into the mandible. The wound is closed. A bulky dressing is applied.

Anesthetic

MAC with local anesthesia is often used.

GETA is used, but be aware that intubation may be difficult. A thorough preoperative airway exam is necessary in these patients. An oral RAE may be placed or an endonasal intubation done to minimize intrusion into the surgical field.

Positioning

The patient is placed in a supine, reverse Trendelenburg position, with the head of the bed elevated 20–25 degrees, with bilateral arms tucked at the sides.

Anesthetic Implications

Electrocautery is used, so airway fire is possible. See the discussion of safety concerns in Chapter 1 for more information.

A local anesthetic and epinephrine solution is usually infiltrated to decrease swelling and to prevent bleeding. Monitor the total amounts of local anesthesia and epinephrine given. *See the local anesthetic chart at the beginning of this chapter.* The amounts of local anesthetic and epinephrine given for a mentoplasty are usually small.

Whenever epinephrine is given, anticipate an increase in the patient's blood pressure and monitor for EKG changes. Anticipate hypertension and *pretreat* (i.e., labetalol) to prevent blood pressure increases, especially in any patient who has a history of cardiovascular problems such as hypertension. The goal is to prevent blood pressure spikes, not just to treat the blood pressure once it has become elevated. Mild controlled hypotension may be requested to facilitate hemostasis.

Give antiemetics to prevent nausea and vomiting (see Chapter 4 and "Plastic Surgery Pearls" section in this chapter for more information).

The patient should be wide awake before extubation is attempted.

Otoplasty (Ear Pinning)

Otoplasty involves correction of a protruding pinna of the ear or correction of other congenital deformities of the ears, including microtia (abnormal smallness of the auricle/pinna) and absent external ears (anotia). It may also seek to reduce the size of large ears or reshape the cartilage of the ear. This surgery is performed for cosmetic reasons—to improve the shape or proportion, or the position of the ear, or to correct a defect in the ear structure.

Operative Procedure

One or more incisions may be made, depending on what needs to be done. For "ear pinning," the only incision is the one behind the ear. The attempt is made to place each incision in a naturally occurring skin fold. Cartilage from the ear or rib is commonly used for reconstruction. Other ear changes may be made by moving or weakening ear structures. A bulky dressing is applied to the ear at the end of the surgery.

Anesthetic

In adults, MAC with local anesthetic is used. In patients who are younger than 16 years of age, general anesthesia with an OETT or LMA is usually done. If the patient is placed in the supine position, tape the endotracheal tube on the opposite side of the mouth from the surgical ear.

Positioning

The patient is placed in a supine or lateral decubitus position, with the operative ear in the upright position. Reverse Trendelenburg position, with the head of the bed elevated 20–25 degrees, may also be useful.

Anesthetic Implications

Otoplasty is usually performed on younger patients. Preoperative PO midazolam can help to decrease their anxiety about the surgical procedure.

Mild controlled hypotension may be requested to facilitate hemostasis. Anticipate hypertension and *pretreat patients* with, for example, labetalol, as bleeding is possible with surgery to this very vascular area.

Local anesthetics with epinephrine are given very frequently during otoplasty to decrease the risk of bleeding and swelling. Whenever epinephrine is given, anticipate an increase in the patient's blood pressure. *Pretreat patients* to prevent blood pressure increases, especially when surgery involves very vascular areas such as the face and scalp. Also, pretreatment is appropriate for any patient who has a history of cardiovascular problems such as hypertension. The goal is to prevent blood pressure spikes, not just to treat the blood pressure once it has become elevated.

Antiemetics should be given (see Chapter 4 and "Plastic Surgery Pearls" section in this chapter for more information). Avoid coughing, bucking, vomiting on emergence from anesthesia or postoperatively to avoid suture line strain and bleeding.

Rhinoplasty

Rhinoplasty is the surgical correction of the external appearance of the nose. Three steps may be done: tip remodeling (reduction or augmentation), hump removal, and narrowing of the nose. Other surgeries may also be done in combination with a rhinoplasty:

- *Alarplasty:* narrows the wide flaring and large opening of the nasal nostrils by wedge resection of the lateral nostrils with primary closure.
- *Septoplasty:* provides for surgical correction of any deformity of the nasal septum, the wall between the two nostrils.
- *Septorhinoplasty:* repairs the deviated septum in combination with a rhinoplasty

Rhinoplasty may be performed for cosmetic reasons; for traumatic, congenital, or developmental nasal malformations; or to alleviate nasal airway problems caused by a deviated septum that is unable to be fixed by closed reduction.

Operative Procedure

The postoperative difference between closed and open procedures is that the open procedure produces one small external incision at the base of the nose.

In the *closed* approach, the surgeon makes endonasal incisions, which are invisible after healing. These incisions are made into the nostril along the rim of the lower lateral cartilage bilaterally; the skin is then freed over the dorsal septum and the columella is freed anteriorly. Prominent septal, lateral, and alar cartilage is excised and retrimmed as necessary. The nasal bones are osteotomized laterally and medially and compressed to infracture (break without displacement) the bones, creating a more normal contour. The anterior septum, columella, alar, and marginal rim incisions are all sutured, and the septum is aligned.

In the *open* approach, an incision is made at the columella of the nose. This approach allows the surgeon to lift the skin off the nose for direct exposure of nasal anatomy and to shape the cartilage. It leaves an almost unnoticeable scar on the underside of the nose.

Augmentation can be done with synthetic material, cadaveric tissue, or autologous cartilage or bone (usually a piece of the nasal septum, ear concha, iliac crest, or rib). Skin tissue for grafting can be taken from the groin or temporoparietal region.

Intranasal packing is inserted, and a plastic splint is placed. A mustache dressing is placed under the nares.

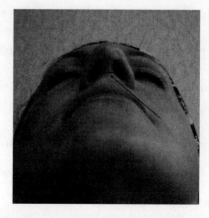

Figure 23-1 *Collumella Incision for Rhinoplasty*

Anesthetic

General anesthesia is used with an OETT with cuff; the ETT is taped to the middle of the bottom lip/jaw. The surgeon may prefer an oral RAE tube to keep the ETT out of the surgical area.

Local anesthetic (usually 4% cocaine) and epinephrine-soaked pledgets are placed in the operative nares before all nasal surgery begins. This measure is intended to decrease mucosal size and lower the risk of bleeding.

Keep the patient asleep until the nose splint is put on top of the nose or in the nares.

Positioning

The patient is placed in a supine, reverse Trendelenburg position, the head of the bed elevated 20–25 degrees, with a shoulder roll and arms tucked at the sides bilaterally. The head of the table may be turned away at least 90 degrees, if not 180 degrees, from the anesthetist.

Anesthetic Implications

A local anesthetic and epinephrine solution (vasoconstrictor-soaked nasal pack and/or infiltrated local anesthetic) is placed into the nares to decrease mucosal swelling and to minimize bleeding. Watch for an increase in heart rate or blood pressure.

Whenever epinephrine is given, anticipate an increase in the patient's blood pressure. *Pretreat patients* to prevent blood pressure increases, especially when surgery is done on very vascular areas such as the face and scalp. Also, pretreatment is appropriate for any patient who has a history of cardiovascular problems such as hypertension. The goal is to prevent blood pressure spikes, not just to treat the blood pressure once it has become elevated.

Mild controlled hypotension may be requested to facilitate hemostasis.

Lubricate both of the patient's eyes. They may need to be relubricated several times during the case.

A throat pack is usually placed to help prevent blood from entering the posterior pharynx. Document its insertion and removal times. A cuffed endotracheal tube should also be used in these cases.

These patients are at high risk of having postoperative nausea and vomiting. Smooth emergence from anesthesia is important with these surgeries. The goal is to avoid coughing, bucking, or nausea/vomiting or retching so as to prevent increased risk of bleeding, hematoma formation, or suture line disruption from the increased head, neck, chest, and abdominal pressures. Give antiemetics prophylactically (see Chapter 4 and "Plastic Surgery Pearls" section in this chapter for more information).

Suction the back of the patient's throat gently with a soft suction catheter before extubating him or her.

Postoperative oxygenation should be delivered by facemask or face tent, as the nose is usually packed. No pressure should be placed on the nose.

NECK

Neck Lift

A neck lift seeks to lift and resuspend the soft tissues of the neck for cosmetic rejuvenation purposes. This procedure is usually done in conjunction with a facelift and/or liposuction.

Operative Procedure

If the neck lift is done in conjunction with a facelift, the inferior incision (curving behind the posterior aspect of the ear) is dissected more inferiorly to just below the jaw line. A second incision in the submental crease is also used to allow for a platysmaplasty—tightening of the platysma to correct platysmal bands and improve the contour of the neck and also permits access to the subplatysmal space for direct fat removal.

A drain may be placed, and the skin is sutured closed. A full neck/face wrap is placed before the patient awakens.

Anesthetic

General anesthesia is used with an OETT, which should consist of a straight endotracheal tube. Muscle relaxation should not be needed.

Positioning

The patient is placed in a supine, reverse Trendelenburg position, with the head of the bed elevated 20–25 degrees, with bilateral arms tucked at the sides.

Anesthetic Implications

These patients are often men and women older than 50 years of age, who commonly have a history of hypertension and possibly cardiovascular disease. A local anesthetic and epinephrine solution is usually infiltrated to decrease swelling, for intraoperative hemostasis/avoidance of hematoma formation, and for postoperative pain control, especially when surgery is done on very vascular areas such as the face and neck. Monitor the total amounts of local anesthesia and epinephrine given. *See the local anesthetic chart at the beginning of this chapter.*

Whenever epinephrine is given, anticipate an increase in the patient's blood pressure and monitor for EKG changes. Anticipate hypertension and *pretreat* (with i.e., labetalol) to prevent blood pressure increases, especially in any patient who has a history of cardiovascular problems such as hypertension. The goal is to prevent blood pressure spikes, not just to treat the blood pressure once it has become elevated.

Mild controlled hypotension may be requested to facilitate hemostasis.

These patients are at high risk of having postoperative nausea and vomiting. Smooth emergence from anesthesia is important with these surgeries. The goal is to avoid coughing, bucking, or nausea/vomiting or retching so as to prevent increased risk of bleeding, hematoma formation, or suture line disruption from the increased head, neck, chest, and abdominal pressures. Give antiemetics prophylactically (see Chapter 4 and "Plastic Surgery Pearls" section in this chapter for more information).

BREAST

Breast Implants

Surgical augmentation of one or both breasts with (an) implant(s) is performed to enlarge the breasts.

Operative Procedure

Either an inframammary, periareolar or axillary incision is used and then either a retromammary or subpectoral pocket is created for the implant. Prior to placement of the implant a sizer is placed and inflated. Once the pocket is sufficient, a saline or silicone implant is placed. The saline implants are then filled with saline (the silicone implants come prefilled).

Once the surgeon places the implant, the anesthetist will need to raise the head of the bed to a high Fowler's position; this allows the breasts to fall into a more natural position to check for symmetry and placement on the chest. Before raising the head of the bed, deepen the anesthetic to prevent bucking or movement. Hypotension can occur when the head of the bed is raised; a fluid bolus may be used to maintain blood pressure. Implants are placed one at a time, the head of the bed may need to be raised more than once.

These cases commonly last from 45 to 75 minutes.

Anesthetic

The most common method of anesthesia is MAC with local anesthesia and epinephrine. An example regimen is midazolam given preoperatively and intraoperatively; fentanyl IV given based on the respiratory rate; and propofol and ketamine given as a continuous infusion. For example, propofol 50 mL (500 mg) may be mixed with ketamine 50 mg infusion. Start the infusion at a rate of 120–140 mcg/kg/min as soon as monitors are on the patient; maintain that rate through local anesthetic infiltration by the surgeon. Decrease the infusion rate to approximately 100 mcg/kg/min during periods of low stimulation. Increase the infusion rate before insertion of the other breast implant and decrease the rate after the implant has been seated. If more propofol is needed (more than 500 mg), it is not mixed with ketamine.

General anesthesia with a LMA may be needed if the patient cannot tolerate MAC anesthesia. If a LMA is inserted, increased volatile agent can be given with less narcotic.

A third anesthetic option is GETA with insertion of an OETT.

Short-acting narcotics should be used, as these patients are almost always treated on an outpatient basis.

Positioning

The patient is placed in a supine position, with bilateral arms on padded armboards. The feet should be supported on a padded footboard. The arms must be secured so that they do not fall off the armboards when the head of the bed is put into high Fowler's position.

Anesthetic Implications

The FDA guidelines approve silicone implants for woman at least 22 years of age and saline implants for women at least 18 years of age.

A local anesthetic and epinephrine solution is usually infiltrated to decrease swelling and to prevent bleeding during breast implant surgery. Monitor the total amounts of local anesthesia and epinephrine given. *See the local anesthetic chart at the beginning of this chapter.*

Whenever epinephrine is given, anticipate an increase in the patient's blood pressure and monitor for EKG changes. Anticipate hypertension and *pretreat* (i.e., labetalol) to prevent blood pressure increases, especially in any patient who has a history of cardiovascular problems such as hypertension. The goal is to prevent blood pressure spikes, not just to treat the blood pressure once it has become elevated.

Mild controlled hypotension may be requested to facilitate hemostasis.

Is this patient post-mastectomy? If so, she may be post-chemotherapy and/or radiation therapy. Tissues in such cases may be friable; the patient may have had or be having multiple procedures. Depression, heightened sensitivity to pain, and other issues must be considered in these patients.

The surgeon will mark the skin while the patient is in an upright position in the preoperative area.

Have an extra-long length of ventilator circuit tubing available to accommodate putting the head of the bed in the high Fowler's position.

These patients are at high risk for having post-operative nausea and vomiting. Smooth emergence from anesthesia is important with these surgeries. The goal is to avoid coughing, bucking, or nausea/vomiting or retching so as to prevent increased risk of bleeding, hematoma formation, or suture line disruption from the increased head, neck, chest, and abdominal pressures. Give antiemetic prophylaxis (see Chapter 4 and "Plastic Surgery Pearls" section in this chapter for more information).

A bulky dressing and a surgical bra are applied at the end of the case. Sitting the patient up, after extubation but while she is still on the operating room table, will help position the bra around the patient's back.

Complications

Potential complications include bleeding, seroma, infection, scarring, fat or clot pulmonary emboli, and pneumothorax.

Capsulotomy

Capsulotomy is the surgical removal or release of thickened scar tissue that has formed around a breast implant. It can be a unilateral or bilateral procedure.

All breast implants, and any implantable device for that matter, (a vascular port, pacemaker, etc) will be walled off from the body by a thin capsule shortly after placement. Usually the capsule remains thin and is not noticed by the patient; however, in some instances the capsule may become firm and calcified—called capsular contracture. This condition has an unknown etiology, but is thought to be related to an autoimmune cause. It is believed that the use of perioperative antibiotics as well as irrigation of the pocket prior to implant placement with an antibiotic solution will decrease the risk of capsular contraction. Silicone implants are associated with significantly higher rates of scar formation, as silicone can microscopically leak through the implant shell, causing calcification and hardening of the surrounding breast tissue. Placing the implants under the pectoralis muscle will reduce scar formation.

Operative Procedure

- *Open capsulotomy:* the capsule is incised and the implant is removed. The entire capsule, except that affixed to the chest wall or pectoralis major muscle, is removed and a new implant is placed. The new implant may be returned to the original pocket or placed in a new location. Women who have experienced capsular contracture are at a higher risk of forming a hard capsule again.

A bulky dressing and a surgical bra are applied at the end of the case.

Anesthetic
Local anesthetic with IV sedation may be used if the capsule is small, although GETA may be better option. Removing a capsule is very stimulating and painful.

Positioning
The patient is placed in a supine position.

Anesthetic Implications
The blood pressure cuff and the peripheral IV will both be placed on the nonoperative side arm. If the capsulotomy is done bilaterally, place the blood pressure cuff and IV on the leg.

The surgeon will mark the skin while the patient is in an upright position in the preoperative area.

Pretreat patients to prevent blood pressure increases. In addition, pretreatment is indicated for any patient who has a history of cardiovascular problems such as hypertension. The goal is to prevent blood pressure spikes, not just treat to the blood pressure once it has become elevated.

Make sure to have an extra-long length of ventilator circuit tubing to accommodate putting the head of the bed into high Fowler's position if breast positioning is checked.

These patients are at high risk of having postoperative nausea and vomiting. Smooth emergence from anesthesia is important with these surgeries. The goal is to avoid coughing, bucking, or nausea/vomiting or retching so as to prevent increased risk of bleeding, hematoma formation, or suture line disruption from the increased head, neck, chest, and abdominal pressures. Give antiemetics prophylactically (see Chapter 4 and "Plastic Surgery Pearls" section in this chapter for more information).

A bulky dressing and a surgical bra are applied at the end of the case. Sitting the patient up, after extubation but while she is still on the operating room table, will help position the bra around the patient's back.

Excision of Male Gynecomastia

This procedure provides for excision of excessive breast tissue (gynecomastia) in the male that has become feminized (round areola, inframammary fold, and larger breasts).

Operative Procedure
May be performed strictly by liposuction (usually by ultrasound); liposuction and resection of some breast gland in a pattern similar to a female breast reduction depending on the extent of the gynecomastia.

Anesthetic

GETA is used.

Positioning

The patient is placed in a supine position, with bilateral arms on padded armboards. The feet should be supported on a padded footboard. The arms must be secured so that they do not fall off the armboards when the head of the bed is put into high Fowler's position.

Anesthetic Implications

The surgeon will mark the skin while the patient is in an upright position in the preoperative area.

Extra anxiolytics may be needed, especially in a young male patient.

These patients are at a large risk of having postoperative nausea and vomiting. Smooth emergence from anesthesia is important with these surgeries. The goal is to avoid coughing, bucking, or nausea/vomiting or retching so as to prevent increased risk of bleeding, hematoma formation, or suture line disruption from the increased head, neck, chest, and abdominal pressures. Give antiemetics prophylactically (see Chapter 4 and "Plastic Surgery Pearls" section in this chapter for more information).

Anticipate hypertension and *pretreat* patients with, for example, labetalol. Both bleeding and hematoma are possible with surgery to this vascular area.

A bulky dressing and a surgical bra are applied at the end of the case.

Mammoplasty: Breast Augmentation

This type of mammoplasty seeks to enlarge the breast(s) by implanting a prosthesis. This procedure is performed in patients with small breasts, unilaterally or bilaterally; sagging of the breast tissue; ptosis; and postsurgical deformity.

Operative Procedure

The breast implant(s) are placed under either the mammary gland or the pectoral muscle. Either of

these pockets (implant positions) can be accessed by the following three incisions:

- *Inframammary:* A 2.5–5 cm incision is made just below the inframammary crease. The implant is then placed either under the mammary gland, or a pocket is created beneath the pectoralis major muscle to house the implant. Meticulous hemostasis is obtained, and the incisions are closed. Intercostal nerve damage is possible with the inframammary technique.
- *Peri-areolar:* The incision is made around the inferior border of the areola. The subcutaneous tissue is cut away to the inferior border of the breast, and a pocket is created to hold the prosthesis in the retromammary or subglandular space. The prosthesis is inserted, meticulous hemostasis is obtained, and the areolar incision is closed.
- *Transaxillary:* The incision (oblique or vertical) is made in the axilla and cut down through the subcutaneous tissue. The prosthesis is inserted, meticulous hemostasis is obtained, and the incision is closed. A suction unit may be applied.

Before placing the permanent implant, a "sizer" is inserted into the space created for the implant. The sizer is filled with fluid, and then the breasts are temporarily sutured closed.

During this part of the procedure, the surgeon will ask for the head of the bed to be raised to a high Fowler's position, which allows the breasts to fall into a more natural position, to check for symmetry and placement on the chest. Before raising the head of the bed, deepen the anesthetic to prevent bucking or movement. Hypotension can occur when the head of the bed is raised; fluid boluses can be administered to maintain blood pressure.

Once symmetry, size, and placement of the sizers are checked, the head of the bed will be lowered to a flat, supine position. The sizers are removed and the prostheses are inserted. Meticulous hemostasis is obtained, and the incision is closed in layers. A bulky dressing and a surgical bra are applied at the end of the case.

Anesthetic

Anesthesia options include either GETA or local anesthesia with sedation.

Positioning

The patient is placed in a supine position, with bilateral arms on padded armboards. The feet should be supported on a padded footboard. The arms must be secured so that they do not fall off the armboards when the head of the bed is put into high Fowler's position.

Anesthetic Implications

The surgeon will mark the skin while the patient is in an upright position in the preoperative area.

A local anesthetic and epinephrine solution is usually infiltrated to decrease swelling and to prevent bleeding during breast surgery. Monitor the total amounts of local anesthesia and epinephrine given. *See the local anesthetic chart at the beginning of this chapter.*

Whenever epinephrine is given, anticipate an increase in the patient's blood pressure and monitor for EKG changes. Anticipate hypertension and *pretreat* (i.e., labetalol) to prevent blood pressure increases, especially in any patient who has a history of cardiovascular problems such as hypertension. The goal is to prevent blood pressure spikes, not just to treat the blood pressure once it has become elevated.

Mild controlled hypotension may be requested to facilitate hemostasis.

These patients are at high risk of having postoperative nausea and vomiting. Smooth emergence from anesthesia is important with these surgeries. The goal is to avoid coughing, bucking, or nausea/vomiting or retching so as to prevent increased risk of bleeding, hematoma formation, or suture line disruption from the increased head, neck, chest, and abdominal pressures. Give antiemetics prophylactically (see Chapter 4 and "Plastic Surgery Pearls" section in this chapter for more information).

Make sure to have an extra-long length of ventilator circuit tubing to accommodate putting the head of the bed up in high Fowler's position.

A bulky dressing and a surgical bra are applied at the end of the case. Sitting the patient up, after extubation but while still on the operating room table, will help position the bra around the patient's back.

Complications

Monitor the patient for hematoma formation.

Mammoplasty: Breast Reduction

This procedure involves excision of excessive breast tissue and reconstruction of the breasts. The principal indication for this procedure is alleviation of symptoms associated with breast weight.

Operative Procedure

In general, there are two types of procedures performed: a Wise pattern incision which leaves an inverted "T" pattern on the breast (also known as an anchor incision pattern), and a vertical reduction pattern, also known as a lollipop incision pattern. In the latter, only an incision around the nipple and a vertical incision to the inframammary crease is used. The nipple is kept on a breast pedicle to preserve its blood supply and ensure its survival as it is relocated to a more superior location on the chest. Less commonly, the nipple is removed and reapplied after the lift as a free nipple graft in patients that have very long, pendulous breasts where a pedicle would not survive.

An incision circumscribes the areola, which is usually left attached to the underlying tissue as a pedicle graft. Tissue and skin flaps are developed under the nipple, with the surgeon excising a wedge of breast skin and adipose tissue inferiorly in an anchor shape. Excess skin and breast tissue are excised; breast tissue is weighed as it is removed so that an equivalent amount is taken from each breast. The breast is reconstructed by approximating the medial and lateral breast tissue with skin flaps inferior to the nipple site and transversely, in the inframammary fold.

During this part of the procedure, the surgeon will ask for the head of the bed to be raised to a high Fowler's position, which allows the breasts to fall into a more natural position, to check for symmetry and placement on the chest.

Once symmetry, size, and placement of the breasts are checked, the head of the bed will be lowered to a flat, supine position. Meticulous hemostasis is obtained, and the incision is closed in layers. A suction unit is applied. A bulky dressing and a surgical bra are applied at the end of the case.

Anesthetic

General anesthesia is used with insertion of an OETT or LMA.

Positioning

The patient is placed in a supine position, with bilateral arms on padded armboards. The feet should be supported on a padded footboard. Once the surgeon removes the anticipated amount of breast tissue and temporarily sutures the breasts closed, the anesthetist will need to raise the head of the bed to high Fowler's position to allow the breasts to fall into a more natural position, to check for symmetry. The arms must be secured so that they do not fall off the armboards when the head of the bed is put into high Fowler's position.

Anesthetic Implications

The surgeon will mark the skin while the patient is in an upright position in the preoperative area.

A local anesthetic and epinephrine solution is usually infiltrated to decrease swelling and to prevent bleeding during breast surgery. Monitor the total amounts of local anesthesia and epinephrine given. *See the local anesthetic chart at the beginning of this chapter.*

Whenever epinephrine is given, anticipate an increase in the patient's blood pressure and monitor for EKG changes. Anticipate hypertension and *pretreat* (i.e., labetalol) to prevent blood pressure increases, especially in any patient who has a history of cardiovascular problems such as hypertension. The goal is to prevent blood pressure spikes, not just to treat the blood pressure once it has become elevated.

Mild controlled hypotension may be requested to facilitate hemostasis.

These patients are at high risk of having postoperative nausea and vomiting. Smooth emergence from anesthesia is important with these surgeries. The goal is to avoid coughing, bucking, or nausea/vomiting or retching so as to prevent increased risk of bleeding, hematoma formation, or suture line disruption from the increased head, neck, chest, and abdominal pressures. Give antiemetics prophylactically (see Chapter 4 and "Plastic Surgery Pearls" section in this chapter for more information).

Make sure to have an extra-long length of ventilator circuit tubing to accommodate putting the head of the bed up in high Fowler's position.

Before raising the head of the bed, deepen the anesthetic to prevent bucking or movement. Hypotension can occur when the head of the bed is raised; fluid boluses may be administered to maintain blood pressure.

A bulky dressing and a surgical bra are applied at the end of the case. Sitting the patient up, after extubation but while still on the operating room table, will help position the bra around the patient's back.

A single peripheral IV may be placed in the foot for bilateral breast surgery.

Complications

Potential complications include decreased blood supply and/or decreased sensation to the nipple and possible hematoma formation.

Mastopexy

Mastopexy is done to lift the breast on the chest wall. This procedure may be done in combination with breast augmentation for women who also want larger breasts. It is also done to treat breast ptosis.

Operative Procedure
This surgery resembles reduction mammoplasty, except that the breast tissue is usually not removed.

- *Periareolar:* a crescent-shaped incision above the nipple
- *Circumareolar:* an incision made around the nipple
- *Vertical:* a "V-shaped" incision that extends around the top of the areola and down the midline of the breast
- *Anchor:* an "anchor-shaped" incision that extends around the top of the areola and laterally across the lower portion of the breast

The areola is incised, skin flaps are made, and the nipple is then moved to a higher position on the chest wall. If breast augmentation is to be done with a mastopexy, sizers are placed first. The skin is redraped and temporarily sutured closed. Once the surgeon lifts the breast tissue, the anesthetist will need to raise the head of the bed to high Fowler's position to allow the breasts to fall into a more natural position, so that the surgeon can check for symmetry and placement on the chest.

Before raising the head of the bed, the anesthetic should be deepened to prevent bucking or movement. Hypotension can occur when the head of the bed is raised; fluid boluses can be administered to maintain blood pressure.

Meticulous hemostasis is obtained, and the incision is closed in layers.

Anesthetic
GETA is used with insertion of an OETT or LMA.

Positioning
The patient is placed in a supine position, with bilateral arms on padded armboards. The feet should be supported on a padded footboard. The arms must be secured so that they do not fall off the armboards when the head of the bed is put into high Fowler's position.

Anesthetic Implications
The surgeon will mark the skin while the patient is in an upright position in the preoperative area.

A local anesthetic and epinephrine solution is usually infiltrated to decrease swelling and to prevent bleeding during breast surgery. Monitor the total amounts of local anesthesia and epinephrine given. *See the local anesthetic chart at the beginning of this chapter.*

Whenever epinephrine is given, anticipate an increase in the patient's blood pressure and monitor for EKG changes. Anticipate hypertension and *pretreat* (i.e., labetalol) to prevent blood pressure increases, especially in any patient who has a history of cardiovascular problems such as hypertension. The goal is to prevent blood pressure spikes, not just to treat the blood pressure once it has become elevated.

Mild controlled hypotension may be requested to facilitate hemostasis.

These patients are at high risk of having postoperative nausea and vomiting. Smooth emergence from anesthesia is important with these surgeries. The goal is to avoid coughing, bucking, or nausea/vomiting or retching so as to prevent increased risk of bleeding, hematoma formation, or suture line disruption from the increased head, neck, chest, and abdominal pressures. Give antiemetics prophylactically (see Chapter 4 and "Plastic Surgery Pearls" section in this chapter for more information).

Make sure to have an extra-long length of ventilator circuit tubing to accommodate putting the head of the bed up in high Fowler's position.

A bulky dressing and a surgical bra are applied at the end of the case. Sitting the patient up, after extubation but while still on the operating room table, will help position the bra around the patient's back.

A single peripheral IV may need to be placed in the foot for bilateral breast surgery.

ABDOMEN

Abdominoplasty

Abdominoplasty is the surgical removal of loose, redundant abdominal skin and underlying subcutaneous fat, with repair of the rectus abdominus muscle as necessary.

This procedure is performed for cosmetic rejuvenation and improved function. It is often done in combination with liposuction of the upper abdominal area or flanks.

The incision usually extends from hip to hip (often in a previous scar from a hysterectomy or C-section). The rectus abdominus are paired muscles (create the "six-pack" in thin patients) that extend from the xiphoid region to the symphysis pubis; these paired muscles can separate from the midline and widen with aging and after pregnancy. Plastic surgeons can suture the fascia overlying the rectus abdominus muscles and relocate them to the midline thereby restoring a patient's waist and flattening their abdominal wall. Occasionally, the plastic surgeon will repair a small umbilical or ventral hernia at the time of the abdominoplasty. A new umbilicus is made (the umbilicus is preserved on its original stalk and just brought out through a new aperature in the skin).

Abdominoplasty is not to be confused with a panniculectomy. A *panniculectomy* is performed in the hospital to remove the pannus or "apron" that hangs down off the abdominal wall over the pubic region and occasionally down to the knees. It is performed for patients with recurrent infections of the pannus (panninculitis) and does not involve any muscle work and usually the umbilicus is not saved. Sometimes performed in conjunction with a general surgeon who repairs a ventral or umbilical hernia.

Operative Procedure

Partial (modified) abdominoplasty (mini tummy tuck) is usually done on patients who are within 10% of their ideal body weight and have a good waist contour and just a little lower bulge of redundant skin and a small amount of localized fat that needs to be removed to flatten their abdomen. This procedure utilizes a smaller incision made transversely above the pubis bone; the navel is left in its natural position.

Full abdominoplasty is done on patients who are usually greater than 20% above their ideal weight; it is frequently undertaken in combination with liposuction. A diamond-shaped incision is made around the navel and preserved for later replacement through the flap. A low-transverse abdominal incision is made above the mons, extending out bilaterally to the anterior iliac spines. Dissection is begun at the lower portion of the incision and progressed upward to the inferior aspect of the ribs; the amount of tissue removed is carefully selected with the patient in a beach-chair position to permit the maximum amount of tissue removal. The skin flap and subcutaneous tissue are raised and placed up on the chest, while the rectus abdominus is repaired or folded over (plication) to provide tight musculature. (In plication, the lateral edges of a muscle are both folded over toward the middle and secured.) Electrocautery is used to stop any bleeding. A hernia affecting the rectus muscle may be repaired with mesh.

The deep fat is closed with heavy absorbable suture, while the skin is closed with a subcuticular running suture. The umbilicus is located and brought through to the skin surface and drains are placed. An abdominal binder or compression garment may be placed.

Anesthetic

General endotracheal anesthesia (GETA); rapid-sequence induction is needed if the patient is obese. Muscle relaxation is required for abdominal muscle plication. An abdominoplasty is frequently performed as an outpatient; panniculectomy patients are admitted. If done on an outpatient basis, use short-acting narcotics.

Positioning

The patient is placed in a supine position, with bilateral arms extended on armboards; the arms should be padded and wrapped to prevent movement when flexing the bed for closure. The patient is placed in a slightly flexed, semi-Fowler's position to prevent strain on suture lines; the patient should stay in this position from the OR table, into recovery, and postoperatively. Educate the patient to stay in the "granny" position when walking upright and lying in bed for several days.

Anesthetic Implications

The surgeon will mark the skin while the patient is in an upright position in the preoperative area.

These cases are usually 3–5 hours long, so patient body temperature is a major concern. Use warming blankets over nonsurgical areas, warm fluids, and keep the room temperature warm.

Third-space loss and fluid shifts can occur with this surgery. Have two peripheral IVs in place for infusion of warmed fluids.

Anticipate hypertension and *pretreat* the patient (i.e., labetalol) to prevent blood pressure increases. Also, pretreatment is indicated for any patient who has a history of cardiovascular problems such as hypertension. The goal is to prevent blood pressure spikes, not just to treat the blood pressure once it has become elevated.

There is an increased risk for deep venous thrombosis (DVT) and pulmonary embolism with abdominoplasty. Patients should have compression stockings as well as inflation sleeves throughout the perioperative period. It is also very important to get the patient up and ambulating as soon as possible after surgery. Consider Lovenox administration prior to incision.

Abdominal and truncal contouring is commonly performed in post-bariatric surgery patients who have large areas of redundant skin. These patients often have comorbid chronic conditions such as hypertension and Type-2 diabetes and might still be obese. They may require a medical clearance before having office-based surgery. These individuals tend to have a high body mass index (BMI) and can have vascular access issues.

Sometimes the abdominoplasty will extend all around the patient: a circumferential belt lipectomy. During a belt lipectomy, an entire conically shaped amount of tissue is removed so the incision line extends 360 degrees around the patient. These case are longer than traditional abdominoplasties and require two position changes during the case. Most patients begin supine and then move onto one lateral side, and finally a flip to the other lateral side. Liposuction of the lateral thigh is frequent with this type of surgery.

Avoid coughing, bucking, and vomiting on emergence from anesthesia or postoperatively to avoid suture line strain and bleeding. Antiemetics should be given (see Chapter 4 and "Plastic Surgery Pearls" section in this chapter for more information).

LIPOSUCTION

Liposuction (Lipectomy)

Liposuction is the removal of subcutaneous fat deposits through use of a high-pressure suctioning device or ultrasonic emulsifying suction device. This procedure is performed for cosmetic rejuvenation and to improve body contour. It is best performed in patients who are not obese, but rather have localized, resistant adipose deposits. It is not a weight-loss procedure.

Operative Procedure

The surgeon will first infiltrate a wetting solution of local anesthetic and epinephrine to reduce bleeding and provide postoperative analgesia. The wetting solution usually consists of a local anesthetic (i.e., lidocaine) and epinephrine or just epinephrine that is added to one liter of lactated Ringer's solution. One milliliter of wetting solution is instilled into the body tissues for every one milliliter of fat to be resected. This solution can continue to be absorbed over a 36- to 48-hour period, so patients may need to be monitored for pulmonary edema perioperatively. Careful intake and output measurements must be made in surgery.

Through a small incision, a blunt suction tip is inserted and used to tunnel under the skin, separating it from the subcutaneous and connective tissues. By inserting and withdrawing the suction tip, the surgeon removes the fat by suction. The amount of fat that can be removed depends on the total amount of local anesthetic that is put into the wetting solution. If *only* epinephrine is added to the liter of lactated Ringer's solution, there is no limit to the amount of fat that can be suctioned off. It is important to monitor the percentage of local anesthetic and document how much is added to the wetting solution. There is a limit to how much wetting solution can be instilled in an office-based setting.

The ultrasonic liposuction procedure liquefies fat before its removal, allowing greater amounts of fat to be removed with less bleeding.

The incision is closed and a compression dressing is applied. A special "girdle" (a compression garment named depending on the area of the body where liposuction performed) is placed to reduce swelling and risk of bleeding.

Anesthetic
For liposuction of small areas, IV sedation local anesthetic and epinephrine is used. A spinal or epidural may also be given, or GETA is used with insertion of an OETT or LMA.

Positioning
The patient's position is selected so as to allow the surgical area to be upright and accessible. A flexed position is useful to decrease the strain on the surgical area or on incision lines.

Anesthetic Implications
It is very important to tally the running total of local anesthetic used by the surgeon. *See the local anesthetic chart at the beginning of this chapter.*

The surgeon will mark the skin while the patient is in an upright position in the preoperative area.

Limit the amount of peripheral IV fluid administered during this procedure, as the patient is being instilled with large amounts of wetting solution. Diuretics may need to be given if the patient absorbs the wetting solution. Patients who have absorbed wetting solution and any patients undergoing large-volume liposuction (greater than 5 liters of wetting solution instilled) should be observed overnight. Watch for fluid shifts, pulmonary edema, and a decreasing hematocrit level.

IV steroids can be given to help decrease swelling, unless otherwise contraindicated.

These patients are at high risk of having postoperative nausea and vomiting. Smooth emergence from anesthesia is important with these surgeries. The goal is to avoid coughing, bucking, or nausea/vomiting or retching so as to prevent increased risk of bleeding, hematoma formation, or suture line disruption from the increased head, neck, chest, and abdominal pressures. Give antiemetics prophylactically (see Chapter 4 and "Plastic Surgery Pearls" section in this chapter for more information).

Whenever epinephrine is given, anticipate an increase in the patient's blood pressure and monitor for EKG changes. Anticipate hypertension and *pretreat* (i.e., labetalol) to prevent blood pressure increases, especially in any patient who has a history of cardiovascular problems such as hypertension. The goal is to prevent blood pressure spikes, not just to treat the blood pressure once it has become elevated.

Mild controlled hypotension may be requested to facilitate hemostasis.

Complications
Multiple serious complications are associated with liposuction, including moderate blood loss, fat emboli, pulmonary emboli, pulmonary edema with fluid overload, local anesthetic toxicity, and pneumothorax or body cavity perforation from suction

cannula insertion. While less serious, hypothermia is a common complication of liposuction. To guard against this problem, wetting solutions should be warmed and warming blankets placed over all non-operative areas.

EXTREMITY

Palmar Fasciectomy

Palmar fasciectomy is the excision—either partial or total—of the fascia of the palm. It is indicated to treat Dupuytren's contracture, a hereditary condition caused by hyperplasia of fibrous tissue in the palmar subcutaneous tissues with nodules fixed to the palmar fascia. Subsequent contracture results in deformity and/or contractures of the dermis or digits limiting full extension.

Operative Procedure

For less involved presentations, a short longitudinal palmar incision is made adjacent to the restrictive band, which is resected. For more extensive disease, a longer incision with a Z-plasty arrangement is employed (zig-zag), resecting the palmar fascia distally. Wound closure may be done by primary suture or full-thickness free skin graft. An anterior splint is applied.

Anesthetic

Anesthetic options include either IV sedation and local anesthetic or a regional block.

Positioning

The patient is placed in a supine position, with the nonoperative arm secured on a padded armboard with the shoulder at an angle less than 90 degrees.

Anesthetic Implications

A compression tourniquet is used, with a setting of 250–300 mm Hg. It must be released after 2 hours to prevent injury. Chart both the tourniquet time and setting. Maintain anesthesia until the splint is applied.

SKIN AND FLAP GRAFTING

Composite Graft

A composite graft is composed of multiple structures from either synthetic or natural sources, such as skin and cartilage. Most commonly, a composite skin and cartilage graft is used to repair skin defects after cancer is resected.

Split-Thickness and Full-Thickness Skin Grafts

A skin graft is a surgical procedure in which a piece of skin from one area of the patient's body is transplanted to another area of the body. In addition, skin from another person or animal may be used as temporary cover for large burn areas in an attempt to decrease fluid loss. The skin is taken from a donor site, which has healthy skin, and implanted at the damaged recipient site.

Skin grafts and flaps are more serious than other scar revision surgeries such as dermabrasion. They are usually performed in a hospital under general anesthesia. The treated area, depending on its size and the severity of the injury, will determine the amount of time needed for healing; this time may range from 6 weeks to several months. Within 36 hours of the surgery, new blood vessels will begin to grow from the recipient area into the transplanted skin. Most grafts are successful, but some may require additional surgery if they do not heal properly.

Split-thickness grafts are done only for non-weight-bearing parts of the body. A graft of the epidermis and part of the dermis in sheets of various thickness is taken. Each graft contains only the mucosal layer—no subcutaneous tissues. The grafts may be up to 4 inches wide and 12 inches long. Grafts are placed at the recipient site and then a temporary bolster is applied (sometimes a wound "vac") and kept in place until the graft has taken, usually 5 to 7 days.

Full-thickness grafts are done for weight-bearing parts of the body in friction-prone areas and areas of greater cosmetic concern (face). Such a graft contains all the layers of the skin as well as the arteries and veins. The blood vessels will grow into the transplanted tissue in as little as 36 hours.

During any flap or graft procedure, the patient's blood pressure should be tightly controlled. The blood pressure should not be allowed to rise too high, as it may cause bleeding. A too-low blood pressure is also dangerous, as the graft may not get adequate perfusion. If the patient develops hypotension, give crystalloids and colloid IV fluids, rather than a vasoconstrictor.

During periods of high stimulation, plan for hypertension and *pretreat* the patient—for example, with labetalol.

Types of Flap Procedures

- Commonly used muscle flaps: latissimus dorsi, pectoralis major, trapezius, rectus abdominus, soleus, gluteus maximus
- Common bone flaps: fibula, scapular spine, iliac spine, and rib

Free Flap Procedure

A free flap procedure is considered microsurgery; it involves moving tissue from one body site to another. In general, when local tissue is not available to reconstruct a defect, a free flap is required. A muscle (with or without adjacent bone or skin) is harvested along with its blood supply; the pedicle is preserved with the muscle and is completely removed from the body. These vessels are then anastomosed to a new blood supply in the area of injury and the flap is inset to close the defect. They are usually very reliable flaps but require close post-operative monitoring in case of thrombosis; in which case an emergency return to surgery would be necessary to save the flap. Donated tissue, which can be skin, muscle, and/or bone, is molded and shaped to replace the missing anatomy.

A free flap procedure may be performed following trauma; as part of a surgical resection with cancer or chronic infection, burns, or wounds; or to remedy soft-tissue loss due to congenital defects. It can be done anywhere on the body.

Operative Procedure

See the discussion of transverse rectus abdominus myocutaneous (TRAM) flaps in Chapter 13 in relation to breast surgery. There are too many areas of the body that can give and receive a free flap to outline specifics here.

Anesthetic

GETA is used. Check with the surgeon before giving muscle relaxation. Spinal anesthetics can reduce the sympathetic response for lower extremity reconstruction with free flaps and are preferred.

Keep the patient asleep until the dressing and splints (applied with bone flaps) are applied.

Positioning

Patient positioning depends on the site that is to *receive* the tissue donation.

Anesthetic Implications

Monitor for hematoma formation.

Keep nonoperative sites covered with warming blankets, and administer warm fluids. These cases can be very long.

A tourniquet may be used when tissue donation is taken from an extremity.

Type and cross-match the patient's blood preoperatively. There is a potential for a moderate amount of blood loss with a free flap procedure.

There is a potential for fluid shifts and large third-space shifts with free flap procedures. Monitor urinary output to assess for these complications.

Monitors and IV Access

Have a discussion with the surgeon about anticipated flap sites *before* placing peripheral lines, central lines, or an arterial line.

An arterial line should be placed for long cases or if the patient has cardiac history.

Have two 18-gauge catheters peripheral IVs.

IV Vasoactive Agents

Vasoconstrictors (Neosynephrine) should not be used unless absolutely necessary and only after discussing their use with the surgeon. Treat hypotension with IV crystalloids and colloids. Ephedrine and calcium chloride may be helpful.

Other drugs to have available include dextran 40 and heparin.

IV Fluids and Volume Requirements

Keep the patient euvolemic but not overhydrated. Dehydration can lead to flap tissue ischemia from vasoconstriction. Overhydration can cause stress on the flap, too.

Emergence

Avoid coughing, bucking, and vomiting on emergence from anesthesia or postoperatively to avoid suture line strain and bleeding. Antiemetics should be given (see Chapter 4 and "Plastic Surgery Pearls" section in this chapter for more information).

Postoperative pain control is important to help prevent sympathetic-induced vasoconstriction.

NEONATE SURGERY PEARLS

- The functional residual capacity (FRC) in neonatal patients is decreased until the child is approximately 24 hours old, after which it reaches normal infant levels. Oxygen consumption of a neonate may be twice that of an adult: 6–8 mL/kg/min as compared to the adult rate, which is 3 mL/kg/min.
- Neonates are obligate nose breathers.
- Neonates are highly vagotonic (they have an overactive vagus nerve). They depend on an increased heart rate to increase their cardiac output (myocardium has less contractile muscle, which reduces compliance of the ventricle and limits the ability to increase stroke volume). To help meet increased oxygen requirements in neonates, cardiac output increases 30–60%.
- The neonatal glottic opening is at the C3–C4 level. The narrowest portion of the neonate's airway is the cricoid ring.
- An immature central nervous system, as seen in a premature infant, predisposes the child to irregular breathing patterns and periods of apneas and bradycardias.
- A neonate with one congenital anomaly often has other coexisting anomalies.
- Newborns of diabetic mothers have an increased tendency to develop hypoglycemia and hypocalcemia (with an elevated potassium) in the perinatal period. These babies must be treated with an intravenous glucose infusion.
- Hypoglycemia:
  - Glucose is the major energy source for the fetus and neonate. The newborn brain depends upon glucose almost exclusively.

    Preterm infant hypoglycemia: serum glucose < 30 mg/dL

    Full-term infant hypoglycemia: serum glucose < 40 mg/dL

    Give 250–500 mg/kg of glucose to treat hypoglycemia

- If arterial hypoxemia or acidosis occurs in the neonate, a return to a fetal pattern of circulation can result, leading to pulmonary artery vasoconstriction and pulmonary hypertension. This return, which is also termed *persistent fetal circulation* or *persistent pulmonary hypertension (PPHN)*, further exacerbates the hypoxemia and acidosis. Neonatal preoperative oxygen saturation levels are commonly in the range of 88–95%. Maintain FiO_2 levels to keep these saturation levels steady and to avoid hyperoxemia, which may predispose the baby to retinopathy of prematurity with subsequent blindness.
- Retinopathy of prematurity (ROP) is due to an immature retina that is deficient in a number of enzymes, which makes it more susceptible to the deleterious effects of O_2. Predisposing factors for ROP include low birth weight, gestational age immaturity, and extended duration of supplemental oxygen.
- Infants who had perinatal asphyxia should be identified, because this condition can lead to impaired autoregulation of the cerebral circulation and depressed myocardial function. Decreased perfusion to the gut, shock, and a variety of metabolic derangements, such as hypoglycemia, hypocalcemia, hyperkalemia, and clotting disorders, can also result.

NEONATE ANESTHESIA AND ISSUES

Neonates have a reduction in protein binding that causes a larger volume of distribution (in comparison to adults). Total body water, extracellular fluid, and blood volumes are also larger in a neonate than in a child or an adult. This difference explains why the neonate requires a higher per-kilogram dose of a drug to reach the desired effect.

Hepatic enzyme systems are incompletely developed or absent at birth, which is another factor affecting drug metabolism in the neonate. Phase 1 and 2 processes are limited but develop within a few days after birth. Conjugation reactions are developed by 3 months. Preoperative lab tests for neonates should include clotting studies (due to the immature hepatic clotting system).

Some neonates—especially those born prematurely, with birth weights less than 1.0 or 1.5 kg—may require specialized mechanical ventilation or complex hemodynamic support with infused dopamine, dobutamine, and epinephrine. In such situations, following preoperative discussions involving the anesthesia team, the surgeon, and the neonatologist, it may be deemed safer to perform the surgical procedure "at the bedside" in the neonatal intensive care unit (NICU). In such situations, anesthesia care providers and NICU physicians typically work together at the bedside to coordinate appropriate anesthetic management.

Pre-induction Measures
Provide preoxygenation.

Monitors
Monitors for a neonate are generally the same as for an adult, albeit adapted to the smaller size of the patient.

Induction
Induction may consist of fentanyl 2–5 mcg/kg or ketamine 0.5–1.0 mg/kg.

The choice of induction agent depends on the neonate's cardiovascular function, presence of acidosis, and severity of hypoxemia. Generally a balanced technique is recommended. Isoflurane is an agent of choice and usually maintained at less than 1 MAC. (The MAC requirement is decreased in neonates up to 1 month old.) N_2O is avoided due to the potential for development of a patent foramen ovale (PFO). Fentanyl IV is used for maintenance at a rate of 5–30 mcg/kg during general anesthesia and PRN. Use of an air filter in the IV line is highly recommended.

Maintenance
Provide standard maintenance with muscle relaxation. Avoid drugs and diluents containing benzyl

alcohol (a bacteriostatic preservative found in many IV medicines); there is an association between large doses of benzyl alcohol and intraventricular hemorrhage (kernicterus). You can reconstitute vecuronium with sterile water or normal saline; give a dose of 0.1 mg/kg, and repeat it every 30–45 minutes as needed. Pancuronium and rocuronium may contain benzyl alcohol.

Monitor for hypoglycemia, electrolyte abnormalities, and metabolic acidosis.

Mechanical ventilation for the neonate is generally accomplished with pressure-controlled ventilation or high-frequency ventilation in an effort to prevent barotrauma and to attenuate the hemodynamic effects of positive-pressure ventilation. In some institutions (especially those with a large number of premature neonates), protocols may exist for transport of specialized neonatal ventilators from the NICU to the OR, and for use during the surgical procedure.

Emergence

In some facilities, the child remains intubated and is sent to NICU without reversing the muscle relaxant, allowing for a slow and monitored emergence and extubation by NICU staff.

IV Fluids and Blood in Neonates

Fluid and blood replacement boluses are given at a rate of 5–10 mL/kg over 5–10 minutes.

When considering blood replacement, remember that the estimated blood volume (EBV) of a premature neonate is approximately 90–100 mL/kg (80–85 mL/kg for a full-term neonate). Therefore, a 2-kg neonate may have an EBV of approximately 200 mL. As a rule of thumb, most surgeons consider a "unit of blood" in children to be 10 mL/kg, and this blood transfusion will raise the HCT by 3–4%.

Maintaining adequate fluid balance is extremely important, as the neonate may experience significant third spacing, especially with bowel procedures. Maintain adequate intravascular volume status; urinary output should be 1–2 mL/kg/hr. Because the smallest commercially available Foley

catheters may be only a 6 French size, 5 French pediatric feeding tubes may be utilized as urethral catheters for intraoperative urine output monitoring.

- Volume expansion can be done with normal saline, lactated Ringer's solution, 5% albumin, fresh frozen plasma (FFP), and/or packed red blood cells (PRBCs).
- *Maintenance IV fluid* for neonate consists of $D_5\frac{1}{2}$ NS($\pm$KC1); it is given via a 100-mL bag or syringe infusion.
- *Replacement IV fluid* consists of lactated Ringer's solution or normal saline.

Neonate Hemoglobin Levels

A preterm infant has an Hgb level of approximately 13 g/dL. A minimum of at least 10 g/dL is highly recommended.

A full-term newborn has an Hgb level in the range of 18–20 g/dL. The nadir (when the Hgb will normally fall) in a term infant occurs at 10–12 weeks, though this decline is generally well tolerated. This condition is called the normal "physiologic anemia of infancy." In the premature infant, the Hgb may decline more rapidly (at 4–6 weeks), fall to lower levels (to 8.0 g/dL), and not be well tolerated.

Fetal Hgb has a greater affinity for oxygen, leading to an oxy-hemoglobin dissociation curve shift to the left, where Hgb holds onto the oxygen without releasing it to the tissues as readily.

Emergency Medications and Equipment to Take When Transporting a Neonate

- Atropine 0.02 mg/kg with IM needle.
- Epinephrine 0.01 mg/kg. Take 1 mL of 100 mcg/mL and dilute it into 9 mL preservative-free normal saline to make a 10 mcg/mL solution; you can then put 1 mL in a tuberculin (TB) syringe for more precise dosing. Most often cardiac events in the neonate are attributed to respiratory events. When the hypoxia is corrected, the cardiac event usually resolves.

- Emergency airway equipment: oxygen source with full O_2 cylinder, pediatric-size stethoscope, and neonatal-size ambu bag with pressure-limiting relief valves. Pediatric laryngoscope handle, ML 0 and 00 blades, appropriate-size face masks and oral airways, and 2.0, 2.5, and 3.0 uncuffed endotracheal tubes (ETTs).

Neonate Spinal Anesthesia

Spinal anesthesia may be used for lower abdominal procedures in neonates, such as inguinal hernia repairs. Neonatologists often prefer this technique, especially in ex-premature infants with chronic lung disease (defined as the need for continued intubation/mechanical ventilation and/or supplemental inhaled oxygen at 37–38 weeks corrected gestational age).

Use the standard spinal tray but with 1.0- to 1.5-inch neonatal/pediatric spinal needle. In our facility, we use tetracaine (Pontocaine) 1% (10 mg/mL) diluted in 10% dextrose. The dosage for tetracaine is 1 mg/kg. Example: For a 2-kg neonate, the dose would be 2 mg, which is 0.2 mL of the 1% tetracaine. We take the 0.2 mL (2 mg) and mix it with equal parts of 10% dextrose, drawn up in a small TB syringe. The child is positioned and supported in a sitting, upright position in the same posture as an adult would be for a spinal. A 1–2% lidocaine skin infiltrate is given to numb the skin before inserting the spinal needle. After administration of spinal anesthesia, the child may be placed supine. Be careful not to lift the child's legs up for at least 3–5 minutes to prevent a high spinal effect. Have an emergency airway, supplemental O_2, and emergency medication ready.

Neonate Epidural Anesthesia

Often a caudal epidural block will be used as a primary anesthetic in newborns for pelvic procedures, such as perinatal testicular torsions, or cystoscopy with ablation of urethral valves. The caudal catheter is positioned between the cornu of the sacrum, with the tip of the needle placed below the filum termanale externum. A caudal anesthetic may also be given for postoperative pain control. When this technique is used as the primary anesthetic, having a pacifier with Sweet-eese 50% sucrose may help calm the infant. Alternatively, ketamine can be used if needed. When giving a caudal block, Marcaine with epinephrine is administered; peaked T waves are a warning of an undesired intravascular position of the caudal catheter. The advantage of a caudal catheter is that you cannot have an epidural leak, because it is positioned inferiorly to the thecal sac.

PEDIATRIC SURGERY PEARLS

- Bradycardia (heart rate of less than 80 beats per minute) should be treated in any child younger than 12 years old. Atropine IV is typically given prior to or during induction of anesthesia to prevent bradycardia. The recommended dose is 0.01–0.02 mg/kg, with a minimum dose of 0.1 mg, and a maximum dose of 1.0 mg in a child and 2.0 mg in an adolescent.
- Three structures that are unique to the fetal circulation:
  - *Ductus venosus:* vessel between the umbilical vein and the inferior vena cava; blood bypasses the liver
  - *Foramen ovale:* opening between the right and left atria
  - *Ductus arteriosus:* between the pulmonary trunk and descending aorta
- Resumption of fetal circulation is caused by hypoxia, hypercarbia, hypothermia, hypoglycemia, hypomagnesemia, and hypocalcemia.
- Pediatric patients tend to lose their teeth between the ages of 5 and 12. Assess for loose teeth preoperatively. Parents should be informed when there is a possibility of tooth dislodgement. It is probably best to pull

easily removable loose teeth, once general anesthesia is induced, rather than risk aspiration of teeth into the trachea or bronchi.

- Postoperative hypoxemia may occur in the pediatric population due to upper airway obstruction. Children should be given supplemental oxygen (face mask or blow-by), and oxygen saturation should be monitored continuously during surgery, transfer to the surgical stretcher, and transport to recovery. Pediatric patients should be positioned on their sides with the head of the bed lifted slightly, if possible. Many practices maintain portable pulse oximetry throughout the transfer of the pediatric patient to the recovery room.

PEDIATRIC ANESTHESIA AND ISSUES

Pharmacologic maturation occurs between 3 and 6 months of age.

Pre-induction Measures
Provide atropine 0.01–0.02 mg/kg IV, with a minimum dose of 0.1 mg, before laryngoscopy to prevent bradycardia and to decrease secretions.

Monitors
Monitors for a pediatric patient are generally the same as for an adult, albeit adapted to the child's smaller size.

IV Induction
- STP 4–7 mg/kg, or
- Propofol 2–3 mg/kg, or
- Ketamine 1–2 mg/kg

A combination of barbiturates with ketamine can be used for induction.

Inhalation Induction
A Bain circuit or pediatric circle tubing with humidified and warmed gases may be needed.

- Oxygen at 30% with 70% nitrous oxide
- Sevoflurane (preferred) or
- Halothane

If nitrous oxide is contraindicated, oxygen and air may be used to maintain the lowest possible FiO_2 to maintain an oxygen saturation of more than 95%.

Depolarizing Muscle Relaxation on Induction
The use of succinylcholine in the pediatric population is very controversial, especially in young boys who may have undiagnosed Duchenne's dystrophy. However, a syringe containing a weight-specific IM dose of succinylcholine should be available for every pediatric case if the need for emergency intubation and paralysis arises. Atropine can also be given IM at a 0.2 mg/kg dose; you may want to preemptively administer this agent if a second dose of succinylcholine is needed.

Maintenance
Avoid high FiO_2 levels. Use oxygen and air/oxygen and nitrous oxide mixtures to maintain oxygen saturation at more than 95%. Sevoflurane, isoflurane, halothane, or desflurane are all acceptable volatile maintenance anesthetics.

When an epidural is used, the epidural anesthesia is dosed with local anesthetic and opioids, and supplemented with a low-dose inhalation agent.

Without an epidural, use high-dose narcotics: fentanyl 10–25 mcg/kg IV total.

Nondepolarizing muscle relaxants include the following agents:

- Vecuronium 0.1 mg/kg (intermediate-acting nondepolarizing muscle relaxant [NDMR])
- Cisatracurium 0.1 mg/kg (intermediate-acting NDMR)
- Rocuronium 0.6–1.2 mg/kg (intermediate-acting NDMR)
- Pancuronium 0.1 mg/kg (vagolytic; long-acting NDMR)

Train of four monitoring of the neuromuscular junction in the infant is the same as with an adult. Due to the infant's larger volume of distribution and longer elimination half-life, neuromuscular blocking agents can be given in smaller doses and less frequently.

Emergence
Reversal drugs consist of neostigmine 0.05 mg/kg with glycopyrrolate 0.007 mg/kg IV.

IV Fluids in Pediatric Patients

- 1 month to 1 year old: D_5LR with minidrip tubing or a Buretrol chamber
- 1 year old: hang 500 mL lactated Ringer's solution
- Lactated Ringer's solution: used for deficit volume replacement

Fluid maintenance follows the 4-2-1 rule:

- 4 mL/kg/hr for first 0–10 kg, then
- 2 mL/kg/hr for 10–20 kg, then
- 1 mL/kg/hr for weight in excess of 20 kg.

The NPO-derived fluid deficit is calculated as the number of hours NPO × hourly fluid maintenance.

Emergency Medications and Equipment to Take When Transporting a Pediatric Patient

- Atropine 0.02 mg/kg with IM needle.
- Epinephrine 0.01 mg/kg. Take 1 mL of 100 mcg/mL and dilute it into 9 mL preservative-free normal saline to make a 10 mcg/mL solution. Most often, cardiac

events in the child are attributed to respiratory events. When the hypoxia is corrected, the cardiac event is resolved.

- Emergency airway equipment: oxygen source with full O_2 cylinder, pediatric stethoscope, and pediatric-size ambu bag with pressure-limiting relief valves. Pediatric laryngoscope handle, 1–3 blades, appropriate-size face masks and oral airways, and 4.0, 4.5, and 5.0 uncuffed and cuffed ETTs.

One-Lung Ventilation in Pediatric Patients

In one-lung ventilation, a single-lumen ETT is advanced into the bronchus of the nonoperative lung. A bronchial-blocker is advanced under fiberoptic visualization, and a balloon may be placed in the operative lung in the mainstem bronchus. The balloon is inflated, and the lung deflated. Suction may be needed to assist in lung collapse.

Selective mainstem intubation with a single-lumen ETT can also be done with a microlaryngeal tracheal tube (MLT). This device is a longer than usual ETT; it is the same length as an adult ETT but comes in much smaller sizes. MLTs are stiffer and less prone to compression. They come in sizes 4.0, 5.0, and 6.0. The MLT must be large enough to seal the bronchus but small enough to avoid mucosal damage owing to excessive pressure.

Single-lung ventilation is often requested by pediatric surgeons for thoracoscopic procedures. Because double-lumen tubes are typically available only for children ages 8 years and older, surgeons

AGE	ENDOTRACHEAL TUBE	DOUBLE-LUMEN ENDOBRONCHIAL TUBE
8–10 years	6 cuffed	26 Fr
10–12 years	6.5 cuffed	26–28 Fr
12–14 years	6.5–7 cuffed	30–32 Fr
14–16 years	7.0 cuffed	32 Fr
16–18 years	7.0–7.5 cuffed	35 Fr

may need to make use of valved trocars and gentle insufflation with CO_2.

A double-lumen endobronchial tube (DLEBT) can be inserted for one-lung ventilation. After insertion of a DLEBT, a pediatric fiberoptic scope is inserted through the tube to visualize and confirm correct placement.

TEMPERATURE ISSUES WITH NEONATE AND PEDIATRIC PATIENTS

Children are particularly prone to heat loss because they have very little subcutaneous fat, an inability to shiver (to increase their metabolism), and a relatively large body surface to total weight ratio. Therefore, prior to the induction of anesthesia, children should be covered with warm blankets (or other warming measures used). Even after short procedures, a child's temperature may be markedly reduced. Thus heat loss must be countered by warming through conduction, radiation, and convection.

Heat preservation is a very big issue with pediatric surgeries: Keep the infant warm! Warm the operating room to approximately 70–75°F, use warming lamps and a warming mattress, use a heated humidifier, warm fluids, wrap the child's extremities and head in plastic, use neonatal/pediatric warming blankets, and use warm, low-flow gases.

Do not attempt to extubate a hypothermic child. The body temperature should be at least 36°C to extubate a pediatric patient. A body temperature of less than 36°C can place demands on the child that exceed cardiopulmonary compensation, resulting in acidosis and hypoventilation.

ETT and LMA Size: (Age + 16)/ 4
- Carina T5: 13-cm lip to carina
- Uncuffed ETT: may use in a child who is less than 8–10 years old
- Should have an air leak at 15–25 cm H_2O

WEIGHT(KG)	ETT ID (MM)	LMA
1–2.5	3.0	
2.5–3.5	3.5	
3.5–5.0	3.5	
5–8	3.5–4.0	1
8–11	4.0–4.5	1.5
10–20		2
20–30		2.5
> 30		3
50–79		4
> 70		5

DOWN SYNDROME: ANESTHETIC IMPLICATIONS

Anatomic and physiologic characteristics may affect anesthetic delivery in the patient with Down syndrome.

- Airway: congenital subglottic stenosis, narrow nasopharynx, large tonsils and adenoids, large tongue, poor function of laryngeal and pharyngeal reflexes, and mid-face hypoplasia
- Heart: increased incidence of congenital heart disease (CHD), especially atrial and ventricular septal defects
- Pulmonary: higher pulmonary vascular resistance related to chronic hypoxemia
- Musculoskeletal: atlanto-axial instability; can result in C1–C2 subluxation with spinal cord injury

It is of utmost importance to keep *all* air bubbles out of the IV lines. Any air can cross over a septal defect into the left atrium and/or ventricle and result in an arterial air embolism.

Antibiotic prophylaxis is important in these patients if they have CHD.

Avoid heavy or unsupervised sedation due to these patients' predisposition to upper airway obstruction. Patients with Down syndrome often have obstructive sleep apnea; their airways may become obstructed and desaturation occurs quickly. Effective mask ventilation may require manual displacement of the mandible and placement of an oral airway.

To prevent cervical subluxation, maintain the head and neck in a neutral position. Provide manual in-line stabilization (with a second provider holding traction cephalad to the patient's head during intubation). Avoid flexion, extension, and rotation of the neck and head.

Choose a smaller than predicted ETT size due to the potential for subglottic stenosis. Measure airway leak pressure to avoid unnecessary tracheal pressure.

Extubate the patient with Down syndrome only when he or she is wide awake and protective airway reflexes are intact. Careful postoperative monitoring should be done owing to these patients' predisposition for airway obstruction.

CEREBRAL PALSY: ANESTHETIC IMPLICATIONS

Cerebral palsy (CP) is a nonprogressive injury to the brain that is caused before, during, or shortly after birth. Children with CP have damage to the area of the brain that controls muscle tone; this tone may be tight, too loose, or a combination of both. The abnormalities in muscle tone affect these patients' movements, which are classified into three categories: spastic (stiff and jerky movements), ataxic (unsteady, shaky), or athetoid (mixed; intermittently tight and loose). Approximately 50% of CP patients also have seizures.

When positioning a child with CP during surgery, ensure that careful padding is performed and joints are placed in a natural position due to contractures.

Anesthetic management of a patient with CP includes tracheal intubation due to the propensity for gastrointestinal reflux and poor function of laryngeal and pharyngeal reflexes. Owing to the increased risk for aspiration, rapid-sequence induction should be done. An anti-sialagogue may be given to decrease oral/airway secretions.

Despite the muscle spasticity in these patients, succinylcholine does not produce an abnormal potassium release in children with CP. Their response to NDMRs is normal.

Opioids may impair the airway reflexes of patients with CP.

Many of these patients are taking antiseizure medications; they should take these agents the day of surgery. These drugs can also cause the patient to need more frequent drug dosing of muscle relaxants or narcotics. Some patients may also be taking dantrolene or baclofen to counteract muscle spasticity.

Body temperature should be monitored, as these patients are susceptible to hypothermia in the perioperative period.

Emergence from anesthesia may be slow due to the presence of hypothermia and the cerebral damage from CP.

Extubation should not be attempted until the patient is fully awake and normothermic.

Careful observation must be carried out in the postoperative period, as these patients have a higher incidence of airway obstruction and pulmonary complications.

MANDIBULAR HYPOPLASIA (MICROGNATHIA): ANESTHETIC IMPLICATIONS

Mandibular hypoplasia is a prominent feature in craniofacial abnormalities and includes the Pierre Robin, Treacher Collins, and Goldenhar syndromes. With micrognathia, the small mandible leaves little room for the tongue, leading to a propensity for upper airway obstruction and difficult intubation of the trachea.

- *Pierre Robin syndrome:* micrognathia, glossoptosis (posterior displacement of tongue), and cleft palate. Feeding difficulties, failure to thrive, and cyanotic episodes are common.

Associated congenital heart defects are also common.

- *Treacher-Collins syndrome:* micrognathia, with cleft palate occurring approximately 30% of time. Congenital heart disease, external auditory canal gross deformities, and ossicular chain abnormalities frequently accompany this syndrome. Feeding difficulties, failure to thrive, and cyanotic episodes are common.
- *Goldenhar syndrome:* characterized by unilateral mandibular hypoplasia. Associated anomalies include ear, eye, and vertebral abnormalities on the affected side.

A thorough evaluation of the upper airway and development of a plan for intubation must be completed before coming to the operating room. These patients may have chronic airway obstruction and chronic arterial hypoxemia with pulmonary hypertension.

A preoperative dose of an anticholinergic agent can reduce upper airway secretions as well as increase the heart rate (thereby preventing bradycardia on induction). Sedation is avoided preoperatively. A histamine blocker can be given if there is a risk of regurgitation with pulmonary aspiration.

A rapid-sequence induction should be done, after a longer than usual pre-oxygenation period. A volatile anesthetic is given while the patient breathes spontaneously, until an adequate depth of anesthesia is obtained. Forward traction of the tongue (an oral airway may suffice) may facilitate maintenance of a patent upper airway. Nondepolarizing muscle relaxants should not be given until the ETT placement is confirmed. Direct laryngoscopy should be attempted, but emergency airway equipment should be readily available in case this effort fails. A tracheostomy may be required if all other attempts to intubate and maintain an airway have been attempted.

Extubation should not be attempted until the child is fully awake and moving purposefully.

Equipment for reintubation must be readily available.

NEUROSURGERY
Craniectomy for Craniosynostosis

Craniectomy is the removal of fused sutures of the skull. The normal skull consists of several plates of bone that are separated by sutures. In craniosynostosis, some or all of the skull sutures close too early, creating problems with brain growth and potentially leading to increased intracranial pressure. Not only can the skull become deformed, but facial bones may also be affected. (See the discussion of craniofacial surgery later in this chapter.)

Operative Procedure

The goal of surgery is to decrease the intracranial pressure and correct the deformities of the face and skull bones. The fused sutures of the skull must be separated; this surgery may be combined with other surgeries (plastic, oral, and maxillofacial surgery) to treat facial deformities. The incision usually involves a zigzag incision from ear to ear over the top of the head. The scalp is peeled back to expose the skull, with either total or subtotal removal of the affected skull. Multiple holes are drilled into the skull; these holes connected, and then the skull is separated into several pieces and removed. Next, the skull is rebuilt with a variety of materials, including the removed pieces of the patient's own skull. Sutures, plates, and screws help to hold the bones together; bone protein is often used to fill the gaps around the bones, thereby encouraging new bone growth. The incision is closed with sutures.

For children younger than 6 months of age, an endoscopic-assisted procedure has recently been described, and can be done to remove the fused suture. One or two very small incisions (1 inch in length) are made in the scalp (the site on the head depends on where the fused suture is located), and the affected suture is removed. The endoscopic approach is associated with significantly less blood loss, swelling, and pain. The length of this procedure is usually about 1 hour and the child can be discharged after 24-hour monitoring. Postoperatively, the child will need to wear a custom-made "molding helmet" to help ensure proper bone growth as the brain develops.

Anesthetic

General anesthesia is used with an oral endotracheal tube (OETT); muscle relaxation is usually given. These patients may be considered "difficult airway" cases due to their facial deformity.

Positioning

The patient is placed in a supine position for coronal synostosis. He or she is placed in a prone position for sagittal and lambdoidal synostosis.

Anesthetic Implications

After taping the eyelids shut, securely tape eye pads over both of the patient's eyes to protect them. Depending on the area of planned incision, occlusive tape (Tegaderm) may be placed over the eyes to keep prep solution from getting into the eye(s).

Prior to the induction of anesthesia, children should be covered with warm blankets (or other warming measures used). Heat loss must be counteracted by warming through conduction, radiation, and convection. Keep the room warm, use warming lamps and mattress, use a heated humidifier, warm fluids, wrap the child's extremities and head in plastic, and use warm, low-flow gases.

This surgery can last from 3 to 7 hours and will usually involve multiple groups of specialists, including pediatric neurosurgeons and plastic surgeons.

Most children have central venous catheters placed following induction of anesthesia. Many have invasive arterial monitors placed.

There can be considerable blood loss in these cases, and patients usually require blood transfusions. Closely monitor blood loss from the scalp and skull; monitor the drapes around the surgical site; and communicate closely with the surgeon regarding blood loss. Catastrophic blood loss can occur if the dural venous sinuses are opened.

Craniofacial Surgery

Craniofacial surgery is a broad term used to refer to reconstructive procedures of the skull and face. These procedures are performed to correct hereditary conditions such as cranial dysostosis or craniofacial dysmorphism—conditions with developmental disturbance of the cranial bones and parts of the face. Acrocephaly (a high, pointed skull), exophthalmos (bulging of the eye), hypertelorism (having an increased distance between the two eyes), parrot-beaked nose, hypoplastic maxilla, and Treacher-Collins syndrome are all examples of maldevelopment of the cranial/facial bones.

Operative Procedure

The precise procedure depends on the condition and its severity. See the earlier discussion of "craniectomy for craniosynostosis" for more information.

Anesthetic

General anesthesia is used with an OETT. Muscle relaxants may be needed.

Positioning

The patient may be placed in a supine or prone position, depending on the site of the deformity.

Anesthetic Implications

Check with the surgeon regarding the surgical field and the need to tape the eyelids shut. You may need to securely tape eye pads over both of the patient's eyes to protect them.

Some craniofacial conditions are associated with airway abnormalities and, therefore, may require flexible bronchoscopy for difficult endotracheal intubations. Some of these children may have already undergone tracheostomy prior to craniofacial reconstruction.

Prior to the induction of anesthesia, children should be covered with warm blankets (or other warming measures used). Heat loss must be counteracted by warming through conduction, radiation, and convection. Keep the room warm, use warming lamps and mattress, use a heated humidifier, warm fluids, wrap the child's extremities and head in plastic, and use warm, low-flow gases.

Correction of Spinal Dysraphism

This procedure comprises surgical closure of the spinal column. If needed, untethering of the spinal cord is done to allow movement with growth.

Spinal dysraphism is the failure of the spinal column to properly close (in utero), which causes neural tube defects; this broad term encompasses a group of anomalies of the spinal column. Spinal dysraphism may cause progressive neurologic deterioration, including the absence of some of the neural arches, and defects of the skin, filum terminale, nerves, and spinal cord.

Operative Procedure

If a cerebrospinal fluid (CSF) leak is present, the surgery is urgent and occurs immediately after birth. If no leak is present, the surgery is typically performed in the first 24–48 hours of life. Multiple procedures can be done because of the range of defects possible with spinal dysraphism, including placement of a ventriculoperitoneal shunt, spinal stabilization, or tendon excisions (for club foot).

Anesthetic

General endotracheal anesthesia (GETA) is used with muscle relaxation.

Positioning

The patient is placed in a prone position.

Anesthetic Implications

This procedure carries a risk of damage to the spinal cord or nerves.

Prior to the induction of anesthesia, children should be covered with warm blankets (or other warming measures used). Heat loss must be counteracted by warming through conduction, radiation, and convection. Keep the room warm, use warming lamps and mattress, use a heated humidifier, warm fluids, wrap the child's extremities and head in plastic, and use warm, low-flow gases.

Most children with spinal dysraphism have bladder dysfunction. For this reason, a urinary catheter is usually inserted preoperatively for intraoperative management.

Myelomeningocele/Meningocele Closure (Myelodysplasia)

This procedure consists of the surgical closure of a congenital disorder of the spinal canal; it is performed when a sacular protrusion, usually in the thoracolumbar spine, presents in the newborn child. Surgery is usually done within 24 hours of birth after screening for other potential associated congenital anomalies (atrial or ventricular septal defects, hydronephrosis, malrotation of the gut).

Myelodysplasia is the failure of neural tube closure, which can result in abnormalities ranging from spina bifida to myelomeningocele.

Myelomeningocele is a congenital disorder that is characterized by the failure of the spinal canal to close during fetal development. It can result in the spinal cord (neural components) and its covering membranes protruding out of the infant's back. This protrusion may be small and localized, or it may be extensive and severe, involving multiple vertebral levels. Myelomeningocele results in nerve root abnormalities below the defect, which may be associated with neuromuscular, bladder, and bowel dysfunction. In addition, the fourth ventricle may be obstructed due to a Chiari malformation (structural defects in the cerebellum); often a ventriculoperitoneal shunt is placed for treatment of hydrocephalus.

With *meningocele,* neurological function is usually intact. In this case, the sac contains only CSF.

Operative Procedure

Infants with myelomeningocele require prompt closure of the defect to prevent infection and sepsis. Surgery involves placement of the spinal cord and/or nerve roots in a normal position and suturing of the overlying meninges and other structures closed. In approximately 90% of cases, a ventriculoperitoneal shunt is required to drain excess fluid from the brain as well. The shunt may be placed at the time of the original surgery or several days later.

Closure is largely palliative: It protects the child from infection but probably does not reverse preexisting damage.

Intrauterine endoscopic techniques are currently being studied for myelomeningocele repair.

Anesthetic

General anesthesia is used with insertion of an OETT; succinylcholine is not contraindicated but not usually given in the pediatric population. Muscle relaxants with vecuronium or rocuronium may be needed, but check with the surgeon regarding his or her preferences and the need for lower-extremity neuromuscular monitoring.

Positioning

Patients should come to the operating room in the prone position. While the child is in the supine position for induction and intubation, protect the spinal defect from any pressure. In our practice, we have placed these babies on a foam head ring so that the defect fits down into the hole. If the defect is too large for the ring, firm rolls or sterile towels can be used along both sides of the defect, holding the baby still while not putting any pressure on the defect.

Anesthetic Implications

Often latex precautions are utilized to prevent development of latex allergy with subsequent procedures.

After taping the eyelids shut, securely tape eye pads over both of the patient's eyes to protect them.

Hypovolemia and hypothermia are both concerns with this surgery.

Most children with myelodysplasia have bladder dysfunction. For this reason, a urinary catheter is usually inserted preoperatively for intraoperative management.

Postoperative aspiration and hypoventilation are concerns with myelodysplasia patients.

Ninety percent of myelomeningocele patients have *Arnold-Chiari malformation* with downward displacement of the brain stem and cerebellar tonsils through the cervical spinal canal. This defect blocks the passage of CSF, leading to hydrocephalus.

Prior to the induction of anesthesia, children should be covered with warm blankets (or other warming measures used). Heat loss must be counteracted by warming through conduction, radiation, and convection. Keep the room warm, use warming lamps and mattress, use a heated humidifier, warm fluids, wrap the child's extremities and head in plastic, and use warm, low-flow gases.

EAR, NOSE, AND THROAT SURGERY
Branchial Cleft Cyst Tract Excision

Branchial cleft cyst tract excision is the surgical excision of a congenital epithelial cyst. Branchial cleft cysts arise on the lateral part of the neck during embryonic development.

Although the second listed branchial cleft cysts are, by far, the most commonly encountered branchial cleft anomalies, they may occur in three distinct locations:

- The first is found in the neck just below the jaw (the tract can extend as far as the outer ear canal).
- The second is found between the sternocleidomastoid muscle and the trachea

(the tract can extend to the tonsillar fossa area).

- The third is found a few millimeters deep in the chest wall below the clavicle.

Many branchial cleft cysts are initially asymptomatic but may become tender and enlarged, and even develop abscesses, during periods of upper respiratory tract infection, a sore throat, or ear infection. These effects arise when the lymph tissue located beneath the epithelium becomes infected. Spontaneous rupture of an abscessed cyst may also cause a sinus to form in the skin, which allows the purulent material to drain out. These sinuses, or tracts, may extend out from the cyst itself. If the abscess becomes large enough, dysphagia, dyspnea, and stridor can occur.

Operative Procedure

Excision of these cysts is usually an outpatient procedure. An elliptical incision is made around the branchial cleft cyst, and the cyst is removed. Removal of the tract, extending inward from the cyst, and associated tissues is usually necessary as well. Depending on the location of the cyst(s), major nerves, arteries, and veins may be involved. Methylene blue may be injected into a sinus tract to allow for full visualization, with the tract then being dissected out. A drain may be placed to drain the sinus tract.

In some cases, fistulas can also be excised through the mouth.

Anesthetic

General anesthesia is used with insertion of an OETT; secure the OETT to the opposite side of the mouth from the surgical side. A LMA is rarely used because the surgeon may need to place his or her gloved finger into the mouth so as to palpate the tonsillar fossa.

Muscle relaxants may need to be given. Because the facial nerve may be an area of concern, check with the surgeon before giving any paralytic.

Positioning

The patient is placed in a supine position, with the head turned away from the surgical side.

Anesthetic Implications

After taping the eyelids shut, securely tape eye pads over both of the patient's eyes to protect them.

Prior to the induction of anesthesia, children should be covered with warm blankets (or other warming measures used). Heat loss must be counteracted by warming through conduction, radiation, and convection. Keep the room warm, use warming lamps and mattress, use a heated humidifier, warm fluids, wrap the child's extremities and head in plastic, and use warm, low-flow gases.

Vomiting and coughing should be avoided at the end of the case to prevent strain on suture lines.

Choanal Atresia Repair

Choanal atresia (CA) repair is surgery to reopen the nasal passages; it is performed in case of occlusion of one or both nares. Atresia is usually caused by partial or totally bony occlusion, although membranous tissue may also produce occlusion. Bilateral choanal atresia may cause suffocation if affected infants are not promptly intubated (because neonates are obligate nose breathers until they reach 4–6 months of age), so it is considered a medical emergency. The affected child's mouth must be kept open to oxygenate the patient. The baby will present with respiratory distress and cyanosis relieved by crying. A tracheostomy may be done for bilateral atresia if the child has an unstable airway. Unilateral choanal atresia may not be diagnosed until the child is older; even if it is diagnosed at a very early age, it may not be repaired until a later time.

Diagnosis of CA is made if healthcare providers are unable to pass a catheter down one or both of the child's nostrils.

Operative Procedure

The surgical approach is based on several factors, including the anatomy of the nasal passages. The surgeon enters through the nostrils if the bone is thin (*transnasal*). An incision is made through the roof of the mouth if the nostrils have thick bone blocking the passages (*transpalatal*). Alternatively, the surgeon may enter through the nasal septum (*transseptal*).

Endoscopic approaches for transnasal repair of choanal atresia provide direct visualization of the nasal cavity and posterior choana (the passageway from the back of one side of the nose to the throat).

Anesthetic

General anesthesia is used with insertion of an oral RAE endotracheal tube; muscle relaxants are given. Local anesthesia with epinephrine is usually infiltrated around the surgical site to decrease swelling and bleeding.

Positioning

The patient is placed in a supine position, with a shoulder roll used to extend the head, with bilateral arms tucked at the sides.

Anesthetic Implications

Prior to the induction of anesthesia, children should be covered with warm blankets (or other warming measures used). Heat loss must be counteracted by warming through conduction, radiation, and convection. Keep the room warm, use warming lamps and mattress, use a heated humidifier, warm fluids, wrap the child's extremities and head in plastic, and use warm, low-flow gases.

A CT scan is the preoperative study of choice. It is usually performed to confirm abnormal anatomy of the nasal cavity, posterior nasal choana, and nasopharynx.

The child will have some type of apparatus keeping the mouth open: an oral airway strapped into place, or a large rubber nipple with large holes cut in it that is strapped into the mouth with umbilical tape tied around the neck.

After taping the eyelids shut, securely tape eye pads over both of the patient's eyes to protect them.

Monitor EKG changes and heart rate if local anesthetic with epinephrine is given.

Make sure the child is wide awake before attempting extubation.

Choanal atresia can be related to craniofacial synostosis.

Foreign Body Aspiration or Foreign Body Obstruction or Ingestion

Endoscopic-assisted removal of a foreign body from the throat, airway, esophagus, or stomach is performed in case of foreign body obstruction (FBO), aspiration, or ingestion. This diagnosis is suspected in any patient who presents with wheezing or history of coughing or choking while eating or having anything in the mouth. It is best to remove an object from the airway or lung within 24 hours to minimize the risk of migration of FBO or pneumonia.

If the foreign body has been swallowed and entered the stomach, and is sharp or made of a caustic material, it may need to be removed by an esophagoscopy.

Operative Procedure

These cases are considered an emergency when surgical removal of the object is required. After adequate depth of anesthesia is attained:

- *For airway obstruction:* Direct laryngoscopy is performed and the larynx sprayed with a local anesthetic (LA). Topical LA is helpful in preventing laryngospasm or larynx irritation and coughing during endoscopy.
- *For ingestion:* Endoscopy is used to identify and remove the foreign object.

Depending on the severity of the obstruction, this surgery may take precedence over all other operative procedures in the operating room and, therefore, may "bump" aside all other patients being prepared for surgery.

Anesthetic

Techniques for induction depend on the severity of airway obstruction. If the airway is compromised, spontaneous ventilation with inhalational induction (a volatile agent and oxygen) is appropriate; induction may be prolonged when the airway is obstructed. Vigorous "hand bagging" during anesthesia induction may push the foreign body deeper into the airway and cause complete obstruction of a mainstem bronchus or, worse yet, the airway at the level of the carina, blocking the passage of air to both lungs.

Spontaneous ventilation should be maintained if possible. IV induction with a barbiturate (or comparable) should be done if the airway is not compromised.

Maintenance of anesthesia consists of a volatile anesthetic and oxygen.

Avoid nitrous oxide to minimize the likelihood of air-trapping distal to the obstruction.

Positioning

The patient is placed in a supine position, with a shoulder roll used to extend the head.

Anesthetic Implications

X-rays may not show an object but will indicate air-trapping and or atelectasis.

An anticholinergic can be given preoperatively to help reduce oral and airway secretions and increase the heart rate so as to prevent bradycardia.

Prior to the induction of anesthesia, children should be covered with warm blankets (or other warming measures used). Keep the room warm, use warming lamps and mattress, use a heated humidifier, warm fluids, wrap the child's extremities and head in plastic, and use warm, low-flow gases.

A soft rubber tooth guard is placed over the upper teeth to protect them from the endoscope.

Muscle relaxation may be required to remove an object that is too large to pass through the moving vocal cords. Hand-ventilation should be done while the patient is relaxed; the healthcare provider should take note of any changes in ventilation/airway pressures. Monitor airway pressures throughout the case.

IV steroids (i.e., Decadron) should be given, if there are no contraindications, to reduce swelling of the airway or larynx. If airway edema is present, the patient may need to remain intubated. If the child experiences any subglottic swelling after extubation, aerosolized racemic epinephrine can be given. Steroids are usually given postoperatively to prevent further edema.

Increased mucus production is the body's natural response to a foreign object. Chest percussion will enhance the clearance of any secretions postoperatively.

Myringotomy with Ear Tube Placement (Tympanostomy)

Myringotomy is performed to drain infection or effusion in the middle ear (otitis media). It is intended to remedy the presence of middle ear fluid or pus, or chronic perforation of the tympanic membrane. Middle ear fluid, especially if is present on both sides of the head, can cause some degree of chronic hearing loss. This problem usually occurs because the Eustachian tube is either partially or completely blocked.

In tympanostomy, ear tubes are placed. This procedure is performed because the myringotomy normally closes within 48 hours and the fluid almost always reaccumulates. These ear tubes stent the eardrum open, allowing the remaining fluid to drain and reducing the likelihood of infection.

Operative Procedure

A tiny incision is made in the tympanic membrane to relieve pressure caused by fluid buildup. Suctioning of the middle ear may be done to drain pus.

Antibiotic ear drops are usually instilled after placing the tubes. Cotton balls are placed in the outer ear canal.

Typically, an operating microscope is used as part of this procedure, but is not always necessary.

Anesthetic

General anesthesia with inhaled volatile agents is usually all that is required. Myringotomy/tympanostomy is considered a "mask case"; an oral airway is usually inserted to facilitate bag-mask ventilation or spontaneous ventilation.

Positioning

The patient is placed in a supine position. The head is turned from side to side to allow the surgeon access, with the operative ear in the upright position.

Anesthetic Implications

An IV is usually not started for this procedure. One may need to be placed for a reason other than the surgery (such as reactive airway disease requiring IV medication).

Tape the eyes closed. Eye pads are usually not needed.

At the end of the case, when the inhaled agent has been turned off and the child is breathing spontaneously, you can suction the stomach to remove oral preoperative sedatives to facilitate wake-up and discharge home.

If a myringotomy/tympanostomy is unable to be done or proves unsuccessful in relieving the problem, a mastoidectomy may be required to treat an ear infection.

Keep the child covered and warm.

Tonsillectomy and Adenoidectomy

Tonsillectomy and adenoidectomy (T&A) entail excision of the palatine tonsils and/or nasopharyngeal tonsils (adenoids). The palatine tonsils (posterior pharynx) and nasopharyngeal tonsils (back of nose) are aggregates of lymphoid tissue that may hypertrophy in response to chronic infection. Tonsillar hypertrophy affects the child's ability to swallow due to pain or tonsillar enlargement, whereas adenoid hypertrophy affects the child's ability to breathe through the nose with the mouth closed.

Clinical indications for a T&A include upper airway obstruction, obstructive sleep apnea with snoring, massive hypertrophy, and chronic upper respiratory infection (URI).

In adults, this procedure may be more difficult due to long-standing fibrosis. There has recently been some controversy on the usefulness of tonsillectomies: Far fewer of them are being done now than several decades ago, partly due to the emergence of evolving guidelines for doing a T&A.

Operative Procedure

Following endotracheal intubation, the mouth is retracted open (by a surgical mouth gag, such as the Dingman or McIvor device) and the tongue is depressed.

The adenoids are removed first with an adenotome and/or a curette.

A tonsil is grasped, and the mucosa is dissected free, preserving the posterior tonsil pillar. The capsule of the tonsil is separated from its bed. A snare loop is passed over the free portion of the tonsil, and the tonsil is amputated and removed. The fossa may be packed with a tonsil sponge and should be removed before extubation. Bleeding may be controlled with cautery, ties, and/or suture. The procedure is repeated on the opposite side.

Although this approach is popular in some centers, "laser T&A" is associated with a higher risk of airway fire.

Anesthetic

General anesthesia is used with an OETT; an oral RAE tube may be useful but is selected based on the surgeon's preference. Care must be taken during laryngoscopy with intubation to avoid trauma to the enlarged tonsils. The OETT is secured to the lower lip.

An anticholinergic agent may be given preoperatively to decrease oral secretions.

Muscle relaxation is not needed; spontaneous respirations during general anesthesia with an OETT are acceptable. The surgeon will usually place a throat pack in the hypopharynx to prevent blood or secretions from draining into the lung or stomach; this measure also helps to prevent the volatile agent from blowing up into the surgeon's face.

Positioning

The patient is placed in a supine position, with a shoulder roll used to extend the head. Bilateral arms are tucked at the sides. The head of the bed is moved at least 90 degrees away from the anesthetist.

Postoperatively, the patient is placed in a lateral decubitus position with the head slightly up.

Anesthetic Implications

After taping the eyelids shut, securely tape eye pads over both of the patient's eyes to protect them.

Prior to the induction of anesthesia, children should be covered with warm blankets (or other warming measures used). Keep the room warm, use warming lamps and mattress, use a heated humidifier, warm fluids, wrap the child's extremities and head in plastic, and use warm, low-flow gases.

Monitor for $ETCO_2$ and oxygenation after the mouth gag is placed. Note that the gag can compress the ETT.

If cautery or laser is used, airway fire is a risk. Decrease FiO_2 to 30% and maintain good communication with the surgeon. See the discussion of safety concerns in Chapter 1 for more information.

If a throat pack is placed, chart the time of its placement and its removal.

At the end of the procedure, before the mouth gag is removed, the surgeon, or the anesthetist, can insert an orogastric tube to suction out the stomach. Air from a mask induction, as well as midazolam that is still left in the stomach, can be suctioned out. Suctioning out midazolam can facilitate wake-up in the recovery room.

Smooth emergence from anesthesia is important with this surgery. The goal is to avoid coughing, bucking, or nausea/vomiting or retching so as to prevent increased risk of bleeding, or hematoma formation from the increased throat pressures. Steroids and an antiemetic should be given.

Suctioning the oropharynx (before extubating the patient) is best done with a soft, flexible catheter so as not to disrupt the surgical area and cause bleeding.

All children undergoing T&A should be considered at increased risk for perioperative airway difficulties. Extubate the patient only when the child is fully awake.

Position the child laterally postoperatively to facilitate blood and saliva drainage until the child is fully awake. Laryngospasm is a common complication after any surgery in the throat.

Return to Surgery for Bleeding After Tonsillectomy/Adenoidectomy

In some cases, a return to surgery is needed to stop postsurgical bleeding of the tonsillar or adenoids space after a tonsillectomy and/or an adenoidectomy. This kind of bleeding usually occurs within the first 24 hours after the original procedure (99% within the first 6 hours postoperatively) but can be delayed (occurring 2–3 weeks after surgery); the risk for this complication peaks at 7 days postoperatively. Post-T&A bleeding risk is increased in older patients, patients with inflammation or infection, patients with a history of coagulopathy, and patients who took aspirin or nonsteroidal anti-inflammatory drugs (NSAIDs) preoperatively.

Operative Procedure

If the patient is actively bleeding, an orogastric tube should be placed to suction out the stomach before induction of anesthesia is performed. A nasal or mouth speculum is inserted, and the bleeder is identified and cauterized. Packing is inserted into the nose at the end of the case for adenoid bleeding.

Anesthetic

General anesthesia is used with an OETT; an oral RAE may be used. True rapid-sequence induction should be done.

Positioning

The patient is placed in a supine position, with a shoulder roll used to slightly extend the head. Bilateral arms are tucked at the sides.

Anesthetic Implications

Give an IV anticholinergic agent to reduce airway secretions.

Patients who present from home with post-T&A bleeding may be in shock from hypovolemia and anemia, may still be actively bleeding (leading to poor visualization of the glottis during intubation), and have a stomach full of blood. It is important to assess volume status (urinary output, blood pressure, heart rate, skin turgor) preoperatively. A preoperative hematocrit level should be obtained as well. It may be necessary to establish an IV and rehydrate the patient before going to the operating room. Type and cross-matching of the patient's blood may be necessary, and blood may need to be available in the OR.

Prior to the induction of anesthesia, children should be covered with warm blankets (or other warming measures used). Keep the room warm, use warming lamps and mattress, use a heated humidifier, warm fluids, wrap the child's extremities and head in plastic, and use warm, low-flow gases.

After taping the eyelids shut, securely tape eye pads over both of the patient's eyes to protect them.

With post-T&A bleeding surgery, try to give back up to half of the NPO deficit as a means to attenuate hemodynamic changes that result from bleeding.

Gentle insertion of a soft catheter should be done to suction out the stomach before extubation.

These patients have an even greater risk of perioperative airway difficulties. Make sure the patient is fully awake before attempting extubation.

Position the child laterally postoperatively to facilitate blood and saliva drainage until the child is fully awake. Laryngospasm is a common complication after any surgery in the throat.

Blow-by oxygen is given continuously after extubation and during transport to the recovery room.

Pediatric Tracheostomy

In tracheostomy, an opening is made into the trachea and a cannula is inserted to facilitate breathing. This procedure is performed to relieve upper airway obstruction; for micrognathia, subglottic stenosis, subglottic hemangioma, and laryngotracheomalacia; to provide prolonged ventilatory support with respiratory insufficiency; or in case of craniofacial abnormalities such as Pierre Robin sequence/complex.

Operative Procedure

Although the technical aspects of this procedure differ by surgeon, in general a transverse incision is made one fingerbreadth above the sternal notch (approximately halfway between the cricoid cartilage and the sternal notch). The platysma and deep fascia are incised, the thyroid isthmus is retracted superiorly, and the tracheal rings are exposed. Staying in the midline of the trachea, stay sutures are placed in the tracheal rings and a vertical incision is made through the second and third tracheal rings. The tracheostomy outer cannula is placed, and then the inner cannula is inserted into the outer cannula. The ventilator tubing is then attached to the cannula.

Once $ETCO_2$ is confirmed and the patient's oxygen saturation is acceptable, the surgeon will usually ask the anesthetist to remove the endotracheal tube completely. The outer flange of the tracheostomy tube is usually held in place with umbilical tapes tied around the patient's neck. A split gauze dressing is applied around the bottom part of the tracheostomy cannula and around the wound.

Anesthetic

General anesthesia is used with an OETT; muscle relaxants are given.

Positioning

The patient is placed in a supine position, with a shoulder roll used to extend the head.

Anesthetic Implications

After taping the eyelids shut, securely tape eye pads over both of the patient's eyes to protect them.

Prior to the induction of anesthesia, children should be covered with warm blankets (or other warming measures used). Keep the room warm, use warming lamps and mattress, use a heated humidifier, warm fluids, wrap the child's extremities in plastic, and use warm, low-flow gases.

This procedure requires clear communication between the anesthesia provider and the surgeon, especially after the trachea has been entered by the surgeon. The ETT will be pulled back several centimeters (to the subglottis) under the direction of the surgeon so as to place the tracheostomy tube. Next, rapid confirmation of the tracheostomy tube placement is made via $ETCO_2$, oxygen saturation, and chest movement. The ventilating airway will then be the new tracheostomy site.

To prevent airway fires, use caution with oxygen during this procedure. Airway fire is a risk if cauterization (Bovie) is used. See the discussion of safety concerns in Chapter 1 for more information. Deceasing the FiO_2 levels to 30% while the surgeon is using the Bovie to enter the airway is recommended to prevent airway fire. If the patient's oxygen saturation drops during this level, let the surgeon know. It may be necessary to interrupt the surgery and increase the FiO_2 to get the oxygen saturation up, before decreasing the FiO_2 again to continue the procedure.

Have a tracheostomy flex tube extension available; it connects the tracheostomy and ventilator circuit tubing.

In general, placement of an esophageal stethoscope may get in the way of the surgery.

The ETT tip and balloon will help guide the surgeon in correct placement of the tracheostomy, as a child's neck may be very short.

Note the tracheostomy tube manufacturer and the tube size as part of your hand-off report. The obturator for the tracheostomy tube must accompany the patient out of the operating room; it may be needed to replace the tracheostomy if it becomes dislodged. This device may be taped to the head of the bed or the front of the chart so that it can be readily found in case of tracheostomy dislodgement.

A postoperative chest X-ray is taken to ensure no pneumothorax has occurred.

Complications

Potential complications of tracheostomy include hemorrhage and subcutaneous air in the tissues and pleural space.

PEDIATRIC THORACIC SURGERY

See Chapter 14 on thoracic surgery for more information regarding mediastinal anatomy.

Anesthetic Implications of Pediatric Thoracic Surgery

Preoperative evaluation of pediatric patients undergoing thoracic surgery is crucial—especially assessment for airway obstruction (stridor, wheezing, cyanosis, atelectasis, pneumonia) and signs during a position change such as from the supine or lateral position. CT scans of the chest are invaluable in assessing the mediastinum.

Sympathetic tone is diminished with anesthesia and may cause cardiovascular decompensation.

Mask induction with 100% FiO_2 and a volatile agent while the patient is in a sitting position may be the induction of choice with a patient who has a mediastinal tumor. Ketamine and narcotic-based induction can be used to avoid cardiovascular compromise.

Keeping the child warm during thoracic procedures is crucial, as body heat is easily dissipated when the chest is opened. Prior to the induction of anesthesia, children should be covered with warm blankets (or other warming measures used). Keep the room warm, use warming lamps and mattress, use a heated humidifier, warm fluids, wrap the child's extremities and head in plastic, and use warm, low-flow gases.

Pectus Excavatum or Carinatum Correction

These procedures involve correction of a deformity of the anterior chest wall (sternum and ribs) that progresses in severity as the child develops and grows. With excavatum, there is a depression of the sternum and costal cartilages ("funnel chest"). With carinatum, there is a protrusion of the sternum and ribs ("pigeon chest").

This surgery is performed to relieve respiratory symptoms (restrictive disease and ventilation/perfusion dynamics in the lung) or circulatory symptoms (limited stroke volumes, arrhythmias, right-axis deviation) related to rib cage compression of associated structures. Although it was formerly believed that correction was indicated primarily for cosmetic reasons, it is now known that the primary cardiovascular effect of pectus excavatum is compression of the right atrium and ventricle, with subsequent decreased right heart function/output. Indeed, surgical repair of significant pectus excavatum should be expected to improve right heart output by approximately one third. These chest wall defects may occur in association with scoliosis, spontaneous pneumothorax, mitral valve deformities, and (rarely) Marfan's syndrome.

Operative Procedure
Pectus Excavatum

The *Ravitch-type procedure* was the technique of choice from 1950 to 1999, and is still frequently used. With this approach, a presternal incision is made, with rib cartilages and xiphoid process being separated from the sternum. The mediastinum is entered and the pericardium dissected from the sternum. Depending on the deformity, the sternum may be reshaped and the costal cartilages trimmed as needed. The sternum is fixed in placed with sutures; detached muscles are resutured to their points of division. If the pleural cavity has been entered, a chest tube is inserted and connected to a sealed drainage system.

The *Nuss-type procedure* is the most popular operation now performed; it was introduced in 1997. With this approach, bilateral transverse lateral incisions are made. A stainless steel (or titanium) bar is bent and passed across the mediastinum (between the sternum and the pericardium) and then "flipped" to elevate the sternum off the mediastinum—unilateral or bilateral diagnostic thoracoscopy is usually used to help guide the bar (or bars). Chest tubes are typically used to suction out the bilateral pneumothoraces at the conclusion of the operation, after which the tubes are removed. The bars are typically secured to the lateral chest wall musculature with numerous sutures.

Pectus Carinatum

To repair a pectus carinatum, most surgeons perform a modified version of the Ravitch-type technique.

Anesthetic

GETA is given with insertion of an OETT. Most children also undergo placement of thoracic epidural catheters for postoperative analgesia. Such catheters typically stay in until the fourth or fifth postoperative day. In many institutions, the epidural infusion is controlled by a "pain management team," composed of anesthesia care providers.

Positioning
The patient is placed in a supine position, with a rolled sheet placed between the shoulder blades.

Anesthetic Implications
Preoperatively, assessment of exercise tolerance is important. If the stroke volume is decreased, the child may have symptoms of exercise intolerance.

Patients may have restrictive lung disease with chronic hypoxemia, pulmonary hypertension, and polycythemia. The FEV_1 and FVC may be decreased somewhat, with the FEV_1/FVC ratio being either normal or increased. Residual volume and total lung capacity may also be decreased.

Prior to the induction of anesthesia, children should be covered with warm blankets (or other warming measures used). Keep the room warm, use warming lamps and mattress, use a heated humidifier, warm fluids, wrap the child's extremities and head in plastic, and use warm, low-flow gases.

The goal is to extubate the patient at the end of the case. A chest X-ray in the OR or post anesthesia care unit (PACU) can usually rule out a pneumothorax.

Monitors and IV Access
An arterial line may be needed but is not usually necessary.

Induction
Patients have a decreased FRC with restrictive disease. In such a case, the patient will be induced by inhalation agents faster and lose oxygen reserves faster.

Complications
The most common complications are pneumothorax, pleural effusion, flail chest, and atelectasis.

Thoracotomy: Lobectomy or Pneumonectomy
Thoracotomy is the removal of one or more lobes of the lung (lobectomy) or the entire lung (pneumonectomy). This surgery is performed to treat tumors, trauma, infectious processes, cysts, congenital abnormalities, inflammatory lesions, and bronchiectasis.

Operative Procedure
Although well described in the surgical literature, thoracoscopic lobectomy (also called video-assisted thoracic surgery [VATS]) is offered at only a few select centers by a few pediatric surgeons who are skilled in this advanced thoracoscopic technique. At most institutions, open thoracotomy is performed.

In *lobectomy*, a posterolateral incision is made, and the muscles and ribs of the chest are retracted. The visceral pleura is dissected free from the hilus, and the pulmonary artery and vein of the diseased lobe are ligated and divided. The bronchus is then transected and the stump is sutured closed. The surgeon may test for air leaks by filling the chest with warm saline and observing for bubbles when the anesthesia provider performs a Valsalva maneuver.

In *pneumonectomy*, the surgeon uses the same approach to the lung as in lobectomy. The bronchus, pulmonary artery and superior and inferior pulmonary veins are then isolated. The pulmonary artery and veins are ligated. The bronchial stump is clamped, transected, and sutured closed. Lymph-node tissue is excised.

Lobectomy patients will almost always have a chest tube placed prior to closing. In contrast, pneumonectomy patients may not, because fluid typically "fills up" the empty hemithorax after lung removal.

Anesthetic
General anesthesia is used with an OETT; muscle relaxants are given. A double-lumen tube is impractical in a small pediatric patient younger than age

8–9 years. See double-lumen endobronchial tube chart at the beginning of this chapter for more information on tube sizes.

A generous dose of long-acting local anesthetics, such as bupivicaine, for intercostal nerve blocks, may be given by the surgeon just prior to closing the thoracotomy incision.

Positioning
The patient's position depends on the site of surgery, but is usually lateral on a bean-bag.

Anesthetic Implications
If the patient has a space-occupying lesion, it is important to assess for signs of cardiac and pulmonary dysfunction (e.g., decreased stroke volume, cardiac output, lung volumes, functional residual capacity, and airway compression) preoperatively. Airway compression and cardiovascular depression may occur if the child is placed in the supine position and during anesthesia induction. The child may need to remain intubated in the immediate postoperative period.

Prior to the induction of anesthesia, children should be covered with warm blankets (or other warming measures used). Keep the room warm, use warming lamps and mattress, use a heated humidifier, warm fluids, wrap the child's extremities and head in plastic, and use warm, low-flow gases.

Barotrauma is more likely to occur in pediatric patients with existing lung disease, especially in conjunction with one-lung ventilation. Faster respiratory rates with a decreased tidal volume are used to decrease the peak airway pressures during one-lung ventilation; hand-ventilating can also help assess airway pressures.

Extubation of the patient at the end of the case may be possible if the patient's hemodynamics are stable, if the child is breathing spontaneously and maintaining normal oxygen saturations and end-tidal CO_2 levels, and if the child is fully awake and has a strong cough effort with normal tidal volumes.

Monitors and IV Access
An arterial line may be needed for blood pressure monitoring and blood gas sampling. CVP monitoring may help with fluid management.

Complications
Massive blood loss, pneumothorax, hemopneumothorax, and airway perforation are all possible complications with lung surgery.

Tracheal–Esophageal Fistula Correction in Neonates
In this procedure, a tracheal–esophageal fistula (TEF), also known as a tracheoesophageal fistula, is ligated with anastomosis of the esophagus segments. The infant with such a fistula will usually present with excessive drooling, following by coughing, cyanosis, and choking, all of which occur with the first feeding. As the infant coughs and cries, air enters the stomach through the fistula, resulting in gastric distention. Aspiration pneumonitis can occur from regurgitated gastric fluids.

Diagnosis is made upon failure to pass an orogastric tube into the stomach. An important alternative diagnosis that must be considered when an orogastric tube does not enter the stomach is esophageal perforation. TEF is rarely a surgical emergency if the child is hemodynamically stable and is well oxygenated.

At least five types of congenital tracheal–esophageal anomalies are distinguished. The most frequently encountered type, accounting for 85% of TEF-affected babies, is a "distal fistula" between the trachea (just above the carina) and the *lower* esophageal segment (coming up from the stomach). The proximal esophageal segment ends in a blind pouch. With this type of defect, nothing can get to the stomach from the proximal esophagus, but fluids can back up through the lower esophageal segment and enter the airway and lungs.

The coexistence of other congenital anomalies is common. TEF may be associated with ventricular and atrial septal defects, tetralogy of Fallot, coarctation of the aorta, and a collection of defects known as VATER syndrome (V: missing/abnormal vertebra; A: anal defects such as imperforate anus; T: tracheoesophageal fistula; E: esophageal atresia; R: radial limb hyperplasia or renal abnormalities).

Operative Procedure

It may be necessary to place a gastrostomy tube before the TEF repair is performed, so as to keep the stomach empty and prevent the regurgitation of gastric fluid into the trachea and the lungs. The TEF repair is usually done through a right fourth interspace thoracotomy. The approach may be retropleural (leaving the pleura intact; requires less retraction and a smaller incision; more technically difficult) or transpleural (requires direct retraction of the lung).

This procedure can be done using thoracoscopy. The surgeon may need to stop intermittently to allow the anesthetist to hand-ventilate the patient so as to increase the oxygen saturation.

Ligation of the defect with primary anastomosis of the esophageal segments is undertaken to repair the defect. The fistula to the trachea is closed; the proximal esophageal pouch is opened. Often, the surgeon will direct the CRNA to pass a nasogastric tube (NGT) through the patient's nose and into the upper esophagus. This practice helps the surgeon identify the esophagus in the chest, and the NGT will be in place if the proximal and distal esophageal segments can be anastomosed. The esophagus is anastomosed around the NGT and then secured to the surrounding fascia to stabilize and prevent pressure on the suture line.

If the native esophagus segments are insufficiently long to be brought together, a second (or third) operation may take place at a later date in which a piece of bowel or stomach is used to connect the two segments.

A chest tube is usually left in place after a transpleural thoracotomy.

Anesthetic

An IV should be placed before induction occurs. A rapid-sequence induction with an awake intubation should be done after suctioning the esophageal pouch and oropharynx; maintaining spontaneous ventilation can help to prevent distention of the stomach.

Insert the ETT deeply, with the bevel facing posteriorly, and confirm unilateral breath sounds. Pull the ETT back slowly, and stop pulling as soon as bilateral breath sounds are heard (at this point, the ETT tip is above the carina). The endotracheal tube can be positioned with the Murphy eye at the distal end of the trachea *past the fistula,* with the solid part of the tube occluding the fistula. Proper placement of the endotracheal tube is critical. Hand-ventilate the patient to identify changes in ventilation pressures.

Although it is not usually needed, a Fogarty catheter can be placed through a bronchoscope and used to occlude the fistula.

If possible, use spontaneous ventilation until the fistula is ligated, and then use controlled ventilation.

Frequent endotracheal suctioning is needed.

Use low airway pressures to prevent gastric distention (pushing air through the fistula).

Avoid nitrous oxide so as to prevent gastric distention.

Positioning

The patient is placed in a left lateral decubitus position. Avoid neck extension or instrumentation during or after the repair, as it may disrupt suture lines. The infant should remain in a semi-Fowler's position from preoperatively until after induction.

Anesthetic Implications

These infants are often premature and present with excessive salivation/drooling, inability to feed with cyanotic spells, and coughing relieved by suctioning. Preoperatively, attention to the child's respiratory status is critically important. Preoperative interventions include no feeding, and placement of the neonate in an infant warmer with the head of the bed elevated 30 degrees; the upright positioning will help to prevent fluid reflux through the fistula into the lungs. The upper esophageal pouch should be decompressed with an orogastric tube connected to suction until the repair is done. If saliva is allowed to accumulate in the upper pouch, it can be aspirated into the patient's lungs.

Prior to the induction of anesthesia, children should be covered with warm blankets (or other warming measures used). Keep the room warm, use warming lamps and mattress, use a heated humidifier, warm fluids, wrap the child's extremities and head in plastic, and use warm, low-flow gases.

If a gastrostomy tube is placed, it can be used as a pop-off vent to remove excess air in the stomach.

A thoracic epidural can be placed for postoperative pain control.

A precordial stethoscope is essential, as it is your only source for breath sounds. Placing an esophageal stethoscope is not an option in these cases.

Try to extubate the patient at the end of the case to decrease the stress placed on the suture line by the endotracheal tube. Use smaller amounts of short-acting narcotics.

If transpleural resection is done, a higher oxygen concentration may be needed during right lung compression.

CARDIOVASCULAR SURGERY

Given the vast complexities and institutional-specific guidelines related to pediatric cardiovascular surgery, only the basic disease process and surgical goals are addressed here. For more detailed information, please refer to pediatric cardiology books and your institutional guidelines.

Most congenital heart defects (CHD) require surgery during infancy or childhood. Heart defects can range from an abnormality involving a single part of the heart to very complex defects associated with severe upheaval of cardiac structures.

Pediatric Cardiovascular Defects

Pediatric heart surgery deals with congenital heart defects; the problem in such cases is not a coronary artery perfusion issue. The goal of any pediatric anesthetist is to keep a balance between the pulmonary and systemic blood flow and not over-circulate either system.

Blood goes where resistance is least. As a consequence, the direction of blood flow depends on the balance of pulmonary vascular resistance (PVR) and systemic vascular resistance (SVR). Normally the PVR is much lower than the SVR.

With any abnormal communication between the right and left sides of the heart, blood will flow away from the point of higher resistance (SVR) to the point of lower resistance, increasing pulmonary blood resistance (PVR). This can cause pulmonary edema and right-sided heart failure. Any increase in PVR may cause shunting at the atrial level, with flow going from right to left. This causes a decreased pulmonary blood flow, leading to cyanosis.

The anesthetic management of pediatric patients with CHD requires thorough knowledge of the pathophysiology of the defect. The most important information you can have before starting a pediatric cardiac case is summarized here:

1. What is the problem? Where is the blood going? Is there shunting? If so, in which direction is it going? Can the shunt be manipulated?
   - Cyanotic lesions
   - Acyanotic lesions
   Is this an extracardiac or an intracardiac issue? Is pulmonary blood flow increased or decreased? Is there is a stenosis—that is, an obstruction to normal blood flow? If so, is it a valvular, subvalvular, or pulmonary venous abnormality?
2. Where do you want the blood to go and how do you make that happen? (SVR:PVR)
3. Is the patient compensating or decompensating? Is the patient in congestive heart failure?

Be extremely organized!

A tetracaine with epinephrine spinal can be placed at the beginning of the surgery, creating a "total spinal." This approach blocks the sympathetic nervous system's responses to surgery, allowing for a complete sympathectomy and greater ability to control resistance pharmacologically.

A pulmonary artery catheter is typically not used in pediatric cardiac surgery, but a CVP is routinely placed. Many of these cases have a line placed in the left atrium and a CVP placed in the right atrium; thus a vasopressor may be going to one side of the heart (which can affect the SVR) and a vasodilator may be going to the other side (which can treat the PVR). A radial or femoral arterial line is often placed on the left side, as several procedures use the right-sided vessels as part of the surgical procedure.

The following factors increase PVR and decrease pulmonary blood flow:

- Hypoxemia
- Acidosis
- Hypercapnia/hypercarbia
- Hypothermia

The following factors decrease PVR and increase pulmonary blood flow:

- Nitric oxide
- Oxygen
- Hypocarbia
- Alkalosis
- Anemia
- Amrinone
- Milrinone
- PGE_1

Cyanotic Lesions

A decrease in pulmonary blood flow due to obstruction causes a *right-to-left shunt.* As a result, oxygenated and deoxygenated blood mix together, producing arterial hypoxemia. The unoxygenated blood in the right ventricle is blocked from entering the pulmonary artery and moves through the septum to the left side of the heart, where it mixes with oxygenated blood. Conditions characterized by right-to-left shunt include tetralogy of Fallot, Eisenmenger's syndrome, pulmonary stenosis or atresia with a ventricular septal defect, tricuspid atresia, truncus arteriosus, patent foramen ovale, hypoplastic left heart syndrome, and transposition of the great arteries.

Patients with cyanotic lesions will demonstrate slow uptake of inhaled agents (the blood passes over to the left side of the heart without going into the lung to pick up the volatile agent). Meticulous care must be taken to remove all air bubbles out of IV tubing and IV solution to avoid an arterial air embolism.

A neonate with a cyanotic lesion will require a prostaglandin E_1 infusion to maintain ductus arteriosus patency (also called a ductal dependent lesion). The majority of blood flow goes from the pulmonary artery through the ductus into the descending aorta to ensure adequate lower body perfusion. If the ductus arteriosus is the only connection between the systemic and pulmonary circulations, it must be maintained patent with a prostaglandin infusion or death occurs quickly.

Hypoplastic Left Heart Syndrome (HLHS) Surgery

Hypoplastic left heart syndrome (HLHS) is a complex congenital anomaly of the aorta and left side of the heart. A patient with this condition usually has aortic valve atresia (abnormally closed or absent valve), severe left ventricular (LV) hypoplasia or an absent LV, hypoplasia (incomplete development) of the ascending aorta, mitral valve hypoplasia, and coarctation of the aorta. Although surgeons cannot make another ventricle to remedy HLHS, they can change the physiologic pathways to get oxygenated blood to the aorta.

All blood coming from the pulmonary veins flows first into the right atrium (through the foramen ovale from the left), then into the right ventricle, and finally into the lungs. In the newborn, the child's survival is dependent on a patent ductus arteriosus (PDA) to provide systemic blood flow and a balanced level of PVR to SVR: Both the pulmonary and systemic circulations are supplied from the same ventricle. Said another way, all or nearly all of the cardiac output is ejected from the right ventricle. Premature closure of the PDA results in a progressive decrease in coronary and systemic perfusion leading to metabolic acidosis, myocardial ischemia, and possibly death.

If PVR rapidly decreases, which is a normal occurrence in early neonatal life, a large increase in blood flow will be redirected into the lungs at the expense of the systemic circulation. If systemic circulation decreases, coronary circulation decreases, resulting in metabolic acidosis and potentially death: Increased PVR = decreased pulmonary blood flow (PBF), and vice versa. A prostaglandin E_1 infusion may be given to prevent closure of the PDA.

Anesthetic Implications

Repair of HLHS requires cardiopulmonary bypass. Reconstruction of the aortic arch will require deep hypothermic cardiac arrest (DHCA). Mortality is still approximately 70% in such cases even with surgery; a heart transplant is a possible option in some patients.

Tetralogy of Fallot Correction

The following abnormalities of tetralogy of Fallot are distinguished:

- *Pulmonary stenosis or atresia:* right ventricular outflow tract obstruction (infundibulum); the distal pulmonary artery may be hypoplastic or absent
  - Stenosis of the infundibulum (50% of cases)
  - Stenosis of the pulmonary valve (10%)
  - Stenosis of the pulmonary artery (10%)
  - Stenosis of the pulmonary valve and infundibulum (30%)
- Overriding aorta (over pulmonary outflow tract)

The last two conditions are essential to produce the clinical picture.

- Ventricular septal defect
- Right ventricle hypertrophy

As the right ventricular outflow obstruction increases, right-to-left shunting occurs through the VSD (unoxygenated blood enters the aorta from the right ventricle and through the VSD), resulting in cyanosis along with a reduced pulmonary blood flow.

Pentalogy of Fallot is a syndrome consisting of TOF plus an atrial septal defect.

The child with TOF is cyanotic at rest; this cyanosis increases with activity. The severity of the cyanosis depends on the degree of pulmonary stenosis. In children with less severe pulmonary stenosis, surgery can be done after the child is older than one year of age but usually is performed around 12 months of age.

Operative Procedure

Surgical correction of tetralogy of Fallot (TOF) is achieved by closing the ventricular septal defect (VSD), with placement of a patch to channel blood into overriding aorta (the aorta sits on top of the VSD), resection of hypertrophied infundibulum, and placement of a patch over the right ventricular (RV) outflow tract.

Total correction of the defect is done on cardiopulmonary bypass with aortic cross-clamping. The approach is through either a right atriotomy or ventriculotomy, with the choice depending on the length of the RV outflow tract obstruction. The RV obstruction is resected by opening the pulmonary valve and enlarging the RV outflow tract by a pulmonary valvotomy; a pericardial membrane patch or a synthetic graft is sutured on the margins of the defect to close the VSD. A chest tube is placed and the incision closed.

A *modified Blalock-Taussig shunt* may be performed in the first months of the child's life, with a more definitive surgery following later. This temporary shunt creates a communication between the subclavian artery and the pulmonary artery so as to increase blood flow to the lungs, thereby improving blood oxygenation and relieving cyanosis. The original form of Blalock-Taussig shunt is rarely used today; instead, artificial tubing is sewn between the subclavian artery and the pulmonary artery, making it easier to regulate blood flow to the lungs. Another version, called a *Sano shunt,* involves insertion of a shunt directly from the right ventricle to the pulmonary artery.

Anesthetic Implications

Preoperatively, the child must have a full laboratory investigation with a cardiac catheterization and angiography to determine the precise morphology and size of the pulmonary artery.

Anesthetic Goals

Anesthetic goals of TOF correction include prevention of hypoxemic spells; avoidance of beta-sympathetic drugs (they cause RV infundibular spasm, leading to increased shunt and cyanosis); avoidance of increased PVR and decreased SVR; and avoidance of isoflurane and enflurane, as these agents decrease SVR, which in turn increases shunt and cyanosis. Manipulation of conduction tissues in the heart can occasionally cause dysrhythmias; atrioventricular pacing capabilities should be readily available. Prostaglandin E_1 infusion is used to keep the PDA open.

The severity of RV outflow tract obstruction affects the magnitude of the shunt through the VSD. Severe obstruction of blood into the pulmonary artery decreases pulmonary blood flow and increases right-to-left shunt, so that unoxygenated blood goes directly into the left heart and causes cyanosis. Maintaining systemic vascular resistance by reducing the magnitude of the right-to-left shunt with low pulmonary vascular resistance and maintaining atrioventricular synchrony is very important. Ketamine 3–4 mg/kg IM or 1–2 mg/kg IV can help to improve pulmonary blood flow by increasing SVR.

Some children may have an acute cyanosis crisis called a "tet spell." If the child is stressed or crying, changes in pulmonary vascular resistance are likely to occur, right-to-left shunt increases, oxygen demand increases significantly, and the child becomes extremely cyanotic. This is a life-threatening event but can be treated in a hospital. Treatment of a tet spell involves attempts to increase the preload and afterload with IVF, Neosynephrine, epinephrine, and use of the "knee to chest" position.

Preoperative Measures

Preanesthetic assessment of cyanosis, shunting, and RV outflow tract obstruction is important. The amount of right-to-left shunt depends on (1) the degree of right ventricular outflow tract obstruction; (2) SVR; and (3) PVR.

Monitors and IV Access

Arterial and central venous lines are needed, and possibly a left atrial catheter. TEE monitoring is required

IV Vasoactive Agents

These agents include epinephrine, nitroprusside (need to maintain SVR to prevent hypotension and right ventricular dysfunction), and milrinone.

Transposition of the Great Arteries Correction

Correction of transposition of the great arteries (TGA) is a staged procedure. The first goal is to increase mixing of blood between the two circulations so as to improve systemic oxygenation (see the discussion of balloon atrial septostomy later in this section). The second goal is complete surgical correction of the defect; this procedure, which requires cardiopulmonary bypass, is usually done when the child is 1–2 weeks of age.

TGA is suspected when the infant has persistent severe cyanosis. An echocardiogram and cardiac catheterization are done in the first hours of life. The catheterization is both diagnostic and therapeutic, as the atrial septostomy can be done in the same procedure where TGA is diagnosed.

In TGA, the aorta arises from the *right ventricle* and the pulmonary artery arises from the *left ventricle* (the opposite of normal anatomy). As a consequence of this switch, desaturated venous blood returning from the periphery is pumped back into the systemic circulation, while oxygenated pulmonary venous blood is pumped back into the pulmonary artery (lungs). If the TGA is a complete transposition, the systemic and pulmonary circulations are split and function independently. This condition is incompatible with life (it causes profound hypoxemia) unless there are associated shunts—as with patent foramen ovale (PFO), patent ductus arteriosus (PDA), or ventricular septal defect (VSD)—that permit mixing of oxygenated and unoxygenated blood between the systemic and pulmonary systems. The VSD must be large enough to permit unobstructed mixing and to equalize pressures in the RV and LV. Persistent pulmonary hypertension (PPHN) and increased PVR decrease mixing and lead to cyanosis, dyspnea, and/or congestive heart failure.

A *balloon atrial septostomy* may be done to temporarily enlarge an atrial septal ovale and allow mixing of the blood until the definitive surgery can be done. The complete switch and translocation of the aorta and the pulmonary artery may not be done until the second week of life.

Operative Procedure
Both cardiopulmonary bypass and aortic cross-clamping are done. The proximal portions of both the aorta and the pulmonary artery are transected. The left and right coronary artery ostia are removed from the aortic root and implanted into the main pulmonary artery root. The pulmonary artery is brought over the aorta (in the normal position). The aorta is attached to its root; the pulmonary artery is reconstructed with a cryopreserved homograft and attached to its pulmonary root. The atrial septal defect (ASD) is then closed.

Anesthetic Implications
Third-degree atrioventricular block can occur after the initial procedure of creating an ASD. Chronotropic drugs (atropine) should be available to counteract this complication.

Anesthetics given IV will have minimal dilution to the heart and brain in patients with TGA, and their dosages should be reduced. The effects of inhaled anesthetic will be delayed, as only small amounts will reach the systemic circulation. Induction and maintenance can be done in TGA with ketamine, muscle relaxation, and opioids. Prostaglandin E_1 infusion is given to keep the PDA open.

Monitors and IV Access
A right atrial catheter (central venous pressure line), left atrial catheter (vasoactive infusions), arterial line, and pulmonary artery catheter (to monitor cardiac output and heart pressures) are required. TEE monitoring is performed as well.

IV Vasoactive Agents
These agents include epinephrine, nitroprusside, nitroglycerin, milrinone, and phenoxybenzamine (an antihypertensive that blocks the alpha-adrenergic response to epinephrine and norepinephrine).

Tricuspid Atresia Surgery
Tricuspid atresia surgery aims to create a way for blood to flow into the pulmonary artery. This surgery is commonly referred to as a Fontan procedure; many variations of the procedure exist. It is usually performed in two stages, and the goal is to direct systemic venous return to the pulmonary

arteries without an intervening heart (pumping) chamber and to prevent increased PVR. A low PVR is essential for blood to flow into the pulmonary vasculature without being pumped in.

Tricuspid atresia is a rare condition in which there is no direct communication between the right atrium and the right ventricle because the tricuspid valve did not develop in utero. This defect is frequently associated with varying degrees of right ventricular and pulmonary artery hypoplasia. Successful repair depends on the presence of functional anatomy.

For the infant to survive, there must be associated lesions, including an atrial septal or ventricular septal defects, or patent ductus arteriosus. In such a case, unoxygenated venous blood moves in a right-to-left shunt to mix with oxygenated blood, resulting in systemic arterial oxygen desaturation.

The infant with tricuspid atresia is cyanotic at birth. The EKG shows left-axis deviation and left ventricular hypertrophy.

Operative Procedure

In a Fontan procedure, the surgeon creates a passageway that allows unoxygenated blood from the body to bypass the heart and go directly to the pulmonary artery (PA). The resulting circulation to the lungs is considered passive, as a ventricle does not pump blood into the PA.

Multiple variations of the Fontan procedure exist. In one approach, the superior vena cava is anastomosed directly to the distal right pulmonary artery. In another approach, an extracardiac shunt is constructed that sends blood flow returning to the heart (via the superior vena cava or inferior vena cava) directly to the right pulmonary artery.

If the pulmonary artery is fully formed and can be used, it is disconnected from the rudimentary right ventricle and connected directly to the right atrium, creating a venous right-sided pumping chamber. The patient must have a decreased PVR for this technique to work, because the right atrial

force is limited. An increase in the PVR can lead to right heart failure.

Anesthetic Implications

Careful monitoring of the transpulmonary gradient (central venous pressure [CVP] and the left atrial pressure) and its individual components is important. CVP should be kept at less than 18 mm Hg and transpulmonary gradients should be kept at more than 10 mm Hg. Assessment for adventitious lung sounds, hepatomegaly, and ascites should be done.

PEEP, increased pulmonary artery pressures, and prolonged inspiratory phase must be avoided.

These patients have limited hemodynamic reserves and may require vasoactive infusions.

Cardiac dysrhythmias are common in patients with tricuspid atresia, and atrioventricular pacing equipment should be readily available.

Normal PaO_2 levels after a Fontan procedure are in the range of 88–93%.

Have heparin and protamine available for these cases, as anticoagulation therapy is usually given to prevent thrombus formation in the shunts.

Monitors and IV Access

A right atrial catheter (central venous pressure line), left atrial catheter (vasoactive infusions), arterial line, and pulmonary artery catheter (to monitor cardiac output and heart pressures) are required. TEE monitoring is performed as well.

IV Vasoactive Agents

These infusions may include epinephrine, nitroprusside, nitroglycerin, and milrinone.

Truncus Arteriosus Repair

In truncus arteriosus, the normal separation of the aortic and pulmonary circulations does not occur in utero, leading to a single arterial trunk with a semilunar valve leaving the heart. Outflow from both ventricles is directed into the common trunk; this one artery carries both oxygenated and unoxygenated blood out through the pulmonary artery and the aorta to the lungs and the body. This is a very rare, congenital lesion. The single vessel leaving the heart typically straddles a defect in the interventricular septum that almost always contains a VSD, this allows both ventricles to empty into the arteriosus trunk. While an arteriosus valve exists, it is usually incompetent.

In rare cases, the truncus can originate from either the right or left ventricle.

Because of this anatomy, the pulmonary arterial blood has a higher oxygen saturation than the systemic venous blood and, therefore, the systemic arterial blood has a lower oxygen saturation than the pulmonary venous blood.

Surgery is performed in early infancy to prevent severe pulmonary hypertension.

Operative Procedure

Truncus arteriosus surgery is to close a ventricular septal defect (VSD) and separate blood flow to the body from blood flow to the lungs. This type of repair is one of the more extensive pediatric cardiac procedures done in early infancy.

Surgery is done to close the ventricular septal defect (a synthetic patch or pericardial membrane) and separate blood flow to the lungs from blood flow to the body. The pulmonary arteries are then disconnected from the truncus, and a conduit with a valve is placed from the right ventricle to the pulmonary arteries (also known as Rastelli repair).

Surgical repair with a long period of cardiopulmonary bypass, aortic cross-clamping, and hypothermic circulatory arrest is done. Banding of the pulmonary artery is necessary if pulmonary blood flow is excessive.

The VSD can be closed so that only LV output enters the single arterial trunk. A valved conduit is placed between the right ventricle and the pulmonary artery, allowing blood flow to the lungs.

Anesthetic Implications

Neonates with truncus arteriosus usually develop congestive heart failure (CHF) because of the abundant pulmonary blood flow. Positive-pressure ventilation can be helpful in decreasing the symptoms of CHF.

The anesthetic choice will depend on the pulmonary blood flow.

The conduit and valve will need to be replaced several times as the child grows. It may also need to be replaced in adulthood.

Monitors and IV Access

A right atrial catheter (central venous pressure line), left atrial catheter (vasoactive infusions), arterial line, and pulmonary artery catheter (to monitor cardiac output and heart pressures) are required. TEE monitoring is performed as well.

IV Vasoactive Agents

These infusions may include epinephrine, nitroprusside, nitroglycerin, and milrinone.

Acyanotic Lesions

In acyanotic lesions, the increased pulmonary flow is due to a *left-to-right shunt*. Conditions causing this problem include atrial septal defect, ventricular septal defect, and patent ductus arteriosus.

The increase in pulmonary blood flow causes the pulmonary vascular bed to change, increasing PVR over time and leading to pulmonary hypertension. Ultimately, the volume overload causes pulmonary edema, along with right ventricular and right atrial dilation, with eventual failure.

A reduction in pulmonary vascular resistance (with hypocarbia) or increased systemic vascular resistance (with vasopressors, such as phenylephrine) can create or worsen a left-to-right shunt.

Uptake of inhaled anesthetic agents is faster when the patient has a left-to-right shunt. A left-to-right shunt results in delivery (to the lungs) of a higher partial pressure of anesthetic than that present in venous blood from the tissues.

Atrial Septal Defect Repair

This surgery is undertaken to repair a defect (hole) in the septum between the right and left atria.

Such a congenital defect is caused by improper formation of the septal wall. Normally, right atrial pressure is lower than left atrial pressure, which causes a left-to-right shunt, moving oxygenated blood back over into the right side of the heart. The severity of the shunt depends on the size of the defect.

This condition is referred to as "acyanotic" when it involves a left-to-right shunt because oxygenated blood is shunted to the right atrium. It eventually leads to right-sided heart failure, and possible pulmonary hypertension, if the defect is large and remains uncorrected.

A patient with pulmonary hypertension can lead to a right-to-left shunt that sends unoxygenated blood from the right heart to the left heart and ultimately to the systemic circulation.

Small ASDs may heal spontaneously over time.

Operative Procedure

Three main types of ASDs are distinguished: *primum*, *secundum*, and *sinus venosus*. With any of these forms, the surgeon may be able to close the defect with a direct suture or, if it is too large, with a patch. ASD repair done in the operating room requires cardiopulmonary bypass and aortic cross-clamping.

Primum ASD

A layer of tissue in the lower part of the atrial wall, called the septum primum, acts as a valve over the foramen ovale during fetal development. If it does not close properly, it is a primum ASD.

The right atrium is opened, the leaflet is repaired, and the ASD is sutured closed. A pericardial membrane patch or a synthetic graft is always used with this repair. A patient with a primum ASD has a first-degree heart block with a left-axis deviation on EKG. Arrhythmia is a common complication, as sutures are placed near to the atrioventricular conduction tissues. Atrioventricular pacing equipment should be readily available.

Secundum ASD

The most common type of ASD, the secundum atrial septal defect usually arises from an enlarged foramen ovale or inadequate growth of the septum secundum in the central part of the septal wall. Twenty percent of individuals with secundum ASDs also have mitral valve prolapse.

The secundum ASD may be able to be repaired with a septal occluder (a round, self-expanding, self-centering, double-disc device constructed of a dense mesh of wires). This device is placed into the ASD via a catheter inserted into the femoral artery by a pediatric cardiologist in the cardiac catheterization lab.

If repair is done in the operating room, the right atrium is opened, and the defect is closed by suture. If the defect is exceptionally large, a pericardial membrane patch or a synthetic graft is used.

Sinus Venosus ASD

A sinus venous ASD is a defect in the upper atrial septal wall, involving the venous inflow of either the inferior or the superior vena cava and is the least common type of ASD. It is frequently associated with anomalous drainage of pulmonary blood into the right atrium (pulmonary blood normally drains into the left atrium). This type of repair requires surgical intervention.

The right atrium is opened. With this type of ASD, there is abnormal pulmonary vein drainage into the right side of the heart. The abnormal pulmonary vein is redirected through the ASD so that the venous drainage empties into the left atrium. A pericardial membrane patch or a synthetic graft is used to close the defect.

Anesthetic Implications

It is of utmost important to keep *all* air bubbles out of the IV lines. Any air can cross over into the left atrium and result in an arterial air embolism.

If an ASD is not diagnosed, eventually the pulmonary vascular pathology may worsen, with excessive blood flow to the RV and PA, leading to a PVR that is higher than the SVR.

These children may already be taking diuretics or digoxin.

Monitors and IV Access

A pulmonary artery catheter is not placed during ASD repair, as it would be in the way during this surgery. An arterial line and a central line are needed, however. A left atrial catheter may be required as well.

Closure (Ligation) of Patent Ductus Arteriosus

In the fetus, the ductus arteriosus (DA) is a normal connection between the pulmonary artery and the aorta. It moves the blood from the right ventricle directly into the aorta bypassing the fluid-filled lungs.

When a newborn takes its first breaths, the increase in arterial oxygen tension stimulates pulmonary arterial vasodilation; pulmonary vascular resistance decreases while the pulmonary blood flow increases. These changes cause the ductus to contract and functionally close; bradykinin and prostaglandins also aid in closure. The DA usually closes to a significant extent within 12–24 hours after birth and completely closes within the first few weeks of life. Hypoxia or acidosis in the first few days of life can prevent or reverse these changes. Surgical closure/ligation of a patent ductus arteriosus (PDA) may be necessary if this defect fails to close spontaneously after birth.

A PDA may allow left-to-right shunting from the high-pressured aorta to the main pulmonary artery with turbulent flow back through the patent ductus. This abnormality leads to increased pulmonary blood flow to the lungs, which may result in pulmonary hypertension and volume overload to the left atria and ventricle. A large PDA can result in systemic hypoperfusion.

Signs of PDA include a continuous systolic murmur, tachycardia, tachypnea, and evidence of cardiomegaly on chest X-ray. If the condition is allowed to continue, pulmonary congestion and eventually pulmonary edema may develop.

Most children currently undergoing PDA ligation operations are premature infants, with gestational ages between 24 and 32 weeks and birth weights between 500 and 1500 g (occasionally even smaller). These infants typically have respiratory distress syndrome (RDS), such that preoperative intubation and mechanical ventilation are required. Some infants are considered critically ill prior to surgery and may be considered high-risk cases for transport to the operating room. As a result, surgical repair in the NICU may be necessary.

Operative Procedure

Access in the open procedure is achieved through a left thoracotomy via the third or fourth intercostal space (left posterolateral thoracotomy). Left lung retraction is done to expose the ductus; bradycardia and hypotension (vagal stimulation) may occur during this maneuver. A FiO_2 of 100% may be necessary during retraction to maintain adequate oxygenation. The PDA is identified and either ligated or divided. This extracardiac intervention does not require cardiopulmonary bypass or cross-clamping of the aorta.

Although the technique remains somewhat controversial, some authors suggest that a gradual closure of the PDA, over 50–75 seconds, may help minimize the sudden increase in systemic blood pressure associated with repair of this defect, thereby decreasing the risk of intraventricular hemorrhage. Vasodilators may be needed to control hypertension as well.

A chest tube may be placed. The incision is closed in layers.

A PDA ligation can be done by video-assisted thoracoscopic surgery in the operating room, as an endovascular closure in the heart catheterization lab (detachable intravascular coils are used more frequently), or in the neonatal ICU.

Anesthetic

General anesthesia is used with an OETT; muscle relaxants are given.

Positioning

The patient is placed in a right lateral decubitus position.

Anesthetic Implications

No matter where the surgery is performed, careful attention to temperature and fluid management, oxygenation/intubation, and de-airing of all IV lines with fluid, boluses, and flushes is crucial.

Maintain maintenance IV fluids during surgery. Although some surgeons prefer that total parenteral nutrition (TPN) be held during the surgical procedure, most recommend that it be continued, so as to avoid sudden decreases in serum glucose concentrations during surgery.

The use of indomethacin (Indocin; an NSAID) inhibits the production of prostaglandin and is an important part of the medical management of PDA. Surgery is usually performed only if indomethacin fails to close the ductus, or if there are contraindications to the use of this medication, such as gastrointestinal bleeding/perforation or renal insufficiency.

Femoral pulses are often bounding in patients with PDA. These children have a widened pulse pressure, and a "machinery murmur" is commonly heard at the left sternal border.

Avoid hypoxia and hypoxemia, as these imbalances can reverse the shunt.

In the NICU, the following supplies and monitors are needed (and may be placed on a neonatal cart that is taken to the unit):

- Albumin
- Blood in room; 10–20 mL/kg if needed
- Normal saline flushes (syringes)
- Fentanyl or morphine (Fentanyl up to a 50 mcg/kg total dose is used as high-dose TIVA anesthetic. The morphine dose is 0.05–0.1 mg/kg total dose.)

- Pancuronium (vagolytic) or vecuronium
- Peripheral nerve stimulator
- Atropine 1 mg/mL and epinephrine 10 mcg/mL
- Dopamine drip
- Arterial line and central venous line (usually both umbilical)

Positioning

The patient is placed in a right lateral decubitus position, as the incision is made at the third or fourth intercostal space.

Pre-induction Measures

If the baby is not already intubated, atropine 0.01–0.02 mg/kg IV (minimum dose, 0.1 mg) is given before laryngoscopy to prevent bradycardia. Fentanyl 2–5 mcg/kg IV is given for intubation. Consider giving midazolam 0.5 mg/kg.

Antibiotic prophylaxis for protection against infective endocarditis is recommended. It may consist of either a single dose of a first-generation cephalosporin, such as cephalexin, or a single dose of ampicillin and gentamycin, depending on surgeon/intensivist preference.

Monitors and IV Access

Preductal oxygenation measurements are done on the upper extremities (the ear lobe may be used as well) and reflect the oxygen level moving into the heart; this is the oxygen level in the blood to the retina. A postductal pulse oximeter is placed on the lower extremity (i.e., foot) to monitor for inadvertent ligation of the aorta. Saturation levels should be maintained in the range of 85–90%. Preductal and postductal measurements are monitored to ensure that the PDA is ligated—*not* the ascending or descending aorta. Document the pulse oximetry levels/differences upon ligation of the PDA.

An esophageal stethoscope may be used to monitor the heart sounds, as the heart murmur often disappears with PDA ligation.

$ETCO_2$ monitoring is performed as well.

Induction

The choice of induction agent depends on the patient's level of cardiovascular instability.

Volatile inhaled anesthetic agents decrease the systemic vascular resistance. This effect may improve systemic blood blow by decreasing the magnitude of the left-to-right shunt.

Intraoperative Measures/Maintenance

Preterm infants—that is, those younger than 44 weeks corrected gestational age (CGA)—should have the lowest possible FiO_2 to maintain oxygen saturation. These patients have a high risk of developing retinopathy of prematurity (ROP) when exposed to high oxygen levels. Use an oxygen and air mixture. Use of nitrous oxide should be avoided.

Fentanyl (high dose: up to 50 mcg/kg) is given with muscle relaxation (vecuronium or pancuronium; the latter has vagolytic effects). Titrate the doses based on the blood pressure response.

Monitor for hypoglycemia, electrolyte abnormalities, and metabolic acidosis. Maintain adequate intravascular volume status. Urinary output should be in the range of 1–2 mL/kg/hr.

Inadvertent PA occlusion will be evidenced by a decreased SpO_2 and a decreased $ETCO_2$.

Inadvertent aortic occlusion will be evidenced by decreased lower extremity pulses and perfusion (decreased postductal oxygen saturation).

Bradycardia may occur during manipulation of the ductus.

Emergence from Anesthesia

Maintain ventilatory support. Most neonates are already intubated and usually stay intubated after the surgery ends. Diastolic blood pressure will increase post-ligation.

Vasoactive infusions are usually not needed.

Complications

Potential complications of PDA closure include recurrent laryngeal, vagus, or phrenic nerve injury; inadvertent aortic or pulmonary artery occlusion; and hemorrhage. Because blood volume in the neonate may be roughly 80 mL/kg, a premature neonate weighing 500 g may have a total blood volume of only 40 mL (roughly 3 tablespoons). As a result, even the slightest intraoperative blood loss may prove rapidly fatal. For this reason, most anesthesia care providers choose to have blood for transfusion immediately available, in an ice chest, at the patient's bedside, when these surgical procedures are performed.

Pulmonary Artery Banding

Pulmonary artery banding is a palliative or temporizing procedure that is performed in patients with large left-to-right shunts and excessive pulmonary blood flow associated with complicated malformations: single ventricle, truncus arteriosus, or common AV canal. Banding is done when pulmonary blood flow and pressures are excessively elevated, but complete surgical repair of the malformation poses too high a risk in the neonate.

This surgery seeks to reduce blood flow and lower pulmonary artery pressure to less than 40 mm Hg distal to the banding. PA pressures should be one-half to two-thirds of the systemic pressures. When the child is older, the band can be removed and the malformation corrected with an open heart procedure.

Operative Procedure

Cardiopulmonary bypass is not required. The approach is through a median sternotomy or left thoracotomy. A pulmonary artery pressure catheter is inserted into the distal PA. A band is sutured around the mid-portion of the pulmonary artery, without impingement on either the pulmonic valve or coronary arteries proximally or the branch pulmonary arteries distally. The band is then tightened until the pulmonary artery pressure falls.

Anesthetic Implications

Give anesthetic agents that do not depress cardiac function.

If bradycardia or systemic hypotension develops during banding, it may be necessary to remove the band promptly. If the band is too tight on the PA, it will cause a right-to-left shunt and a drop in arterial oxygen saturation; PaO_2 should be 90% or greater. If the band is too loose, systemic hypoperfusion will occur.

Monitors and IV Access

An arterial line is needed.

Ventricular Septal Defect Repair

Surgical closure is used to repair a ventricular septal wall defect. Such a defect allows blood flow to move through the ventricular septum from the higher-pressure side of the heart to the lower-pressure side—usually through left-to-right shunting. The amount of shunt is related to the size of the defect.

The larger the gradient between the right and left ventricles, the greater the flow to the pulmonary artery. The risk of surgery increases once the pulmonary vascular resistance increases.

The decision to do surgery on a VSD is based on the patient's pulmonary pressures and VSD size. Very small defects may heal spontaneously during infancy. Smaller VSDs that do not heal spontaneously can be repaired in a cardiac catheterization procedure (an umbrella-like device can be passed across the VSD and opened to stop the flow of blood); an open heart procedure is not required in these cases.

Operative Procedure

Open heart surgery is required for larger VSDs and requires both cardiopulmonary bypass and aortic cross-clamping. A right atriotomy is done, and visualization of the defect occurs through the tricuspid valve. A pericardial or synthetic polytetrafluoroethylene (PTFE; Gortex) graft can be used, or the defect may be stitched closed. Some surgeons prefer to use bovine pericardium or other material for the graft.

Anesthetic Implications

Arrhythmia is a common complication with VSD repair, as sutures are placed near to the atrioventricular conduction tissues. Atrioventricular pacing equipment should be readily available. In some centers, temporary pacemaker (epicardial) wires are usually placed, as these patients can develop third-degree AV block.

Inhaled nitric oxide can be used to decrease pulmonary artery pressures.

Spontaneous closure of a small VSD often occurs by the time the child reaches 2 years of age. Congestive heart failure can develop with a large VSD.

Antibiotic prophylaxis against bacterial endocarditis is recommended.

The pharmacokinetics of volatile or injected drugs are not significantly altered in a VSD repair.

Monitors and IV Access

A right atrial catheter (central venous pressure line), left atrial catheter (for vasoactive infusions), arterial line, and pulmonary artery catheter (to monitor cardiac output and heart pressures) are required. TEE monitoring is especially helpful to assess the repair.

IV Vasoactive Agents

Agents for infusion may include epinephrine, nitroprusside, nitroglycerin, and milrinone.

Stenosis: Coarctation of the Aorta and Pulmonary Stenosis

Stenosis is a constriction that obstructs normal blood flow. As a consequence of the stenosis, the ventricle must increase its pressure to get blood through the obstruction.

Repair of Coarctation of the Aorta

Repair of a congenital constriction of the aorta is usually done when the child is between 1 and 2 years of age. Coarctation of the aorta is common in neonates, who often present in congestive heart failure.

This constriction occurs in varying degrees. It usually appears distal to the origin of left subclavian artery (*postductal coarctation*), but can present in the lower thoracic aorta. *Preductal coarctation* occurs just proximal to the ductus arteriosus. Diagnosis in postductal coarctation may not be made until the child is older and may be found due to upper extremity hypertension.

The blood pressure over the constriction increases but the pulse is notably weaker in the femoral artery at the groin.

Operative Procedure

A left thoracotomy without cardiopulmonary bypass is usually done to access the aortic stricture.

- *Aortic resection with end-to-end anastomosis:* The narrowed section of the aorta is excised and the exposed edges of the aorta are brought together and sutured closed. This approach is the most commonly used.
- *Left subclavian patch angioplasty:* The subclavian artery is sacrificed to provide a flap that is sutured over the aortic narrowing to remove the narrowed area of the aorta. Transient hypoperfusion of the left arm can occur but rarely causes limb ischemia.
- *Subclavian translocation:* The subclavian artery is transected at its origin at the aorta. An incision is made along both the subclavian artery and the aorta (cutting away the narrowed portion) to anastomose the opened artery to the open edges at the aorta.

Anesthetic Implications

Maintaining a slightly lower than normal blood pressure can help to decrease blood loss, minimize operative time, and facilitate manipulation of the aorta. A too-low mean arterial pressure, however, may decrease blood flow to the spinal cord or kidneys. Renal failure and paraplegia are potential complications in this event.

As in adult cardiovascular surgery, blood pressure control during aortic cross-clamping is essential (see the discussion of aortic cross-clamping in Chapter 3). The application of the cross-clamp may precipitate left ventricular failure.

Femoral pulses are decreased with coarctation of the aorta—even more so if LV failure exists, because of restriction of blood flow to the lower body. There is a marked difference in blood pressures measured in the upper and lower body.

Extracardiac malformations can accompany coarctation—for example, Turner's syndrome, hypospadius, clubfoot, cerebral aneurysms, and ocular defects.

Blood loss when the surgeon enters the chest can be quite large due to the development of collateral circulation.

A neonate with critical coarctation may require a prostaglandin E_1 infusion to maintain ductus arteriosus patency because a majority of blood flow goes from the pulmonary artery through the ductus into the descending aorta. This flow provides for adequate lower body perfusion.

Cardiac depressive anesthetics should be avoided.

Prevent hypertension and tachycardia on induction and intubation. To do so, you can use lidocaine 1.5 mg/kg, give a preoperative beta blocker, and deepen the anesthetic level.

When the patient has coarctation of the aorta, the gastrointestinal bed is used to a somewhat decreased flow of blood. After repair of this defect, the bowels can actually become damaged if a "reperfusion injury" occurs with the increased blood flow.

The recurrent laryngeal nerve of the vagus nerve is near the operative site. If it is damaged during this procedure, the patient may develop vocal hoarseness.

Induction

- *Infant induction:* narcotics and paralytics (especially pancuronium or vecuronium)

- *Older child induction:* thiopental or volatile inhaled agent with narcotic supplementation

Monitors and IV Access

The arterial line, and the blood pressure cuff, should be placed on the patient's right arm, as the left subclavian artery is often clamped or otherwise occluded during this surgery. A central venous line is usually placed.

One peripheral IV is needed in an upper extremity and at least one in a lower extremity.

Repair of Pulmonary Stenosis

Pulmonary stenosis can be a purely valvular problem (90% of cases), a valvular and infundibular problem (*infundibular* refers to the outflow tract of the right ventricle), or an infundibular only issue. Pulmonary valve occlusion can vary from asymptomatic stenosis to severe stenosis causing right ventricular failure requiring surgical relief.

Surgery is required if a balloon valvuloplasty is ineffective. A balloon valvuloplasty is done in the heart catheterization lab; a catheter is threaded up into the right heart and placed through the pulmonary valve. The balloon is inflated to enlarge the pulmonary valve.

Operative Procedure

Surgical repair of pulmonary valve stenosis is done with the patient on cardiopulmonary bypass. An open valvulotomy is performed under direct vision. Infundibular pulmonary stenosis is treated by resecting the excess right ventricular muscle.

Anesthetic Implications

The severity of symptoms reflects the degree of reduction in pulmonary blood flow and cardiac output. In severe stenosis, the right ventricle cannot produce the pressure necessary to overcome the obstruction. The contraction becomes less efficient, the right ventricle dilates, and the clinical features of heart failure (liver enlargement, peripheral edema) occur.

In a patient with a patent ductus, pulmonary blood flow must be maintained by preventing an increase in PVR and decrease in SVR. A prostaglandin E_1 infusion is given to maintain ductal arteriosus patency. It is important to maintain a stable heart rate in a normal pediatric range, as sinus tachycardia can increase outflow obstruction, decreasing RV filling and cardiac output.

Overall, the goal is to minimize increases in right ventricular oxygen requirements. Maintaining adequate filling volume and myocardial contractility is essential.

RV failure/hypertrophy can develop due to a fixed obstruction that causes a gradient between the right ventricle and the pulmonary artery.

GASTROINTESTINAL DISORDER REPAIR

Temperature control is extremely important with any child, but especially in pediatric patients who are having open abdominal surgery.

Abdominal Tumor Resection or Biopsy: Wilms' Tumor, Hepatoblastoma, and Neuroblastoma

Some pediatric abdominal tumors (such as neuroblastoma and pheochromocytoma) may arise from the sympathetic chain and produce catecholamines. It may be necessary to give a preoperative adrenergic blockade in such cases. In addition, beta blockers may be given intraoperatively for blood pressure control.

Wilms' tumor is a rare abdominal tumor. It may be accompanied by congenital malformations and may be bilateral. Metastasis may occur in the lung, liver, and lymph nodes. Wilms' tumors may produce hypertension or cause anemia, due to preoperative bleeding into the tumor and blood into the urine. This kind of tumor is sensitive to chemotherapy and radiation, and the prognosis for a patient with this condition can be quite good.

Hepatoblastoma affects approximately 80 children in the United States each year. Two-thirds of these children have hepatoblastomas that are unresectable at presentation. Such patients may require preoperative chemotherapy to cause tumor shrinkage prior to definitive resection.

Neuroblastoma may be found anywhere along the sympathetic chain, including the neck, chest, abdomen, and pelvis. These tumors may be small and localized (such as those affecting the adrenal gland) or diffuse and invasive, involving multiple arteries and veins throughout the peritoneal cavity.

Operative Procedure

Usually a large incision is made—either transverse, midline, or thoracoabdominal. The incision may be extended into the thorax if control of the suprahepatic vena cava is necessary. Transverse incisions for Wilms' tumor surgery may need to be extended to the contralateral side to carefully inspect or palpate the contralateral kidney.

The blood supply to the tumor is identified and ligated. The tumor is then separated from its surrounding structures and removed with as little tumor contamination as possible.

Lymph nodes are inspected and removed as needed. In addition, all of the abdominal viscera is examined for evidence of metastasis.

Anesthetic

A rapid-sequence induction may be necessary. General anesthesia is used with an OETT. Muscle relaxants are given to facilitate surgical exposure.

Positioning

The patient is placed in a supine position. A folded towel is placed under the hip on the affected side to facilitate surgical access.

Anesthetic Implications

Patients with abdominal tumors present with varying degrees of hematuria, weight loss, hypertension, and anemia.

Preoperative Measures

Assessment for pulmonary metastasis is important due to the decreased functional residual capacity that accompanies compromised respiratory function. In addition, preoperative chemotherapeutic agents may have toxic effects on the heart or other organs, so some patients may require preoperative pulmonary function testing or echocardiography.

Assessment for liver metastasis is also important because a large abdominal mass can delay gastric emptying. If the abdomen is distended, the child should be considered a "full stomach" case.

If liver involvement is present, the patient may be thrombocytopenic and may have a history of congestive heart failure or portal hypertension.

Prior to the induction of anesthesia, children should be covered with warm blankets (or other warming measures used). Keep the room warm, use warming lamps and mattress, use a heated humidifier, warm fluids, wrap the child's extremities and head in plastic, and use warm, low-flow gases.

Intraoperative blood loss can be very large with resection of abdominal tumors. For this reason, type and cross-match the patient's blood preoperatively, with 2 units of packed cells being made available in the OR. (Each pediatric "unit" is typically 10 mL/kg body weight.)

Multiple sites of intravenous access must be available; preferably a central line is placed. IV sites should typically be located above the diaphragm, as an abdominal tumor can compromise the inferior vena cava.

For large tumors, cardiopulmonary bypass may be needed.

Colostomy

Colostomy is the formation of a temporary or permanent opening into the colon, which is brought out on the abdominal wall as a stoma and diverts stool from the distal colon. This procedure may be performed in cases involving intestinal perforation, necrotizing enterocolitis, Hirschsprung's disease, imperforate anus, bowel obstruction, and necrotizing enterocolitis.

Operative Procedure

A large, transverse abdominal incision is made—in the right upper quadrant for a transverse colostomy or in the left lower quadrant for a sigmoid colostomy. Any dead bowel is resected and a proximal stoma is created.

Anesthetic

General anesthesia is given with insertion of an OETT. Muscle relaxants are given to facilitate surgical access.

Positioning

The patient is placed in a supine position; bilateral arms tucked at the sides.

Anesthetic Implications

These infants may be septic, have thrombocytopenia, and have coagulopathy. Other issues commonly observed with these patients include temperature instability, respiratory and circulatory instability, oliguria, and bleeding problems. There is a high risk of aspiration.

Prior to the induction of anesthesia, children should be covered with warm blankets (or other warming measures used). Keep the room warm, use warming lamps and mattress, use a heated humidifier, warm fluids, wrap the child's extremities and head in plastic, and use warm, low-flow gases.

Intraoperative blood loss can be very large with a colostomy. For this reason, you should type and cross-match the patient's blood preoperatively and have 2 units of packed cells available. (Each pediatric "unit" is typically 10 mL/kg body weight.) Multiple sites of intravenous access must be available—preferably a central line is placed. It is essential to maintain an adequate circulating blood volume; third-space fluid replacement must be aggressive.

Congenital Diaphragmatic Hernia Repair

Congenital diaphragmatic hernia (CDH) surgery seeks to replace displaced viscera back into the abdominal cavity and to repair the hole in the diaphragm, thereby preventing further herniation of abdominal contents into the pleural space in the chest.

During in utero development, the diaphragm does not close completely in some fetuses, allowing the abdominal visceral contents to herniate into the pleural cavity, and affecting the development and maturation of the lungs. The earlier the herniation occurs, the more severe the pulmonary hypoplasia. Herniation occurring later in utero is associated with more mature, well-developed lungs. Babies with CDH have a reduction in lung tissue, alveoli, bronchioles, and pulmonary branching (decreased total size of the pulmonary vascular bed) due to pulmonary hypoplasia (on the affected side) and marked elevations in pulmonary hypertension. Only a small amount of surfactant is present, compounding the respiratory insufficiency.

This congenital defect usually occurs on the left posterolateral side of the diaphragm (85% of cases). Depending on the severity of the herniation, there can be a mediastinal shift away from the side with the defect, with compression of the heart and opposite lung. This effect causes a marked reduction in the volume of the contralateral lung, along with a marked decrease in the number of alveoli. Hypoplasia of the left ventricle can also occur, contributing to postnatal cardiac insufficiency.

Functionally, lungs are noncompliant and cannot be inflated with volumes in excess of normal. Many alveoli remain closed even at increased pressures; increased pressures reach already open alveoli instead, resulting in their rupture and pneumothorax.

Infants with CDH may exhibit symptoms immediately upon delivery, or they may present with symptoms within 24 hours after birth. The abdominal cavity is small and underdeveloped, remaining scaphoid after birth. A triad of signs and symptoms is usually seen: dextrocardia, dyspnea, and cyanosis. Hallmarks of CDH include profound arterial hypoxemia, scaphoid abdomen, barrel-shaped chest, and loops of bowel in the thoracic cavity seen on chest X-ray.

Causes of mortality in this population include respiratory insufficiency, associated cardiac dysfunction, and persistent pulmonary hypertension. Bilateral herniation is rare, and usually fatal. Herniation can also occur after birth.

Immediately after birth, most infants with CDH develop immediate respiratory distress due to hypoxia, hypercarbia, and acidosis. Pulmonary hypertension with elevated pulmonary vascular resistance is the most significant cause of neonatal respiratory distress in these infants. Pulmonary hypoplasia, with fewer alveoli, also prevents good air exchange. In addition, the air-filled bowel in the chest compresses against the mediastinum, pushing it into the opposite chest and lung.

Immediate treatment of CDH consists of cardiopulmonary stabilization by preventing or reversing the pulmonary hypertension, minimizing barotrauma to the lungs, and optimizing oxygen delivery. Chest decompression is accomplished by decompressing the stomach with a orogastric or nasogastric tube; this measure may help to oxygenate the child. Avoid positive-pressure mask ventilation to avoid distending the bowel. If a sudden increase in cyanosis or dyspnea occurs, a pneumothorax on the contralateral side should be considered, to be resolved with insertion of a chest tube.

The infant with CDH should be immediately intubated (mask ventilation should be avoided) and ventilated at settings that prevent over-inflation of the non-involved lung. Peak airway pressures should not exceed 25–30 cm H_2O. "Permissive hypercapnia" is recommended: $PaCO_2$ levels should be maintained greater than or equal to 50–60 mm Hg and the pH maintained greater than or equal to 7.25. This can be done by conventional tidal volume ventilation, high-frequency oscillatory ventilation (HFOV), or jet ventilation. Inhaled nitric oxide (NO) can be given to treat the pulmonary hypertension. Extracorporeal membrane oxygenation (ECMO) may be needed for infants who remain severely hypoxic; veno-venous or veno-arterial bypass is used in such cases.

Operative Procedure
Most surgeons perform repair of the CDH once the child's hemodynamic status has been optimized; this can be hours or days after birth. Most of these hernias are approached through a left subcostal incision, although a thoracic approach is sometimes used. Through the chest incision, the abdominal viscera are withdrawn from the chest, exposing the defect in the diaphragm. The diaphragmatic defect is sutured closed; mesh may be placed to give extra support to the defect. Care must be taken when reducing the spleen and liver, as bleeding from these structures can be fatal.

Repair may involve primary closure if adequate muscle for closure is available; a single layer of nonabsorbable suture is used to close the defect. Many children require patch closure, using PTFE (Gortex) or other similar material. A staged procedure may need to be done if anatomic closure of the abdominal wall is impossible after the viscera are placed back in the abdominal cavity.

A gastrostomy tube may be placed to deflate the stomach and for postoperative access for feedings.

A chest tube may be placed. A chest X-ray should be taken after the chest tube is inserted.

Laparoscopic or thoracoscopic repair is possible for smaller defects.

Anesthetic
After providing preoxygenation, intubate the patient while he or she is awake, if the newborn was not already intubated in the delivery room. Anesthesia consists of general anesthesia with an OETT, muscle relaxants, oxygen, and narcotic agents. Nitrous oxide is contraindicated. Use a low oxygen delivery pressure, and maintain airway pressures at less than 25–30 cm H_2O to minimize risk of pneumothorax.

Positioning

Place the patient in a supine position for the sub-costal approach. Many surgeons place a rolled towel beneath the flank to lift the affected side up off the table slightly. A lateral decubitus position is used for the thoracic approach.

Anesthetic Implications

There is no effective treatment or intervention for pulmonary hypoplasia other than keeping the infant alive with the hope the lung will mature. Do *not* give higher airway or ventilatory pressures in the hopes of opening the alveoli; instead, keep airway pressures at less than 25–30 cm H_2O.

Prior to the induction of anesthesia, children should be covered with warm blankets (or other warming measures used). Keep the room warm, use warming lamps and mattress, use a heated humidifier, warm fluids, wrap the child's extremities and head in plastic, and use warm, low-flow gases.

Monitors and IV Access

An arterial line is advised for continuous blood pressure monitoring and access to blood for labs and arterial blood gases. The temporal artery (preductal) is often cannulated.

A central line (which should *not* be placed below the diaphragm because the inferior vena cava may be compressed after the hernia repair) is especially helpful to monitor heart filling pressures; an increase in CVP of 4 mm Hg during the abdominal defect closure can indicate visceral compression with respiratory compromise.

Preoperative Measures

These infants present with cyanosis, dyspnea, and apparent dextrocardia. Signs and symptoms include a scaphoid abdomen, bulging chest, decreased breath sounds on the affected side, or bowel sounds on the affected side of the chest.

Orogastric tube decompression of the stomach is crucial to prevent further intestinal distention and subsequent increased intrapleural pressures.

Preoperative supportive measures include rapid-rate jet ventilation (i.e., high-frequency oscillation) and ECMO (which works like a heart–lung machine) to prevent respiratory failure from persistent pulmonary hypertension.

Pre-induction Measures

These infants should be stabilized medically before surgery is attempted.

Atropine 0.02 mg/kg IV (minimum dose, 0.1 mg) can be given to prevent bradycardia on induction.

Induction

Positive-pressure mask ventilation may be dangerous.

If the newborn was not emergently intubated in the delivery room or ICU, intubate the awake child using a rapid-sequence induction; use general anesthesia with an OETT, and give muscle relaxants. The lowest possible peak airway pressures (less than 30 cm H_2O) are used to prevent pneumothorax, but pressures must always be sufficient to achieve oxygenation. Jet ventilation is useful with this defect.

The choice of induction agent depends on the patient's cardiovascular function, acidosis, and severity of hypoxemia. High-dose fentanyl and pancuronium (a vagolytic agent) muscle relaxation can be used.

Intraoperative Measures

Use standard maintenance anesthesia with volatile agents, narcotics, and muscle relaxation. Monitor for hypoglycemia, electrolyte abnormalities, and metabolic acidosis.

Maintain mean arterial blood pressure and optimize cardiac contractility with inotropic support (e.g., epinephrine).

Maintain adequate intravascular volume status. The urinary output should be in the range of 1–2 mL/kg/hr. Excess intravenous fluid will worsen the degree of cardiac failure.

A sudden decline in lung compliance, heart rate, blood pressure, or oxygenation may signal a contralateral pneumothorax. A chest tube should be promptly inserted if these signs appear. Some experts have recommended a preoperative prophylactic contralateral chest tube be placed.

Hyperventilation is recommended to decrease PVR and minimize right-to-left shunting. Do *not* attempt to forcefully inflate the lung after the hernia is reduced.

Emergence

The patient should remain intubated with paralysis postoperatively. Ventilation is continued to maintain preductal arterial oxygenation of 80–100 torr.

Approximately 40–50% of these infants have associated anomalies, most commonly involving the heart, brain, craniofacial structures, genitourinary system, and limbs.

Gastroschisis Repair: Abdominal Wall Defect

This emergency procedure is performed to reduce the protruding viscera and repair the abdominal wall defect. In such cases, herniation of the intestines occurs through a defect (usually less than 2 cm in size) in the anterior abdominal wall lateral and to the right of the umbilicus. No peritoneal sac is present, so that the internal viscera are exposed to amniotic fluid while in utero. The bowel is unprotected, rendering it vulnerable to peritonitis, intestinal ischemia, edema, and heat loss. Associated congenital anomalies are far less common than in omphaloceles. See the discussion of omphaloceles later in this chapter for more information.

Operative Procedure

A recent dramatic change in management has occurred with the development of commercially produced spring-loaded silos, which can be placed in the neonatal intensive care unit with conscious sedation. Viscera can be placed into the silo, which can then be gradually reduced over a period of several days, followed by definitive fascial closure in the operating room.

Some surgeons choose the traditional midline abdominal incision, with urgent repair in the operating room occurring within several hours of birth. The abdominal viscera that are protruding are gently replaced into the abdominal cavity and the abdominal wall is repaired.

Anesthetic

General anesthesia is given with insertion of an OETT; muscle relaxants are given. An awake intubation or muscle relaxation with cricoid pressure is recommended. Nitrous oxide should be avoided to prevent gastric distention. Muscle relaxation must be given judiciously, however, as it may make it difficult to determine whether abdominal wall closure is feasible or if respiratory embarrassment will occur due to a tight closure with compression of the inferior vena cava and reduction in diaphragmatic function.

Positioning

The patient is placed in a supine position, with arms at the sides bilaterally.

Anesthetic Implications

Heat preservation is a major issue with this surgery: Keep the infant warm! Keep the room warm, use warming lamps and mattress, warm fluids, wrap the child's extremities and head in plastic, and use warm, low-flow gases.

Anesthesia Goals

- Protect the sac with warm saline-soaked gauze.
- Prevent cold stress.
- Decompress the stomach with a gastric tube.
- Establish a reliable IV in an upper extremity.
- Be aware that the sac may compress IVC flow and impede venous return.

Preoperative Measures

Care must focus on prevention of heat loss, avoidance of direct trauma to the protruding viscera, prevention of infection and sepsis, and prevention of fluid loss.

Pre-induction Measures

Orogastric tube decompression of the stomach is important to prevent regurgitation and pulmonary aspiration.

Atropine 0.02 mg/kg IV (minimum dose, 0.1 mg) may be given to prevent bradycardia.

Induction

Intravenous induction is preferred to an inhalation induction to help prevent gastric distention with positive-pressure ventilation. Inhalation induction can be done with an air/oxygen combination; nitrous oxide is avoided to prevent bowel distention. Intubate the patient while he or she is awake or relaxed with cricoid pressure.

Intraoperative Measures

Full muscle relaxation is required to close the abdomen. During abdominal closure, monitor airway pressures and watch for decreased lung compliance. Monitor airway pressures throughout the case.

Replace third-space fluid losses aggressively. With large amounts of exposed bowel, fluid replacement needs may approach 15–25 mL/kg to ensure stabilization of vital signs. Placement of a Foley catheter helps with evaluation of fluid status. Metabolic acidosis can result from hypovolemia. To maintain normal oncotic pressure, colloid solutions should make up 25% of the replacement fluids given.

Emergence

Extubation is possible if the repair was done on a small defect; however, the infant usually remains intubated for 24–48 hours following surgery. ICU monitoring will be important postoperatively.

Monitors and IV Access

An arterial line is advised for continuous blood pressure monitoring and easy access to blood for frequent labs and arterial blood gases. Maintain an appropriate blood glucose and acid–base balance.

A central line is especially helpful to monitor heart filling pressures. An increase in CVP of 4 mm Hg during the abdominal defect closure can indicate visceral compression with respiratory compromise.

Monitor for hypoglycemia, electrolyte abnormalities, and metabolic acidosis. Maintain adequate intravascular volume status; urinary output should be in the range of 1–2 mL/kg/hr.

Pull-through for Hirschsprung's Disease: Colorectal Resection

Treatment for Hirschsprung's disease (HD) often requires the surgical removal of a section of colon that has a total absence of ganglion cells. The level of removal depends on the results of multiple intraoperative biopsies, which reveal the locations along the intestinal tract where ganglion cells are found.

Normally, innervations in the bowel wall consist of Auerbach's and Meissner's plexuses that form the myenteric nerve complex. Hirschsprung's disease, also called "congenital megacolon," is a congenital anomaly caused by a malformation in the pelvic parasympathetic system; it results in the total absence of ganglion cells (gangliosis) in both plexuses of the intrinsic nerve supply. This problem usually occurs in a segment of the sigmoid colon (distal colon) but occasionally affects the proximal segment of the large colon.

The absence of ganglion cells causes a condition resembling spasm of the affected area, causing the normal bowel proximal to the spastic portion to fill with feces from lack of peristalsis. Stool is then unable to pass beyond the spasm, and the proximal colon becomes distended. Signs include abdominal distention and failure to pass meconium in the first 48 hours of life.

Rarely, patients with HD develop a condition known as Hirschsprung's enterocolitis, which is an inflammatory condition similar to necrotizing enterocolitis (NEC). See the discussion of necrotizing enterocolitis later in this chapter for more information.

Patients with HD may have a distal obstruction and may be quite distended, with a tense/swollen abdominal exam. In an acute situation, a colostomy is created to relieve the obstruction. If the patient remains stable and can tolerate the condition, a more definitive pull-through procedure may be performed. Although this surgery has traditionally been done after the child has reached more than 10 kilograms in weight, many pediatric surgeons now perform the pull-through procedure in the neonatal period.

Operative Procedure

A large, transverse right upper abdomen incision is usually made; alternatively, a left lower quadrant incision may be used. HD patients require multiple intraoperative biopsies of the colon, with frozen section analysis, to determine the level of the HD. The goal is to excise the aganglionic bowel. At that point, the colon that has a normal intrinsic nerve supply is pulled through ("pull-through" for Hirschsprung's disease) the pelvis and sewn to the anorectal junction.

If a colostomy is needed, it is placed in the most distal portion of the colon that contains ganglion cells.

This procedure can be done laparoscopically.

Anesthetic

General anesthesia is given with insertion of an OETT; muscle relaxants are given. Do not use nitrous oxide.

Positioning

The patient is placed in a supine position.

Anesthetic Implications

Approximately 10% of these infants also have Down syndrome.

These infants may be dehydrated but are usually hemodynamically stable.

Preoperative medical treatment includes rehydration, systemic antibiotics, and nasogastric decompression.

Prior to the induction of anesthesia, children should be covered with warm blankets (or other warming measures used). Keep the room warm, use warming lamps and mattress, use a heated humidifier, warm fluids, wrap the child's extremities and head in plastic, and use warm, low-flow gases.

This surgery is not typically associated with major blood loss unless the patient has Hirschsprung's enterocolitis. The latter patients may be septic and have diffuse peritonitis.

Complications

Potential complications include damage to the parasympathetic nerves that lie adjacent to the rectum. To avoid this problem, some surgeons prefer to perform the Soave procedure, which involves stripping the rectal mucosa from the muscular sleeve. The aganglionic portion of bowel is then brought through the sleeve and anastomosed to the anus. This procedure may be performed completely through the rectum.

Repair of Imperforate Anus

This procedure seeks to establish colorectal continuity when there is an absence of an anal opening.

Although there are multiple ways to classify anorectal congenital anomalies, most pediatric surgeons now attempt to use this simplified grouping:

- *Low imperforate anus:* either a membranous barrier at the anus, treated with simple incision of the membrane, or an abnormal anal opening somewhat anterior to the usual location.
- *High imperforate anus:* rectus ends above the perineum. May be associated with various fistulae (rectovesical, rectourethral, rectovaginal) that may allow the passage of the fecal stream by way of the genitourinary tract. Correction depends on the type of

fistulae present. May also end in a blind pouch proximally, without a fistula. A rare finding, it is treated with preliminary colostomy, with definitive repair several months later by direct anastomosis.

In female infants, a rectovaginal fistula may help to prevent the development of distention, allowing the surgery to be postponed up to several weeks. A male infant with an imperforate anus may require surgery immediately after birth.

Operative Procedure

Low imperforate anus is usually repaired by a perineal approach. An incision is made into the anal dimple; the rectal pouch can then be dissected free from the surrounding structures and brought to skin level without tension. The full thickness of the rectal wall is sutured to the skin.

If the rectal pouch is high, most surgeons perform a colostomy in the neonatal period, followed by a definitive repair at a later date. A left lower oblique or paramedial abdominal incision is made. Stool is aspirated from the distal portion of the colon, and a divided colostomy is created.

For the definitive repair, most surgeons perform a posterior sagittal anorectoplasty (PSARP) in the prone position. The rectal pouch can be dissected free from surrounding tissue until it can be brought to skin level without tension. The rectal wall is sutured to the skin around the sphincter.

Anesthetic

A rapid-sequence induction with an awake intubation is recommended. General anesthesia is used with an OETT; muscle relaxants are given.

Positioning

The patient is placed in a modified lithotomy or frog-legged position for a perineal approach. A supine position is used for an abdominal incision.

Anesthetic Implications

Type and cross-match the patient's blood preoperatively; make sure blood products are ready for immediate use. This infant may have thrombocytopenia and coagulopathy.

Patients with imperforate anus may have a distal obstruction and be quite distended, as revealed by a tense and/swollen abdomen on exam. Intestinal distention can cause respiratory compromise with the risk of pulmonary aspiration of gastric contents. The infant may also be septic.

Prior to the induction of anesthesia, children should be covered with warm blankets (or other warming measures used). Keep the room warm, use warming lamps and mattress, use a heated humidifier, warm fluids, wrap the child's extremities and head in plastic, and use warm, low-flow gases.

Preoperative Measures

Care must focus on airway management, fluid and electrolyte imbalance, and sepsis. Volume resuscitation is usually necessary before anesthesia can be induced. Most infants are hemodynamically stable.

Pre-induction Measures

Give atropine 0.02 mg/kg IV (minimum dose, 0.1 mg) to prevent bradycardia on induction.

Monitors and IV Access

An arterial line and central line can be helpful if the child is severely compromised.

Induction

Intravenous or inhalation induction can be done with an air/oxygen combination. Nitrous oxide should be avoided to prevent bowel distention.

Intraoperative Measures

Use a volatile agent along with narcotics, and intermediate- or long-acting neuromuscular blockers.

Emergence

Extubation can be done if the repair involved a small defect. ICU monitoring will be important postoperatively.

Monitor for hypoglycemia, electrolyte abnormalities, and metabolic acidosis. Maintain adequate intravascular volume status; urinary output should be in the range of 1–2 mL/kg/hr. This operation is not typically associated with major blood loss.

Reduction of Intussusception

Reduction of intussusception seeks to relieve the obstruction and reestablish blood flow to the obstructed bowel. With this defect, a segment of intestine becomes drawn into the lumen of the more distal bowel. The problem usually begins in or around the terminal ileum and can extend distally into the ascending, transverse, or descending colon. The normal peristaltic movement of the intestine then causes the bowel to invaginate into itself. Intussusception has an unknown etiology, although viral infection or a growth in the intestine (polyp, tumor) may contribute to its development.

Operative Procedure

In the *open* procedure, a right lower abdominal quadrant incision is usually made. Reduction is usually accomplished by the surgeon applying gentle pressure to the distal colon. If the bowel is gangrenous, resection is done and primary anastomosis is usually performed. Rarely, creation of a temporary diverting ileostomy may be necessary.

Reduction can occasionally be performed *laparoscopically,* even in very young babies. An incidental appendectomy is usually performed in such cases.

Anesthetic

GETA is used, along with muscle relaxation.

Positioning

The patient is placed in a supine position, with bilateral arms tucked at the sides.

Anesthetic Implications

Preoperatively, an air or barium enema is done; this measure may be both diagnostic and (often) curative. Air (some radiologists use barium or other liquid contrast material, rather than air) is

introduced into the bowel with a manometer; the pressure should not exceed 120 mm Hg.

Prior to the induction of anesthesia, children should be covered with warm blankets (or other warming measures used). Keep the room warm, use warming lamps and mattress, use a heated humidifier, warm fluids, wrap the child's extremities and head in plastic, and use warm, low-flow gases.

"Currant-jelly" stool (bloody mucus) may indicate gangrene of the intussusception. Perforation of the bowel can follow. If peritonitis is present, urgent laparotomy is indicated.

Recurrent intussusception occurs in approximately 10% of patients.

Necrotizing Enterocolitis Repair

To treat necrotizing enterocolitis (NEC), removal of necrotic or perforated bowel is required. The procedure may result in stoma placement.

Multiple risk factors have been associated with the development of NEC, including prematurity (less than 32 weeks gestation and weight less than 1500 g), initiation of enteral feeding, bacterial infection, intestinal ischemia resulting from birth asphyxia, persistence of a patent ductus arteriosus, cyanotic heart disease, and maternal cocaine abuse. The commonly encountered clinical situation is a stressed infant who is fed enterally.

The common feature in all cases of NEC is hypoperfusion and ischemia of the gastrointestinal tract, leading to necrosis and perforation. NEC may involve single or multiple segments of the intestine, most commonly the terminal ileum. The gross findings in NEC include bowel distention, and gangrene or frank perforation. In the most severe form of NEC, patients have intestinal perforation and develop progressive peritonitis, acidosis, sepsis, disseminated intravascular coagulopathy (DIC), and death. Metabolic acidosis occurs secondary to peritonitis.

Operative Procedure

A large, transverse abdominal incision is usually made. Frankly gangrenous or perforated bowel is resected, and the intestinal ends are brought out as stomas.

Anesthetic

GETA is used, and muscle relaxation is given. Avoid administration of nitrous oxide in the presence of free air in the portal venous or gastrointestinal systems.

Positioning

The patient is placed in a supine position.

Anesthetic Implications

Infants with NEC may be septic, have thrombocytopenia, and have coagulopathy. Most of these patients have diffuse peritonitis and/or perforation. They are usually hypovolemic and require vigorous fluid resuscitation with both crystalloid and colloid solutions to maintain an adequate circulating blood volume. Despite the risk of massive third spacing during fluid resuscitation, replacement must be aggressive.

Type and cross-match the patient's blood preoperatively, and ensure that blood is available in the room. Multiple sites of intravenous access are preferred, and preferably a central line is placed.

Prior to the induction of anesthesia, children should be covered with warm blankets (or other warming measures used). Keep the room warm, use warming lamps and mattress, use a heated humidifier, warm fluids, wrap the child's extremities and head in plastic, and use warm, low-flow gases.

Monitor patients for congestive heart failure and signs of patent ductus arteriosus.

Hemorrhage from thrombocytopenia is a risk. To counteract this problem, infusion of RBCs, platelets, or FFP may be needed.

Monitors and IV Access

Central venous and arterial lines are placed. Have multiple IV sites available.

Preoperative Measures

Care must focus on airway management, fluid and electrolyte imbalance, and sepsis. Volume resusci-

tation is usually necessary before anesthesia can be induced.

Pre-induction Measures

Give atropine 0.02 mg/kg IV (minimum dose, 0.1 mg) to help prevent bradycardia on induction.

Medical management consists of gastric decompression with a nasogastric tube, intravenous fluids, and antibiotics.

Induction

An intravenous induction is commonly done with an air/oxygen combination. Induction of anesthesia will most likely cause hypotension, especially if volatile anesthetics are used. Nitrous oxide should be avoided to prevent bowel distention. Induction with ketamine, an opioid, and a nondepolarizing muscle relaxant may be used.

Intraoperative Measures

A volatile agent is used, along with a narcotic, and intermediate- or long-acting neuromuscular blockers.

Emergence

The child will remain intubated postoperatively. ICU monitoring will be needed.

Monitor for hypoglycemia, electrolyte abnormalities, and metabolic acidosis. Maintain adequate intravascular volume status; urinary output should be in the range of 1–2 mL/kg/hr.

Laparoscopic Nissen Fundoplication

Nissen fundoplication consists of laparoscopic wrapping of the gastric fundus (upper rounded curve of stomach) around the intra-abdominal esophagus (also called gastroesophageal [GE] junction) so that the distal esophagus passes through a tunnel of muscle. This procedure, which is done to create an adequate barrier between the stomach and the esophagus, is performed almost exclusively by laparoscopy.

Nissen fundoplication is indicated to correct severe gastroesophageal reflux disease (GERD) and hiatal hernia. It helps to strengthen and reinforce the GE junction, which in turn stops acid from backing up into the esophagus. A hiatal hernia is associated with GERD; it is caused by an opening in the diaphragm that allows a portion of the stomach to protrude up into the chest, weakening the GE junction. The Nissen procedure prevents protrusion of the stomach into the chest.

Operative Procedure
Laparoscopic trocars are inserted into the abdominal cavity and a pneumoperitoneum is established. An esophageal dilator is passed through the esophagus, and the esophagus is dissected while protecting the vagal nerve. (The vagal nerve controls movement of food from the stomach into the small intestine; damage to it can impair gastric motility.) The esophagus and gastric fundus are mobilized. A Nissen wrap (or partial wrap) is created by forming a wrap of fundus around the esophageal junction with two or three nonabsorbable sutures to create a barrier. The fundus can then be secured to surrounding fascia.

Anesthetic
General anesthesia is given with insertion of an OETT; muscle relaxants are given.

Positioning
The patient is placed in a supine position, with both arms beside the body.

Anesthetic Implications
Patients may have preexisting motility difficulties. Unwrapping is a possibility, such that the repair may need to be tightened or redone completely.

Prior to the induction of anesthesia, children should be covered with warm blankets (or other warming measures used). Keep the room warm, use warming lamps and mattress, use a heated humidifier, warm fluids, wrap the child's extremities and head in plastic, and use warm, low-flow gases.

Tape the eyelids shut to protect the cornea from being scratched or the eye from drying. Place eye pads over both eyes to prevent accidental injury

when the esophageal dilator is placed or other movement around the face.

The anesthetist should hold the OETT securely when the esophageal dilator is inserted and positioned to prevent moving the OETT into a right mainstem position or inadvertently extubating the patient.

Omphalocele Repair: Abdominal Wall Defect
This emergency procedure seeks to reduce the protruding viscera and repair the abdominal wall defect in cases of omphalocele; a small defect can be repaired in one surgical procedure. A large defect (which can contain the liver, stomach, bladder, spleen, intestines, and reproductive organs) may require a staged surgical repair for complete defect closure.

An omphalocele consists of herniation of the intestine into the base of the umbilical cord (through a defect in the umbilical ring), with viscera protruding through an abdominal wall defect. A peritoneal sac is always present but may be ruptured, with abdominal contents exposed through the sac. Associated congenital anomalies occur in two-thirds of these infants, especially in the gastrointestinal, diaphragmatic, genitourinary, and cardiovascular systems.

Operative Procedure
A midline abdominal incision is made. The abdominal viscera that are protruding are gently replaced into the abdominal cavity, and the abdominal wall is repaired. A large defect may be left open and covered with a sterile occlusive dressing.

Anesthetic
General anesthesia is used with insertion of an OETT; muscle relaxants are given. Intubation should be done while the patient is awake or muscle relaxed with cricoid pressure. Nitrous oxide should be avoided to prevent gastric distention. Near the time of abdominal closure, muscle relaxation must be given judiciously; it may make it difficult to determine whether abdominal wall closure

is feasible or if respiratory embarrassment will occur due to a tight closure with compression of the inferior vena cava and reduction in diaphragmatic function.

Positioning

The patient is placed in a supine position, with arms at the sides.

Anesthetic Implications

Heat preservation is a major issue with omphalocele repair surgery: Keep the infant warm! Keep the room warm, use warming lamps and mattress, warm fluids, wrap the child's extremities and head in plastic (after induction and intubation), and use warm, low-flow gases.

Anesthetic Goals

- Protect the sac with warm saline-soaked gauze or "lap sponges."
- Prevent cold stress.
- Decompress the stomach with a nasogastric tube.
- Establish a reliable IV in an upper extremity for fluid and antibiotic therapy.
- Be aware that the sac may compress IVC flow and impede venous return.

Preoperative Measures

Care must focus on prevention of heat loss (cover exposed viscera with sterile plastic to limit evaporation), avoidance of direct trauma to the protruding viscera, prevention of sepsis, and prevention of fluid loss (replace fluids and electrolytes aggressively). Treat hypoglycemia with a slow glucose infusion.

Pre-induction Measures

Orogastric tube decompression of the stomach is important to prevent regurgitation.

Give atropine 0.02 mg/kg IV (minimum dose, 0.1 mg) to prevent bradycardia on induction.

Monitors and IV Access

An arterial line is advised for continuous blood pressure monitoring and access to blood for frequent labs and arterial blood gases.

A central line is especially helpful to monitor heart filling pressures. An increase in CVP of 4 mm Hg during the abdominal defect closure can indicate visceral compression with respiratory compromise.

Induction

Intravenous induction is preferred to inhalation induction to help prevent gastric distention with positive-pressure ventilation. Inhalation induction can be done with an air/oxygen combination; nitrous oxide should be avoided to prevent bowel distention. Intubate the patient while he or she is awake or relaxed with cricoid pressure.

Intraoperative Measures

During abdominal closure, monitor airway pressures and watch for decreased lung compliance. Full muscle relaxation may be needed to facilitate abdominal closure.

Replace third-space fluid losses aggressively. With large amounts of exposed bowel, fluid replacement needs may approach 15–25 mL/kg to ensure stabilization of vital signs. A urethral catheter helps with evaluation of fluid status. Metabolic acidosis can result from hypovolemia. To maintain normal oncotic pressure, colloid solutions should make up 25% of the replacement fluids.

Maintain blood glucose and acid–base balance.

Emergence

Extubation may be done if the repair involved a small defect. ICU monitoring will be important postoperatively.

Monitor for hypoglycemia, electrolyte abnormalities, and metabolic acidosis. Maintain adequate intravascular volume status; urinary output should be in the range of 1–2 mL/kg/hr.

Pyloromyotomy for Hypertrophic Pyloric Stenosis

Pyloromyotomy is a procedure in which the surgeon cuts the pylorus muscle, removing an obstruction caused by pyloric stenosis, so that food can pass into the duodenum. It is indicated for idiopathic hypertrophy of the circular smooth muscle of the pylorus in the distal stomach. This condition results in a gradual obstruction of the gastric outlet at the pylorus. Hypertrophic pyloric stenosis usually becomes symptomatic in infants between the ages of 2 and 8 weeks of life; they present with a history of forceful, projectile, nonbilious vomiting. Diagnosis is often made on physical examination by palpation of an olive-sized mass in the right upper quadrant. Ultrasound will definitively diagnose the condition in 95% of affected children.

Operative Procedure

If an orogastric tube has not already been inserted, one should be passed orally up to three times to suction out the stomach before induction and intubation. After the endotracheal tube has been secured, an orogastric tube is inserted and left in place during the surgery.

With the *open* approach, either a right upper quadrant incision is made or a periumbilical incision is done.

This procedure can also be done *laparoscopically*. In such a case, three laparoscopic incisions are made for port access.

With either approach, after the pyloric muscle is cut, the orogastric tube is used to inject a bolus of air to test the integrity of the pyloric wall after pyloromyotomy. The surgeon will instruct that 20–30 mL of air be injected slowly and will watch for air bubbles around the pyloric incision: If any air escapes, the incision line is not intact and will be reinforced.

Anesthetic

A true rapid-sequence induction is preferred, as there is still a risk of aspiration even after the orogastric tube has been used to suction the stomach before induction and intubation. General anesthesia is given with insertion of an OETT. Nondepolarizing muscle relaxants can be given, but are not usually necessary.

Use a pediatric circle or Bain circuit with warmed, humidified gases.

Muscle relaxation reversal is given at the end of the case, as the goal is to extubate the patient. The child should be fully awake prior to extubation, as these patients are prone to postoperative respiratory depression due to pre-existing central alkalosis.

Positioning

The patient is placed in a supine position. In our institution, after intubation, the child is turned laterally in the bed, with the baby's feet toward the surgeon (not the bed, just the baby is turned). This position allows the surgeon access to the abdomen and the anesthetist access to the airway/head of the infant.

Anesthetic Implications

Pyloric stenosis is a medical emergency, not a surgical one. These children are usually severely dehydrated and have metabolic *alkalosis* (hyponatremic, hypokalemic, hypochloremic) from projectile nonbilious vomiting; they must be stabilized preoperatively with IV fluids and electrolyte replacements. Severely dehydrated babies can present with metabolic *acidosis* secondary to hypoperfusion. Jaundice may occur in association with this condition.

Preoperatively, fluid resuscitation with electrolyte abnormality correction is essential before general anesthesia is given. Give IV fluids containing sodium, potassium chloride, and glucose ($D_5$1/2 normal saline with 40 mEq/L of potassium chloride) for 12–48 hours preoperatively. The perioperative urinary output should be more than 1 mL/kg/hr.

An orogastric tube may have already been inserted so that the stomach has been kept empty to avoid regurgitation and aspiration. *Aspiration of gastric juices into the lungs is a primary concern.* Some surgeons leave an orogastric tube in place for 24 hours postoperatively, but most do not.

Prior to the induction of anesthesia, children should be covered with warm blankets (or other warming measures used). Keep the room warm, use warming lamps and mattress, use a heated humidifier, warm fluids, wrap the child's extremities and head in plastic, and use warm, low-flow gases.

Induction
- Have an IV in place.
- Give O_2 by mask.
- Give atropine 10–20 mcg/kg IV (minimum dose, 0.1 mg) to prevent bradycardia with induction.
- Suction the stomach with a large-bore (14 Fr) catheter at least three times, giving O_2 between each suction catheter insertion.
- Perform rapid-sequence induction with thiopental or propofol, succinylcholine, and an ETT with stylet.

Local anesthetic may be injected at the incision site by the surgeon. Short-acting narcotic administration (no long-acting narcotics should be given) should be kept to a minimum: Once the surgery is done and the local anesthetic has minimized any painful stimulation, narcotics may make it difficult to arouse the child for extubation.

Have available a 60-mL syringe (for air bolus) with a tip that can be secured into the proximal end of the orogastric tube—either a catheter tip or a Luer lock.

Position the child laterally, in a slight head-up position, postoperatively for transport to the recovery room. Give blow-by oxygen.

Biliary Atresia Correction: Hepatoportoenterostomy (Kasai Procedure or Kasai Portoenterostomy)

Hepatoportoenterostomy is performed to correct biliary atresia by creating an intestinal conduit to allow bile to drain. In extrahepatic biliary atresia, the bile cannot drain normally from the liver to the gastrointestinal tract owing to progressive destruc-tion of the biliary tree. The net result is neonatal jaundice due to bile stasis, with subsequent hepatocellular damage and eventual hepatic fibrosis and cirrhosis.

Biliary atresia presents in the first few weeks of life, and can progress to portal hypertension, splenomegaly, esophageal varices, and liver failure. If left untreated, death is inevitable within 2 years. Even when the Kasai procedure is performed, two-thirds of these patients require liver transplantation because of progressive liver failure; one-third will need a liver transplant within the first year of life, and the other two-thirds will usually need a transplant prior to reaching school age.

Operative Procedure
The surgical goal is to promote bile flow into the intestine.

A right upper abdominal quadrant incision is made. Fibrous tissues are transected to expose the porta hepatic (the area of the liver from which bile should drain), and part of the small intestine (usually a Roux-en-Y limb of the jejunum) is attached to the exposed liver surface.

Bile flow may be established when these channels are opened. Radiopaque contrast dye is used to visualize the gallbladder. A liver biopsy is usually performed to assess the degree of liver degeneration/change.

Anesthetic
GETA and muscle relaxation are used.

Positioning
The patient is placed in a supine position.

Anesthetic Implications
This surgery has the best success rate when it is performed before the child reaches two months of age. The prognosis becomes worse the later the surgery is done.

Ask the parents if either has an allergy to contrast dye. Although the infant will not have been exposed to the allergen, the allergy itself may have a familial origin. Monitor for any signs of allergic response if dye is given.

Prior to the induction of anesthesia, children should be covered with warm blankets (or other warming measures used). Keep the room warm, use warming lamps and mattress, use a heated humidifier, warm fluids, wrap the child's extremities and head in plastic, and use warm, low-flow gases.

Use a volatile agent with an oxygen/air combination. Avoid the use of nitrous oxide to prevent bowel distention.

Extubation is possible at end of the case with uncomplicated patients.

ORTHOPEDIC SURGERY

Syndactyly Repair

This procedure entails separation of webbed or fused digits of the hands or feet. Syndactyly can be bilateral. The surgery to repair it is usually done when the child is between 6 months and 2 years of age.

Operative Procedure
Z-plasty (zigzag) incisions are made in the interdigital space to avoid contracture and provide flaps for the web-spacing reconstruction. Full-thickness grafts, if required, usually come from the skin of the abdomen or the medial aspect of the arm or thigh. Stents are usually sutured over the grafts. A bulky dressing and splint are applied.

Anesthetic
General anesthesia is given with insertion of an OETT. Muscle relaxants are not needed.

Positioning
The patient is placed in a supine position.

Anesthetic Implications
Prior to the induction of anesthesia, children should be covered with warm blankets (or other warming measures used). Keep the room warm, use warming lamps and mattress, use a heated humidifier, warm fluids, wrap the child's extremities and head in plastic, and use warm, low-flow gases.

Maintain anesthesia until the splint is on.

Club Foot Surgical Correction

This procedure is the surgical correction of a foot (or feet) that is pointed downward and rotated inward. The club foot abnormality includes plantar flexion with twisting of the ankle, an unusually high arch in the foot, an inversion of the heel that causes the front of the foot to turn inward, and adduction of the forefoot where the forefoot is pulled downward. The initial treatment for this defect, which is begun in the first days of life so as to take advantage of favorable connective tissue elasticity, is usually nonoperative. Manipulation and casting can help the ligaments, joint capsules, and tendons be molded into a better position before surgical correction is done.

Operative Procedure
The surgeon rearranges tendon insertions or performs soft-tissue releases to straighten the foot.

Anesthetic
General anesthesia is given with insertion of an OETT, along with caudal anesthesia. Inhalation induction with intubation is performed, and then a caudal epidural is given. For example, injection of 0.25% bupivacaine 1 mL/kg helps with pain control for 4–6 hours postoperatively.

Positioning
The patient is initially placed in a supine position. After intubation is done, the baby is usually repositioned down to the far end of the OR table. Make sure you know where the IVs and ETT are, and have plenty of slack on all of the tubes to prevent anything from being pulled out during the repositioning.

Anesthetic Implications

A tourniquet is typically used on the affected leg. After the tourniquet is released, cold blood perfuses the area and body temperature can drop.

An increase in body temperature can be an issue as most of the baby is covered and a warming blanket is used. Monitor the child's temperature, and keep the baby warm but not too warm.

Surgical repair may be very painful, so give appropriate narcotics.

Casting is applied at the end of the surgical correction procedure. Keep the child fully asleep until the cast material is hardened.

Spica Cast Application (Body Cast)

A spica cast is an orthopedic cast that is form-fitted to immobilize the hips or thighs to maintain their correct positions so that the acetabulum will stay in the hip bone. The orthopedic cast can begin at the trunk, and may extend down to cover one leg, both legs, or the majority of the leg on one side and only down to the hip or knee of the other side. The cast is left on until the healing is complete.

A body cast is applied in case of dislocated hip and to promote healing of a damaged hip joint or fractured femur. In *hip dysplasia,* the femur acetabulum becomes dislodged from the hip bone socket; this condition can range from joint laxity, where ligaments are stretched, to irreducible displacement. Hip dysplasia may not become apparent until the child starts to walk. Most children are assessed for this condition both immediately after birth and at each check-up for the first year. If it is detected early, the majority of children can be successfully treated with a splint or harness (Pavlick harness). This method helps to place the hip in the socket and hold it there until the ligaments tighten. If splinting is unsuccessful, a spica cast may be needed. In rare cases, the child may need to have the hip replaced.

Operative Procedure

After the skin is coated with a protective cream, a layer of specially made plastic is placed between the skin and the plaster cast. The cast is then formed.

Anesthetic

General anesthesia is used with an OETT or LMA.

Positioning

The patient is initially placed in a supine position, but will be moved into multiple positions for cast application.

Anesthetic Implications

When the cast is being formed around the thigh and pelvis, the child will be lifted off the bed. Extubation is the major risk when moving and lifting child. Often, the child is laid on an elevated platform that has been placed on the OR table. When the child is lifted, the arms are abducted away from where the cast is being placed to keep them out of the way. Stabilize the ETT and maintain the neck to keep it from flexing or extending when the child is lifted into the air. Keep the child covered as much as possible to maintain body temperature during these position changes.

Taping the tube (ETT or LMA) very securely will help keep the airway secure. Disconnect the circuit during movement to prevent ETT/LMA dislodgement but give 100% FiO_2 before doing so. Keep the child in Stage III anesthesia while moving him or her. Monitor breath sounds continuously with an esophageal stethoscope.

Prior to the induction of anesthesia, children should be covered with warm blankets (or other warming measures used). Keep the room warm, use warming lamps and mattress, use a heated humidifier, warm fluids, wrap the child's extremities and head in plastic, and use warm, low-flow gases.

The child's body temperature should be at least 36°C before extubation takes place.

GENITOURINARY SURGERY

Bladder Exstrophy Repair

Bladder exstrophy encompasses a spectrum of birth defects of the lower abdominal wall, bladder (in which the bladder is inside out and is herniated out of the abdominal wall), anterior bony pelvis (the pelvic bones are also usually separated), and external genitalia. This congenital malformation results in herniation of the open bladder and, in many children, the urethra exits the body on the front lower abdomen (because the skin of the lower abdominal wall that normally covers the bladder also does not form properly). There is usually multisystem involvement.

Bladder exstrophy occurs most often in boys and is associated with, among many defects, epispadius of the penis.

The goal of bladder exstrophy surgery is to separate the bladder plate from the abdominal wall and close it along with the epispadic penis in one sitting, if possible. This procedure can involve, in many children, moving the urethra to its normal position. Often orthopedic surgeons will start the case by performing anterior sacroiliac osteotomies. This facilitates closure of the pubis at the end of the abdominal wall closure.

Surgery is usually performed within 24–48 hours of birth and may be a staged approach or a primary repair.

Operative Procedure

Bladder exstrophy repair may involve anterior or pelvic osteotomies—which are typically performed by a pediatric orthopedist—to allow the pelvis to "fold in" anteriorly so as to allow for better bladder closure. If this approach is used, patients with exstrophy may be initially positioned prone on the operating room table, and then flipped over for the bladder repair.

Multiple surgical approaches to these anomalies have been advocated:

- The bladder, posterior urethra (epispadias repair), and abdominal wall are (preferably) all closed during the newborn period.
- The urethral closure may be done at 6 months to 1 year of age if the size of the penile urethral plate is a limiting factor in the original surgery.

- The bladder neck reconstruction for urinary continence and bilateral ureteral reimplantation are usually performed at 4 to 5 years of age.

Anesthetic

GETA is used, along with muscle relaxation.

Positioning

The patient is placed in a supine position.

Anesthetic Implications

Blood loss, evaporative losses, and third-space losses are all possibilities with this surgery. For this reason, an arterial line is usually placed, along with two peripheral IVs or a central line.

Prior to the induction of anesthesia, children should be covered with warm blankets (or other warming measures used). Keep the room warm, use warming lamps and mattress, use a heated humidifier, warm fluids, wrap the child's extremities and head in plastic, and use warm, low-flow gases.

Repair of bladder exstrophy may require approximation of the symphysis pubis by an orthopedist. Often the patient will be placed in Buck's traction and remain intubated and paralyzed for a few days to allow initial wound healing.

Circumcision

Note: While circumcision can be performed in an adult patient, it is most often done in the pediatric population and is only detailed in the pediatric surgery chapter. Some details listed here relate to adult patients.

Circumcision is the surgical cutting away of the penis foreskin (prepuce). It is indicated for phimosis (inability to retract the foreskin in the male penis), paraphimosis (where the foreskin is retracted back and cannot be replaced, which causes severe pain and swelling of the glans), balanoposthitis (infection and inflammation of the glans penis and foreskin in uncircumcised males, usually due to poor hygiene), severe infection, trauma, condyloma (genital warts), and cancer.

Circumcision may also be done for cultural or religious reasons. In addition, removal of the foreskin is thought to decrease the incidence of penile cancer.

Operative Procedure

The foreskin is released from the glans. A circumferential incision is made around the inner preputial layer, and the foreskin is removed. The remaining penile skin edge is sewed to the mucosal collar below the glans.

- *Guided forceps technique:* The foreskin is pulled over the glans and clamped with long forceps. The foreskin is then cut along the outside edge of the forceps.
- *Dorsal slit technique:* the foreskin is pulled taut over the glans, and a slit is made along the top of the foreskin. Dissection scissors are then used to cut in a circle from the slit, and the foreskin is excised at its base. Hemostasis is achieved with electrocautery. The proximal and distal edges of the foreskin are circumferentially approximated with absorbable suture.

Petroleum jelly–impregnated gauze is wrapped around the penis and suture line and covered with a sterile, clear plastic wrap (leaving the urethral meatus open).

Anesthetic

In adult patients, IV sedation and local anesthetic *without epinephrine* can be given by penile block, followed by a ring block once the patient is asleep. In pediatric patients, general anesthesia is given with a mask, LMA, or OETT. A penile block with local anesthetic without epinephrine can be given for postoperative pain control.

Positioning

The patient is placed in a supine position.

Anesthetic Implications

Postoperative bleeding is a common complication. In rare cases, hematoma formation occurs or intravascular injection of local anesthetic can occur.

Prior to the induction of anesthesia, children should be covered with warm blankets (or other warming measures used). Keep the room warm, use warming lamps and mattress, use a heated humidifier, warm fluids, wrap the child's extremities and head in plastic, and use warm, low-flow gases.

Newborn boys whose parents have requested a circumcision may ask for local anesthetic to be used to decrease the pain in an elective circumcision. In such a case, penile block or a local anesthetic crème (EmLa) can be placed 20 minutes before the procedure (and wrapped in plastic wrap to prevent it from rubbing off).

Epispadias Repair

An epispadias is a congenital anomaly in which the urethra terminates at a point on the dorsal (upper) surface of the penis. It may be associated with bladder exstrophy (discussed earlier in this chapter). An epispadias is most often associated with deformities of the bladder and urinary sphincter and occurs at the abdominopenile junction. A complete deformity results in urinary incontinence.

Operative Procedure

The penis is disassembled to correct this deformity. The urethral plate is rolled into a tube and transposed ventrally in the glans, while the corpora cavernosum is rolled internally so that the dorsal curvature is corrected.

If the patient is already circumcised, a segment of vein, ureter, or skin (a non-hair-bearing area) may be used to patch the urethral defect. A suprapubic cystostomy may be created with placement of a urinary catheter for temporary urinary diversion.

Repair is required to provide for continence and ability to copulate.

Anesthetic

GETA is given with insertion of an OETT. A penile or caudal block is done at the end of the case to manage postoperative pain.

Positioning

The patient is placed in a supine, frog-legged position, with arms at the sides.

Anesthetic Implications

Prior to the induction of anesthesia, children should be covered with warm blankets (or other warming measures used). Keep the room warm, use warming lamps and mattress, use a heated humidifier, warm fluids, wrap the child's extremities and head in plastic, and use warm, low-flow gases.

Hypospadias Repair

A hypospadias is a congenital anomaly in which the urethral opening is on the underside (ventral surface) of the penis rather than at the end; the severity of the condition may vary. The urethra can exit the penis and occur distally (near the glans) or all the way up to the perineum. Surgery is performed to allow normal urination and to correct the deformity.

Operative Procedure

A mild defect may be repaired in a primary procedure, while a severe defect may require several procedures to correct. The surgical goal is to reconstruct the missing urethra, widen the urethral meatus, and correct chordee, if present. Chordee is a condition in which the penis bends downward during erection due to a strand of connective tissue between the urethral opening and the glands.

The penis may need to be de-gloved (skin separated from shaft) to cut the chordee and construct a new urethra that will reach to the head of the penis.

The urethra is typically reconstructed out of the foreskin. If the patient is already circumcised, a segment of vein, ureter, or skin (a non-hair-bearing area) may be used.

A urinary catheter (or pediatric feeding tube) is passed, with the reconstructed urethra added to the natural urethra. The patient is usually continent postoperatively.

Anesthetic

GETA is given with insertion of an OETT. A caudal or penile block can be done to help with postoperative pain.

Positioning

The patient is placed in a supine, frog-legged position, with arms at the sidees.

Anesthetic Implications

Correction of hypospadias may be done in single procedure, but many patients need multi-staged repair.

Prior to the induction of anesthesia, children should be covered with warm blankets (or other warming measures used). Keep the room warm, use warming lamps and mattress, use a heated humidifier, warm fluids, wrap the child's extremities and head in plastic, and use warm, low-flow gases.

Orchiopexy (Orchidopexy)

Orchiopexy is the repair of an undescended testicle (cryptorchidism). In this procedure, the surgeon moves an undescended testicle into the scrotum and fastens it there with absorbable sutures. Orchiopexy may be performed in patients ranging in age from infants to older males. If left untreated, undescended testicles in adult men are usually removed because of the increased risk of testicular cancer.

Operative Procedure

Depending on the location of the testicle (how low or high in the inguinal canal or in the abdomen), a surgeon will make one or two small incisions in the groin, scrotum, or abdomen to reach the testicle and move it to the scrotum. This procedure can be done laparoscopically, but is performed as an open abdominal procedure if the testicle cannot be located in the inguinal area. A "hybrid" approach may also be employed that incorporates both traditional open and laparoscopic maneuvers.

Usually, an orchiopexy can be done in one stage. Occasionally, if the testicle cannot be easily moved into the scrotum, a two-stage procedure (Fowler-Stephens operation) may be performed, wherein the testicular blood vessels are clipped/divided at the first operation to promote the development of collateral vessels along the vas deferens. Rarely, an undescended testicle is removed and then reimplanted in the scrotum. The blood vessels are then reattached microsurgically.

Anesthetic

GETA is given with insertion of an OETT or LMA. Caudal or ilioinguinal/iliohypogastric nerve blocks are helpful with postoperative pain. This procedure may also be done with epidural block in an adult (caudal block in a child).

Positioning

The patient is placed in a supine, frog-legged position.

Anesthetic Implications

Prior to the induction of anesthesia, children should be covered with warm blankets (or other warming measures used). Keep the room warm, use warming lamps and mattress, use a heated humidifier, warm fluids, wrap the child's extremities and head in plastic, and use warm, low-flow gases.

Vesicoureteral Reflux (Ureteral Reimplantation)

This procedure involves the reimplantation of one or both ureters into the bladder. It is indicated in case of congenital ureteral reflux (which can cause pressure on the kidneys from the backup of urine) or repeated urinary tract or kidney infections.

In this procedure, the surgeon changes the way a ureter connects with the bladder. Normally, the ureters attach to the posterior surface of the bladder. If the ureters are dilated (resulting in the absence of the normal valve-like function of the ureter) or have abnormal peristalsis (moving urine from the kidneys to the bladder even when the patient is in a supine position), vesicoureteral reflux—the backflow of urine from the bladder into the ureter and up to the kidney—can occur. Kidney damage may result from pressure-related changes from urine backflow or movement of bacteria from the urethra backward to the kidney.

Operative Procedure

The ureters may be approached either intravesically (within the bladder) or extravesically.

A small incision is made into the lower abdomen. The bladder is opened in a midline abdominal (intravesical) approach; the ureters are removed from their natural positions. They are then angled in at a more diagonal direction and tunneled through the bladder wall between the inner mucosa and the detrusor muscle until they emerge into the bladder. The new position has more bladder muscle around the ureter, preventing further reflux. One or more stents may be placed. The bladder is closed. A urethral catheter and a small Penrose drain in the incision are placed. The incision is closed with absorbable sutures.

Robotic-assisted ureteral reimplantation is also done.

Anesthetic

General anesthesia is given with insertion of an OETT; muscle relaxants are given. A caudal or lumbar epidural catheter is used to minimize the amount of general anesthesia required and to control postoperative pain and bladder spasm.

Positioning

The patient is placed in a supine position, with bilateral arms at the sides.

Anesthetic Implications

This procedure is associated with a potential risk of significant blood loss. Two intravenous catheters should be placed because of this risk.

Prior to the induction of anesthesia, children should be covered with warm blankets (or other warming measures used). Keep the room warm, use warming lamps and mattress, use a heated humidifier, warm fluids, wrap the child's extremities and head in plastic, and use warm, low-flow gases.

If this procedure is performed intravesically, a brisk urine output is desired postoperatively. In such a case, run fluids at 1.5 times the calculated maintenance rate.

PLASTIC AND RECONSTRUCTIVE SURGERY

Cleft Lip Repair: Unilateral or Bilateral

Cleft lip—a congenital deformity of the lips and face—results from a fusion failure during the embryonic processes. It can be unilateral or bilateral. The defect appears as a narrow gap in the skin of the upper lip that extends all the way to the base of the nose. Although it can be closed in the neonate, repair at age 3 months is preferable, as growth of the tissue facilitates the initial detailed surgery.

Four categories of cleft lip are distinguished:

- Clefts of the lip only
- Clefts of the palate only
- Clefts of lip, alveolus, and palate
- Clefts of lip and alveolus

When cleft lip occurs in combination with a cleft palate, its repair usually requires only one reconstructive surgery, especially if the cleft is unilateral.

Operative Procedure

An incision is made on each side of the cleft from the lip to the nostril, and the edges are then anastomosed. If the other side is also clefted, a second surgery is usually done approximately one month later.

Proper restoration of the philtrum and shape of the bow of the lip is sought. Palatal deformities are repaired as required for feeding requirements and tissue growth. The cheeks are splinted with a Logan's bow to counter the effects of crying. If needed, secondary repairs may be done months or years later.

Anesthetic

General anesthesia is given with insertion of an OETT. An oral RAE tube may be taped to the center of the lower lip to minimize facial distortion. These patients can be induced by either mask or IV technique.

Induction depends on the degree of airway abnormality. If there are no airway abnormalities, induction can be done by IV barbiturate, followed by a muscle relaxant to facilitate tracheal intubation. If the child has airway abnormalities, a volatile inhaled anesthetic can be given while the child breathes spontaneously.

Positioning

The patient is placed in a supine position.

Anesthetic Implications

Prior to the induction of anesthesia, children should be covered with warm blankets (or other warming measures used). Keep the room warm, use warming lamps and mattress, use a heated humidifier, warm fluids, wrap the child's extremities and head in plastic, and use warm, low-flow gases.

After taping the eyelids shut, securely tape eye pads over both of the patient's eyes to protect them.

A high index of suspicion for endotracheal tube dislodgement must be maintained during the surgery.

Patients with cleft lip are at risk for unrecognized blood loss if blood goes down the trachea or esophagus. A throat pack may be placed; if it is, chart both its placement and its removal.

Local anesthetic with epinephrine will be infiltrated locally to aid in hemostasis. Monitor the EKG for changes in heart rate or rhythm.

Patients with cleft lip can have an increased risk of aspiration.

Cleft Palate Repair (Palatoplasty)

A cleft palate is a congenital defect in which there is an opening between the roof of the mouth and the nasal cavity; it results from lack of embryonic development of elements of the prepalate and the palate. The split can be unilateral or bilateral. It may involve only the uvula or extend through the entire palate. A cleft palate may also occur in conjunction with a cleft lip.

Palatoplasty is intended to create a functional palate to reduce the chance of fluid developing in the middle ear and to help the teeth and facial bones develop properly. Depending on the severity of the cleft, its shape, and the thickness of available tissues, additional surgeries may be required to improve the appearance of the lip and nose and to stabilize the jaw (the cleft palate can also create a split in the upper jaw).

Multiple defects can occur, and repair of these problems is desirable prior to 2 years of age to minimize speech difficulties. Palatoplasty is usually performed in children between 9 and 14 months of age. Secondary repairs may be needed to correct a residual fistula, to remedy speech problems, and to facilitate dental restoration.

Owing to velopharyngeal insufficiency (the opening between the oral and nasal cavity), these patients may have swallowing problems and are at risk for aspiration. The tongue can prolapse into the airway, causing obstruction. Many have frequent upper respiratory tract infections and otitis media. In severe defects, nursing and respiratory problems may be present and may demonstrate poor nutrition or anemia. Some children may benefit from preoperative placement of a feeding tube (gastrostomy tube) to provide supplemental caloric intake.

Operative Procedure

A device such as a Dingman gag is used to support mouth open. Surgery involves pulling tissue from either side of the mouth to rebuild the palate.

At the end of the case, because postoperative airway problems are common in these patients, the surgeon may place a suture in the tongue and tape it to the cheek to pull the tongue out of the mouth and away from the palate. In case of airway obstruction, the tongue can be pulled forward and patency of the airway restored. Tongue swelling can occur.

Anesthetic

General anesthesia is given with insertion of an OETT. An oral RAE tube may be taped to the center of the lower lip to minimize facial distortion. A reinforced RAE tube reduces the likelihood of tracheal tube occlusion by the Dingman gag during palatoplasty. Nitrous oxide may be used in these patients.

The induction approach depends on the degree of airway abnormality. If there are no airway abnormalities, induction can be done by IV barbiturate, followed by a muscle relaxant to facilitate tracheal intubation. If the child has airway abnormalities, a volatile inhaled anesthetic can be given while the child breathes spontaneously.

Positioning

The patient is placed in a supine position, with bilateral arms at the sides.

Anesthetic Implications

Prior to the induction of anesthesia, children should be covered with warm blankets (or other warming measures used). Keep the room warm, use warming lamps and mattress, use a heated humidifier, warm fluids, wrap the child's extremities and head in plastic, and use warm, low-flow gases.

Moderate to significant blood loss can occur during palatoplasty. Check with the surgeon regarding the need for a type and cross-match of the patient's blood.

After taping the eyelids shut, securely tape eye pads over both of the patient's eyes to protect them from accidental injury.

Intubation may be especially difficult in an infant with a large defect in the palate. The laryngoscope blade can slip into the cleft, presenting problems. To avoid this possibility, place a small roll of gauze in the palate to fill the gap.

Local anesthetic with epinephrine will be infiltrated locally to aid in hemostasis.

A high index of suspicion for endotracheal tube dislodgement must be maintained during the surgery. The Dingman gag sits on top of the tongue, with the ETT in the center. If this arrangement is disrupted, it can completely obstruct the ETT.

Patients with cleft palate are at risk for unrecognized blood loss if blood goes down the trachea or esophagus. A throat pack should be placed; chart both its placement and its removal.

Extubation is usual at end of case. The patient should be fully awake during this process to avoid airway obstruction. Airway edema may occur.

Arm restraints are used in the postoperative period to keep the child's hands away from the face.

HERNIA SURGERY PEARLS

Etiology of hernias:

- Caused by a congenital defect. May occur prenatally or early on in life; internally or externally; and unilaterally or bilaterally.
- Caused by infection, trauma, or inadequate suturing. Predisposing factors include pregnancy, constipation, or chronic muscular effort (coughing, vomiting).

Complications of hernias:

- Strangulation: Pressure from the hernia can compromise surrounding tissue and its blood flow, causing ischemia and possibly becoming fatal.
- Obstruction: Pressure on surrounding structures can block their normal function.

Hernia repair (herniorraphy):

- *Open surgical method:* An incision is made over the hernia. Any protruding tissue is returned to its original placement, and the hernia sac that has formed is cut away. The surrounding muscle is used to sew the defect closed.
- *Mesh method:* An incision is made over the hernia, and a piece of mesh larger than the defect is collapsed and inserted through the incision. It is stapled or sewn to surrounding tissues to secure it; the mesh covers and reinforces the defect. Sewing the muscle is not done during mesh repair.
- *Laparoscopic:* Several laparoscopic ports are inserted into the abdominal cavity through small incisions. One of the ports contains a small camera connected to a TV monitor where the surgeon can view the surgery. The hernia is repaired through these ports.

HERNIA SURGERY

Diaphragmatic (Adult) Hernia Repair

Repair of a diaphragmatic hernia in an adult may become necessary when a congenital diaphragmatic hernia goes undetected in childhood or a traumatic diaphragmatic hernia occurs. The diaphragm is a major muscle of respiration, so any interruption in this muscle's function will affect respiratory exchange. The abdominal contents travel upward through a diaphragmatic hernia, pushing on the lung parenchyma.

Operative Procedure

A large midline abdominal incision is made; the surgeon dissects upward, gently pulling back all the abdominal contents that are above the diaphragm. The hole is closed with suture. Sometimes mesh is needed to close the opening completely.

Anesthetic

General anesthesia is used with insertion of an oral endotracheal tube (OETT); a double-lumen endobronchial tube (DLEBT) is used if one-lung ventilation is required. Muscle relaxants are required.

Multiple large-bore IVs are placed, and an arterial line is usually needed.

Positioning

The patient is placed in a supine or lateral decubitus position.

Anesthetic Implications

The potential for blood loss with this procedure is enormous, as the liver, stomach, spleen, or lungs may need to be retracted and may be inadvertently damaged.

Large third-space fluid shifts are common. Consider giving albumin/hetastarch fluid boluses to counteract this effect.

Temperature loss is common with an open-abdomen procedure. Upper- and lower-body warming blankets are needed as well as fluid warmers.

The ambient temperature in the room may also need to be increased.

Hand-ventilation of the patient may be needed during part of the dissection. If maintaining ventilator respirations, decreasing the tidal volumes with an increase in respiratory rate may be helpful for the surgeon when accessing the lung space.

Do not use nitrous oxide.

A chest tube will most likely be inserted at the end of the case to assist in full expansion of the lung on the affected side.

Give antiemetics to prevent vomiting postoperatively and avoid coughing and straining on emergence from anesthesia to prevent repair disruption and strain on suture lines.

Hiatal Hernia Repair

A hiatal hernia is a variant presentation of a diaphragmatic hernia. In this case, there is a defect in the normal passageway where the esophagus meets the stomach. This defect allows part of the stomach to intermittently bulge, or herniate, into the chest. A "sliding" hiatal hernia allows the gastroesophageal (GE) junction (also known as the cardiac sphincter or cardia—it is not a valve but actually more of a stricture) to slide up into the chest. In a "non-sliding" hiatal hernia, the GE junction does not slide up into the chest. This condition is considered more dangerous because the stomach can actually rotate and obstruct other organs. Potentially, rupture of the stomach can occur, with fatal results.

Operative Procedure

A hiatal hernia can be repaired through an incision or by laparoscopy; the latter is becoming the preferred option. Through laparoscopic ports, the surgeon can pull the hernia sac down out of the chest and then sew the hole in the diaphragm. If the defect is large, mesh may be stapled over the repair to supplement and strengthen the repair.

Anesthetic

General anesthesia is used with insertion of an OETT; muscle relaxants are given. An epidural block to the T4 level may be done for postoperative pain control.

Positioning

The patient is placed in a supine position.

Anesthetic Implications

Give antiemetics to prevent vomiting postoperatively and avoid coughing and straining on emergence from anesthesia to prevent repair disruption and strain on suture lines.

Incisional (Ventral) Hernia Repair

This procedure seeks to repair and strengthen an abdominal hernia, where the hernia is usually the result of an incompletely healed surgical wound after a midline incisional laparotomy. The problem is called a ventral hernia if a previous abdominal surgery did not create the problem; it is called a congenital ventral hernia if it has been present from birth.

Operative Procedure

A midline incision is made over the hernia, the fascial edges are freed, and the pieces brought together to close the hole. Large defects may require mesh to secure the wound.

Anesthetic

General anesthesia is used with insertion of an OETT; muscle relaxants are given. An epidural block to the T4 level may be done for postoperative pain control.

Positioning

The patient is placed in a supine position.

Anesthetic Implications

Give antiemetics to prevent vomiting postoperatively and avoid coughing and straining on emergence from anesthesia to prevent repair disruption and strain on suture lines.

Inguinal Hernia Repair

A hernia in the groin is characterized by defects in the transverse abdominal fascia; it is the most common hernia in both women and men. A "direct" inguinal hernia comes through a weak point in the posterior wall of the inguinal canal; an "indirect" inguinal hernia protrudes through the inguinal ring.

Operative Procedure

For an open procedure, an incision is made in the affected groin, and the hernia sac is ligated. The spermatic cord structure in the male patient is protected. A piece of mesh may be used to help close the edges.

This procedure can also be done laparoscopically, with the mesh being stapled over the defect from the inside. The patient may have a section of strangulated bowel in the hernia, which will require an emergency laparotomy and a bowel resection to repair.

Anesthetic

Local anesthesia with sedation is provided; a spinal block to the T6 level may be done. Alternatively, general anesthesia is used with insertion of an OETT if muscle relaxation would be helpful.

Positioning

The patient is placed in a supine position with at least one arm tucked at the side.

Anesthetic Implications

Traction on the viscera can cause vagal stimulation with resultant bradycardia, hypotension, nausea, and vomiting.

Give antiemetics to prevent vomiting postoperatively and avoid coughing and straining on emergence from anesthesia to prevent repair disruption and strain on suture lines.

Spigelian Hernia Repair

A hernia of the spigelian fascia (lateral ventral hernia) penetrates between the muscles of the abdominal wall; thus there is often no notable swelling with this type of hernia. Spigelian hernias are usually small but should be surgically repaired due to their high risk of bowel strangulation. Large defects may require mesh prosthesis.

Operative Procedure

In an *open* repair, a horizontal incision is made down to the external oblique muscle. The peritoneal cavity is entered, and the hernia sac is located and circumferentially dissected away. A piece of mesh, larger than the hernia defect, is fixed with sutures on the inside of the abdominal cavity. The incision is then closed.

In a *laparoscopic* approach, multiple laparoscope ports are inserted through several small incisions. The mesh is collapsed and inserted through one of the ports. It is secured in the patient in the same way as in the open approach.

Anesthetic

With the open approach, an epidural with sedation is used. With either the open or laparoscopic approach, general anesthesia is used with an OETT; muscle relaxants are required.

Positioning

The patient is placed in either a lateral decubitus position or a supine position with a bump-up on the surgical side.

Anesthetic Implications

Patients typically present with either an intermittent mass, localized pain, or signs of bowel obstruction. An ultrasound or CT scan can establish the diagnosis.

Give antiemetics to prevent vomiting postoperatively and avoid coughing and straining on emergence from anesthesia to prevent repair disruption and strain on suture lines.

Umbilical Hernia Repair

An umbilical hernia usually involves protrusion of intra-abdominal contents through an abdominal wall weakness at the umbilical cord.

Operative Procedure

A midline incision is made over the hernia and the pieces brought together to close the hole. Mesh is used to close and supplement large umbilical hernias. This material should extend well beyond the edges of the defect to reduce pressure on the hernia opening.

In a *laparoscopic* approach, multiple laparoscope ports are inserted through several small incisions. The mesh is collapsed and inserted through one of the ports. It is secured in the patient in the same way as in the open approach.

Anesthetic

General anesthesia is used with insertion of an OETT. Muscle relaxants are given in cases involving larger umbilical hernias; local anesthetic and sedation can be used for repair of very small umbilical hernias.

Positioning

The patient is placed in a supine position with at least one arm tucked at the patient's side.

Anesthetic Implications

Give antiemetics to prevent vomiting postoperatively and avoid coughing and straining on emergence from anesthesia to prevent repair disruption and strain on suture lines.

ELECTROCONVULSANT THERAPY

Electroconvulsant therapy (ECT) involves the stimulation of an electrically induced grand mal seizure for its cognitive and behavioral side effects. The therapeutic effect of ECT is caused by the grand mal seizure, not the electrical stimulus. The precise mechanism of therapeutic action is unknown.

ECT is indicated for severe major depressive states that are unresponsive to medical treatments, acute psychosis, acute schizophrenic states, and mania. Treatment usually takes place three times per week. Approximately 80% of patients who receive ECT have a favorable response to it.

Operative Procedure

An electrical shock is given to one or both cerebral hemispheres to elicit a grand mal seizure. The quality of the ECT seizure is crucial. The goal is to have a seizure last 30–60 seconds (total of both tonic and clonic phases). A seizure less than 30 seconds is ineffective.

- The *tonic phase* lasts 20 seconds. It comprises the rigid contracture of muscles and stiffening of limbs; breathing may decrease or cease altogether, producing cyanosis of the lips, nail beds, and face.
- The *clonic phase* lasts 40 seconds. It involves a rhythmic shaking and jerking of the limbs and face.

In *unilateral ECT,* the plan is to hold the patient's lips tight around a mouth guard; the jaw is held up tight to the face, and pressure is placed against the opposite temple. Electrical stimulation is then delivered to one cerebral hemisphere.

In *bilateral ECT,* the plan is to hold the patient's lips tight around a mouth guard, pull up on the lower jaw, and press down on the top of the head. Electrical stimulation is then delivered to both cerebral hemispheres. Bilateral shocks are better for depression and amnesia, but tend to produce decreased cognition.

Anesthetic

The anesthetic goals for ECT are a rapid induction, decreased consciousness, limited physiologic effects of the seizure, no seizure inhibition, and a rapid recovery.

Once the patient is sedated, place an oral airway to maintain a patent airway. To prepare for shock, hyperventilate the patient and make sure the mouth guard is in place. Right before shock occurs, stop oxygen delivery.

Induction anesthetics used for ECT include the following agents:

- Methohexital 0.75–1.5 mg/kg: associated with fewer dysrhythmias and minimal anticonvulsant activity
- Etomidate 0.15–0.3 mg/kg: associated with seizures of longer duration
- Thiopental 1.5–2 mg/kg: increases bradycardia and shortens the duration of the seizure
- Ketamine: has low anticonvulsant effects and may possibly reduce cognitive side effects

Succinylcholine (Anectine) 0.3–1 mg/kg may be given to prevent injury during ECT; otherwise, potentially dangerous skeletal muscle contractions or bone fractures may occur during the tetany associated with the seizure. To avoid tonic and clonic movements over the entire body, a tourniquet can be placed on one of the lower legs to isolate an extremity for seizure activity quantification. Immediately after induction of anesthesia, the tourniquet is inflated before giving succinylcholine. Because the succinylcholine cannot get past the inflated leg cuff, the lower leg will have seizure activity and permit visual confirmation that the seizure has occurred, thereby allowing for timing and effectiveness of seizure activity.

Seizure duration may be increased by administration of caffeine 125–500 mg IV and hyperventilation (which produces alkalosis).

Do not give propofol, as it tends to shorten seizures.

Dexmedetomidine (Precedex) has been shown to blunt hyperdynamic responses to ECT without altering seizure duration. If this agent is used, you can give 1 mcg/kg IV slowly over 10 minutes before induction.

Drugs with anticonvulsant properties, such as benzodiazepines and anticonvulsants, are counter-productive and should not be given to patients undergoing ECT.

An undesirably long seizure (i.e., one that last more than 2–3 minutes) can be terminated by giving a benzodiazepine (diazepam 10 mg) and/or a long-acting barbiturate. Longer seizures lead to increased cerebral metabolic rate without additional behavioral benefits.

Immediately post-shock, a *parasympathetic nervous system* response occurs: first hypotension, and bradycardia to asystole. Next, a *sympathetic nervous system* response occurs that is characterized by increased heart rate and/or hypertension. Tachycardia usually lasts about 2 minutes. EKG changes can occur during this period.

Cerebral effects of ECT include vasoconstriction, cerebral blood flow increases 100–400% with increased intracranial pressure (ICP). *Neuroendocrine* effects include ACTH release, increased cortisol levels, catecholamine release with tachycardia, hypertension, dysrhythmias, increased levels of glucagon, and inhibition of insulin production. *Gastric* effects include increased gastric pressures.

Treat the *parasympathetic response* with atropine (at occurrence) or glycopyrrolate (pre-procedure). Treat *sympathetic nervous system signs* with nitroglycerin, labetalol, esmolol (Brevibloc), hydralazine, and/or nicardipine. In case of *emergence delirium*, you can give midazolam in 1 mg increments or diazepam.

Positioning

The patient is placed in a supine position, with arms at the sides. The head of the bed is usually raised slightly.

Anesthetic Implications

Acidosis increases seizure threshold (decreasing convulsant activity). For this reason, the patient should be hyperventilated by face mask just before ECT is done.

Electroconvulsive therapy often generates strong myopotentials (muscle electrical activity) that may interfere with pacemaker sensing in the same manner as does electrocautery. Have an external magnet available to convert the pacemaker to asynchronous mode if the unit is negatively affected by ECT.

Relative contraindications to ECT include unstable angina, severe osteoporosis or major bone fracture, glaucoma, retinal detachment, congestive heart failure, pregnancy, thrombophlebitis, and severe pulmonary disease. *Absolute contraindications* include pheochromocytoma, brain mass or aneurysm, stroke within 3 months, increased ICP, recent myocardial infarction, and recent intracranial surgery.

ORGAN DONOR MANAGEMENT

When the brain dies, the body organs try to die, too. A storm of catecholamines is released, which floods and affects all organs in the body. Some organ systems are more sensitive to this flood due to age, health history, genetics, and other factors and cannot survive despite intervention. Medical personnel intervention consists of the use of vasoactive medications to maintain the blood pressure within very specific parameters, maintain a urinary output at a rate of more than 30 mL/hr, and mechanical ventilation and oxygen to maintain arterial blood gases within normal limits and a pulse oximetry saturation greater than 92%.

Following the declaration of brain death in the donor, both preoperatively and intraoperatively:

- Mean arterial blood pressure (MAP) must be maintained within the range of 70–90 mm Hg. If the blood pressure falls, the first-line choice to increase it with an inotrope (e.g., dopamine). Peripherally acting vasopressors (phenylephrine [Neosynephrine]) are used if the inotrope is not effective.
- Hypertension should be vigorously treated with sodium nitroprusside (SNP) or nitroglycerin.
- ABGs should be maintained within normal limits with FiO_2 at 100% and PEEP if necessary.

- Fluids and diuretics should be given to maintain the urinary output of more than 30 mL/hr.
- Maintain CVP within the range of 5–10 mm Hg.
- Crystalloids and albumin may be used for volume resuscitation.
- The hematocrit level should be more than 20, with a transfusion being performed if it falls to less than 20.

The goal is to keep the donor's organs in good condition during procurement, specifically avoiding hypotension, hypovolemia, hypoxemia, and hypothermia.

Have all emergency medications and IV drips available to maintain stable hemodynamics. Have crystalloids, colloids, and blood products available as well.

Antibiotics are given. Maintain sterile technique, as organ recipients are considered to be immunocompromised.

An arterial line is an absolute requirement, and placement of a central line and pulmonary artery catheter should be considered.

Donor Facts

The United Network of Organ Sharing (UNOS) is national organization that develops a common ground of policies and procedures and facilitates sharing of information for the betterment of public health.

In the United States, organ procurement organizations (OPO's) are funded by Medicare and regulated by the federal government. They must maintain strict standards to maintain eligibility for reimbursement. Some OPOs are hospital based, whereas other are independent and have their own revenues and policies.

Any hospital in a city with a transplant organization can call and inform the OPO of a possible donor. Each city has its own RN coordinator for its donor program. Several very large OPOs operate in the United States, including those based in Pittsburgh, Nebraska, and Alabama.

When a hospital contacts the OPO regarding a potential donor, the OPO's RN coordinator comes to the contacting hospital and begins a process of information gathering regarding transplant suitability. Usually, the donor's family is not approached until the coordinator is involved and present. The OPO coordinator is an advanced care RN who is specifically schooled and certified in organ procurement.

The OPO nurse coordinator becomes the team member orchestrating potential donor care at the patient's bedside. At this time, a very detailed flow sheet of donor health information begins to be filled out; this information-gathering process continues until all organs are procured or the donor is deemed unsuitable. Pertinent information includes all past and present medical and surgical history, test results, current vital signs and condition, and all medical interventions—in short, anything that may affect the organs.

When a recipient hospital is notified of a suitable organ, the recipient hospital's transplant team travels to the donor hospital, arriving at a scheduled time. The transplant team consists of the transplanting physician and his or her associates. Once there, the transplant surgeon reviews the actual tests (not just the reports of their results) and examines all of the history available. The transplant surgeon is an active part of actual organ retrieval and assesses the organ status (e.g., function, color) while it is still in the donor's body.

The transplant team communicates with the recipient hospital regarding appropriateness of donor organ. The ultimate decision maker regarding donor organ appropriateness for transplantation is the receiving surgeon.

If the donor organ is deemed suitable for transplant, its surgical removal begins. The donor chest and abdomen are opened through a large midline incision (suprasternal notch to pubis). If the heart is to be donated, it is mobilized, and heparin is given into the superior vena cava before it is ligated. The ends of the superior and inferior vena cava are clamped; the heart is allowed to beat empty for 30 seconds before cold cardioplegia is administered through a catheter inserted into the ascending aorta. The procured organ is placed in a bag filled with a sterile solution called UW (developed at the University of Wisconsin) to maintain the organ. The organ is then placed in a container that sits in a bed of ice inside a cooler. Cooling an organ causes stress but should not cause tissue death.

The recipient will have been notified of organ availability and brought to the receiving hospital's operating room and prepped for transplant. Once the donor transplant team has flown into its home-base city and landed, the recipient's diseased organ is removed. This second-by-second orchestration is necessary because the donated organ has a limited number of hours of viability outside a body. The time needed is different for each particular organ.

While the term "harvest" has been used for many years to describe the donation of organs, people working within the field typically refer to "recovery" of organs.

Order of Organs Affected by Time Without Perfusion

Heart (4–6 hours)

Lungs (4–6 hours)

Pancreas (12 hours)

Small bowel (12 hours)

Liver (12 hours)

Kidneys (24–48 hours depending on receiving surgeon requirements; usually placed on a "kidney pump" which keeps preservation fluid circulating through the organ until transplant)

SHOCK STATES

Cardiogenic Shock

- Preload: increased
- Afterload: increased (vasoconstricted)
- Cardiac output: very decreased

CAUSES	SIGNS AND SYMPTOMS	TREATMENT
Massive AMI	Decreased BP	Give oxygen
Pericardial tamponade	Tachycardia and arrhythmias	Correct acid–base imbalances
Pulmonary emboli	Gallop S_3 and S_4	Relieve pain
Tachycardia or bradycardia	Absent/decreased peripheral pulses	Treat arrhythmias
Ventricular aneurysm	Cool and clammy skin	Fluid PRN
	Pulmonary crackles	Inotropes
	Respiratory alkalosis	Decreased myocardial demand
	(hyperventilation)	Decreased heart rate
	Decreased level of consciousness	
	Distended jugular vein	

Neurogenic Shock

- Preload: decreased
- Afterload: decreased
- Cardiac output: decreased

CAUSES	SIGNS AND SYMPTOMS	TREATMENT
Severe damage to the brain and spinal cord	Hypotension	Large volumes of fluid may be needed to restore
• Spinal anesthesia	Bradycardia	normal hemodynamics.
• Spinal cord injury	Warm, dry extremities	Dopamine often used either
• Head injury	Peripheral vasodilation	alone or in combination
• Barbiturate overdose	Venous pooling	with other inotropic agents.
	Decreased cardiac output	Vasopressors (e.g., epinephrine)
		Atropine speeds up heart
		rate and cardiac output.

Hypovolemic Shock

- Preload: decreased
- Afterload: increased (vasoconstriction)
- Cardiac output: decreased

CAUSES	SIGNS AND SYMPTOMS	TREATMENT
Hemorrhage/trauma	Skin: cool and clammy	Life support
Trauma: tissue/blood loss	Lowered body temperature	Identify underlying cause
Thirst	Dilated pupils	and fix it
Burns: plasma loss	Nausea	Restore volume:
Dehydration: vomiting	Altered level of consciousness	crystalloids and colloids
Third spacing	Tachycardia	Mast trousers
	Arrhythmia	
	Flat neck veins	

Septic Shock

- Preload: within normal limits
- Afterload: decreased
- Cardiac output: very increased

When the patient is in the cold stage, preload is decreased and afterload is increased due to vasoconstriction.

CAUSES	SIGNS AND SYMPTOMS	TREATMENT
Infectious disease Inadequate immune response	Fever and chills Increased CO Blood pressure rise and fall Respiratory alkalosis Change in level of consciousness Hyperventilation Warm, flushed skin Bounding pulse	Volume replacement Antibiotics Steroid treatment Restore acid–base balance

Anaphylactic Shock

- Preload: decreased
- Afterload: decreased
- Cardiac output: decreased (pooled blood)

CAUSES	SIGNS AND SYMPTOMS	TREATMENT
Food	Difficulty breathing	Epinephrine SQ
Drugs	Bronchospasm	Benadryl
IV contrast dye	Swelling	Tagamet
Insect stings	Vascular shock	Racemic epinephrine
Blood transfusions	Hives	Hydrocortisone

TRAUMA RESUSCITATION

Any patient who is considered an emergency surgical case will also be considered to have a full stomach. A rapid-sequence induction is needed with these patients. Insert an endotracheal tube only—do not use a laryngeal mask airway (LMA).

Throughout the entire assessment and resuscitative process, recognize the potential for cervical spine injury. Maintain the spine in a safe neutral position until clinical examination and radiological findings exclude injury.

Primary Survey

A * B * C * D * E: should take 2–3 minutes.

Airway

While you are delivering high-flow 100% oxygen, assess the airway.

- Open the airway with a chin-lift or jaw-thrust maneuver. Do *not* extend the patient's head.
- Is the airway patent?
- Is the airway obstructed?

Possible Causes of Airway Obstruction

- Tongue: most common cause of obstruction in unconscious patients.
- Bilateral mandibular fracture: creates a "flail mandible" with loss of support of the tongue muscles, resulting in obstruction of the upper airway. *This airway obstruction requires immediate attention.*
- Debris: teeth, blood, and other tissues.
- Neck hematoma: causes compression and deviation of the neck anatomy.
- Laryngeal trauma: trauma leading to hemorrhage and/or edema.
- Tracheal tear: air cannot get to the lungs in full.

Signs and Symptoms of Airway Obstruction

- Stridor
- Accessory muscle use
- Cyanosis
- Subcutaneous emphysema
- Agitation, confusion
- Gasping
- Panic
- Unconsciousness
- Apnea

Intubation

If there is *any* doubt, *intubate*. Use manual in-line stabilization to protect the neck during intubation.

Cricothyrotomy (cricothyroidotomy) may be performed in case of failed intubation or inability to intubate.

Other reasons to intubate are as follows:

- Glasgow Coma Scale score that is less than 9
- Combative patient
- Uncooperative patient requiring CT, aortography, or other imaging studies

Breathing
- Assess the effort and effectiveness of breathing.
- Inspection
  - Check for midline trachea.
  - Oxygen saturation adequate?
  - Paradoxical respirations?
  - Accessory muscle use?
- Palpation
  - Subcutaneous emphysema?
- Percussion
  - Tympany?
- Auscultation
  - Equal, bilateral breath sounds?

You cannot always wait for the chest X-ray: Treat the patient!

Tension Pneumothorax

- Suspect with penetrating or blunt chest trauma
- After intubation, patient has high airway pressures

Signs and symptoms:

- Decreased breath sounds on one side
- Tracheal deviation away from decreased breath sounds
- Respiratory distress
- Shock

Tension pneumothorax occurs when air builds up on one side of the pleural cavity due to accumulation of air or gas in the pleural cavity. It causes an increase in intrathoracic pressure that results in massive shifts of the mediastinum away from the affected lung, compressing intrathoracic vessels. The artery compression causes hypotension.

Air in the thorax appears as black areas on a chest X-ray. The hemidiaphragm is depressed from the intrathoracic pressure.

Tension pneumothorax can lead to death. Needle decompression must be performed immediately. Insert the needle at the second or third intercostal space at middle clavicular line (MCL) over the *top* of the rib; nerves and arteries run under the rib. After air escapes and the patient is stable, a chest tube will need to be inserted.

Open Pneumothorax

In an open pneumothorax, air moves in and out of an open chest wall.

To treat this condition, place Vaseline gauze over the wound, tape three of the four sides of the gauze to help air come out and prevent air from going in. The patient will eventually need surgery to repair the defect in the chest wall and placement of a chest tube.

Hemothorax

A hemothorax appears as a white area on the chest X-ray.

If the hemothorax is small, it may simply be watched. If it is large, a chest tube should be inserted. Thoracotomy may be necessary.

Flail Chest

Flail chest occurs with the fracture of two or more ribs in two or more places. Look for paradoxical respirations: deflation of the ribcage during inspiration, and inflation during expiration.

Support the chest with a tight chest wrap or temporarily position the patient with the flail segment down against the exam table.

Circulation

- Stop obvious bleeding.
- Assess blood pressure, heart rate, and rhythm.
- Observe skin color, skin temperature, and capillary refill.
- Place at least two large-bore peripheral IVs.

Cardiac Tamponade

Cardiac tamponade is an acute distention of the pericardial sac with blood; the pericardial sac does not stretch. Any fluid or blood filling this potential space prevents the heart's ventricles from filling properly, leading to low stroke volume. The end result is ineffective pumping of blood, shock, and often death.

Causes of acute tamponade include penetrating trauma involving the pericardium, blunt chest trauma, and myocardial rupture.

Classical cardiac tamponade is associated with three signs known as *Beck's triad:*

- Hypotension: decreased stroke volume
- Jugular venous distention (JVD): impaired venous return to the heart
- Muffled heart sounds: fluid inside the pericardium

Pulsus paradoxus occurs when the SBP decreases by more than 10 mm Hg during inspiration. If a pulmonary artery catheter is present, the patient will demonstrate equal right and left heart pressures, plus elevated and equal CVP and wedge pressures.

Assess for cardiac tamponade with **f**ocused **a**bdominal **s**onography for **t**rauma (FAST). This modality is sensitive and specific in the determination of traumatic pericardial effusion, and can effectively guide emergent surgical decision making.

Treatment for cardiac tamponade consists of the following measures:

- Intubate the patient, oxygenate, and give volume.
- If the patient is stable, non-emergency surgery is performed for the pericardial window.
- If the patient is in extremis, attempt pericardiocentesis. In this blind procedure, a needle is inserted under the xiphoid process, and blood is "sucked" out of the pericardium into the syringe.
- If pericardiocentesis is unsuccessful in an acutely compromised patient, emergency thoractomy for surgical pericardectomy is needed.

The overall risk of death depends on the speed of diagnosis, the treatment provided, and the severity of the tamponade.

Disability

Glasgow Coma Scale

The Glasgow Coma Scale (GCS) is discussed in depth in Chapter 5. Each item on this scale is assigned a value ranging from 3 (no response) to 5 (awake/oriented); total scores range from 3 to 15.

Trauma Score

Also known as the Revised Trauma Score (RTS), this value is calculated as follows:

- Respiratory rate: $10-29 = 4$, $> 29 = 3$, $6-9 = 2$, $1-5 = 1$, $0 = 0$
- Systolic blood pressure (mm Hg): $> 89 = 4$, $76-89 = 3$, $50-75 = 2$, $1-49 = 1$, $0 = 0$
- Glasgow Coma Scale: $13-15 = 4$, $9-12 = 3$, $6-8 = 2$, $4-5 = 1$, $3 = 0$

The maximum "good" score is 12.

The RTS provides an indication of the chance of survival:

Greater than $7.84 = 98.8\%$ probability of survival

$7 = 96.9\%$ probability of survival

$6 = 91.9\%$ probability of survival

5 = 80.7% probability of survival

4 = 60.5% probability of survival

3 = 36.1% probability of survival

2 = 17.2% probability of survival

1 = 7.1% probability of survival

0 = 2.7% probability of survival

The difference between the patient's RTS on arrival and the best RTS after resuscitation will give a reasonably clear picture of the patient's prognosis.

Exposure/Environmental Factors

Expose the patient so that an adequate complete examination can be performed. Prevent the patient from becoming hypothermic by giving warmed fluids, using warming blankets, and increasing the room temperature as necessary.

Secondary Survey

The secondary survey is a complete assessment of the patient, from head to toe. It lasts as long as needed and covers the following areas:

- Examine the head and face.
- Examine the neck.
- Examine the chest.
- Examine the abdomen.
- Turn the patient to examine the back. You can log roll the patient if five people are available—three at the body, one at the head, and one examining the back. Examine the extremities.
- Perform a neurological examination (repeat the GCS scoring).
- Look for any localizing or lateralizing signs.
- Look for signs of spinal cord injury.

Diaphragmatic Injury

Blunt trauma usually causes a large and posterolateral diaphragmatic injury. While a penetrating trauma causes a smaller defect, this smaller defect usually gets larger and will need surgical repair.

Diagnose by this type of injury with a chest X-ray. A hemidiaphragm elevation will be seen on the affected side.

Surgical repair consists of a laparotomy.

Esophageal Injury

Suspect an esophageal injury with any upper chest/abdomen penetrating injury. A subcutaneous emphysema may be seen, and mediastinal or peritoneal air or blood may be evident on chest X-ray. An esophagoscopy may be needed to make a definitive diagnosis. Repair is by surgical closure.

Blunt Cardiac Injury

Blunt chest trauma can cause myocardial contusion. Arrhythmias are common in such cases, and the injury can cause cardiac rupture (think cardiac tamponade) or heart failure. To diagnose this kind of injury, perform an echocardiogram, check for hypokinesis by assessing wall motion, and run serial serum CPK and troponin levels.

Treatment is to watch the patient, monitor the EKG, and give antiarrhythmics if needed. Rhythms to watch for include sinus tachycardia, premature atrial contraction, premature ventricular contraction, and atrial fibrillation.

Traumatic Aortic Rupture

Traumatic aortic rupture may occur with rapid deceleration injuries (e.g., high-speed auto accidents, falls). In this injury, the aorta is separated from the heart. Approximately 80% victims die at the scene.

Signs and symptoms include hypotension, which may respond to fluid resuscitation. Other signs and symptoms include unequal upper-extremity blood pressures, widened pulse pressure, chest wall contusion, and posterior scapular pain.

Diagnosis is made by chest CT, TEE, and/or aortography. The most consistent sign is a widened mediastinum and hypotension.

The main concern is to control SBP, keeping it at 100 mm Hg or less to prevent bleeding from getting worse. A strong muscular chest can actually limit bleeding by compressing a small tear.

If patients are in extremis, the case is considered a surgical emergency. The goal is to open the chest and try to get control of the bleeding.

Pulmonary Contusion

Pulmonary contusion is the biggest concern of the "hidden six" delayed concerns. It arises when patients have bruising or hemorrhage in the lung parenchyma. These patients will have worsening hypoxia over 24–48 hours with hemoptysis as the only presenting symptom.

Major Tracheobronchial Disruption

Tracheobronchial disruption injuries are rare but potentially lethal; they are caused by blunt or penetrating trauma. The disruption occurs for two reasons:

- Reflex closure of glottis along with the compression of the tracheobronchial tree causes a rapid rise in the intraluminal pressure, which is too high for airway elasticity.
- Shearing forces produced by sudden deceleration and rotation of the lung on the relatively fixed carina may exceed elasticity of the bronchus and result in rupture.

Respiratory distress, hemoptysis, and subcutaneous emphysema are common with tracheobronchial disruption; flail chest may also be seen. Bronchial disruption can be manifested by massive air leak and intrapleural pneumothorax. Pneumomediastinum extending into the cervicothoracic soft tissues (usually the first through fifth ribs) is the most consistent radiological sign of a breach of airway integrity

Diagnosis is confirmed by bronchoscopy.

Treatment is to immediately place an endotracheal tube into the bronchus of the non-injured lung. Primary surgical repair is usually done but lung resection may also be needed.

FLUID RESUSCITATION IN TRAUMA PATIENTS

Adequate volume therapy appears to be a cornerstone of managing the trauma patient. In addition to apparent blood loss in the trauma patient, fluid deficits may occur secondary to generalized alterations of the endothelial barrier, resulting in diffuse capillary leakage and fluid shift from the intravascular system to the interstitial compartment. These effects may result in the development of post-trauma multiple-organ failure on the intensive care unit.

Crystalloids

Common crystalloids for trauma patients include lactated Ringer's solution and normal saline.

- The half-life of crystalloid solution is 20–30 minutes.
- Hypotonic, isotonic, and hypertonic solutions are available to treat trauma-related volume deficits.

A 0.9% sodium chloride solution contains 9 g/L sodium chloride (NaCl):

- pH 5.0
- 154 mEq/L sodium
- 154 mEq/L chloride
- 308 mOsmol/L

"Too much" normal saline (NS) can cause metabolic hyperchloremic acidosis.

Lactated Ringer's solution contains potassium, calcium, and lactate in addition to sodium chloride, which causes volume expansion. It is metabolized to bicarbonate, so avoid its use in alkalotic patients.

- pH 6.5
- 273 mOsmol/L

Colloids

Colloids are non-oxygen-carrying fluids. They include albumin, plasma protein fraction (PPF), dextran, and Hespan. Indications for colloid resuscitation include the following circumstances:

- Fluid resuscitation in severely dehydrated patients (e.g., hemorrhagic shock)
- Fluid resuscitation in patients with hypoalbuminemia
- Conditions involving a loss of large amounts of proteins (e.g., burns)

The half-life of a colloid is 16 hours. Two types of colloids are used: blood-derived colloids and synthetic colloids.

Blood-Derived Colloids

Blood-derived colloids include albumin and plasma protein fraction 5% (PPF). Albumin is derived from pooled human plasma. It is available as 5% and 25% solutions. Albumin has a much higher cost than crystalloid solutions. There is a small but significant incidence of adverse reactions (especially anaphylactoid reactions) with its use.

There is no risk of transmission of hepatitis or HIV with albumin or plasma protein fractions because these fluids are subjected to heat treatment to 60°C for 10 hours.

Synthetic Colloids

Synthetic colloids include dextrose starches.

- *Dextran:* improves microcirculation by decreasing blood viscosity and having antiplatelet effects. Antigenic: associated with both anaphylactic and anaphylactoid reactions. Maximum dose: 20 mL/kg/day.
- *Hetastarch:* less expensive than albumin. Associated with urticarial and anaphylactoid reactions. Do not exceed 1500 mL/day IV or give at a rate faster than 20 mL/kg/min.
  - *Hespan (Hetastarch in sodium chloride):* half-life for 90% of the Hespan particles is 17 days, whereas that of remaining 10% is 48 days. Can increase serum amylase levels for up to 5 days after administration. Contraindicated in patients with severe bleeding disorders (can interfere with platelet function and increase bleeding times), severe CHF (danger of fluid overload with fluid expander), or renal failure with oliguria or anuria.
  - *Hextend (Hetastarch in lactated Ringer's)*

Blood Products

- Fresh autologous blood: ideal resuscitative fluid
- Stored allogenic blood (donated blood)
- Blood substitutes

O negative is the universal donor type; AB positive is the universal recipient type (can receive any blood type).

CPDA is added to blood products as a preservative during storage:

- C: citrate (Ca^{++} binds to citrate)
- P: phosphate
- D: dextrose (food for cells)
- A: adenine (extender)

Mass transfusion causes citrate toxicity, which is characterized by acidity and hyperkalemia. Hypocalcemia also occurs because citrate binds to calcium to prevent the stored blood from clotting.

Metabolic problems due to use of stored blood may include decreased 2,3-DPG production.

Trauma Packs

Trauma packs include non-cross-matched, O-negative blood. After receiving 2 units of non-cross-matched blood, a patient should *not* be given patient-type-specific blood until the blood bank determines that the patient's levels of transfused anti-A and anti-B antibodies have decreased low enough to allow this use.

Some institutions send a range of products in the pack for a trauma case—for example, 6 units packed red blood cells, 3 units plasma (FFP), and 1 pack platelets.

Blood Substitutes

Blood substitutes are oxygen-carrying fluids that can be hemoglobin based.

- Because hemoglobin has no "blood type," the resultant *hemoglobin-based oxygen carrier (HBOC)* would be a universal donor.
- *Perfluorocarbons* are IV carbon–fluorine emulsions that carry large amounts of O_2. They have not been proven to increase survival and cannot be given in amounts sufficient to compensate for critical RBC losses. Because the antigen-bearing RBC membrane is not present, these substances do not require cross-matching. They also can be stored up to 2 years, providing a more stable source than banked blood.

HBOC products are divided into those that use outdated human blood as their hemoglobin source and those that use bovine hemoglobin. They were developed by veterinarians who noted that a dog can give blood to another dog—no cross-matching is needed.

- Prototype: stroma-free hemoglobin
  - High O_2 affinity
  - Rapid clearance
  - Nephrotoxic
  - Produces hypertension
  - Lacks ATP and 2,3-DPG
- *Hemopure*
  - Polymerized bovine hemoglobin
  - Available from Biopure Corporation
  - Extensive veterinary use
  - Can be stored for 24 months at room temperature
  - Can cause vasoconstriction
- *Hemassist*
  - Diaspirin cross-linked hemoglobin from expired human blood
  - Available from Baxter Corporation
  - Can be stored for 9 months if frozen, and for 24 hours if refrigerated
  - Can cause vasoconstriction and gastrointestinal distress
- *Optro*
  - Recombinant engineered cross-linked hemoglobin
  - Available from Somatogen Corporation
  - Can be stored for 18 months if refrigerated
  - Can cause vasoconstriction and gastrointestinal distress
- *Polyheme*
  - Pyridoxylated hemoglobin polymerized from expired human blood
  - Available from Northfield Labs
  - Can be stored for 12 months if refrigerated
  - Usually causes no major side effects

RESUSCITATION MARKERS

Base Deficit

The base deficit (BD) has been regarded as the standard end point of resuscitation in trauma patients. This value, which is derived from blood gas analysis, gives an approximation of tissue acidosis—an indirect evaluation tissue perfusion. However, it has been shown to be an insensitive and slowly responsive indicator of changes in intravascular volume.

Lactate

The base excess is closely related to blood lactate levels. Increased blood lactate levels warn the physician that the patient is at risk of increased morbidity and has a decreased chance of survival. Prompt therapeutic measures to restore the balance between oxygen demand and supply are warranted in these patients. There is a relationship between increased blood lactate levels and the presence of oxygen debt (tissue hypoxia).

The normal serum lactate level is approximately 1 mmol/L, with a range up to 2 mmol/L. Values greater than 4–5 mmol/L are indicative of lactic acidosis.

In hypoperfused states, persistent lactate elevation is associated with excessive mortality. If circulatory failure develops, serial lactate values are helpful in following the course of a hypoperfusion state and determining the response to therapeutic interventions.

Capnometry

Esophageal or sublingual capnometry may prove to be a useful tool for monitoring the adequacy of resuscitation in trauma victims.

Sublingual Capnometry

Sublingual capnometry (SC) is a rapid, minimally invasive bedside test. It allows assessment of end-organ perfusion and, therefore, provides additional information about circulatory failure.

Sublingual PCO_2 ($SLCO_2$) is a regional marker of microvascular perfusion and tissue hypoxia that holds great promise for the risk stratification and determination of the end point of goal-directed resuscitation in critically ill patients. It is measured using a disposable CO_2 sensor. This device incorporates a CO_2-specific fluorescent dye in a buffer solution encased in a silicone capsule that is permeable to CO_2 gas. The sensor is attached to an instrument that measures the amount of CO_2 present by projecting light onto the sensor with an optical fiber. Changes in the projected light are used to calculate the amount of CO_2 present. For clinical measurements, the sensor is placed under the tongue, with the sensor element facing the sublingual mucosa.

TRAUMA RESUSCITATION RECOMMENDATIONS

Use a team approach: Everything should be done at once.

- Start with the primary survey: A * B * C * D * E. Complete it within 2–3 minutes.
- Start multiple, large-bore peripheral IVs.

- Start warmed IV fluids.
- Keep the patient warm—use warming blankets, fluid warmers, and increased room temperature as necessary.
- Oxygenate the patient. Perform intubation or cricothyroidotomy if needed.
- Maintain cervical precautions.
- Evaluate the clinical response to IV fluids.
- Get baseline lab and ABG results.
- Initiate invasive monitoring if there is an inappropriate response to volume replacement.

End-Point Resuscitation

- Respiratory rate: 10–29 breaths per minute
- Systolic blood pressure: greater than 89 mm Hg
- Glasgow Coma Scale score: 13–15
- Capillary refill: normal return to pink in 2–3 seconds

ANESTHESIA ON TRAUMA PATIENTS

- The patient's blood pressure may indicate that he or she will not be able to tolerate opioids or inhaled agents. In such cases, give scopolamine 0.4 mg IV and/or Versed (midazolam) 1 mg increments during surgery for amnesia.
- If possible, have one person do all the charting in the OR.
- Establish peripheral IV lines. An arterial line is almost always needed in trauma cases. Do you need CVP? The answer to this question depends on how many peripheral/femoral lines have already been placed and condition of the patient.
- Place warming blankets over body parts that aren't being operated on.
- Draw frequent ABGs that monitor pH, PCO_2, PO_2, base levels, HCO_3, and oxygen saturation, along with H&H, potassium, calcium, and blood sugar levels.

- Maintain blood glucose levels in the range of 80–120 mg/dL; keep tight controls.
- Have sodium bicarbonate in the room and give as needed, based on base deficit, while you are giving IV fluids, colloids, and blood products.

Anesthesia Hints

- Lay a folded bath blanket on the floor, and place piles of used IV fluid bags and all empty blood product bags on it. This helps to keep tabs of all the fluids and blood products you are giving.

- If you need extra room for notes, ask your circulator for several pages of progress notes. You will have plenty of room to list all the drugs given and interventions undertaken.
- Make stacks of your blood products papers: cryoprecipitate products in one stack, PRBCs in another stack, FFP papers in another stack, and so on. This helps you keep track of exactly what has been given in the operating room.

Abbreviations

±: plus or minus; add or not

abd: abdominal

ABG: arterial blood gas

AC: acromioclavicular

ACL: anterior cruciate ligament

ACP: anterior cerebral perfusion

ACT: activated clotting time (measurement)

ACTH: adrenocorticotropic hormone

ADH: antidiuretic hormone

AFib: atrial fibrillation

AFl: atrial flutter

AICD: automatic implantable cardioverter-defibrillator

AMI: acute myocardial infarction

ANS: autonomic nervous system

ARDS: adult respiratory distress syndrome

ASA: acetylsalicylic acid (aspirin)

ASD: atrial septal defect

BAEP: brain stem auditory evoked potentials

BAER: brain stem auditory evoked responses

BBB: blood–brain barrier

BID: twice a day

BIS: bispectral analysis monitor

BMI: body mass index

BMP: bone morphogenic protein

BP: blood pressure

BRAT: scavenged cell saver blood

BSO: bilateral salpingo-oophorectomy

C: Celsius/centigrade

C: cervical

Ca^{++}: calcium

CABG: coronary artery bypass graft

C-arm: a type of x-ray machine used in an operating room that has a "C-shaped" arm.

CAT scan: computed axial tomography scan

CBC: complete blood count

CBD: common bile duct

CBF: cerebral blood flow

CBV: cerebral blood volume

CCU: coronary care unit

CEA: carotid endarterectomy

Chem: chemistry

CHF: congestive heart failure

CI: cardiac index

cm: centimeter

CMRGI: cerebral metabolic rate of glucose consumption

$CMRO_2$: cerebral metabolic rate of oxygen; brain oxygen consumption

CN: cranial nerve

CNS: central nervous system

CO: cardiac output

CO_2: carbon dioxide

COPD: chronic obstructive pulmonary disease

CPAP: continuous positive airway pressure

CPB: cardiopulmonary bypass

CPK: creatine phosphokinase

cpm: cycles per minute

CPP: cerebral perfusion pressure

CRNA: certified registered nurse anesthetist

cryo: cryoprecipitate

CSE: combined spinal-epidural

CSF: cerebrospinal fluid

C-sxn: cesarean section

CT: computed tomography

CTSU: cardio-thoracic surgical unit

CVA: cerebrovascular accident

CVL: central venous line

CVP: central venous pressure

CXR: chest X-ray

DBP: diastolic blood pressure

D&C: dilation and curettage

DEP: dermatome evoked potentials

DHCA: deep hypothermic cardiac arrest

DIC: disseminated intravascular coagulation

dL: deciliter

DLEBT: double-lumen endobronchial tube

DMR: depolarizing muscle relaxant

dopa: dopamine

DVT: deep venous thrombosis

EBL: estimated blood loss

ECMO: extracorporeal membrane oxygenation

ECT: electroconvulsant therapy

EDV: end diastolic volume

EEG: electroencephalography

EF: ejection fraction

EGD: esophagoduodenoscopy

EKG: electrocardiogram

EMG: electromyography

ENT: ear, nose, and throat

EP: evoked potential

epi: epinephrine

ESU: electrical surgical unit

$ETCO_2$: end-tidal carbon dioxide

ETOH: alcohol

ETT: endotracheal tube

F: factor

f: French

FES: fat embolism syndrome

FFP: fresh frozen plasma

FHT: fetal heart tones

FiO_2: fraction of inspired oxygen

Fr: French

FRC: functional residual capacity

g: gram

GA: general anesthetic

GCS: Glasgow Coma Scale

GERD: gastro-esophageal reflux disease

GETA: general endotracheal anesthesia

GI: gastrointestinal

glu: glucose

GU: genitourinary

GYN: gynecological

H: histamine

H_2O: water

HBOC: hemoglobin-based oxygen carrier

HCG: human chorionic gonadotropin

HCT: hematocrit

HFJV: high-frequency jet ventilation

HFOV: high-frequency oscillatory ventilation

Hgb: hemoglobin

H&H: hemoglobin and hematocrit

HOB: head of the bed

HOTN/hotn: hypotension

HR: heart rate

HTA: hydrothermal ablation

HTN: hypertension

IABP: intra-aortic balloon pump

ICD: implantable cardioverter-defibrillator

ICP: intracranial pressure

ICU: intensive care unit

I:E: inspiratory-to-expiratory ratio

IM: intramuscular

IM: intramedullary

INR: International Normalized Ratio

IPTH: intact parathyroid hormone

ISD: intrinsic sphincter deficiency

ITP: idiopathic thrombocytopenic purpura

IUD: intrauterine device

IV: intravenous (catheter)

IVC: inferior vena cava

IVF: intravenous fluid

kg: kilogram

KVO: keep vein open

L: liter

L: lumbar

LA: local anesthesia

LAP: left atrial pressure

LES: lower esophageal sphincter

LIMA: left internal mammary artery

LMA: laryngeal mask airway

LOC: level of consciousness

LR: lactated Ringer's solution

LV: left ventricle

m: meter

MAC: minimal alveolar concentration

MAC: monitored anesthesia care

MAO: monoamine oxidase

MAP: mean arterial pressure

mcg: microgram

MEP: motor evoked potentials

mEq: milliequivalent

mg: milligram

MI: myocardial infarction

MIDCAB: minimally invasive coronary artery bypass

min: minute

mL: milliliter

MLT: microlaryngeal tracheal tube

mm: millimeter

MMA: methylmethacrylate

mm Hg: millimeters of mercury

mmol: millimole

mOsm: milliosmole

MPAP: mean pulmonary artery pressure

MRI: magnetic resonance imaging

MVO_2: mixed venous oxygen

N_2O: nitrous oxide

NaCl: sodium chloride

NDMR: nondepolarizing muscle relaxant

NEC: necrotizing enterocolitis

Neo: Neo-Synephrine

NGT: nasogastric tube

NICU: neonatal intensive care unit

NICU: neurologic intensive care unit

NPO: nothing by mouth

NS: normal saline

NSAID: nonsteroidal anti-inflammatory drug

NSR: normal sinus rhythm

NTG: nitroglycerin

O_2: oxygen

OETT: oral endotracheal tube

OGT: orogastric tube

OPCAB: off-pump coronary artery bypass

OPO: organ procurement organization

OR: operating room

ORIF: open reduction with internal fixation

OSA: obstructive sleep apnea

PA: pulmonary artery

PAC: pulmonary artery catheter

PAC: premature atrial contraction

$PaCO_2$: partial pressure of carbon dioxide

PACU: post anesthesia care unit (recovery room)

PAD: pulmonary artery diastolic (pressure)

PaO$_2$: partial pressure of oxygen
PAP: pulmonary artery pressures
PAS: pulmonary artery systolic (pressure)
PBF: pulmonary blood flow
PCWP: pulmonary capillary wedge pressure
PDA: patent ductus arteriosus
PE: pulmonary embolism
ped: pediatric
PEEP: positive end-expiratory pressure
PFO: patent foramen ovale
PFT: pulmonary function tests
PIV: peripheral IV
plt: platelet
PNB: peripheral nerve block
PO: by mouth
PONV: postoperative nausea and vomiting
postop: postoperatively
POVL: postoperative visual loss
PPHN: persistent pulmonary hypertension of newborn
PRBC: packed red blood cells
preop: preoperatively
PSARP: posterior sagittal anorectoplasty
PT: prothrombin time
PTCA: percutaneous transluminal angioplasty
PTH: parathyroid hormone
PTT: partial thromboplastin time
PVC: premature ventricular contraction
PVR: pulmonary vascular resistance
RAE: type of preformed "U-shaped" endotracheal tube
RAP: right atrial pressure
RBC: red blood cell
RCP: retrograde cerebral perfusion
RIJ: right internal jugular
RIMA: right internal mammary artery
RIS: rapid infusion system
ROP: retinopathy of prematurity
RVP: right ventricular pressure
S: sacral
SaO$_2$: saturation of oxygen
SBP: systolic blood pressure
SCM: sternocleidomastoid muscle

sec: second
SIADH: syndrome of inappropriate antidiuretic hormone
SNP: sodium nitroprusside
SNS: sympathetic nervous system
S/S: signs and symptoms
SSEP: somatosensory evoked potentials
ST: sinus tachycardia
SV: stroke volume
SVG: saphenous vein graft
SVO$_2$: saturated venous oxygen content
SVR: systemic vascular resistance
T: thoracic
T&A: tonsillectomy and adenoidectomy
TAH: total abdominal hysterectomy
TB: tuberculosis
T&C: type and cross
TEE: transesophageal echocardiography
TEG: thromboelastogram
TID: three times a day
TIPS: transjugular intrahepatic portosystemic shunt
TIVA: total intravenous anesthesia
TMP: transmural pressure
TOF: train of four
TPN: total parenteral nutrition
T&S: type and screen
TUR: transurethral resection
TURB: transurethral resection of lesions of the bladder
TURP: transurethral resection of the prostate gland
UNOS: United Network of Organ Sharing
V$_T$: tidal volume
Ua: urine
UGI: upper gastrointestinal
UTI: urinary tract infection
VAE: venous air embolism
VATS: video-assisted thoracic surgery
VEP: visual evoked potentials
V/Q: ventilation-perfusion ratio
VVB: veno-venous bypass
WBC: white blood cell count
WNL: within normal limits

Spanish–English Anesthesia Translator

While this guide can be used for general questions and commands, it is a legal requirement to have a Spanish interpreter for any patient consent for surgery or anesthesia or to sign a legal document.

GENERAL RULES OF SPANISH LANGUAGE

Don't pronounce "h."
The noun before the adjective.
Pronunciation of vowels:

 a = ah

 e = a

 i = e

 o = o

 u = oo

General Questions	*Preguntas Generales*

The phonetic pronunciation appears in parentheses. Emphasis is placed where word is all capitalized.

How tall are you?
¿Qué alto es usted?
(cay alto es oo-stead)

See the height chart later in this section.

How much do you weigh?
¿Cuánto usted pesa?
(coo-AHN-toe oo-stead pass-a)

See the weight chart later in this section.

Do you take any medications?
¿Toma usted algún medicamento?
(toe-mah oo-stead al-goon medicah-MAN-toe)

Are you allergic to any medicines?
¿Es usted alérgico(a) a medicinas?
(es oostead alER-heeco ah med-ah-cee-nas)

Last food eaten?	¿Cuándo comió por última vez?
	(coo-ahn-doe co-mio por ool-TEEM-a vaz)
Last drink?	¿Cuándo bebió por última vez?
	(coo-ahn-doe ba-BEE-o por ool-TEEM-a vaz)
Did you eat or drink today?	¿Usted comió o bebió hoy?
	(oostead co-mio o ba-BEE-o hoy)
How much?	¿Cuánto?
	(quanto)
Where?	¿Donde?
	(DON-day)
When?	¿Cuándo?
	(quando)
Why?	¿Por qué?
	(poor cay)
How many times?	¿Cuántas veces?
	(coo-AHN-tah-s veh-sass)
What is your name?	¿Cuál es su nombre?
	(coo-ahl s soo NOM-bray)
How old are you?	¿Cuántos años tiene usted?
	(coo-AHN-tah-s anyos tea-en-ye oostead)
How are you?	¿Cómo esta usted?
	(como aystah oostead)
Where does it hurt?	¿Dónde le duele?
	(done-day lah due-ELL-a)
Point to the pain.	Muestre dónde le duele.
	(mwestrey donda lay due-ELL-a)
Do you drink alcohol?	¿Toma usted bebidas alcohólicas?
	(toma oostead bay-BEE-das al-co-lake-us)
Do you smoke?	¿Fuma?
	(FOO-ma)
Almost finished?	¿Casi terminamos?
	(cah-see termin-OH-mos)

Medical History

Historial Médico

Do you have pain?	¿Tiene usted dolor?
	(tea-n oostead doe-lore)
Point.	Señala.
	(see-NYAH-la)
Where?	¿Dónde?
	(done-day)

Do you have chest pain?

¿Tiene usted dolor en el pecho?
(tea-EN oostead doe-lore n al paycho)

Do you have any breathing
problems such as asthma?

¿Tiene problemas respiratorios tales como asma?
(tea-EN pro-BLE-mahs respeera-sea-own tahl-ass co-mo ass-mah)

Do you have any kidney or bladder problems?

¿Tiene ustéd problemas de los riñones o de la vejiga?
(tea-EN oostead pro-BLE-mahs da los reen-YO-nass vah-HEE-ga)

Do you have many infections?

¿Sufre usted de muchas infecciones?
(soofrah oostead da moochass infexx-see-o-nas)

Do you have any heart problems?

¿Tiene usted problemas del corazón?
(tea-EN oostead pro-BLE-mahs core-a-zone)

High blood pressure?

¿Presión alta?
(press-see-own alta)

Do you bleed easily from your nose or gums?

¿Sangra usted fácilmente de la nariz o las encías?
(sangra oostead fah-sill-a-mentey da lah nareese o las en-SEE-us)

Have you ever had a seizure?

¿Ha tenido usted alguna vez un ataque de epilepsia?
(ah ta-NEED-o oostead al-GOO-nah base oon attack-a da ep-a-LEP-see-a)

Do you have muscle weakness?

¿Tiene usted debilidad muscular?
(tea-EN oostead day-bill-e-dad MOOSE-cool-ahr)

Do you have stomach problems like ulcers?

¿Tiene usted problemas del estómago como úlceras?
(tea-EN oostead pro-BLE-mahs dall est-AH-mago co-mo ool-CER-ahs)

Have you had any diseases of the liver or blood?

¿Ha tenido usted enfermedades del hígado o de la sangre?
(ah ta-NEED-o oostead ahn-fer-mahd-ah-des del ee-GAH-doe o da lah san-grah)

Do you have diabetes or blood sugar problems?

¿Tiene usted problemas de diabetes o del azúcar en la sangre?
(tea-EN oostead pro-BLE-mahs dah dee-a-bay-tees o dall as-u-car da san-grah)

Anesthesia Questions and Teaching

I'm with the group of anesthesia.

Yo estoy con el grupo de anestesia.
(yo astoy con al groupo da ahh-nah-STAY-see-ah)

Have you had other operations?

¿Usted ha tenido otras operaciones?
(oostead ah taneedo o-tras oh-per-a-see-o-neys)

Have you had problems with anesthesia?

¿Usted ha tenido problemas con la anestesia?
(oostead ah taneedo pro-BLE-mahs con l ah ahh-nah-stay-cee-ah)

Have you had an allergic reaction to anesthesia?

¿Usted ha tenido reacciones alérgicas a la anestesia? (oostead ah taneedo ree-ack-see-o-nass alER-heeco ah lah ahh-nah-stay-cee-ah)

Nausea, vomiting

Náusea, vómitos (naw-z-ah, vo-MEE-toes)

Obstetrics

Has this been a normal pregnancy?

Have you ever had a spinal injection for pain?

Would you like a spinal injection for the pain?

I need your permission for this injection. There is one chance in one hundred that you could get a bad headache. There are other much rarer complications that are possible. These complications include infection, bleeding, and nerve damage. These risks are rare, perhaps greater than one in ten thousand.

Directions

Take a deep breath.

Tell me when it feels cold the same way.

Sit up.

More.

Relax.

Lean.

Open your mouth, please.

Lie down.

Obstetricia

¿Ha sido normal este embarazo? (ah see-doe nor-mall estay em-bar-a-zoe)

¿Le han puesto alguna vez una inyección en la columna para el dolor? (lay ahn PUAY-stow al-goon-ah base oona in-YEXX-ee-own en lah co-loom-nah pah-rah el doe-lor)

¿Le gustaría a usted una inyección en la médula espinal para el dolor? (lah goo-star-ee-ah ah oostead oo-nah in-YEXX-ee-own ahn lah KO-lum-nah pair-a el doe-lor)

Necesito su permiso para darle esta inyección. Existe la posibilidad del un por ciento que le pueda dar un dolor fuerte de cabeza. También es posible que hayan otras complicaciones más raras. Estas incluyen infección, hemoragia y daño al nervio. Estos riesgos son raros, tal vez uno en diez mil casos.

Instrucciones (instruck-tee-OWN-as)

Respire profundo. (res-PEER-a pro-foon-da)

Dígame cuando sienta el frío de la misma manera. (de-gah-ma coo-ahn-do see-en-tay al freeo da lah mis-mah mah-nar-ah)

Siéntese. (see-EN-ten-sey)

Mas. (mahs)

Cálmese. (cahl-may-sey)

Inclínese. (in-CLEAN-asay)

Abra su boca, por favor. (ah-bra soo boca poor fa-voor)

Mire hacia abajo. (meeday AH-see-ah a-bah-ho)

Look up.	Mire hacia arriba.
	(meeday AH-see-ah a-REE-bah)
Breathe naturally.	Respire normal.
	(res-peer-ah nor-MALL)
Hold your breath.	Aguante la respiración
	(a-wan-tay lah res-PEER-a-see-own)
Don't move.	No se mueva.
	(no say moo-way-vay)
Move over here.	Muevase para aca.
	(MWAY-vah-say PAH-rah ah-KAH)
Move up.	Muevase hacia arriba.
	(MWAY-vah-say AH-see-ah ah-RRHEE-bah)
Move down.	Muevase hacia abajo.
	(MWAY-vah-say AH-see-ah ah-BAH-hoh)
Good-bye.	Adiós.
	(ah-dee-OS)
Thank you.	Gracias.
	(GRA-see-os)

Symptoms / Síntomas

Cold	Frío (freeo)
Very cold	Mucho frío/muy frío (moo-ee freeo)
Mild/little/small	Suave/poco/poquito (swa-vay/poko/po-kee-toe)
Moderate	Moderado (mow-day-ado)
Severe	Severo o fuerte (sah vee-do foo-ER-tay)
Ear ache	Dolor de oído (doe-lor day o-EE-doe)
Sore throat	Dolor de garganta (doe-lor day gar-gan-tah)
Difficulty swallowing	Dificultad para tragar (diff-a-cul-tad para tra-GAR)
Shortness of breath	Falta de respiración (FAL-tah da res-peer-ah-see-own)
Chest pain	Dolor de pecho (doe-lor da PAY-cho)
Cough	Tos (toe-s)
Abdominal pain	Dolor abdominal (doe-lor ab-DOM-en-al)
Back pain	Dolor de espalda (doe-lor day es-PAL-da)
Weak	Débil (day-bill)
Dizzy	Mareado(a) (mah-ray-ah-doe)
Loss of consciousness	Pérdida de conocimiento (per-DEE-dah day con-o-sah-mee-ento)
Fever/chills	Fiebre/escalofríos (fee-ah-bra/es-cala-frios)

Miscellaneous / Misceláneas

Medications	Medicamentos (med-ah-seen-a)
Antibiotics	Antibióticos (ante-bee-ot-ah-coes)
Pain pills	Pastillas para dolor (pas-TEE-yas pah-ra doe-lor)

Narcotics	Narcóticos (nar-COT-i-cos)
Penicillin	Penicilina (pen-ah-sill-en-nah)
Operation	Operación (op-er-ACE-e-own)
Oxygen	Oxígeno (oxy-HAY-no)
Cast	Yeso (yay-so)
Splint	Entablillado (enta-blee-yado)
Stitches	Puntos (poon-tos)
Hospital	Hospital (hos-PEE-tahl)
Doctor	Doctor (doc-toor)
Yes	Sí (see)
No	No (no)

Body Parts	***Partes del Cuerpo***
Right	Derecho(a) (day-RAY-cho)
Left	Izquierdo(a) (iss-KEY-erdo)
Skull	Cráneo (CRAHN-ee-o)
Brain	Cerebro (say-RAY-bro)
Face	Cara (CAR-ah)
Ears	Orejas (ore-A-hose)
Eyes	Ojos (OH-hose)
Open your eyes	Abra su ojos (ah-bee-EN-toe oh-hose)
Nose	Nariz (nare-ee-say)
Mouth	Boca (bow-cah)
Open your mouth	Abra su boca (ah-bee-EN-toe bow-cah)
Tongue	Lengua (leng-wah)
Tooth/teeth	Diente/dientes (dee-en-tay)
Throat	Garganta (gar-gan-tah)
Tonsils	Amígdalas (a-MIG-dall-as)
Neck	Cuello (coo-way-o)
Chest	Pecho (peh-cho)
Bronchus	Bronquio (bronk-ee-o)
Lungs	Pulmones (pool-mon-us)
Heart	Corazón (COR-ah-zon)
Ribs	Costillas (co-stee-yas)
Abdomen	Abdomen (ab-DOE-man)
Skin	Piel (pee-EL)
Liver	Hígado (ee-GA-low)
Gallbladder	Vesícula (veh-sick-u-lah)
Stomach	Estómago (es-TOM-a-go)
Intestines	Intestinos (in-tes-TEEN-os)
Appendix	Apéndice (a-pen-dee-say)
Bladder	Vejiga (veh-hee-ga)
Kidney or kidneys	Riñón/riñones (ree-nnones)

Colon	Colon (CO-lawn)
Rectum/anus	Recto/ano (recto/ah-no)
Penis	Pene (pey-ney)
Testicles	Testículos (tes-tick-you-los)
Vagina	Vagina (vah-hee-nah)
Ovary	Ovario (oh-vah-rio)
Uterus	Útero (oo-ter-ah)
Back	Espalda (es-PAL-dah)
Arm	Brazo (BRA-sew)
Leg	Pierna (pee-ER-nah)
Shoulder	Hombro (home-bro)
Elbow	Codo (coe-doe)
Wrist	Muñeca (moo-NAY-cah)
Hand	Mano (mah-no)
Finger	Dedo (day-do)
Hip	Cadera (cah-DAY-rah)
Knee	Rodilla (row-DEE-ha)
Ankle	Tobillo (toe-BEE-hoe)
Foot	Pie (PEE-ah)
Toe	Dedo del pie (day-doe del PEE-ah)
Fetus	Feto (FAY-toe)

Numbers	*Números*
1	Uno (OOO-no)
2	Dos (dose)
3	Tres (trays)
4	Cuatro (coo-ON-tro)
5	Cinco (SINK-o)
6	Seis (cease)
7	Siete (see-EH-tay)
8	Ocho (O-cho)
9	Nueve (noo-WEV-eh)
10	Diez (DEE-ez)
11	Once (OWN-say)
12	Doce (DOE-say)
13	Trece (TRAY-say)
14	Catorce (ca-TORE-say)
15	Quince (KEEN-say)
16	Dieciséis (dee-es-sea-says)
17	Diecisiete (dee-es-sea-sea-ET-tay)
18	Dieciocho (dee-es-sea-OH-cho)
19	Diecinueve (dee-es-sea-noo-EV-ey)
20	Veinte (VEIN-tay)

30	Treinta (TRAIN-tah)
40	Cuarenta (coo-are-EN-tah)
50	Cincuenta (seen-coo-EN-tah)
60	Sesenta (ses-EN-tah)
70	Setenta (seh-TEN-tah)
80	Ochenta (o-CHEN-tah)
90	Noventa (no-VENT-tah)
100	Cien (see-EN)

Height and Weight

Altura y Peso

Your height is?

¿Tu altura es?
(too al-TOO-rah es)

How tall are you?

¿Qué alto es usted?
(cay alto es oo-stead)

Point here.

Señala aqui.
(seh-NYAH-la ah-KEY)

Six feet seven inches 6' 7"

Seis pies y siete pulgadas
2 metros

Six feet six inches 6' 6"

Seis pies y seis pulgadas
1 metro 98 centímetros

Six feet five inches 6' 5"

Seis pies y cinco pulgadas
1 metro 99 centímetros

Six feet four inches 6' 4"

Seis pies y cuatro pulgadas
1 metro 93 centímetros

Six feet three inches 6' 3"

Seis pies y tres pulgadas
1 metro 98 centímetros

Six feet two inches 6' 2"

Seis pies y dos pulgadas
1 metro 88 centímetros

Six feet one inch 6' 1"

Seis pies y una pulgada
1 metro 85 centímetros

Six feet 6'

Seis pies
1 metro 83 centímetros

Five feet eleven inches 5' 11"

Cinco pies y once pulgadas
1 metro 80 centímetros

Five feet ten inches 5' 10"

Cinco pies y diez pulgadas
1 metro 78 centímetros

Five feet nine inches 5' 9"

Cinco pies y nueve pulgadas
1 metro 75 centímetros

Five feet eight inches 5' 8"

Cinco pies y ocho pulgadas
1 metro 73 centímetros

Five feet seven inches 5' 7"

Cinco pies y siete pulgadas
1 metro 70 centímetros

Five feet six inches 5' 6"

Cinco pies y seis pulgadas
1 metro 68 centímetros

Five feet five inches 5' 5"	Cinco pies y cinco pulgadas
	1 metro 65 centímetros
Five feet four inches 5' 4"	Cinco pies y cuatro pulgadas
	1 metro 63 centímetros
Five feet three inches 5' 3"	Cinco pies y tres pulgadas
	1 metro 60 centímetros
Five feet two inches 5' 2"	Cinco pies y dos pulgadas
	1 metro 57 centímetros
Five feet one inch 5' 1"	Cinco pies y una pulgada
	1 metro 55 centímetros
Five feet 5'	Cinco pies
	1 metro 52 centímetros
Four feet eleven inches 4' 11"	Cuatro pies y once pulgadas
	1 metro 50 centímetros
Four feet ten inches 4' 10"	Cuatro pies y diez pulgadas
	1 metro 47 centímetros
Four feet nine inches 4' 9"	Cuatro pies y nueve pulgadas
	1 metro 45 centímetros
Four feet eight inches 4' 8"	Cuatro pies y ocho pulgadas
	1 metro 42 centímetros
Four feet seven inches 4' 7"	Cuatro pies y siete pulgadas
	1 metro 40 centímetros
Four feet six inches 4' 6"	Cuatro pies y seis pulgadas
	1 metro 42 centímetros
Four feet seven inches 4' 5"	Cuatro pies y cinco pulgadas
	1 metro 35 centímetros

How much does your baby weigh?	¿Cuánto su bebé pesa?
	(coo-AHN-toe sue beh-BAY pass-a)
How much do you weigh?	¿Cuánto usted pesa?
	(coo-AHN-toe oo-stead pass-a)
Mark here.	Marque aqui.
	(mar-kay ah-KEY)

Baby   *Bebé*

KILOGRAMS/ KILOGRAMAS	POUNDS/ LIBRAS
1	2
2	4
3	7
4	9
5	11
6	13

KILOGRAMS/ KILOGRAMAS	POUNDS/ LIBRAS
7	15
8	18
9	20
10	22
11	24
12	26

(continues)

KILOGRAMS/ KILOGRAMAS	POUNDS/ LIBRAS	KILOGRAMS/ KILOGRAMAS	POUNDS/ LIBRAS
13	29	27	59
14	31	28	62
15	33	29	64
16	35	30	66
17	37	31	68
18	40	32	70
19	42	33	73
20	44	34	75
21	46	35	77
22	48	36	79
23	51	37	81
24	53	38	84
25	55	39	86
26	57	40	88

Adult   *Adulto*

POUNDS/ LIBRAS	KILOGRAMS/ KILOGRAMAS	POUNDS/ LIBRAS	KILOGRAMS/ KILOGRAMAS
40–45	18–20	120–125	54–57
45–50	20–28	125–130	57–59
50–55	23–25	130–135	59–61
55–60	25–27	135–140	61–64
60–65	27–30	140–145	64–66
65–70	30–32	145–150	66–68
70–75	32–34	150–155	68–70
75–80	34–36	155–160	70–73
80–85	36–39	160–165	73–75
85–90	39–41	165–170	75–77
90–95	41–43	170–175	77–80
95–100	43–45	175–180	80–82
100–105	45–48	180–185	82–84
105–110	48–50	185–190	84–86
110–115	50–52	190–195	86–89
115–120	52–54	195–200	89–91

(continues)

POUNDS/ LIBRAS	KILOGRAMS/ KILOGRAMAS	POUNDS/ LIBRAS	KILOGRAMS/ KILOGRAMAS
200–205	91–93	275–280	125–127
205–210	93–95	280–285	127–130
210–215	95–98	285–290	130–132
215–220	98–100	290–295	132–134
220–225	100–102	295–300	134–136
225–230	102–105	300–305	136–139
230–235	105–107	305–310	139–141
235–240	107–109	310–315	141–143
240–245	109–111	315–320	143–145
245–250	111–114	320–325	145–147
250–255	114–116	325–330	147–150
255–260	116–118	330–335	150–152
260–265	118–120	335–340	152–155
265–270	120–123	340–345	155–157
270–275	123–125	Mas de 345	(greater than 345)

Sources

American Academy of Orthopaedic Surgeons (AAOS). (2004). *Paramedic: Anatomy and physiology*. Sudbury, MA: Jones & Bartlett Learning.

American College of Cardiology & American Heart Association. (2002). *ACC/ AHA guideline update on perioperative cardiovascular evaluation for noncardiac surgery*.

American Society of Regional Anesthesia and Pain Medication (ASRA). (n.d.). *Publications: Consensus statements*. Retrieved September 10, 2010, from http://www.asra.com/publications.php

Barash, P. G., Cullen, B. F., & Stoelting, R. K. (2006). *Clinical anesthesia* (5th ed.). Philadelphia, PA: Lippincott, Williams & Wilkins.

Bhatti, M. T., & Enneking, F. K. (2003). Visual loss and ophthalmoplegia after shoulder surgery. *Anesthesia and Analgesia, 96,* 899–902.

Bhatti, M. T., & Enneking, F. K. (2004). Hypotensive technique and sitting position in shoulder surgery [Letter to the editor]. *Anesthesia and Analgesia, 97,* 1199–2003.

Brown, D. L. (1999). *Atlas of regional anesthesia* (2nd ed.). Philadelphia, PA: W. B. Saunders.

Chiras, D. (2008). *Human biology* (6th ed.). Sudbury, MA: Jones & Bartlett Learning.

Clark, R. K. (2005). *Anatomy and physiology: Understanding the human body*. Sudbury, MA: Jones & Bartlett Learning.

Cubbon, R. M., & Witt, K. K. A. (2009, May 2). Cardiac resynchronization therapy for chronic heart failure and conduction delay. *British Medical Journal, 338,* 1265.

Donnersberger, A. B. (2010). *A laboratory textbook of anatomy and physiology: Cat version* (9th ed.). Sudbury, MA: Jones & Bartlett Learning.

Dutton, R. P., & Goldstein, A. D. (1995). *The anesthesiologist's guide to the OR*. Philadelphia, PA: Lippincott, Williams & Wilkins.

ECRI Institute. (2009). *Only you can prevent surgical fires*. Plymouth Meeting, PA: Author.

Ezekiel, M. R. (2008). *Handbook of anesthesiology*. Laguna Hills, CA: Current Clinical Strategies.

Ferschl, M., & Gelb, A. (2008, January 17). Pathophysiology and anesthetic management of cerebral aneurysms. *Current Reviews for Nurse Anesthetists, 30,* 18.

Frost, E. (2007, April 12). "He can't be blind, it's only back surgery." *Current Reviews for Nurse Anesthetists, 29,* 249.

Hensley, F. A., Goldman, M. A. (1996). *Pocket guide to the operating room* (2nd ed.). Philadelphia, PA: F. A. Davis.

Horlocker, T. T., Wedel, D. J., Benzon, H., Brown, D. L., Enneking, F. K., Heit, J. A., et al. (2003). Regional anesthesia in the anticoagulated patient: Defining the risks (The second ASRA consensus conference on neuraxial anesthesia and anticoagulation). *Regional Anesthesia and Pain Medicine, 28*(3), 172–197. Retrieved September 10, 2010, from http://www.asra.com/pdf/RAPM-nticoagulation.pdf

Jaffe, R. A., & Samuels, S. I. (Eds.). (2004). *Anesthesiologist's manual of surgical procedures* (3rd ed.). Philadelphia, PA: Lippincott Williams & Wilkins.

Joyce, J. A. (2006, December 21). "Postoperative vision loss." *Current Reviews for Nurse Anesthetists, 29,* 16.

Kirby, R. R., & Cullen, D. J. (2008, April 10). The beach chair position: Anatomic and physiologic concerns. *Current Reviews for Nurse Anesthetists, 30,* 24.

Martin, D. E., & Gravlee, G. P. (2008). *A practical approach to cardiac anesthesia.* Philadelphia, PA: Lippincott Williams & Wilkins.

May, L. E. (2008). *Pediatric heart surgery: A ready reference for professionals* (4th ed.). Milwaukee, WI: maxiSHARE.

Miller, R. D., Eriksson, L. I., Fleisher, L. A., Wiener-Kronish, J. P., & Young, W. L. (2009). *Miller's anesthesia* (7th ed.) London, UK: Churchill Livingstone (Elsevier Science).

Olyaei, A. (2004). *Perioperative steroid coverage (stress dose).* Retrieved September 10, 2010, from http://www.ohsu.edu/medicine/residency/handouts/pharmpearls/Endocrine/SteroidsStressDose.pdf

Ouellette, R. G. (2009, February 12). Robotic-assisted radical prostatectomy: Anesthetic considerations and management. *Current Reviews for Nurse Anesthetists, 31,* 20.

Rothrock, J. C. (2007). *Alexander's care of the patient in surgery* (13th ed.). St. Louis, MO: Mosby Elsevier.

Soper, N. J.,Swanström L. L., & Eubanks, W. S. (2004). Upper extremity sympathectomy thoracic laparoscopic approach to sympathectomy. In *Mastery of endoscopic and laparoscopic surgery.* Philadelphia, PA: Lippincott Williams & Wilkins.

Stoelting, R. K., & Dierdorf, S. F. (2008). *Anesthesia and coexisting disease* (3rd ed.). City: Philadelphia, PA: Saunders.

Troianos, C. (2002). *Anesthesia for the cardiac patient.* St. Louis, MO: Mosby.

Young, W. L. (2009, January 1). Anesthesia for neurointerventional procedures. *Current Reviews for Nurse Anesthetists, 31,* 17.

WEBSITES

American Society of Regional Anesthesia and Pain Medicine: http://www.asra.com/consensus-statements/2.html

Chronic steroid therapy: http://www.ohsu.edu/medicine/residency/handouts/pharmpearls/Endocrine/SteroidsStressDose.pdf

Endoscopy and small bowel enteroscopy: http://www.gi.org/patients/gihealth/smallbowel.asp

Frameless stereotaxy: http://www.sd-neurosurgeon.com/practice/image_guided_neuro.html

Perioperative anticoagulation: http://hematology.im.wustl.edu/education/hemerefs/NEJM_336_1506.pdf

SSEP neurophysiologic monitoring: http://www.biotronic.com/html/ssep.html#types

Stapedectomy: http://www.earsurgery.org/surgoto.html

SVO_2: http://rnbob.tripod.com/svo2monitoring.html

Tourniquets: http://www.tourniquets.org/complications_preventive.html

Tympanoplasty: http://www.earsurgery.org/tympan.html

Index

A

AAA. *See* Abdominal aortic aneurysm
Abciximab (ReoPro), 60, 65
Abdomen, awake *vs.* anesthetized, 54*f*
Abdominal aortic aneurysm (AAA)
    emergency surgery, 771–772
    endovascular repair, 770–771
    open resection, 767–770
Abdominal approach, gynecological
    surgery, 696–703
Abdominal diversion reservoir, 669
Abdominal surgery. *See also specific abdominal
    surgeries*
    abdominoplasty, 807–808
    laparoscopy, 34–35, 589–590
    laparotomy, 589
    pearls, 589
    postoperative nausea and vomiting, 590
    tumor resection or biopsy, 849–850
Abdominal wall defects
    gastroschisis repair, 854–855
    omphalocele repair, 860–861
Abdominoperineal resection (APR), 608–609
Abdominoplasty, 807–808
Abdominothoracic esophagectomy, 592–593
Abducens nerve (CN VI), 338, 420
Abortion, therapeutic, 689
Absorption atelectasis, 53
Acetabulum fracture reduction, open, 733–734
Achilles tendon repair, 743
Acidosis, 58
Acoustic nerve (CN VIII), 338
Acoustic neuroma removal, 449–451
ACP (antegrade cerebral perfusion), 26–27
Acromioclavicular joint
    anatomy, 713, 714*f*
    separation, correction of, 713–714
Activated clotting time (ACT), 58
Acyanotic lesions, pediatric, 842

Adenoidectomy
    bleeding after, return to surgery for, 829–830
    procedure, 828–829
Adenosine diphosphate receptor inhibitors
    (ADP receptor inhibitors), 60, 64–65
Adenosine reuptake inhibitors, 61, 65
Adjustable gastric banding, 602–603
ADP receptor inhibitors (adenosine diphosphate
    receptor inhibitors), 60, 64–65
Adrenalectomy, 482
Adrenalin (epinephrine), 84. *See also under*
    Cardiovascular drug table
Aggrastat (tirofiban), 61, 65
AICD. *See* Automatic implantable cardioverter-
    defibrillators
Airway
    assessment, in trauma patients, 882–883
    fires, management of, 3
    obstruction
        causes, 882
        foreign body, pediatric, 826–827
        signs/symptoms, 882
    safety, with laser and cautery use, 1–3
Alfentanil, total intravenous anesthesia, 68–69
Alkalosis, 58
Allergies, 25–26
Allograft, 395
ALS (amyotrophic lateral sclerosis), 76
Alzheimer's disease, anesthesia and, 76
Aminocaproic acid (Amicar), 62, 82
Aminophylline, 82. *See also under* Cardiovascular
    drug table
Amiodarone, 82. *See also under* Cardiovascular drug table
Amputation
    above-the-knee, 749
    below-the-knee, 749–750
    disarticulation of hip, 748–749
    foot, 750
    toe, 750

Amrinone (Inocor), 82–83. *See also under*
   Cardiovascular drug table
Amyotrophic lateral sclerosis (ALS), 76
Anaphylactic shock, 882
Anaphylactoid reactions, 61, 765
Anaphylaxis, 25, 61, 765
Andrews frame, prone position on, 12
Anectine (succinylcholine), 420, 428, 878
Anesthetics. *See also specific anesthetics*
   body states influencing intraoperative neurologic
      monitoring and, 45–46
   contraindicated for neurological conditions, 346
   for endoscopy surgery, 617–618
   histamine-releasing, 25
   implications
      for AICD, 548–549
      for cerebral palsy patients, 820
      for Down syndrome patients, 819–820
      for mandibular hypoplasia patients, 820–821
   inhalational
      airway resistance and, 52
      ventilatory response to hypoxemia and, 52
   liver disease and, 627–628
   liver surgery and, 627–628
   mechanisms of action, 44
   neonates and, 814–816
   for orthopedic surgery, 712–713
   renal disease and, 646–649
   SSEP monitoring and, 41–42
   on trauma patients, 889–890
   types, respiratory patterns/function and, 52–53
   volatile, 42, 52, 345
Ankle
   arthrodesis, 745
   arthroscopy, 756
   fracture, open reduction of, 744–745
   total arthroplasty, 751
Antacids, 57
Antegrade cardioplegia perfusion, 560
Antegrade cerebral perfusion (ACP), 26–27
Anterior cruciate ligament tear repair, 739–740
Anterior mediastinoscopy, 520–521, 520f
Anterior resection of sigmoid colon, 609–610
Anterior retropharyngeal approach, 396
Anterior seromyotomy, vagotomy with, 599–601, 600f
Anterior vitrectomy, 443–444
Anticoagulants, 58–62
   chronic usage of, 59
   neuraxial anesthesia and, 62
   oral, 59
   parenteral, 59–60
Antiemetics
   for nausea/vomiting, 56–57
   for plastic surgery, 789–790

Antifibrinolytics
   aminocaproic acid, 62, 82
   for coronary artery bypass grafting, 558–559
   indications, 62
Antiphogistic iridectomy, 439–440
Antiplatelet drugs
   neuraxial anesthesia and, 64
   pharmacology, 60–61
Antithrombin III (AT III; thrombate III), 59–60, 83
Anzemet (dolasetron), 56
Aorta, coarctation of. *See* Coarctation of aorta
Aortic cross-clamping
   for AAA resection, 769–770
   application/withdrawal, 18
   removal effects, 19
   spinal cord injury and, 19
   spinal cord protection, 19–20
Aortic resection with end-to-end anastomosis, for
   coarctation of aorta repair, 848
Aortic rupture, traumatic, 885
Aortic shunt, 20
Aortic valve
   regurgitation, 570, 572
   repair, 572–573
   replacement, 573
   stenosis, 570, 571–572
Aortobifemoral bypass graft, 782
Apneic oxygenation, 519
Appendectomy
   laparoscopic, 606
   open, 605–606
APR (abdominoperineal resection), 608–609
Aqueous humor
   definition of, 417
   drainage of, 447
Arfonad (trimethaphan), 86. *See also under*
   Cardiovascular drug table
Arnold-Chiari malformation, 824
Arterial blood pressure transducer levels, patient
   positioning and, 10–11
Arterial occlusive disease, surgical interventions, 767
Arteriovenous fistula or shunt, 772–773
Arteriovenous malformation (AVM)
   anesthesia goals, 349
   grading, 349
   surgical resection/embolization, 351–354
Artery of Adamkiewicz, 19
Arthotomy, 711
Arthrodesis
   ankle, 745
   definition of, 711
   hip, 734–735, 734f
   knee, 739
   wrist, 730–731

Arthrofibrosis, knee, 740
Arthroplasty, total
    ankle, 751
    elbow, 751–752
    hip, 752–753
    knee, 754–755
    minimally invasive hip, 753–754
    shoulder, 755–756, 755f
Arthroscopy
    ankle, 756
    definition of, 711
    elbow, 756–757
    hip, 757–758
    knee, 758
    rotator cuff tear correction, 719–720, 720f
    shoulder, 758–759
ASD. See Atrial septal defect
Aspirin, neuraxial anesthesia and, 64
Asthmatic patients, histamine and, 25–26
Atherosclerotic arterial insufficiency, 766–767
AT III (antithrombin III; thrombate III), 59–60, 83
Atlas (C1), 392, 392f
Atrial reflex, 340
Atrial septal defect (ASD)
    primum, 843
    repair, 842–844
    secundum, 843
    sinus venosus, 843
Atrioventricular blocks (AV blocks), 550
Auditory nerve (CN VIII), vestibular neurectomy, 457
Augmentation cystoplasty, 665
Autograph, 395
Automatic implantable cardioverter-defibrillators
    (AICD)
    anesthetic implications, 548–549
    contraindications, 550
    ESUs and, 4
    insertion, 553–554
    safe procedures with, 550
Autoregulation, 341
AV blocks (atrioventricular blocks), 550
AVM. See Arteriovenous malformation
Axillary block, 713
Axillary node dissection. See Lymphadenectomy
Axillobifemoral bypass graft, 782
Axillofemoral bypass graft, 782
Axis (C2), 392, 393f

B
Backer's cyst excision, 742–743
BAEP (brain stem evoked potentials), 42–43
Balloon atrial septostomy, 840
Balloon dilation, esophageal, 590–591
Bankart procedure, 715

Barbiturates
    for cerebral protection, 23
    EEG burst suppression and, 23, 39
    MEPs and, 45
Bariatric surgery, 601–605, 604f
    adjustable gastric banding, 602–603
    Roux-en-Y gastric bypass, 603–604, 604f
    vertical banded gastroplasty, 604–605
Baroreceptors
    cardiac, 543
    definition of, 339
Baroreflex, 543
Bartholin duct cyst or abscess, marsupialization
    of, 693
Basal iridectomy, 439–440
Base deficit, as resuscitation marker, 888
Battery insertion, deep brain stimulation for, 368–369
BBB (blood-brain barrier), 336
Beach-chair position, 13–14
Bier block, 713, 728
Bifascular block, 551
Bilateral salpingo-oophorectomy, with total abdominal
    hysterectomy, 697–698
Biliary atresia correction, 863–864
Biliary tract surgery, 636–638
Billroth II procedure (gastrojejunostomy),
    595–596, 596f
Billroth I procedure (gastroduodenostomy), 595–596
Biopsy
    abdominal tumor, pediatric, 849–850
    breast, 504
    cervical, 686–687
    hepatoblastoma, 849–850
    lung, 528–529
    neuroblastoma, 849–850
    sentinel lymph node, 508–510
    testicular, 654
Bispectral analysis (BIS; BISMonitor), 39
Biventricular pacing, 551–552
Bladder
    perforation, 659
    surgery, 665–668
        augmentation, 665
        bladder substitution surgery, 669
        exstrophy repair, 865–866
        radical cystectomy, 666–667
        sacral nerve stimulator implantation, 668
        simple cystectomy, 665–666
        suprapubic cystolithotomy, 667
        suprapubic cystostomy, 667–668
        transurethral resection of lesions of bladder,
            657–659
        urinary diversions, 668–669
        for urinary incontinence, 669–672

Blalock-Taussig shunt, modified, 839
Bleb excision, lung, 523
Blepharoplasty, 790–792
Blepharoptosis repair, 421–422
Blood-brain barrier (BBB), 336
Blood-derived colloids, 887
Blood flow
    cerebral. *See* Cerebral blood flow
    distribution, 53
    liver, 626*f*
Blood glucose
    concentration, for cerebral protection, 25
    management, 57–58
Blood pressure
    elevation, 344
    mean arterial. *See* Mean arterial pressure
Blood pressure cuff, vertical distance to brain, 11
Blood products
    for neonates, 815
    for trauma patients, 887–888
    types of, 20–21
    usage. *See also under specific surgeries*
Blood substitutes, 887–888
Blood vessels, distal, acute blockage of, 766
Blood viscosity, for cerebral protection, 25
BMI (body mass index), 601
BMP (bone morphogenic protein), 395
Body, dependent portions, compression injury risk, 9
Body cast (spica cast application), 865
Body mass index (BMI), 601
Body weight
    ideal, 601
    obesity, 601–602
Bone morphogenic protein (BMP), 395
Bougie dilation, esophageal, 590–591
Bovie electrocautery, 548
Bowel surgery
    large. *See* Large bowel surgery
    operating room fires and, 6
    reduction of intussusception, 858
    small. *See* Small intestine surgery
Brachial plexus surgery, 716–718, 717*f*
Brachytherapy, with interstitial radiotherapy, 664–665
Brain
    anatomy, 332–333, 333*f*, 335*f*
    ascending sensory pathways, 40–42, 41*f*
    blood pressure difference between base and top, 11
    descending motor pathways, 43–44
    edema/swelling, 336–337
    intracranial neurosurgery. *See* Intracranial
        neurosurgery
    neurosurgical approaches, 349–350
    patient positioning
        semi-Fowler, 13–14
        Trendelenburg, 12
    physiology, 332
    vertical distance to blood pressure cuff, 11
Brain stem evoked potentials (BAEP), 42–43
Brain tumors
    anesthetic management goals, 346–347
    craniotomy, 354–357
    infratentorial masses, 348
    supratentorial masses, 347–348
Branchial cleft cyst tract excision, 824–825
Breast surgery, 503–514
    augmentation or implants, 800–801, 803–804
    axillary node dissection or
        lymphadenectomy, 504
    biopsy
        with needle localization, 504
        open, 504
    breast biopsy with needle localization, 504
    breast reconstruction
        tissue expanders, 513–514
        using transverse rectus abdominis myocutaneous
            flaps, 511–512
    capsulotomy, 801–802
    excision of male gynecomastia, 802–803
    lumpectomy, 505
    mastopexy, 805–807
    modified radical mastectomy, 506–507
    nipple reconstruction, 512–513
    open breast biopsy, 504
    pearls, 503
    postoperative nausea and vomiting, 503–504
    radical mastectomy, 507–508
    reconstruction of breast, 510–514
    reduction, 804–805
    sentinel lymph node biopsy, 508–510
    simple mastectomy, 505–506
    subcutaneous mastectomy, 506
Brevibloc (Esmolol), 83. *See also under* Cardiovascular
    drug table
Bristow procedure, 715
Bronchoplastic resection, 523
Bronchopleural fistula, 524
Bronchopulmonary lavage, 524–526
Bronchoscopy
    flexible, 517
    lung biopsy, 528–529
    rigid, 517–519
Brow lift, 792–794
Buerger's disease (thromboangiitis obliterans), 766
Bullae excision, lung, 523
Bunionectomy, with/without fusion, 745–746
Bupvacaine (Marcaine; Sensorcaine), 787
Burch retropubic colposuspension, 671
Burns, muscle relaxants and, 79
Burr holes, 349–350
Burst suppression, EEG, 23–24, 38–39

C

CABG. *See* Cardiopulmonary bypass
CAD. *See* Coronary artery disease
Calcium-channel blockers, 17, 24
Calculi removal, from ureter, renal pelvis and
    kidney, 678
Caldwell-Luc procedure, 461
Canthorrhaphy, 422
Canthotomy, 422–423
CAPD (continuous ambulatory peritoneal dialysis),
    679–680
Capnometry, 889
Capsule endoscopy, 624
Capsulotomy, 801–802
Carbon dioxide
    gas embolism, 31–32
    hypercarbia, 24
    responsiveness, 343
Carbon dioxide laser, for blepharoplasty, 790–792
Carcinoid crisis, 21–22
Carcinoid syndrome, 21
Carcinoid tumor resection, 22
Cardene (nicardipine), 83. *See also under*
    Cardiovascular drug table
Cardiac conduction pathway, 550f
Cardiac index formula, 544
Cardiac mapping and ablation, 556
Cardiac output formula, 544
Cardiac resynchronization (biventricular pacing),
    551–552
Cardiac surgery, 543–587
    anesthetics and, 545
    conduction disturbances, 545–556
    coronary artery disease, 556–569
    definitions for, 543
    formulas, 544–545
    heart pressures, 543–544
    heart transplantation, 582–587
    heart valves, 570–576
    minimally invasive, 569
    pearls, 543
    pericardial, 576–577
    permanent pacing and AICD, 551–554
    temporary pacing, 554–556
    thoracic aorta, 577–582
Cardiac tamponade, 884
Cardiogenic shock, 880–881
Cardioplegia, 560
Cardiopulmonary bypass (CABG)
    full-flow, for heart transplant, 584–586
    off-pump issues, 22
    on-pump issues, 22
Cardiovascular drugs, 82–87. *See also specific drugs*
    dosage calculations. *See under* Cardiovascular
        drug table

IV infusion calculations, 88
    loading doses, 88
Cardiovascular drug table, 88–330
Cardiovascular system surgery. *See also specific*
    cardiovascular surgeries
    deep hypothermic circulatory arrest and, 28
    drugs for, 82–87. *See also specific drugs*
    heart setup, 87
    heart surgery. *See* Cardiac surgery
    patient positioning, 9–14
    pediatric, 836–849
Cardizem (Diltiazem), 83. *See also under* Cardiovascular
    drug table
Carotid/aortic bodies, 340
Carotid arteries, anatomy, 773–774, 773f, 774f
Carotid bodies, 773, 773f
Carotid endarterectomy (CEA), 774–779
Carotid shunt, 775
Carotid sinus, 773, 773f, 774f
Carpal bone fracture, open reduction, 727
Carpal tunnel release, 728–729
Cataract extraction with intraocular lens implant,
    441–442
Cautery usage in airway, safety considerations for, 1–3
CBF. *See* Cerebral blood flow
CCPD (continuous cycling peritoneal dialysis), 679–680
CEA (carotid endarterectomy), 774–779
Central nervous system, heart rate control, 340
Cerebral aneurysm, intraoperative rupture, 379
Cerebral aneurysmal repair, 377–379
Cerebral blood flow (CBF)
    autoregulation, 22–23
    cerebral oxygen-metabolism flow coupling and, 342
    decrease, 332, 343
    determinants, 341–342
    electroencephalography and, 38
    increase, factors in, 342–343
    normal, 332
Cerebral effects, from deep hypothermic circulatory
    arrest, 27–28
Cerebral embolectomy, craniotomy, 357–359
Cerebral metabolic rate of glucose consumption
    (CMRGl), 58, 332
Cerebral monitoring, for carotid endartectomy, 775–776
Cerebral oxygen-metabolism flow coupling
    (CMRO$_2$), 342
Cerebral palsy
    anesthesia implications, 820
    muscle relaxants and, 79–80
Cerebral perfusion pressure (CPP)
    during carotid endarterectomy, 775
    definition of, 340
    EEG effects, 340–341
    mean arterial blood pressure and, 10–11
    patient positioning and, 10–11

Cerebral protection
     deep hypothermic circulatory arrest for, 25, 26–27
     formula, 22–23
     interventions, 24–25
     pharmacologic, 23–24
Cerebrospinal fluid (CSF)
     circulation, 335–336, 335*f,* 336*f*
     drainage, for cerebral protection, 25
     formation, 335
     leak repair, 359–361
     Monroe-Kelly hypothesis and, 334
     normal values, 335
Cerebrum, anatomy, 41*f*
Cervical biopsy, 686–687
Cervical cerclage (cervical ligature), 703
Cervical conization, 686–687
Cervical decompression and fusion
     anterior and posterior approaches, 399
     anterior approach, 396–397
     posterior approach, 397–399
Cervical mediastinoscopy, 520–521, 520*f*
Cervical vertebrae
     anatomy, 393–394, 393*f,* 394*f*
     surgical approaches, 396
Cervicothoracic spine surgery, 405–408
Cesarean section birth, 703–706
Cetacaine (tetracaine), 787
Chalazion excision, 423
Chemical labyrinthectomy, 453
Chemoreceptors
     cardiac, 543
     definition of, 340
Chest trauma, blunt, 885
Chest tube (thoracostomy), 535
Chest wall disorders, 515
Chin prosthesis (mentoplasty), 796–797
Chloroprocaine (Nescaine), 787
Choanal atresia repair, 825–826
Cholangiogram, intraoperative, 636
Cholecystectomy
     laparoscopic, 637–638
     open, 636–637
Chorioid, 417
Cilostazol (Petal), 65
Circle of Willis, 332, 333*f,* 774
Circumcision, 866–867
Cirrhosis, 627
Clavicular fracture repair, 718
Cleft lip repair, 870
Cleft palate repair, 871–872
Closed reduction, 711
Club foot surgical correction, 864–865
CMRGI (cerebral metabolic rate of glucose
     consumption), 58, 332
CMRO₂ (cerebral oxygen-metabolism flow coupling), 342

Coagulation tests
     neuraxial anesthesia and, 63–65
     types of, 58–59
Coarctation of aorta
     preductal *vs.* postductal, 848
     repair, 847–849
     stenosis repair, 847
Cochlea, anatomy, 452*f*
Cochlear implantation, 451
Colectomy, 611–612
Collateral ligament tear repair, 739–740
Colloids, 886–887
Colonoscopy, 618–619
Colorectal resection, for Hirschsprung's disease,
     855–856
Colostomy
     adult, 610–611
     closure method, 611
     pediatric, 850–851
Colporrhaphy, anterior and/or posterior, 687
Colpotomy
     for uterine fibroid removal, 698–699
     for visualization of pelvic structures, 687–688
Common carotid, 774, 774*f*
Compartment syndrome
     causes, 710, 711
     fasciotomy for, 710–711
     rhabdomyolysis and, 710
     treatment, 711
Composite graft, 810
Compression injury risk, 9
Conduction disturbances, cardiac, 545–556
     AICD. *See* Automatic implantable cardioverter-
          defibrillators
     heart blocks, 550–551
     operating room issues, 547–550
     pacemakers and. *See* Pacemakers
Conduit harvesting, for coronary artery bypass graft, 559
Condylomata acuminata excision
     penile, 650
     vulvar, 684–685
Congenital anomalies. *See* Congenital heart defects;
     specific congenital anomalies
Congenital diaphragmatic hernia repair, 851–854
Congenital heart defects, 836–849
     acyanotic lesions, 842
     atrial septal defect repair, 842–844
     cyanotic lesions, 837
     hypoplastic left heart syndrome, 837–838
     patent ductus arteriosus closure, 844–846
     pulmonary artery banding, 846–847
     pulmonary stenosis repair, 849
     stenosis repair, 847
     teralogy of Fallot, 838–839
     transposition of great arteries correction, 839–840

tricuspid atresia surgery, 840–841

truncus arteriosus repair, 841–842

ventricular septal defect repair, 847

Conization, cervical, 686–687

Conjunctiva, 417

Continent urinary diversion, 669

Continuous ambulatory peritoneal dialysis (CAPD), 679–680

Continuous cycling peritoneal dialysis (CCPD), 679–680

Continuous positive airway pressure (CPAP), 52

Corectomy (iridectomy), 439–440

Corlopam (fenoldapam), 84. *See also under* Cardiovascular drug table

Corneal laceration repair, 437

Corneal transplantation, 437–439

Coronary artery bypass graft, 557–568

    antifibrinolytics, 558–559

    bypass termination requirements, 561

    coming off bypass support, 562

    conduits, 557

    gradual rewarming, 561

    induction/maintenance, 558

    minimally invasive direct, 566–568

    off-pump, 563–566

    post-bypass period, 562–563

    pre-bypass period, 558

    procedure, 559–561

    redo, 563

    separation, 562

    sternotomy, 559, 563

Coronary artery disease (CAD), 556–569

    coronary artery bypass graft, 557–568

    coronary artery bypass graft conduits, 557

    laser transmyocardial revascularization, 568–569

    minimally invasive cardiac surgery, 569

    percutaneous transluminal angioplasty, 556–557

Coronary perfusion pressure (CPP), 544

Corticosteroids, 24, 66

Coumadin (warfarin), 59, 63

CPAP (continuous positive airway pressure), 52

CPDA, 887

CPP. *See* Cerebral perfusion pressure

CPP (coronary perfusion pressure), 544

Cranial nerves

    description of, 337–339

    microvascular decompression, 361–363

Craniectomy

    for craniosynostosis, 821–822

    definition of, 350

    for posterior fossa exploration, 384–386

Craniofacial surgery

    LeFort osteomy, 409–412, 410f–411f

    mandibular fracture reduction, 412–413

    mandibular osteotomy, 413–414

    maxillary fracture reduction, 414

orbital floor fractures, open reduction of, 414

    pearls, 409

    pediatric, 822–823

    zygomatic fracture reduction, 415

Craniopharyngioma surgical resection, 363–366, 364f

Cranioplasty, 366–368

Craniosynstosis, craniectomy for, 821–822

Craniotomy

    for brain tumor, 354–357

    for cerebral embolectomy, 357–359

    definition of, 350

    for intracranial aneurysm, 372–377

    for meningioma, 379–381

    for posterior fossa exploration, 384–386

Crawford classification of thoracic aorta dissection, 577

Cretinism, 482

Creutzfeldt-Jakob disease, 77

Cruciate ligament tear repair, 739–740

Cryoablation, 690

Cryoprecipitate, 21

Cryosurgery

    cervical conization, 686–687

    transrectal ablation of prostate gland, 656–657

Crystalloids, 886

CSF. *See* Cerebrospinal fluid

Culdocentesis, 688

Culdoscopy, 688

Culdotomy, 687–688

Cushing response, 340

Cutaneous ureterostomy, 678–679

Cutaneous urinary diversion, 668–669

Cyclooxygenase inhibitors, 60, 64

Cyclophotocoagulation, laser, 444–445

Cystectomy, simple, 665–666

Cystocele, 687

Cystolithotomy, suprapubic, 667

Cystoplasty, augmentation, 665

Cystoscopy, 649–650

Cystostomy, suprapubic, 667–668

D

Dacryocystorhinostomy, 426–427

DBS (deep brain stimulation), 368–369

D&C (dilation and curettage), 686, 688–689

DDAVP (desmopressin), 61. *See also* Cardiovascular drug table

D&E (dilation and evacuation), 689

Dead space increase, 55

DeBakey classification of thoracic aorta dissection, 577

Decortication (pleural stripping), 526

Deep brain stimulation (DBS), 368–369

Deep hypothermic circulatory arrest (DHCA)

    anesthesia considerations, 27

    for cerebral protection, 25, 26–27

surgical considerations, 27
systemic effects, 27–28
Demylinating diseases, anesthesia and, 74–75
Dentistry, operative, 471–473
Dentoalveolar procedures, 471–473
DEP (dermatome evoked potentials), 43
Dermabrasion, 796
Dermatome evoked potentials (DEP), 43
Dermatomes, 333
Desflurane, wake-up test, 44
Desmopressin (DDAVP), 83. *See also under*
    Cardiovascular drug table
Dexmedetomidine (Precedex), 878
Dextran, 887
Dextran 40/70, 60, 64
DHCA. *See* Deep hypothermic circulatory arrest
Diabetes insipidus, 332
Dialysis access, 679–680
Dialysis catheter placement, venous access, 778
Diaphragm
    disorders, 516
    hernia repair, adult, 874
    traumatic injuries, 885
Dilation and curettage (D&C), 686, 688–689
Dilation and evacuation (D&E), 689
Dilators, for esophageal dilation, 590–591
Diltiazem (cardizem), 83. *See also under* Cardiovascular
    drug table
Direct thrombin inhibitors, 60
Discectomy, lumbar, 403–404
Dislocation, 711
Distal revascularization, 780–781
Distal vessels, acute blockage of, 766
Diuretic agents, 644
DIVER mnemonic, 3
Diverticulectomy, 606–607
Diverticulum
    esophageal, excision of, 593–594
    Meckel's, 606–607
DLBET (double-lumen endobronchial tube), 28–30, 818
Dobutamine (Dobutrex), 83–84. *See also under*
    Cardiovascular drug table
Dolasetron (Anzemet), 56
Dopamine (Intropin), 84. *See also under* Cardiovascular
    drug table
Dorsal root rhizotomy, 399
Double-barrel colostomy, 610–611
Double-lumen endobronchial tube (DLBET), 28–30, 818
Down syndrome, anesthetic implications, 819–820
Drapes, oxygen buildup under, 2–3
Droperidol (Inapsine), 57
Drug index number, 88
Drugs, for gynecological surgery, 684
Duchenne muscular dystrophy, anesthesia and, 70–71
Ductus arteriosus, 816

Ductus venosus, 816
Duranest (etidocaine), 787
Dyes, IV, 684

E
Ear, inner, anatomy of, 452*f*
Ear surgery, 449–457
    acoustic neuroma removal, 449–451
    cochlear implantation, 451
    ear tube placement, 827–828
    facial nerve decompression, 452–453
    labyrinthectomy, 453
    mastoidectomy, 453–454
    myringotomy, 454–455, 827–828
    operative approaches
        middle fossa, 450, 452
        retrosigmoid or suboccipital, 450
        translabyrinthine, 450
        transmastoid, 452
    ossicular chain reconstruction, 455–456
    pearls, 449
    pinning, 797–798
    postoperative nausea and vomiting, 449
    stapedectomy, 456
    tympanoplasty, 456–457
    tympanostomy, 457
    vestibular neurectomy, 457
Ear tube placement, with myringotomy, 827–828
ECT (electroconvulsant therapy), 877–879
Ectopic tubal pregnancy, 701–702
Ectropion correction, 423–424
Edecrin, 644
EEG. *See* Electroencephalography
EGD (esophagogastroduodenoscopy), 620–621
Eisenmenger's syndrome, cyanotic lesion correction, 837
Ejection fraction, 544
Elbow
    arthroscopy, 756–757
    fracture repair, 724, 724*f*
    total arthroplasty, 751–752
    ulnar nerve transposition, 391–392, 726–727
Electric surgical unit (ESU), 2–4
Electrocautery
    bipolar, 3
    electrosurgical unit for, 2–4
    monopolar or unipolar, 3
Electroconvulsant therapy (ECT), 877–879
Electrode insertion, deep brain stimulation for, 368–369
Electroencephalography (EEG), 37–39
    burst suppression, 23–24, 38–39
    cerebral blood flow and, 38
    description of, 37–38
Electrohydraulic lithotripsy, 674
Electromagnetic interference (EMI), 548

Electromyography (EMG), 44
Embolectomy, femoral, 779–780
Embolism
    carbon dioxide gas, 31–32
    fat embolism syndrome, 32–33, 710
    venous air, 30–31
Emergence. *See under specific surgeries*
Emergency medications, for infants 3–6 months, 818
Emergency surgery
    for abdominal aortic aneurysm, 771–772
    cesarean section birth, 705–706
    compartment syndrome, 710–711
    obstetrical hysterectomy, 708
    orthopedic, 712
EMG (electromyography), 44
EMI (electromagnetic interference), 548
"Empty nose syndrome," 466
Empyema drainage, 527
Endobronchial tubes, double-lumen, 28–30, 818
Endocrine disorders
    cretinism, 482
    hyperparathyroidism, 479–480
    hyperthyroidism, 480
    hypoparathyroidism, 480
    hypothyroidism, 481
    myxedema coma, 481–482
    thyroid storm, 480–481
Endocrine surgery
    adrenalectomy, 482
    parathyroidectomy, 483–484
    pearls, 479
    pheochromocytoma removal, 484–486
    thyroidectomy
        substernal or intrathoracic, 488
        subtotal or total, 486–488
Endocrine system, 479
Endocrinopathy, with craniopharyngiomas, 364–365
Endodontic procedures, 471–473
Endometrial ablation, 689–690
Endoscopic retrograde cholangiopancreatography
    (ERCP), 619–620
Endoscopic sinus surgery, 462–463
Endoscopy surgery, 617–624
    anesthesia, 617–618
    colonoscopy, 618–619
    endoscopic retrograde cholangiopancreatography,
        619–620
    esophagogastroduodenoscopy, 620–621
    gastroscopy, 622–623
    pearls, 617
    sigmoidoscopy, 623
    small bowel enteroscopy, 623–624
    thoracic, 517–523
        flexible bronchoscopy, 517
        mediastinoscopy, 519–521, 520*f*

        rigid bronchoscopy, 517–519
        thoracic sympathectomy, 522–523
        thoracoscopy, 521–522
    upper gastrointestinal, 621–622
Endothelial keratoplasty, 437–439
Endotracheal tubes (ETT)
    fire prevention considerations, 1–2
    intubation for operative dentistry, 472
    laser-retardant or flexible metal, 1–2
    migration, 10
    NIM EMG, 483, 486–487
    sizes, pediatric, 818, 819
Endovascular procedures, 350
End-tidal carbon dioxide (ETCO$_2$), 31, 53
Enflurane, 80, 346
Enoxaparin (low-molecular-weight heparin), 60, 63
Enterocele, 687
Enterostomy, 607
Entropion correction, 424–425
EP. *See* Evoked potentials
Ephedrine, 84
Epicardial pacing electrode insertion, 555
Epididymectomy, 652–653
Epidural anesthesia, neonatal, 816
Epidural hematoma, evacuation, 369–371
Epilepsy
    muscle relaxants and, 80–81
    treatment, 351
Epinephrine (Adrenalin), 84. *See also under*
    Cardiovascular drug table
Epispadias repair, 867–868
Epistaxis treatment, 467
Eptifibatide (integrilin), 61, 65
ERCP (endoscopic retrograde
    cholangiopancreatography), 619–620
Esmolol (brevibloc), 83. *See also under* Cardiovascular
    drug table
Esophageal surgery
    abdominothoracic esophagectomy, 592–593
    dilation, 590–591
    esophageal diverticulum excision, 593–594
    Nissen laparoscopic fundoplication, 594–595,
        859–860
    transhiatal esophagectomy, 591–592
    transthoracic esophagectomy, 592–593
    for traumatic injuries, 885
Esophagogastroduodenoscopy (EGD), 620–621
Esophagoscopy (upper gastrointestinal endoscopy),
    621–622
ESU. *See* Electric surgical unit
ESU (electric surgical unit), 2–4
ESWL (extracorporeal shock wave lithotripsy), 672–674
ETCO$_2$ (end-tidal carbon dioxide), 31, 53
Ethmoidectomy, 463
Etidocaine (Duranest), 787

Etomidate, 23, 45, 80, 878
ETT. *See* Endotracheal tubes
Evoked potentials (EP), 39–44
   brain stem, 42–43
   dermatome, 43
   motor, 43–44
   sensitivity of, 40
   somatosensory, 40–42, 41*f*
   visual, 43
Exosectomy (bunionectomy), 745–746
External auditory meatus, arterial blood transducer
   zeroing and, 11
External carotids, 774, 774*f*
External fixation, 711–712
Extracapsular method for cataract extraction, 441–442
Extracorporeal shock wave lithotripsy (ESWL)
   with water bath, 672–674
   without water bath, 673–674
Eyebrow lift, 792–794
Eyelid surgery, 421–426
   blepharoptosis repair, 421–422
   canthorrhaphy, 422
   canthotomy, 422–423
   chalazion excision, 423
   cosmetic, 790–792
   ectropion correction, 423–424
   entropion correction, 424–425
   laceration repair, 425
   lesion excision, 425–426
   tarsorrhaphy, 426
Eye surgery
   enucleation, 428–429
   evisceration, 429–430
   exenteration, 430–431

F
Facelift (rhytidectomy), 794–796
Facial block, 419
Facial injuries, from ventilator mask strap, 35–36
Facial laser resurfacing, 796
Facial nerve (CN VII), 338
   blocks, 420, 420*f*
   decompression, 452–453
   injuries, from ventilator mask strap, 35–36
Facial surgery, cleft lip repair, 870
Factor VII, 84
Fallopian tubes
   ectopic tubal pregnancy, 701–702
   postpartum tubal ligation, 706
   removal, by salpingo-oophorectomy, 700
   tuboplasty, 702
Familial periodic paralysis, anesthesia and, 73–74
Famotidine (Pepcid), 56
Fasciotomy, 710–711

FAST assessment, for cardiac tamponade, 884
Fat embolism syndrome (FES), 32–33, 710
Femoral and sciatic block, 713
Femoral artery, cannulation, 559
Femoral block, 713
Femoral fracture
   femoral shaft fracture, open reduction and internal
      fixation, 737
   intertrochanteric, 736
   open reduction and internal fixation, 736
   proximal femur fracture, open reduction and
      internal fixation, 736
   supracondylar, open reduction and internal fixation,
      737–738
Femoral thrombectomy/embolectomy, 779–780
Femorofemoral bypass graft, 782–783
Femoropopliteal bypass graft, 783
Femorotibial bypass graft, 783
Femur
   prosthetic replacement of femoral head, 735–736
   proximal, anatomy of, 735*f*
   shaft fracture, 735
   subtrochanteric fracture, 735
Fenoldapam (Corlopam), 84. *See also under*
   Cardiovascular drug table
Fentanyl, total intravenous anesthesia, 68–69
FES (fat embolism syndrome), 32–33, 710
FFP (fresh frozen plasma), 21
Fibrinolytics, 61
Filtration surgery (trabeculectomy), 440–441
Finger surgery
   replantation, 731
   syndactyly repair, 864
Fire extinguishers, types of, 5–6
Fires
   airway, management of, 3
   in operating room, 4–6
Fistulas, bronchopleural, 524
Fistulotomy, 614
Flail chest, 883
Flap procedures, 811–812
Flexed lateral decubitus position, 15
Flexible bronchoscopy, 517
Flexor tendon laceration repair, 729
Fluid restriction, 23
Fluid resuscitation, IV
   for infants 3-6 months, 818
   markers, 888–889
   for neonates, 815
   in neuroanesthesia, 346
   in trauma patients, 886–888
Foot bones, anatomy of, 547*f*
Foot surgery, 745–748
   amputation, 750
   bunionectomy, with/without fusion, 745–746

for club foot correction, 864–865
hammer toe correction, 746
metatarsal fracture repair, 746–747
metatarsal head resection, 747
tendon lengthening, 748
Foramen ovale, 816, 843
Foraminotomy, 400–401, 400f
Foreign bodies
  aspiration, pediatric, 826–827
  intraocular, extraction of, 431–432
  magnetic resonance imaging and, 7
  obstruction/ingestion, pediatric, 826–827
Fracture. *See also specific types of fractures*
  definition of, 712
Fracture table, patient positioning on, 16, 16f
FRC. *See* Functional residual capacity
Free flap procedure, 811–812
Fresh frozen plasma (FFP), 21
Frontal craniotomy, 371–372
Frontal sinus drainage, 463–464
Fuel sources in operating room, 4, 5
Full-thickness skin grafts, 810–811
Functional endoscopic sinus surgery, 462–463
Functional neurosurgery, 351
Functional residual capacity (FRC)
  decrease, induction of anesthesia and, 51
  patient positioning and, 10
  PEEP and, 51
  postoperative, anesthesia and, 51
Fundoplication, laparoscopic (Nissen procedure)
  adult, 594–595
  pediatric, 859–860
Furosemide, 644

G
Gallbladder surgery, 636–638
Ganglion cyst excision, 729–730
Gastrectomy
  subtotal, 595–596
  total, 596–597, 597f
Gastric acidity, intraoperative testing of, 600
Gastric banding, adjustable, 602–603
Gastric bypass, Roux-en-Y, 603–604, 604f
Gastroduodenostomy (Billroth I procedure), 595–596
Gastrointestinal surgery, 589–615. *See also specific gastrointestinal surgeries*
  bariatric, 601–605, 604f
  esophageal, 590–595
  large bowel, 608–613
  pediatric disorders, repair of, 849–864
    abdominal tumor resection or biopsy, 849–850
    biliary atresia correction, 863–864
    colostomy, 850–851
    congenital diaphragmatic hernia repair, 851–854

gastroschisis repair, 854–855
imperforate anus repair, 856–858
laparoscopic Nissen fundoplication, 859–860
necrotizing enterocolitis repair, 858–859
omphalocele repair, 860–861
pull-through for Hirschsprung's disease, 855–856
pyloromyotomy for hypertrophic pyloric stenosis, 861–863
reduction of intussusception, 858
  rectal, 613–615
  small intestine, 605–608
  stomach, 595–601
Gastrojejunostomy (Billroth II procedure), 595–596, 596f
Gastroschisis repair, pediatric, 854–855
Gastroscopy, 622–623
Gastrostomy, percutaneous endoscopic tube placement, 598–599
Gastrostomy tube insertion, 597–598
GCS (Glasgow Coma Scale), 343, 884
General anesthesia
  EEG burst suppression and, 38–39
  in opthalmic surgery, 420
  for renal disease patients, 647–648
Genitourinary irrigating solutions, 648–649
Genitourinary surgery
  abbreviations, 644
  cystoscopy, 649–650
  for non-renal disease patients, 646
  pearls, 643
  pediatric, 865–870
Giant cell arteritis (temporal arteritis), 767
Glasgow Coma Scale (GCS), 343, 884
Glaucoma surgery, 439–441
Glenoid fossa, anatomy, 715f
Globe immobilization, 419
Globe surgery, 428–436
  extraction of intraocular foreign body, 431–432
  eye enucleation, 428–429
  eye evisceration, 429–430
  eye exenteration, 430–431
  rupture repair, 434–435
  strabismus correction, 435–436
Glossectomy, partial or total, 473–474
Glossopharyngeal nerve (CN IX), 338
Glucocorticosteroids, 66
Glycoprotein IIB/IIIA inhibitors, 60–61, 65
Glycosylated hemoglobin (HbA$_{1C}$), 57
Goldenhar syndrome, 821
Grafts, for distal revascularization, 780–781
Graves' disease (hyperthyroidism), 480
Great arteries transposition, correction of, 839–840
Guillain-Barré syndrome, anesthesia and, 74–75

Gynecological surgery, 683–703
  abdominal
    for ectopic tubal pregnancy, 701–702
    laparoscopic-assisted hysterectomy with
        transvaginal manipulation, 696
    myomectomy, 698–699
    pelvic exenteration, 699–700
    radical hysterectomy, 696–697
    salpingo-oophorectomy, 700
    total abdominal hysterectomy, 697–698
    tubal ligation, 701
    tuboplasty, 702
    uterine artery embolization, 702–703
    uterine fibroid embolization, 702–703
  abdominal approach for, 696–703
  drugs for, 684
  pearls, 683
  postoperative nausea and vomiting, 683–684
  preemptive analgesia, 684
  vaginal, 686–696
  vulvar, 684–686
Gynecomastia, male, 802–803

H
Hallux abductus valgus repair, 745–746
Hammer toe deformity correction, with/without
    fusion, 546
Hand
  surgery, 727–731
    digit and hand replantation, 731
    flexor tendon laceration repair, 729
    ganglion cyst excision, 729–730
    palmar fasciectomy, 810
    syndactyly repair, 864
  "swimmer position," 11
Harrington rod procedure, 761–763
Hartmann procedure, 612
HbA$_{1C}$ (glycosylated hemoglobin), 57
HBOC (hemoglobin-based oxygen carrier), 887–888
Heart
  anesthetics and, 545
  blunt cardiac injury, 885
  cardiac conduction pathway, 550f
  conduction disturbances, 545–556
  congenital defects. See Congenital heart defects
  surgery. See Cardiac surgery
Heart blocks, 550–551
Heart transplantation, 582–587
  full-flow cardiopulmonary bypass for, 584–586
  organ donor management, 879–880
  post-bypass period, 586–587
Heart valves
  aortic, 570–573
  mitral, 570, 573–576

Helium (Heliox), for pediatric patients, 55–56
Hemassist, 888
Hematologic effects, of deep hypothermic circulatory
    arrest, 28
Hemiarthroplasty
  hip, 735–736
  shoulder, 755–756
Hemiblocks, 550f, 551
Hemicolectomy, right, 612–613
Hemilaryngectomy (partial laryngectomy), 492–494
Hemiplegia, muscle relaxants and, 81
Hemodialysis catheter
  access, 33
  flushing, 33
Hemoglobin
  glycosylated or HbA$_{1C}$, 57
  neonatal levels, 815
Hemoglobin-based oxygen carrier (HBOC), 887–888
Hemopure, 888
Hemorrhoidectomy, 614–615
Hemostatics, topical, 61–62
Hemothorax, 883
Heparin
  dosage calculations. See under Cardiovascular
      drug table
  neuraxial anesthesia and, 63
  pharmacology, 59, 84
  reversal, 61
  vascular surgery and, 765
Hepatic resection, 628–629
Hepatitis A, 628
Hepatitis B, 628
Hepatitis C, 628
Hepatoblastoma resection or biopsy, 849–850
Hepatoportoenterostomy, 863–864
Hepspan, 887
Herbal agents, 789
Hernia repair (herniorraphy), 873–876
  abdominal, 875
  abdominal, incisional or ventral repair, 875
  complications, 873
  congenital diaphragmatic, 851–854
  diaphragmatic, adult, 874
  etiology, 873
  hiatal, 874–875
  inguinal, 875
  laparoscopic method, 873
  mesh method, 873
  open method, 873
  spigelian, 875
  umbilical, 875
Herniation, brain, ICP elevation and, 334–335
Hetastarch, 887
Hextend, 887
HFJV (high-frequency jet ventilation), 33–34

Hiatal herniorraphy, 874–875
High-frequency jet ventilation (HFJV), 33–34
Hip joint, anatomy, 734f
Hip surgery, 733–735, 734f
    arthrodesis, 734–735, 734f
    arthrodesis of hip, 734–735
    arthroscopy, 757–758
    disarticulation, 748–749
    hemiarthroplasty, 735–736
    minimally invasive total arthroplasty, 753–754
    open reduction of acetabulum fractures, 733–734
    total joint replacement, 752–753
Hirschsprung's disease, pull-through for, 855–856
Histamine, asthmatic patients and, 25–26
HLHS (hypoplastic left heart syndrome), 837–838
HOCM (hypertrophic cardiomyopathy), 570–571
Homocysteinemia, 767
Hot water balloon, for endometrial ablation, 690
HPV (hypoxic pulmonary vasoconstriction), 54
Humerus fracture
    closed reduction, 722
    distal, repair of, 723
    epicondylar, repair of, 723
    head, open reduction, 719
    intercondylar, repair of, 723
    open reduction, 722–723
    supracondylar, repair of, 723
Hunsaker tube, 491
Hunt and Hess clinical grading system, 377–378
Huntington's chorea (disease), 77
Hydrocelectomy, 653
Hydrocephalus, ventricular catheter/shunt placement
    for, 386–389
Hydrochlorothiazide, 644
Hydrothermal ablation, 690
Hypercapnia, during anesthesia, 54–55
Hypercarbia, 24
Hyperglycemia, treatment, 58
Hyperkalemia, 58, 73, 549
Hyperparathyroidism, 479–480
Hyper-perfusion syndrome, 778
Hypertension, 344
Hyperthyroidism (Graves' disease), 480
Hypertrophic cardiomyopathy (HOCM), 570–571
Hypertrophic pyloric stenosis, pyloromyotomy for,
    861–863
Hyperventilation
    for cerebral protection, 24–25
    EEG burst suppression and, 39
Hypocapnia, during anesthesia, 55
Hypoglossal nerve (CNXII), 338–339
Hypoglycemia
    neonatal, 813
    treatment, 57
Hypoglycemic agents, preoperative guidelines, 57

Hypokalemia, 74, 549
Hypoparathyroidism, 480
Hypophysectomy, 371–374
Hypoplastic left heart syndrome (HLHS), 837–838
Hypospadias repair, 868
Hypotension, controlled, 377
Hypothermia, EEG burst suppression and, 39
Hypothyroidism, 481
Hypoventilation, 54–55
Hypovolemic shock, 881
Hypoxemia, signs of, 55
Hypoxic pulmonary vasoconstriction (HPV), 54
Hysterectomy
    emergency obstetrical, 708
    laparoscopic-assisted with transvaginal
        manipulation, 696
    radical, 696–697
    total abdominal, 697–698
    vaginal, 691
Hysteresis, 546
Hysteroscopy, 691–692

I
ICP. See Intracranial pressure
Ignition sources, in operating room, 4–5
Ileal conduit diversion, 668–669
Ileocolostomy, 612–613
Ileostomy, 607
Iliofemoral bypass graft, 782
Immune arteritis, 766
Imperforate anus repair, 856–858
Implantable cardiac devices, manufacturers, 549
Implants, for breast augmentation, 800–801, 803–804
Indigo carmine, 509, 684
Induction anesthetics. See also under specific surgeries
    for electroconvulsant therapy, 878
    for infants 3–6 months, 817
    intravenous, 45
    neonates and, 814
Inferior vena cava filter insertion, 785
Infiltration anesthesia, for ophthalmic surgery, 419
Inflow reconstruction, 781–783
Infraclavicular block, 713
Infratentorial masses, 348
Inguinal hernia repair, 875
Inhalation induction, for infants 3–6 months, 817
Inhaled nitric oxide (INO), 55
Inhibited pacemaker, 546
INO (inhaled nitric oxide), 55
Inocor (amrinone), 82–83. See also under
    Cardiovascular drug table
Insulin
    pharmacology, 57–58, 85
    preoperative guidelines, 57

Integrilin (eptifibatide), 61, 65
Intercostobrachial block, 713
Internal carotids, 774, 774*f*
Interscalene block, 712–713
Interstitial radiotherapy with brachytherapy, 664–665
Interventional neuroradiology, 381–383
Intracapsular method for cataract extraction, 441–442
Intracranial aneurysm
    anesthetic management goals, 348
    craniotomy, 372–377
Intracranial neurosurgery, 351–383
    atriovenous malformation resection/embolization, 351–354
    cerebral aneurysmal repair, 377–379
    craniopharyngoma resection, 363–366, 364*f*
    cranioplasty, 366–368
    craniotomy. *See* Craniotomy
    CSF fluid leak repair, 359–361
    deep brain stimulation, 368–369
    evacuation of epidural or subdural hematoma, 369–371
    hypophysectomy, 371–374
    microvascular cranial nerve decompression, 361–363
Intracranial pressure (ICP)
    definition of, 333
    increased, 334–335
    supratentorial masses and, 347–348
Intracranial-space-occupying lesions
    brain tumors, 346–347
    infratentorial masses, 348
    intracranial aneurysms, 348
    supratentorial masses, 347–348
    vasospasm, 348–349
Intramedullary nailing (intramedullary rods), 712
Intranasal antrostomy, 461–462
Intraocular foreign body, extraction of, 431–432
Intraocular pressure (IOP), 417
Intraoperative cholangiogram, 636
Intraoperative neurologic monitoring
    by electrophysiologist, 37
    influence of body states and anesthetics on, 45–46
Intropin (dopamine), 84. *See also under* Cardiovascular drug table
Intubation, of trauma patients, 883
Intussusception, reduction of, 858
IOP (intraocular pressure), 417
Iridectomy (corectomy), 439–440
Iridotomy, laser, 445–446
Irrigating solutions
    absorption, factors affecting, 658
    genitourinary, 648–649
Ischemic brain damage, EEG burst suppression and, 39
Isopreterenol (Isuprel), 85. *See also under* Cardiovascular drug table

Isosulfan blue dye (Lymphazurin 1%), 508–509
Isuprel (isopreterenol), 85. *See also under* Cardiovascular drug table

J
Jack-knife position, 14
Jejunostomy, 607
Jejunostomy tube insertion, 597–598
Jet ventilation, 519

K
Kasai portoenterostomy procedure, 863–864
Keratoplasty, 437–439
Ketamine, 45, 346, 878
Kidney
    anatomy, 644
    disease, 644
        anesthesia and, 646–649
        anesthesia considerations for, 647
        complications, 644–645
    failure
        drug alterations from, 647
        risk factors, 645–646
    functions, 643
    surgery transplantation, 680–682
Kidney surgery, 672–679
    abbreviations, 644
    cystoscopy, 649–650
    electrohydraulic lithotripsy, 674
    extracorporeal shock wave lithotripsy, 672–674
    laparoscopic nephrectomy, 675
    laser lithotripsy, 674–675
    nephrolithotomy, 678
    nephrostomy, 677
    open nephrectomy, 675–676
    pearls, 643
    pyelolithotomy, 678
    radical nephrectomy, 676–677
    ultrasonic lithotripsy, 675
Knee joint, anatomy, 738*f*
Knee surgery
    arthrodesis, 739
    arthroscopy, 758
    cruciate or collateral ligament tear repair, 739–740
    manipulation under anesthesia, 740
    menisectomy, lateral or medial, 740–741
    patella dislocation correction, 741
    patellar fracture reduction, 742
    patella tendon rupture repair, 741
    patellectomy, 741–742
    popliteal cyst excision, 742–743
    total arthroplasty or replacement, 754–755
K-pouch, 607

L

Laboratory tests, preoperative. *See under specific surgeries*

Labyrinthectomy, 453

Lacrimal duct probing, 427–428

Lacrimal gland surgery
    dacryocystorhinostomy, 426–427
    lacrimal duct probing, 427–428

Lactate, as resuscitation marker, 888

LAH (left anterior hemiblock), 550*f*, 551

Lambert-Eaton syndrome (myasthenic syndrome), 70

Lamellar keratoplasty, 437–439

Laminectomy, with or without disectomy, 401–402, 401*f*

Laminotomy, 402–403, 402*f*

LAP (lateral arterial pressure), 544

Laparoscopic-assisted hysterectomy with transvaginal manipulation, 696

Laparoscopic surgery
    abdominal, 34–35, 589–590
    appendectomy, 606
    bariatric, 603–604, 604*f*
    cholecystectomy, 637–638
    for ectopic tubal pregnancy, 701–702
    fundoplication or Nissen procedure, 594–595
    herniorraphy, 873
    myomectomy, 698–699
    nephrectomy, 675
    Nissen fundoplication, pediatric, 859–860
    robotic-assisted prostatectomy, 661–663

Laparotomy, abdominal, 589

Large bowel surgery, 608–613
    abdominoperineal resection, 608–609
    anterior resection of sigmoid colon, 609–610
    colectomy, 611–612
    colostomy, 610–611
    colostomy closure, 611
    Hartmann procedure, 612
    right hemicolectomy and ileocolostomy, 612–613
    transverse colectomy, 613

Laryngologic surgery. *See also* Neck and laryngologic surgery
    laryngectomy, 492–494
    laryngoscopy, 490–491

Larynx, anatomy, 491*f*

Laser surgery
    blepharoplasty, 790–792
    cervical conization, 686–687
    cyclophotocoagulation, 444–445
    facial laser resurfacing, 796
    iridotomy, 445–446
    laser-assisted in situ keratomileusis or LASIK, 448
    lithotripsy, 674–675
    ophthalmic, 444–447
    photocoagulation, 446
    photodynamic therapy, 446–447

trabeculoplasty, 447

transmyocardial revascularization, 568–569

transurethral resection of prostate or lesions of bladder, 657–659

use in airway, safety considerations, 1–3

LASIK (laser-assisted in situ keratomileusis), 448

Lateral arterial pressure (LAP), 544

Lateral decubitus position
    for anesthetized, non-spontaneous breathing patient, 15
    for awake, spontaneous breathing patient, 15
    flexed, 15
    functional residual capacity and, 10
    issues associated with, 15
    precautions, 14
    ventilation/perfusion matching and, 53–54

Lateral internal sphincterotomy, 613–614

Lateral meniscectomy, 740–741

Lateral rectus resection, 435

Latissimus dorsi myocutaneous flaps, for breast reconstruction, 510–511

LBBB (left bundle branch block), 550, 550*f*

LDLT (live donor liver transplantation), 635, 636*f*

LEEP (loop electrosurgical excision procedure), 692–693

LeFort osteomy, 409–412, 410*f*–411*f*

Left anterior hemiblock (LAH), 550*f*, 551

Left bundle branch block (LBBB), 550, 550*f*

Left posterior hemiblock (LPH), 550*f*, 551

Left subclavian patch angioplasty, for coarctation of aorta repair, 848

Left-to-right shunt, pediatric, 842

Left uterine displacement (LUD), 17

Left ventricle, 543

Left ventricular vent use, 570

Leg, vascular system, 766*f*

Lens surgery, 441–442

Levophed (norepinephrine), 85–86. *See also under* Cardiovascular drug table

Lid lift, 790–792

Lidocaine, 85, 787. *See also under* Cardiovascular drug table

Ligature, cervical (cerclage), 703

Liposuction (lipectomy), 808–810

Lithotomy position, 10, 13

Lithotripsy
    electrohydraulic, 674
    extracorporeal shock wave, 672–674
    laser, 674–675
    ultrasonic, 675

Live donor liver transplantation (LDLT), 635, 636*f*

Liver
    blood flow, 626*f*
    disease, 627

anesthetics and, 627–628
  end-stage, comorbidities in, 633
  viral hepatitis, 628
functions, 625–626
sphincter of Oddi spasm, 626
Liver surgery, 625–636
  anesthetics and, 627–628
  hepatic resection, 628–629
  pearls, 625
  transjugular intrahepatic porto-systemic shunt, 629–630
  transplantation. *See* Liver transplantation
Liver transplantation, 630–635, 631*f*, 636*f*
  live donor, 635, 636*f*
  organ donor management, 879–880
  recipient, 630
    anhepatic stage, 631
    prehepatic stage, 630–631, 631*f*
    reperfusion syndrome, 632–633
    revascularization/reperfusion posthepatic stage, 631–632
LMA sizes, pediatric, 819
LMWH (low-molecular-weight heparin), 60, 63
Lobectomy
  adult, 527–528
  pediatric, 833–834
Local anesthetics, for plastic surgery, 787
Loop colostomy, 610–611
Loop diuretics, 23, 644
Loop electrosurgical excision procedure (LEEP), 692–693
Lou Gehrig's disease, 76
Lovenox (low-molecular-weight heparin), 60, 63
Lower extremity, vascular system, 766*f*
Low-molecular-weight heparin (LMWH; Enoxaparin; Lovenox), 60, 63
LPH (left posterior hemiblock), 550*f*, 551
LUD (left uterine displacement), 17
Lumbar discectomy and microdiscectomy, 403–404
Lumbar fusion and instrumentation
  anterior approach, 405–406
  posterior approach, 404–405
Lumbar sympathectomy, 390
Lumpectomy, 505
Lung
  anatomy, shunt and dead space conditions, 52*f*
  surgery, 523–537
    bleb excision, 523
    bronchoplastic resection, 523
    bronchopleural fistula, 524
    bronchopulmonary lavage, 524–526
    bullae excision, 523
    decortication or pleural stripping, 526
    empyema drainage, 527
    lobectomy, 527–528

lung biopsy, 528–529
    pediatric, lobectomy or pneumonectomy, 833–834
    pneumonectomy, 530–531
    pneumonectomy with extrapleural resection, 531–532
    segmental resection, 532–533
    thoracostomy, 535
    thoracotomy, 535–536
    transplantation. *See* Lung transplantation
    video-assisted thoracoscopic surgery or VATS, 536–537
    volume reduction, 529–530
    volume reduction or reduction pneumoplasty, 529–530
    wedge resection, 533–535
Lung transplantation, 540–542
  organ donor management, 879–880
  recipient, 540–542
Luxury perfusion, 342
Lymphadenectomy (axillary node dissection)
  groin, with radical vulvectomy, 685–686
  with mastectomy, 504
  pelvic, with radical cystectomy, 666–667
  pelvic/retroperitoneal, with nerve-sparing radical prostatectomy, 660–661
Lymphazurin 1% (isosulfan blue dye), 508–509
Lymph node
  axial dissecction. *See* Lymphadenectomy
  mapping, 508–510
  sentinel biopsy, 508–510

M
Macular degeneration, wet, laser therapy for, 446–447
Mad cow disease, 77
Magnesium, 17, 24
Magnetic resonance imaging (MRI), 6–7
Maintenance. *See also under specific surgeries*
  pediatric, 814–815, 817–818
Male gynecomastia, excision of, 802–803
Mammoplasty
  breast augmentation or implants, 803–804
  breast reduction, 804–805
Mandibular fracture, reduction, 412–413
Mandibular hypoplasia, anesthesia implications, 820–821
Mandibular osteotomy, 413–414
Mannitol, 23, 644
MAP. *See* Mean arterial pressure
Marcaine (bupvacaine), 787
Marshall-Marchetti-Krantz procedure (vesicourethral suspension), 670–672
Marsupialization of Bartholin duct cyst or abscess, 693

Mask strap (ventilator), facial injuries, 35–36
Mastectomy
    modified radical, 506–507
    radical, 507–508
    simple, 505–506
    subcutaneous, 506
Mastoidectomy, 453–454
Mastopexy, 805–807
Maxillary fracture reduction, 414
Maxillectomy, 464–465
Mean arterial pressure (MAP)
    cerebral perfusion pressure and, 10–11
    CPP and, 341
    electroencephalography and, 38
    formula, 544
Mean pulmonary artery pressure (MPAP), 544
Meckel's diverticulum, 606–607
Medial collateral ligament tear repair, 739–740
Medial menisectomy, 740–741
Medial rectus recession, 435
Mediastinal anatomy, 537–538
Mediastinal disorders, 515
Mediastinal masses, 519
Mediastinoscopy, 519–521, 520f
Meningioma, craniotomy for, 379–381
Meningocele closure, 823–824
Menisectomy, lateral or medial, 740–741
Mentoplasty (chin prosthesis), 796–797
Mepivacaine, 787
MEPs. See Motor evoked potentials
Metabolic effects, of deep hypothermic circulatory
    arrest, 28
Metatarsal fracture repair, 546–547, 547f
Metatarsal head resection, 547, 547f
Methohexital, 45, 80, 878
Methotrexate, for ectopic pregnancy, 701–702
Methylene blue dye, 509, 684
Methylmethacrylate (MMA) bone cement, 36
Metoclopramide (Reglan), 56
Microdiscectomy, lumbar, 403–404
Microvascular decompression, of cranial nerves,
    361–363
Midazolam, intraoperative neurologic monitoring
    and, 45
MIDCAB (minimally invasive direct coronary artery
    bypass graft), 566–568
Milrinone (primacor), 86. See also under Cardiovascular
    drug table
Mineralocorticoids, 66
Minimally invasive surgery
    direct coronary artery bypass graft, 566–568
    neurosurgical, 350–351
    total hip arthroplasty, 753–754
MITHA (minimally invasive total hip arthroplasty),
    753–754

Mitral valve
    prolapse, 843
    regurgitation, 570, 574–575
    repair, 575
    replacement, 575–576
    stenosis, 570, 573–574
    surgery, 570
Mixed venous oxygen content or saturation (MVO_2),
    36–37, 544
MMA (methylmethacrylate) bone cement, 36
Modified neck dissection, 494–495
Modified radical mastectomy, 506–507
Monroe-Kelly hypothesis, 334
Motor evoked potentials (MEPs)
    anesthesia during, 44
    barbiturates and, 45
    for cranial nerve monitoring, 44
    definition of, 43
Mouth surgery, 471–477
    glossectomy, 473–474
    operative dentistry, 471–473
    oral cavity lesion excision, 474–476
    pearls, 471
    uvulopalatopharyngoplasty, 476–477
MPAP (mean pulmonary artery pressure), 544
MRI (magnetic resonance imaging), 6–7
Multiple sclerosis, anesthesia and, 75
Multiple system atrophy, 79
Muscle denervation, muscle relaxants and, 81
Muscle relaxants
    altered response, conditions with, 79–81
    chest wall compliance and, 52–53
    contraindications, 346
    depolarizing, 345, 817
    infants and, 817
    nondepolarizing, 345
Muscular dystrophy, anesthesia and, 70–71
MVO_2 (mixed venous oxygen content or saturation),
    36–37, 544
Myasthenia gravis, anesthesia and, 71–72
Myasthenic syndrome (Lambert-Eaton
    syndrome), 70
Myelodysplasia, 823–824
Myelomeningocele closure, 823–824
Myelopathy, 395
Myocardial oxygen balance, 545
Myomectomy, 698–699
Myotonia (myotonic dystrophy), anesthesia and, 73
Myringotomy
    adult, 454–455
    pediatric, with ear tube placement, 827–828
Myxedema coma, 481–482

N

Narcotics, respiratory rate and, 52

Nasal cannula, 2f
 "blending" gases with, 2
 placement, for ophthalmic surgery, 419, 419f
 using with laser or cautery procedure, 1

Nasal fracture repair, 467–468

Nasal intubation, for operative dentistry, 472

Nasal packing, 467

Nasal polypectomy, 465–466

Nasolacrimal duct probing, 427–428

Naso-Rae, 472

Nasoseptoplasty, 468–469

Nausea, postoperative. *See also* Postoperative nausea
 and vomiting
 antiemetics for, 56–57
 risk factors, 57
 surgery associated with, 57

Neck and laryngologic surgery
 branchial cleft cyst tract excision, 824–825
 laryngectomy, 492–494
 laryngoscopy, 490–491
 modified neck dissection, 494–495
 neck dissection
  modified, 494–495
  radical, 495–497
 neck lift, cosmetic, 799–800
 panendoscopy, 497
 parotidectomy, 497–498
 pearls, 489–490
 postoperative nausea and vomiting, 490
 radical neck dissection, 495–497
 submandibular gland excision, 498–499
 thyroglossal duct cyst resection, 499–500
 tonsillectomy, 828–829
 tracheal-esophageal fistula correction, 834–836
 tracheostomy, 500–502

Necrotizing enterocolitis repair, 858–859

Needle biopsy, lung, 528–529

Neonates
 anesthesia and, 814–816
 emergency medications/equipment, 815–816
 epidural anesthesia, 816
 hemoglobin levels, 815
 spinal anesthesia, 816
 surgical pearls, 813–814
 temperature issues, 819
 tracheal-esophageal fistula correction, 834–836

Neosynephrine (phenylephrine), 86. *See also under*
 Cardiovascular drug table

Nephrectomy
 laparoscopic, 675
 open, 675–676
 radical, 676–677

Nephrolithotomy, 678

Nerves, patient positioning
 flexed lateral decubitus, 15
 on fracture table, 16
 jack-knife, 14
 lithotomy, 13
 prone, 12
 reverse Trendelenburg, 13
 semi-Fowler, 14
 supine, 12
 Trendelenburg, 13

Nerve-sparing, radical retropubic prostatectomy with
 pelvic/retroperitoneal lymphadenectomy, 660–661

Nescaine (chloroprocaine), 787

Neuraxial anesthesia, anticoagulants and, 62–65

Neuroanesthesia
 cases, types of, 346–349
 goals, 343–346
 for intracranial-space-occupying lesions, 346–348

Neuroblastoma resection or biopsy, 849–850

Neurodegenerative diseases, anesthesia and, 76–79

Neurogenic shock, 881

Neurointerventional procedures, 381–383

Neuromuscular blocking agents, intraoperative
 neurologic monitoring and, 45

Neuromuscular diseases, anesthesia and, 70–81

Neuroperipheral nerve surgery, 389–390

Neurophysiologic monitoring, 37

Neuroradiology, interventional, 381–383

Neurosurgery
 approaches, 349
  to brain, 349–350
  minimally invasive procedures, 350–351
 diseases associated with, 332
 functional, 351
 intracranial. *See* Intracranial neurosurgery
 pearls, 331
 for pediatric patients, 821–824
 postoperative nausea and vomiting, 331
 vascular, 349

Neurovascular surgery
 for posterior fossa pathology. *See* Posterior fossa,
  surgery
 sympathectomy, 390–392

Nicardipine (cardene), 83. *See also under*
 Cardiovascular drug table

NIM (Nerve Integrity Monitor) EMG endotracheal tube,
 483, 486–487

Nipple reconstruction, 512–513

Nissen fundoplication, laparoscopic
 adult, 594–595
 pediatric, 859–860

Nitric oxide (NO), 55

Nitric oxide synthase (NOS), 55

Nitroglycerin (Tridil; NTG), 85. *See also under*
 Cardiovascular drug table

Nitroprusside, 85. *See also under* Cardiovascular drug table
Nitrous oxide
contraindications, 80, 346
intraoperative neurologic monitoring and, 45–46
NO (nitric oxide), 55
Noncontinent urinary diversion, 668–669
Nonsteroidal anti-inflammatory drugs (NSAIDS), 60, 64, 66
Norepinephrine (Levophed), 85–86. *See also under* Cardiovascular drug table
Normotension alterations, for cerebral protection, 25
NOS (nitric oxide synthase), 55
Nose surgery
adenoidectomy, 828–829
choanal atresia repair, 825–826
nasal fracture repair, 467–468
nasal polypectomy, 465–466
rhinoplasty, 798–799, 798*f*
Novasure system, for endometrial ablation, 690
Novocaine (procaine), 787
NSAIDS (nonsteroidal anti-inflammatory drugs), 60, 64, 66
NTG (nitroglycerin), 85. *See also under* Cardiovascular drug table

O
Obesity, 601–602
O'Brien block, 420
Obstetric surgery, 703–708
cervical cerclage, 703
cesarean section birth, 703–706
emergency obstetrical hysterectomy, 708
postpartum tubal ligation, 706
retained placenta removal, 706–707
uterine inversion management, 707–708
Oculocardiac reflex, 420–421
Oculomotor nerve (CN III), 337, 420
Odansetron (Zofran), 56
Off-pump coronary artery bypass graft (OPCABG), 563–566
Olecranon fracture repair, 724, 724*f*
Olfactory nerve (CN I), 337
Oliguria
post-renal, 644
pre-renal, 644
renal, 644
Ommaya reservoir, 364
Omphalocele repair, 860–861
Oocyte retrieval, transvaginal, 694
OPCABG (off-pump coronary artery bypass graft), 563–566
Open appendectomy, 605–606
Open biopsy
breast, 504
lung, 529

Open cholecystectomy, 636–637
Open nephrectomy, 675–676
Open pneumothorax, 883
Open splenectomy, 642
Open thoracotomy, 529
Operating room
fires, 4–6
common sites, 1
patient burns and, 6
surgeries associated with, 6
issues, conduction disturbances and, 547–550
Operative dentistry, 471–473
Ophthalmic surgery, 417–448
anatomic terminology, 417–418
anesthesia for, 419–420, 419*f*
conjunctival, 436–437
conjunctival approach, 423
cornea, 437–439
eyelids, 421–426
glaucoma, 439–441
globe and orbit, 428–436
lacrimal gland, 426–428
laser therapy, 444–447
lens, 441–442
oculocardiac reflex, 420–421
pearls, 418–419
postoperative nausea and vomiting, 421
refractive eye surgery, 447–448
retina, 442–443
skin approach, 423
vitreous, 443–444
Opioids
cerebral blood flow and, 345
contraindications, 346
intraoperative neurologic monitoring and, 46
Optical iridectomy, 439–440
Optic nerve (CN II), 337
Optro, 888
Oral cavity lesion excision, 474–476
Oral intubation, for operative dentistry, 472
Orbital floor fractures, open reduction of, 414
Orbit fracture repair, 432–434
Orbit surgery, 428–436
Orchiectomy, 653–654
Orchiopexy (orchidopexy), 868–869
Organ donor management, 879–880
Oropharyngeal surgery, operating room fires and, 6
Orthopedic surgery, 709–763
amputation of lower extremity, 748–750
anesthetics for, 712–713
ankle/foot, 744–748
arthroscopy, 756–759
definitions for, 711–712
digit and hand replantation, 731
fat embolism syndrome, 710

femur, 735–738, 735*f*
of hand/wrist, 727–731
hip, 733–735, 734*f*
of humerus, radius and ulna, 722–727, 724*f*
knee, 738–743, 738*f*
levels of, 712
lower leg, 743–744
pearls, 709–710
pediatric, 864–865
pelvis, 731–733
rhabdomyolysis, 710
shoulder girdle, 713–722
    acromioclavicular joint separation correction,
       713–714, 714*f*
    anterior shoulder dislocation repair, 714–716, 715*f*
    brachial plexus, 716–718, 717*f*
    clavicular fracture repair, 718
    open reduction of humeral head fracture, 719
    recurrent anterior shoulder dislocation
       correction, 720–721
    rotator cuff tear correction, 719–720, 720*f*
    sternoclavicular dislocation, correction of, 721, 722*f*
spinal column, 759–763, 760*f*
total joint replacement, 750–756, 755*f*
Osmotic diuretics, for cerebral perfusion, burst
    suppression, 23
Ossicular chain reconstruction, 455–456
Osteotomy, 712
Otoplasty (ear pinning), 797–798
Outflow reconstruction, 783–785
Ovary removal, by salpingo-oophorectomy, 700
Oxygen
    minimizing concentrations in field, 2–3
    sources, in operating room, 4, 5
       patient protection methods, 5
Oxygenation, for cerebral protection, 25
Oxygen consumption, of heart, 545
Oxygen prongs, during facial surgery, 2
Oxygen tanks, in MRI suite, 7
Oxytocics, 684

P
Pacemakers
    biventricular pacing, 551–552
    contraindications, 550
    ESUs and, 4
    general information, 546
    lead types, 546
    naming functions, 547
    operating room issues, 547–549
    permanent, insertion of, 552–553
    safe procedures with, 550
    terminology, 546
    types of, 546

Pacing, temporary, 554–556
Packed red blood cells (PRBCs), 20
PAD (pulmonary artery diastolic), 543
Pain
    sympathetic, 390
    tourniquet
Palatoplasty (cleft palate repair), 871–872
Palebral, 417
Pallidotomy, 351
Palmar fasciectomy, 810
Pancreas transplantation
    organ donor management, 879–880
    procedure, 641
Pancreatectomy
    complete or total, 638–639, 639*f*
    partial, 638–639, 638*f*
Pancreaticoduodenectomy (Whipple procedure),
    640–641, 640*f*
Panendoscopy, 497
PAP (pulmonary artery pressures), 543
Paranasal sinuses, anatomy, 460*f*
Paraplegia, 394
Parathyroidectomy, 483–484
Parathyroid hormone (PTH), 643
Parkinsonism (Parkinson's disease), 78, 351
Parotidectomy, 497–498
Pars plana, 418
Partial maxillectomy, 464–465
Partial thromboplastin time (PTT), 58
PAS (pulmonary artery systolic), 543
Passy-Muir valve, 490
Patella dislocation correction, 741
Patellar fracture reduction, 742
Patella tendon rupture repair, 741
Patellectomy, 741–742
Patent ductus arteriosus closure, 844–846
Patent foramen ovale (PFO), 30
Patient positioning. *See also under specific surgeries*
    arterial blood pressure transducer levels and, 10–11
    cardiovascular system and, 9
    cerebral perfusion pressure and, 10–11
    endotracheal tube migration, 10
    flexed lateral decubitus, 14–15
    on fracture table, 16, 16*f*
    functional residual capacity and, 10
    jack-knife, 14
    lateral decubitus, 14–15
    lithotomy, 13
    peripheral nerves and, 10
    prone, 11–12
    pulmonary system and, 10
    reverse Trendelenburg, 13
    semi-Fowler, sitting or beach-chair, 13–14
    supine, 11
    Trendelenburg, 12–13

Patient state analysis (PSA 4000), 39
PCWP (pulmonary capillary wedge pressure), 544
Pectus carinatum correction, 832–833
Pectus excavatum correction, 832–833
Pediatric surgery, 813–872
    anesthesia issues
        for ages 3–6 months, 817–818
        neonatal, 814–816
    cardiovascular, 836–849
    with cerebral palsy, anesthesia implications, 820
    congenital heart defects, 836–849
    with Down syndrome, anesthetic implications of,
        819–820
    for ear, nose and throat, 824–831
    endoscopic, anesthesia for, 618
    gastrointestinal disorder repair, 849–864
        abdominal tumor resection or biopsy, 849–850
        biliary atresia correction, 863–864
        colostomy, 850–851
        congenital diaphragmatic hernia repair, 851–854
        gastroschisis repair, 854–855
        imperforate anus repair, 856–858
        laparoscopic Nissen fundoplication, 859–860
        necrotizing enterocolitis repair, 858–859
        omphalocele repair, 860–861
        pull-through for Hirschsprung's disease, 855–856
        pyloromyotomy for hypertrophic pyloric
            stenosis, 861–863
        reduction of intussusception, 858
    genitourinary, 865–870
    helium (Heliox) usage, 55–56
    mandibular hypoplasia, anesthesia implications,
        820–821
    neonates
        anesthesia and, 814–816
        surgical pearls, 813–814
    neurosurgery, 821–824
    one-lung ventilation, 818–819
    orthopedic, 864–865
    pearls, 816–817
    plastic and reconstructive, 870–872
    remifentanil dosage and, 67
    temperature issues, 819
    thoracic, 831–836
Pedicle fixation, spine, 759–761, 760f
Pedicle TRAM flap, for breast reconstruction, 511–512
PEEP (positive end-expiratory pressure), functional
    residual capacity and, 51
Pelvic exenteration, 699–700
Pelvic fracture
    closed reduction and external fixation of, 731–733
    realignment and fixation, 733–733
Pelvic lymphadenectomy, with radical cystectomy,
    666–667

Pelvis, closed reduction and external fixation of pelvis,
    731–733
Penectomy, partial or total, 650–651
Penile implant, 651
Penis surgery, circumcision, 866–867
Pentalogy of Fallot, 838
Peptic ulcer closure, 599
Percutaneous endoscopic tube placement,
    gastrostomy, 598–599
Percutaneous nephrolitotomy, 678
Percutaneous transluminal angioplasty, 556–557
Perfluorocarbons, 888
Perfusionist role, in coronary artery bypass
    graft, 560
Peribulbar block, 419
Pericardial tamponade, 570, 576
Pericardial window, 576–577
Pericardiectomy, 576–577
Perineal prostatectomy
    radical or total, 660
    simple, 659–660
Periodic paralysis, anesthesia and, 73–74
Periodontic procedures, 471–473
Periorbital, 418
Peripheral iridectomy, 439–440
Peripheral nervous system (PNS)
    nerve blocks, 712
    nerve repair, 389–390
    patient positioning and, 10
    vascular tone and, 340
Peripheral vascular disease (PVD),
    766–767, 766f
Peritoneal dialysis
    catheter placement, 679
    phases, 679–680
    types of, 680
Petal (cilostazol), 65
PFO (patent foramen ovale), 30
Phacoemulsification, 441–442
Phenylephrine (Neosynephrine), 86. See also under
    Cardiovascular drug table
Pheochromocytoma removal, 484–486
Phlebostatic axis, 11
Phosphodiesterase inhibitors, 60
Photocoagulation, laser, 446
Photodynamic therapy, laser, 446–447
Pierre Robin sequence, 820
Piggyback modification, for liver transplantation,
    630–631, 631f
Pilonidal cyst and sinus excision, 615
Pitressin (vasopressin), 86–87. See also under
    Cardiovascular drug table
Placenta, retained, removal of, 706–707
Plastic and reconstructive surgery, pediatric patients,
    870–872

Plastic surgery, 787–812
    abdomen, 807–808
    antiemetics for, 789–790
    breast, 800–807
    ear, 797–798
    extremity, 810
    facial, 790–799, 798f
    herbal agents and, 789
    liposuction, 808–810
    neck lift, 799–800
    pearls, 787–789
    skin and flap grafting, 810–812
Platelet function test, 58–59
Platelets, 21
Plavix (clopidogrel), neuraxial anesthesia and, 64
Pleural disorders, 515
Pleural stripping (decortication), 526
Pneumonectomy, 530–531
    with extrapleural resection, 531–532
    pediatric, 833–834
Pneumothorax, 883
PNS. See Peripheral nervous system
Polyheme, 888
PONV. See Postoperative nausea and vomiting
Popliteal block, 713
Popliteal cyst excision, 742–743
Popliteal entrapment syndrome, 767
Popliteal-tibial bypass graft, 783–784
Portal hypertension, 627
Portosystemic shunt (portocaval shunt), 784
Positive end-expiratory pressure (PEEP), functional
    residual capacity and, 51
Positive-pressure ventilation, 519
Posterior cruciate ligament tear repair, 739–740
Posterior fossa
    pathology, 383
    surgery, 383–389
        craniotomy or craniectomy, 384–386
        ventricular catheter/shunt placement for
            hydrocephalus, 386–389
Posterior vitrectomy, 443–444
Postoperative nausea and vomiting (PONV)
    breast surgery, 503–504
    ear surgery, 449
    gynecological surgery, 683–684
    neck and laryngologic surgery, 490
    ophthalmic surgery, 421
    risk factors, 331
    sinus and rhinologic surgery, 461
Postoperative visual loss (POVL)
    prone position, 12
    risk factors, 46–47
Postpartum tubal ligation (PTL), 706
Postural changes, for cerebral protection, 25
Potassium-sparing diuretics, 644

POVL. See Postoperative visual loss
PRBCs (packed red blood cells), 20
Precedex (dexmedetomidine), 67, 68, 878
Precordial Doppler, for venous air embolism, 30–31
Preemptive analgesia, for gynecological surgery, 684
Pregnant patients
    anesthetics and, 17–18
    blood products for, 20–21
    elective surgery and, 17
    left uterine displacement and, 17
    tocolytics and, 17
Preliminary iridectomy, 439–440
Preoperative measures. See under specific surgeries
Presacral rectopexy, 615
Prilocaine, 787
Primacor (Milrinone), 86. See also under
    Cardiovascular drug table
Primum atrial septal defect, 843
Procaine (Novocaine), 787
Prone position, 11–12
Propofol
    cerebral protection and, 23
    EEG burst suppression and, 39
    intraoperative neurologic monitoring and, 45
Prostatectomy
    nerve-sparing radical, pelvic/retroperitoneal
        lymphadenectomy, 660–661
    radical or total perineal, 660
    robotic-assisted laparoscopic, 661–663
    simple perineal, 659–660
    simple retropubic, 663
    suprapubic or transvesical, 663–664
Prostate gland surgery, 656–665
    nerve-sparing, radical retropubic prostatectomy
        with pelvic/retroperitoneal lymphadenectomy,
        660–661
    radical or total perineal prostatectomy, 660
    robotic-assisted laparoscopic prostatectomy,
        661–663
    simple perineal prostatectomy, 659–660
    simple retropubic prostatectomy, 663
    suprapubic prostatectomy, 663–664
    transrectal crysurgical ablation, 656–657
    transrectal seed implantation, 664–665
    transurethral resection of prostate or lesions of
        bladder, 657–659
Prosthetic replacement, of femoral head, 735–736
Protamine, 61, 86, 765
Prothrombin time (PT), 58
Prothrombotics, 61
Proximal femur fracture, open reduction and internal
    fixation, 736
PSA 4000, 39
PT (prothrombin time), 58

Pterional approach (frontotemporosphenoidal), 363–364, 364*f*

Pterygium excision, 436–437

PTH (parathyroid hormone), 643

PTL (postpartum tubal ligation), 706

PTT (partial thromboplastin time), 58

Pubovaginal sling, for urinary incontinence treatment, 669–670

Pull-through for Hirschsprung's disease, 855–856

Pulmonary artery banding, 846–847

Pulmonary artery diastolic (PAD), 543

Pulmonary artery pressures (PAP), 543

Pulmonary artery reflex, 340

Pulmonary artery systolic (PAS), 543

Pulmonary atresia
  cyanotic lesion correction, 837
  definition of, 838

Pulmonary atresia, cyanotic lesion correction, 837

Pulmonary capillary wedge pressure (PCWP), 544

Pulmonary contusion, 885–886

Pulmonary disorders, 515

Pulmonary hypertension, 47

Pulmonary stenosis
  cyanotic lesion correction, 837
  definition of, 838
  surgical repair repair, 847, 849

Pulmonary system
  patient positioning, 10
    flexed lateral decubitus, 15
    on fracture table, 16
    jack-knife, 14
    lateral decubitus, 15
    lithotomy, 13
    prone, 12
    reverse Trendelenburg, 13
    semi-Fowler, 14
    supine, 12
    Trendelenburg, 12–13
  surgery. *See specific surgeries*

Pulmonary vascular resistance (PVR)
  congenital heart defects and, 836–837
  formula, 544

Puttii-Platt procedure, 715

PVD. *See* Peripheral vascular disease

PVR. *See* Pulmonary vascular resistance

Pyelolithotomy, 678

Pyloromyotomy for hypertrophic pyloric stenosis, 861–863

Pyroplasty, with vagotomy, 599–601, 600*f*

Q

Quadriplegia, 393, 394

R

Radial keratomy (RK), 447–448

Radiation exposure
  occupational limit, 7
  sources, 7

Radical cystectomy, with or without pelvic lymphadenectomy, 666–667

Radical hysterectomy, 696–697

Radical mastectomy, 507–508

Radical neck dissection, 495–497

Radical nephrectomy, 676–677

Radical or total perineal prostatectomy, 660

Radical parotidectomy, 497–498

Radical trachelectomy, 693

Radical vulvectomy, with groin lymphadenectomy, 685–686

Radiculopathy, 395

Radiofrequency ablation, 549

Radiofrequency endometrial ablation, 690

Radius fracture
  closed reduction, 722
  open reduction, 724–725

RAP (right atrial pressure), 543

Rate adaptive pacing, 546–547

RBBB (right bundle branch block), 550, 550*f*

RBC leukocyte poor, 20

RBC washed, 20

RCP (retrograde cerebral perfusion), 27

Realignment, patellar, 741

Rectal prolapse, 615

Rectocele, 687

Rectosigmoidostomy, 609–610

Rectum surgery, 613–615
  fistulotomy, 614
  hemorrhoidectomy, 614–615
  lateral internal sphincterotomy, 613–614
  pilonidal cyst and sinus excision, 615
  rectal prolapse, 615

Reduction pneumoplasty (lung volume reduction surgery), 529–530

Reflexes
  atrial, 340
  cranial nerve, 339
  pulmonary artery, 340

Refractive eye surgery, 447–448

Refractive keratoplasty, 447–448

Regional anesthesia, for renal disease patients, 648

Reglan (metoclopramide), 56

Remifentanil (Ultiva) infusion, 67–68

Renal disease. *See* Kidney, disease

Renal surgery. *See* Kidney surgery

ReoPro (abciximab), 60, 65

Reperfusion syndrome, 632–633

Replacement total hip, 752–753

Resuscitation markers, 888–889

Retained placenta removal, 706–707
Retina, 418
Retinal detachment repair, 442–443
Retina surgery, 442–443
Retrobulbar block, 419–420
Retrograde cardioplegia perfusion, 560
Retrograde cerebral perfusion (RCP), 27
Retrograde pyelogram, 650
Retroperitoneal procedure, for lumbosacral fusion, 405–406
Retropubic prostatectomy, simple, 663
Reverse steal phenomenon, 342
Reverse Trendelenburg position, 13
Revised Trauma Scale (RTS), 884–885
Rhabdomyolysis, 645, 710
Rhinologic surgery
    epistaxis treatment, 467
    nasal fracture repair, 467–468
    nasoseptoplasty, 468–469
Rhinoplasty, 798–799, 798f
Rhytidectomy (facelift), 794–796
Right atrial pressure (RAP), 543
Right bundle branch block (RBBB), 550, 550f
Right hemicolectomy and ileocolostomy, 612–613
Right-to-left shunt, neonatal cyanotic lesions and, 837
Right ventricle, 543
Right ventricular pressure (RVP), 543
Rigid bronchoscopy, 517–519
Ritodrine, 17
RK (radial keratomy), 447–448
Robin Hood effect, 342
Robotic-assisted laparoscopic surgery
    myomectomy, 698–699
    prostatectomy, 661–663
Ropivacaine (Naropin), 787
Rotator cuff tear correction, 719–720, 720f
Roux-en-Y gastric bypass, 603–604, 604f
RTS (Revised Trauma Scale), 884–885
RVP (right ventricular pressure), 543
R-wave sensitivity, 546

S
Sacral nerve stimulator implantation, 668
Safety considerations, magnetic resonance imaging, 6
Sano shunt, 839
Saphenous vein grafts, for distal revascularization, 780–781
Saphenous veins, varicose vein excision and stripping, 784–785
Sciatic nerve block, 713
Scleral buckling, 442–443
Scoliosis, surgical treatment, 761–763
Sctrotum and testicles surgery, 652–656
Second-look laparotomy, 699

Sector iridectomy, 439–440
Secundum atrial septal defect, 843
Sedatives
    intravenous, 45
    preoperative, 344
Segmental resection, 532–533
Segmental resection (lumpectomy), 505
Selective vestibular neurectomy (SNV), 453
Semi-Fowler position, 13–14
Sensorcaine (bupvacaine), 787
Sentinel lymph node biopsy, 508–510
Septic shock, 881–882
Septum, submucous resection, 468–469
Septum secundum, 843
Sevoflurane, 80
Shock
    from aortic cross-clamp removal, 19
    states of, 880–882
Shoulder
    anatomy, 713, 714f, 715f
    arthroscopy, 758–759
    total arthroplasty, 755–756, 755f
Shoulder girdle surgery, 713–722
    acromioclavicular joint separation correction, 713–714
    anterior shoulder dislocation repair, 714–716, 715f
    brachial plexus, 716–718, 717f
    clavicular fracture repair, 718
    open reduction of humeral head fracture, 719
    recurrent anterior shoulder dislocation correction, 720–721
    sternoclavicular dislocation, correction of, 721, 722f
Shunt and dead space conditions, lung, 52f
Shunt placement, for hydrocephalus, 386–389
Shy-Drager syndrome, 79
SIADH (syndrome of inappropriate antidiuretic hormone), 332
Sigmoid colon, anterior resection, 609–610
Sigmoidoscopy, 623
Sinus and rhinologic surgery, 459–469
    paranasal sinus anatomy, 460f
    pearls, 459–460
    postoperative nausea and vomiting, 461
Sinus surgery, 461–467
    endoscopic, 462–463
    ethmoidectomy, 463
    frontal sinus drainage, 463–464
    intranasal antrostomy, 461–462
    maxillectomy, 464–465
    nasal polypectomy, 465–466
    sphenoidotomy, 466
    turbinectomy, 466–467
Sinus venosus atrial septal defect, 843
Sitting position, 13–14
Skin and flap grafting, 810–812

Skin grafts, split- and full-thickness, 810–811
Slew rate, 546
Sling creation, for urinary incontinence treatment, 669–670
Small intestine surgery (small bowel surgery), 605–608
    diverticulectomy, 606–607
    enterostomy, 607
    laparoscopic appendectomy, 606
    nteroscopy, 623–624
    open appendectomy, 605–606
    organ donor management, 879–880
    resection, 608
SNS (sympathetic nervous system), 340, 390
Soft-tissue lesion excision, in oral cavity, 474–476
Somatosensory evoked potentials (SSEP), 40–42, 41f
Spermatocelectomy, 654
Spetzler and Martin grading system, for arteriovenous malformations, 349
Sphenoidotomy, 466
Sphincter of Oddi spasm, 626
Sphincterotomy, lateral internal, 613–614
Spica cast application (body cast), 865
Spigelian hernia repair, 875
Spinal accessory nerve (CN XI), 338–339
Spinal anesthesia, neonatal, 816
Spinal column
    anatomy, 760f
    surgery, 759–763, 760f
    vertebrae, 393–395
Spinal cord
    anatomy, 332, 333f
    aortic cross-clamping and, 18–19
    injury, from aortic cross-clamping, 19
    perfusion, 20
    protection, during aortic cross-clamping, 19–20
Spinal surgery, 396–408
    cervical decompression and fusion
        anterior and posterior approaches, 399
        anterior approach, 396–397
        posterior approach, 397–399
    dorsal root rhizotomy, 399
    dysraphism correction, 823
    foraminotomy, 400–401, 400f
    laminectomy with or without disectomy, 401–402, 401f
    laminotomy, 402–403, 402f
    lumbar disectomy and microdisectomy, 403–404
    lumbar fusion and instrumentation
        anterior approach, 405–406
        posterior approach, 404–405
    pearls, 392–393
    pedicle fixation, 759–761, 760f
    reconstruction, 405–408
    stapling technique, 761
    tumor resection of spine, 408

Spironolactone, 644
Splenectomy, open, 642
Split-thickness skin grafts, 810–811
Spongiform encephalopathy, 77
SSEP (somatosensory evoked potentials), 40–42, 41f
Stanford classification of thoracic aorta dissection, 577
Stapedectomy, 456
Stenopeic iridectomy, 439–440
Stenosis repair, for aortic coarctation, 847
Stereotaxy
    frame-based, 350
    frameless, 350
    procedures, 350
        hypophysectomy, 372
        radiosurgery, 350–351
Sterilization (tubal ligation), 701
Sternoclavicular joint
    anatomy, 721, 722f
    dislocation, correction of, 721
Sternotomy
    for coronary artery bypass, 559, 563
    for heart transplantation, 584
Stimulator placement, for chronic pain and movement disorders, 351
Stomach stapling (vertical banded gastroplasty), 604–605
Stomach surgery, 595–601
    gastrostomy, percutaneous endoscopic tube placement, 598–599
    gastrostomy tube insertion, 597–598
    jejunostomy tube insertion, 597–598
    peptic ulcer closure, 599
    subtotal gastrectomy, 595–596
    total gastrectomy, 596–597, 597f
    vagotomy, 599–601
Strabismus correction, 435–436
Stroke volume, formula, 544
Stroma-free hemoglobin, 888
Subarachnoid hemorrhage, 378–379
Subclavian translocation, for coarctation of aorta repair, 848
Subcutaneous mastectomy, 506
Subdural hematoma, evacuation, 369–371
Sublingual capnometry, 889
Sublingual PCO$_2$, 889
Subluxation, 712
Submandibular gland excision, 498–499
Subtotal gastrectomy, 595–596
Succinylcholine (Anectine), 420, 428, 878
"Sucker bypass," 563
Superaclavicular block, 713
Superficial parotidectomy, 497–498
Supine position (dorsal position), 10, 11
Supracervical hysterectomy, 696

Supracondylar femoral fracture, open reduction and internal fixation, 737–738
Supraglottic laryngectomy, 492–494
Suprapubic cystolithotomy, 667
Suprapubic cystostomy, 667–668
Suprapubic prostatectomy (transvesical prostatectomy), 663–664
Supratentorial masses, 347–348
Surgical field, minimizing oxygen concentrations in, 2–3
Surgical positioning. *See* Patient positioning
SVR. *See* Systemic vascular resistance
Sympathectomy, 390–392
    lumbar, 390
    thoracic, 522–523
    upper-extremity, 390–391
Sympathetic nervous system (SNS), 340, 390
Syndactyly repair, 864
Syndrome of inappropriate antidiuretic hormone (SIADH), 332
Synovectomy, 712
Synthetic colloids, 887
Systemic vascular resistance (SVR)
    congenital heart defects and, 836–837
    formulas, 544

T

T&A (tonsillectomy & adenoidectomy), 828–829
TAH (total abdominal hysterectomy), 697–698
Takayasu's arteritis, 767
Tarsal (Meibomian) gland, 418
Tarsal plate, 418
Tarsorrhaphy, 426
Technetium, 509
TEE (transesophageal echocardiography), for venous air embolism, 30
TEG (thromboelastography), 59
Temporary pacing, 554–556
Tenckhoff catheter placement, 679
Tendon lengthening, foot, 748
Tenon's capsule, 418
Tension pneumothorax, 883
Teralogy of Fallot
    correction, 838–839
    cyanotic lesion correction, 837
Terbutaline, 17
Terminal colostomy, 610–611
Testicular biopsy, 654
Testicular torsion, 654–655
Tetracaine (Cetacaine), 787
"Tet spell," 839
Thalamotomy, 351
Therapeutic abortion (dilation and evacuation), 689
Therapeutic iridectomy, 439–440
Thermachoice balloon, for endometrial ablation, 690

Thiazide diuretics, 644
Thiopental, 45, 878
Thoracic aorta dissection
    classification, 577
    clinical presentation, 577–578
    medical management, 578
    surgical repair, 578
        of arch, 580
        of ascending portion, 578–580
        of descending portion, 580–582
Thoracic surgery, 515–542
    anesthesia key points, 516–517
    aortic, 577–582. *See also* Thoracic aorta dissection
    endoscopy, 517–523
    lung. *See* Lung, surgery
    lung transplantation, 540–542
    mediastinal anatomy, 537–538
    mediastinal tumor excision, open approach, 538
    pearls, 515–516
    pediatric, 831–836
        anesthetic implications for, 831–832
        pectus carinatum correction, 832–833
        pectus excavatum correction, 832–833
        thoracotomy, 833–834
    sympathectomy, 522–523
    thymectomy, 538–539
    tracheal tumor resection, 539–540
Thoracic vertebrae, 394
Thoracoabdominal aortic aneurysm or dissection repair, 580–582
Thoracoscopic minimally invasive correction, for scoliosis, 761
Thoracoscopy, 521–522
Thoracostomy (chest tube), 535
Thoracotomy
    adult, 527, 535–536
    pediatric, 833–834
Thrombate III (AT III; antithrombin III), 59–60, 83
Thrombectomy, femoral, 779–780
Thrombolytics, 61
Thymectomy, 538–539
Thyroglossal duct cyst resection, 499–500
Thyroidectomy
    substernal or intrathoracic, 488
    subtotal or total, 486–488
Thyroid storm, 480–481
Tibial fracture
    open reduction, 743–744
    plateau type, 743
Ticlid, neuraxial anesthesia and, 64
"Tinctures," 5
TIPS (transjugular intrahepatic porto-systemic shunt), 629–630
Tirofiban (Aggrastat), 61, 65
Tissue expanders, for breast reconstruction, 513–514

TIVA (total intravenous anesthesia), 68–69

TMP (transmural pressure), 341

Tocolytics, 17, 684

Toe amputation, 750

Tonsillectomy

bleeding after, return to surgery for, 829–830

procedure, 828–829

Topical anesthesia, for ophthalmic surgery, 419

Toradol (Ketorolac), 69

Total abdominal hysterectomy (TAH), 697–698

Total gastrectomy, 596–597, 597f

Total intravenous anesthesia (TIVA), 68–69

Total joint replacement

ankle, 751

elbow, 751–752

hip, 752–753

knee, 754–755

minimally invasive hip, 753–754

shoulder, 755–756, 755f

Total laryngectomy, 492–494

Total maxillectomy, 464–465

Total parotidectomy, 497–498

Tourniquet use, 48–49

Trabeculectomy (filtration surgery), 440–441

Trabeculoplasty, laser, 447

Tracheal//bronchial disorders, 515

Tracheal-esophageal fistula correction, in neonates, 834–836

Tracheal tumor resection, 539–540

Trachelectomy, radical, 693

Tracheleorrhaphy, 693–694

Tracheobronchial disruption, major, 886

Tracheostomy, 6, 490, 500–502

Tracheostomy, pediatric, 830–831

TRAM flap, for breast reconstruction, 511–512

Transcutaneous pacing, 554–555

Transesophageal echocardiography (TEE), for venous air embolism, 30

Transesophageal pacing, 555

Transhiatal esophagectomy, 591–592

Transjugular intrahepatic porto-systemic shunt (TIPS), 629–630

Transmural pressure (TMP), 341

Transoral surgical approach, for cervical decompression and fusion, 396

Transperitoneal procedure, for lumbosacral fusion, 405–406

Transplantation

digit and hand, 731

heart. *See* Heart transplantation

kidney, 680–682

liver, 630–635, 631f, 636f

organ donor management, 879–880

pancreas, 641

Transposition of great arteries correction, 839–840

Transrectal cryosurgical ablation of prostate gland, 656–657

Transrectal seed implantation, 664–665

Transsphenoidal approach, to brain, 350

Transsphenoidal hypophysectomy, 372

Transthoracic esophagectomy, 592–593

Transurethral resection of lesions of bladder (TURB), 657–659

Transurethral resection of prostate gland (TURP), 657–659

Transvaginal anchor, 670

Transvaginal oocyte retrieval (TVOR), 694

Transvenous pacing electrode insertion, 555

Transverse colectomy, 613

Transverse rectus abdominis myocutaneous flaps, for breast reconstruction, 511–512

Transvesical prostatectomy (suprapubic prostatectomy), 663–664

Trauma packs, 887

Trauma patients

airway assessment, 882–883

anesthesia on, 889–890

breathing assessment, 883

circulation assessment, 883–884

disability assessment, 884–885

resuscitation, 882–886

markers, 888–889

recommendations, 889

secondary survey, 885–886

shock states, 880–881

Treacher-Collin syndrome, 821

Trendelenburg position, 12–13

functional residual capacity and, 10

steep, effects on body systems, 662

Trephination, 350

Tricuspid atresia surgery, 837, 840–841

Tridil (nitroglycerin), 85. *See also under* Cardiovascular drug table

Trifascular block, 551

Trigeminal nerve (CN V), 337–338

Triggered pacemaker, 546

Trimethaphan (Arfonad), 86. *See also under* Cardiovascular drug table

Trochlear nerve (CN IV), 337, 420

Truncus arteriosus repair, 841–842

Tubal ligation (sterilization), 701

Tuboplasty, 702

Tumor resection. *See also specific tumors*

abdominal, pediatric, 849–850

carcinoid, 22

of spine, 408

tracheal, 539–540

TURB (transurethral resection of lesions of bladder), 657–659

Turbinectomy, 466–467

TURP (transurethral resection of prostate gland), 657–659
TUR syndrome, 658–659
TVOR (transvaginal oocyte retrieval), 694
Tympanoplasty, 456–457
Tympanostomy, 455, 457, 827–828

U

UAE (uterine artery embolization), 702–703
UFE (uterine fibroid embolization), 702–703
Ulnar fracture
    closed reduction, 722
    open reduction, 724–725
    of proximal third, repair of, 725–726
Ulnar nerve transposition, 391–392, 726–727
Ultiva (remifentanil) infusion, 67–68
Ultrasonic lithotripsy, 675
Umbilical hernia repair, 875
Upper-extremity sympathectomy, 390–391
Upper gastrointestinal endoscopy, 621–622
UPPP (uvulopalatopharyngoplasty), 476–477
Ureter surgery, 672–679
    cutaneous ureterostomy, 678–679
    reimplantation, for vesicoureteral reflux, 879–870
    ureterectomy, 678
    ureterolithotomy, 678
Urethral bulking agents, 671–672
Urethral surgery
    meatotomy, 651–652
    sling creation, 695
Urethra surgery, 665–668
Urinary diversions, 668–669
Urinary incontinence surgery, 669–672
Urinary sphincters, artificial prosthetic, 671–672
Urinary stress incontinence operation, 694–695
Uterine artery embolization (UAE), 702–703
Uterine fibroids
    embolization, 702–703
    removal, myomectomy for, 698–699
Uterine inversion management, 707–708
Uvea, 418
Uvulopalatopharyngoplasty (UPPP), 476–477

V

VAE (venous air embolism), 30–31
Vaginal approach, vesicovaginal fistula repair, 695–696
Vaginal hysterectomy, 691
Vaginal surgery, 686–696
    cervical biopsy, 686–687
    cervical conization, 686–687
    colporrhaphy, 687
    colpotomy, 687–688
    culdotomy, 687–688
    dilation and curettage, 686, 688–689
    dilation and evacuation, 689
    endometrial ablation, 689–690
    hysteroscopy, 691–692
    loop electrosurgical excision procedure, 692–693
    marsupialization of Bartholin duct cyst or abscess, 693
    radical trachelectomy, 693
    tracheleorrhaphy, 693–694
    transvaginal oocyte retrieval, 694
    urinary stress incontinence operation, 694–695
    vaginal hysterectomy, 691
    vaginotomy, 687–688
    vesicovaginal fistula repair, 695–696
Vaginal tape, tension free, 670
Vaginotomy, 687–688
Vagotomy, with or without pyloroplasty, 599–601, 600*f*
Vagus nerve (CN X), 338–339
Valsalva maneuver, 384, 393
Van Lint block, 420
Varicocelectomy, 655
Varicose vein excision and stripping, 784–785
Vascular bypass grafts, 780–781
Vascular surgery, 765–785
    abdominal aortic aneurysm resection
        emergency, 771–772
        endovascular repair, 770–771
        open, 767–770
    for arterial occlusive disease, 767
    arteriovenous fistula or shunt, 772–773
    carotid arteries, anatomy of, 773–774, 773*f*, 774*f*
    carotid endarterectomy, 774–779
    for dialysis catheter placement, venous access, 778
    distal revascularization, 780–781
    femoral thrombectomy/embolectomy, 779–780
    inflow reconstruction, 781–783
    outflow reconstruction, 783–785
    pearls, 765
Vascular system, lower extremity, 766*f*
Vascular tone, 340
Vasectomy, 655–656
Vasoactive drugs, for neurologic anesthesia, 346
Vasoconstrictors, cerebral, 23
Vasodilators, 345
Vasomotor center, 340–343, 340*f*
Vasopressin (Pitressin), 86–87. *See also under* Cardiovascular drug table
Vasospasm, 348–349
Vasovastomy, 656
VATS (video-assisted thoracoscopic surgery), 527, 529, 530, 536–537
Vena cava filter insertion, 785
Venous air embolism (VAE), 30–31
Venous cannulation, for coronary artery bypass graft, 559–560
Veno-venous bypass, for liver transplantation, 630, 631*f*

Ventilation, distribution, 53
Ventilation/oxygenation, EEG burst suppression and, 39
Ventilation/perfusion matching, 53–54, 54*f*
Ventilator mask strap facial injuries, 35–36
Ventricular catheter/shunt placement, for hydrocephalus, 386–389
Ventricular septal defect, cyanotic lesion correction, 837
Ventricular septal defect closure, 570
Ventricular septal defect repair, 847
Ventricular system, 333–337, 335*f*, 336*f*
VEP (visual evoked potentials), 43
Vertebrae, spinal
    anatomy, 393*f*–395*f*, 760*f*
    assessment, 394–395
    cervical, 393–394, 393*f*, 394*f*
    thoracic, 394, 760*f*
Vertical banded gastroplasty (stomach stapling), 604–605
Vesicoureteral reflux, ureteral reimplantation for, 879–870
Vesicourethral suspension, 670–672
Vesicourethral suspension (Marshall-Marchetti-Krantz procedure), 670–672
Vesicovaginal fistula repair, 695–696
Vestibular neurectomy, 457
Vestibular schwannoma removal, 449–451
Video-assisted thoracoscopic surgery (VATS), 527, 529, 530, 536–537
Visual evoked potentials (VEP), 43
Vitrectomy, anterior and posterior approaches, 443–444
Vitreous humor, 418
Volatile anesthetics, 42, 52, 345

Vomiting, postoperative. *See also* Postoperative nausea and vomiting
    antiemetics for, 56–57
    risk factors, 57
    surgery associated with, 57
V/Q ratio, lateral decubitus position and, 15
Vulva surgery, 684–686
    condylomata cuminata excision, 684–685
    marsupialization of Bartholin duct cyst or abscess, 693
    simple vulvectomy, 685
    vulvectomy
        radical with groin lymphadenectomy, 685–686
        simple, 685

W
Wake-up test, 44–45
Warfarin (Coumadin), 59, 63
Weber-Ferguson procedure, 464
Wedge resection, lung, 533–535
Whipple procedure (pancreaticoduodenectomy), 640–641, 640*f*
Whole blood, 20
Wilm's tumor resection or biopsy, 849–850
Wire dilation, esophageal, 590–591
Wire-loop resection, for endometrial ablation, 690
Wrist surgery, 727–731
    arthrodesis, 730–731
    carpal tunnel release, 728–729
    ganglion cyst excision, 729–730
    open reduction of carpal bone fracture, 727

Z
Zenker's diverticulum, excision of, 593–594
Zygomatic fracture reduction, 415